CLINICAL
PHARMACOLOGY

CLINICAL PHARMACOLOGY

Editor-in-Chief
CESARE R. SIRTORI, MD, PhD
Professor of Clinical Pharmacology
Institute of Pharmacological Sciences
University of Milano and
Niguarda Hospital
Milano – Italy

Editors
JOCHEN KUHLMANN, MD, PhD
Professor of Pharmacology and Toxicology
Institute of Clinical Pharmacology
Pharma Research Center
Bayer AG
Wuppertal – Germany

JEAN-PAUL TILLEMENT, Pharm.D
Professor of Pharmacology
Department of Pharmacology
University of Paris XII
Créteil Intercommunal Hospsital (CHIC)
Créteil – France

BOŽIDAR VRHOVAC, MD
Professor of Medicine and Clinical Pharmacology
Section of Clinical Pharmacology, Dept. of Medicine
University Hospital Centre Zagreb
Zagreb – Croatia

Consulting Editor
MARCUS M. REIDENBERG, MD
Professor of Pharmacology and Medicine
Division of Clinical Pharmacology
Weill Medical College of Cornell University
New York, New York – USA

McGraw-Hill International (UK) Ltd.

London • New York • San Francisco • St. Louis • Auckland • Bogotá • Caracas • Lisbon • Madrid • Mexico City • Milan • Montréal • New Delhi • San Juan • Singapore • Sydney • Tokyo • Toronto

CLINICAL PHARMACOLOGY

McGraw·Hill

A Division of The McGraw·Hill Companies

Editors-in-Chief: J. Dereck Jeffers, Fulvio Bruno
Acquisition Editor: Sandra Fabiani
Production Manager: Gino La Rosa
Copyediting and proof-reading: Lorenza Dainese, Jim Madru, Faith Voit
Preparation of index: Marji Toensing
Typesetting: Cse srl, Milano, Italy
Printing and binding: Stiav, Firenze, Italy

Cover illustration courtesy of: Pascoli Perugino a. *Il Corpo Umano*, Fidenza: Casa Editrice Mattioli, 1991; edition published exclusively for Master Pharma (Parma, Italy)

ISBN 0-07-709522-7
Printed in Italy

CONTENTS

SECTION 15
EMERGENCIES

SECTION 16
DRUGS AND SPECIAL
POPULATION GROUPS

SECTION 17
PHARMACOECONOMICS

CONTRIBUTORS

Numbers in brackets refer to chapters written or co-written by the contributor

IRMA B. ADAMS
Division of Forensic Science
Department of Criminal Justice Services
Richmond, Virginia - USA [84]

ANTONIO ADDIS
Laboratory of Clinical Pharmacology
Mario Negri Institute for Pharmacological Research
Milano – Italy [88]

CATIA ANGIOLINI
Department of Medical Oncology
National Institute for Cancer Research
Genova – Italy [50]

SANDRO ARDIZZONE
Department of Gastroenterology
University of Milano
Luigi Sacco Hospital
Milano – Italy [35,37]

WALTER ARTIBANI
Professor of Urology
Department of Urology
University of Modena
University Hospital
Modena – Italy [19]

LUC V.M. BAERT
Department of Urology
Catholic University of Leuven
Gasthuisberg Hospital
Leuven - Belgium [18]

IVAN BAKRAN
Professor of Medicine
Section of Clinical Pharmacology
Department of Medicine
University of Zagreb
University Hospital Centre Rebro
Zagreb - Croatia [28]

LUC P. BALANT
Professor of Pharmacotherapy
Clinical Research Unit, Department of Psychiatry
University of Geneva
Geneva – Switzerland [2]

EFFIE A. BALANT-GORGIA
Therapeutic Drug Monitoring Unit
Department of Psychiatry
University of Geneva
Geneva – Switzerland [2]

BERNARD BANNWARTH
Professor of Therapeutics
Department of Rheumatology
Victor Segalen University
Pellegrin Hospital
Bordeaux – France [46]

JÉRÔME BARRÉ
Pharmacology Unit
Intercommunal Hospital Centre
Créteil Cedex – France [4]

PIERRE R. BECHTEL
Professor of Clinical Pharmacology
Department of Clinical Pharmacology
University Hospital
Jean Minjoz Hospital
Besançon Cedex – France [3]

YVETTE C. BECHTEL
Assistant Professor of Clinical Pharmacology
Department of Clinical Pharmacology
University Hospital
Jean Minjoz Hospital
Besançon Cedex – France [3]

GABRIELE BIANCHI PORRO
Professor of Gastroenterology
Department of Gastroenterology
University of Milano
Luigi Sacco Hospital
Milano – Italy [35,37]

HOWARD BIRD
Professor of Pharmacological Rheumatology
Clinical Pharmacology Unit
University of Leeds
Chapel Allerton Hospital
Leeds – United Kingdom [44]

MAURIZIO BONATI
Laboratory for Mother and Child Health
Mario Negri Institute for Pharmacological Research
Milano – Italy [88]

CRISTINA BORGHI
Consultant Phamacologist
Centre for Clinical and Therapeutic Pharmacology Research
University of Milano
Milano – Italy [Appendix]

EMILIO BOUZA
Professor of Clinical Microbiology and Infectious Diseases
Department of Clinical Microbiology and Infectious Diseases
University Hospital Gregorio Maranon
Madrid - Spain [39]

STEFAN BRACHT
Department of Research and Development
LTS Lohmann Therapie-Systeme AG
Andernach – Germany [5]

LISA H. BRAUER
Assistant Research Professor
Department of Psychiatry and Behavioral Sciences
Duke University Medical Center
Durham, North Carolina – USA [83]

GERD D. BURCHARD
Professor of Tropical Medicine
Department for the Research of Tropical Diseases
Bernard Nocht Institute for Tropical Medicine
Hamburg – Germany [42]

VLADIMIR ČAJKOVAC
Professor of Dermatology
Department of Dermatology
University of Zagreb
Clinical Hospital "Sestre milosrdnice"
Zagreb – Croatia [76,77,78]

CHRISTOPHER P. CANNON
Professor of Medicine
Cardiovascular Division, Department of Medicine
Harvard Medical School
Brigham and Women's Hospital
Boston, Massachusetts – USA [25]

MARIA GRAZIA CANTÚ
Clinic of Obstetrics and Gynecology
University of Milano Bicocca
San Gerardo Hospital
Monza - Italy [60]

PIERUGO CARBONIN
Professor of Gerontology
Department of Gerontology
Catholic University "Sacro Cuore"
Gemelli Hospital
Rome – Italy [89]

ANNA CARIELLO
Department of Oncology and Hematology
Santa Maria delle Croci Hospital
Ravenna - Italy [61]

LUCA CASTAGNA
Department of Medical Oncology
Institute Gustave Roussy
Villejuif - France [59]

FABIO CELOTTI
Professor of General Pathology
Institute of Endocrinology
University of Milano
Milano – Italy [67]

RACHELE CICCOCIOPPO
Department of Internal Medicine
University of L'Aquila
L'Aquila – Italy [34]

FRANCESCO CLEMENTI
Professor of Pharmacology
Department of Pharmacology, Chemotherapy
and Medical Toxicology
University of Milano
Milano – Italy [16]

GINO R. CORAZZA
Professor of Gastroenterology
Department of Internal Medicine
University of Pavia
San Matteo University Hospital
Pavia – Italy [34]

WILLIAM M. CORRAO
Professor of Medicine
Division of Pulmonary, Sleep
and Critical Care Medicine, Department of Medicine
Brown University School of Medicine
Rhode Island Hospital
Providence, Rhode Island – USA [30]

SVEIN G. DAHL
Professor of Pharmacology
Department of Pharmacology, Institute of Medical Biology
University of Tromsø
Tromsø - Norway [13]

RAFFAELE DE CATERINA
Associate Professor of Cardiology
Department of Clinical Sciences and Bioimaging
Gabriele D'Annunzio University of Chieti
Chieti - Italy [74]

GILLES-LOUIS DEFER
Professor of Neurology
Déjerine Neurologic Unit
Hospital CHU Côte de Nacre
Caen – France [11]

JAMES A. DE LEMOS
Professor of Medicine
Cardiovascular Division, Department of Medicine
Harvard Medical School
Brigham and Women's Hospital
Boston, Massachusetts – USA [25]

TIMOTHY A. DENTON
Associate Professor of Medicine
Divisions of Cardiothoracic Surgery and Cardiology
Cedars-Sinai Medical Center
Los Angeles, California – USA [73]

BEN E. DE PAUW
Professor of Medicine
Clinical Mycology Unit, Departments of Haematology and
Blood Transfusion Service
Medical Center St. Radboud
Nijmegen – The Netherlands [41]

HARRIET DE WIT
Associate Professor of Psychiatry
Department of Psychiatry
University of Chicago
Chicago, Illinois – USA [83]

PIERRE DUCHÊNE-MARULLAZ
Emeritus Professor of Pharmacology
Clermont-Ferrand – France [1]

ULLA FELDT-RASMUSSEN
Professor of Endocrinology
Department of Medical Endocrinology
National University Hospital
Copenhagen - Denmark [65]

GILLES FENELON
Neurologic Unit
University of Paris
Tenon Hospital
Paris - France [11]

JÜRGEN C. FRÖLICH
Professor of Clinical Pharmacology
Department of Clinical Pharmacology
Hannover School of Medicine
Hannover - Germany [48]

CLAUDIO GALLI
Professor of Experimental Pharmacology
Institute of Pharmacological Sciences
University of Milano
Milano - Italy [72]

ANDRES AVILA GARAVITO
Department of Medical Oncology
Institute Gustave Roussy
Villejuif - France [59,62]

MARIANNE GEX-FABRY
Clinical Research Unit, Department of Psychiatry
University of Geneva
Geneva – Switzerland [2]

FRANCO GIADA
Cardiology Unit
Umberto I Hospital
Mestre - Italy [85]

ANNE-MARIE GLENNY
Cochrane Oral Health Group
University Dental Hospital of Manchester
Manchester – United Kingdom [70]

LARS F. GRAM
Professor of Clinical Pharmacology
Institute of Public Health
University of Southern Denmark
Odense – Denmark [13]

SEBASTIAN HARDER
Assistant Professor of Clinical Pharmacology
Institute for Clinical Pharmacology
Johann Wolfgang Goethe University of Frankfurt
University Hospital
Frankfurt am Main – Germany [27]

BEATE M. HENZ
Professor of Dermatology and Allergy
Department of Dermatology and Allergy
Humboldt University of Berlin
Charité Hospital
Berlin - Germany [79]

HELGE HOHAGE
Associate Professor of Internal Medicine
Department of Internal Medicine
University of Münster
Münster – Germany [23]

TROELS S. JENSEN
Professor of Neurology and Pain
Department of Neurology
University of Aarhus
Aarhus University Hospital
Aarhus – Denmark [9]

G. DENNIS JOHNSTON
Professor of Clinical Pharmacology
Department of Therapeutics and Pharmacology
The Queen's University of Belfast
Belfast City Hospital
Belfast, Northern Ireland – United Kingdom [17]

RALPH E. KAUFFMAN
Professor of Pediatrics and Pharmacology
Department of Medical Research
University of Missouri at Kansas City
Children's Mercy Hospital
Kansas City, Missouri – USA [87]

GABRIELA V. KORNEK
Department of Clinical Oncology
University of Wien
General Hospital
Wien – Austria [54]

STEPHAN KRÄHENBÜHL
Professor of Clinical Pharmacology and Internal Medicine
Department of Clinical Pharmacology
University of Basel
University Hospital
Basel – Switzerland [36]

GUNNAR KROESEN
Professor of Anesthesiology
Department of Anesthesiology and Critical Care Medicine
Leopold Franzens University of Innsbruck
University Hospital
Innsbruck - Austria [86]

JOCHEN KUHLMANN
Professor of Pharmacology and Toxicology
Institute of Clinical Pharmacology, Pharma Research Center
Bayer AG
Wuppertal – Germany [8]

RON C. KUPERS
PET Center
University of Aarhus
Aarhus University Hospital
Aarhus – Denmark [9]

BORIS LABAR
Professor of Medicine
Division of Hematology, Department of Medicine
University Hospital Rebro
Zagreb – Croatia [52,63]

HARALD LABISCHINSKI
Professor of Chemistry
Pharma Research Center
Bayer AG
Wuppertal - Germany [43]

CORNELIS B.H.W. LAMERS
Professor of Medicine
Department of Gastroenterology - Hepatology
University of Leiden
Leiden University Medical Center
Leiden – The Netherlands [33]

FRANÇOIS LE DOZE
Déjerine Neurologic Unit
Hospital CHU Côte de Nacre
Caen – France [11]

PIERRE J. LEFÈBVRE
Professor of Internal Medicine
Division of Diabetes, Nutrition and Metabolic Disorders,
Department of Medicine
University of Liège
CHU Sart Tilman
Liège - Belgium [68]

ROBERT J. MACFADYEN
Department of Cardiology
University of Aberdeen
Raigmore Hospital
Inverness – United Kingdom [24]

BRANKO MALENICA
Assistant Professor of Immunology
Department of Immunology
University of Zagreb
Clinical Hospital Center Zagreb
Zagreb - Croatia [55]

ANDREA MANEO
Clinic of Obstetrics and Gynecology
University of Milano Bicocca
San Gerardo Hospital
Monza - Italy [60]

COSTANTINO MANGIONI
Professor of Obstetrics and Gynecology
University of Milano Bicocca
San Gerardo Hospital
Monza - Italy [60]

PIER FRANCESCO MANNAIONI
Professor of Toxicology
Department of Preclinical and Clinical Pharmacology
University of Firenze
Careggi General Hospital
Firenze – Italy [80,81]

LAJOS MATOS
Department of Clinical Pharmacology
Hungarian Institute of Cardiology
Budapest – Hungary [22]

JACQUES F.G.M. MEIS
Assistant Professor of Medical Microbiology
Clinical Mycology Unit
Department of Medical Microbiology
University Medical Center St. Radboud
Nijmegen – The Netherlands [41]

MARCO MONCINI
Department of Preclinical and Clinical Pharmacology
University of Firenze
Careggi General Hospital
Firenze – Italy [80,81]

JAMES S. MORRIS
Consultant in Medical Information and Software
Rugeley, Staffs – United Kingdom [6]

PHILIPPE NACACHE
Department of Medical Oncology
Institute Gustave Roussy
Villejuif - France [62]

NORBERT NIEDERLE
Professor of Internal Medicine
Department of Oncology and Hematology
University of Köln
Leverkusen Teaching Hospital
Leverkusen - Germany [56]

SUSAN O'MEARA
NHS Centre for Reviews and Dissemination
University of York
York - United Kingdom [70]

GIUSEPPE OPPIZZI
Division of Endocrinology
University of Milano
Niguarda Hospital
Milano - Italy [66]

PAOLO PALATINI
Professor of Internal Medicine
Medical Clinic IV
University of Padova
University Hospital
Padova - Italy [85]

CARLO PATRONO
Professor of Pharmacology
Department of Medicine and Aging
Gabriele D'Annunzio University of Chieti
Chieti - Italy [74]

STEVEN Z. PAVLETIC
Associate Professor of Medicine
Section of Oncology, Department of Medicine
University of Nebraska Medical Center
Omaha, Nebraska – USA [63]

FRANCO PAZZUCCONI
Assistant Professor of Clinical Pharmacology
Institute of Pharmacological Sciences
Enrica Grossi Paoletti Center
University of Milano
Niguarda Hospital
Milano - Italy [49,69]

EMILIO PERUCCA
Associate Professor of Clinical Pharmacology
Clinical Pharmacology Unit
Department of Internal Medicine and Therapeutics
University of Pavia
San Matteo University Hospital
Pavia – Italy [10]

FRANCESCO PESCE
Assistant Professor of Urology
Department of Urology
University of Modena
University Hospital
Modena – Italy [19]

ZBIGNIEW PETROVICH
Department of Radiation Oncology
University of Southern California School of Medicine
Los Angeles, California - USA [18]

JOSÉ-LUIS PICO
Department of Medical Oncology
Institute Gustave Roussy
Villejuif - France [59,62]

SHIBLEY RAHMAN
Research Neuropsychologist
Department of Psychiatry
University of Cambridge
Addenbrooke's Hospital
Cambridge – United Kingdom [12]

KARL HEINZ RAHN
Professor of Medicine
Department of Medicine D
University of Münster
University Hospital
Münster – Germany [23]

JÜRG REICHEN
Professor of Medicine
Department of Clinical Pharmacology
University of Bern
Bern – Switzerland [36]

MARCUS M. REIDENBERG
Professor of Pharmacology and Medicine
Division of Clinical Pharmacology
Weill Medical College of Cornell University
New York, New York – USA

WILLEM J. REMME
Professor of Cardiology
STICARES Cardiovascular Research Foundation
Rotterdam/Rhoon – The Netherlands [26]

RICCARDO ROSSO
Professor of Chemotherapy
Department of Medical Oncology
National Institute for Cancer Research
Genova – Italy [50]

GIOVANNI ROSTI
Department of Oncology and Hematology
Santa Maria delle Croci Hospital
Ravenna - Italy [61]

RENÉ J. ROYER
Professor of Pharmacology
Department of Pharmacology
Faculty of Medicine
CNRS 1288
Vandoeuvre lès Nancy - France [7]

RICHARD SACHSE
Peptor GmbH
Erkrath – Germany [20]

BARBARA J. SAHAKIAN
Professor of Clinical Neuropsychology
Department of Psychiatry
University of Cambridge
Addenbrooke's Hospital
Cambridge – United Kingdom [12]

ANDRÉ J. SCHEEN
Professor of Internal Medicine
Division of Diabetes, Nutrition and Metabolic Disorders
Department of Medicine
University of Liège
CHU Sart Tilman
Liège - Belgium [68]

REINHOLD E. SCHMIDT
Professor of Medicine and Immunology
Department of Clinical Immunology
Hannover School of Medicine
Hannover - Germany [47,75]

GÖRAN C. SEDVALL
Professor of Psychiatry
Department of Clinical Neuroscience
Karolinska Institute
Karolinska Hospital
Stockholm - Sweden [14]

PRAMOD M. SHAH
Professor of Internal Medicine
Department of Internal Medicine
Johann Wolfgang Goethe University of Frankfurt
University Hospital
Frankfurt am Main - Germany [38,39]

SALVATORE SIENA
Chief, Department of Oncology
Niguarda Hospital
Milano - Italy [57]

ROSELLA SILVESTRINI
Department of Experimental Oncology
National Institute for the Research and Treatment of Cancer
Milano – Italy [64]

CESARE R. SIRTORI
Professor of Clinical Pharmacology
Institute of Pharmacological Sciences
University of Milano and
Niguarda Hospital
Milano - Italy [15,21,23,38,49,69,71]

J.M. AD SITSEN
Professor of Clinical Pharmacology
Department of Medical Pharmacology
University of Utrecht
Utrecht – The Netherlands [82]

JURIJ ŠORLI
Professor of Internal Medicine
Department of Respiratory Diseases and Allergology
University of Ljubljana
University Clinic of Respiratory Diseases and Allergology
Golnik – Slovenia [29]

HAIKO SPROTT
Department of Rheumatology and
Institute of Physical Medicine
University of Zürich
University Hospital
Zürich - Switzerland [45]

THOMAS STAMMINGER
Professor of Virology
Institute for Clinical and Molecular Virology
University of Erlangen-Nürnberg
Erlangen - Germany [40]

ROY STEIN
Assistant Professor of Psychiatry
Department of Psychiatry
Duke University
Durham Veterans Affairs Medical Center
Durham, North Carolina – USA [83]

DIRK O. STICHTENOTH
Department of Clinical Pharmacology
Hannover School of Medicine
Hannover - Germany [48]

IVAN STOCKLEY
School of Biomedical Sciences
University of Nottingham Medical School
Queen's Medical Centre
Nottingham – United Kingdom [6]

GEROLD STUCKI
Professor of Physical Medicine and Rehabilitation
Department of Physical Medicine and Rehabilitation
University of München
München – Germany [45]

ERHARD SUESS
Assistant Professor of Neurology
Department of Clinical Neurology
University Clinic for Neurology
University of Wien
General Hospital
Wien - Austria [53]

THOMAS D. SZUCS
Professor of Health Economics
Department of Medical Economics
University of Zürich
Zürich - Switzerland [90]

JEAN-PAUL TILLEMENT
Professor of Pharmacology
Department of Pharmacology
University of Paris XII
Créteil Intercommunal Hopsital (CHIC)
Créteil – France

NEVEN TUDORIĆ
Assistant Professor of Medicine
Section of Pulmunology, Department of Medicine
University of Zagreb School of Medicine
University Hospital Dubrava
Zagreb - Croatia [31]

SAÏK URIEN
Pharmacology Unit
University of Paris XII
Créteil Cedex – France [4]

HEIN VAN POPPEL
Professor of Oncologic Urology
Department of Urology
Catholic University of Leuven
Gasthuisberg Hospital
Leuven - Belgium [18]

FRANCESCO VISIOLI
Assistant Professor of Experimental Pharmacology
Institute of Pharmacological Sciences
University of Milano
Milano - Italy [72]

WOLFGANG VOELCKEL
Department of Anesthesiology and Critical Care Medicine
Leopold Franzens University of Innsbruck
University Hospital
Innsbruck - Austria [86]

BOŽIDAR VRHOVAC
Professor of Medicine and Clinical Pharmacology
Section of Clinical Pharmacology, Department of Medicine
University Hospital Centre Zagreb
Zagreb – Croatia

GEORGE WADE
The European Agency for the Evaluation of Medicinal
Products (EMEA)
London – United Kingdom [Appendix]

BERND WEIDMANN
Department of Oncology and Hematology
University of Köln
Leverkusen Teaching Hospital
Leverkusen - Germany [56]

THOMAS R. WEIHRAUCH
Associate Professor of Internal Medicine
and Gastroenterology
Department of Internal Medicine and Gastroenterology
University of Düsseldorf
Düsseldorf - Germany [32]

J. ALFRED WITJES
Department of Urology
University Medical Center St. Radboud
Nijmegen - The Netherlands [58]

TORSTEN WITTE
Division of Clinical Immunology
Department of Internal Medicine
Hannover School of Medicine
Hannover - Germany [47,75]

NADIA ZAFFARONI
Department of Experimental Oncology
National Institute for the Research and Treatment of Cancer
Milano – Italy [64]

CHRISTOPH C. ZIELINSKI
Professor of Medicine and Medical Experimental Oncology
Clinical Division of Oncology, Department of Medicine I
University of Wien
General Hospital
Wien – Austria [53,54]

GIUSEPPE ZUCCALÁ
Assistant Professor of Gerontology
Department of Gerontology
Catholic University "Sacro Cuore"
Gemelli Hospital
Rome – Italy [89]

HEINZ ZWIERZINA
Professor of Internal Medicine
Institute for Internal Medicine
Leopold Franzens University of Innsbruck
University Hospital
Innsbruck – Austria [51]

ACRONYMS

A

AAG: α_1-acid glycoprotein
ABMT: autologous bone marrow transplantation
ACE: angiotensin converting enzyme
AD: Alzheimer's disease
ADME: absorption, distribution, metabolism, excretion
ADR: adverse drug reaction
AIDS: acquired immunodeficiency syndrome
ALG: antilymphocyte globulin
ALL: acute lymphoblastic leukemia
ALT: alanine aminotransferase (also GPT)
AMI: acute myocardial infarction
AML: acute myelogenous leukemia
APC: antigen presenting cells
APD: action potential duration
APL: acute promyelocytic leukemia
APTT: activated partial thromboplastin time
ARA: American Rheumatism Association
ARDS: adult respiratory distress syndrome
ASA: acetylsalicylic acid
AST: aspartate aminotransferase (also GOT)
AT: angiotensin
AT_1: angiotensin I
ATIII: antithrombin III
ATRA: all-trans retinoic acid
AUC: area under the curve (generally of drug concentrations)
AV: atrioventricular
AVP: arginine vasopressin
AZT: azidothymidine (ziduvidine)

B

BCG: bacillus Calmette-Guerin
BCNU: bischloroethyl nitrosourea
bid: bis in die (twice a day)
BMI: body mass index
BOO: bladder outlet obstruction
BPH: benign prostatic hyperplasia
BRM: biological response modifier

C

CAD: coronary artery disease
CAMP: cyclic adenosine monophosphate
CABG: coronary artery bypass graft
CBC: complete blood count
CBZ: carbamazepine
CC: combination contraceptive
CCB: calcium channel blocker
CD: computed tomography
CDDP: cis diaminodichloroplatinum (cisplatin)
CEA: carcinoembryonic antigen
CGD: chronic granulomatous disease
CGRP: calcitonin gene-related peptide
CFC: chlorofluorocarbons
CFU: colony forming units
CHD: coronary heart disease
CHF: congestive heart failure
CIOMS: Council of International Organizations of Medical Sciences
CK: creatine kinase
CLL: chronic lymphocytic leukemia
C_{max}: maximal concentrations in body fluids after drug intake
CML: chronic myelogenous leukemia
CMV: cytomegalovirus
CNS: central nervous system
CO: cardiac output
COMT: catechol-O-methyl-transferase
COPD: chronic obstructive pulmonary disease
COX-1: cyclooxygenase 1

COX-2: cyclooxygenase 2
CPAP: continuous positive alveolar pressure
CPMP: Committee of Proprietary Medicinal Products
CR: complete response
CRP: C reactive protein
CsA: cyclosporine A
CSF: cerebrospinal fluid
CSF: colony stimulating factor
CT: computed tomography
CYP: cytochrome P (generally 450)

D

DAS: disease activity score
dc: direct current
DHA: docosahexaenoic acid
DHT: dihydrotestosterone
DMARD: disease modifying antirheumatic drug
DAT: dementia Alzheimer type
DPH: diphenylhydantoin (phenytoin)
DRG: dorsal root ganglion
DSM: diagnostic and statistical manual
DTIC: dimethyl-triazenyl-imidazole-carboxamide (dacarbazine)

E

EBV: Epstein-Barr virus
EC: European Community
ECG: electrocardiogram
ECT: electroconvulsive therapy
ED: extensive disease
EEG: electroencephalogram
EFTA: European Free Trade Area
EGF: endothelial growth factor
EH: hepatic extraction ratio
ELISA: enzyme linked immunosorbent assay
EMEA: European Medicines Evaluation Agency

EM: extensive metabolizers
EPA: eicosapentaenoic acid
EPO: epoietin, eritropoietin
EPS: extrapyramidal side effects
ESR: erytrocyte sedimentation rate
ET: endothelin
EXP: exponential

F

FDA: Food and Drug Administration (US)
FEV1: forced espiratory volume in 1 second
FGF: fibroblast growth factor
FH: familial hypercholesterolemia
5-FU: 5-fluorouracil

G

GABA: gamma-aminobutyric acid
GCP: Good Clinical Practice
GERD: gastroesophageal reflux disease
GFR: glomerular filtration rate
GH: growth hormone
GHRH: growth hormone releasing hormone
GI: gastrointestinal
GCP: Good Clinical Practice
GLP: Good Laboratory Practice
GMP: Good Manufacturing Practice
GST: glutathione S-transferase
GvHD: graft versus host disease

H

Hb: hemoglobin
HCL: hairy cell leukemia
HD: Hodgkin disease
HD: Huntington disease
HDL: high density lipoproteins
HGPRT: hydroxyguanine phosphoribosyl transferase
HIV: human immunodeficiency virus
HL: Hodgkin lymphoma
HMG CoA: hydroxyl methylglutaryl coenzyme A
HPA: hypophysis pituitary axis
HPLC: high pressure liquid chromatography
HRT: hormone replacement therapy
HSA: human serum albumin
HSV: herpes simplex virus
HTN: hypertension
Ht: hematocrit

I

ia: intraarterial
IBD: inflammatory bowel disease
IBS: irritable bowel syndrome

ICD: International Classification of Diseases
ICH: International Conference on Harmonization
ICP: intracranial pressure
ICU: Intensive Care Unit
IDC_{50}: inhibitory dose 50%
IDDM: insulin dependent diabetes mellitus
IEC: Independent Ethical Committee
IFN: interferon
IGF: insulin-like growth factor
IL: interleukin
im: intramuscular
IM: intermediary metabolizer
INR: International Normalized Ratio
ip: intraperitoneal
IRB: Independent Review Board
ISA: intrinsic sympathetic activity
it: intrathecal
ITP: idiopathic thrombocytopenic purpura
iv: intravenous

L

LAK: lymphokine activated killer cell
LAAM: L-acetylmethadol
LBBB: left bundle branch block
LCAT: lecithin cholesterol acyltransferase
LD: limited disease
LDH: lactate dihydrogenase
LDL: low density lipoproteins
LES: lower esophageal sphincter
LH: luteinizing hormone
LL: lymphocytic leukemia
LMWH: low molecular weight heparin
LNG: levonorgestrel
LPL: lipoprotein lipase
LpX: lipoprotein X
LV: left ventricular

M

MAB: monoclonal antibody
MALT: mucosa-associated lymphoid tissue
MAOI: monoamino oxidase inhibitor
MBC: minimum bactericidal concentration
MCBC: monocytoid B cells
MDI: metered dose inhaler
MDMA: methylenedioxy-methyamphetamine (ecstasy)
MDR: multi-drug-resistance
MDS: myelodysplastic syndrome
MEGX: monoethylglycinexylidide
MHC: major histocompatibility complex
MESNA: sodium-2-mercapto-

ethanesulphonate
MI: myocardial infarction
MIC: minimum inhibitory concentration
MMSE: Mini Mental State Examination
6-MP: 6-mercaptopurine
MPA: mycophenolic acid
MPA: medroxyprogesterone acetate
MRI: magnetic resonance imaging
MRT: mean residence time
MTD: maximum tolerated dose
MTX: methotrexate
MW: molecular weight

N

NA: nicotinic acid
NAT: N-acetyl transferase
NCE: new chemical entity
NCI: National Cancer Institute (USA)
NEP: neutral endopeptidase
NIDDM: non insulin dependent diabetes mellitus
NHL: non Hodgkin's lymphoma
NKA: neurokinin A
NK: natural killer
NMDA: N-methyl-D-aspartate
NNT: number needed to treat
NMR: nuclear magnetic resonance
NMS: neuroleptic malignant syndrome
NNRTI: non-nucleoside reverse transcriptase inhibitors
NO: nitrous oxide
NOS: nitric oxide synthase
NQMI: non Q wave myocardial infarction
NR: non response
NSCLC: non-small cell lung cancer
NSAID: non steroidal antiinflammatory drug

O

OA: osteoarthritis
OR: odds ratio
OTC: over-the-counter

P

PABA: para-aminobenzoic acid
PAH: para-amino-hippurate
PBP: penicillin binding protein
PCR: polymerase chain reaction
PcP: *Pneumocystis carinii*
PD: progressive disease
PD: Parkinson's disease
PDE: phosphodiesterase
PEF: peak expiratory flow
PET: positron emission tomography
PEEP: positive end-expiratory pressure

PGI_2: prostacyclin
PGE_1: prostaglandin E_1
PGE_2: prostaglandin E_2
$PGF_{2\alpha}$: prostaglandin$F_{2\alpha}$
PK: pharmacokinetics
PK-PD: pharmacokinetics - pharmacodynamics
PMDI: pressurized metered-dose inhaler
PM: poor metabolizer
po: per os (oral)
PPAR: peroxisome proliferator-activated receptor
PPI: proton pump inhibitor
PR: partial response
PRL: prolactin
PSA: prostate specific antigen
PTCA: percutaneous transluminal coronary angioplasty
PT: prothrombin time

Q

QALY: quality adjusted life years
qd: once a day
qid: quater in die (four times a day)
Q_H: hepatic blood flow
QL: quality of life
QTc: electrocardiographic Q-T interval corrected for heart rate

R

RA: rapid acetylator
RA: rheumatoid arthritis
RAST: radioallergosorbent test
RCT: randomized controlled trial
RDA: recommended dietary allowance
RIA: radioimmunoassay
RT: radiation therapy

S

SA: slow acetylator
SBS: short bowel syndrome
sc: subcutaneous
SCLC: small cell lung cancer
sl: sublingual
SLE: systemic lupus erythematosus
SOD: superoxide dismutase
SPET: single-photon-emission-tomography
SSRI: selective serotonin reuptake inhibitors
SVR: systemic vascular resistance
SSZ: sulphasalazine
ss: steady-state
SU: sultamicillin

T

TBG: thyroxine binding globulin
TCA: tricyclic antidepressants
TCR: T-cell receptor
TD: tardive dyskinesia
TDM: therapeutic drug monitoring
TDS: transdermal delivery system
TFT: thyroid function tests
$t_{1/2}$: half-life
TG: triglycerides
THC: tetrahydrocannabinol
TIA: transient ischemic attack
tid: ter in die (three times a day)
T_{max}: time to the attainment of C_{max}
TNF: tumor necrosis factor
TNM: tumor, node, metastasis (classification)
TOTPAR: total pain relief
tPA: tissue-type plasminogen activator
TPR: total peripheral resistance
TRH: thyrotropin releasing hormone

TSH: thyroid stimulating hormone
TURP: transurethral resection of the prostate
TZ: tazobactam
TXA_2, B_2: thromboxane A_2, B_2

U

UE: untoward effects
UGT: UDP-glucuronyl transferase
UM: ultrarapid metabolizer
UPDRS: Unified Parkinson's Disease Rating Scale
URTI: upper respiratory tract infection
UTI: urinary tract infection
UVA: ultraviolet A

V

V_d (or V): volume of distribution
V_{dss}: volume of distribution at steady state
VEGF: vascular endothelial growth factor
VF: ventricular fibrillation
VIP: vasoactive intestinal peptide
VLDL: very low density lipoproteins
VSCC: voltage-sensitive calcium channels
VT: volume, tissue
VP: volume, plasma
VT: ventricular tachycardia
VW: Vaughan Williams
VZV: varicella zoster virus

W

WHO: World Health Organization

FOREWORD

Medicine changes rapidly, making it difficult for those of us who treat a broad range of patients to keep current. New scientific knowledge changes our concept of how we treat disease. For example, peptic ulcer was treated in the past with surgical procedures to suppress gastric acid secretion. Then, potent medications were given to suppress acid secretion. Now, antimicrobials are given to eradicate *H. pylori*.

The introduction of new and effective drugs with sub-classification categories, such as beta adrenergic blockers being either selective or nonselective and each either with or without intrinsic sympathomimetic activity, provides opportunities to individualize therapy. Having so many choices also makes the decision-making process much more complex. What one needs today is a readily available authoritative reference about drugs that is well organized for the practicing physician.

This is the intent of this book. The Editor-in-Chief, Professor Cesare R. Sirtori, has assembled an international group of editors and contributors who have produced a book that is both authoritative and useful. The text focuses on drug facts organized by therapeutic class and often presented in tables that facilitate comparison of similar drugs. This book will be of particular benefit to physicians who want specific drug information quickly, clearly, and comparatively.

One of the themes of clinical pharmacology is individualization of therapy. By making drug facts accessible in a practical format, CLINICAL PHARMACOLOGY helps the physician prescribe the best modern therapy for each individual patient.

Marcus M. Reidenberg, MD
New York, USA

PREFACE

Clinical pharmacology was born in the twentieth century, although frequent efforts have been made to recognize forerunners way back to Galen or to James Lind, who carried out a randomized trial on the antiscury activity of citrus juice. Middle-aged clinical pharmacologists of today have had the unique privilege of sharing their birth with their profession and of knowing that concepts such as the "placebo effect" and the "controlled randomized trial" have led to modern clinical pharmacology. The path to maturity has been at times dramatic and traumatic. Experiences of adverse drug effects have occurred, a prime example being that of thalidomide. Witnessing these events taught clinical pharmacologists a lesson: drugs are never just good or bad – usefulness and safety depend on the therapeutic circumstances. The recent revival of thalidomide as an effective treatment for multiple myeloma is a good example.

During the 1970s and 1980s clinical pharmacologists widened their interest in basic research and in the development of therapeutic services. They also aspired to play a central role in human therapy. Advances in the development of clinical pharmacokinetics and therapeutic drug monitoring, greater understanding of drug interactions, and improvements in the methods designed to assess drug responses hastened the progression of clinical drug development. But defeat also ensued. Clinical pharmacologists failed in their attempt to be recognized as obligate leaders in large clinical trials. Rarely do clinical pharmacologists attain a leading role either in very large randomized trials with a variety of indications (from coronary disease to cancer), or in the establishment of therapeutic guidelines. These exclusions at times may be the result of pharmacologists exhibiting an elitist or superior attitude over "ordinary physicians." On the other hand, young clinical pharmacologists are finding an appropriate role in their hospitals. Some indeed may find it shocking now to see a new actor on the clinical scene – a pharmacologist – acting as a team member between a patient and his or her physician in the patient's behalf. Clinical pharmacologists performing as well-respected consultants in the complex field of drug use have made major contributions in understanding the genetic diversity in drug responses and in developing well-structured analytical approaches to evaluating new medications, providing a thorough knowledge of comparative efficacy, side effects, and individual characteristics, thus benefiting both physician and patient.

It was indeed an honor when McGraw-Hill approached me to develop and organize a multiauthored textbook of clinical pharmacology with a major emphasis on European practice. The pool of clinical pharmacologists, however, is not large, and I was gratified to welcome the help of first-class specialists from the United States.

My co-editors, Jochen Kuhlmann from Wuppertal, Božidar Vrhovac from Zagreb, Jean-Paul Tillement from Paris, and Boris Labar from Zagreb, who was responsible for the Anticancer Section, were helpful in establishing some major structural formats for the book. Interests in clinical pharmacology have become very wide. We knew we wanted to include a chapter on pharmacoeconomy, on international drug regulations, and to introduce for the first time in this type of book, a chapter on male impotence. Sacrifices were necessary, in our case eliminating a chapter on anesthesiology, now a highly specialized field of limited interest to the majority of our readers.

Each chapter follows a well-defined sequence: from clinical presentation to evidence-based medical criteria for drug evaluation, to analysis of major drug classes, and in specific cases to selected major agents. Kinetics, interactions, and P450 handling are presented in each chapter, thus offering clues to problems encountered in therapy. Nowadays, studies describing randomized trials appear daily in print. We believe, however, that clinical pharmacology is a doctrine and that we have discussed and described this approach clearly and completely in the book so that readers can readily made a judgment of whatever new or less new becomes available in the literature.

Each author deserves my personal gratitude for the ability to condense enormous amounts of information into instructive and readable material. Our message must be accessible and beneficial for every practitioner in the health sciences. This was our goal, and we hope we have come as close as possible to attaining it.

We must, of course, acknowledge a number of individuals who were directly or indirectly responsible for this publication. Professor Marcus Reidenberg, a world leader among clinical pharmacologists, was kind enough to advise us on parts of the text and to prepare a laudable

Foreword. I personally would like to thank Liliana Francavilla for her extreme patience in enduring three years of ordeals ranging from tracking down texts to finding authors themselves, always with a pleasant spirit and outstanding scientific communication expertise. Fulvio Bruno of McGraw-Hill Medical Publishing Europe was the leader throughout the birth and growth of this medical series, and Sandra Fabiani provided help and often patience during corrections, revisions, and occasional mishaps. I wish also to thank Dereck Jeffers of McGraw-Hill US for his advice and encouragement, despite innumerable difficulties. Finally, it is my personal hope that a number of colleagues will find this text useful and that the vision of clinical pharmacology by professionals and nonprofessionals will be illuminated and appreciated.

Cesare R. Sirtori, MD, PhD
Milano, Italy

Clinical pharmacology: the fundamentals

1

Drug definition

Pierre Duchêne-Marullaz

Drugs were once an unreliable aspect of therapy but are now increasingly effective. Prescribing drugs has become a science more than an art. It also carries rapidly evolving financial implications due to the increasingly huge investment required for new drug development, which in turn has prompted a series of takeovers and mergers among the major drug manufacturers. In addition, the number of potential consumers can be expected to increase along with the improvement in economic conditions and lifespan in many countries. The number of new products has decreased in recent years, but the genetic engineering revolution has opened new avenues of research.

HISTORICAL OVERVIEW

A brief history

No one can be sure when drugs – or medicines, remedies, potions, or cures – first made their appearance or when a line was first drawn between food and medicine. The first text known to mention therapy is thought to be a Chinese treatise by Daode Jing – *The Book of the Yellow Emperor* – dating from around 2600 B.C., whereas at approximately the same point in time the Sumerian tablets excavated at Nippur were incised with the names of herbs having medicinal properties, such as henbane, poppy, mandrake, and so on.

Thirteen papyri, the best known being that bought by Ebers in 1873, give an idea of the medicines used by the Egyptians in 1536 B.C. They include not only sedatives, purgatives, and diuretics (e.g., spring squill) but also blood, powdered bone, animal fats, and certain plants. Medicine was closely connected to magic (even the West has a history of combatting plague with processions, among other examples). Greek physicians were greatly prized by barbarians and later by the Romans. The writings of Hippocrates of Kos (460-370 B.C.) deal mainly with fractures, dislocations, and "intestinal wind." Dioscorides Pedanius also was a major figure. As an army doctor under Nero, he identified over 600 plants and remedies, including various minerals, describing their uses and the illnesses that they could cure. His book, written in Greek and extensively quoted by Galen, was subsequently translated into Arabic and later, in the fifteenth century, into Latin as *De Materia Medica*.

Initially, Roman physicians would go into the countryside themselves to collect the plants that they used. However, as the preparation of medicines became more and more complex, fully fledged laboratories – *tabernae* – were opened. They tended to compete with physicians, and fakes were not uncommon. For example, Pliny mentions a false opium sold in Alexandria.

Apothecaries first appeared in Europe in the thirteenth century. In France, Louis IX granted them the right to prepare and sell medicines. The Swiss physician Paracelsus (1493-1541), in an encyclopedic work, became known in particular for his theory of signatures. This theory hypothesized that because many plants resembled human organs, they were therefore a natural treatment for the resembled organ. Thus plants with yellow sap were indicated in the treatment of jaundice. Similarly, the resemblance of the autumn crocus to a big toe justified its use in the treatment of gout. The discovery of the New World introduced new substances such as cocoa, cinchona bark, and ipecacuanha.

In France in 1777, following a decree by Louis XVI, the Apothecaries' Garden was replaced by the College of Pharmacists. The groundwork for this change had been provided by such works as the *Royal Galenical and Chemical Pharmacopoeia* by Charras (1676) and the *Universal Treatise on Drugs* by Nicolas Lémery (1698).

Scientific study of the effects of drugs began with Withering (1741-1799) in England. Withering spent 10 years collecting observations on the action of foxglove powder before publishing *An Account of the Foxglove* (1785), which has remained a classic in medical literature. A crucial turning point came in the nineteenth century with the development of chemistry and the biological sciences. Many active principles were isolated from plant sources: Sertürner isolated morphine (1805); Pelletier and Caventou isolated strychnine and quinine (1818, 1820); and Robiquet isolated codeine (1832). These were followed by cocaine, atropine, acetylsalicylic acid, papaverine, and digitoxin. Chloroform was synthesized. Each new discovery was a story in itself, an uncharted adventure. One in particular is especially noteworthy – the Pasteur revolution, which led the way to vaccines, to sera, and above all, perhaps, to asepsis.

In the twentieth century, synthetic chemistry came into

its own, giving birth to the barbiturates and sulfonamides, whose appearance marked the first effective treatment of infectious disease. Various hormones were isolated and, in some cases, were followed by synthetic: insulin (Banting and Best, 1921), follicle-stimulating hormone (Doisy, 1929), and cortisone (1942). They were followed shortly by the antibiotics.

Pharmaceutical forms

The history of pharmaceuticals follows the evolution from apothecary preparation to industrial manufacture. At the end of the nineteenth and the beginning of the twentieth centuries, many pharmaceutical companies grew out of apothecaries' premises or chemical plants' effects. The apothecaries' craft was long symbolized by the mortar and pestle used to pulverize plants into mixtures with honey and various syrups. This resulted in large, soft pills, the preferred dosage form in the eighteenth century. These soft pills were followed by cachets, shells of gelatinized starch paste made from maize or wheat which were used to hide unpleasant-tasting substances. For example, quinine was first administered enclosed within two communion wafers.

Tablets and capsules followed. Tablet manufacture can be dated to the British patent entitled, "Shaping pills, lozenges and blacklead by pressure in dies," granted on December 8, 1843, to Brockedon. Tablets were a very rapid success not only in England but also in Germany, Russia, and above all, America. They were ignored or disregarded, however, by French pharmacists and physicians, who preferred the pills and cachets that were more suited to magistral preparations (i.e., in accordance with a physician's prescription). Effervescent tablets made their appearance in the last 20 years of the nineteenth century.

Capsules were invented by Lehuby, a pharmacist on the rue Saint Lazare in Paris (1846-1850). Injectable preparations went through a number of vicissitudes. Harvey's description of the circulation of the blood (1628), opened the way to the idea of introducing drugs into the circulation. Louis XIV actually ordered the Royal College of Medicine (who were reluctant to depart from the doctrines of Hippocrates and Galen) to teach Harvey's theory. Astonishing as it may now seem, and against all reason, the first medicines to be injected were purgatives. However, in the absence of even the most basic asepsis, this route of administration was brought to a temporary halt by catastrophes, including septicemia and tetanus, most probably never reported.

In the early nineteenth century, Pravaz, a French physician in Lyon, had a craftsman make a syringe fitted with a hollow needle for some experiments in rabbits and horses. By 1852, the syringe was being manufactured by a Parisian medical equipment company. Under the influence of Pasteur, the use of syringes became widespread, especially after 1885. At the same time a cautious resumption of intravenous injection began, starting with normal saline during the July 1884 cholera epidemic in Paris. Injectable medicines were introduced slowly but gradually increased in number, particularly with the use of vaccination in World War I.

Registration

For a long time drugs were used solely under the personal responsibility of the provider. For example, in 1879 Murrell gave nitroglycerin to his friends and one of his children before taking it himself. The only risk incurred was that of being accused of poisoning. In the United States, however, the deaths of over 100 Oklahoman children in 1937 from an elixir of sulfanilamide in a toxic solvent, diethylene glycol, led the Food and Drug Administration (FDA), which had been set up in 1906, to require that a toxicology test be performed and a report submitted before approving a new drug application (NDA). Therapeutic research could then proceed without further formalities. However, another disaster occurred in 1960-1961. Thalidomide, a tranquilizer that caused severe fetal deformity when given to pregnant women, revealed that drugs could be teratogenic. Shortly afterward, the discovery of carcinoma of the vulva in girls whose mothers had received diethylstilbestrol in pregnancy further revealed that drugs could also be mutagenic. The FDA responded in 1962 by setting up a new approval procedure. Before any study could take place with an investigational new drug (IND) in humans the FDA must grant its approval after expert assessment of the animal experimentation dossier.

Health authority requirements thus increased considerably. Extended toxicology studies in at least two animal species became mandatory, together with tests for mutagenicity, teratogenicity, and carcinogenicity. Over the next 30 years, preclinical drug studies increased fivefold in duration and cost. To remain competitive, the major pharmaceutical manufacturers steadily increased their research and development budgets, up to 20% of their total turnover. The downside, though, was a fall in research productivity. For example, in 1960, 34 new drugs were introduced in France as opposed to only 5 in 1996. There is obviously no question of turning back the clock, but given the current requirements, which have vastly increased the difficulty and cost of experimentation in humans, it could well be asked whether drugs such as neuroleptics and antidepressants would have been discovered had their testing been conducted under the current rules. And what research director would have pressed ahead with aspirin (whose annual consumption now runs at 50,000 tons) after discovering that it was ulcerogenic and teratogenic in animals and only a weak analgesic in animal pharmacology models? Valuable compounds have no doubt been consigned to the bottom drawers and trash cans of synthetic chemistry laboratories.

Yet, despite all the legal requirements, drugs are still being withdrawn every year because of serious adverse effects. All the long and costly preclinical studies came to nothing. Human beings are a unique animal.

The Council Directive 65/65/EEC (Chap. 1, Article 1, Paragraph 2) defines a medicinal product or drug as "any substance or combination of substances presented for treating or preventing disease in human beings or animals; any substance or combination of substances which may be administered to human beings or animals with a view to making a medical diagnosis or to restoring, correcting or modifying physiological functions in human beings or in animals is likewise considered a medicinal product."

This definition covers, in particular, cosmetics and toiletries containing toxins in doses exceeding preset limits and nutritional products containing chemical or biological substances that are not foods in their own right but whose presence confers on these products either special properties required in nutritional therapy or properties of test meals.

Pharmaceutical forms

Oral ingestion remains the most common route of administration. Capsules are tending to supplant tablets, but some drugs are available in both forms. Any drug taken by mouth has to pass through the liver to reach the general circulation, which will take it to its sites of action. Some drug is destroyed by hepatic enzymes — the proportion varies among individuals and sometimes within the same individual. This first-pass effect makes it difficult to determine the effective dose. Sometimes the transcutaneous route can be used or even the intranasal route. There is considerable ongoing research on possible oral formulations of fragile drugs such as insulin. Parenteral administration has been facilitated by the use of electric pumps for controlled intravenous infusion.

Origins of drugs

Minerals Aluminum salts are still widely used as gastric coating agents, in ointments, and as vaccine excipients. There is little use nowadays for the bactericidal effect of silver. Bismuth was a widely used gastrointestinal agent, but after more than 100 years of use, it caused some fatal poisonings that were never properly explained but which considerably reduced its sales. Many products are based on a calcium salt, whether ascorbate, carbonate, gluconate, or phosphate. Iron-deficiency anemia is still treated with ferrous iron. Discovery of the activity of lithium in manic depression transformed the lives of those affected. Magnesium-based products are commonly used, although the criteria for their use are not always strictly scientific. Manganese is used mainly as a trace element. Despite the difficulties associated with its use, gold is still employed as a slow-acting antirheumatic agent. Platinum salts are effective against cancer at several sites. Potassium remains essential in the deficiency states. Zinc is indicated in various forms of malnutrition and is used as a trace element.

Plants Herbal teas – or whole-plant infusions – are still a useful form of self-medication. However, the focus of current demand is for pure chemical products. The active principles of medicinal plants are therefore isolated and extracted. Although they often can be synthesized, this method can be more expensive than extraction. A great number of compounds thus continue to be extracted from plants cultivated precisely for that purpose. The discovery of penicillin drew attention to the potential of molds and led to the discovery of other active medicines, in particular for typhoid and tuberculosis. More recently, a mold also was the source of cyclosporine, which has transformed the prognosis of organ transplantation.

The potential of plant sources is far from exhausted. It is estimated that there are approximately 250,000 plant species, of which only 5% have been screened to date for therapeutic activity. It is unrewarding work. The only active anticancer agents isolated in a 30-year plant-screening program by the U.S. National Cancer Institute were paclitaxel and topotecan. The program was suspended in 1980 and resumed in 1990, still focused on cancer but including the acquired immune-deficiency syndrome (AIDS). A dozen private companies in the United States, the United Kingdom, and Italy have specialized in this research. Many plant species fall into extinction each year.

Animals Although mummy powder was dropped from the French Pharmacopoiea only at the end of the nineteenth century, many other relics of the past persist in popular medicine. In some parts of the world rhinoceros horn is still credited with aphrodisic properties. The discovery of organ extract therapy (opotherapy) by Brown-Séquard paved the way for hormone therapy. Some hormones were synthesized from an early date and often underwent some structural improvements in the process. Some insulin, however, is still extracted from porcine pancreases, and until recently growth hormone was extracted from human cadaver pituitaries. Calcitonin is also obtained by extraction. Heparin is still extracted from porcine intestinal mucosa or cattle lung. AZT, the first medicine to be effective in AIDS, comes from herring spermatozoa.

Synthetic chemistry Synthetic chemistry was responsible for most of the major therapeutic innovations of the twentieth century. Its first exponents began by copying the plant world, concentrating on molecules extracted from plants with recognized therapeutic effects. Acetylsalicylic acid differs little from the salicin in willow bark, which was known to be an antipyretic. Serendipity played a role in some cases. Thus verapamil, the first known calcium antagonist and still in extensive use, was modeled on papaverine. Tacrine, which offerts a glimmer of hope in the treatment of Alzheimer's disease, is similar in formula and biological properties to the eserine isolated in 1915 from the Calabar bean.

Chemists also succeeded in modifying molecules of plant origin in order to reduce their unwanted effects, permit or improve their absorption, or enhance their resistance to breakdown in the stomach. Penicillin therapy originally required one intramuscular injection every 4 hours with a product stored in a cold room. The antibiotic was fragile and rapidly destroyed at acid pH, so it could not be used via the oral route. The molecule was modified to decrease its instability. Subsequently, after bacteria learned how to destroy penicillin by secreting penicillinase, the site of penicillinase action was identified to make the antibiotic less vulnerable.

Some molecules that are expensive to synthesize can be extracted from plants and then modified. Thus an alkaloid simply can be converted to a salt, as with the anticancer agents vinblastine and vincristine. In other cases, when the bulk of the extraction product forms the skeleton of the new molecule, the process can be described as *semisynthesis.*

Another common approach was to copy molecules of animal origin. Thus the derivatives of norepinephrine (noradrenaline), the physiologic neurotransmitter of the sympathetic nervous system, include the reference bronchodilator isoproterenol (isoprenaline), as well as the adrenergic beta blockers. In 1942, 28 different steroids were isolated from the adrenal cortex. Less than 10 years later, hydrocortisone was discovered to have spectacular effects in rheumatoid arthritis. Synthetic chemists later prepared several dozen structural analogues, some of which were 25-fold more anti-inflammatory than the native molecule. The discovery of testosterone and ovarian estrogens allowed the synthesis of analogues and, in particular, of effective oral contraceptives.

Systematic synthetic chemistry The development of synthetic chemistry showed that many structures had activity in living organisms. The idea arose that systematic screening of molecules in pharmacologic models would sooner or later lead to therapeutic breakthroughs. Initial triage had to be wide ranging enough to include all substances of potential interest. Some companies were not content simply with the products of their own synthetic chemistry departments but included university laboratories in their screening net. Some drugs were born of this approach.

Recent research has been conducted on a more scientific and rational basis involving the characterization of the crystalline structure of specific targets. This has led to the discovery of the molecular structure of several hundred enzymes. Sites of action have been patented. Robots are used for the flash synthesis of thousands of peptides from amino acids, one of which is then picked out by computer as having the right structure to block the designated target. Intellectually, the approach is highly satisfying, but it must not be forgotten that the underlying purpose is to find new drugs and not to have a paper accepted by a prestigious journal.

A breach, once made quickly becomes an avenue. The following antimigraine agents have been consecutively introduced: sumatriptan, naratriptan, and zolmitriptan. Rizatriptan, clotriptan, and almotriptan are ready and waiting in the wings. Although enhanced therapeutic benefit is always possible, and one formulation may be better tolerated than another, the obvious driving force behind this approach is primarily commercial.

Genetic engineering Many diseases, both inborn and acquired, result from a genetic defect. We are constantly learning more about the genes that need to be introduced to treat these conditions. The main difficulty is in developing reliable vectors to carry them to the cells.

Bacterial gene pools also can be modified to produce foreign proteins. Insulin was the first such genetically engineered medicine to be approved by the FDA. The same operation can be performed in plants. Thus tobacco has been made to synthesize hemoglobin, although admittedly in too small quantities.

The development of transgenic animals also has helped in the development of medicines. Since 1997, several products have been undergoing evaluation in humans: an antithrombin III, an α_1-antitrypsin designed for the treatment of cystic fibrosis, and a C-peptide with an intended antithrombotic effect. An exciting area is represented by humanized monoclonal antibodies.

Bacterial gene mapping also provides targets for drugs. Thus staphylococci have only 2000 genes, of which no more than 5% are important. These can be targeted and microbial proliferation blocked.

Discovery in humans The experimental models developed by pharmacologists have become increasingly more sophisticated predictors of clinical effect thanks to the results of finely tuned therapeutic trials. Forty years ago, it was easy to test a new drug on patients; thus chlorpromazine, which was to revolutionize psychiatric therapy, was introduced in 1950, only 2 years after it was synthesized and after brief toxicity testing in a single animal species. At that time, of course, it was only possible to discover neuroleptic activity in humans. Another clinical discovery was the antidepressant effect of imipramine, initially thought to be an antihistamine rather than a neuroleptic.

Other discoveries in humans include the antiarrhythmic activities of cinchona bark, quinine, lidocaine, and later, amiodarone; the hypotensive effects of clonidine and propranolol; the anti-inflammatory activities of phenylbutazone and penicillamine; and the hypoglycemic effects of the sulfonamides. Current requirements have reduced the frequency of such discoveries, but not eliminated them altogether.

Clinical trials

Clinical trials are the crucial phase in new drug development. The costs involved have become so great that before proceeding, not only must risk assessment have shown a favorable ratio between therapeutic efficacy and unwanted effects, but there must also be a prior agreement with the company that subsequently will be responsible for marketing the drug. Therapeutic risk is low and commercial risk rather obvious when, as is often the case, the drug is a new member of an already established therapeutic class.

In virtually all countries, clinical trials follow four phases (see Chap. 8):

- Phase I is confined to clinical pharmacology centers. It is performed in a small number of closely observed healthy volunteers, with the preclinical results in hand. The aim is as far as possible to confirm the animal data in humans: tolerance to gradually increasing doses, metabolic fate, nature of metabolites, and, where possible, pharmacodynamic properties. Safety is more likely to be ensured if the metabolites identified in humans are the same as in one of the animal species used for toxicology testing.
- Phase II, mainly based on comparative, double-blind studies, aims to determine the dose having the best efficacy/safety ratio in the target disease.
- Phase III involves large patient populations, from several hundred to several thousand. In chronic diseases, trials should run for at least 1 year. Many health authorities insist on numerous studies so that findings can be consolidated by matching results. However, in June of 1997, the Labor and Human Resources Committee of the US Senate requested that some applications be accepted by the FDA after only one correctly conducted clinical trial. A positive phase III trial leads to a marketing licence application.
- Phase IV refers only to medicines already on the market and can run for the entire product life. For example, clinical trials are still running on aspirin. The justification for phase IV is that phase III is inadequate either for absolutely guaranteeing safety or for evaluating a new drug's full potential. A phase III population is by definition limited and homogeneous. It will reveal only the most frequent unwanted effects. Phase IV is best suited to full risk evaluation.

Phase IV studies include large-scale surveys such as those in which patients are randomized to answer a specific question. After myocardial infarction, is it better to be treated by an antivitamin K or by aspirin (EPSIM Study)? Do class I antiarrhythmics decrease mortality after a myocardial infarction (CAST Study)? Such studies are becoming more and more numerous. They are highly protracted, taking up to 10 years, and can be very expensive, costing many millions dollars. They can benefit the sponsor by justifying the extension of a drug's indications, e.g., in supporting the use of a lipid-lowering drug to prevent the complications of coronary atherosclerosis. However, greater involvement by the authorities is needed in this kind of research, focused on low-return products, where companies are insufficiently motivated to make the necessary effort.

Marketing authorization in Europe

Marketing authorization procedures were uniformly fixed for European Economic Community (EEC) countries in two directives, in 1965 and 1975, whose requirements put European authorizations on much the same level as those of the FDA. The European Medicines Evaluation Agency (EMEA) was established in London on July 22, 1993, with each country maintaining its own evaluation system. As a result, there are now three possible types of registration procedures for a new drug (see Chap. 91): (1) A national procedure that is either limited to the requirements of local interests or is the first stage in a decentralized European Community (EC) procedure; (2) In the decentralized EC procedure, a country that has agreed to grant a marketing licence to a medicine becomes the reporter and defender of the dossier to the EMEA. This ensures coordination between member states and the drug company. Introduction onto the market is then authorized by the Brussels Commission on the recommendation of the EMEA and is valid for all EC states; (3) The centralized procedure is mandatory for all new chemical entities and medicines derived from biotechnology, such as recombinant DNA, hybridomas, monoclonal antibodies, cell cultures, and so on. The appropriate national authorities confer within the Committee of Proprietary Medicinal Products (CPMP) before first authorization. The committee's recommendation is mandatory.

Prescribing practice

Knowledge and understanding of medicines area constantly increasing, in particular thanks to the health authority requirements that have become practically the same all over the world. It therefore would be natural to suppose that national prescribing habits are broadly similar and that the same disease, e.g., hypertension, is similarly treated, at least throughout Europe. In fact, however, not only do the percentages of the population treated for hypertension differ, but there is an astonishing degree of international disparity in the treatments used. There is no clear reason why, of the 50 highest-selling medicines in Germany, France, Italy, and the United Kingdom, only 7 should be common to all four countries.

To incorporate the results of major trials into the daily practice of all countries is difficult. In addition, the problem of alternative treatments without claim to scientific rigor remains. In many countries, considerable effort is required to retain such alternative practices. One key to this imperative is to give therapy its rightful place in the medical school curriculum. The general public also needs education. An introduction to medicines should be included in the secondary school curriculum.

The economics of drugs

The economics of drugs (see Chap. 90) has become a discipline in its own right. Evaluation is becoming systematized based not only on risk versus efficacy but also on the ratio between expenditures on pharmaceuticals and the savings engendered in shorter hospitalizations and less time – off work.

Pharmaceutical production is concentrated essentially in seven countries: United States, Great Britain, Germany, Switzerland, France, Italy, and Japan. Worldwide, 40 pharmaceutical groups account for more than half of production. However, unlike other industries, multinational companies dominate only a small share of the world market, but they tend to specialize in a product range in which they hold a dominating position. The estimated world market in 1995 was $ 283 billion. However, there are huge regional differences in consumption. OECD countries account for 73% of world consumption, Latin America for 5%, and Africa for only 3%.

Pharmaceutical companies face spectacular international competition and if they are to survive must devote a large part of their budgets to research. This is only possible if they make enough profit. Profitability varies among countries. Efforts to contain or decrease the level of expenditure on pharmaceuticals continue. One solution promoted the production of *generic drugs*, which are copies of an original drug whose patent has expired after the 20 regulatory years. The EC has instituted a supplementary certificate of protection prolonging the duration of a patent by a further 5 years, although not more than 15 years may elapse between the marketing authorization and its expiration. The generic drug argument is based on the fact that because a generic drug is much cheaper to develop than the original, it can be sold for considerably less.

The advantage is less striking in countries where medicines are not expensive. Frank disadvantages, however, include undisputed overconsumption of the medicine in question together with reduced profits for research investment by the drug companies responsible for therapeutic progress in the first place. Several large firms developed generics alongside their original drugs. Some have very recently given up this approach. In fact, all the figures show that the savings expected from generics are far lower than are needed to solve the problem.

Increasing pharmaceutical consumption is common to all developed countries and is accelerating, particularly in the elderly who are responsible for the greatest expenditure and whose life expectancy is steadily increasing. However, health economics must take into account not only the expenditure on pharmaceuticals but also on the savings involved. Drugs have changed life.

As evidence, think of the havoc wreaked in the recent past by tuberculosis, smallpox, syphilis, and other infectious diseases. Thanks to drugs, peptic ulceration no longer requires major surgery and expensive hospitalization. The spectacular advances in surgery, in particular transplantation, were made possible only by the development of increasingly well-tolerated anesthetics and highly effective drugs, including antibiotics, anticoagulants, and immunosuppressants. The development of contraceptives changed patterns of social behavior. New challenges continue to emerge, including the treatment of cancer and, of course, AIDS.

Drugs have become an essential ingredient of our civilization. However, uncommon diseases, with a correspondingly small market, attract little research, and diseases such as leprosy, for which effective treatment is available, have still not been totally eradicated. The broader economics of pharmaceuticals prevails.

2

Pharmacokinetics: from genes to therapeutic drug monitoring

Luc P. Balant, Marianne Gex-Fabry, Effie A. Balant-Gorgia

In order to exert its effect, a pharmacologically active substance must reach its site of action and remain there for an adequate period of time before being excreted (Fig. 2.1). Experience has shown that the fate of the active principle in the organism (pharmacokinetics) is as important as its intrinsic pharmacologic activity. *Pharmacokinetics* is defined as the study of absorption, distribution, metabolism, and excretion (ADME) of drugs in living organisms as a function of time. Pharmacokinetics also implies that the fate of metabolites must be considered (Fig. 2.2). *Pharmacodynamics* is the study, as a function of time, of the nature, intensity, and duration of action or effect of the active compound. In the clinical setting, knowledge of pharmacokinetics helps to minimize the frequency of unwanted side effects and to optimize the therapeutic

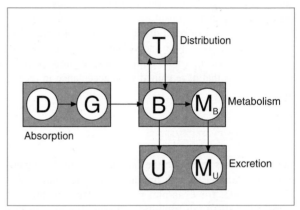

Figure 2.2 Schematic representation of the processes included in the definition of pharmacokinetics. D is the administered drug product. G is the drug in solution in the gastrointestinal tract. B is the parent drug in the central, or blood, compartment. T is the parent compound in the peripheral, or tissue, compartment. U is unchanged drug in urine. M_B and M_U are metabolites in the central compartment and in urine, respectively. Arrows indicate drug transfer, generally by "first order" kinetics.

effect of the drug. Until recently, it was usual to study kinetics and dynamics separately. In recent years, however, new methods have been developed that integrate the two approaches into the field of pharmacokinetics/pharmacodynamics. This chapter is restricted essentially to the pharmacokinetic side of this field.

It is usual to present pharmacokinetics as separated into *absorption, distribution, metabolism, and excretion* (ADME) of drugs in living organisms. This separation has the advantage of delineating areas of interest that are macroscopically different, but it ignores common features, such as the passage through biologic membranes, that underlie all these phenomena. This chapter is an attempt to present pharmacokinetics as an integrated discipline starting at the molecular level and ending with

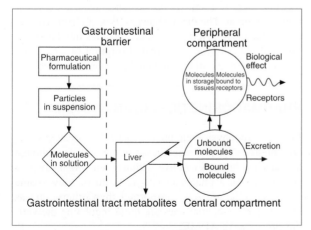

Figure 2.1 Schematic representation of the fate of a drug after oral administration. In most cases, the receptors are not located in the "central", or blood, compartment but in a "peripheral", or tissue, compartment, sometimes called the *biophase*. However, in many instances, it is possible to consider that the body behaves kinetically as if these two compartments were one single compartment.

populations of patients – without, however, neglecting organ systems and the assets of classic pharmacokinetics.

This "inverted Russian doll" point of view is based on the acceptance that most processes governing the fate of drugs in the body occur at the cellular level either because enzymes convert drugs to metabolites or because cells excrete substances into urine, bile, perspiration, milk, or pulmonary gases. This means that drugs must pass through cellular membranes either to exert their effect at receptor sites or to be biotransformed and/or excreted.The next degree of integration level is organs or organ systems. Indeed, the understanding of the mechanisms and kinetics of drug handling in different organ systems serves as a basis for the construction of models that integrate the different phenomena of ADME. One further level of abstraction is provided by equations underlying these models. Such equations allow reduction of large amounts of experimental data to a few relevant pharmacokinetic parameters. They represent the usual means to describe the behavior of drugs in the body and allow the study of the influence of physiologic variables such as gender, age, genetic constitution, and pathologic conditions such as liver or renal disease. The fate of drugs also can be studied not only in individual healthy or diseased subjects but also in whole populations, leading to more global models that have gained wide acceptance in recent years.

GENES AND ENZYMES

Some processes related to the fate of drugs in the organism are common to both humans and other mammals. They include, for example, passive diffusion through membranes, tissue distribution and equilibration, and to some extent, protein binding and urinary secretion. At the other extreme, hepatic metabolism shows extreme interspecies, interethnic, and interindividual variability. Clearly, all processes regulating the behavior of drugs in the organism are, at least to some extent, controlled by genes, and directly or indirectly, enzymes play an important role. However, it is usual to restrict the term *pharmacogenetics* to metabolic processes that display genetic regulation. Pharmacogenetic knowledge is very important for the adaptation of dosage regimen in individual patients (see Chap. 3).

CELLS AND CELLULAR MEMBRANES

Cells can be considered to perform four basic tasks: uptake of molecules, storage, biotransformation, and release of the parent compound or its metabolic transformation products. By analogy, it can be proposed that individual cells perform "micro-ADME" tasks, even if cell specialization tends to distinguish between cells involved in storage, biotransformation, and excretion. In any case, movement through membranes is a common feature.

Cell membranes are composed of a central lipid matrix covered on each side by more hydrophilic proteins. Narrow aqueous channels exist between some cells, and cell membranes contain small, water-filled pores and carrier systems. A major component of the ease with which substances pass through membranes is their lipophilicity. Lipid-soluble drugs tend to penetrate lipid membranes with ease and thus express high permeability, whereas polar neutral molecules or ionized compounds pass through membranes with greater difficulty. Other important factors are size and shape of transported molecules. Since most drugs are weak acids or weak bases, they exist in biologic fluids as an equilibrium between un-ionized and ionized forms. The un-ionized, lipophilic form is assumed to be preferentially transported through membranes. In the body, such considerations are of minor relevance because most tissues display a pH close to 7.4. However, such equilibria are of importance for the transport of drugs through the gastrointestinal membrane and for their excretion in urine by tubular secretion, since the pH of the gastric fluids varies between 1.5 and 7.0 and the pH of urine fluctuates between 4.5 and 7.5 (see Chap. 4).

Most drugs pass through cellular membranes by *passive diffusion*. The driving force for drug transfer is the difference between concentrations in two neighboring cells. Drug transport continues toward an equilibrium in which the concentrations in the two cells (or compartments) are the same in both aqueous phases. In living organisms, elimination of substances from the body starts immediately, and such an equilibrium is never reached unless drug loss is continuously compensated by new drug input.

Functioning of cellular life does not rely only on equilibrium conditions; for many substances or ions, gradients between intracellular and extracellular water are a vital necessity. To achieve this goal, membranes contain specialized carrier-mediated transport systems. Two types of transport processes have been described: *passive facilitated diffusion* and *active transport*. Only the latter is of importance for drugs. Active transport is characterized by saturability, specificity, competitive inhibition, and the fact that there is a transfer of substance against a concentration gradient. The maintenance of this gradient requires metabolic energy. Active transport includes tubular secretion and reabsorption, intestinal absorption of some substances, and transport through the blood-brain barrier.

PHARMACOKINETIC ORGAN SYSTEMS

From a pathophysiologic point of view, all organ systems are important for the maintanance of normal life, although animals and humans can live without some organs (e.g., a finger). From a pharmacokinetic point of view, some organ systems are more important than others, and as expected, the essential ones are those regulating the various processes of ADME:

- *absorption*: gastrointestinal tract and, to a lesser extent, skin, lung, nose, and eyes;
- *distribution*: fat and muscle but also erythrocytes and sometimes bone;

- *metabolism*: essentially the liver, but on occasions lung, kidney, gastrointestinal tract, blood, muscle;
- *excretion*: kidney, but on occasions lung (for volatile compounds), skin through sweat, and milk in lactating mothers.

One organ system that plays a crucial role in the transport of drugs is plasma and plasma water and, to a minor extent, lymph. Blood, plasma or serum, and plasma water represent the biologic matrix most often used to take samples, but urine, bile, and feces are also useful matrices.

Gastrointestinal system

It is usual to consider that the "pharmacokinetic" gastrointestinal system consists of the mouth, the stomach, the intestine, and the liver. Drugs may be absorbed in the mouth (e.g., sublingual administration of nitrates), from the stomach, and essentially from the intestine. They may be presystemically destroyed by the acid environment in the stomach, bacteria present in the lower part of the intestine, and enzymes present in the intestinal wall and the liver. Gastrointestinal absorption is a prerequisite for activity. In addition to passage through cellular membranes, gastric emptying, intestinal transit time, and dissolution for solid pharmaceutical forms also may play an important role in the rate and extent to which a drug reaches the systemic circulation.

The fraction of dose reaching the systemic circulation (*systemic availability*, or F) can be defined as the product of the fraction of dose escaping loss in the stomach (F_G), passing through the wall and escaping loss on passing through this membrane (F_I), and escaping loss on passing through the liver (F_H).

The fraction of drug escaping loss across the liver is:

$$F_H = 1 - \varepsilon_H$$

where ε_H is the hepatic extraction ratio, which is a measure of the capacity of the liver to extract substances from the incoming blood. Accordingly, for a drug with a high hepatic extraction ratio, the systemic availability is low, whereas for a drug with a low extraction ratio, F_H tends toward 1. Enzyme induction, for example, can modify the systemic availability of drugs with moderate to high hepatic extraction ratios.

From a pharmacokinetic point of view, the systemic availability defines the amount of drug absorption and, if deemed interesting, the rate at which this phenomenon occurs. For the quantitative description of pharmaceutical formulations, the concepts of bioavailability and bioequivalence have been developed.

Protein and tissue binding

Distribution or *tissue distribution* refers to the reversible transfer of substances between different organs of the body (for more details, see Chap. 4). At equilibrium (Fig. 2.3), the substance in plasma can bind to various proteins; in tissues, it can partition into adipose masses and bind to a variety of cellular components. In plasma, acidic drugs usually bind to albumin and basic drugs to α_1-acid-glycoprotein or to lipoproteins.

Drug concentration in blood, plasma, or plasma water depends on the amount of drug in the body and on how the drug is distributed. The proportionality constant relating amount in the body and concentration measured in a biologic matrix is the *apparent volume of distribution*. This volume of distribution (V) depends on binding to plasma proteins (albumin, α_1-acid-glycoprotein) as well as to tissue components (muscle, fat, etc.). The following simple model may be used to describe this double dependency:

$$V = V_P + V_T(f_u/f_{u,T})$$

where V_P is the true plasma volume (usually 3 liters), V_T is the true water present in tissues (usually 40 liters), and f_u and $f_{u,T}$ are the fractions of drug unbound in plasma and tissue, respectively. This model is based on the assumption that tissue equilibrium is achieved when the unbound concentrations in plasma and tissues are equal.

This model shows that when a drug has a high affinity for components in the tissues, the volume of distribution may be much greater than the volume of the body. As a consequence, plasma concentrations are low. As an example, for very lipophilic drugs, large amounts distribute in adipose tissue and relatively low concentrations are measured in blood. This may correspond to V values exceeding 1000 liters. The apparent volume of distribution thus has no specific physiologic value. In other situations, tissue binding is low, whereas plasma protein binding is high, resulting in a small V. Finally, plasma and tissue binding may both be high. The value of V then depends on the respective affinities of the drug for binding sites in

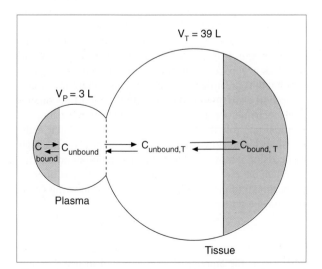

Figure 2.3 Schematic representation of the distribution of drug between plasma and tissue. At equilibrium, the plasma concentration $C_{unbound}$ (i.e., unbound to plasma proteins) is equal to the tissue concentration $C_{unbound,T}$ (i.e., unbound to tissue components). Equations have been derived to calculate the apparent volume of distribution V from the fractions of unbound drug in plasma and tissues, assuming the actual plasma volume (V_P) and tissue volume (V_T) are constants.

and outside plasma. Thus, even a drug that is highly bound to plasma proteins may display a high apparent volume of distribution.

The concepts of binding and distribution refer to systems at equilibrium. However, if a drug is introduced into an organism, its tissue concentration is first equal to zero, and some time is needed for an equilibrium or pseudo-equilibrium to be reached. Numerous factors determine the distribution rate of drugs from plasma to various body tissues. These factors include the rate of delivery (i.e., blood flow) to the tissue, the ability of the drug to pass through biologic membranes, and the binding of the drug to both plasma proteins and tissue components. If equilibrium is reached very quickly throughout the body, it is said that the body behaves as a *one-compartment open-body system,* whereas if the time to reach distribution equilibrium is relatively long as compared with the process of drug input, the body is said to behave as a *multicompartmental system.* With the exception of prolonged intravascular perfusions, seldom is a true (i.e., static) equilibrium reached. In most situations, drugs start to be eliminated as soon as the first molecules enter the organism, and accordingly, if distribution is rate-limited (going into or coming out of the tissues), only a pseudoequilibrium will be reached. This, however, does not impede pharmacokinetic concepts from remaining valid, and different means exist to take these phenomena into account.

The liver

Among all organs, the liver has the highest metabolic capacity. The ability of the liver to eliminate drugs from the body is described by a parameter called *hepatic clearance* (CL_H). Hepatic clearance includes metabolic clearance and biliary excretory clearance. Substances in blood may be bound to plasma proteins, partitioned into blood cells, or free (or unbound) in plasma. Only unbound molecules can be taken up by the liver, but it appears that for some substances the time to partition out of the blood cells, dissociate from the plasma proteins, pass through the hepatic membranes, and be either metabolized by enzymes and/or transported into bile is so short that it appears that all the drug delivered to the liver is irreversibly extracted. In this situation, the hepatic *extraction ratio* E_H is said to be high (i.e., close to 1), and the hepatic clearance based on blood concentrations approaches hepatic blood flow (i.e., around 1.5 liters/min). If the extraction rate is low (i.e., close to 0), one must assume that one or more of the following processes is rate limiting: slow diffusion out of the blood cells or dissociation from plasma proteins, poor diffusion into hepatocytes, slow enzymatic reactions or biliary transport. In theory, when E_H is close to 1, hepatic clearance is limited by the perfusion rate because changes in blood flow directly influence the value of hepatic clearance. When E_H is low, two main phenomena are known to modify clearance: changes in plasma protein binding (e.g., drug-drug interactions) and changes in enzymatic activity (e.g., enzyme induction or inhibition).

Clearance may be viewed as a measure of substance loss across an organ of elimination or as a measure of drug loss from the organism. The hepatic clearance may be defined as a function of the hepatic blood flow (Q_H) and the hepatic extraction ratio (ε_H):

$$CL_H = Q_H \cdot \varepsilon_H$$

The hepatic extraction ratio is equal to 1 if all drug is irreversibly extracted and 0 if no extraction occurs at all. The extraction concept is valuable because it allows assessment of the effects of changes in blood flow, protein binding, or enzyme activity. The intrinsic clearance may be considered as the sum of all enzymatic processes involved in the elimination of the drug. This concept allows us to explain how the hepatic extraction ratio is influenced by changes in hepatic blood flow, protein binding, and enzymatic activity.

The kidneys

The basic anatomic and functional unit of the kidney is the nephron, composed of the glomerulus, the proximal tubule, the loop of Henle, the distal tubule, and the collecting tubule (see Chap. 21). The glomerulus filters about 120 ml of plasma water per minute; this is called the *glomerular filtration rate* (GFR). Most of the water is reabsorbed in the tubule, and only 1 or 2 ml/min leaves the kidneys and goes into the urine. Only unbound substances in plasma water are filtered through the glomerulus. As a consequence, the efficiency of drug removal by this mechanism is highly sensitive to changes in plasma protein binding. *Tubular secretion* may provide additional urinary excretion. Separate mechanisms exist for secreting acids and bases. These are active processes. *Tubular reabsorption* is the third factor controlling renal handling of substances. It varies from being almost absent to being virtually complete. For most drugs, reabsorption occurs by passive processes. Passive reabsorption is possible because of water reabsorption in the tubule, which concentrates the drug in the glomerular filtrate up to 100 times as compared with the unbound concentration in plasma, thus creating the necessary concentration gradient for passive diffusion. As expected, depending on the physicochemical nature of the drug, urinary pH may play an important role in controlling the extent of tubular reabsorption. Urine flow usually plays a minor role, although on occasion it may influence renal clearance significantly.

When the rate of urinary excretion of a drug is directly proportional to plasma concentration, the following equation may be written:

$$dA_e/dt = CL_R \cdot C$$

where A_e is the amount of drug excreted in urine. *Renal clearance* is usually expressed on the basis of concentrations measured in plasma or plasma water. If protein binding is saturable, CL_R is not constant but varies as a function of the plasma concentration.

The appearance of drugs in urine is the net result of filtration, secretion, and reabsorption. Each process contributes to renal clearance in an additive manner. In theory, secretion is inferred when the rate of excretion exceeds the rate of filtration or if renal clearance exceeds clearance by filtration. On the other hand, reabsorption necessarily occurs if renal clearance is less than the calculated clearance by filtration. In reality, secretion and reabsorption may coexist, and calculation of the magnitude of each process is then far from evident.

PHARMACOKINETIC MODELS

Pharmacokinetics addresses issues related to the study of pharmacologically active substances in living organisms. For this purpose, pharmacokinetic methods organize *data pairs* (i.e., blood or tissue concentrations versus time or amount excreted versus time) to determine parameters that are at higher levels of abstraction than the actual data and are used to summarize the behavior of drugs in the body. These parameters characterize a mathematical model that can be challenged with new doses, routes of administration, and/or dosage schedules. Ideally, models also should be able to reflect changes in plasma protein binding and blood or urine flow in order to be used in both healthy volunteers and patients.

Pharmacokinetic models may be considered to be either empiric or explicative. *Empiric* models are purely mathematical descriptions of the time course of drug concentration in a sample of biologic tissue or fluid. An example is provided by the classically used sum of exponentials. *Explicative* models incorporate physiologic hypotheses. The classic compartmental models have been considered to be explicative because they require compartments for absorption, distribution, and elimination. The same applies to the simple clearance-based models. However, the term explicative probably should be restricted to the full physiologic models that separate

the body into a number of anatomic compartments, each of them interconnected through the body fluid system.

Compartmental models were the first models and are still valuable, in particular if computers are used for nonlinear regression analysis. It is thus possible to use compartmental models for data analysis and to derive, in a second step, clearance values, or to use the clearance approach directly to determine such parameters as clearance or volume of distribution.

If equilibration between blood and tissues is very fast as compared with absorption, metabolism, and excretion, the body can be visualized as a single entity in which all drug molecules have the same probability to be eliminated (Fig. 2.4). This system behaves as if it were at equilibrium for all its components at any time following drug administration. The basic assumption underlying the one-compartment open-body model is that the rate of decline of the amount of drug (A) or of plasma concentration (C) is proportional to a rate constant termed the *elimination rate constant* (k_e) according to

$$-dA/dt = k_e \cdot A \text{ or } -dC/dt = k_e \cdot C$$

The proportionality constant between A and C is the *volume of distribution* (V) such as V = A/C.

Clearance-based models have been developed as an alternative to compartmental models in order to incorporate more physiologic concepts into pharmacokinetic data analysis. These models are sometimes called physiologic models, although, in our opinion, this term should rather be used for models that incorporate various organs and their respective blood flows, as discussed later in this chapter. The clearance-based model makes no specific assumption regarding the structure of the model in terms of number of compartments but assumes that the rate of elimination of drug from the body is proportional to a parameter termed the *clearance* according to

$$-dA/dt = CL \cdot C \text{ or } -dC/dt = (CL/V) \cdot C$$

It is immediately apparent that these equations are similar to the equation describing the one-compartment open-body model and that $CL = k_e \cdot V$.

When the drug is equilibrating between plasma and other tissues at a rate appreciably slower than the absorption and elimination processes, more complex models must be used to quantify the time course of drug and metabolites in the body and to estimate the distribution in the body tissues. Classically, two- and three-compartment models have been used (Fig. 2.5). The number of compartments, however, is limited by the number of distinguishable disposition phases. In addition, it is seldom possible to attribute physiologic meaning to these compartments, and the calculated "compartment concentrations" are fraught with errors.

Physiologic pharmacokinetic models attempt to use basic physiologic and biochemical information to deter-

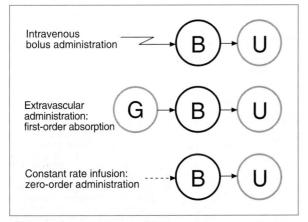

Figure 2.4 The one-compartment open-body model. The central, or blood, compartment B is assumed to be an isomorphic space, with each molecule present at one time in the compartment having the same probability to be eliminated. Elimination, depicted as U, may include urinary excretion and/or metabolism. The three classic modes of drug administration are also illustrated. For extravascular administration, G is the drug in solution in the gastrointestinal tract.

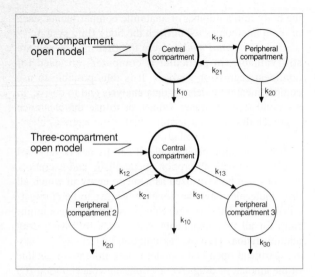

Figure 2.5 The two- and three-compartment models. The number of exponentials needed to describe the concentration-versus-time curve following intravenous injection determines the number of compartments. Elimination may occur either from the central compartment only, from one of the peripheral compartments, or from a combination of both central and peripheral compartments. k_{ij} are first-order transfer rates from compartment i to compartment j; k_{io} are elimination rates from compartment i.

mine drug distribution and disposition. They have been developed with the hypothesis that compartmental models can be misleading because they do not provide insight into the concentration history of a drug at the local site of a target organ or tissue, which is not always reflected by blood concentrations. Physiologic models usually are based on the principle of mass conservation and on all the knowledge available concerning mass transport and physiology of mammalian systems.

Models may be used to simulate the behavior of drugs in organisms with one or more compartments. Their main interest lies in data analysis. All procedures of pharmacokinetic data analysis use one of the models briefly described above. Accordingly, the term *model-free pharmacokinetics*, sometimes used to describe a strategy of data analysis based on noncompartmental models, is not correct because some underlying model is always assumed.

Bolus intravenous injection

When a drug is administered to an a healthy volunteer or a patient and blood samples are collected at adequate time points, the concentration of the parent compound can be measured in whole blood or plasma. When a single dose of a drug is injected as a bolus, it is frequent to observe a monoexponential decline in blood concentrations as a function of time. When a logarithmic scale is used for concentrations, a straight line is obtained. These are the two classic modes of data representation in pharmacokinetics (Fig. 2.6). From such a graph, the half-life of the drug is calculated easily. The *half-life* ($t_{1/2}$) is the time necessary for the concentration to decrease to one-half. When the decline is monoexponential, the half-life is independent of the reference concentration. As a basic rule, it takes 7 half-lives for drug concentration to reach a value lower than 1% of any reference concentration.

Compartmental models may be used to describe the decline in the blood (plasma or serum) concentrations as a function of time. In the present case, one would use a one-compartment open-body model as depicted in Figure 2.4 because only one exponential phase is visible on the semilogarithmic plot. The equations describing the fate of the drug in the organism (or its concentration C_t in blood as a function of time) are derived by integration of equation

$$-dC_t/dt = k_e C_t$$

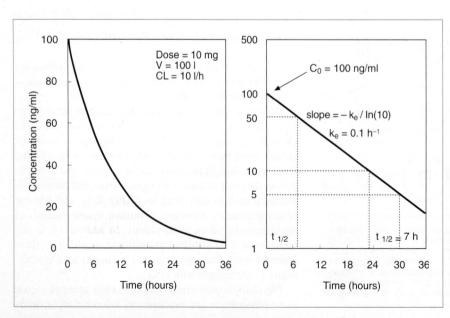

Figure 2.6 Blood (or plasma or serum) concentration as a function of time following bolus intravenous injection. As indicated in the right panel, the elimination rate constant k_e is calculated from the slope of the curve in semilogarithmic coordinates. The elimination half-life $t_{1/2}$ is the time needed for the concentration to decrease to one-half its initial value, independently of the reference concentration. The concentration measured immediately after injection C_0 allows one to calculate the volume of distribution because $C_0 = dose/V$. In this case $V = \dfrac{10\ mg}{100 ng/ml} = 100$ liters.

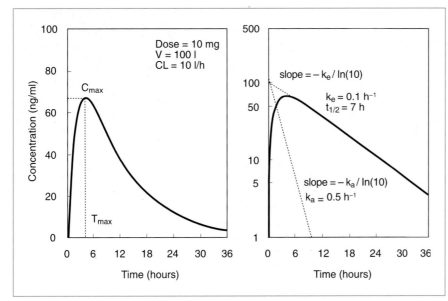

Figure 2.7 Blood (or plasma or serum) concentration as a function of time following first-order absorption. As indicated in the right panel, the elimination rate constant k_e is calculated from the slope of the terminal portion of the curve in semilogarithmic coordinates. The absorption rate constant k_a can be estimated from the slope of the curve resulting from subtraction of the actual concentration-versus-time curve from the extrapolated line corresponding to the elimination phase (method of residuals, also called *peeling* or *stripping method*). In the present case, and for many drugs, absorption occurs relatively rapidly when compared with elimination.

$$C_t = C_0 \cdot \exp(-k_e \cdot t) \text{ or } \ln C_t = \ln C_0 - k_e \cdot t$$

where C_0 is the concentration in blood immediately after bolus injection, k_e is the apparent elimination rate constant, and t is time; exp represents an exponential function $[\exp(x) = e^x]$, and ln is the natural logarithm. The slope of the line obtained when plotting $\ln C_t$ versus time is thus equal to $-k_e$. When using the common logarithm (i.e., base 10 logarithm), as is usually done for semilogarithmic plots, the slope becomes equal to $-k_e/\ln(10)$, with $\ln(10) = 2.303$.

If the drug equilibrates very rapidly between blood and tissues, the concentration measured immediately after injection (C_0) allows one to calculate the volume into which the drug distributes because, at this time, the amount of drug present in the organism is equal to the administered dose. More generally, as described earlier, the apparent volume of distribution (V) is a parameter defining the relationship between measured concentration and amount (A) of drug in the body at any given time (i.e., V = A/C). In the case of a bolus intravenous injection, it is assumed that the amount of drug present in the body is equal to the injected dose, and the theoretical concentration at that time is back-calculated from the measured plasma concentrations (see C_0 in Fig. 2.6).

The main organs of drug elimination are the liver and the kidney, and their capacity for drug elimination per unit of time is described by the hepatic and renal clearances (CL_H and CL_R). Metabolism is the most important route of drug elimination from the body. However, biotransformation does not always lead to inactivation of endogenous or exogenous substances. In many instances, active and even toxic metabolites are formed. In addition, inactive pro-drugs are activated in vivo to the active principle. Since drug metabolism occurs mainly in the liver, pharmacokinetic concepts have been developed to describe biotransformation in this organ, but the same principles apply for the description of metabolism in other tissues. Hepatic clearance includes not only clearance of drugs by metabolism but also biliary excretory clearance. In practice, it is often difficult to distinguish between metabolic and biliary clearance if no bile concentration measurements are available. Clearance is an additive term; accordingly, the total-body clearance is the sum of all partial clearances (e.g. hepatic, renal, etc.). It is thus possible to define the rate of elimination of the drug from the body as

$$-dAt/dt = CL \cdot C_t$$

If the drug behaves according to a one-compartment open-body model (Fig. 2.4), this equation becomes

$$-d(Ct \cdot V)/dt = CL \cdot C_t \text{ or } -dC_t/dt = (CL/V) \cdot C_t$$

Integration of this equation leads to the following expression:

$$C_t = C_0 \cdot \exp(-t \cdot CL/V)$$

Comparing these expressions, it appears that the elimination rate constant k_e is equal to CL/V. The higher the CL, the faster is the elimination, whereas for constant clearance, a high volume of distribution leads to a slower elimination of the drug from the body.

From the preceding paragraphs and equations it can be shown that the time necessary for concentration C_t to decrease to half of its value (i.e., the apparent half-life of elimination $t_{1/2}$) is equal to

$$t_{1/2} = \ln 2 \cdot V/CL \text{ or } t_{1/2} = \ln 2/k_e$$

This concept is strictly valid only when the drug behaves according to a one-compartment open-body

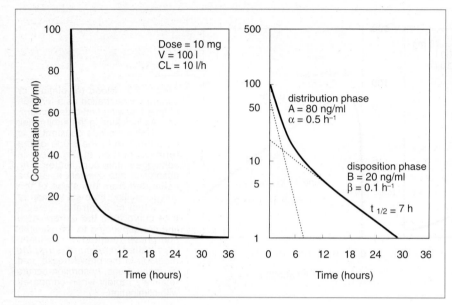

Figure 2.8 Blood (or plasma or serum) concentration as a function of time following bolus intravenous injection of a drug that distributes in the body according to a two-compartment open-body model. The curve can be described as a sum of two exponentials with parameters A, α, B, and β. As indicated in the right panel, the constants B and β can be calculated from the terminal portion of the curve in semilogarithmic coordinates. The constants A and α can be estimated from the residual curve.

model. In other situations it may be necessary to define distribution and elimination half-lives. Similarly, it is possible to define an absorption half-life if the drug is given orally. The apparent half-life of elimination is a very useful parameter for the choice of optimal dosage regimens.

First-order absorption

Gastrointestinal absorption is a complex physiologic phenomenon. However, from a pharmacokinetic point of view, absorption often can be described by a first-order process similar to elimination of a drug from the body after a bolus intravenous injection, as described in the preceding subsection. The oral drug is supposed to be at once fully available at its site of absorption in the gastrointestinal system. The equation describing the time course of drug absorption (absorption rate constant = k_a) and elimination (elimination rate constant = k_e) is the *Bateman function:*

$$C_t = (F \cdot Do/V)[k_a/(k_a - k_e)] \cdot [\exp(-k_e \cdot t) - \exp(-k_a \cdot t)]$$

where F is the systemic availability of the drug, and Do is the administered dose. The systemic availability is a number indicating the fraction of the administered dose reaching the general (or systemic) circulation. The *absorption rate constant* indicates the rate of drug entry into the central compartment of the model (Fig. 2.7) but also the rate of exit from the gastrointestinal system, which is then believed to behave as a homogeneous compartment.

Normally (Fig. 2.7), the rising phase is the absorption phase and the decreasing phase is the elimination phase (i.e., $k_a \gg k_e$). In this case, when time increases, the term $\exp(-k_a \cdot t)$ tends to decrease faster than $\exp(-k_e \cdot t)$, and the Bateman function is reduced (during the "elimination phase") to

$$C_t = (F \cdot Do/V)[k_a/(k_a - k_e)] \cdot [\exp(-k_e \cdot t)]$$

This equation is similar in its form to the equation describing elimination after a bolus intravenous injection. The apparent elimination half-life must be calculated from the elimination phase.

In some cases, k_a is smaller than k_e. This is the *flipflop situation* where the decreasing phase is the absorption phase. When a drug can be given only orally, it is not possible to decide whether the normal or the flipflop situation prevails if only blood concentrations are available. Other factors must then be used for decision making. On the contrary, if the drug also can be administered parenterally, the decision is easily made on the basis of the intravenous profile.

Maximal blood or plasma concentrations (C_{max}) are important parameters in the field of bioequivalence testing. The same applies for the time (T_{max}) at which C_{max} is observed.

For many drugs, the time course of concentration in blood shows a *time lag* between the moment of oral administration and the apparent onset of gastrointestinal absorption. This lag may be the result of delayed release of the active principle from the dosage form or delayed gastric emptying or other intestinal phenomena.

BASIC PHARMACOKINETIC METRICS

Intravenous administration

As described earlier, knowing the amount of drug reaching the systemic circulation, and assuming that the drug behaves according to a one-compartment open-body model, it is possible to calculate the apparent half-life of elimination and the elimination rate constant (k_e) from the slope of the concentration versus time curve in semilogarithmic coordinates. The *area under the blood concentration versus time curve* (AUC) from time zero to infinity (Fig. 2.6) can be calculated. The analytical solution of this integral is obtained by dividing the plasma concentration at time zero by the elimination rate constant:

$$AUC = C_0/k_e$$

Using the relationship $CL = k_e \cdot V$, the preceding equation becomes

$$AUC = Do/(k_e \cdot V) \text{ or } AUC = Do/CL$$

With these equations it is then possible to calculate the volume of distribution and the clearance. These parameters fully describe the time course of drug in the body if the "body" is considered to be a one-compartment model. AUC is an important pharmacokinetic metric, and great care must be taken to estimate it correctly. Usually, AUC is calculated using the trapezoidal rule from time zero to the last measured point and then extrapolated to infinity using the calculated slope of the elimination phase.

Oral administration

The Bateman function upon integration from time zero to infinity gives the following relationship:

$$AUC = F \cdot Do/k_e \cdot V \text{ or } AUC = F \cdot Do/CL$$

The area under the blood concentration curve for a given drug in a given subject depends on its elimination characteristics CL and on the amount of drug reaching the general circulation $F \cdot Do$. In this case, AUC characterizes the extent of absorption and is independent of the rate of absorption *ka*. As stated earlier, when the drug is administered only orally, it is generally not possible to calculate F. As a consequence, CL and V cannot be determined. However, if the drug also has been administered intravenously, F can be determined from the ratio of the *AUCs* after oral and intravenous administration according to

$$F = (AUC_{po}/AUC_{iv}) \cdot (Do_{iv}/Do_{po})$$

As indicated earlier, in order to fully describe the blood concentration versus time profile, for regulatory purposes, it is usual to indicate also the maximum concentration (C_{max}) and the time (T_{max}) at which this maximum occurs. The parameters C_{max} and T_{max} are then considered as valid surrogate points to characterize the rate of absorption (k_a) and possible absorption lag time.

Two-compartment open-body models

For most drugs under distribution pseudoequilibrium conditions, the calculated apparent volume of distribution is within 10% of the "true" steady-state volume, and therefore, either value is appropriate as long as it is clearly indicated on which basis it was calculated. Often, when a

drug is administered intravenously as a bolus, equilibrium between the central compartment and the peripheral compartment takes some time to be reached (Fig. 2.8). It is then possible to distinguish between a *distribution phase* (or α phase) and a *disposition phase* (or elimination or β phase). The equation describing the concentration versus time curve is

$$C_t = A \cdot \exp(-\alpha \cdot t) + B \cdot \exp(-\beta \cdot t)$$

The model describing this type of behavior is the two-compartment open-body model (Fig. 2.5), and its equation is biexponential. For comparison, the Bateman function is also biexponential, but it relates to the one-compartment model. It is thus important to clearly state what kind of compartmental model and what kind of equation is to be used to describe the behavior of a drug.

During the distribution phase, concentrations in the central compartment are higher than in the peripheral compartment. The reverse is true during the disposition phase. It is thus only a pseudoequilibrium that is reached during this latter phase. However, concentrations in the central and peripheral compartments run in parallel. When distribution between the central and peripheral compartments is relatively rapid, the latter is termed a *shallow compartment*. When distribution is slow, the term *deep compartment* is used. This distinction may be of relevance when the drug is administered over prolonged periods of time.

When a drug behaves according to a two-compartment model and is administered orally, two situations may arise: (1) a distribution phase is clearly observed if absorption is fast compared with distribution, and (2) no distribution phase is observed if absorption is slow compared with distribution. In the latter case, the two-compartment model collapses into a one-compartment model.

ADMINISTRATION OVER TIME

Drugs are usually not administered as single doses, although during drug development this type of administration is quite common. As discussed in the following paragraphs, constant-rate infusion or prolonged iterative dosing eventually leads to a *steady state or plateau*. Although in clinical practice infusions usually are restricted to hospital settings and iterative oral administration is the common way of administering medications in outpatients, the two modes of administration are very similar from a pharmacokinetic point of view. Indeed, it can be considered that constant-rate infusion is an iterative dosing where the time between doses (τ) is infinitely small.

Constant-rate infusion

If a drug is administered at a constant rate (e.g., 100 mg per day or 1 mg per 10 minutes), a constant plasma concentration is eventually reached. This is usually achieved by infusing the drug intravenously by intravenous drip or a pump. The drug does not reach this constant concentration faster when given by the intravenous route rather than the oral route, but possible first-pass metabolism can be avoided, and thus higher concentrations may be reached. A constant plasma concentration also can be achieved orally if specific formulations that mimic infusion are used.

If a drug is infused continuously at a fixed infusion rate (K_0), a plateau will be reached (Fig. 2.9). The plateau is characterized by a steady-state concentration (C_{ss}). In this situation, the amount of drug eliminated per unit time is exactly the same as drug input into the system per unit time. If the drug behaves according to a one-compartment model, simple relations exist between C_{ss}, K_0, CL, $t_{1/2}$, and duration of infusion. At any time during infusion the rate of change of the amount of drug in the body (dA/dt) is given by the difference between the infusion rate (K_0) and its elimination rate:

$$dA/dt = K_0 - CL \cdot C$$

On starting a constant-rate infusion, the amount of drug in the body is zero. At steady state, the change in the amount in the body is zero, and as a consequence, the steady-state concentration is given by

$$C_{ss} = K_0/CL$$

Accordingly, C_{ss} depends on the rate of infusion and CL and not (as instinctively perceived) on the volume of distribution. As seen in the following paragraphs, the volume of distribution influences the time needed to reach steady state. Sometimes it is desirable to reach steady state rapidly. It is then necessary to administer a *loading dose*, e.g., as an intravenous bolus. In clinical practice, loading doses are sometimes useful for drugs with very long half-lives in order to reach a therapeutic concentration earlier than with a constant-rate infusion.

During infusion, the concentration-versus-time curve is described by the following equation:

$$C_t = C_{ss} [1 - \exp(-k_e \cdot t)]$$

It is interesting to note that the exponential term is the same as the one describing drug elimination after a bolus injection. This is not surprising because at any time (during and after an infusion) the drug is eliminated according to the exponential rules governing the one-compartment model. Intuitively, it also can be understood that different equations are needed to describe the blood concentration profile during and after an infusion. If time is expressed in half-lives (i.e., N is the number of half-lives elapsed since the start of the infusion), it is possible to derive the following expression:

$$C_t = C_{ss}(1 - 0.5^N)$$

It becomes apparent (Fig. 2.9) that after 1 half-life, half the increase from zero to C_{ss} has been made; after 2 half-lives, 0.75 of the way is made; and it needs 4 half-lives to reach more than 90% of C_{ss}. In clinical practice, one accepts that steady state is reached when the drug has been administered at a constant rate over 4 half-lives. The same rule applies for iterative dosing. It thus appears that if clearance determines C_{ss}, the apparent volume of distribution modulates $t_{1/2}$ and influences the time to reach steady state; for constant clearance, the larger the volume of distribution, the longer is the time to reach steady state. The same rules can be applied for any change in infusion rate, as depicted in Figure 2.10. Finally, it is intuitively apparent that steady state is also reached in multicompartmental systems, even if the kinetic processes are different from those of the rapidly equilibrating one-compartment model.

Iterative dosing

Although not a classic mode of administration, neither in toxicology nor in clinical practice, multiple intravenous bolus administrations are interesting in terms of understanding the cumulation process. It can be shown that steady state is reached (Fig. 2.11) in a way fundamentally similar to that

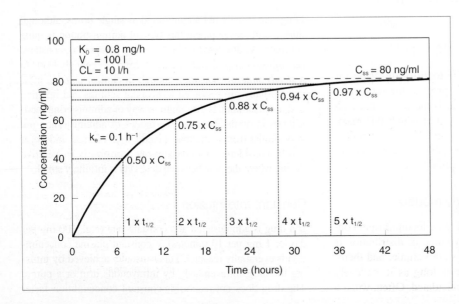

Figure 2.9 Blood (or plasma or serum) concentration as a function of time following constant-rate intravenous infusion. Steady state is characterized by a plateau concentration C_{ss}. One half-life is needed to reach half this plateau value, and 4 half-lives are needed for drug concentrations to be within 10% of steady state.

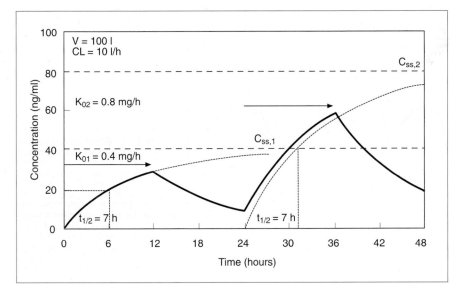

Figure 2.10 Blood (or plasma or serum) concentration as a function of time following two infusions with different rates and separated by a constant time interval. The first infusion is characterized by a plateau concentration $C_{ss,1}$, and 1 half-life is needed to reach half this plateau value. The second infusion is characterized by a steady-state value $C_{ss,2}$. The time to reach a certain fraction of this plateau is calculated from the start of the second infusion.

in the constant-rate infusion described in the preceding subsection. The major difference is that the time between administrations (τ) is now different from zero, leading to fluctuations in the blood concentration profile, with maximal ($C_{ss,max}$) and minimal ($C_{ss,min}$) steady-state concentrations being observed. If the concentrations at steady state are compared with the corresponding values after the first dose, it can be shown that

$$C_{ss,max}/C_{1,max} = C_{ss,min}/C_{1,min}$$

This ratio is called the *accumulation index*. As a practical rule, if $\tau = t_{1/2}$, the accumulation index equals 2. If the dosing interval is longer than the half-life, the index is lower

than 2; if the converse is true, the index is higher than 2. It is thus important to see that the accumulation index from zero to steady state is not an intrinsic property of a drug but is a function of the chosen mode of application. This is particularly important in therapeutics. The average steady-state concentration $C_{ss,av}$ can be defined as $C_{ss,av} = \text{dose}_\tau/CL \cdot \tau$, where τ is the time between each dose.

Multiple oral administrations

Drugs usually are given orally over a period of time and not as repeated injections. Under these conditions, steady state also may be reached, characterized by maximal ($C_{ss,max}$) and minimal ($C_{ss,min}$) concentrations over one dos-

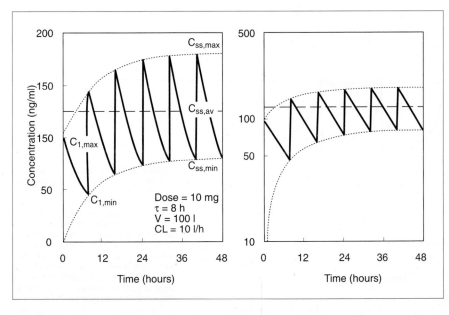

Figure 2.11 Blood (or plasma or serum) concentration as a function of time following repeated bolus intravenous injections. As a result of accumulation from one dosing interval to the next, the maximum and minimum concentrations observed over one dosing interval increase toward steady-state values $C_{ss,max}$ and $C_{ss,min}$. As for a constant-rate infusion, 4 half-lives are needed for concentrations to be within 10% of steady-state values. $C_{ss,av}$ is the average plasma concentration at steady state, and τ is the time interval between two consecutive doses.

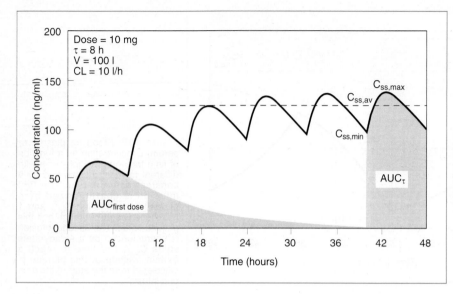

Figure 2.12 Blood (or plasma or serum) concentration as a function of time following repeated extravascular administrations. $C_{ss,max}$, $C_{ss,min}$, and $C_{ss,av}$ are the maximum, minimum, and average concentrations at steady state. The area under the concentration-versus-time curve during a dosing interval at steady state (AUC_τ) is equal to the area under the curve after a single dose. It is also equal to the area of a rectangle of height $C_{ss,av}$ and width τ.

ing interval (Fig. 2.12). The average steady-state concentration $C_{ss,av}$ can be defined as $C_{ss,av} = F \cdot dose_\tau/CL \cdot \tau$.

Multicompartmental systems

In the simplest case of the two-compartmental model, when tissues and blood reach equilibrium relatively rapidly, multiple-dose administration (Fig. 2.13) is not fundamentally different from the situation depicted for the one-compartment model, as described in the preceding subsection. However, if a deep compartment is present (Fig. 2.14), the possibility of accumulation of large amounts of substance in this slowly equilibrating deep compartment must be taken into account. The slow release of substance from this deep compartment manifests itself as an increased apparent half-life of the drug.

BIOAVAILABILITY AND BIOEQUIVALENCE

If instead of considering the behavior of an active substance without any reference to a pharmaceutical form one is interested in the characteristics of this substance administered as a precise pharmaceutical formulation, it is more appropriate to use the term *bioavailability* instead of systemic availability (see also Chap. 5). The *absolute bioavailability* defines the rate and extent at which the parent compound reaches the systemic circulation as compared with intravenous administration. The *relative bioavailability* defines the rate and extent at which the parent compound reaches the systemic circulation as compared with a formulation administered via the same route (e.g., tablet versus oral solution).

Two drug products are considered *bioequivalent* when

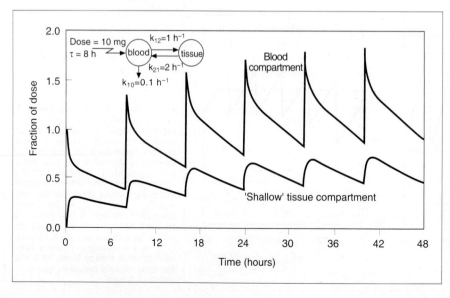

Figure 2.13 Blood (or plasma or serum) concentration as a function of time following repeated bolus intravenous injections for a two-compartment open-body model with rapid distribution between blood and tissues. The peripheral, or tissue, compartment is called a *shallow compartment*. The distribution and elimination phases are clearly distinguishable from the concentration-versus-time curve in the central compartment.

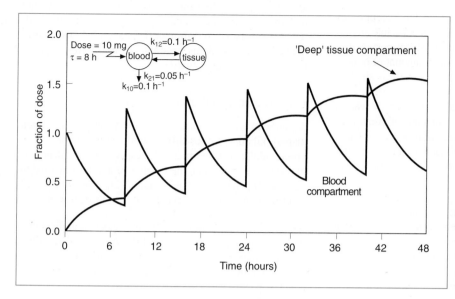

Figure 2.14 Blood (or plasma or serum) concentration as a function of time following repeated bolus intravenous injections for a two-compartment open-body model with slow distribution between blood and tissues. The peripheral, or tissue, compartment is called a *deep compartment*. The slow release of substance from this compartment may lead to accumulation of large amounts of drug in the tissues. This may lead to organ-specific toxicity.

they display the same bioavailability (i.e., identical rate and extent of absorption). Bioavailability and bioequivalence testing is usually performed in young, healthy volunteers in order to try to minimize inter- and intraindividual variability. The new pharmaceutical form (i.e., test drug) and a reference formulation are administered to the same volunteers in a crossover design. The *identity of clearance* is a prerequisite for correct estimation of bioavailability. AUC, C_{max}, and T_{max} are then compared between test and reference formulations. For bioequivalence studies, formal statistical procedures have been devised. Bioequivalence issues are very important from a regulatory point of view because they allow a new drug product to be substituted for a product already on the market.

MISCELLANEOUS TOPICS IN PHARMACOKINETICS

The preceding section illustrate the basic concepts of pharmacokinetics. These concepts are valid for studies conducted in animals or humans and constitute the fundamental part of the areas that must be investigated for the registration of a new drug. However, it is evident that pharmacokinetics is not limited to these topics and encompasses many other aspects of drug development and clinical use. The following subsections give a brief outline of some other important aspects of pharmacokinetics.

Metabolite kinetics

Metabolites of drugs can be very important for their clinical use or their impact on animals or ecosystems if they show therapeutic or toxic effects. Their kinetics thus should be investigated during drug development, and sometimes metabolites are included in therapeutic drug monitoring programs. Prodrugs represent special cases of metabolites

and, accordingly, must be developed with methodologies that take into account their double nature as "parent compound" and "inactive precursor" of "active moieties".

Urinary excretion

Urinary excretion is an important process for many (essentially) hydrophilic drugs. Renal clearance (CL_R) can be calculated from the urinary excretion rate (dA_e/dt) and the related plasma concentration. The excretion rate is the amount of unchanged drug excreted in urine per unit time.

Nonlinear kinetics

Three types of linearities and nonlinearities are known in pharmacokinetics, and they have fundamentally different meanings. Linear and nonlinear equations are types of equations encountered for the description of pharmacokinetic models. Linear and nonlinear regressions are methods used to calculate pharmacokinetic parameters using a model that must be fitted to a set of experimental data. Finally, linear and nonlinear models are used to describe different types of behaviors of drugs in living organisms. This subsection focuses on the latter type of nonlinearities.

Linear models frequently are applicable in pharmacokinetics, and their mathematics are relatively simple. They require first-order transfers of an amount A of a drug from one compartment to another, into and out of the body (Figs. 2.4 and 2.5). First-order transfers necessitate direct proportionality between a transfer rate (dA/dt) and the amount of drug (A) in a compartment. The proportionality factor (k_{ij}) is a rate. Such constants in linear models do not vary with time or as a function of the concentration of the drug in the body. Adherence of a drug to a linear model means that all transfer rates within or out of the body must be of first order, with the exception of drug input, which can be of zero order for a bolus injection.

Nonlinear models do not exhibit direct proportionality between transfer rate and concentration or amount of drug in a compartment. The best known nonlinear process is elimination by Michaelis-Menten kinetics. Nonlinearities are encountered each time a saturable process operates or when a process is modified, for example, as a function of duration of exposure to the drug under consideration. Representative causes of dose- or time-dependent kinetics can be encountered at all levels of ADME, as shown by the following examples:

- *absorption*: saturable transport in gut wall; drug close to insoluble; saturable gut wall or hepatic metabolism on first pass;
- *distribution*: saturable plasma protein binding; saturable tissue binding;
- *metabolism*: capacity-limited kinetics, cofactor limitation, etc.; enzyme induction; hepatotoxicity; saturable plasma protein binding; decreased hepatic blood flow; inhibition by metabolite;
- *excretion*: active secretion (saturable); active reabsorption (saturable); decrease in urine pH; saturable plasma protein binding; nephrotoxicity; increase in urine flow.

The effects of saturable protein binding and enzyme induction are discussed in more details in the context of drug-drug interactions.

Integration of pharmacokinetics and pharmacodynamics

When an acute pharmacologic effect can be measured after administration of a drug, it can be interesting to link a pharmacokinetic model describing the time course of drug concentrations to a pharmacodynamic model describing the time course of drug effects. This is called *PK/PD modeling*.

Stereoselective metabolism

A number of drugs exist as molecules having at least one asymmetric center. Enantiomers are stereoisomers that are related to each other like nonsuperimposable mirror images, and diastereomers are stereoisomers that do not mirror each other. In addition, many drugs are marketed as racemates, i.e., equimolar mixtures of enantiomers. Such enantiomers often differ in their pharmacokinetic and/or pharmacologic activity.

KINETICS IN SPECIAL POPULATIONS

Patients are usually not healthy, fasting, young male volunteers. Accordingly, volunteer (or phase 1) kinetic studies must be followed by studies in subjects (healthy or not) aimed at exploring clinically relevant sources of variability in kinetics or dynamics. Such studies are important

to define the "pharmacokinetic fingerprint" of the new drug under well-defined conditions. In this context, clearance, volume of distribution, systemic availability, and half-life are calculated, and inter- as well as intraindividual variability is determined. This section only briefly delineates the problems encountered in different physiologic and pathologic situations.

Physiologic situations

Kinetics in neonates and children Young infants often display kinetic profiles different from those observed in young adults. Ad hoc methods respecting ethical principles must be used when the kinetics of a drug is studied in very young patients (see Chap. 87). The concept of healthy "volunteers" is not applicable in this case.

Kinetics in elderly patients Renal and metabolic functions tend to decrease with age. In addition, drug distribution also may be modified. Kinetic modifications in subjects older than 70 or 75 years are frequently observed (see Chap. 89). The study of the kinetics of new drugs in elderly patients is now a necessity for drug registration if such patients are to be found in the target population.

Pharmacogenetics Some enzymes such as *N*-acetyltransferase or cytochrome P450 CYP2D6 show a *genetic polymorphism*. This means that some subjects are able to rapidly metabolize substrates for these enzymes (extensive metabolizers = EMs), whereas other subjects lack this possibility (poor metabolizers = PMs). This topic is developed in detail in Chapter 3. The frequency distribution of EMs and PMs is not necessarily the same in different populations (e.g., Caucasians, Mongoloids, etc.), and this diversity is the basis of *interethnic differences* in drug metabolism.

Drug-drug interactions When two or more drugs are given simultaneously, they may compete at the level of drug absorption (e.g., formation of poorly soluble complexes), distribution (e.g., protein binding), metabolism (e.g., inhibition or induction of enzymatic systems), or renal excretion (e.g., tubular secretion or reabsorption). This may lead to lower or higher than expected drug concentrations. If preclinical data indicate that a drug might provoke or suffer from drug-drug interactions, ad hoc studies must be performed before registration. Such studies are often performed in healthy volunteers. The interaction of drug formulations with food is an important aspect of bioavailability and bioequivalence testing, especially for so-called controlled-release formulations. This subsection focuses mainly on changes in plasma protein binding, enzyme inhibition, and induction, since these phenomena allow a better understanding of some basic principles presented in that are more directly related to drug metabolism (for more details, see Chap. 6).

If a drug binds to plasma proteins, saturation of the binding sites may occur at higher concentrations because of the limited number of such sites. In this case, the fraction of drug unbound in plasma (f_u) is concentration dependent, and a nonlinearity in the kinetic behavior is observed. For such drugs, the volume of distribution increases with plasma concentration because f_u increases. Similarly, if two drugs compete for the same binding sites on plasma proteins, their fraction unbound in plasma tends to increase. If only the volume of distribution is affected, this leads to an increase in the apparent elimination half-life. With an increase in f_u, however, liver and renal clearances might increase, with a consequent decrease in elimination half-life that could compensate for the increase produced by modification of the volume of distribution. Because of the possible dependence on the fraction unbound in plasma of both volume of distribution and clearance in opposite directions, dose dependence in plasma protein binding and displacement of drugs in the context of drug-drug interactions may be difficult to detect and to quantify unless plasma protein binding is measured at different concentrations of the drug or drugs.

When two drugs compete for the same enzyme (i.e., *enzymatic inhibition*) for their biotransformation prior to being excreted from the body, capacity limitation may occur. As a consequence, the clearance of one of the two substances may be drastically diminished. Among the consequences of such an interaction, prolonged half-life and higher steady-state concentrations are the most clinically relevant modifications that may be observed.

The mechanisms by which *enzyme induction* occurs are numerous. From a pharmacokinetic viewpoint, enzyme induction increases the hepatic intrinsic clearance of a drug. As a consequence, the half-life of elimination decreases, as do steady-state concentrations. The systemic clearance of drugs with a low extraction ratio is particularly sensitive to enzyme induction, since an increase of ε_H from 0.1 to 0.2 doubles CL_H. On the contrary, for a drug with a high extraction ratio, an increase of ε_H from 0.8 to 0.9 induces a negligible change in the hepatic clearance. In the latter case, systemic availability is mainly affected, since $F_H = 1 - \varepsilon_H$. Thus, for a drug essentially eliminated from the body by biotransformation in the liver, enzyme induction manifests itself after both intravenous and oral administration if the substance has a low ε_H. Induction has noticeable consequences only after oral administration if a substance has a high ε_H. A measured change in clearance is often an indirect measure of the effect of an inducer. The direct effect is an increase in the synthesis rate of the drug-metabolizing enzyme. Accordingly, there is a delay between the first administration of the inducer and modifications in blood concentration profiles. The same delay may be observed when the inducer is removed because it takes some time for the hepatic enzymes to decrease to basal level.

Pathologic situations

Renal insufficiency For drugs essentially eliminated unchanged by renal excretion, renal insufficiency or renal failure may cause a serious reduction in total-body clearance if renal function is severely impaired. This may result in higher than wanted steady-state concentrations. Dosage adjustments by reduction of the dose and/or an increase in the interval between doses must then be proposed after car-

rying out studies in patients with varying degrees of renal insufficiency. Dosage adjustment is usually based on creatinine clearance. Renal failure also may have an influence on drug metabolism, and more information on dosage adjustment in patients with kidney disease is found in Chap. 21.

Liver failure Many drugs metabolized in the liver display modified kinetics in patients with hepatitis or cirrhosis. Under these conditions, the systemic clearance may be reduced, and first-pass metabolism also may be diminished, leading to higher than wanted concentrations (see Chap. 36). As opposed to the case with renal insufficiency, there is no specific physiologic indicator such as creatinine clearance to guide dosage adjustment in specific patients or patient subgroups suffering from liver disease.

SPARSE DATA KINETICS

Most pharmacokinetic studies (with the notable exception of studies performed in young children) imply the collection of many concentration and time pairs per subject. This is called the "data rich" situation. In recent years, new approaches have been proposed for the "data poor" situation, i.e., when only a few data pairs are available per subject.

Pharmacokinetic screen

This type of study implies that one or two drug concentrations are measured per subject during phase 2 and 3 clinical trials. Data are then analyzed in order to detect patients who show excessively high or low concentrations and to try to relate these modifications to covariables such as age, concomitant drug therapy, or disease. This approach thus leads to the detection of "subpopulations" at risk. It is also possible to correlate these kinetic findings with efficacy or side effects in order to try to define dose-concentration-response relationships. Such studies usually can be performed with standard statistical approaches.

Population approaches

If the pharmacokinetic screen approach is extended to allow modeling of pharmacokinetic and, possibly, pharmacodynamic behavior, it is usual to speak of *population methods*. These approaches require relatively sophisticated mathematical techniques and are still subjects of intensive development both in academia and in the pharmaceutical industry. The aim of population PK/PD methods is to describe the relationship of physiologic parameters to pharmacokinetic metrics and drug effects.

THERAPEUTIC DRUG MONITORING

Therapeutic drug monitoring (TDM) is an integration of pharmacokinetics and pharmacodynamics (PK/PD) aimed at improving pharmacotherapy. If a drug has a narrow therapeutic margin and displays high interindividual variability, it may be useful to measure the concentration of the active principle during therapy at steady state. This may facilitate dosage individualization. TDM basically should be restricted to drugs with narrow therapeutic margins, with high inter- and/or intraindividual variability, and for which therapeutic or toxic endpoints are difficult to measure. TDM also may be used in situations where compliance is of crucial importance and there are no clinical endpoints (e.g., arterial pressure, blood sugar, pain) that may lead the physician.

Optimization of dosage regimen in individual patients is closely related to the population approach. The Bayesian method integrates already available informa-tion regarding population behavior of the drug with information from observed drug concentrations in individual patients. Since dosage adjustment is of particular concern for clinical pharmacologists, hospital pharmacists, and interested therapists, a number of software programs have been developed to their intention. Data obtained from therapeutic drug monitoring also may be analyzed using "screen" or "population" methods.

As seen from this discussion, pharmacokinetics is not limited to studies performed in limited numbers of healthy subjects or patients. On the contrary, it starts at the level of genes controlling the synthesis of enzymes or membrane proteins and ends in the general patient population susceptible to be treated with a given medicine. Therapeutic drug monitoring combines knowledge of both the behavior in the organism of the drug, as presented in this chapter, and actions and effects on the body, as presented in other chapters in this book.

Pharmacogenetics of biotransformations

Pierre Bechtel, Yvette Bechtel

Biotransformation (drug metabolism) is probably the main source of variability in human pharmacologic and/or therapeutic response. At the beginning of the 1960s, B. B. Brodie stated that if there were no such processes as drug metabolism or elimination, the action of pentobarbital, a particularly lipid-soluble drug, would last a hundred years.

The transformation of the lipid into a water-soluble drug requires the action of specialized enzymes mainly located, for this purpose, in the liver. These catalyze two kinds of reactions: (1) functionalization reactions and (2) conjugation reactions.

The quantities of enzymes in the hepatocytes are regulated by specific genes according to the "one gene, one enzyme" rule. Thus the metabolic capacity of a subject depends on his/her genome and on the various environmental or host factors that might influence the regulation of gene expression and hence the quantity of enzymes and/or the activity of existing enzymes. In theory, all the enzymes

involved in drug metabolism, their functioning, and the consequences of their functioning fall into the field of *pharmacogenetics,* a term coined by W. Kalow in 1962.

In practical terms, however, only a few of these enzymes have been studied properly in this respect. This is due to the difficulties of clinical research and to the fact that the techniques allowing a molecular approach to the problem have been developed only recently. The cellular receptors responsible for the activities of drugs also exhibit a protein structure, and as such, their synthesis depends on genes. This last decade has witnessed the publication of numerous reports linking the variability, or part of the variability, of drug responses to a modification of gene receptor expression. This opens up a new field of research in pharmacogenetics. At present, however, these results cannot be used directly in therapeutic situations. Data therefore will be presented on the specific enzymes whose pharmacogenetic studies have been completed, taking into account

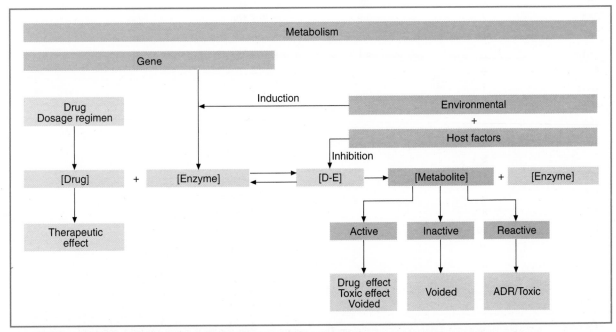

Figure 3.1 General outline of drug metabolism (for explanation, see text).

their relative importance and relevance in the field of drug metabolism as a whole. The consequences of pharmacogenetic knowledge on new drug development and drug use in patients will then be analyzed.

Using these pharmacogenetic concepts as a basis, it will be possible to show to what extent this approach allows us to forecast the metabolic behavior of a patient and thus to manage the interindividual and/or intraindi-

vidual variability of drug response by a judicious and acknowledged choice of dosage regimens designed to improve efficacy and avoid adverse drug reactions (ADRs).

ENZYMES OF DRUG METABOLISM

As shown in Figure 3.1 , enzymes play a central and dominant role in drug metabolism. On each occasion, once it has been diffused in the hepatocyte according to its

Table 3.1 Families of the cytochrome P450 acting in humans

CYP450	Chromosome localization	Liver content %	Variability (fold)	Polymorphism
1A1	15	< 1	~ 100	+
1A2	15	12	40	(+)
1B	2	<1	–	–
2A6	19	4	30	+
2A7	19	?	?	
2B6	19	<1	50	
2C8	10	–	–	
2C9	10	20	25	
2C10	10	–	–	
2C17	10	–	–	
2C18	10	–	–	
2C19	10	–	~ 100	+
2D6	22	4	> 1000	+
2E1	10	6	~ 20	(+)
2F1	19	–	–	
3A4	7	28	~ 20	
3A5	7	0-8	> 100	(+)
3A7	7	< 1	–	
4A1	–	< 1	–	–
4A9	–	–	–	
4A11	1	–	–	
4F2	–	–	–	
4F3	–	–	–	
5	–	–		
7	8	–		
11A1	15		Constant	
11B1	8		Constant	
11B2	8		Constant	
17	10		Constant	
19	15		Constant	
21A2	6		Constant	
27	2		Constant	
21A2	6		Constant	

(Families 1, 2, and 3 are mainly involved in xenobiotic metabolism. The activity of the others families is mainly directed to endobiotic metabolism.)

extraction coefficient, the quantity of drug that is metabolized (and thus not available to produce a therapeutic effect) depends only on the quantity and activity of the involved enzymes in the liver; the metabolites produced may lose all their activity, maintain the same activity as the parent drug, exhibit a slightly different activity from that of the parent drug, or display a toxic effect. Usually, but not always, the conjugation reactions inactivate the metabolites produced.

Various environmental or host factors are able to modify the activity of the enzymes present, usually by reducing this activity. Above all, however, the variability of drug metabolism depends on the structure of the genes coding for the enzymes and on the factors capable of modifying the regulation of their expression.

Cytochromes P450. Cytochromes P450 are coded by a superfamily of genes. Their ubiquitous presence throughout the animal and vegetable kingdom has prompted many studies that have resulted in extensive knowledge in this particular field. The major cytochromes P450 present in humans are listed in Table 3.1. Families 1, 2, and 3 are mainly, if not exclusively, involved in the metabolism of xenobiotics.

The genetic polymorphism of enzymes of drug metabolism Genetic polymorphism may be defined as the simultaneous existence in a given population of two or more alleles at a specific gene locus at frequencies that cannot be maintained solely by mutation. The rarest polymorphisms occur at a frequency lower than 0.01. When the frequency drops below 0.01, it is considered to be a rare genetic trait.

The discovery of a genetic polymorphism affecting an enzyme responsible for the metabolism of one or more drugs was and still is the result of clinical observation. Thus, it was discovered in the late 1950s that certain subjects in the general population were unable to metabolize an antituberculosis drug named isoniazide (INH) by acetylation. Certain groups of patients seemed to resist treatment, while others presented adverse reactions despite the similarity of the INH doses used in both groups. The genetic origin of this difference was established at the beginning of the 1960s. Subjects may be classified as slow acetylators (SAs) and rapid acetylators (RAs).

About 50% of Caucasian subjects are carriers of the SA genetic trait, and this was recognized as being transmissible in autosomal recessive fashion. This genetic polymorphism was considered to be a quite exceptional phenomenon until the end of the 1970s, when the oxidation polymorphism of debrisoquine, sparteine, and bufuralol, *CYP2D6*-dependent,

Table 3.2 Major mutations, described in Caucasian populations, associated with the absence of an enzyme or a completely inefficient CYP2D6

Mutation	Location on the gene	Consequence	Effect	Frequency in PM %
188 C → T	Exon 1	34 Pro→ ser	Null allele	65.8
212 G → A	Exon 1	4 Gly → Arg	Null allele	0,7
971 G → C	Intron I, exon 2	Splicing defect	Null allele	0.7
1062 C → A	Exon 2	91 Leu → Met	Null allele	60.3
1072 A → G	Exon 2	94 His → Arg	Null allele	60.3
1085 C → G	Exon 2	Silent	Null allele	60.3
1127 C → T	Exon 2	Silent	Null allele	4.8
1749 G → C	Exon 3	Silent	Null allele	69.3
1795 T del.	Exon 3	Frameshift	Null allele	6.2
1837 A → G	Exon 3	166 Asn → Asp	Null allele	0.7
1846 G → T	Exon 3	169 Gly stop codon	Null allele	0.7
1934 G → A	Intron 3, exon 4	Splicing defect	Null allele	65.8
2064 G → A	Exon 4	212 Gly → Glu	Null allele	4.8
2627-30 AACT del.	Exon 5	Frameshift	Null allele	0.7
2637 Adel	Exon 5	Fframeshift	Null allele	4.8
2938 C → T	Exon 6	296 Arg → Cys	Null allele	4.9
3023 A → C	Exon 6	324 His → Pro	Null allele	0.7
3376 G → A	Exon 7	373 Gly → Ser	Null allele	0.7
4268 G → C	Exon 9	486 Ser → Thr	Null allele	70
CYP2D6 deletion		No CYP2D6	Null allele	16.9

(The frequencies of these alleles in poor metabolizers are also reported.)

Table 3.3 A nonrestrictive list of drugs metabolized by cytochrome P450 2D6

Cardiovascular drugs	Psychotropic drugs	Miscellaneous
Propafenone	Haloperidol	Codeine
Encainide	Perphenazine	Dextromethorphan
Flecainide	Thioridazine	Phenformin
Sparteine	Clozapine	Perhexiline
Mexiletine	Amitriptyline	MDMA (ecstasy)
Timolol	Nortriptyline	
Metoprolol	Clomipramine	
Propranolol	Desipramine	
Bufuralol	Imipramine	
Indoramine	Paroxetine	
Debrisoquine	Methoxyphenamine	
Guanoxan	Minaprine	

was discovered; in this case, 7 to 10% of the Caucasian population was unable to oxidize these three drugs. This was the signal for a spate of research on this topic and the birth of a new discipline: pharmacogenetics.

ENZYMES OF DRUG METABOLISM OF DRUGS AFFECTED BY A POLYMORPHISM OF GENETIC ORIGIN

Polymorphism of cytochrome P450

Over the last 20 years, the genetic polymorphism of drug-metabolizing enzymes to which most study has been devoted is that of *CYP2D6*. At present, it serves as an example to which reference may be made in studying the causes and consequences of any polymorphisms affecting other enzymes of drug metabolism.

Cytochrome P450 2D6

Molecular basis of the genetic polymorphism of CYP2D6: the genotype The CYP2D6 gene has been mapped to chromosome 22. It forms a cluster, along with two pseudogenes, *CYP2D8P* and *CYP2D7P*, situated upstream of *CYP2D6*. Thanks to polymerase chain reaction (PCR) and SSCP (single strand conformation polymorphism) methods, 48 point mutations have at the present time been identified at the 9 exons and 8 introns of the gene. These mutations are associated with a normal, diminished, or zero expression of the gene corresponding, respectively, to extensive metabolizers (EMs), intermediary metabolizers (IMs), and poor metabolizers (PMs). The

mutations may be associated on the same allele in different ways. At the present time, 53 different alleles have been characterized, also associated with EMs, IMs, and PMs.

Table 3.2 lists all the mutations that, when present on the two alleles at the locus of *CYP2D6*, lead to modifications or an inability to transcribe the mRNA structure. In these conditions, the information is either not transmitted to the ribosomes or is transmitted incorrectly. In the former case, there is no synthesis of CYP2D6; in the latter, the protein produced is nonfunctional. Carriers of these mutations are classified as PMs and will find it difficult, even impossible, to biotransform the drug whose metabolism depends exclusively or mainly on CYP2D6 (Tab. 3.3).

In vivo exploration of CYP2D6 activity: the phenotype As we have just seen, the genotype enables us to analyze the information contained in the *CYP2D6* gene and to predict the existence or the lack of a functional protein in a given subject. When the protein is expressed, it does not allow us to prejudge the current activity of *CYP2D6* and its evolution over a period of time as a function of the subject's condition and environment. The phenotype is a measure of the genotype expression for existing conditions in a given time interval. However, it is difficult to know exactly all the factors liable to act on the enzyme activity present at the time of phenotyping, and its stability or variation over time can only be confirmed through repeated measurements.

For the purposes of interpretation, the following factors therefore must be taken into account: (1) the quantity of enzyme present at the time of its determination (depending on the gene expression) and (2) the activity of the enzyme depending on its environment at the time of its measurement. The determination of the phenotype requires a probe drug whose pharmacokinetic characteristics are known and for which there are specific and sensitive analytical methods capable of characterizing and quantifying the parent drug and its metabolites. Lastly, the probe drug must, of course, be devoid of any relevant toxic effect in humans at the dosage used.

Three probe drugs have been used widely over the past 20 years: debrisoquine, sparteine, and dextromethorphan. The general principle is simple: the probe drug is given orally, after the subject has voided his bladder. Urine is collected over 8-hour periods, and the parent drug and oxidized metabolite(s), are determined by gas chromatography or by high-pressure liquid chromatography (HPLC). The parent drug-metabolite urinary metabolic ratio is calculated. Thus, the value of the ratio of debrisoquine to 4-hydroxydebrisoquine (D/4-OHD) establishes the phenotype of a patient or a healthy subject when this value is compared with the curve of the frequency distribution of the ratio in a population of the same ethnic/racial origin (Fig. 3.2). Irrespective of the probe drug used, a bimodal distribution of the ratio is always observed. The lack of normality of the distribution is checked either by a probit analysis, as shown in Figure 3.2, or by a more sophisticated approach such as the maximum-likelihood method. On the strength of the distribution antimode, those subjects who eliminated debrisoquine exclusively in the urine after 8 hours and

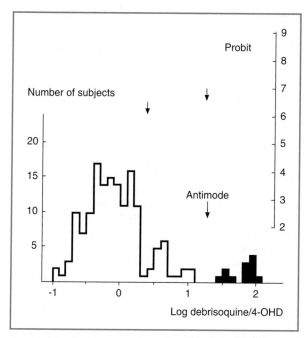

Figure 3.2 Graphic representation of the distribution of the debrisoquine/4-OHD ratio in 163 healthy subjects of Caucasian origin. The value of the log D/4-OHD at the antimode of the distribution is 1.12. Above this value, 7.4% of the population is classified as poor metabolizers (PMs). Two groups of subjects can be detected below this value, as shown by the arrows on the probit plot. IMₛ-intermediary metabolisers; EMₛ-extensive metabolisers (for more explanation, see text).

thus exhibited a metabolic ratio in excess of 1.2 are classified as PMs. In contrast, subjects are classified as EMs when the values of their metabolic ratios were less than 1.2 due to the fact that the quantity of debrisoquine eliminated in the urine is lower than that of 4-OHD.

With Caucasians, 7.4% of the population exhibit a PM phenotype. However, the classification of subjects as EMs and PMs is inadequate for the purpose of taking into account the interindividual variability of CYP2D6 activity. The EM group includes subjects who are highly efficient, moderately efficient and (close to the antimode), poorly efficient. In the case of the last-mentioned category, the use of recommended dose regimens may be the cause of adverse reactions identical to those observed in subjects classified as PMs if the drug used has a low chemotherapeutic index.

In contrast, therapeutic failures have been described in patients whose metabolic ratio was very low, commonly below 0.14, when sparteine was used as a probe drug. These ultrarapid metabolizers (UMs) have an amplified functional *CYP2D6* gene. At present, alleles with 2, 3, 4, 5, and 13 *CYP2D6*2* genes in tandem have been described. Ultrarapid metabolic capacity occurs even if only one allele exhibits the gene amplification, whatever the type of the other allele.

Relationship between phenotypes and genotypes Is the genotype capable of predicting the phenotype? Is the genotype able to forecast an individual's metabolic capacity? Subjects presenting the PM phenotype are all homozygous for two alleles carrying mutations associated with an

absence of gene expression. Subjects presenting the EM phenotype are homozygous for two alleles that, even if mutated, express a functional CYP2D6 protein. EM subjects also may be heterozygous when one allele expresses a functional protein and the other allele has a mutation modifying expression of the gene. The genotype determined from known mutations is thus capable of predicting the EM or PM phenotype, except, of course, in the case of a subject presenting with a rare mutation that renders the gene inactive and which has not yet been described. The observed discrepancy between the EM genotype and the PM phenotype is thus the spur for a new set of molecular investigations seeking to identify a "new" mutation. It is unlikely that there are many such new mutations, at least in the Caucasian population that has been screened extensively.

A number of studies tend to suggest that certain mutations, alone or associated on one allele, may be responsible for a decreased expression of *CYP2D6*. This may be explained by interindividual variability in *CYP2D6* activity, as shown in Figure 3.2. If such a hypothesis were proven to be correct, it might be possible to predict the metabolic capacity, in a simple way, through an individual's *CYP2D6*. Unfortunately, we can as yet discern no more than a trend, and many factors may interfere, not with a patient's gene expression, but with his enzyme activity. Genotyping of an individual remains a sound basis for classifying him as an EM or a PM of debrisoquine/sparteine and, when used carefully, also would give meaningful but incomplete indications as to the choice of an adapted dosage regimen – at least for drugs with narrow chemotherapeutic indexes. For the moment, however, and no doubt for some time to come, there is no alternative to therapeutic drug monitoring as a means of patient follow-up.

Interethnic/racial differences in the expression of CYP2D6 genetic polymorphism As we have seen, the frequency of the PM phenotype in Caucasians is on the order of 7.4%. With the exception of a few special ethnic groups, the frequency is much the same for people of African descent. In contrast, the frequency drops to under 1% in Asians, thereby making PM status a rare genetic trait.

On the other hand, certain molecular studies carried out in Asians living either outside or within their countries of birth have shown that they were carrying more *CYP2D6* alleles associated with decreased activity. A comparison of Caucasian and Asian populations reveals that, in addition to the absence of the PM phenotype, the interindividual variability being identical in EMs, there is a shift of the D/4-OHD metabolic ratio to higher values in Asian populations. We thus may expect a lower metabolic capacity in such populations. The recommended dosage regimen of a drug that is mainly or exclusively metabolized by CYP2D6, as determined in Caucasians, may prove to be too high in the case of Asians. Of course, the clinical consequences should be evaluated in light of the known toxic effect of the drug when the toxic effect depends on blood concentrations. This fact ought perhaps to be taken into account in the worldwide development of a new drug.

The issue is quite different in the case of UMs. Not only inter- but intraethnic/racial differences have been described. Thus, in the Caucasian populations, 1 to 2% of Swedish, 7% of Spaniards, 3.6% of Germans, and 0.8% of Danish are classified as UMs. Moreover, 29% of Ethiopians and 20% of Saudi Arabians are of this genotype. It becomes less easy to propose a clear-cut dosage regimen of CYP2D6-metabolized drugs to prescribe to EMs, a significant percentage of whom may be UMs. Clinicians aware of these differences should watch not only the occurrence of ADRs linked to the PM status but also the possible lack of expected therapeutic responses in EM patients.

Polymorphism of cytochrome P450 2C19

These molecular bases have been established only recently (they were not described before the early 1990s). In contrast to CYP2D6, PM frequency is greater among Asians (20%) than among Caucasians (3%). Eighty percent of PM-classified subjects in both Caucasians and Asians present a mutant allele (*m1*) on which the single substitution of a base pair provokes an aberrant splicing site. A second allele, also presenting the substitution of a single base pair (*m2*), leads to the appearance of a stop codon. This mutation is especially frequent among Asians. In both cases the allele is inactive and the enzyme protein absent. The metabolism of amitriptyline, citalopram, clomipramine, diazepam, hexobarbital, imipramine, mephobarbital, moclobemide, omeprazole, proguanil, propranolol, and mephenytoin are reduced in PMs. The last-named product acts as a probe drug and makes it possible to establish the phenotype of CYP2C19.

Among this nonexhaustive list of drugs biotransformed by CYP2C19, special mention should be made of proguanil. This antimalarial is absorbed in the form of a prodrug of limited efficacy. It is transformed by cyclization into an active metabolite by CYP2C19. PM subjects therefore are unable to perform this cyclization, and the drug is relatively ineffective. The malarial regions are mostly situated in the Middle and Far East, where races of Mongoloid origin are located. Since PMs make up 20% of these populations, it may readily be imagined that the use of proguanil may give rise to problems.

The induction of drug-metabolizing enzymes is in most cases dose-dependent or "rather" concentration-dependent. Omeprazole, a well-known inducer of CYP1A2, is metabolized by CYP2C19. When recommended dosage regimens are used in patients who are PMs of mephenytoin, there is a probability that its inducing capacity will be increased. The consequences may be an increased risk of biotransformation of poly-cyclic aromatic hydrocarbons (PAHs) from the procarcinogen to the carcinogen state by induced CYP1A2. PAHs are components of tobacco smoke. However, the hypothesis for a direct link between omeprazole use and indirectly increased carcinogenesis risk is as yet unproven.

Polymorphism of CYP2C9

Many important therapeutic agents are metabolized by this cytochrome: tolbutamide, ibuprofen, diclofenac, mefenamic acid, naproxen, phenytoin, piroxicam, tenoxicam, tienilic acid, sodium warfarin, fluvastatin, and tetrahydrocannabinol. Several of these drugs exhibit a narrow therapeutic index and, in the case of phenytoin, a nonlinear pharmacokinetics. Several point mutations have been found at the *CYP2C9* locus resulting in amino acid changes in CYP2C9, and two of them – Arg_{144}-Cys and Ile_{359}-Leu – have proved particularly significant. Replacement of Arg by Cys in position 144 of the protein causes a major decrease in K_m and V_{max} for sodium warfarin hydroxylation and a lower effect on V_{max} for tolbutamide and phenytoin. In marked contrast, Leu instead of Ile in position 359 causes an increased biotransformation of phenytoin by CYP2C9.

At present, information on the frequency of these mutations in Caucasian or Asian populations is scarce. The Cys_{144} mutation has not yet been detected in Chinese people, and Leu_{359} occurs at a very low frequency (no higher than 0.02%). Few studies have been carried out in vivo in Caucasian populations. Moreover, those which have been conducted involved fewer than 150 people, and tolbutamide (which is also metabolized by CYP2C19) was used as probe drug. Under these conditions, the 0.02% frequency of PMs can be no more than an approximation. CYP2C9 is a polymorphic enzyme that requires further investigation because of the interest of metabolized drugs, particularly warfarin.

Polymorphism of CYP2E1

CYP2E1 is inducible by ethanol. It metabolizes almost exclusively compounds of low molecular weight such as ethanol, acetone, and the nitrosamines. It also could play a part in transforming acetaminophen into quinones (toxic products) in the event of overdose. Numerous mutations, for the most part located at the *CYP2E1* introns, have been described. They do not seem to affect the activity of the protein. In the 5'-flanking region, on the other hand, there is a mutation at the possible mooring site of HNF-1, a factor regulating gene expression. The frequency of subjects homozygous for this mutated allele is 0.027% and 0.02% in Japanese and Caucasian populations, respectively. It is thus a rare genetic trait. It is not possible, on the strength of the phenotype-genotype relationship, to state categorically that this mutation affects the metabolism of CYP2E1 substrates. This is due in part to the fact that the probe drug used to establish the phenotype is chlorzoxazone, which is metabolized not only by CYP2E1 but also by CYP1A1 and CYP1A2, thereby introducing a confounding factor in the phenotype expression.

CYP2A6 catalyzes the 7-hydroxylation of coumarin and is also involved in procarcinogen activation and the metabolism of nicotine. Analysis of the cDNA has revealed an inactive allele: CYP2A-6v. Subjects homozygous for this allele are unable to biotransform coumarin or any other molecule that might depend on CYP2A6 for its metabolism. Although there would seem to be interethnic differences, further epidemiologic studies are needed before the consequences of such differences can be established.

CYP1A1, CYP1A2, and CYP3A4

A certain amount of controversy surrounds the various publications concerning the search for a polymorphism affecting these cytochromes P450 for which a bi- or tri-modal distribution has not been found consistently. Above all, most of the studies have failed to take into account, for CYP1A2, such confounding factors as the inducing power of PAHs (such as those produced by tobacco combustion) or the inhibiting power of estrogens (such as those associated with progesterone in contraceptive pills). In the case of CYP3A4, the main cytochrome P450 present in the human liver, the large and varied number of inducing and inhibiting factors introduces bias into the different studies published up to now. The clinical relevance of a possible polymorphism is thus far from being established. On the contrary, these cytochromes present great interindividual variability, precisely because of all the factors capable of inducing or inhibiting their activity. This should be in the forefront of the physician's mind when prescribing low-index chemotherapeutic drugs metabolized by cytochromes P450.

The use of therapeutic drug monitoring (TDM) thus becomes essential, as opposed to in vivo phenotyping, which would have to be repeated regularly in order to keep track of the variations in activity of the CYP in question. This would give rise to restrictions that conflict with current imperatives concerning treatment of patients.

PHASE I ENZYMES

Noncytochrome P450-mediated oxidations

Drug oxidation does not depend exclusively on cytochromes P450. Xanthine oxidase, monoamine oxidases, and flavin-containing monooxygenases are capable of oxidizing a number of substrates. Thus, chlorpromazine, morphine, nicotine, and propranolol, which all contain secondary or tertiary amino groups, are metabolized by flavin-containing monooxygenases.

Monoamine oxidases are of two types – type A and B. Their activity varies considerably in the Caucasian population, but it is difficult at present to attribute a clinical relevance to this variability. Indeed, although monoamine oxidase A is responsible for the oxidative deamination of sumatriptan, its major role is the deamination of neurotransmitters carrying an amino function. The existence of genetic polymorphisms affecting these enzymes is poorly documented. Their role in the endogenous metabolism

may explain the rarity of a polymorphic expression of these enzymes, whose existence may be lethal in subjects homozygous for zero expression of their genes. However, mention should be made of a rare inborn metabolic error affecting xanthine oxidase. Less than 2% of Caucasians have very weak or even zero activity of this enzyme. The consequences can be serious when this characteristic is associated with zero activity of thiopurine methyl transferase and the patient must be treated with azathioprine. We shall consider the consequences of this polymorphism later.

Esterases such as paraoxonase and acetylcholinesterase, epoxide hydrolase, and dehydrogenases such as aldehyde and alcohol dehydrogenase present interindividual differences in activity that may be related to a genetic polymorphism. However, their activity in drug metabolism remains limited. In subjects homozygous for zero activity of acetylcholinesterase, the use of succinylcholine outside a general anesthetic may lead to paralysis of the diaphragm and death through asphyxia. Succinylcholine is used mainly to obtain myorelaxation in the course of general anesthesia, during which, even in the event of zero acetylcholinesterase activity, assisted respiration leads to complete elimination of the product or at least to blood concentrations free of pharmacologic activity.

PHASE II ENZYMES

N-Acetyltransferases: NAT-1, NAT-2

There are two types of *N*-acetyltransferase: NAT-1, whose role is the acetylation of endogenous substrates, and NAT-2, responsible for the acetylation of xenobiotics. Among the latter, isoniazide (INH), the antibiotic that made it possible to overcome tuberculous endemia, is inactivated by NAT-2. Very soon after its launch in 1953, INH at recommended doses was inactive in certain subjects or, on the contrary, caused serious hepatic or neurologic side effects. The existence of rapid acetylators (RAs) and slow acetylators (SAs) in the population came to light at the end of the 1950s, and the RA or SA genetic status could then provide an explanation for the lack of therapeutic efficacy or the appearance of toxic effects.

Slow acetylators represent about 60% of the Caucasian population. There are some very pronounced differences between races, ranging from 90% of RAs among the Eskimos of northern Canada and Asians to less than 10% in Marocco populations. It has proved difficult, in light of these interethnic variations, to standardize a daily dose of INH in countries with a high RA percentage and where access to treatment centers is made difficult by the considerable distances involved. Relatively few drugs are biotransformed by acetylation besides INH, and these include amrinone, clonazepam, dapsone, dipyrone, endralazine, hydralazine, nitrazepam, prizididol, procainamide, sulfamethazine, and sulfapyridine.

Research on the molecular bases of this polymorphism did not provide results in terms of identification of the responsible mutations until the mid 1990s. At the present time, 15 different alleles have been described, carriers of point mutations at the level of a pair of nucleotides, and are associated with a normal or reduced expression of the gene. Unlike *CYP2D6*, there are in fact no zero-expression alleles. The most commonly encountered mutated alleles in Caucasians are *NAT2*5A* and *NAT2*6A*. Though present, *NAT2*7A* is much less frequent. These mutated alleles are also encountered in Mongoloid populations, *NAT2*7A* being the most frequent. It would seem that the *NAT2*14A* allele, also associated with reduced activity, is specific to black African populations. In all, these alleles are encountered in over 95% of SA subjects, irrespective of their ethnic/racial origin, and provide a perfect explanation of their reduced acetylation potential.

UDP-glucuronyltransferases (UGTs)

These enzymes play a key role in the metabolism of drugs and endogenous substrates; irrespective of their origin, they are transformed into extremely polar compounds and thus may be eliminated totally by the natural emunctories: bile, urine, and feces. There are two general families of genes in humans, coding for UGT1 and UGT2, and there are mutations at gene level that modify the activity of the enzymes produced. Two inborn errors of metabolism are expressed by hyperbilirubinemia, reaching a lethal threshold in Criggler-Najjar's disease, and moderate (and usually well-tolerated) hyperbilirubinemia in Gilbert's disease. Further study is needed on the consequences of these polymorphisms for drug metabolism.

We are still far from being in a position to provide certain proof of the existence of a polymorphic conjugation of fenofibric acid, acetaminophen, or codeine. On the other hand, interethnic variations appear to be relevant. When compared with Caucasians, Asians appear to have reduced conjugation of codeine or its active metabolite morphine. However, it is difficult to pinpoint the clinical consequences in terms of analgesia, since the conjugated metabolites of morphine are as active as morphine itself. On the other hand, morphine production by *O*-demethylation, depending on CYP2D6, seems more critical in this respect. We have recorded the differences between Caucasian and Asian populations. The latter's PM frequency is virtually zero, and it follows that the risk of codeine inefficacy is greater in Caucasians, 7.4% of whom are PMs of debrisoquine.

Glutathione S-transferases (GSTs)

There are four different classes of GSTs in mammals: α, μ, π, and θ. A polymorphism has been described for classes μ and θ. The consequences of the mutations at the origin of the polymorphism relate above all to the hepatic detoxication capacity in mammals and, in particular, humans rather than to drug metabolism.

Sulfotransferase (ST)

Four different enzymes that catalyze *O*-sulfation reactions have been discovered in humans, and their genes have been cloned. Further studies, with a view to determining the exact role of these enzymes and the effect of mutations on their genes, will be needed before clinical use in the human can be contemplated.

Thiopurine methyltransferase (TPMT)

There are no known instances of endogenous substrates metabolized by TMPT. However, azathioprine and its active metabolite 6-thioguanine nucleotide are inactivated to 6-methylthioguanine by the transfer of a methyl group in the presence of TMPT. This is an important reaction inasmuch as it limits the therapeutic activity of 6-thioguanine nucleotide and thus prevents the appearance of agranulocytosis. In the population as a whole, 1% of subjects are homozygous for mutated alleles of *TMPT* associated with zero expression. It has been shown that the concentration of 6-thioguanine nucleotide in these subjects remained high and was associated with an increased risk of agranulocytosis. Nevertheless, it should be noted that there is a very wide interindividual variability in TMPT activity and that the risk of agranulocytosis also exists in subjects expressing protein, albeit with a weak activity. Here again, therapeutic drug monitoring of 6-methylthioguanine, the inactive metabolite, in erythrocytes is a definite aid in the surveillance of patients receiving treatment. There is an increased risk of this adverse event when the subject associates a reduced or zero TMPT activity with a reduced xanthine oxidase activity. This enzyme is also capable of metabolizing thioguanine nucleotide into inactive urate in the liver, thus supporting an inactive TMPT.

REVIEW OF THE ANALYSIS OF ENZYMES PRESENTING WITH A POLYMORPHISM

In all, it emerges clearly that only a few enzymes responsible for drug metabolism (Tab. 3.4) are affected by a polymorphism whose clinical consequences have been clearly established. CYP2D6 is responsible, either on its own or in association with other cytochromes P450, for the metabolism of many low-chemotherapeutic-index drugs. In the case of a large number of them, adverse drug reactions observed for recommended doses are encountered essentially in PMs but also in EMs presenting a very low activity of CYP2D6. On the other hand, in the case of UM subjects, i.e., those with a gene amplification, therapeutic inactivity is in most cases observed at recommended doses. Above all, thanks to the considerable work carried out over the past 15 years, we have been able to build up a comprehensive picture of the *CYP2D6* gene with its multiple alleles and its relationship with phenotypes and to explain the interindividual and interethnic/racial variability. If it ever proved possible to extend the same degree of knowledge to all other enzymes responsible for drug metabolism, we could be sure of controlling this source of variability. CYP2C19, CYP2C9, and CYP2E1

Table 3.4 List of the enzymes able to metabolize xenobiotics

Phase I enzymes

Alcohol dehydrogenases
Aldehyde dehydrogenases
Aldehyde oxidase
Aldo-Keto reductases
Arylesterases
Arylsulfatases
Carboxylesterases
Cholinesterase
Cytochromes P450
Copper-containing amine oxidases
Dihydrodiol dehydrogenases
Dopamine B-mono-oxygenase
Endo - and exo-peptidases
Epoxide hydrolases
FAD-containing monooxygenases
Glucuronidases
Monoamine oxidase
Myeloperoxidase and other peroxidases
Xanthine oxidase
Phosphatases
Thiolester hydrolases
Quinone reductase

Phase II enzymes

Alcohol sulfotransferases
Amine sulfotransferases
Arylformamidases
Catechol O-methyltransferase
Cysteine-S-conjugate β-lyase
Glucuronyltransferases
Glutathione S-transferases
Lyases
N-Acetyltransferases
N-Acyltransferases
N-Methyltransferase
O-Acetyltransferases
O-Acyltransferases
Phenol sulfotransferases
Phosphotransferases
S-methyltransferase
Steroid sulfotransferases

are also responsible for the metabolism of low-chemotherapeutic-index drugs, but there have been fewer fundamental studies devoted to them, and the clinical consequences of their polymorphisms are, in some cases, largely a matter of conjecture.

NAT-2 and TPMT

Given that these enzymes metabolize two essential and widely used drugs (INH in the treatment of tuberculosis and azathioprine in the prevention of organ or tissue transplant rejection), their polymorphisms can have serious consequences for the vital prognosis of patients if this factor is not taken into account. Awareness of the patient's genetic status for these enzymes makes it possible to choose appropriate doses and in particular to provide clinical surveillance that secures efficacy with a minimal risk of ADRs.

In the case of all other enzymes for which the existence, or the suspected existence, of a genetic polymor-

phism has been suggested, it is difficult at present to assess the clinical consequences. From a general point of view, whatever the interest for the drug industry or the clinician at the bedside, the dissemination of pharmagenetic concepts collected during the two past decades has been at best slowed down and sometimes impeded. Drawbacks linked to methodologic difficulties in genotyping and phenotyping, the individuals, were and, to some extent, are always important brakes to their dissemination.

To date, some of these drawbacks remain present, but in the field of genotype determination, recent developments of semiautomatic methods may help to generalize *CYP450* genotyping. The system is composed of a cell that contains millions of copies of a specific oligonucleotide probe that can hybridize a single strand of fluorescently labeled DNA target. The GeneChip CYP450 assay is used in conjunction with the GeneChip analysis system. Thus, the main gene mutations of *CYP2D6* and *CYP2C19* can be detected in less than 5 hours. Extension of this method should allow easier pharmacogenetics screenings in the very near future.

PHARMACOGENETICS AND DRUG DEVELOPMENT

Pharmacogenetics and drug variability

The major concept, clearly established and verified, from 30 years of research in clinical pharmacology is the existence of inter- and intraindividual variability in patient therapeutic response for recommended drug doses. Drug metabolism may be considered as a major, but not the exclusive, cause of this variability. Despite the technical and methodologic obstacles, in particular the lack of simple methods for exploring all causes of variability, much work has been and continues to be devoted to metabolism. In the context of the development of a new drug, as soon as a new molecule has been chosen, chemists are able to predict the potential metabolites. Notwithstanding their limitations, the various in vitro methods employing hepatocytes or microsomes of animal or human origin, associated with effective analytical methods, make it possible (qualitatively speaking at least) to establish which metabolites are in fact produced. The incubation of the drug with transfected cells expressing a specific isoform of cytochrome P450 permits pinpointing of one or more of these isoforms as being responsible for drug metabolism.

It is thus possible to recognize at a very early stage the biotransformation of a drug by a cytochrome P450 affected by a genetic polymorphism. In such circumstances, and in the case of phase I studies on healthy volunteers, the influence of the polymorphic metabolism on drug pharmacokinetics may be evaluated. It is simply a question of determining, for the healthy volunteers included in the study, the phenotype and genotype of the P450 in question. Characterization of healthy volunteers also opens the door to more relevant tolerability studies and helps to explain why a subject classified as a PM presents a poorer tolerance of a dose well tolerated by most subjects classified as EMs. On the contrary, a subject classified as a UM will be able to tolerate far higher doses than the average subject classified as an EM.

Similarly, it will be easier to find the dose-concentration-effect relationships if the metabolic characteristics of the healthy subjects or patients included in the study have been determined. In phase II or III studies involving patients, any variability of the therapeutic response, and the extent of this variability for a given dose, can be related to the polymorphism of the metabolism, once again explaining the differences in behavior between a PM and a UM compared with that of average EMs. Once the drug has been launched on the market, i.e., once it is used in common therapeutic situations, quite different from the circumstances of clinical trials, it will be a great help to make use of the known, qualified, and quantified role of metabolism in the variability of response when choosing individual doses and monitoring therapeutic or toxic effects.

Pharmacogenetics and interethnic variability

Drugs are nowadays developed at world level, and it is abundantly clear that the interethnic differences, with reference to mutations, PM and EM status, and SA and RA status, need to be taken into account. For example, the PM characteristic for CYP2D6 is a rare genetic trait in Asian populations. In the case of a new drug, it is highly unlikely that the pharmacokinetic consequences of CYP2D6 polymorphisms would come to light during trials conducted exclusively with populations of Asian origin. The opposite could apply in the case of a drug metabolized by CYP2C19 and developed exclusively in Caucasian populations, where the PM status of mephenytoin is rare (less than 3%). In such cases, provision should be made for specific interethnic phase I studies.

However, the variability problem cannot be overcome exclusively by making allowances for PM or EM status. Even when drug metabolism depends exclusively or principally on a polymorphic enzyme, there is still a very great interindividual variability in EM subjects. No study has so far succeeded in establishing beyond doubt the existence of a correlation between genotype and phenotype, which would make it possible to predict an individual metabolic capacity on the strength of genotype alone. In addition to the genomic factor, variability also depends on environmental factors such as illness, drug associations, diet, and climate. Thus, in the case of CYP2D6, mutations associated with a reduced gene expression suggest a reduction in the enzyme metabolic capacity measured in vivo. But the adjustment of the expression of *CYP2D6* and/or the activity of CYP2D6 may be modified by environmental factors. The genotype, therefore, can do no more than give a presumption of metabolic capacity, and accurate knowledge of the patient's current metabolic capacity can only be obtained by determining the phenotype or TDM of the drug.

A subject's metabolic capacity, at any given moment, is the result of gene structure, gene expression, amount of enzyme proteins present, and influence of various environmental factors on activity.

PHARMACOGENETICS AND DRUG USE IN PATIENTS

The clinician is confronted with a large body of knowledge emanating from virtually all current fields of biology: (1) molecular and biochemical bases of the functioning of a few enzymes responsible for the biotransformation of drugs such as CYP2D6 and NAT-2, (2) physiologic bases of the pharmacokinetics of a probe drug allowing the in vivo exploration of the activity of these enzymes, (3) physiopathologic bases of the molecular, biochemical, or physiologic modifications of drug metabolism in patients, and (4) epidemiologic bases exploring drug metabolism through a genetic approach of populations, making it possible to affirm or rule out the existence of interethnic/racial variations.

As we have shown in the preceding paragraphs, all these data may be taken into account by drug companies and regulatory authorities. Guidelines for the exploration of drug metabolism and its consequence have been put forward in Europe, the United States, and Japan, and their adoption has been very strongly advocated. Almost by definition, such guidelines cannot be other than exceedingly directive and categoric. There is little room for nuance, despite the fact that any biologic study of living beings will reveal the interindividual variability in a species and the intraindividual variability of an individual in a species. Genetically speaking, every human being, with the exception of identical twins, is unique. In view of the fact that knowledge in terms of drug use in patients is at the present time limited to a few enzymes of drug metabolism, can pharmacogenetics be anything else but a paradigm, a frame of reference?

Pharmacogenetics and variability of patient response for recommended doses

Therapeutic response

It is quite clear that all substrate drugs of CYP2D6, CYP2C19, or NAT-2, when prescribed at recommended doses, are potentially ineffective in patients with very high enzyme activity. Reports detailing these facts can be found in the literature, but there is no organized epidemiologic study establishing the degree of risk for a drug or therapeutic class whose metabolism cosegregates with debrisoquine, dextromethorphan, mephenytoin, or dapsone. In real-life situations, a genotyping procedure investigating *CYP2D6* amplification will be required, for example, in the case of a lack of response in a patient receiving standard doses of a drug metabolized by CYP2D6. Confirmation of the existence of the UM genotype will explain the lack of effective response and will make it possible to increase doses or to change drugs entirely without risk.

Although the polymorphic metabolism of INH was

discovered some time ago, dose adjustments are still made empirically (in the absence of large-scale studies) and backed up by either (1) an "INH test," which consists of taking measurements of INH and acetyl-INH in plasma in the third hour following drug intake (analytical conditions for determining INH and acetyl-INH are, however forbidding, and there is a substantial risk of error), or (2) in vivo phenotyping with caffeine or dapsone as the probe drug. Depending on whether the patient is classified as an SA or an RA, the INH dose will be reduced to 3 mg/kg or increased to 6 mg/kg in relation to the recommended dose (4-5 mg/kg in adults).

Notwithstanding the lack of controlled studies, the illustrative value of cases of inefficacy associated with a high metabolic capacity reported in the literature is sufficiently conclusive to confirm the advantage of using TDM for a few "difficult" drugs such as antiepileptics, immunosuppressants, and antidepressants.

Adverse drug reactions (ADRs)

Without doubt, it is in the explanation, if not the prevention, of ADRs associated with the variability of drug metabolism that concepts of pharmacogenetics have proved most useful.

ADRs related to blood concentration Toward the end of the 1960s and thanks to TDM, the relationship between the blood concentration of phenytoin (DPH) and the onset and/or worsening of therapeutic accidents was discovered and clearly recognized. The mechanism of nonlinear kinetics of DPH was attributed more to the possible saturation of enzyme(s) responsible for its metabolism than to the exceedingly rare deficiency in DPH parahydroxylase depending on CYP2C9. The hepatic and neurologically serious ADRs observed with perhexiline and the relationship with the polymorphism of *CYP2D6* had a major impact on pharmacovigilance by virtue of the increased frequency of the metabolic error. These ADRs were observed mainly in patients classified as PMs. They were not confined to this category, however, because patients classified as IMs also presented the same adverse events. The simplistic EM-PM classification therefore would seem insufficient, in this case, to predict subjects at risk. Allowance must be made for the interindividual variability in CYP2D6 activity, partially explained by the different alleles encountered in EM subjects. Patients classified as EMs may have a low CYP2D6 activity, and the toxic risk of perhexiline at usual doses may be as high as for patients classified as PMs. Although it is impossible to define the value limits of the debrisoquine/4-OHD ratio, which would make it possible to predict the risk in EM patients. This is nonetheless a therapeutic condition, where an influence of the CYP2D6 activity can be anticipated and the risk avoided.

Drug-drug interactions The single intake of 75 mg of quinidine transforms an EM subject into a PM subject for a period of 8 days. Quinidine has a very strong affinity for CYP2D6, and although it is metabolized by CYP3A4 (and not CYP2D6), it irreversibly occupies the active site of CYP2D6 and competitively inhibits the metabolism of all usual substrates. Numerous publications have shown that CYP2D6 substrates could all, to greater or lesser degree, behave as competitive inhibitors when associated with each other. The quantitative extent of the inhibition then depends on the respective values of their K_m (affinity constant) and K_i (inhibition constant) determined in vitro for CYP2D6. Tricyclic antidepressants (TCAs), selective serotonin reuptake inhibitors (SSRIs), and antipsychotics are frequently associated and thus may influence the depressive illness, for example, resulting in resistance to therapy or suicide risk when inhibition is removed by treatment. In such cases, the risk of ADRs could well be increased: (1) dry mouth, increased perspiration, or orthostatic syndromes with nortriptyline; (2) cardiotoxicity, arrhythmias, or cardiac arrest with nortriptyline, imipramine, and desipramine; and (3) sedation with thioridazine, perphenazine, and haloperidol.

These interactions have been well documented in in vitro studies of human liver microsomes, but the relevance of clinical consequences needs (or would need) to be confirmed in vivo. In the case of healthy subjects, we may point to the modification of kinetic parameters resulting in increased blood concentrations of the drug whose metabolism is inhibited. However, when patients are concerned, it is difficult to relate, with certainty, clinical modifications to kinetic modifications due to interactions, without allowing for the existing possible pharmacodynamic interactions. Whatever the case, any association of drugs metabolized by CYP2D6 or, more generally, of drugs metabolized by the same cytochrome P450 must be the signal for the prescribing physician to exercise extra care in surveillance of the patient.

Idiosyncratic ADRs These reactions are independent of the drug dosage or concentration. They are usually consequent to the production of a reactive metabolite that fails to find the efficient detoxification system inside the cell, where it is produced. Thus the metabolites of acetaminophen or metronidazole appear more prone to induce lymphocyte damages in subjects with an inherited deficiency in glutathione-S-transferase class μ or θ. Similarly, the defective detoxification of hydroxylamine metabolites may be responsible for hypersensitivity reactions to sulfonamide. In this case, the SA phenotype may be a marker of higher risk. This is another area where further investigation would be welcome.

Ever since the pioneering work of B. B. Brodie, drug metabolism has remained a research field of paramount importance. Even if we confined our inquiry to that part of pharmacogenetics touching on drug metabolism, and despite the fact that only a few enzymes have as yet been investigated, there is still enough basic knowledge to fill the pages of a book. It is therefore all the more disappointing that so few clinical studies have resulted and that pharmacogenetics continues to constitute more an abstract frame of reference, a paradigm than a pragmatic and technical tool for treating patients. As a paradigm, it is, however, extremely useful. It helps to improve knowledge on new, licensed drugs by urging the drug industry to stimulate investigations capable of detecting and, in some cases, managing pharmacokinetic variability associated not only with polymorphic enzymes but also with all enzymes involved in xenobiotic metabolism.

During drug treatment, pharmacogenetics also validates the interest of TDM for drugs with a low therapeutic index. In many cases, it provides an explanation for some serious ADRs and proves that these adverse events may be the result of a potential toxic effect of the drug, expressed in an individual who presents either with an inborn error of metabolism or with a decreased metabolic capacity following drug-drug interaction or whose metabolic capacity is impaired by environmental and/or host factors. This might create the basis for forecasting "subjects at risk" as well as "drugs at risk".

In addition to the issue of drug metabolism, there are other aspects of pharmacogenetics. There appears to be polymorphisms in the genetics of drug transfer and drug transport. This may be another source of pharmacokinetic variability to be detected, explained, and managed. Finally, the importance of genetic factors governing the pharmacodynamic response should not be overlooked. At present, available data on genetic polymorphism of drug receptors are sketchy, and the clinical consequences, in terms of therapeutic efficacy, are not established. In the not-too-distant future, however, there may be reasonable hope to see in vitro and in vivo investigational procedures used for polymorphic enzymes, extended to the majority of the relevant enzymes of drug metabolism. Simultaneously, we can look to a significant increase in available data on the genetics of drug transport and receptors. Thus, all these data might be used in the so-called population approach of the pharmacokinetic/pharmacodynamic relationship as a means of acquiring greater knowledge about drugs in development and about their quality, efficacy, and safety as treatments for patients.

Suggested readings

ALVAN G, BALANT LP, BECHTEL PR, et al (eds). European Consensus Conference on Pharmacogenetics, Vol. 1. ECSC-AEC Brussels, Luxembourg: Office for Official Publications of the European Communities, 1990.

BATHUM L, HOHANSSON I, INGELMAN-SUNDBERG M, et al. Ultrarapid metabolism of sparteine: frequency of alleles with duplicated CYP2D6 genes in a Danish population as determined by restriction fragment length polymorphism and long polymerase chain reaction. Pharmacogenetics 1998;8:119-25.

DALY AK, BROCKMOLLER J, BROLY F, et al. Nomenclature for human CYP2D6 alleles. Pharmacogenetics 1996;3:193-203.

JOHANSSON JI, LUNDQVIST E, BERTILSSON E, et al. Inherited amplification of an active gene in the cytochrome P450 CYP2D locus as a cause of ultrarapid metabolism of debrisoquine. Proc Natl Acad Sci USA 1993;90:11825-9.

KALOW W, BERTILSSON L. Interethnic factors affecting drug response. Adv Drug Res 1994;25:1-59.

KROEMER HK, EICHELBAUM M. It's the genes, stupid: molecular bases and clinical consequences of genetic cytochrome P450 2D6 polymorphism. Life Sci 1995;56:2285-98.

MAREZ D, LEGRAND M, SABBAGH N, et al. Polymorphism of the cytochrome P-450 CYP2D6 gene in a European population: Characterization of 48 mutations and 53 alleles, their frequencies and evolution. Pharmacogenetics 1997;7:193-203.

MICHALETS EL. Update: Clinically significant cytochrome P450 drug interactions. Pharmacotherapy 1998;18:84-112.

PACIFICI GM, FRACCHIA GN (eds). Advances in drug metabolism in man, Vol. 1. ECSC-EAEC Brussels, Luxembourg: Office Official Publications of the European Communities, 1995.

QUINN DI, O'DAY R. Drug interactions of clinical importance: an updated guide. Drug Safety 1995;12:393-452.

RENDI S, DI CARLO FJ. Human cytochrome P450 enzymes: a status report summarizing their reactions, substrates, inducers and inhibitors. Drug Metab Rev 1997;29:413-80.

SACHSE S, BROCKMOLLER J, BAUER S, ROOTS I. Cytochrome P450 2D6 variants in a Caucasian population: allele frequencies and phenotypic consequences. Am J Hum Genet 1997; 60:284-95.

Distribution of drugs

Jérôme Barré, Saïk Urien

Once a drug has been absorbed or injected into the blood, it may be distributed into interstitial and cellular fluids and interact with macromolecules present in the various body fluids and tissues. The diffusion into fluids and the binding of drugs to macromolecules influence both pharmacodynamics and pharmacokinetics.

Binding to specific receptors is an essential step in eliciting the action of many drugs. Proteins form the most important class of drug receptors. Examples are the receptors for hormones, neurotransmitters, growth factors, the enzymes involved in essential metabolic and regulatory pathways, and the proteins participating in transport processes or serving structural roles. Cellular constituents other than proteins, such as nucleic acids, also can act as specific drug receptors.

Binding of drugs to carrier proteins and tissue components (e.g., lipids, mucopolysaccharides, etc.) often leads to drug inertness because the bound drug does not initiate a pharmacologic effect and is transiently unavailable for interaction with receptors. These proteins and tissue components are known as *acceptors*. Finally, binding to enzyme systems in the liver or in any tissue with metabolic activity and involved in the biotransformation of drugs can be responsible for metabolism and excretion. All these considerations imply that appreciable amounts of a drug in the body may be reversibly bound to proteins and tissue constituents without resulting in a pharmacologic effect. This type of binding is a major determinant of drug distribution that influences the pharmacokinetics of a drug.

The distribution process results from an interaction between a drug and the body components. Consequently, the pattern of this distribution is determined, on the one hand, by the physicochemical properties of the drug such as the pK_a value or the degree of ionization, lipid solubility, and molecular weight and, on the other hand, by physiologic factors such as pH, plasma protein binding, permeability of membrane barriers, blood flow, tissue, and composition.

FACTORS INFLUENCING DRUG DISTRIBUTION

Permeability of capillaries

When a drug has reached the bloodstream, the major pathway for its distribution, it usually diffuses within the body by crossing one or more biologic barriers to reach its ultimate site of action. Since the capillary is the initial barrier to distribution, its permeability characteristics will be our first concern.

Three major types of capillary endothelia have been described: continuous, discontinuous, and fenestrated. Capillaries with *continuous* endothelium are found in the brain, retina, muscle, lung, and adipose tissue. Adjacent endothelial cells in these capillary beds are connected by continuous intercellular tight junctions and no breaks in the vessel wall. The degree of functional permeability in this subclass varies from the characteristic tight blood-brain barrier functions of brain and retinal capillaries to the relatively more permeable functions of muscle, lung, and adipose tissue capillaries. *Discontinuous,* or *sinusoidal,* endothelium, characteristic of the liver, spleen, and bone marrow, has gaps between adjacent endothelial cells. In these vascular beds, the endothelium is not thought to play a major role in impeding the flow of blood-borne substances to the surrounding tissue. *Fenestrated* endothelium exhibits *fenestrae,* specialized intracellular pores that have been proposed to play a major role in transport and filter functions. Fenestrated endothelium can be found in the capillaries of all endocrine glands, the renal glomeruli and renal tubules, and the intestinal mucosa.

After passing the endothelial barrier, the drug penetrates into the interstitial fluid and may further bind to or diffuse through tissue cell membranes that consist of a lipid bilayer matrix.

Lipid solubility and ionization of drugs

In addition to passing through the pores of the capillaries and tissues cells (see below), lipid-soluble drugs dissolve in the plasma membranes of cells and thus may pass through the endothelial cells of the capillaries and then into tissue cells. However, most drugs are either weak acids or weak bases, and their extent of passage through the capillary endothelial cells and into tissue cells also depends on their degree of ionization at the pH values of the blood, of the extracellular spaces, and within tissue cells. Because of the fact that most drugs are absorbed by passive diffusion of the nonionized moiety, the extent to which a drug is in its ionized and nonionized forms at a certain pH is of great importance. The pH of the environment and the pK_a of the drug will determine the degree of ionization of weak acids and bases according to the Henderson-Hasselbach equation as follows:

$$\log \left(\frac{\text{ionized form}}{\text{unionized form}}\right) = pK_a - pH$$

$$\log \left(\frac{\text{ionized form}}{\text{unionized form}}\right) = pH - pK_a$$

Drugs are relatively more water soluble when they are ionized and more lipid soluble when they are nonionized.

Passage of drugs across membranes

The movement of drugs through the biologic membranes is accomplished by means of several processes.

Passive diffusion Passive diffusion is characterized by the movement of drug molecules down a concentration or electrochemical gradient without cellular expenditure of energy. Both lipid-soluble or nonionized molecules and lipid-insoluble (water-soluble) molecules of small size may cross body membranes by passive diffusion. The former penetrate through the bimolecular lipoid layer of the cell membrane, whereas the latter diffuse through the channels or pores present in the membrane cells. The rate of diffusion is determined by Fick's law of diffusion:

$$\text{Rate of diffusion} = -\frac{D \cdot SA \cdot K (C_1 - C_2)}{T}$$

where D is the diffusion coefficient of the drug molecule in the membrane, SA is the area across which the diffusion occurs, K is the partition coefficient, C_1 and C_2 are the concentrations of the drug on each side of the membrane, and T is the thickness of the membrane. The minus sign denotes loss of drug from the outside when the concentration on the outside of the membrane is greater than that on the inside ($C_2 > C_1$) . The ratio (D · SA · K)/T is often referred as the *permeability coefficient P.*

Active transport Active transport is mediated by means of carriers through the expenditure of energy (i.e., use of adenosine triphosphate, ATP). This transport proceeds against a concentration gradient and, in the case of ions, against an electrochemical potential. Selectivity can be shown for compounds of the same size, and competitive inhibition can occur among substances handled by the same mechanism.

Facilitated diffusion Facilitated diffusion is a special form of carrier transport that has many of the characteristics of active transport. The only difference is that drug transport occurs with a concentration gradient.

Pinocytosis Pinocytosis refers to the ability of cells to engulf extracellular material within membrane vesicles formed by the epithelial cell. This process may be of some importance in the uptake of large molecules such as polypeptides.

pH partition The pH within cells is slightly lower than that in the extracellular space and the blood. As a result, a weak organic base entering a cell generally becomes ionized. This results in an extracellular to intracellular gradient of the nonionized form that favors penetration of the substance into intracellular space. Therefore, the total concentrations of the ionized and nonionized forms of a weak base will be somewhat higher inside than outside cells. From the foregoing, it follows that alterations in plasma pH can alter the tissue to plasma ratios of weak acids and weak bases by altering their rates of entrance into tissues.

Blood and tissue binding

Drug binding Binding of drugs to blood proteins and tissue components such as macromolecules (e.g., proteins, heteroproteins, or lipid structural components) influences drug distribution. In plasma, circulating proteins can be considered as acceptors that transport and release drugs throughout the body. In tissues, a drug can interact with various macromolecular structures that mediate effects, biotransformations, and/or elimination. Since only the free drug is thought to diffuse through biologic membranes, the free drug concentration in plasma will influence its distribution in the body and reflect the drug concentration available at the site of action, site of metabolism, or site of elimination (Fig. 4.1).

Binding of drugs to macromolecules is generally reversible and obeys the law of mass action. At equilibrium, the concentrations of bound (C_b) and free (C_u) drug are related to the number of protein binding sites n and the corresponding association constant K as follows:

$$C_b = \frac{n K C_u}{1 + K C_u} R$$

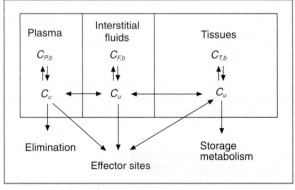

Figure 4.1 Schematic representation of drug interactions and distribution in the body. C_u denotes the unbound (free) drug concentration. C_{Pb}, C_{Fb}, and C_{Tb} denote the bound drug concentrations in plasma, interstitial fluids, and tissues, respectively.

where R stands for the total protein concentration. The curve of C_b versus C_u is a hyperbola; i.e., C_b will reach a plateau when C_u increases. This explains why for some drugs the plasma unbound fraction f_u can increase as the total plasma drug concentration increases. This *saturable binding* is observed when drugs have a high plasma concentration relative to the concentration of binding nR. Interestingly, for some drugs, no saturation occurs within the therapeutic range of drug plasma concentrations. This *nonsaturable binding* is observed when drugs have a low plasma concentration relative to the concentration of binding sites nR. In this case, f_u is related to the total binding protein concentration as follows:

$$f_u = \frac{1}{1 + n\,K\,R}$$

Plasma binding The extent of plasma binding varies widely between drugs. Most drugs are bound, but others are not, at least not detectably. Drugs that do not bind to plasma proteins generally are small molecules that are hydrophilic, whereas highly plasma-bound drugs are usually hydrophobic (Tab. 4.1).

Plasma protein binding of drugs can be classified simplistically according to the binding protein. The chemical structure and the acidic, basic, or neutral properties of the drug generally suggest the plasma protein(s) that will be involved in the binding. The most abundant plasma protein, albumin (human serum albumin, HSA), accounts for the binding of most acidic drugs, whereas plasma lipoproteins (LPs) and α_1-acid glycoprotein (AAG) are the main binding proteins for neutral and basic drugs. However, highly bound drugs generally interact with several proteins in plasma. This is particularly true for lipophilic basic drugs that often distribute among all plasma proteins.

HSA is mainly involved in the transport of free fatty acids, bilirubin, tryptophan, cysteine, pyridoxal phosphate, calcium, and various hormones such as thyroxine and steroids when specific transport proteins are saturated. The plasma binding of acidic drugs can be accounted for by HSA. There are at least two main drug binding sites of relative specificity on the albumin molecule. The warfarin binding site is involved in the binding of most oral antico-agulants, nonsteroidal anti-inflammatory drugs, and such other drugs as furosemide, glibenclamide, iophenoxic acid, tolbutamide, and valproic acid, as well as contrast media. The diazepam binding site is involved in the binding of anti-inflammatory drugs related to propionic acid, benzodiazepines, clofibric acid, ethacrynic acid, and iopanoic acid. However, some drugs such as indomethacin, diclofenac, and valproic acid can bind to the two distinct sites with a different affinity for each. Additionally, HSA is also responsible for the binding of digitoxin and related cardiac glycosides, also ascribed to a third specific binding site. Basic and neutral drugs may be bound by HSA, but they can be bound more avidly to other proteins in plasma. The binding of cardiac glycosides and basic drugs is generally nonsaturable.

Alpha$_1$-acid glycoprotein (AAG) is a globulin with a molecular weight of 40000 and a high carbohydrate content (55%). AAG shows large variations as a result of both biologic and pathologic conditions. AAG plays a major role in the plasma binding of most basic drugs. AAG also may play a role in the binding of certain steroids and acidic drugs and drugs having quaternary ammonium groups. Drugs are bound to a single common site on AAG, and the binding process is saturable in most cases. However, two classes of binding sites have been documented for certain drugs.

Plasma lipoproteins (LPs) are macromolecular complexes that transport water-insoluble plasma lipids in the circulation. The LPs are grouped according to their size, density, and composition: chylomicrons, very-low-density LPs (VLDLs), low-density LPs (LDLs), and high-density LPs (HDLs) (see Chap. 69). Plasma LPs are involved in the binding of basic drugs, but they also play a major role in the transport of highly lipophilic, water-insoluble drugs such as probucol, chloroethyl nitrosoureas, etretinate, amphotericin B, and cyclosporin A. In most cases, the binding is apparently nonsaturable, resembling a partition phenomenon between the LPs and the aqueous dispersion medium.

There is little information about drug binding to gamma globulins. Psychoactive drugs such as chlorpromazine, imipramine, nortriptyline, and some opiate derivatives bind to gamma globulins, but the extent of binding is thought to be too small to be of any significance.

Blood binding In blood, drugs can interact with plasma proteins but also with blood cells, erythrocytes, lymphocytes, neutrophils, and platelets. Erythrocytes are the most abundant cells in the blood and occupy a large and variable fraction of blood volume (between 35 and 50%). Basic drugs are known to penetrate and associate with red blood cells. This association depends on the ionization (pK_a) and lipid solubility of the drug and may involve solubilization in the interior of erythrocyte, binding to erythrocyte proteins, cytosol, or binding to the membrane. For example, more than 60% of cyclosporin A and 90% of chlorthalidone are associated with erythrocytes in blood because of high-affinity binding to cyclophilin and carbonic anhydrase, respectively.

Table 4.1 The variability of drug plasma protein binding

Drug	Plasma binding (%)
Paracetamol	0-10
Gentamicin	<10
Acebutolol	26
Caffeine	36
Phenobarbital	50
Carbamazepine	70
Theophylline	50-80
Valproic acid	85-95
Digitoxin	97
Diazepam	98-99
Warfarin	99
Ibuprofen	>99

Very few data are available on the quantitative binding of drugs to white blood cells or platelets, although many investigations dealing with the binding of certain drugs to specific receptors located on these cells have been performed. Doxorubicin and daunorubicin are associated with white blood cells and platelets to a significant extent, and the concentration of daunorubicin associated with leukemic cells in blood has been reported to be higher than the plasma concentration. Likewise, cyclosporine is significantly associated with leukocytes (15%) in human blood. Anticancer drugs of the *Vinca* alkaloid group are more than 50% associated with platelets in blood.

Plasma versus blood binding Plasma protein binding is the usual reference parameter for circulating drugs. The reason for this is that most pharmacokinetic studies are based on measurement of plasma drug concentration. In this case, the reference to plasma binding is relevant, and blood cells and platelets are included in the tissue compartment. However, for drugs that are highly bound to blood cells or platelets, pharmacokinetic studies are or should be based on blood concentrations of drug, and the drug binding parameter in the circulation should be blood binding of the drug.

Tissue binding In tissues, drugs can interact with various structures, receptors, enzymes, acceptors, and active transport systems that mediate drug effect, drug biotransformation, drug storage, or drug elimination, for example. Drug storage within tissues, i.e., drug binding to acceptors, can quantitatively affect drug distribution in the body. Lipophilic drugs or compounds such as thiopental, diazepam, or beta-carotene can accumulate in fat (adipocytes), where they are solubilized in lipids. Since fat proportion varies widely among individuals, this is a cause of interindividual variability in drug distribution. Some drugs display very high affinities for specific tissues. For example, chloroquine can concentrate in the liver and retina, and tetracycline avidly binds to areas of bone and tooth formation.

Altered plasma binding of drugs Reduced or increased plasma binding of drugs can be caused by specific physiologic conditions, diseases, or drug interactions. HSA concentration is decreased with aging or in the neonatal period, in inflammatory and nephrotic syndromes, and in hepatic impairment. By contrast, AAG or LP concentrations generally are increased. AAG increases considerably in a number of conditions characterized by stress, in myocardial infarction, cancer, and inflammatory syndromes, and in the postoperative period. Hyperlipoproteinemia is determined by the increase in one or several LP groups. The increase may be of unknown origin (i.e., primary hyperlipoproteinemia) or result from diseases such as hypothyroidism, obstructive liver disease, alcoholism, etc. However, AAG and LP concentrations can be diminished by severe hepatic insufficiency. Abnormalities in protein structure, genetically acquired or due to a pathologic condition (e.g., protein glycosylation in diabetes mellitus) also can decrease drug protein binding. Of course, drug-drug interaction can occur at the protein binding level, resulting in drug displacement. The decrease in plasma binding due to drug interaction is generally a transient phenomenon, ending when plasma drug concentrations decrease as a result of increased distribution volume and elimination (the increase in elimination occurs only for drugs with a low extraction ratio). Moreover, endogenous substances may alter drug binding. For example, an increased concentration of nonesterified free fatty acids, bilirubin, or other compounds generally decreases binding of acidic compounds to HSA.

Drug binding and distribution The drug concentration in plasma after distribution is complete is a function of the dose administered and the extent of drug distribution in the tissues. When a distribution equilibrium is achieved between drug in plasma and drug in tissues, an apparent volume into which a drug distributes in the body can be defined:

$$V_d = \frac{A}{C}$$

where V_d is the apparent volume of distribution, A is the amount of drug in the body at equilibrium (i.e., when distribution equilibrium is achieved between drug in tissues and drug in plasma), and C is the plasma drug concentration.

Since volume of distribution is a dilution space with no true physiologic meaning in terms of an anatomic space, the term *apparent volume of distribution* is used. It can be seen as a volume of fluid in which the drug would be distributed at a concentration equal to that in plasma. This parameter is a volume term or a constant relating the amount of drug in the body to plasma concentration, and it depends on the balance between plasma and tissue binding. Using compartments and the principle of mass balance, an equation showing the dependence of the apparent volume of distribution on plasma protein binding and tissue binding has been developed:

$$V_d = V_p + \frac{f_u}{f_{uT}} \cdot V_T$$

where V_p is the plasma volume, f_{uT} is the fraction unbound to tissue components, and V_T is the tissue physical volume of distribution outside the plasma (for the sake of clarity, the interstitial fluid compartment is included entirely in the tissue compartment). This clearly indicates the extent to which drug distribution will vary. An increase in f_u, i.e., a decrease in plasma binding, will involve a proportional increase in drug distribution, and an increase in f_{uT}, i.e., a decrease in tissue binding, will involve a curvilinear decrease in drug distribution. Finally, V_d depends on the ratio f_u/f_{uT}, which can be equated to a tissue-to-plasma binding ratio. That is, the lower this ratio, the higher is the plasma protein binding.

For a hypothetical drug whose plasma and tissue binding are equal, V_d thus equals V_p plus V_T, and total body water equals 0.6 liter/kg, or 42 liters, assuming a body weight of 70 kg and a body water content of 70% of body weight. When the f_u/f_{uT} ratio is greater than 1, tissue binding predominates, and the V_d is higher than 0.6 liter/kg. Conversely, when the f_u/f_{uT} ratio is lower than 1, plasma binding predominates, and the V_d is below 0.6 liter/kg.

Figure 4.2 depicts the concomitant variations in V_d and fraction of drug dose in the plasma compartment as a function of f_u/f_{uT}.

When acute changes in protein binding occur (e.g., a reduction in drug protein binding due to competition of another drug acting as a displacer), an interesting question regarding plasma protein binding is the extent of the increase in the plasma concentration of the unbound drug from C_u to C_u' as a result of binding alterations (increase from f_u to f_u'). Figure 4.3 depicts the instantaneous variation in C_u'/C_u as a function of the relative increase in f_u, that is, f_u'/f_u (a quasi-instantaneous equilibrium between drug concentrations in plasma and tissues is assumed, and f_{uT} is assumed not to change significantly). Actually, the conclusion depends on V_d. For a drug with a small V_d, say, 0.1 liter/kg, a meaningful increase in C_u is observed, although the increase in C_u is far lower than the increase in f_u. In fact, a twofold increase in f_u will result in a 25% increase in C_u. For a V_d of 0.6 liter/kg, there should be fivefold increase in f_u to produce a marginal 5% increase in C_u, whereas for larger V_d values, no significant C_u variation occurs.

Once the distribution of a drug is completed, the variation in unbound concentration after peak level depends on the clearance process. At steady state, for a drug with a low extraction ratio, i.e., a low-clearance drug, an increase in the unbound fraction of drug in plasma that occurs immediately after introduction of the displacing drug results in a transient increase in unbound concentration that gradually returns to its predisplacement steady-state value after redistribution occurs. For a drug with a high extraction ratio, i.e., a high-clearance drug, the variation in unbound concentration is much more complex, depending on whether the drug is administered by the oral or intravenous route.

For drugs with a small V_d, say, below 0.1 to 0.2 liter/kg, i.e., with a small f_u/f_{uT} ratio, plasma protein binding can be viewed as "restrictive" because a significant fraction of the dose is located in plasma. Conversely, plasma protein binding can be viewed as "permissive" for drugs whose V_d is large (0.6 liter/kg is commonly considered a large value), and the fraction in plasma is much lower than in tissues. Plasma binding variations may result in pharmacologic consequences for drugs with a restrictive plasma binding, especially if therapeutic and/or toxic effects depend on changes in unbound concentration. However, in the case of permissive plasma binding, no significant effects will result from alterations in plasma binding because marginal or even no changes in the unbound concentration are observed.

Tissue perfusion rate

For highly lipid-soluble drugs, characterized by a large partition coefficient, penetration is sufficiently rapid that only a single passage of blood through an organ is necessary to establish equilibrium between tissue and plasma. Rate of drug uptake into tissues is then limited by the tissue perfusion rate (i.e., blood flow/volume of tissue). Tissues can be classified into three groups according to their perfusion rates: rapidly perfused tissues such

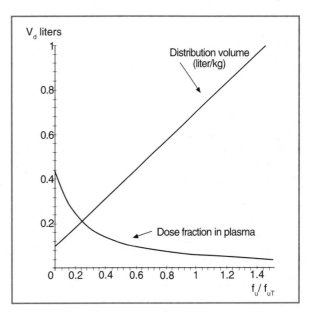

Figure 4.2 Concomitant variations of distribution volume (in liters per kilogram) and dose fraction in plasma as a function of the f_u/f_{uT} ratio that measures the relative tissue-to-plasma binding ratio. For example, when $f_u/f_{uT} = 0.6$, the distribution volume is 0.44 liter/kg and the fraction of the dose in plasma is 8%.

as brain, kidney, liver, heart, spleen, and thyroid gland; less rapidly perfused tissues such as muscle and skin; and poorly perfused tissues such as fat and bone. There is a 500-fold difference between very rapid (e.g., lungs) and very slow (e.g., bone) tissue perfusion rates.

Redistribution

Some highly lipid-soluble drugs acting in the brain may be subjected to a redistribution phenomenon when they are administered rapidly by intravenous or inhalation routes. When the drug reaches its maximum concentration in the blood, it rapidly equilibrates with highly perfused tissues such as brain. Then a rapid fall in blood concentration occurs. This fall is related to redistribution of the drug from the brain and other well-perfused organs to lean tissues. For an anesthetic drug such as thiopental, the redistribution phenomenon results in a rapid decline in the concentration in the brain owing to the uptake into poorly perfused tissues. When the concentration falls below the activity threshold, the effect wears off during the redistribution, accounting for the rapid recovery of consciousness within 20 minutes.

SPECIFIC LOCALIZATIONS OR BARRIERS

Diffusion into extracellular and intracellular spaces

Free drug in the bloodstream will be diluted in about at least 15 liters fluid, the sum of extravascular interstitial fluid (about 12 liters in the adult male) and plasma water

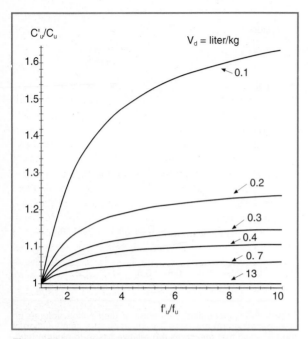

Figure 4.3 The instantaneous variation of unbound drug concentration (C'$_u$) relative to the initial C$_u$ as a function of the variation in plasma free fraction f'$_u$/f$_u$ for different values of V$_d$. The simulation assumes a fast, quasi-instantaneous equilibrium between plasma and tissue drug concentrations and that f$_{uT}$ does not change significantly. For example, for a drug with a 0.1 liter/kg V$_d$ (7 liters for an individual weighing 70 kg), when f$_u$ varies from 3 to 6%, f'$_u$/f$_u$ = 2, and C'$_u$/C$_u$ = 1.3, there is a 30% increase in C$_u$.

volume (about 3 liters). Thus, a drug that can readily leave the capillaries but which cannot enter cells will diffuse into the total extracellular fluid, i.e., 15 liters. Water-soluble and poorly lipid-soluble drugs are mostly distributed within the extracellular fluid.

If the drug is capable of crossing the cell membrane, it will move from the extracellular space into the fluid within the cell. Assuming that no active transport process is involved, the transfer across the cell wall will proceed until the intracellular drug concentration is the same as that outside the cell. Since the permeability characteristics of the cellular membrane are about the same for all cells, it follows that the concentration of the drug will be further diluted by a volume equal to that of the total intracellular water of all cells, approximately 27 liters. Consequently, a drug readily passing all biologic barriers with no binding to any cellular components will dilute in a volume equal to the total water content of the body, about 42 liters.

At this stage it is essential to emphasize again that the pharmacokinetic concept of apparent volume of distribution, i.e., a parameter that relates the amount in the body to plasma concentration, cannot be equated to the anatomophysiologic fluid compartments previously defined in this section, i.e., extravascular interstitial fluids and intracellular fluids. Even if the V_d value resulting of pharmacokinetic calculations corresponds with the value of a physiologic body fluid compartment, one cannot con-

clude unambiguously that the drug distributes only into that volume.

Blood-central nervous system barriers

There are two anatomic barriers to drug transport into the central nervous system (CNS): the blood-brain barrier and the blood-cerebrospinal fluid barrier. The *blood-brain barrier* consists of a monolayer of cells that serve as the interface between the fluids of the CNS and the blood. The capillary bed comprises this monolayer of cells for most of the brain and has been referred to as the *endothelial barrier*. All the endothelial cells of the capillaries of the CNS are connected by high-resistance tight junctions characterized by the absence of fenestrations and of pinocytotic vesicles. Aqueous bulk flow is thus severely restricted. The cell membranes consist of lipids, and hence the property that generally governs passive diffusion and penetration of a compound into brain, via endothelial cells, is the compound's lipid solubility.

The *blood-cerebrospinal fluid barrier* is located in the choroid plexus and circumventricular organ consisting of about a half dozen tiny areas of brain around the ventricules, the site of formation of cerebrospinal fluid (CSF).

The blood-CSF barrier is composed of tight junctions joining the ependyma or epithelial cells that line the ventricular surface at each respective circumventricular organ. As with the blood-brain barrier, only lipid-soluble drugs penetrate the blood-CSF barrier through the choroid plexus. Inflammation increases the permeability of this anatomic barrier, presumably by opening some tight junctions. This phenomenon accounts for the better penetration of some antibiotics in meningitis.

Drugs leave the brain by reverse passage through the blood-brain barrier for lipid-soluble drugs and by clearance into the CSF and eventually into the general circulation via the arachnoid villi.

Placenta

The placenta is an interface between maternal and fetal circulations during pregnancy to provide delivery of oxygen and exchange of nutrients for the fetus. The two circulations are separated by a cellular barrier composed from the fetal to the maternal pole of (1) the syncytiotrophoblast, consisting of a continuous layer of cells lining the intervillous space; (2) the cytotrophoblast, which is initially a continuous layer and later a discontinuous layer; (3) the trophoblastic basal lamina; and (4) the capillary fetal endothelium. As term approaches, fetal-maternal exchanges increase in part because of thinning of the membranes. Since drugs cross the placenta in the same manner as nutrients, it is inevitable that drugs administered to the mother reach the fetus. Thus, the placenta should not be viewed as a barrier to drugs.

The characteristics of drug diffusion from maternal blood to fetal blood are very similar to those of passage across any epithelial barrier. Lipid-soluble, nonionized drugs readily move from mother to fetus in accordance with lipid/water partition coefficients and degree of ionization. Water-soluble drugs move much more slowly and in inverse proportion to their molecular size. The rate and direction of this exchange depend on the concentration gradients and the rate of delivery to the intervillous spaces and villi. This placental transfer of drugs can be harmful to the fetus, giving rise to teratogenic effects, and concerns persist about the numerous substances that reach the fetus during pregnancy. The transfer of drugs across the placenta sometimes can benefit the fetus. Based on the passage of some drugs across the placenta, specific intentional therapy has been devised for several fetal problems such as arrhythmias, congestive heart failure, pulmonary immaturity, adrenal hyperplasia, bacterial infections, and maternal-fetal transmission of human immunodeficiency virus (HIV).

Breast milk

Each breast contains about 20 lobes that are subdivided into lobules. The functional units are composed of secretory cells surrounding an alveolus (a lumen), ducts, and blood supply. Alveoli are connected by large ducts that empty into lactiferous ducts. These ducts have a dilatation prior to their termination at the nipple. The luminal or duct contents are separated from the extracellular space by a biologic membrane composed of basement membrane, myoepithelial cells, and glandular cells. Drugs have to pass from maternal plasma across this biologic membrane to be excreted in the milk. The passage of drugs into milk may be explained by passive diffusion of the nonionized, non-protein-bound fraction. The mean pH of milk (7.2) is lower than that of plasma. The ratio of unbound drug concentration in milk M to unbound drug concentration in plasma P may be predicted on the basis of the Henderson-Hasselbach equation as follows:

$$M/P = \frac{1+10^{\ pH_M - pK_a}}{1+10^{\ pH_P - pK_a}}$$

$$M/P = \frac{1+10^{\ pK_a - pH_M}}{1+10^{\ pK_a - pH_P}}$$

where pH_M is the pH of milk and pH_P is the pH of plasma. These equations predict that for unbound drug, M/P will be less than 1 for acidic drugs, more than 1 for basic drugs, and equal to 1 for neutral drugs.

The passage of drugs from plasma to milk may cause concern about infant exposure. If M/P ratios can be helpful in estimating drug concentrations in milk, they do not provide any indication of the likely infant dose received from human milk, since milk and plasma drug concentrations do not parallel each other throughout the dosing interval. Calculation of the daily infant dose of a drug ingested in milk and from this the dose in milk relative to the maternal dose on a weight-adjusted basis is much more relevant in terms of infant exposure. The problem is that drug package insert information about use during lactation is frequently not informative. Some pharmacokinetic reviews devoted to this specific area, however, provide very helpful information about infant exposure and safety problems resulting from breast feeding (see also Chap. 88).

Adipose tissue

Adipose tissue, or fat, must be considered an important potential storage site for drugs because it contains a high proportion of stored lipid in the form of triacylglycerols. In humans, the average proportion of adipose tissue increases from 18 to 36% of total body weight in males and from 33 to 48% in females with increasing age. In obese persons (i.e., those with a weight exceeding 25% of the ideal body weight), adipose tissue can constitute up to 50% of total body weight. Adipose tissue can serve as an important reservoir for lipid-soluble drugs.

Suggested readings _____

ATKINSON HC, BEGG EJ, DARLOW BA. Drugs in human milk: Clinical pharmacokinetic considerations. Clin Pharmacokinet 1988;14:217-40.

BONATI M, KANTO J, TOGNONI G. Clinical pharmacokinetics of cerebrospinal fluid. Clin Pharmacokinet 1982;7:312-35.

JUSKO WJ, GRETCH M. Plasma and tissue protein binding of drugs in pharmacokinetics. Drug Metab Rev 1976;5:43-140.

ØIE S, TOZER TN. Effect of altered plasma protein binding on apparent volume of distribution. J Pharm Sci 1979;68:1203-5.

PACIFICI GM, NOTOLI R. Placental transfer administered to the mother. Clin Pharmacokinet 1995;28:235-69.

ROWLAND M, TOZER T. Distribution. In: Rowland M, Tozer T (eds). Clinical pharmacokinetics: concepts and applications, 3 ed. Baltimore: Williams & Wilkins, 1995:137-55.

TILLEMENT JP, ZINI R, BARRÉ J, HERVÉ F. Blood binding and drugs. In: Dulbecco R (ed). Encyclopedia of human biology, vol 2, 2nd ed. San Diego. Academic Press, 197:1-8.

TILLEMENT JP, HOUIN G, ZINI R, et al. The binding of drug to blood plasma macromolecules: recent advances and therapeutic significance. Adv Drug Res 1984;13:59-94.

WARD RM. Pharmacological treatment of the fetus: clinical pharmacokinetic considerations. Clin Pharmacokinet 1995;28:343-50.

Methods in drug delivery

Stefan Bracht

Whenever a drug is to be delivered into the human body, it has to pass one of its outer or inner surfaces. The easiest way to achieve this is the mechanical puncture or other local destruction of these barriers, as it is done with injection, infusion, or implantation. Any other method of drug delivery involves passage through biologic barriers by diffusion processes and largely dependent on the physicochemical nature of the barrier and of the drug. Generally, the outer surfaces of the body exhibit protective functions, whereas the inner surfaces are mostly dedicated to the exchange of low-molecular-weight chemical entities with the environment.

In terms of drug application, outer surfaces are comprised of the cornified skin; the mucosa and cornea of the eye; and the mucosae of the nose, mouth, pharynx, vagina (outer part), and penis. Inner surfaces relevant for drug delivery are the lower airways, the complete gastrointestinal tract, and the inner cavities of the vagina, uterus, and penis. In special cases, inner surfaces may be used for delivery that are not directly accessible from the outside, e.g., a peritoneal injection.

Independent of the permeability of barriers for a certain drug, the diffusion process is always ruled by the concentration gradient and the area as well as the thickness of the barrier. Thus an increase in the application area or the applied concentration of the drug always increases absorption as long as other parameters are kept constant.

Today, three major challenges for methods of drug delivery can be identified: (1) the increasing need for time- and rate-controlled delivery of a drug, (2) targeted drug delivery, and (3) the development of peptides and proteins as a new generation of drugs.

These challenges are constantly driving a trend in galenical development from simple dosage forms or units toward complete drug delivery units or systems. In terms of the pharmaceutical sciences, drug delivery usually means that the drug will be delivered in a predetermined way from the unit or system and at a predetermined location of the body. This chapter will focus on trends in drug delivery that are based on new pharmaceutical technologies and does not provide a complete list of all methods.

ORAL DRUG DELIVERY

Typical oral dosage forms are liquids, tablets, and hard and soft gelatin capsules. Soft gelatin capsules are the usual transport vehicle for small single doses of liquid drugs or drug solutions. Hard gelatin capsules are very versatile vehicles that can be filled with a variety of dosage subunits such as granules, pellets, or microcapsules. Additionally, by exterior coating or integrated mechanisms, it can be predetermined where, when, and how the capsule opens or releases its ingredients.

Besides simple one-compartment dosing units, tableting technology allows the production of multilayer systems (all compartments in direct contact with the environment) as well as systems comprising a core covered by one or more coatings.

Zero-order release To avoid plasma peaks, especially for drugs with a narrow therapeutic window, a number of oral systems have been developed that release the drug at a constant rate over time. Underlying techniques involve the use of rate-controlling semipermeable membranes, osmotic or hydrodynamic pumps (e.g., OROS technology), increase in drug-releasing surface area by swelling processes during application (e.g., Geomatrix technology), or increase in drug-releasing surface area by erosion of coating material during application (e.g., Smartrix technology). Obstacles for all these technologies have to be seen in the influence of the fasted or fed state and the variations in transport speed, pH, and ionic strength along the alimentary canal. Last but not least, cost-effective mass production must be possible.

A well-known representative of this group, the OROS system, is depicted schematically in Figure 5.1. In contact with gastric juices, a swellable polymeric compartment takes up water through a semipermeable shape-retaining membrane and drives a drug from a separate reservoir through a small rate-limiting orifice into the environment.

Time-controlled drug release (delayed-action, biphasic, and pulsatile delivery) Especially with chronic diseases, it has been shown that circadian rhythms increasingly play an important role and that homeostasis of drug thera-

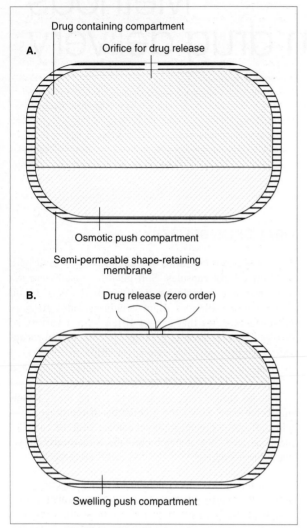

Drug containing compartment

Orifice for drug release

A.

Osmotic push compartment

Semi-permeable shape-retaining membrane

B. Drug release (zero order)

Swelling push compartment

Figure 5.1 OROS system (**A**) before oral intake and (**B**) during contact with gastric juices.

juices, the plug starts to swell with water until it pops off, placing the drug reservoir in the other half of the capsule in contact with the environment.

Gastrointestinal targeting Small intestine targeting by enteric coating has been in use for a long time to protect active compounds from the chemically aggressive environment of the stomach. These coatings are pH-sensitive polymers that do not dissolve below a predetermined pH. With this method, targeting within the proximal part (pH ≈ 6) and the distal part (pH ≈ 7) of the small intestine is also possible.

In recent years the colon has been the most interesting site for targeted oral delivery. This interest is based mainly on peptide delivery (see below). The colon offers a chemically moderate environment with low enzyme activity compared with the small intestine. The surface area for absorption, on the other hand, is much smaller, but this is compensated for in part by longer physiologic residence times. Colon targeting is possible by bacterially triggered systems (enzymatic degradation of protective coating), delayed-action systems (e.g., Pulsincap; see above), and pH-triggered systems.

Prolongation of gastrointestinal residence time Any oral delivery system is subject to the gastrointestinal transport process and thus a maximum passage time of typically 24 hours until excretion can be expected. For

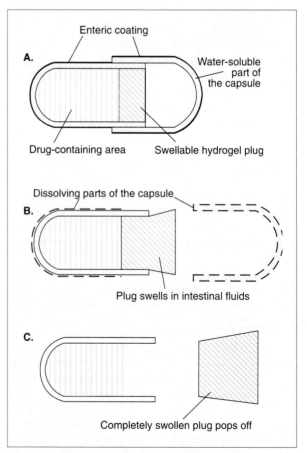

Enteric coating

A.

Water-soluble part of the capsule

Drug-containing area   Swellable hydrogel plug

Dissolving parts of the capsule

B.

Plug swells in intestinal fluids

C.

Completely swollen plug pops off

Figure 5.2 Pulsincap system (**A**) before oral intake, (**B**) after gastric passage, and (**C**) at the start of drug release.

py is not always the ideal treatment. On the other hand, the development of tolerance (e.g., functional tolerance or receptor downregulation) must be avoided when using certain drugs such as organic nitrates. A very typical requirement is the combination of an initial dose and a maintenance dose. The latter situation can be mastered by a large number of systems, e.g., capsules filled with a mixture of sustained- and instant-release pellets or tablets containing a slow-release core covered with an instant-release coating material.

For the treatment of asthma or angina pectoris, it is often desirable to delay the onset of drug release until the early morning hours after oral intake in the evening. This can be accomplished, for example, by the Pulsincap technology, which is already at an advanced stage of development, as depicted in Figure 5.2. A hydrogel plug maintains a drug reservoir within half the capsule. After the first half of the capsule has been dissolved in gastric

most drugs, only a certain interval of this passage is available for absorption. To enable longer residence times including once-a-day systems, gastric retention in particular has attracted interest, and this has led to the development of several retention techniques.

Retention of solid forms of drugs may be achieved by mucoadhesion, flotation, sedimentation, or expansion of the system. The coadministration of drugs that delay gastric emptying is also possible. Mucoadhesion is hardly ever strong enough in the stomach but might be sufficient in the small intestine; flotation requires filling of the stomach and a more or less upright posture; and sedimentation of pellets into the folds close to the pylorus in some cases results in the desired retention. The most reliable method seems to involve expansion of the system or by unfolding or inflation to a size that does not pass the pyloric sphincter. This expansion has to be reversible so that transport ultimately can continue so as to prevent accumulation of these systems in the gastrointestinal tract.

Peptide delivery The main obstacles to peptide delivery are the poor absorption of these polar compounds, their high lumenal degradation, and the brush-border proteolytic activity of the small intestine. Thus, release of peptide and protein drugs in the distal ileum and colon is seen as one of the keys to success. Inhibition of proteolytic activities by suitable polymers that are not absorbable (e.g., polyacrylic acid) may be another. This will have to be done selectively to minimize side effects.

In many cases, existing carrier systems such as the relatively nonspecific di- and tripeptide carrier of the brush border can be used. Even the vitamin B_{12} carrier could be used as specific entry for modified peptides. Other strategies under discussion are the use of enhancers such as bile salts or the widening of tight junctions to increase peptide absorption by the brush border. The latter effect is described for chitosans (cationic polymers derived from chitin) but may be too unspecific.

DERMAL AND TRANSDERMAL DRUG DELIVERY

The main permeation barrier for most drugs is the stratum corneum, which is only 10 to 15 µm thick and made up of several layers of nonviable cornified cells. The interspaces between these corneocytes are filled with several lipid bilayers, and the whole construction is similar to bricks and mortar. Several specialized pathways such as hair follicles and the ducts of different glands interrupt this barrier but are rarely involved in the absorption of drugs.

The intercellular lipid bilayers are the most important pathway for drug absorption.

Topical semisolid drug forms typically include ointments, creams, gels, and pastes. Ointments are often composed of oleagenous or fatty lipophilic excipients only, a cream additionally contains water, and a gel typically consists of a small amount of a polymer dissolved in a mixture of liquid excipients mostly including volatile solvents such as water and isopropyl alcohol. Topical forms often serve as skin care and maintenance products at the same time. Regardless of the composi-

tion of the system, the release of a drug strongly depends on its solubility and the degree of its saturation within the matrix. Only at higher degrees of saturation (or especially at supersaturation) can an optimal release be achieved.

Creams are complex systems, and their microstructures (directly affecting drug release) may change significantly and uncontrollably after application. The topical forms described earlier normally do not enable reliable and reproducible dosage regimens. Transdermal delivery systems (TDSs) were developed as controlled systemic delivery vehicles, but they also can be used for the controlled topical delivery of drugs. The distinction between topical and systemic delivery by the dermal route depends in principle only on the question of whether therapeutically effective plasma levels of a drug can be obtained. The main advantages of TDSs over oral drug delivery systems are the possibility of maintaining therapy with drugs that have a short biologic half-life, to avoid hepatic first-pass effects, the ability to simplify the medication regimen and improve patient compliance, and the potential to reach nearly constant plasma levels for a prolonged period of time.

Some prominent drugs that have been marketed as TDS are clonidine, 17ß-estradiol, fentanyl, nicotine, nitroglycerin, testosterone, and scopolamine. It is important to note that typically not more than 15 to 20 mg per day of a drug can be administered transdermally because higher rates often cause skin irritation regardless of the type of drug.

Membrane-controlled and matrix-controlled TDSs The classic approach in the construction of TDSs includes a drug-containing reservoir (e.g., solution or semisolid preparation of the drug) with an adjacent membrane that controls release rate to provide zero-order release. An additional adhesive layer is used to affix this system to the skin. A simplified (monolithic) matrix construction without a membrane is used in many modern systems in which the drug reservoir makes direct contact with the skin and has self-adhesive properties at the same time. The latter improvement became possible when it was recognized that in many cases the skin itself acts as a rate-controlling membrane. Based on these two concepts, a large number of system designs are possible (Fig. 5.3).

Penetration enhancers, liposomes, and prodrugs Since many drugs lack the ideal physicochemical properties to be absorbed sufficiently by the transdermal route, penetration enhancers have attracted much interest in the field of TDS development. Enhancers mostly work on the lipid biayers in the stratum corneum by disordering of the lipids, extracting the lipids, widening the polar pathways, or increasing solubility of the drug within the barrier, all resulting in accelerated diffusion of the drug through the skin. A large number of enhancers lack the necessary toxicologic expertise, and the risk of skin irritation is usually increased in the presence of enhancers. Thus, enhancement is an essential tool in a limited number of cases and should be used carefully. A welcome permeation-enhanc-

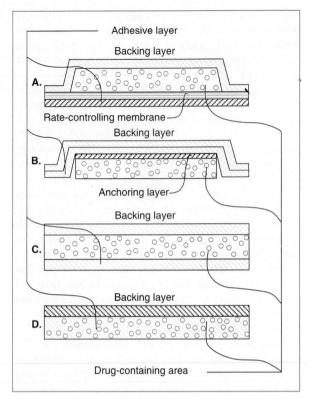

Figure 5.3 Selection of typical TDS designs: (**A**) membrane-controlled reservoir system; (**D**) monolithic matrix system; (**B, C**) intermediate forms between **A** and **D**.

ing effect that works for most drugs is skin occlusion, which results in hydration and swelling of the stratum corneum, along with increased permeability.

Liposomes often have been proposed as vehicles for dermal and transdermal delivery of enclosed drugs. There is evidence for liposomes enhancing drug incorporation into the upper layers of the stratum corneum, but it is generally accepted that liposomes do not permeate the skin as a complete entity.

Electrically assisted transdermal delivery Electric current can be employed within various modalities to facilitate transdermal transport of drug molecules that are inappropriate for passive transport. Among these methods, iontophoresis is the most frequently used, followed by electroporation. While iontophoresis creates an electromotive force that drives charged molecules through the barrier, electroporation nonspecifically and transiently lowers the barrier function for all kinds of otherwise too large or too polar compounds through the application of high-voltage pulses.

Iontophoresis is an interesting tool for the delivery of new classes of drugs such as peptides or oligonucleotides. The development of miniaturized systems to be used by outpatients, however, is complex and costly. At the moment, the huge number of patents in this field is in strong contrast to the market share of iontophoretically

assisted TDSs. Iontophoresis probably will be more a niche within the TDS market than one of the next generation TDS devices.

Phonophoresis The application of ultrasound (typically 200-1000 kHz) is known to lower the permeation barrier of the skin for a number of chemically different compounds. Several underlying mechanisms are being hypothesized, among which is the formation of gaseous bubbles within the stratum corneum by cavitation. The potential of this kind of enhancement with regard to the necessary miniaturization of systems seems to be unclear, and very few developmental efforts have been made in this field.

BUCCAL AND SUBLINGUAL DRUG DELIVERY

The advantages of drug delivery within the oral cavity include elimination of hepatic first-pass effect, rapid onset of action, and protection of drugs from chemical or enzymatic inactivation within the gastrointestinal tract. The latter is of special interest for peptide and protein drugs. Lacking cornified layers, the oral mucosa is much more permeable than skin. On the other hand, oral mucosa lacks the large surface area and absorptive function of the gut.

The sublingual area has the highest permeability and traditionally has been used for rapid-onset delivery, for example, of nitroglycerin. Several bioadhesive formulations and systems for controlled release of drugs have been developed for the oral cavity, including patches (e.g., the Cydot mucoadhesive system) and adhesive tablets. So far the market potential for controlled-release systems is unclear because they seem to cause significant discomfort for the patient.

NASAL DRUG DELIVERY

Nasal delivery, in its most simple form, is a very popular route for the abuse of cocaine and other "street" drugs. The nasal epithelium is unique among other mucous tissues in its easy accessibility, rich vasculature, and low thickness of the epithelium. On the other hand, the ciliary clearance is counterproductive. Certain commercially available products (e.g., desmopressin formulations) already use this route for systemic drug delivery. For the delivery of peptides and proteins in particular, the nasal route has attracted a great deal of interest in recent years, and delivery systems have been developed involving controlled-release powders or microspheres.

In most cases of peptide delivery and especially protein delivery, the normal permeability of human nasal mucosa is too low, and proteolytic activity is also present. Coadministration of enhancers depends on the safety and efficacy of these compounds, especially with respect to normal ciliary function. Cyclodextrins and their derivatives play a role as complexing agents in this field and are promising enhancers for the nasal absorption of oligopeptides and less for polypeptides and proteins such as insulin.

PULMONARY DRUG DELIVERY

The lungs offer a hugh surface area for the absorption of drugs that is approximately 90% attributed to the alveoli. Traditionally, pulmonary delivery has been used in the localized therapy of diseases such as asthma. Pressurized metered-dose inhalers (pMDIs) with chlorofluorocarbons (CFCs) as propellants have been the standard aerosol delivery device for a long time. Technologic changes and advances in recent years have originated mostly from requirements to eliminate or replace CFCs, known to destroy the ozone layer. Within the propellant-based aerosol technology, it was very difficult to develop suitable substitutes due to the unique properties of CFCs as a combined propellant and solvent system. CFC-free products are now based on ozone-friendly hydrofluorocarbons.

Another general problem with propellant-based aerosols has involved patient timing errors based on inaccurate coordination of pMDI use with inspiration. This can be overcome by additional spacers (or holding chambers) that allow the aerosol ejected by the device to mix with a suitable volume of air before the patient inhales the mixture in a second step.

Both the need for CFC-free devices and the interest in breath-activated systems have promoted the development of dry-powder inhalers; e.g., from systems that had to be loaded with a capsule prior to each use; multidose devices are now available. This progress is largely based on advanced pharmaceutical technologies in the formulation and micronization of powders.

There is no doubt that the lungs are a suitable absorption site for the systemic delivery of drugs as long as they can be delivered directly to the alveolar membranes. Pulmonary absorption of interesting peptides and proteins (such as insulin) will strongly depend on the efficiency of powdering and aerosol technologies. For reliable and reproducible alveolar delivery, it will be essential to generate highly monodisperse particles or droplets less than 5 µm in diameter as a vehicle for each individual drug.

OCULAR DRUG DELIVERY

Drug delivery into the eye is complicated by the strong barrier properties of the cornea. Additionally, the constant tear flow usually eliminates drugs quite rapidly from the precorneal area via the lacrimal duct. Thus, the ocular half-life of drugs applied as conventional eyedrops may

only be in the range of a few minutes, and the main part of the dose can cause unwanted effects after drainage into the nose or gut. Drainage delay by viscous or sticky preparations like gels and ointments may cause blurred vision and is acceptable for use only during sleep.

Drug-delivering ocular inserts are another alternative, but the first candidate in the marketplace, the Ocusert system for the delivery of pilocarpine, had only limited success because of complicated application and a high level of irritation. Generally, this strategy, including drug-loaded contact lenses, suffers from discomfort for the patient and difficult application.

Liposomes as well as microspheres and nanoparticles offer the chance to increase both the precorneal residence time of the drug and transcorneal absorption into the eye. At the same time they can be used in solution as easily as eyedrops. The latter two types of microparticulate carriers offer numerous possibilities for controlled and targeted drug delivery to the eye.

INVASIVE PARENTERAL DRUG DELIVERY

Intravasal injection or infusion is still the fastest and most flexible method of systemic drug delivery, but normally it precludes self-administration. It is still an essential method for all drugs that are insufficiently absorbed or not tolerated by other routes (e.g., some antibiotics and most proteins). In fact, the targeting of specific organs, tissues, and cells often demands biochemical or immunochemical modifications of the drug molecule or the use of microcarriers (e.g., liposomes). Parenteral depot preparations generally are supplied by subcutaneous or intramuscular injection. Typical strategies to decrease the solubility of the drug employ complexation, precipitation, microencapsulation, or prodrug formation. Diffusion, dissolution, bioerosion, or biodegradation may work as the rate-limiting step during the sustained drug release from such preparations. Advances in this field are associated with progress in the synthesis of biocompatible and bioerodable or biodegradable polymeric materials.

Two modern parenteral delivery devices are named here as representatives of the whole group of devices. The Medipad is a miniaturized infusion pump for subcutaneous injection that can be worn like a patch on the skin. The device can be (re)charged with drug cartridges and is designed for self-administration by outpatients. In another development, needle-less injection systems use a jet stream of helium gas to accelerate fine drug particles to supersonic speed that subsequently permeate the skin or mucosa with little or no pain.

*Suggested readings*_____

AHUJA A, KHAR RK, ALI J. Mucoadhesive drug delivery systems. Drug Dev Ind Pharm 1997;23:489-515.

ANONYMOUS. Scherer DDS develops "Alarm Clock" dose formulation. Pharm J 1991;247:137-9.

ASMUSSEN B. Transdermal therapeutic systems: actual state and future developments. Methods Find Exp Clin Pharmacol 1991;13:343-51.

BAI JPF, CHANG LL, GUO JH. Targeting of peptide and protein drugs to specific sites in the oral route. Crit Rev Ther Drug Carrier Syst 1995;12:339-71.

BERNER B, JOHN VA. Pharmacokinetic characterization of transdermal delivery systems. Clin Pharmacokinet 1994;26:121–34.

CHIEN YW (ed). Novel drug delivery systems. 2nd ed. Drugs and the pharmaceutical sciences. Vol. 50. New York: Marcel Dekker, 1992:139-96.

KIRJAVAINEN M, URTTI A, JÄÄSKELÄINEN I, et al. Interaction of liposomes with human skin in vitro: The influence of lipid composition and structure. Biochim Biophys Acta 1996;1304:179-89.

LALOR CB, FLYNN GL, WEINER N. Formulation factors affecting release of drug from topical vehicles: II. Effect of solubility on in vitro delivery of a series of n-alkyl-p-aminobenzoates. J Pharm Sci 1995;84:673-6.

MOËS AJ. Gastroretentive dosage forms. Crit Rev Ther Drug Carrier Syst 1993;10:143-95.

RIVIERE JE, HEIT MC. Electrically assisted transdermal drug delivery. Pharm Res 1997;14:687-97.

RUSSELL-JONES G. Utilization of the natural mechanism for vitamin B12 uptake for the oral delivery of therapeutics. Eur J Pharmacol Biopharm 1996;42:241-9.

SWANSON DR, BARCLAY BL,WONG PSL, et al. Nefedipine gastrointestinal therapeutic system. Am J Med 1987;83:3-9.

WATTS PJ, ILLUM L. Colonic drug delivery. Drug Dev Ind Pharm 1997;23:893-914.

ZIMMER A, KREUTER J. Microspheres and nanoparticles used in ocular delivery systems. Adv Drug Del Rev 1995;System:61-73.

6

Fundamentals of drug interactions

James S. Morris, Ivan H. Stockley

A *drug interaction* is said to occur when the effects of one drug taken by a patient are changed by another drug, food, or drink also taken by the patient. Sometimes the term *drug interaction* is used more widely than this definition. Drugs may be involved in physicochemical reactions when mixed in intravenous fluids, creams, etc., causing precipitation or inactivation. A long-established and less ambiguous term for these processes is *pharmaceutical incompatibility.* Drugs may interfere with biochemical assays and other tests carried out on body fluids. The term *drug interaction* is best reserved for reactions that go on within, rather than outside, the body of a patient.

The outcome of an interaction can be harmful, beneficial, or clinically insignificant. For clinicians, the main concern is interactions that have a potentially harmful outcome. It may be possible to represcribe to avoid harmful interactions, especially when a suitable noninteracting alternative is available. For instance, one may wish to treat a patient taking theophylline with ciprofloxacin. Ciprofloxacin causes a two- to threefold increase in theophylline serum levels, which is likely to result in theophylline toxicity. Selecting an alternative quinolone antibiotic such as lomefloxacin or sparfloxacin, which does not interact, can avoid the problem.

However, this type of approach becomes more difficult if patients need to take a large number of drugs or suitable alternatives are not available. Trying to avoid interactions completely may result in a patient being denied appropriate drug therapy. The alternative approach is to manage the interaction using various methods, including monitoring, dosage separation, and dosage alterations as appropriate for the interaction. Some examples can illustrate this. An isolated report describes overwhelming fatigue in a patient taking zidovudine with acyclovir. There is no reason for avoiding concurrent use of these drugs, but the patient should be monitored. The interaction between tetracycline and antacids can be minimized by separating the dosages by 2 to 3 hours. Patients on warfarin who are given rifampin need an increase in the dosage of warfarin to maintain adequate anticoagulation.

Today's prescriber needs to place into perspective and feel comfortable managing interactions as part of the daily workload. Some insight into the incidence and importance of drug interactions is helpful.

INCIDENCE AND IMPORTANCE OF DRUG INTERACTIONS

Many studies have attempted to identify the incidence of drug interactions. Incidence figures of clinically significant interactions as low as 4.7% (general patients), with evidence of interactions observed in only 0.3% of patients, or as high as 88% (geriatric patients), of which 22% were regarded as serious or life-threatening, have been quoted, with a range of values in between. Probably we will never know the true incidence of interactions; underreporting of adverse reactions is well recognized, and presumably, different institutions can vary considerably in preferred therapies, patients, diseases treated, resources, and quality of staff. Nevertheless, a considerable number of patients appear to be at risk when one thinks of the large numbers of drugs prescribed and taken every day.

Worldwide, significant resources have been invested in the study of drug interactions. Most licensing authorities require detailed data on drug interactions as part of the product license application, either as predictions from metabolic research or as clinical studies of combined usage. Significant sums of money have been spent on specific interaction textbooks and computer programs. Large costs can be involved in litigation and damages when a patient suffers a serious adverse drug interaction.

Despite this possible high incidence and perceived importance, it is sensible to keep a balanced view. Concluding that it is extremely risky to treat patients with more than one drug at a time would be an overreaction. The figures quoted earlier illustrate that many drugs that are known to interact in some patients simply fail to do so in others. The figures also suggest that patients apparently tolerate adverse interactions remarkably well and that many experienced physicians compensate for them without being aware of it. Many warfarin interactions will be accommodated automatically if the patient regularly attends an anticoagulation clinic. When an antibiotic does not appear effective, it may be because either the infecting organism is not sensitive or an interaction is lowering serum levels below therapeutic values. Normally, the antibiotic simply would be changed. It is also common for patients simply to discontinue a drug if they feel it is making them ill, without telling their physician.

Variability in patient response has lead to some extreme responses among prescribers. Excessive anxiety can lead to patients being denied useful drugs. At the other extreme, some clinicians who personally have encountered few interactions substantially disregard them so that some of their patients are potentially at risk.

The responsible position lies between these two extremes. A considerable number of interacting drugs can be taken together safely, provided the appropriate precautions are employed, whereas there are relatively few pairs of drugs that must always be avoided. To be able to manage interactions successfully, the clinician needs an appreciation of the characteristics of drug interactions so as to provide a framework for assessing the most beneficial course of action.

CHARACTERISTICS OF DRUG INTERACTIONS

Drug interactions are usually catalogued and retrieved as pairs of interacting drugs. The general format is: This drug + that drug = an interaction. This is only part of the picture. It leaves out possibly the most important component of the interaction as we have defined it – the patient. The preceding format could be regarded as complete only if patients were a homogeneous group, thus allowing them to be disregarded.

Patients are a heterogeneous group. Individuals vary in general health, body weight, sex, genetic makeup, nutritional status, presence of other diseases, renal and hepatic status, other drugs taken, the routes by which these drugs are taken, and many other things. It should not be forgotten that the human body is the most complex self-regulating system known and will automatically try to restore the correct internal balance whenever drugs are taken. The ability to make these corrections is greatly influenced by the individual variations mentioned. This means that the outcome of giving one or more drugs to a particular individual for the first time can never be totally predictable. Even so, an idea of the probable outcome can be based on what has been seen in other patients. The extent and quality of the information available will greatly influence confidence in predications.

The prescriber has to consider the information available and apply it to the particular patient. The clinician is best placed for knowing, or finding out, details about the patient, which is why, ultimately, the action to be taken is a matter for professional judgment. There are no algorithms to easily give the "right" answer. As for all matters of judgment, the soundness of the decisions and the ease by which they are arrived at can improve with experience.

To be able to use interaction information, prescribers need to be able to critically assess it rather than simply accept it.

DRUG INTERACTION INFORMATION

The primary data on drug interactions are of widely varying quality and reliability. Some come from well-designed studies in large numbers of patients. Others may come from individual case reports, and care has to be taken before extrapolating from them. There are also some very poor quality data based solely on speculation or theory.

For general use, prescribers will not be working from these primary data sources but from a reference work on drug interactions or review articles. The primary sources will only be consulted when the prescriber wishes to examine a particular case in more depth. Before using these secondary information sources, prescribers need to be confident that they will meet their needs.

For prescribing, clinical significance will be of prime importance, and the work should be based on evidence. Commonly, especially in condensed information sources, the authors have assigned interactions based on drug families. If one drug from family X interacts with drug Y, the interaction is listed as if all the drugs from family X interact with drug Y. This may be based on extrapolation in the absence of specific evidence. Such an assumption occasionally may be reasonable when the mechanism is well understood. One example of this is the reduction in antihypertensive effect of adrenergic blockers (guanethidine, etc.) by indirectly acting sympathomimetic amines such as amphetamine and ephedrine. Even in this case, there is an exception in that diethylpropion appears not to interact with guanethidine or bethanidine. Often such extrapolation is not justified, and we have already seen that finding a related drug that does not interact is a method of interactions management.

Various charts and other pictorial presentations are available as quick checking devices for interactions. Chart designers rarely intend them to be other than a preliminary screening device and expect those using them to consult more widely before coming to any decision. The constraints of the format tend to force listings to be in terms of drug families, with only the most commonly encountered interactions presented. When an interaction is shown, there may be noninteracting members of the families. When the chart does not show an interaction, never assume that one does not exist. It may be outside the chart, but it may still exist. Importantly, no chart can easily give enough information to allow you to apply it to a particular patient.

Although some charts are very carefully designed, others are "alarmist." They may fail to make a distinction between well-documented, established interactions and those which have been encountered in a single patient, which probably were idiosyncratic reactions. To help in assessing the weight that should be applied to any particular interaction, various coding systems have appeared. First, they need to encompass two concepts, severity and frequency, which have no true relationship. An interaction may be severe but rare, moderate yet frequent or rare, not life-threatening but have serious social consequences.

Imposing an arbitrary code is very difficult; boundaries between the classifications become blurred and can become misleading. The other deficiency with coding systems is that they take no account of the individual patient. Many interactions can be managed by initial close monitoring or dosage adjustments. After the patient is stabilized and taking the combination without any apparent adverse effects, the need for positive action will be decreased dramatically. Beta-blockers and verapamil have been used together very successfully, but sometimes, serious cardiac depression occurs. Initially, the combination should be started only when the patient can be supervised closely, ideally in a hospital setting. Because of this potentially serious initial risk, a high-ranking classification will be assigned. However, for a patient who has been well stabilized over a number of years without untoward effects, the benefits of treatment will far outweigh the risks, which have become small.

The number of recorded interactions is too large for any human to have a complete recollection of, especially under the pressure of the consulting room. Computers offer an ideal solution. It is worth considering the use of computers in interaction information retrieval as a special case.

COMPUTERIZED DRUG INTERACTION INFORMATION

All of us tend to become too passive when we are in front of the computer screen. We quickly begin to respond to its messages like automata, without stopping to ask ourselves, "What does this really mean?" We cannot answer this question unless we first know what the program is designed to do.

In the very early stages of any design, a document known as the System Requirements and Constraints, or SRC, is produced. This states not only what the system will do but, just as important, what it will *not* do. All this is in the context of intended use. A prescribing checking system needs a different SRC than a drug interactions reference database.

There are broadly two different uses of computers for interactions — decision support and reference database. A single program site may deliver both, but it is very important that the designers clearly separate the two functions, because they need very different specifications. An interactions reference database ideally should give details concerning everything known about an interaction pair, including when they are known not to interact. It is a tool intended for use outside patient consultation, when you are researching in more detail. It can be seen as analogous to a search through a virtual library.

Decision support software is very different. When your primary aim is prescribing, returning everything known about a drug pair makes the system unusable. Users immediately will be overwhelmed by large volumes of information, much of which will be irrelevant "noise." When an interaction is detected, the program will automatically warn the user in some way. Numerous methods for alerting are available to program designers, ranging from a warning appearing that the user must acknowledge to an option to "see information" becoming available. These vary in sophistication, but as a minimum requirement, an intrusive presentation should

never be used for interactions that have no clinical significance.

Is the interaction checking based on drug families, generics, or formulation/route? Clearly, those based on drug families will generate numerous false messages. Those based on formulation/route will be the most specific. What distinction does the specification draw between the clinically significant and insignificant? Do the messages offer advice as to how to proceed, or do they only summarize the data? Do the texts provide help to decide which patients are particularly at risk? Are extra noise filters available based on recorded patient details? The most sophisticated will gather missing patient information at the point of interaction checking, to enable faster execution subsequently. If filters are based on the arbitrary codes, they may remove information important for a particular patient and yet still allow considerable noise through.

Before leaving computer systems, it is important to mention an advantage of decision support software that has no equal. Often a prescriber will already have encountered the interaction and may understand it quite well. The computer reliably reminds the prescriber to consider it. The more sophisticated programs will reduce the prominence of messages and the need for acknowledgment for a specific patient + interaction + prescriber trio after it has been marked by the prescriber as "considered." This is probably the most effective noise reduction step available.

Good noise filtration is important for a decision support program. If you constantly have to disregard inappropriate warnings, it becomes very easy to miss something important to your patient hidden within the muddle. However, noise reduction should be concerned with reducing the prominence of messages and the need for prescriber responses. It should never delude the user into thinking no interaction exists when one does.

Knowing the specification will mean you understand the significance of any warnings returned and be able to make prescribing decisions based on them.

MAKING PRESCRIBING DECISIONS

The most difficult decisions concern isolated incidents, many of which only achieved prominence because they were serious. Can these be ignored as idiosyncratic, or is the combination thereafter contraindicated? There is no simple yes or no answer to this question. A simple rule of thumb is that isolated cases with old and well-tried pairs of drugs are unlikely to be of general importance, whereas those with new drugs could possibly be the first reports of a more widespread problem. Treat these more cautiously until more is known. The delicate balance between these two then has to be set against the seriousness of the reaction reported.

Drugs that have a narrow therapeutic window or with which serum levels need to be kept within a specified range, such as anticoagulants, anticonvulsants, cytotoxics, digitalis glycosides, etc., pose special problems. Interactions causing changes in serum levels can easily lead to adverse effects for the patient. Metronidazole markedly increases the anticoagulant effect of warfarin, and the warfarin dose needs to be reduced by about one-third to one-half. If folic acid supplements are given to treat folate deficiency, which can be caused by anticonvulsants, serum anticonvulsant levels may fall, and decreased seizure control can occur. However, with both situations, routine serum monitoring facilities are often already in place.

Serum monitoring has the advantage that results clearly show what is happening for the individual patient. This can be useful if the interaction is seen unpredictably. Carbamazepine serum levels have been increased by fluvoxamine in some patients but not others. Monitoring will identify those patients needing carbamazepine dosage reductions.

It is important that antibiotic serum levels are not reduced below therapeutic concentrations. If the interaction is caused by a reduction in absorption and the patient takes dosages of the two drugs some hours apart, in many cases the effects of the interaction can be reduced. Several interactions involving antibiotics are of this kind, e.g., tetracycline + antacids or ciprofloxacin + didanosine. In contrast, the marked reduction of itraconazole serum levels caused by rifampin is probably due to an effect on metabolism and cannot be controlled in this way.

Ciprofloxacin causes a marked reduction in the clearance of diazepam, but this appears not to be important in most individuals with normal hepatic and renal function. When an interaction is seen rarely and the drug is like diazepam (i.e., relatively nontoxic), it may be possible for suitable patients to monitor themselves. The patient can be told that occasionally the combination leads to excessive drowsiness.

Letting the patient decide may appear as an abdication of duty, but there are occasions when this is appropriate. Very rarely various antibiotics may cause oral contraceptive failure. Does the physician ignore this because it is so rare? If the facts can be explained to the woman so that she can decide if she will use additional barrier methods or not, the decision rests with the person whose life could be greatly affected.

The main concerns normally arise when a pair of drugs is first taken together. After the management has been established, little more than an occasional confirmation of the patient's status is needed. However, some interactions develop over time and require involvement by the physician to continue more intensively. Allopurinol can gradually raise serum carbamazepine levels by about one-third. Some reduction in carbamazepine dosage eventually may be needed.

We have seen that there are numerous ways an interaction can be managed. The method chosen depends mainly on the characteristics of the interaction, but the ability and willingness of the patient to cooperate and the necessity for using those particular drugs have been factors. One of the most important characteristics of an interaction is the mechanism. This may be unknown, but when it is known or strongly suspected, an understanding of the mechanism can help greatly. An understanding of the mechanism also becomes important when a drug interaction is suspected but appears not to have been reported previously. If the same or related drugs are involved in similar and established interactions with mechanisms that are plausible in the new case, a new interaction may be possible. If toxicity was seen, is this similar to the known toxic effects of one of the drugs? None of this is either essential or proves that an interaction has occurred, although it constitutes circumstantial evidence. Confidence will be greater when serum levels can be determined.

Prescribers also should consider other possibilities, such as an adverse or idiosyncratic reaction to a single drug. Consideration also should be given to other drugs the patient may be taking. Could this be an adverse reaction to another drug taken? Is the interaction due to a different pair than you first suspected? If treatment failure is the observation, has the patient simply failed to take the medication? If after due consideration you remain convinced that an interaction has occurred, report it.

MECHANISMS OF DRUG INTERACTIONS

Some drugs interact together in a unique way; other mechanisms are encountered frequently. Interactions are usually discussed as if a single mechanism were taking place in isolation. This is a simplification because both drugs will enter a multitude of alternate processes within the body. The simplification is justified because it empowers understanding and management. However, it is worth remembering that we may be looking at only part of the picture.

Traditionally, interactions are classified into two main groups — pharmacokinetic or pharmacodynamic interactions. *Pharmacokinetic interactions* are those which affect the processes by which drugs are absorbed, distributed, metabolized, or excreted. *Pharmacodynamic interactions* are those in which the effect of one of the drugs is changed at its site of action by the other. Sometimes both drugs compete directly for the same receptor, but often such interactions involve a more complex interference with physiologic mechanisms. These interactions are events such as additive or synergistic effects, antagonistic effects, combined toxicity, etc.

Pharmacokinetic interactions are particularly amenable to quantitative investigation, and a wealth of protocols and data analysis techniques is now available. Many new drugs arrive on the market with studies already completed that confirm either the presence or absence of possible pharmacokinetic interactions. The clear demonstration that a pharmacokinetic interaction does not occur offers valuable reassurance when the drug is coprescribed with newer drugs.

Absorption interactions

In most circumstances, the preferred route for drug administration is oral, where drugs have first to disperse or dissolve in the gut contents and then cross through the mucous membranes of the gastrointestinal tract. This involves a series of chemical and physicochemical processes that offer the potential for an interaction. Most of the interactions that happen in the gut reduce rather than increase absorption.

A clear distinction has to be drawn between interactions that slow the rate of absorption and those which alter the total amount of drug absorbed. For drugs taken chronically (e.g., antidepressants), the rate of absorption is usually unimportant, provided the total amount absorbed does not change appreciably. For drugs given acutely (e.g., analgesics), where a rapid response is needed, reductions in the rate of absorption may result in failure to achieve adequate serum levels. Drugs such as metoclopramide, cisapride, and propantheline, which alter gut motility, have the potential for causing this type of interaction. Some drugs, such as levodopa, can be metabolized in the gastric mucosa. A delay in gastric emptying may offer more time for this "wasteful" metabolism to occur. Anticholinergics will delay gastric emptying, and although the combination is used widely, it is thought that to some extent the effectiveness of levodopa is reduced by such wasteful metabolism. Clinicians should be alert for signs of reduced levodopa response when anticholinergics are added or for signs of levodopa toxicity if anticholinergics are withdrawn.

The mucosa is essentially a lipid-based structure. Drugs will pass through it by simple diffusion if they are in a lipid-soluble form. Drugs vary in their lipid solubility, but in general, non-ionized forms of the drug are far more lipid soluble than ionized forms. Many drugs are weak acids or bases, and therefore, a proportion of the dose will exist dissolved in ionized form and some remains non-ionized, in a dynamic equilibrium. With drugs that are weak acids or bases, the balance of this equilibrium can be shifted dramatically by changes in gastric pH. Drugs, disease, excipients used in formulations, and other gut contents such as food or drink can all cause changes in gastric pH. The ingestion of a meal also causes gastric quiescence. This adds an additional complication. Changes in gut pH caused by antacids would be expected to reduce the absorption of many drugs. In practice, the outcome is uncertain because other processes such as chelation, adsorption, and changes in gut motility also may come into play.

Other mechanisms for one drug interfering with the absorption of another are also known. Cholestyramine is an anionic exchange resin intended to bind with bile acids and cholesterol metabolites in the gut. It also can bind with a number of drugs if coadministered, including digoxin, warfarin, and theophylline, thereby reducing their absorption. Neomycin can cause a malabsorption syndrome similar to tropical sprue. This can impair the absorption of a number of drugs, including digoxin and penicillin V.

Some examples of absorption interactions in more depth illustrate some of the points described above.

Quinolone antibiotics + metallic ions There is a wealth of information about quinolone-antacid interactions. Table 6.1 shows the maximum serum levels (C_{max}) when ciprofloxacin was given at the same time as antacids and when separated by differing time intervals (e.g., 2 hours, +4 hours, etc.) in various studies. There is a considerable variation in the results. The reduced serum levels reflect reduced absorption. It is believed that certain functional groups (3-carbonyl and 4-oxo) on the antibiotics form insoluble chelates with aluminum and magnesium ions within the gut that are not absorbed to any great extent. In addition, these chelates appear to be relatively inactive as antibacterials. The chemical stability of the chelate formed seems to be an important factor in determining the degree of interaction.

This interaction is well established and, depending on the particular quinolone and antacid concerned, often of clinical importance. The risk is that the serum levels of the antibiotic may fall to subtherapeutic concentrations for the infecting organisms so that treatment failures

---

Table 6.1 Ciprofloxacin-antacid interactions

Dose: time (mg: hour[1])	Antacid	C_{max} (µg/ml) alone/with	
250	Magnesium/ aluminum hydroxides	3.69	1.25
500	Magnesium/ aluminum hydroxides	2.1	0.82
500 + 24 h	Magnesium/ aluminum hydroxides	1.7	0.1
500 + 24 h	Magnesium/ aluminum hydroxides	1.9	0.13
750 + 2 h	Magnesium/ aluminum hydroxides	3.01	3.96
+ 0.08 h		3.42	0.68
+ 2 h		3.42	0.88
+ 4 h		3.01	2.62
+ 6 h		2.63	2.64
750 + 0.08 h	Aluminum hydroxide	3.2	0.6
750	Aluminum hydroxide	2.4	0.8
200	Aluminum hydroxide	1.3	0.2
500	Calcium carbonate	2.9	1.8
750 + 0.08 h	Calcium carbonate	3.2	1.7
750 + 2 h	Calcium carbonate	1.25	1.44
500	Oscal (Ca supplement)	2.9	1.8
500	Magnesium citrate	2.4	0.6
500	Bismuth subsalicylate	3.8	2.9
750	Bismuth subsalicylate	2.95	2.57

[1]Time interval between intake of ciprofloxacin and the other agent: and + indicate that ciprofloxacin was administered before and after, respectively, intake of the antacid.
(Modified from Stockley IH. Drug Interactions, 5th ed. London: Pharmaceutical Press, 1999).

occur. From the mechanism, it is predicted that a suitable time interval between the dosages, preventing the two drugs making physical contact with each other, could avoid the interaction.

The overall picture is that the aluminum/magnesium antacids interact to a greater extent than the calcium antacids, and bismuth antacids interact hardly at all. As a very broad rule of thumb, the quinolones should be taken at least 2 hours before and not less than 4 to 6 hours after an aluminum/magnesium antacid. This can be reduced to 2 hours after with calcium antacids, and separation appears unlikely to be important with bismuth antacids.

Since the process is not due to high pH per se, alternative methods of raising gastric pH would not be expected to behave in this way. This seems to be the case. The H_2 blockers cimetidine, famotidine, ranitidine, etc. and the proton pump inhibitors lansoprazole, omeprazole, pantoprazole, etc. do not appear to interact with the quinolones or only to a clinically irrelevant extent. Enoxacin is less soluble as the pH rises, and intravenous ranitidine was found to reduce the absorption of enoxacin by 26 to 40%. This observation does seem to be related to the change in gastric pH. Although the enoxacin pharmacokinetic changes are substantial, this has not been shown to affect the outcome. Nevertheless, it would be prudent to monitor the patient closely if these two drugs are used together.

The formation of insoluble quinolone chelates is also possible with other sources of di- and trivalent cations such as iron and zinc preparations or even enteral feeding solutions. The absorption of ciprofloxacin is markedly reduced by preparations that contain ionic iron. Several studies have clearly demonstrated area under the curve (AUC) reductions and maximum serum level reductions of 30 to 80% with ferrous fumarate, ferrous gluconate, ferrous sulfate, and iron-glycine sulfate. Similarly, ferrous sulfate has caused reductions of between 51 and 96% in norfloxacin bioavailability. Reductions in the absorption of levofloxacin, ofloxacin, and sparfloxacin caused by iron also have been recorded. It is believed that the quinolones form a complex with iron and zinc by chelation between the metal ion and the 4-oxo- and adjacent carboxyl groups that is less easily absorbed by the gut. Fleroxacin, however, appears not to interact.

A new product, iron-ovotransferrin, differs from other iron preparations in being able to combine directly with the transferrin receptors of intestinal cells, and appears to release little ionic iron into the gut to interact with the quinolones. Iron-ovotransferrin does not interact with ciprofloxacin and is not expected to interact with any of the quinolones, but this awaits confirmation.

Ciprofloxacin has been shown to interact with enteral foods containing mineral ions. No treatment failures have been reported, but the interaction is expected to be of clinical importance. For example, if patients were to be switched from parenteral to oral ciprofloxacin, there could be a significant reduction in serum ciprofloxacin levels. Be alert for any evidence that ciprofloxacin is less effective. The effect of the ofloxacin-enteral food interaction is much smaller.

Metal ions may be included as an excipient as with oral didanosine preparations. Didanosine is unstable in acidic medium and therefore is formulated with buffering agents (such as aluminum and magnesium hydroxides) to raise gastric pH and prevent hydrolysis of the drug. This changed environment may not be suitable for absorption of many other drugs, including the quinolones. The didanosine itself seems to take no part in the interaction. Direct information seems limited to three reports involving ciprofloxacin, but it appears to be a clinically important interaction. Drastic reductions (93%) in serum ciprofloxacin levels have been reported when ciprofloxacin was given at the same time as didanosine. However, when ciprofloxacin was given 2 hours before didanosine, the ciprofloxacin AUC was reduced by only 26%. Ciprofloxacin and similar quinolones should be given at least 2 hours before or 6 hours after didanosine

Ketoconazole + antacids, H_2 blockers, sucralfate, and proton pump inhibitors

Some drugs need an acid medium for proper absorption. Ketoconazole is a poorly soluble base that must be transformed by the acid in the stomach into the soluble hydrochloride salt. Agents that reduce gastric acid secretion such as H_2 blockers or antacids raise the pH in the stomach so that dissolution of the ketoconazole and its absorption are reduced. The evidence that this occurs in practice is not extensive, but it has been confirmed that dramatic reductions in ketoconazole serum levels occur when it is given with cimetidine or ranitidine. Very little evidence from formal studies with ketoconazole and antacids is available, but a similar interaction would be expected.

One method for managing this interaction is to give the ketoconazole between dosages of the H_2 blockers or antacids, when the stomach contents are most acidic. Advise patients to separate dosages by not less than 2 to 3 hours. Sucralfate appears to cause a more moderate reduction of about 25% in ketoconazole serum levels. However, it would still seem prudent to separate the dosages. In addition, gastric reacidification may be unpredictably delayed in some patients. It is advisable to monitor the effects of treatment to ensure that ketoconazole is effective. Proton pump inhibitors would be expected to reduce ketoconazole serum levels similarly, and this has been confirmed in a study with omeprazole. Separating the dosages is unlikely to be effective because proton pump inhibitors tend to have a prolonged duration of action. An alternative method for managing these interactions is to use fluconazole instead because its absorption is essentially unaffected by changes in gastric pH. Studies confirm that fluconazole only interacts to a small and clinically irrelevant extent with H_2 blockers or antacids and does not interact with omeprazole.

Some digoxin interactions

The serum level of digoxin may be reduced by about a third if slowly dissolving forms of digoxin are taken with metoclopramide. One study found that this did not happen if the digoxin was taken in capsule form. Although the evidence is limited, it seems that metoclopramide increases the motility of the gut to such an extent that full dissolution and absorption of digoxin are unfinished by the time it is lost in the feces. Fast-dissolving and liquid forms do not require such a long time for full absorption and are unlikely to be affected.

Propantheline, on the other hand, seems to increase digoxin serum levels by about a third if slowly dissolving formulations of digoxin are used. Studies have found that this does not occur with fast-dissolving or liquid forms of digoxin. Propantheline causes a reduction in gut motility, so the time available for the digoxin to pass into solution and be absorbed increases.

Changes in digoxin levels of a third could place the patient outside the desired range for serum levels, since digoxin has a narrow therapeutic index. It may be possible to accommodate either of these interactions by some change in the dosage of the slowly dissolving digoxin formulation, although there are no studies on which to base guidelines and titration of dosages with this type of formulation is rarely easy. Digoxin levels will need to be monitored closely.

Drug displacement (protein-binding) interactions

Much has been written about the mechanism of drug displacement, but in reality, the effects seem to be buffered so effectively by other body processes that the outcome is rarely clinically important. Undoubtedly, the importance of drug displacement interactions has been overemphasized, but such interactions may need to be taken into account in some circumstances.

Following absorption, after passing through the liver, a drug is transported rapidly around the body by the circulation. The drug then will become distributed between the body tissues and plasma. Some drugs are greatly taken up by the tissues, whereas others remain largely in the plasma. This distribution between plasma and tissues can be represented by a parameter, the apparent volume of distribution (V_d). If V_d is low, the drug remains largely in the plasma; if it is high, the drug is largely taken up by the tissues.

Within the plasma, some drugs are completely dissolved in water, but many others have a proportion of their molecules bound to plasma proteins, predominantly albumin. A dynamic equilibrium exists between those molecules which are bound and those dissolved in water. The unbound molecules, free in solution, are pharmacologically active. The bound molecules form a circulating but pharmacologically inactive reservoir. Because there is a dynamic equilibrium, as free molecules are metabolized and excreted, they are replaced by others from the binding sites.

The proportion of bound molecules varies enormously, but some drugs are extremely highly bound. For example, dicumarol at serum concentrations of 5.0 mg/liter has only 4 per 1000 molecules free in solution.

Depending on concentrations and the relative affinities of the drugs for the binding sites, one drug may compete with another for sites and displace it. A new equilibrium is established between all four moieties (i.e., the bound and unbound forms of both drugs). If drugs are highly bound, small reductions in the proportion bound may create large increases in free forms. For example, if one drug is normally 99% bound and another drug reduces this to 95%, the unbound proportion has increased fourfold, from 1 to 4%. When most of the drug is in the plasma (i.e., drugs with a low V_d), the displaced molecules can significantly increase the number of those capable of pharmacologic activity. Such drugs include tolbutamide (96% bound, V_d = 10 liters) and warfarin (99% bound, V_d = 9 liters). If most of the drug is in the tissues (i.e., drugs with a high V_d), more free molecules in the plasma will have minor effects, because most will be in the tissues and play no part in the displacement.

This effect is normally very short-lived because the increased numbers of free molecules become exposed to metabolism as they pass through the liver. Many drugs are protein bound, but it is difficult to find an example of a clinically important interaction due to this mechanism alone. One possible example is the marked diuresis seen in patients with the nephrotic syndrome when they were given clofibrate.

Drug metabolism interactions

A small number of drugs are lost from the body simply by being excreted in the urine unchanged. A large number are chemically changed in the body to more water-soluble compounds, which makes them more easily excreted by the kidneys. Commonly this is by oxidation or glucuronidation. This chemical change is called *metabolism, biotransformation, biochemical degradation,* or sometimes, *detoxification.* Some metabolism goes on in the serum, skin, intestines, and other tissues, but the greatest proportion takes place in the liver. The changes are catalyzed by enzymes found in the membranes of the endoplasmic reticulum of liver cells. If the liver is homogenized and centrifuged, the reticulum breaks down into small sacs called *microsomes.* These enzymes are therefore often called *microsomal enzymes.*

When two drugs have an involvement or an effect on the same range of enzymes, this can lead to changes in the metabolism of either or both, either increasing it or decreasing it, with consequent changes in serum levels. Environmental substances such as the insecticide lindane also may produce these effects. Phase I oxidation is commonly affected. This term covers a number of biotransformations, all requiring the presence of NADPH and the heme-containing protein cytochrome P450.

Various drugs such as aminoglutethimide, barbiturates, carbamazepine, phenytoin, primidone, rifampin, and tobacco smoke can stimulate the activity of different microsomal enzymes so that the pace of metabolism and excretion is increased. This is referred to as *enzyme induction.* It is often possible to accommodate these interactions by suitably increasing the dosage of the affected drug. There are hazards, however, and good monitoring is needed. Induction may take days or weeks to develop fully and may persist when the inducing drug is withdrawn. This means characteristically that these interactions are delayed in onset and ending. In such cases, close patient monitoring therefore will have to be prolonged when drugs are both added and withdrawn. Withdrawal of an inducing drug is a particular risk. Dosages of other drugs may have been increased because of the interaction. If this is forgotten, an overdose may occur when metabolism returns to normal.

Some drugs have the opposite effect on microsomal enzymes and act as inhibitors. The normal pace of metabolism of other drugs that are substrates for the enzymes is reduced, and they begin to accumulate within the body. The degree of inhibition varies according to drug and dosage. The effect is essentially the same as a dosage increase. Unlike induction, which may develop slowly, inhibition is immediate, so within 2 or 3 days drug accumulation in the body can produce toxicity. The clinical significance of an interaction will depend on the extent to which serum levels rise. If they remain within the therapeutic range, the interaction may be advantageous. If not, the interaction becomes adverse, as serum levels climb into the toxic range. There are many examples of this type of interaction. Chloramphenicol inhibits the metabolism of phenytoin, leading to possible phenytoin intoxication. Similarly, azapropazone can increase tolbutamide effects, with possible hypoglycemia the result. Chlorpropamide can inhibit the metabolism of alcohol, leading to a rise in blood acetaldehyde levels causing flushing, etc.

Cytochrome P450 is not a single entity but a family of isoenzymes that exist in human liver tissue. In practice, two specific subfamilies called CYP2D6 (corresponding gene *P450IID6*) and CYP3A4 (corresponding gene *P450IIIA4*) seem to involve in the metabolism of about 90% of commonly used drugs (see Chap. 3). CYP2D6 exhibits what is called *genetic polymorphism*. This means that human populations are divided into two genetically determined groups. Most humans are "fast metabolizers" of drugs metabolized by CYP2D6 and lose these drugs from the body more quickly than the minority of "slow metabolizers". Those who are slow metabolizers need lower doses than fast metabolizers do because they lose the drug more slowly. CYP3A4 does not show this genetic polymorphism, although there is considerable variation within the population. As so often noted, the individual patient is an important factor. Depending on the individual's particular enzyme profile and the existence of alternate metabolic pathways for a drug, some patients may quickly develop toxicity when an interacting pair of drugs is given, whereas others appear unaffected.

Knowing which particular cytochrome P450 isoenzyme is responsible for a drug's metabolism can usefully explain why interactions occur. This can be determined from in vitro tests with human microsomal enzymes. Such testing is particularly valuable with new drugs, when it becomes possible to predict interactions in advance of case reports, clinical trials, and postmarketing surveillance. Although these are theoretical predictions, they are based on sound in vitro evidence and need to be given far greater credence than the "wild speculations" sometimes published. It is prudent to assume that the interactions will occur until other evidence to the contrary becomes available. This being the case, interactions predicted by this method are not always seen. Presumably, other pathways or processes that may not have been identified are able to compensate for the interaction.

Following absorption, drugs and food are taken via the hepatic portal system directly through the liver before passing into the general circulation. A number of highly lipid-soluble compounds undergo substantial metabolism during this "first pass" through the gut wall and liver. First-pass metabolism can remove a considerable proportion of a compound. For instance, tyramine, a potent pressor agent found in many hard cheeses, is substantially removed during first-pass metabolism. Otherwise, such cheeses would be poisonous. Some drugs can cause changes in blood flow through the liver that lead to marked effects on first-pass metabolism. Cimetidine (but not ranitidine) decreases hepatic blood flow, which leads to increased propranolol bioavailability. Propranolol serum levels can be doubled. Surprisingly, this rarely seems to have important clinical consequences. Although not confirmed, patients with impaired hepatic function potentially could be more vulnerable to this interaction, and consideration should be given to this if coadministration is intended in these patients.

We will now look at some examples in more detail to illustrate the points just described. Because the range of metabolism-type drug interactions is so large, these examples cannot be properly representative of what you will encounter in clinical practice. Almost certainly you will think of some others you would have liked discussed. However, these examples should be thought provoking.

Miscellaneous drugs + grapefruit juice

Enzyme inhibition is not confined to drugs. Components of grapefruit juice inhibit the P450 isoenzymes CYP1A2 and CYP3A4. These isoenzymes are involved in the metabolism of many drugs, and therefore, consumption of grapefruit juice is predicted to lead to increases in the serum levels of drugs with a metabolism that depends extensively on these pathways. Table 6.2 gives a list of drugs for which studies have shown that a 200- to 250-ml glass of grapefruit juice has lead to increases in the AUC.

The clinical significance of these interactions is uncertain. In the case of oral contraceptives, the increases are still less than the extent of known variability between individuals, so they are unlikely to be of practical importance. The AUCs for the listed calcium channel blockers are increased two- to threefold. In one study the side effects of felodipine were increased, but this has not been recorded with the others, despite the increase in serum levels. However, it would be worth checking the diet of any patient complaining of side effects with any of the calcium channel blockers known to interact with grapefruit juice. Grapefruit juice can increase the AUC of midazolam and triazolam by as much as 50%. Such an increase would be expected to increase the extent of sedation and amnesia seen with these drugs, particularly when

Table 6.2 Drugs known to interact with grapefruit juice	
Antibiotics	Macrolides
Antihistamines	Terfenadine
Benzodiazepines	Midazolam
	Triazolam
Calcium channel blockers	Felodipine
	Nifedipine
	Nimodipine
	Nisoldipine
	Nitrendipine
Contraceptives (oral)	Ethinylestradiol
	(ethinyloestradiol)
Immunosuppressants	Cyclosporine
Statins	Lovastatin, Simvastatin

there are other factors such as old age or hepatic impairment. However, this still awaits further study. Various studies have found that grapefruit juice increased the AUC of cyclosporine by up to 62%. Monitor the patient if any changes in diet are made (e.g., food and milk also can affect the bioavailability of cyclosporine). Some patients only poorly metabolize terfenadine, leading to an accumulation in the body. In a group of poor metabolizers, grapefruit juice was found to increase terfenadine serum levels, and this was associated with an augmented QT complex prolongation. Most people do not accumulate terfenadine, but these results suggest that the small subset of people who do could be particularly at risk from its cardiotoxic side effects.

Nelfinavir + rifampin or rifabutin Both the new nonnucleoside reverse transcriptase inhibitor nelfinavir and the antitubercular drug rifampin are likely to be used in HIV+ patients. It is important to know what will happen if both drugs are used together. Nelfinavir is partially metabolized by the P450 isoenzyme CYP3A. Rifampin is a very potent inducer for this enzyme and thus is expected to increase the metabolism of nelfinavir, resulting in a greater clearance from the body. Rifampin has been shown to reduce the AUC of nelfinavir by 82%. The manufacturers therefore recommend that this combination be avoided.

An alternative antitubercular drug is rifabutin. This is also an enzyme inducer but is far less potent than rifampin. In one study rifabutin was given with nelfinavir. The AUC of nelfinavir was reduced by 32%, whereas the AUC of rifabutin was increased by 207%. The reduction in nelfinavir AUC was less dramatic, as expected. However, the two drugs are both substrates for CYP3A, and competition for the enzymatic sites leads to a large reduction in rifabutin metabolism. The manufactures suggest halving the rifabutin dosage when both drugs are used together.

Carbamazepine, phenobarbital, and phenytoin are also known inducers for the hepatic isoenzyme CYP3A. The manufactures of nelfinavir therefore predict that a similar reduction will occur with these drugs (and other potent inducers for CYP3A4), and the combinations are best avoided.

Chlormethiazole + alcohol Chlormethiazole is used commonly to treat withdrawal from alcohol. However, alcoholics may readily transfer dependence to chlormethiazole, and tolerance develops, with some patients taking up to 25 g daily. Alcoholics often visit several practitioners to get additional supplies. In addition, alcohol abuse may continue. Both alcohol and chlormethiazole are central nervous system (CNS) depressants, and the effects are additive, large amounts of both together having resulted in coma and fatal respiratory depression. The risk is further increased because alcohol appears to increase the bioavailability of chlormethiazole by a reduction in first-pass metabolism. In patients with alcoholic cirrhosis, bioavailability may be increased tenfold by venous shunting.

Some interactions of the statins Statins competitively inhibit an enzyme found in the liver (HMG CoA reductase) and can cause hepatic side effects. In addition, various statins have been shown to have affinities for various P450 isoenzymes (Tab. 6.3). Because of this, they might be expected to be involved in metabolism-type drug interactions. In practice, mechanisms have been very hard to determine so far.

A limited number of reports have clearly established that the anticoagulant effects of warfarin can be increased in some patients by lovastatin. Bleeding and increased prothrombin times are reported. It is suspected that lovastatin inhibits the metabolism of warfarin, which results in its accumulation in the body. Generally in warfarin drug metabolism interactions, isoenzyme CYP2C9 is involved. However, lovastatin is mainly metabolized by CYP3A4, so the mechanism is puzzling. Fluvastatin has been shown to have a high affinity for the P450 isoenzyme CYP2C9 in vitro. It therefore was expected to interact like lovastatin with warfarin. However, an in vivo study found that fluvastatin had no effect on warfarin serum levels or prothrombin times, and thus no special precautions would seem necessary. Another statin, simvastatin, normally causes only a small, clinically irrelevant increase in the

Table 6.3 Statins and main metabolizing cytochrome P450	
Atorvastatin	CYP3A4
Cerivastatin	CYP3A4, CYP2C8
Fluvastatin	CYP2C9
Lovastatin	CYP3A4
Pravastatin	?
Simvastatin	CYP3A4

anticoagulant effects of warfarin. (However, a single case report of more marked effects and bruising exists, so it would be prudent to monitor patients closely until more is known.) Pravastatin does not interact with warfarin.

A proposed metabolic interaction does offer a satisfactory explanation for an interaction seen with the statin, fluvastatin, and rifampin. In one study, rifampin reduced fluvastatin serum levels by 51%. Rifampin is a well-known hepatic enzyme inducer. Increased fluvastatin metabolism therefore will lead to a fall in serum levels. Probably the fluvastatin dosage will need to be approximately doubled when these drugs are used together, but this needs confirmation.

The potent inhibitor of CYP3A4 itraconazole interacts with some statins in a more predictable manner. Lovastatin and simvastatin are metabolized by CYP3A4, and their serum levels are dramatically increased by itraconazole. Dosage reductions for lovastatin and simvastatin will be required if either are given with itraconazole. Grapefruit juice, another inhibitor for CYP3A4, also has been shown to dramatically increase lovastatin and simvastatin serum levels. Other inhibitors of CYP3A4 such as erythromycin and cyclosporine would be expected to behave similarly, although this awaits confirmation.

Occasionally serious adverse effects (e.g., myopathy, rhabdomyolysis) have been seen with various statins and other drugs, but an explanation is not yet available.

Some succinylcholine interactions As mentioned earlier, not all drug metabolism takes place in the liver. The neuromuscular blocker succinylcholine chloride, used as an adjunct in surgery, is metabolized in the serum by the circulating enzyme pseudocholinesterase. Cyclophosphamide irreversibly inhibits this enzyme; as a result, the metabolism of succinylcholine is reduced. Respiratory insufficiency and prolonged apnea have occurred when these drugs are used together. If the patient is taking cyclophosphamide, succinylcholine should be used with caution at a reduced dosage.

Sometimes systemic absorption of a drug from eye drops can be sufficient to cause a systemic effect. This has been found to occur with ecothiopate iodide eye drops. The absorbed ecothiopate depresses pseudocholinesterase levels. Several cases of prolonged apnea when succinylcholine was given to patients using these eye drops have been reported. The dosage of succinylcholine should be reduced appropriately.

The monoamine oxidase (MAO) inhibitor phenelzine caused a reduction in the serum levels of cholinesterase in 4 of 10 patients studied. This could explain three case reports of patients taking (or having previously taken) phenelzine who developed apnea after being given succinylcholine. Electroconvulsive therapy (ECT), during which succinylcholine is used, is sometimes administered to patients taking phenelzine, and it would be prudent to be alert for the possibility of this interaction. This does not appear to happen with other MAO inhibitors.

Interactions due to changes in excretion

Some marginal drug losses occasionally occur through the sweat or the breath, and this is the basis for alcohol breath tests and drug sweat tests used by many police forces. Inhalation anesthetics are substantially lost in the breath. However, most drugs are excreted mainly in the bile or urine, which is the main concern with interactions (see also Chap. 21).

Blood entering the kidneys is delivered to the glomeruli of the tubules, where smaller molecules such as water, salts, and some drugs pass through the glomerular membrane into the lumen of the tubules. Larger molecules such as plasma proteins and blood cells are retained. The blood flow then passes on to the remaining parts of the tubules. Here, active (energy-using) transport systems are able to transfer drugs and their metabolites into the tubular filtrate. The tubule cells also have active and passive transport systems for the reabsorption of drugs and salts. Drugs that interfere with tubule pH, active transport systems, and blood flow through the kidneys can interact with other drugs by affecting their excretion.

Similar to absorption from the gut, passive reabsorption of drugs in the kidney depends on the extent to which the drug exists in its non-ionized, lipid-soluble form. Only the lipid-soluble form is able to diffuse back. Ionized, water-soluble forms remain in the tubular fluid. Since many drugs are weak acids or bases, the balance between the ionized and non-ionized forms will depend on lumen pH and the particular drug. In alkaline urine, weakly acidic drugs exist mainly as ionized, water-soluble forms and therefore remain in the tubular fluid. The opposite is true for weak bases, which, since they are mainly non-ionized, will be reabsorbed by passive diffusion.

Clinically, the significance of this type of interaction is small because metabolism in the liver produces metabolites that are more water soluble. Few drugs are excreted in the urine unchanged. A handful of drugs may interact in this way. Patients taking large, chronic doses of aspirin may have salicylate serum levels reduced to subtherapeutic levels by some antacids. Aspirin is known to cause gastrointestinal irritation, so be aware of the possibility that patients are self-medicating with antacids without telling the prescriber. In overdose, this interaction can be exploited by deliberately changing the urinary pH to increase the loss of drugs such as phenobarbitone and salicylates.

Drugs may compete with each other for the same active transport system in the tubules. For example, probenecid reduces the excretion of many drugs, including dapsone, indomethacin, nalidixic acid, and penicillin, by competing for the transport mechanism. The serum levels of these drugs then rise, with possible toxicity risks occurring. Sometimes the interaction is exploited to increase urinary antibiotic concentrations when treating urinary tract infections.

Because renal blood flow is controlled in part by local vasodilatory prostaglandins (PGE_2), synthesis inhibitors such as indomethacin may reduce it. The excretion of lithium is reduced by indomethacin, causing lithium levels to rise by about 60%. In such situations, the lithium dosage needs to be reduced and the patient well monitored. Although this mechanism seems plausible, aspirin reduces renal prostaglandin synthesis by 65 to 70% yet does not affect lithium serum levels. Various other nonsteroidal anti-inflammatory drugs (NSAIDs) are reported to increase lithium levels, such as diclofenac, ibuprofen, ketoprofen, naproxen, and others, but lysine acetylsalicylate and sodium salicylate appear not to interact.

The other main route of excretion is in the bile, either unchanged or metabolized. Metabolic products are often conjugates, e.g., glucuronides. Some of these conjugates are metabolized back to the parent drug by gut flora and then reabsorbed. This recycling increases the duration of action of the drug. If gut flora are exposed to antibiotics, this recycling may be reduced or prevented. The normally long duration of action is then reduced. This may be a possible explanation for the rare failure of oral contraceptives reported with concurrent use of some antibiotics such as penicillins and tetracyclines.

We will now look at some examples in more detail to illustrate some of the points raised.

Some methotrexate interactions Methotrexate is excreted mainly unchanged in the urine and therefore is a likely candidate to exhibit excretion-type drug interactions. Table 6.4 shows some of the drugs that have been seen to interact with methotrexate and appear to involve excretion mechanisms.

None of the interactions of methotrexate with NSAIDs is very well documented, but an overall picture seems to be that the risks are greatest with high-dose methotrexate and in patients with impaired renal function but less if the dosage is low and the patient has normal renal function.

Table 6.4 Some drugs that interact with methotrexate by an excretion mechanism

Anion exchange resins	Cholestyramine
NSAIDs	Aspirin and salicylates
	Azapropazone
	Dipyrone
	Flurbiprofen
	Ibuprofen
	Indomethacin
	Ketoprofen
	Diclofenac
	Naproxen
	Phenylbutazone
	Tolmetin
Penicillins	Amoxicillin
	Benzylpenicillin
	Carbenicillin
	Dicloxacillin
	Flucloxacillin
	Mezlocillin
	Penicillin
	Piperacillin
	Ticarcillin
Uricosurics	Probenecid
Urinary alkalinizers	Sodium bicarbonate

The NSAIDs inhibit prostaglandin (PGE_2) synthesis, which results in a fall in renal perfusion. This, in turn, leads to a rise in methotrexate serum levels with increased toxicity. Aspirin, salicylates, and phenylbutazone also competitively inhibit the tubular secretion of methotrexate, which would further reduce its removal from the body. Phenylbutazone and indomethacin also can cause renal failure, which may exacerbate the situation. Phenylbutazone and amidopyrine also can cause bone marrow depression, and this might be additive to that caused by methotrexate itself. It also has been suggested that protein-binding displacement may play a part.

It probably would be best to avoid, aspirin, dipyrone, and salicylates. If the use of the other NSAIDs is thought appropriate, treatment should be monitored closely, and folinic acid rescue therapy should be available. The incidence of serious reactions seems much lower with low-dose methotrexate, and some studies have found that most patients experienced only mild or no untoward effects. Even with low-dose methotrexate, it would be prudent to do regular white cell and platelet counts, especially in the elderly or those with high creatinine levels.

The penicillins cause marked reductions in the clearance of methotrexate from the body. Serious toxicity and deaths have occurred. It is thought that weak acids such as the penicillins compete with methotrexate in the kidney tubules for excretion so that methotrexate accumulates in the body. The methotrexate dosage may need to be halved, and twice-weekly white cell and platelet counts are recommended. Folinic acid rescue therapy should be available. If toxicity is suspected, methotrexate serum levels should be determined.

Two- to fourfold increases in methotrexate serum levels have been reported with patients also given probenecid. Probenecid inhibits renal excretion of methotrexate in animals, and probably this also happens in humans. The methotrexate dosage will need to be reduced to avoid toxicity, and the effects should be monitored well. Animal studies suggest that despite the rise in methotrexate levels, the antitumor effects of methotrexate actually may be reduced in the presence of probenecid.

Because methotrexate is more soluble in alkaline than acid solutions, urinary alkalinizers, with ample fluid, have been given to patients on high-dose methotrexate to prevent precipitation of the drug in the renal tubules, which would cause kidney damage. However, this also will increase the loss of methotrexate in the urine because at high pH more of the drug exists in the ionized, water-soluble form that is not readily reabsorbed by the tubules. This increased loss has been clearly demonstrated in a large number of patients using sodium bicarbonate as the alkalinizer. This needs to be considered if the technique is used.

Methotrexate is also excreted in the bile. It is then reabsorbed further along the gut (the enterohepatic cycle). This happens whether the methotrexate is given orally or by infusion. Marked falls in methotrexate serum levels have been seen in two patients given cholestyramine orally. Almost certainly the methotrexate has bound strongly to the cholestyramine in the gut, thereby preventing reabsorption. Separating the dosages of the two drugs will not necessarily keep them from coming into contact because methotrexate is excreted back into the gut in the bile. Concurrent use should be monitored and dosage adjustments made as necessary.

Pharmacodynamic interactions

When two drugs have the same effects or side effects, when given together, their combined effects may be additive. Alcohol taken in moderate amounts with benzodiazepine hypnotics or tranquilizers may cause excessive drowsiness. Simple addition of effects or side effects does not strictly fit our definition of an interaction, but many publications or programs treat them as if they were interactions because it is important that they are not forgotten. For instance, it may be forgotten that chlorpromazine anticholinergic side effects may be additive with those of the anticholinergic drug benzhexol when they are coprescribed. These drugs are very often given together advantageously, but occasionally, serious anticholinergic toxicity is seen. Prescribers should be aware of the serious conditions (e.g., adynamic ileus) that could develop, especially when high dosages are employed. Both gentamicin and cephalothin have nephrotoxic side effects. Doses that on their own are well tolerated may give rise to serious nephrotoxicity when both drugs are given together. If concurrent use is essential, renal function should be monitored closely and dosages kept to a minimum.

Drugs also may be antagonistic in their effects. It is well recognized that glucocorticoids may oppose the effects of hypoglycemic agents. There have been very few formal studies of this as an interaction. Probably because this effect of glucocorticoids has been known for so long, conducting a formal study does not seem worthwhile. Carbenoxolone can cause fluid retention and raise the blood pressure in some patients. Neither spironolactone nor amiloride can be used to treat this because they antagonise the ulcer-healing properties of carbenoxolone. Carbenoxolone also has a potassium-losing effect, so if thiazides are used, an additive effect is possible, and a potassium supplement may be needed.

Some examples in more detail will help illustrate how pharmacodynamic drug interactions come about.

Digitalis glycosides and electrolyte balance

Several interactions may result from disturbances of fluid and electrolyte balance. An increase in the sensitivity of the myocardium to digitalis glycosides, leading to digitalis toxicity, seems to occur when serum potassium levels fall. This is not fully understood, and the mecha-nism is still being debated, but a partial explanation can be given. The cardiac glycosides inhibit Na^+,K^+-ATPase, involved in the transport of Na^+ and K^+ ions across the membranes of myocardial cells. This is associated with an increase in the availability of calcium ions involved in the contraction of cells. Hypokalemia exacerbates potassium loss from the myocardial cells, thereby increasing the activity and toxicity of digitalis glycosides. Some loss of magnesium also may have a part to play.

Potassium-depleting diuretics such as loop diuretics, thiazides, carbonic anhydrase inhibitors, and similarly acting diuretics therefore would be expected to lead to this interaction. A direct link between the use of potassium-depleting diuretics and the development of digitalis toxicity has not been established beyond doubt, but current thinking favors the belief that it can occur. Ideally, if these combinations are used, serum potassium and magnesium levels should be monitored. If necessary, potassium supplements should be given or some other step to conserve potassium taken (such as using a potassium-sparing diuretic).

Corticosteroids given systemically also can increase potassium loss, particularly naturally occurring corticosteroids like cortisone, deoxycortone, and hydrocortisone. Corticosteroids also cause sodium and water retention, resulting in edema and hypertension, which can lead to cardiac failure in some individuals. If these drugs are used with digitalis glycosides, it is therefore important to monitor the patient well.

Predicting the outcome for electrolyte balance interactions can be complicated because often the patient is already receiving a potassium-depleting drug with either a potassium-sparing diuretic or a potassium supplement. Many manufacturers provide both in a single tablet. There are also products combining ACE inhibitors with diuretics or beta-blockers with diuretics and other combinations. This means that there are three drugs to consider. Is the electrolyte balance already well controlled within normal limits? Will the electrolyte balance be likely to move, and if so, which way? Consider the characteristics of the particular interaction, the third drug, and the patient. Subsequently monitor the electrolyte balance closely and adjust dosages as needed. Also, watch digitalis glycoside serum levels closely if appropriate. Spironolactone can interfere with some digoxin assay methods, so first check that the method used will be reliable if the patient is taking both these drugs.

Neuromuscular blockers and/or anesthetics + aminoglycoside antibiotics

In addition to the recognized main, clinically utilized activity, drugs often have additional pharmacologic effects. These also can become involved in pharmacodynamic interactions. The aminoglycoside antibiotics possess significant neuromuscular blocking activity. Appropriate measures must be taken to accommodate this property during surgery. There are many reports of prolonged, even fatal respiratory depression due to the neuromuscular blocking effect of the aminoglycosides. It appears that the aminoglycosides cause an impairment of calcium influx leading to a reduction in the release of the transmitter acetylcholine at the neuromuscular junction. They also may lower the sensitivity of the postsynaptic membrane. These effects are additive to the conventional neuromuscular blockers that act on the postsynaptic membrane. All aminoglycosides seem to show this activity, although their potencies differ.

Concurrent use need not be avoided, but anesthetists need to be alert for the increased and prolonged neuromuscular blockade. The postoperative period also should be monitored closely. There is an additional risk of the neuromuscular blockade returning during the postoperative period if a dose of antibiotic is given during surgery. Attempts to treat the increased blockade with anticholinesterases and calcium have met with variable success.

Antihypertensives + phenothiazines

Some of the phenothiazines, particularly chlorpromazine, promazine, and methotrimeprazine, can cause postural hypotension. This reaction may be exaggerated if the patient is also taking an antihypertensive drug. This has been reported with various antihypertensive agents, including captopril, clonidine, furosemide, hydrochlorothiazide, nadolol, nifedipine, and prazosin. Because the interaction seems to depend on a generalized rather than a specific mechanism, potentially this can occur with any antihypertensive agent. The exception seems to be the andrenergic blocking drugs like guanethidine. In this case, a different pharmacodynamic interaction appears to happen. Adrenergic blocking drugs need to be taken into sympathetic nerve endings by a transport mechanism before they exert their effect of diminishing transmitter release, leading to a fall in blood pressure. Chlorpromazine, haloperidol, thiothixene, various indirectly acting sympathomimetic amines, and tricyclic antidepressants block the uptake of guanethidine. In the case of this type of antihypertensive agent, the drug does not reach its site of action, and the effect of chlorpromazine on guanethidine is therefore antagonistic.

Corticosteroids + NSAIDs

Both corticosteroids and NSAIDs can cause gastrointestinal irritation, leading to bleeding and ulceration. A large retrospective study of more than 20 000 patients who had taken corticosteroids found that the incidence of upper gastrointestinal bleeding was no greater in these patients than in the control group. However, the risk was greater if patients had been taking aspirin or other NSAIDs in addition to corticosteroids. It would seem that the widely held belief that combined use increases the risks of gastrointestinal side effects is vindicated. Presumably, this is a simple additive effect. During concurrent use, patients should be monitored. Eventually, some treatment for gastrointestinal damage

may be required. The overall risks to the patient associated with upper gastrointestinal damage caused by these drugs either alone or combined should not be underestimated. One survey of emergency hospital admissions for gastrointestinal crises and deaths linked to NSAIDs suggested that 62000 emergency admissions and 4000 deaths could be expected annually if its findings were extrapolated to the United Kingdom as a whole.

In addition to this effect, it appears that indomethacin and naproxen can have a "steroid sparing" effect. It seems that this is a protein-binding displacement interaction. It appears that it may be possible to reduce the steroid dosage while maintaining its effect; for example, one study found that paramethasone dosage could be reduced by almost 60% when naproxen also was given.

Predicting pharmacodynamic interactions: the difficulties

Understanding the mode of action of drugs allows theoretical predictions to be made about which drugs might interact pharmacodynamically. Indirectly acting sympathomimetics such as amphetamine, phenylpropanolamine, and tyramine exert their effects by displacing norepinephrine from storage granules in sympathetic nerve endings. This is in contrast to directly acting sympathomimetics, which exert effects directly on the receptors for norepinephrine. Drugs such as ephedrine have both direct and indirect activity (mixed action).

The tricyclic antidepressants block the reuptake of released transmitter amines (principally serotonin and norepinephrine) back into nerve endings. They also reduce the effects of the indirectly acting sympathomimetic tyramine. It was expected, therefore, that tricyclics would reduce the activity of other indirectly acting sympathomimetics. Apart from a single case report involving amitriptyline and ephedrine, this has not been seen.

The problem with predicting interactions this way is that although our understanding about how drugs act might be extensive, it is rarely complete. Possibly the flaw in the preceding prediction is the assumption that the mechanism that facilitates entry of the indirectly acting drugs into the nerve endings is identical to that carrying norepinephrine back. Tyramine is probably an exception and probably does share the same mechanism as norepinephrine, so its actions are reduced by the tricyclics. Either the others use a different mechanism to enter the nerve endings or a further, unidentified process compensates.

Generally, predicted pharmacodynamic interactions need to be tested clinically to confirm or disprove them. If the combination has been used many times and no reports have appeared, then it is likely that the interaction does not occur or is not clinically significant.

Suggested readings

Committee on Safety of Medicines. Current Problems in Pharmacovigilance. 1995, chap. 21, 3.

GRASELA TH, SCHENTAG JJ, SEDMAN AJ, et al. Inhibition of enoxacin absorption by antacids or ranitidine. Antimicrob Agents Chemother 1989;33:615-7.

KANTOLA T, KIVISTO KT, NEUVONEN PJ. Grapefruit juice greatly increases serum concentrations of lovastatin and lovastatin acid. Clin Pharmacol Ther 1998; 63:397-402.

KERR B, YUEP G, DANIELS R, et al. Strategic approach to nelfinavir mesylate (NFV) drug interactions involving CYP3A metabolism. In: Proceedings of the 6th European Conference on Clinical Aspects and Treatment of HIV Infection. 1997, p. 256.

KNUPP CA, BARBHAIYA RH: A multiple-dose pharmacokinetic interaction study between didanosine (Videx) and ciprofloxacin in male subjects seropositive for HIV but asymptomatic. Biopharm Drug Dispos 1997;18:65-77.

LEBSACK M, NIX D, RYERSON B, et al. Effect of gastric acidity on enoxacin absorption. J Clin Pharmacol Ther 1992;53:252-6.

MIZUKI Y, FUJIWARA I, YAMAGUCHI T. Pharmacokinetic interactions related to the chemical structures of fluoroquinolones. J Antimicrob Chemother 1996;37(suppl A):41-55.

NEUVONEN PJ, JALAVA KM. Itraconazole drastically increases plasma concentrations of lovastatin and lovastatin acid. Clin Pharmacol Ther 1996;60:54-61.

NEUVONEN PJ, KANTOLA T, KIVISTO KT. Simvastatin but not pravastatin is very susceptible to interaction with CYP3A4 inhibitor itraconazole. Clin Pharmacol Ther 1998;63:332-41.

PAZZUCCONI F, BARBI S, BALDASSARRE D, et al. Iron-ovotransferrin preparation does not interfere with ciprofloxacin absorption. Clin Pharmacol Ther 1996;59:418-22.

ROGERS JD, ZHAO J, LIU L, et al. Grapefruit juice has minimal effects on plasma concentrations of lovastatin-derived 3-hydroxy-3-methylglutaryl coenzyme A reductase inhibitors. Clin Pharmacol Ther 1999;66:358-66.

STOCKLEY IH. Drug interactions, 4th ed. London: Pharmaceutical Press, 1996.

Side effects of drugs and pharmacovigilance

René J. Royer

Pharmacovigilance – integrated into a public health system, on the one hand, and into a process of drug discovery and development, on the other – has as its mission to train and to inform. Any drug introduced into an organism behaves as an alien substance; it tends to be rejected as it is or after it is metabolized. Frequently, this leads to favorable reactions in terms of the patient's health but also, at times, unfavorable reactions. An isolated prescriber may never be able to detect a rare adverse drug reaction. To be well informed, such a prescriber has to participate in the collective compilation of cases, the coordination of which is the field of pharmacovigilance.

Pharmacovigilance is a term proposed in 1970. It is not exactly synonymous with *postmarketing surveillance*. It is more than a simple regulatory system for spontaneous notification. It encompasses concepts, methods, means, techniques, and systems, adopted mainly by consensus, that together allow the surveillance of unexpected drug effects. It is an active discipline that is useful to public health. Some authors limit the role of pharmacovigilance to a study of postmarketing adverse drug reactions. Instead, however, pharmacovigilance can be adapted and applied successfully to clinical drug trials, drug overdoses, and even unexpected beneficial drug effects.

Pharmacovigilance, a term adopted by the European Community (EC), is part of clinical pharmacology. It is as old as medicine itself, therapeutics being a compromise between the risks undertaken because of illness and those linked to the use of drugs. Pharmacovigilance has been inseparable from therapy for as long as the number of active products has been stable and limited, together with the long experience of practitioners. It grew rapidly in the 1950s, when chemical entities were identified by appropriate screening.

The modern history of pharmacovigilance has its origins in the failure of organized medicine to provide early detection of the thalidomide disaster. It took 4 years (1957-1961), in fact, for the teratogenicity of thalidomide to be recognized despite the appearance of a large number of cases of a previously rare syndrome, phocomelia. The oculomucocuta-neous syndrome associated with practolol (1978), the back pain associated with benoxaprofen (1982), and the myelooptic neuropathy associated with clioquinol all have proven the need for an international postmarketing surveillance system in the Anglo-American countries. At the same time, drugs withdrawn from the market in European nations were mainly national products. For a long time, unfavorable price conditions delayed the introduction of drugs internationally, and adverse drug reactions were detected elsewhere, despite the fact, particularly in France, that a structured pharmacovigilance system was already in place. Isoxicam, which was withdrawn because of European experience, is one of the rare exceptions.

Since the thalidomide disaster, many national authorities, taking into account the World Health Organization (WHO) General Assembly's recommendations, have enacted regulations to improve postmarketing surveillance and sometimes have developed safety regulatory systems, which are the first steps toward a true system of pharmacovigilance.

Approval processes, based primarily on animal studies and clinical trials, are not well adapted to the detection of adverse drug reactions (ADRs). Animals have physiologic and biomedical processes that are different from those of humans. Clinical trials can neither be large enough nor of sufficient duration to detect rare side effects appearing in particular subsets of patients. Such trials are capable of linking ADRs occurring after long-term use or with specific drug-drug interactions (see Chap. 6).

Pharmacovigilance is a part of medical diagnosis. Any physician has to refer to the influence of drug treatment when he/she tries to define the pathology shown by his patient. Use of the term *pharmacovigilance* therefore has spread worldwide. In the United States, it is sometimes improperly spelled *pharmacovigilence;* the Latin root is, in fact, *vigilancia.* The main definitions were proposed first by the WHO and then by the Council of International Organisations of Medical Sciences (CIOMS), but the definition of the EC will be used here in order to try to point out the differences that may exist between them.

DEFINITION

Pharmacovigilance is a discipline that aims to detect, evaluate, understand, and prevent adverse drug reactions (ADRs). The term pharmacovigilance comprises the following points (75/319/EEC and 93/39/EEC):

- Collection and notification about reports of suspected ADRs by marketing authorization (MA) holder(s) and competent authorities.
- Scientific evaluation of these reports and of available data with intensive interactions between MA holder(s) and competent authorities in order to fully evaluate the potential risk of the medicinal product(s), especially taking into account the reported suspected ADR(s) and the sales figures.
- Appointment of a person responsible for pharmacovigilance by the MA holder(s).
- Possible decisions on pharmacovigilance measures taken by MA holder(s) on their own, e.g., as variations made or as "urgent safety restrictions" [Regulations (EC) 541/95 and 542/95].
- Decisions on pharmacovigilance measures by the competent authorities.
- Implementation of pharmacovigilance measures.
- Postauthorization studies as a condition of marketing authorization.

In pharmacovigilance, several standard expressions are used, and they are described in Table 7.1.

Classification of adverse drug reactions

There are several ways to classify ADRs, e.g., whether they are considered frequent or rare, predictable or not, serious or not. The method that is used most frequently is the one proposed by Rawlins and Thomson. They proposed to divide ADRs into two classes: type A, which is dose-related, and type B, which is nondose-related (bizarre). Smith and Royer have proposed adding two further subgroups, i.e., type C, which is long-term effects (continuous), and type D, which is delayed effects.

Type A ADRs (dose-related) are induced by the pharmacodynamic properties of the drug or by the direct toxicity of the parent drug or its metabolites. The metabolic or pharmacokinetic changes are related either to the environment, to a drug-drug interaction, to known genetic factors, or to certain diseases, such as hepatic or renal disease. Since it is possible to identify all these factors, type A ADRs are considered predictable.

Type B ADRs (nondose-related) are produced mainly by an immunoallergic mechanism, itself induced by the parent drug or by some of the drug's normal or pathologic metabolites. Genetic factors, phenotypes, and ethnic differences may play a major role in this category, and type B ADRs are thus considered unpredictable.

Type C ADRs (continuous) are induced by the long-term effect of the parent drug or its metabolites, leading to adaptive modifications and in turn to pharmacodynamic or toxicologic consequences, e.g., transformations of

immune mechanisms. Long-term toxicity (as with amiodarone or phenacetin), hormone feedback, rebound reactions (as with prazosin), and tolerance, addiction, and withdrawal syndromes (as with barbiturates, opioids, etc.) are included in this group.

Type D ADRs (delayed) are of the same kind as type C ADRs, but the delay to the unpredicted hidden biologic effects is longer and often more serious clinically. Bladder cancer in patients taking long-term mutagenic agents (e.g., cyclophosphamide), breast cancer as a result of teratogens, vaginal carcinomas in the daughters of mothers treated with stilbestrol, and others may be included in this subgroup.

ADRs thus can be predictable or unpredictable. Toxicity, pharmacokinetics, pharmacodynamic effects, drug-drug interactions, drug-environment interactions, and drug-disease interactions are the major etiologic factors in predictable ADRs. Immunoallergic mechanisms, genic disturbances that have not been categorized yet, intolerance, and idiosyncratic phenomena are the main factors in unpredictable ADRs. Idiosyncratic ADRs

Table 7.1 Commonly used concepts in pharmacovigilance

Adverse event (or experience)
Any undesirable experience occurring in a group of patients treated with one or several pharmaceutical products, whether or not considered related to the medicinal product. An *adverse drug reaction* (ADR) is an event that can be attributed to one or several drugs

Adverse drug reaction/adverse reaction
A reaction that is harmful and unintended that is attributed to a drug a patient receives or has received. For the EC, only normal daily doses are considered

Expected or unexpected adverse drug reactions
The ADR can be *expected* when it is related to a pharmacologic property of the drug, also called a *side effect*. An ADR can be *unexpected* when it could not be foreseen in relation to the properties of the drug concerned. For the EC, unexpected ADRs are all the effects that are not listed in the Summary of Product Characteristics (SPC)

Serious adverse reaction
The WHO, the EC, and different countries define this roughly the same way. In English, no difference is made between *grave* and *serious*. In French, *grave* is characteristic of the consequence of the side effect of the drug, and *serious* is characteristic of its intensity. Subtle differences can be noted among the different languages of the EC. A serious ADR is an adverse reaction that is fatal, life-threatening, disabling, incapacitating, or which results in, or prolongs, hospitalization

Causality assessment
Evaluation of the causal relationship between an event and a drug, taking into account the degree of probability or plausibility that is responsible for the observed ADR

Consistency of data, completeness of data
Value, in volume and quality, of the collected data that allow an assessment of imputability

Case report
Case reported (*reporting:* action to report one or several cases to a pharmacovigilance system) by health professionals to a health authority

include a heterogeneous group of unpredictable adverse effects and often are the consequence of pharmacogenetic variations in drug bioactivation and metabolite detoxification. The reaction depends more often on the individual than on the drug. This subgroup can be rated as a "waiting box" until the mechanisms of actions are better known or elucidated.

METHODOLOGY

Spontaneous notification

Spontaneous notification covers a set of information exchanges concerning the side effects of drugs between practitioners (i.e., doctors, dentists, midwives, chemists), pharmaceutical companies, and the authorities in charge of pharmacovigilance. This term covers different modes of transmission: (1) voluntary notification on a preestablished schedule, (2) compulsory notification through the same type of organization, and (3) sporadic information (e.g., communications, publications, etc). The aim is to obtain as many notifications as possible and at the same time to take care that the notifiers do not get tired in the process. Many people think that it would be ideal to have 100% notifications of side effects. This obviously is utopic. If this were the case, the mass of notifications would be such that it would jam the collecting organization. Indeed, the essential aim of systems based on spontaneous notification is to detect signals, as early as possible, so as to set up appropriate security measures. If the percentage of notifications is low, it is necessary to widen the range of the population explored – a region, a nation, a continent, the world. The WHO with its databank and pharmacovigilance collaborating centers would like to fill this role.

The main drawback to spontaneous notification is underreporting. Underreporting makes it difficult to estimate the frequency of a side effect because it is impossible to identify the denominator. Frequency is often described as fluctuating in relation to time and to the different periods in the commercial life of a product. However, French studies on such major drug classes as nonsteroidal anti-inflammatory drugs (NSAIDs) and the quinolones frequently have shown that the apparent frequencies of the side effects of these drugs are quite stable. It must be remembered, however, that in France, up to now, a selective notification (black triangle in the United Kingdom, for instance) has not been requested, in order to protect the spontaneous nature of the notification for a given drug class. Another drawback of spontaneous notification is its low efficiency in identifying delayed ADRs (e.g., from carcinogenic substances, growth hormone) or those which skip one or more generations (e.g., stilbestrol).

Finally, guaranteeing the quality of information collected is essential for the analysis of a signal if we do not want to waste time studying the background noises created by cases that provide little information and for which causality is poorly analyzed. The selective French system generates few background noises as compared with the American system, which operates little selection.

The perception of the need to notify, furthermore, differs according to country. Diagnostic uncertainty, difficulty with the notification process, lack of time, insufficient criteria for defining what is to be changed, and fear that the notifications would be used in lawsuits are evoked in decreasing order. Some of the causes also are related to patients and the pharmacologic drug class. Some patients follow prescriptions blindly, up to death if necessary, and say nothing. Others attribute any sensation or particular symptom to the drug that has been prescribed. This latter case is the most frequent.

Drugs often produce side effects peculiar to their class: cough with conversion enzyme inhibitors and blood dyscrasias and liver disorders with analgesics and some antidepressants. These effects generally are recognized and often are the subjects of notifications at least in the first years of a product's life. Others are sparse and sometimes ignored by practitioners who do not recognize them. Others are so common that it appears superfluous to send out a notification. Finally, some side effects can appear as a symptom in the evolution of the illness and not be recognized as such. Mortality and morbidity statistics thus can be very useful in pharmacovigilance.

Walker and Lumley in 1987 and Rawlins in 1988 in the United Kingdom as well as workers at some French regional centers in the 1990s have tried to evaluate undernotification. The figures vary, but it can be estimated that global notification addresses 3 to 5% of reported ADRs and 10 to 25% of serious ADRs. Media intervention or repeated publication also can alter the notification rates.

Despite what has been said, spontaneous notification has important advantages. It is the only approach that allows a simultaneous and continuous overview of all the products taken by a population. It is easy to set up, does not interfere with medical habits, and provided that the subject population is important enough, can rapidly generate a signal or an alert.

In 1992, a group meeting organized by the EC to establish the objectives of pharmacovigilance estimated that spontaneous notification had proved its validity to generate hypotheses and/or signals to allow identification of unknown side effects, to test data thus identified, to search for a predisposition in population subgroups (e.g., by age, sex, or associated pathologies), and to identify drug interactions.

Whatever the drawbacks, spontaneous notification has to be maintained and even developed. Moreover, once an alert is launched, it is sometimes impossible to wait for results of an appropriate epidemiologic study. When the quality of data is satisfactory, emergency decisions can be and have been taken. In France, decisions about restriction or withdrawal taken in view of spontaneous notifications have at times been confirmed by more targeted international studies (e.g., isoxicam, triazolam, phenylbutazone and oxyphenbutazone), but more often, spontaneous notification has been sufficient to convince the authorities in charge to mandate restriction or withdrawal.

Epidemiology

When a hypothesis generated by spontaneous notification has to be confirmed, or when the frequency and impact of side effects have to be evaluated, it is necessary to use other methods, in particular, epidemiology. Epidemiology in pharmacovigilance examines the relationship between the occurrence of an ADR and the use of one or several drugs in order to evaluate frequency, distribution, and evolution in large populations or defined subgroups of these populations. The aim is rarely to generate hypotheses or to discover still unknown effects but mostly to check or test a hypothesis that most often stems from spontaneous notification.

The first exploration consists of establishing a chart of contingencies (Tab. 7.2) that takes into account the number of subjects observed, i.e., the number of people (n_1) who present with a symptom in a treated group (a) and a reference group (c) and the number of people (n_2) who do not present with the symptom under the same conditions in the treated group (b) and the reference (d) group. The excess risk for the people treated will be represented by the formula:

$$(a/n_1) - (c/n_2)$$

whereas the relative risk associated with the treatment will be represented by the formula

$$(a/n_1)/(c/n_2)$$

where $n_1 = a + b$ and $n_2 = c + d$.

It is clear that to obtain information on risk, all the data are needed – hence the use of a reference group. A simple cohort will give only a and b. Spontaneous notification provides only a fraction of the values a and b. Other methods of data collection therefore become necessary.

Cohort A cohort is a group of subjects selected and followed in time to identify and quantify an effect in a subgroup treated with a drug and another that is untreated (reference) and to possibly confirm or evaluate the causal relationship existing between drug and effect. There are three main types of cohorts: historical, prospective, and retrospective. Generally, the reference or control group is organized and selected in order to be as similar as possible to the study group.

Reference cases An epidemiologic study compares drug exposure rates in a group of patients presenting with an ADR with a group that does not present with the ADR. Characteristics of the two groups must be as comparable as possible, and it is probably this comparability that constitutes the major difficulty in case-control studies (cases-controls group chart, Tab. 7.3).

The *odds ratio* (OR) quantifies the strength of the association between exposure to a drug and occurrence of an ADR. If, when compared, the two risks are low, the OR can be assimilated to a relative risk (RR).

Records Records are set up by the exhaustive and systematic registration of all the cases of a given event (an illness more often than an ADR) in a specific geographic area. Records are a priceless source of data in the gathering of groups for a case-control study. Records of malformations, cancers, metabolic illnesses (Reye's syndrome), and degenerative diseases (Creutzfeld-Jacob disease) can implicate drugs.

The preparation of registers demands an efficient organization that often is expensive. Files may be exhaustive or not, and they may have more or less interest for practitioners of pharmacovigilance. Databases are comprised of computerized records of cases, such as the WHO databank, the French databank of pharmacovigilance, and Medwatch in the United Sates. Databases on drug exposure can be gathered from health care system records, such as the VAMP system in the United Kingdom. Record linkage allows interesting information to be obtained from records from different sources. For ethical reasons, this may not be allowed in some European countries, e.g., France.

Population databases Population databases provide systematic and exhaustive health data for a particular region (e.g., Saskatchewan, Canada) or for an insured population (e.g., Medicaid participants in the United States). Theoretically, these records cannot be linked, since all data are included. In northern European countries, population databases can be achieved by use of the electronic health cards.

Meta-analysis This statistical method evaluates data coming from different studies on the side effects of a suspected drug. It sorts out studies carried out by different

Table 7.3 Cases chart, reference group

	Event, ADR Yes	Event, ADR No	Total
Exposed to the drug	a	b	$a + b = n_1$
Not exposed to the drug	c	d	$c + d = n_2$

Odds ratio = $(a/c)/(b/d)$ = ad/bc.

Table 7.2 Contingency chart

	Symptom Yes	Symptom No	Total
Subject treated	a	b	$a + b = n_1$
Reference subject not treated	c	d	$c + d = n_2$

methods (e.g., cohort studies, case-control studies with or
without randomization, etc.) and reevaluates them accord-
 SIDE EFFECTS OF DRUGS AND PHARMACOVIGILANCE • **69**

ing to specified statistical criteria. It rejects cases coming
from insufficient series, as well as cases not collected
according to the specified methodologies. This method
has the advantage of pooling very large numbers of cases.
The statistical methodology is complex, but it is not that
major a difficulty.

Other methods   Other epidemiologic methods have been
proposed for special situations, such as the *capture-recapture method.* This method derives its name from studies of
wildlife populations. In medical practice, this method
allows the number of cases in a defined population to be
estimated by using two or more sources of cases. These
could include records from hospitals or general practices
or any other points of contact. Taken alone, each of these
sources may undercount the actual number of cases, as
indeed would a simple aggregate of the sources that
excluded duplicate cases (cases identified at more than
one source). The capture-recapture technique uses information provided by duplicate cases to allow the number
of people not identified at any of the sources to be calculated, thus allowing expected incidence data to be derived
(with appropriate confidence intervals). Signal generations using a Bayesian neural network, in experimental
work at the Uppsala Collaborating Centre, also may be
included among these ancillary methods.

ORGANIZATION

National structures

In 1972, a WHO technical report presented a model for
the design of a national pharmacovigilance center. Not
surprisingly, pharmacovigilance centers through the years
have evolved differently in different countries according
to their medical and regulatory traditions, health care
organizations, and size and wealth. In all countries, governmental agencies are responsible for the national pharmacovigilance centers, but the competencies and tasks
may be delegated to regional structures, hospitals, universities, or national groups.

In some countries, decentralization is the predominant
feature (e.g., France, Spain, Italy, and Sweden). In others,
centralization is at the core of the system (e.g., Germany,
Belgium, and Ireland). Some structures are mixed, such as
those in the United Kingdom, Canada, and even the
United States (using Medwatch). The regionalized network of reporting centers organized by LAREB in the
Netherlands on behalf of the national center also can be
considered to be a mixed structure. Whatever the system,
it is essential today to have a compilation of notifications
that is as large and as extensive as possible, i.e., at least
national. More extended data gathering may be set up
later. The position of the national agency takes precedence in the definition of rules, methods of data collection, and treatment of information and data storage in
standard computerized systems accessible to satellite
structures. Whether centralized or decentralized, pharma-

covigilance systems have to abide by general rules. The
advantage of decentralized systems is that they consist of
small centers spread throughout the nation that are close
to practitioners who know their patients personally. This
situation allows for a discussion of the data collected and
permits the exchange of information and training, if necessary.

Systems designed to collect and analyze information
also exist for the pharmaceutical industry. Collected data
are then transmitted to national agencies according to different procedures, whether the adverse drug reaction is
severe or not. Pharmaceutical companies possess the
largest amount of information concerning the safety of
products. They must reappraise this information periodically and inform and alert, if necessary, national authorities and health care professionals for the benefit and protection of patients. They must develop modern systems of
communication and information and complement the
available databases as much as possible. Pharmaceutical
companies are often international and take advantage of
international regulations.

The French system as an example of decentralization

The French system is a compromise between mandatory
notification and semi-intensive hospital surveillance. The
causal relationship between drugs and adverse events is
systematically established using an algorithm index
accepted by both the public and private partners in pharmacovigilance. The special features of the system are (1)
the medicalization, (2) the quality of the reported data,
and (3) the training and notification of physicians by systematic feedback.

The country is covered by 31 regional centers located
in the departments of clinical pharmacology or the poison
centers of university hospitals. The centers are linked in a
national network coordinated by the drug agency in a
Technical Committee that includes all the executives of
the regional centers and some civil servants from the
Ministry of Health and the Medical Research Institute
(INSERM).

Every month, during a full-day meeting, discussions
are carried out on:
• interesting cases selected by the regional centers;
• relevant issues in the literature;
• the report of one regional center acting as an expert for
  an inquiry following an alert;
• the decision to present such a report to the National
  Committee;
• pharmacovigilance policy matters.

The National Committee is comprised of representatives of general practitioners, pharmacists, research
institutes, and regional centers. It has the duty to examine reports prepared by the Technical Committee and to
give advice to the director of the drug agency concerning drug safety.

The main duties of a regional center are, of course, to
register physician reports of ADRs, to check their quality

and improve it, if necessary, to establish the causal relationship, and finally, to enter cases into the databank (Tab. 7.4). A regional center also should explore clinical wards to discover unnotified ADRs, answer the queries of consulting physicians and pharmacists about ADRs, provide documents or relevant papers concerning those queries, coordinate postgraduate training in the field of pharmacovigilance, and do research on iatrogenic mechanisms and other aspects of drug safety.

International harmonization

The WHO collaborating center (Uppsala Collaborating Center)

The need to raise the number of notifications and to establish an efficient worldwide alert system to improve patient safety has led the WHO to create a collaborating center for international drug monitoring. The main responsibility of this center is to pool domestic data received and transmitted by national authorities.

After a difficult and uncertain beginning, this center became a clearinghouse for information exchange and consultation for all national pharmacovigilance centers. It has developed a nomenclature and methods to detect signals and has made professionals aware of the need to work together. It also helps countries that do not yet have a pharmacovigilance structure to develop their national centers and provides training to executives of these centers. An annual meeting allows interested parties to synthesize information and develop exchanges. This collaborating center is now situated in Uppsala, Sweden.

The Council for International Organisation of Medical Sciences

The Council for International Organisation of Medical Sciences (CIOMS) is a nonprofit organization established in 1949 under the auspices of the WHO and the United Nations Educational, Scientific, and Cultural Organization (UNESCO). CIOMS engages in a wide range of actions: coordination of conferences and medical congresses, development of human resources for health, drug development and use, establishment of an international nomenclature of diseases, and examination and application of bioethics and health policy ethics. The

purpose of CIOMS was described as to facilitate the exchange of views and scientific information in the medical sciences. The scope of these activities was broadened to include various forms of international collaboration in the medical sciences, not only those with a direct impact on society or progress in medical science but also those with implications in such fields as bioethics, health policy, drug development, and medical education.

In 1986, CIOMS set up the working group on international reporting of adverse drug reactions, more commonly known as CIOMS-1. This working group is made up of independent experts from national centers and the pharmaceutical industry, and it carries out analyses of existing national systems for international ADR reporting. It also has proposed a harmonization of terminologies with the aid of the CIOMS form, which serves as a model for most national forms at present. This allows an easier exchange of information in international reporting. The CIOMS-2 working group has worked on the proposals that have led to periodic safety updates.

International Conference on Harmonization

The International Conference on Harmonization (ICH) is in charge of harmonizing regulatory procedures in reference to specific products from the viewpoints of basic research and preclinical and clinical trials in order to obtain marketing authorization and consequently to ensure maximal patient safety. Japan, the United States, and the EC participate in it, their aim being to translate national regulations into proposals of the conference.

Concerning pharmacovigilance, the ICH E2A report, *Clinical Safety Data Management: Definitions and Standards for Expedited Reporting,* has undergone all stages from 1 to 5 and has been implemented in Europe, the United States, and Japan. The definitions contained in the report were inspired directly by the definitions established by consensus at the WHO collaborating center in 1994. The ICH E2B report, *Clinical Safety Management,* follows a format established by precedence. The ICH E2C report, *Clinical Safety Management: Periodic Safety Update Reports for Marketed Drugs,* largely was inspired by the work of CIOMS-1 and CIOMS-2 and was approved by the EC in December of 1996.

Pharmacovigilance appears to be well structured throughout the world and close to being fully harmonized. It is not possible to describe here all the national peculiarities. The analysis will be limited to the regulations that apply within the European Community because these are close to those applied in Japan and the United States.

European regulations on pharmacovigilance

The legal framework of pharmacovigilance of medicinal products for human use in the EC is given in Council Regulation (EEC 2309/93, Title 2, Chap. III) and Council Directive 75/319/EEC, as amended by 93/39/ECC, Chaps. V_a and VI_a, as well as by the Council Regulation CE540/95 complementing the EEC 2309/33 regulation. Some articles are important for pharmacovigilance (Directive 75/319/EEC, consolidated version):

Table 7.4 Some results of French regional center activity

	1990	1991	1996
Notifications to the centers*	10 967	11 537	17 394
Queries	22 494	23 337	26 171

*To obtain the total number of national notifications, the cases notified by pharmaceutical companies must be added to this figure.

- *Article 29 a:* "…the Member States shall establish a pharmacovigilance system…to collect information… with particular reference to Adverse Drug Reactions (ADRs) and to evaluate such information scientifically."
- *Article 29 c:* "The person responsible for placing the medicinal product on the market shall have permanently and continuously at his disposal an appropriately qualified person responsible for pharmacovigilance." Among other things, such a person should be responsible for the collection of worldwide safety data and evaluation of these collected data, ensuring that all requests from authorities are answered fully and promptly.
- *Article 29 d:* "Establishing detailed records of all suspected ADRs occurring within and outside the EU and which are reported to him by a health care professional. When the suspected ADR is serious, to record and to report to competent authorities immediately and in any case within 15 days of their receipt at the latest. When the suspected ADR is not serious, it shall be submitted in a safety update report every 6 months during the first 2 years, once a year for the following 3 years after marketing authorization, [and] at 5-yearly intervals thereafter immediately upon request."
- *Article 29 e:* "The Member States shall take appropriate measures to encourage doctors and other health care professionals to report suspected adverse reactions to competent authorities."
- *Article 29 f:* "The Member States shall ensure that reports of suspected serious ADRs are immediately brought to the attention of the Agency and of the person responsible for placing the medicinal product on the market, and in any case within 15 days of their notification, at the latest."
- *Article 29 h:* "…in case of urgency, the Member State concerned may suspend the marketing of a medicinal product, provided the Agency is informed at the latest on the following working day."

Regulation and directives are completed according to guidelines that have no legal force but can be assisted by EC regulatory applications. These guidelines must be updated regularly based on new decisions or regulatory recommendations. Completion of the ICH reports will demand numerous modifications because they will be accommodated in the EC guidelines.

Among the fundamental guidelines of pharmacovigilance, I should mention the guidelines relating to periodic safety updates. These are published periodically by the Commission of the European Union.

CAUSALITY ASSESSMENT: IMPUTABILITY

The logic of a standardized assessment to define the relationship between a drug and an ADR was underlined by a number of authors in the 1970s. In 1978, Dangoumeau et al. published an algorithm-type method that was to become official in France after being modified in 1985. This work clearly demonstrates the importance of an analysis of case histories of patients who present with ADRs after receiving one or several drugs. A well-analyzed observation, a seriously built up imputability, makes the analysis of cases gathered in national and international databanks easier.

At face value, it would seem easier to ask the WHO, the CIOMS, and then the ICH to define a general methodology that could be applied to the entire world. A certain number of obstacles have prevented the launching of such an initiative. It has been observed that with a single method there may still be differences in evaluation by different observers. The quality control methods proposed by several authors are different and obviously imperfect. The terms used to define the causal relationship differ according to method and do not share the same correlation powers. Countries have developed habits that are difficult to change. Finally, it appears that a single method of imputability is a useful but relatively basic approach to reality. Over the years it appears that a fine analysis of causal relationships must be evaluated in terms of the pathologies in question. Partial answers have been given to these different points. Concerning the variability of answers, several studies have shown this reality; algorithms may allow us to achieve a higher constancy. It is clear that a minute analysis of the ADR by an expert is safer than one carried out by a practitioner in a hurry.

However, an algorithmic approach can still be very useful when we are dealing with a large amount of data. In face of the fact that methods and terms differ, it is not impossible to define equivalents. Two studies have shown this. The first, a study by Lagier et al. in 1983, proposed a numbered comparison of the 10 most important methods as well as equivalent terms. The second has as its objective the standardization of terms without modification of specific national methods. It is called the *Meyboom and Royer method* for the European Community data. It proposes equivalencies between the different terms used by various countries and an ABC approach to make analysis of international data easier for a common evaluation:

- *category A:* Reports that include good reasons and sufficient documentation to assume a causal relationship, in the sense of plausible, conceivable, likely, but not necessarily highly probable;
- *category B:* Reports that contain sufficient information to accept the possibility of a causal relationship, in the sense of not impossible and not unlikely, although the connection is uncertain and may even be doubtful, e.g., because of missing data, insufficient evidence, or the possibility of another explanation;
- *category 0:* Reports in which causality is, for one or another reason, not assessable, e.g., because of missing or conflicting data.

Up to the present, only a few studies have been carried out using this method. Its field of application should be defined clearly (UE III/3235/92, III/3445/91). ICH E2A, *Clinical Safety Management,* states that imputabiliy methods can be a global introspection, an algorithm, or a Bayesian calculation.

Moreover, there is no controlled vocabulary yet. The terms recommended by the WHO collaborating center are *certain, probable* or *likely, possible, unlikely, conditional* or *unclassified,* and *inaccessible* or *unclassifiable.* As pointed out previously, a fine analysis of imputability according to a specialized analysis of adverse events was first proposed by the WHO and the CIOMS for liver diseases and hematology. A series of consensus meetings presented by Benichou has allowed a better definition of adverse events and of their elements of evaluation. An extension to other pathologies is in progress, the beginning of which can be found in the *Practical Guide to Diagnosis and Management* published by Benichou.

To summarize, there has been a lot of talk about imputability since 1976, but international pharmacovigilance would certainly improve considerably if universal terminologies and methods were adopted.

EVALUATION OF THE RISKS AND BENEFITS OF DRUGS

Pharmacovigilance is not restricted to the reporting of ADRs; the analysis of individual cases; the collection of information from practitioners, health professionals, and the general public; and the promotion of research. It also evaluates the risks compared with the benefits of a particular drug. To do so, pharmacovigilance employs epidemiologic methods to evaluate the frequency and incidence of a suspected event, to establish the causal relationship between the ADRs and the suspected drug, to measure the severity of the effects, and to try to weigh the benefit in terms of disease recovery and quality of life. Premarketing studies, and clinical trials in particular, have to be considered. However, errors in the prescription scheme should not be forgotten.

As far as physicians are concerned, potential problem areas include choice of an inappropriate medication, prescription of incorrect doses, insufficient or inappropriate explanations offered to the patient, and excessive prescriptions given to the patient.

From the perspective of patients, problems result from confusion produced by a lack of knowledge about the proper use of prescribed drugs, undeclared over-the-counter drug use, drug abuse and misuse, and self-prescription of drugs purchased previously and not used at the time of prescription.

COMPUTERIZED DATABANK

They correspond to different aims and are of different nature.

Terminology databanks

ICD 9 for the classification of the diseases.
ICD 10 for the classification of the diseases.
WHOART Adverse Reactions Terminologies.

COSTART Adverse Reactions Terminology, peculiar to the United States and depending on countries.
WHOART and COSTART possess a system elaborated by the WHO that makes them partially compatible.
MEDDRA is an ADR dictionary developed first in the United Kingdom. It seems well adapted and will be introduced soon in the countries of the European Community. It is compatible with WHO and COSTART.
The Uppsala Collaborating Center has developed a new computer software called WHOART ACCESS that helps users to follow the hierarchical structure, to look for terms and synonyms, to choose among the available languages of the WHO Adverse Reactions Terminology. The center also has developed a product to help WHO Drug Dictionary users to take into account the additions and the changes regularly made.

Databanks

MEDLINE, MEDLARS, MICRO, and MEDEX are among the best known and are classic databanks for the research of published information.
IMS, VAMP, IMS, MEDIPlus, MEMO in the United Kingdom, NIVEL in Holland, GLOSTRUP Population Studies in Denmark, MEDICAID in the United States, and SASKATCHEWAN in Canada contain medical and population information.
A certain number of countries have national databanks on ADRs: THERIAQUE, BIAM in France, for instance. In the world, EC EUROCAT is an attempt at coordination. ISPRA is more a databank of products than of pharmacovigilance.
Databanks for the recording and compiling of ADRs. Nowadays the only worldwide structured bank is the WHO collaborating center's. It collects adverse events transmitted by the participating countries.
On a national scale, the U.S. databank is the biggest, and its development is increased by the setting up of the MEDWATCH system. European countries, Japan, and other countries around the world possess less developed systems for their domestic use.
The EMEA wishes to set up a community bank of this type. Experimental trials are in progress.

Telematic systems

To stay in touch safely, agencies or countries need their own safe networks. They must be able to select the persons or the organizations authorized to question the databank.
INTDIS for the WHO databank is working. The EC has several projects that will constitute ENScare, EDIFACT, MEDPHV, MEDADR, EUROSCAPE.
It is clear that in the field of computer sciences, evolution is quick. The projects will be more and more numerous, and there will be a need to choose an intermediate state satisfactory to all. Needless to say, national and international ethical regulations concerning the collection, storage, and broadcast of data will have to be strictly respected (see also Internet, adresses on Chap. 91).

Acknowledgments

I would like to thank Dr. F. Wagniart from the Pharmacovigilance Department of IRIS France for proofreading this paper and providing helpful advice. I would also like to thank Isabelle Royer for helping in the translation of this paper.

Suggested readings

ALBENGRES E, GAUTHIER R, TILLEMENT JP. Current French system of post-marketing drug surveillance. Int J Clin Pharmacol Ther Toxicol 1990;28:312-4.

BENICHOU C. Adverse drug reactions. A practical guide to diagnosis and management. Chichester, England: Wiley, 1994.

GRAHAME-SMITH DG, ARONSON JK. Oxford Textbook of clinical pharmacology and drug therapy. New York: Oxford University Press, 1992.

LAGIER G, VINCENS M, LEFEBURE B, FRELON JH. Imputation médicament par médicament en pharmacovigilance. Essai de comparaison des différentes méthodes. Therapie 1983;38:295-302.

MEYBOOM RHB, ROYER RJ. Causality classification at pharmacovigilance centres in the European Community. Pharmacoepidemiol Drug Safety 1992;1:87-97.

MEYBOOM RHB. Good practice in the post marketing surveillance of medicines. Pharmaceut World Sci 1997;119:186-90.

NONY P, CUCHERAT M, HAUGH MC, BOISSEL JP. Standardization of terminology in meta-analysis: A proposal for working definitions. Fundament Clin Pharmacol 1997;11:481-93.

RAWLINS MD. Spontaneous reporting of adverse drug reactions. Br J Clin Pharmacol 1988;26:1-13.

RAWLINS MD, FRACCHIA GN, RODRIGUEZ-FARRE. EURO-ADR: Pharmacovigilance and research. A European perspective. Pharmacoepidemiol Drug Safety 1992;1:261-8.

ROYER RJ. Pharmacovigilance: the French system. Drug Safety 1990;5(suppl 1):137-40.

Clinicopharmacologic aspects of drug evaluation

Jochen Kuhlmann

The development of drugs is a lengthy and large-scale multidisciplinary process as a result of the requirements of today's scientific standards regarding quality, efficacy, and safety. Between 1960 and 1980, development time of a substance from its synthesis to its introduction to the market almost quadrupled, and this has remained relatively unchanged since 1980, with a present time-to-market period of 9 to 13 years. Among the reasons for this prolonged development time are the increasingly rigorous demands on clinical studies, such as:

- a higher degree of scientific knowledge about the drug;
- the performance of controlled studies and intervention trials;
- regulations for clinical quality assurance;
- changes in professional regulations for physicians;
- more time-consuming administrative work for health authorities.

Accordingly, costs for research and development have risen dramatically. Whereas in 1987 expenses for the development of a new chemical entity (NCE) amounted to around 300 to 450 million German marks, these costs have nearly doubled during the last 10 years, amounting to 600 to 800 million German marks today. If the expenses for all the failures that have to be carried along the way are included, costs for a successfully developed product rise to 1 billion German marks. Moreover, the market itself is becoming intensely competitive. Thus it has become necessary to plan the preclinical and clinical investigations of an NCE at an early stage and organize them on a tight schedule so as to reach registration within a reasonable amount of time.

DRUG DISCOVERY

The path of a new drug from concept to product may be divided into two phases, namely, drug discovery and drug development. In drug discovery, a dramatic change is taking place. In the past, drug discovery usually depended on experimental protocols in which compounds synthesized by medicinal chemists were administered to experimental animals in the hope that biologic activity would be observed that could be separated from unwanted actions by further chemical manipulation of the lead structure, thereby producing a compound with therapeutic utility.

As a result of the remarkable progress in understanding and explaining the underlying causes of many diseases by identifying and sequencing the genes encoded within DNA, it has become possible with such new methods as molecular biology or gene technology to develop simple test assays to determine the biologic efficacy of a large number of compounds. In particular, molecular targets, i.e., proteins or enzymes, directly connected to an illness can be defined and used in the search for a biologic effect of a substance in a test tube or a petri dish. Today, automation of these test systems using computer-controlled robots in so-called high-throughput screening (HTS) methods has made it possible to evaluate up to 1 million substances per robot per year. Of these numerous tested substances, only those interacting with these targets, as shown, for example, by releasing a fluorescent dye, are potential candidates for further investigation. These lead structures must then be optimized to fulfill the required profile for a development candidate.

However, the discovery of such lead structures requires testing an average of 50 000 to 100 000 compounds. Whereas for the past century the biologic test was the limiting step during drug discovery, today chemists are the notch. In recent years, the technology of combinatorial synthesis or chemistry has offered for the first time an opportunity to screen large numbers of novel compounds rapidly.

DRUG DEVELOPMENT

From the day of the discovery of new targets and new lead structures, including their optimization, to the decision to undertake development, 5 to 6 years generally have passed. Then development begins, and this may be divided into two partly overlapping phases, namely, the preclinical and clinical phases. Already in 1878 Buchheim wrote in his *First Manual of Pharmacology*, "Long before a drug is used to cure an illness it must be our effort to receive the greatest possible amount of knowledge regarding the illness to be treated as well as the drug to be used. Equipped with this knowledge the observation of the effect on the patient must then lead us to the correct use of the drug". This is still true today.

Preclinical phase

During the first part of drug development, the necessary requirements for first use in humans are met by performing preclinical pharmacologic, toxicologic, and pharmacokinetic investigations in animals and in vitro. Animal studies are still the best way to set up a pharmacologic-toxicologic profile of a new substance. A number of biochemical in vitro methods as well as investigations on microorganisms, cell cultures, and isolated organs can be used to deliver information on the pharmacodynamic properties of substances. However, these methods generally do not reveal information on the pharmacokinetic behavior of a substance nor on the effect of functional mechanisms in the organism. In addition, animal studies are mandatory in toxicology. Damage recognized during an animal study may be avoided in humans. Before clinical work begins, the health authorities require that the drug be administered to, and its short-term effects be studied in, laboratory animals. Data from these studies are used to decide if the drug is sufficiently safe for initial administration to humans.

Pharmacologic investigations

Modern pharmacologic and biochemical research has developed a number of models that allow conclusions to be drawn about a drug's pharmacologic effect, the minimum and maximum doses to reach this effect, the duration of effect, and the underlying working mechanisms. Based on these investigations, it is then possible to establish a working profile of a new drug that allows the development of first concepts on indication(s), dose, and impact in humans. However, the choice of models must be justified. Suitability and validity of these models should be controlled by appropriate methods and by parallel investigations with known substances if necessary. Despite great efforts in the field of pharmacology, a suitable animal model has not been found so far for a multitude of illnesses affecting humans.

On the other hand, besides toxicologic and pharmacokinetic investigations for the risk-benefit evaluation of new drugs, studies concerning safety and general pharmacology are moving to center stage. In contrast with toxicology, to date there are no internationally valid guidelines for pharmacologic safety studies. The German drug law (*Arzneimittelgesetz*) requires the performance of pharmacologic safety investigations in accordance with

the actual standards of science and technology. In the name of harmonization at the international level, first guidelines are presently being developed regarding minimal requirements and the methods of these investigations. During the planning of pharmacologic safety investigations, one must consider in each individual case whether the new substance belongs to a new or rather a chemically and pharmacologically well-known class of substances, what organs or organ systems are involved, which method is suitable for testing, and which animal species, dose, and route of administration are to be employed, as well as the size of the test group necessary to ensure statistical reliability. In general, within the range of pharmacologic safety investigations, the study should examine the effect of a new substance on the major organ systems such as the cardiovascular system, the respiratory system, the endocrine system, the gastrointestinal system the excretory system, and the autonomous and central nervous system. Furthermore, the influence on blood coagulation and hematologic as well as metabolic parameters should be determined. The unimpaired function of these organs and organ systems is vitally important, and reliable, validated methods are available for the study of their function. In addition, special investigations then depend on the knowledge gained from these studies of the pharmacodynamic effects and working mechanisms of the new drug. For recombinant proteins and biotechnology products, for example, tests of pyrogenicity, immunotoxicity, and hypersensitivity are recommended.

Routinely, reports on results of pharmacologic safety testing must be available at two stages in the course of drug development. First, safety data concerning a new agent must be submitted to health authorities and ethics committees before phase I clinical trials are started. The second critical stage at which pharmacologic safety data must be available is when a new drug application (NDA) is filed. Detailed data on the parent compound as well as any additional studies on the effects of the main metabolites, and occasionally of important by-products, must be provided. All studies must be performed according to good laboratory practice. At present, standard pharmacologic safety testing normally is carried out after single-dose administration of a drug; however, special problems may necessitate repeated dosing. Safety pharmacology assists in the identification of side effects, antidotes, and appropriate critical care strategies in close cooperation with pharmacology, toxicology, and pharmacokinetics.

Toxicologic investigations

Toxicologic studies in animals are performed to elucidate the hazards and to estimate the risks of new drugs before they are administered to humans. There will never be absolute safety in the sense of freedom from risk and total harmlessness of drugs. However, extensive toxicologic studies may minimize the risk for patients and physicians alike. The use of animals as a substitute for humans during drug development is morally and ethically justified in the Helsinki declaration by the World Medical Association (1964) and the extended versions of Tokyo (1975), Venice (1983), Hong Kong (1989), and Somerset

West (1996) and is also mandatory according to the German drug law and international guidelines. With respect to animal welfare, it must be kept in mind that animal experiments should be reduced to a minimum in accordance with state-of-the-art risk assessment. This applies to the type and number of experiments, the number of species, the number of individual animals, and the amount of suffering involved. The species generally used are rats and mice as rodents and dogs, monkeys, and occasionally rabbits or minipigs as nonrodents. Studies aimed at elucidating general systemic tolerability after single and multiple doses are distinguished from those looking specifically at effects on reproduction, genotoxicity, or carcinogenic potential. Toxicologic studies should be accompanied by a determination of plasma concentrations (toxicokinetics) in order to facilitate interpretation of findings and thus the transferability of study results to humans.

During the past, international requirements on toxicologic investigations for the registration of new drugs varied considerably. Recently the process of international harmonization (ICH) has led to an adjustment and standardization of study regulations in parts of Europe, the United States and Japan. In principle, the duration of the animal toxicity studies conducted in two mammalian species should be equal to, or exceed, the duration of the human clinical trials up to the maximum recommended duration of the repeated, dose toxicity studies. Under certain circumstances, where significant gain has been shown, trials may be extended beyond the duration of supportive repeated-dose toxicity studies on a case-by-case-basis.

A repeated-dose toxicity study in two species for a minimum duration of 2 weeks would support phase I and II studies in Europe and phase I to III studies in the US and Japan up to 2 weeks in duration. In the US, as an alternative to 2-week studies, single-dose human trials and multiple-dose up to 2 weeks. Beyond this, 1-3, or 6-month toxicity studies would support these types of human clinical trials for up to 1, 3 or 6 months, respectively.

For phase III studies in Europe and marketing in all regions, a 1-month toxicity study in two species (rondent and non-rodent) would support clinical trials up to 2 weeks' duration. Three-month toxicity studies would support clinical trials for up to 1 month duration, whereas 6-month toxicity studies in rodents and 3-month toxicity studies in nonrodents would support clinical trials up to 3 months. For phase III, up to 6 months in Europe, 6-month toxicity studies in rodents and 6 to 9 months in non-rodents are necessary. Six-month studies in rodents and chronic studies (6 to 9 months in Europe; 9 months in US and Japan) in nonrodents would support clinical trials of longer duration than 6 month.

As already pointed out for pharmacologic safety investigations, all studies must be performed strictly according to standards of Good laboratory practice. For this reason, toxicologic institutions are under permanent supervision and are inspected at regular intervals by federal authorities. While the study guidelines only provide the framework for toxicity studies, it is the toxicologist's responsibility to decide which study is necessary, in what type of animal, and which

method should be applied depending on the substance and its proposed use. The preconditions for toxicologic investigation are that the pharmacologic effects, including any undesired effects, are demonstrated, that the substance is available in a pure and stable form, and that an optimal galenic formulation has been found. The quality of the substance and its formulation ideally should be the same in the different experiments and comparable with the formulation intended for use in humans to ensure actual exposure comparisons for better definition of the therapeutic index.

Pharmacokinetic investigations

The aim of preclinical pharmacokinetic investigations is to gather first-hand information regarding the rate and extent of absorption and bioavailability, distribution, metabolism, and elimination of a new substance. These studies generally are carried out in at least two different animal species and after single and multiple intravenous and oral administrations. A further goal is to look for any signs of clinically relevant interactions with other drugs. These investigations may be carried out with the aid of physical, chemical, or biologic methods, as well as by observing the pharmacodynamic properties of the substance. In large part, they are performed before actual clinical trials are begun, but they must be continued during the clinical phase of drug development. In addition, if the new substance consists of a mixture of stereoisomers, it is also desirable to examine the pharmacokinetic and pharmacodynamic properties of each isomer.

The choice of animal species, the route and method of administration, the dose, the dosing interval, and the duration of administration should be chosen so that they may be interpreted in connection with pharmacologic and toxicologic investigations. Furthermore, the first target objectives of the galenic formulation should be developed in light of the pharmacokinetic and eventual pharmacologic studies so as to optimize them up to the beginning of the clinical trial. During this time period, the analytical methods have to be optimized to the point where, at the start of phase I, it is possible to measure unchanged substance as well as active and inactive metabolites in blood and other body fluids versus tissues at the concentrations expected in humans. Analytical methodology employed to generate these data include high-pressure liquid chromatography, gas chromatography, mass spectrometry, and radio- or enzyme-immunoassays.

If from the pharmacologic, pharmacokinetic, and toxicologic points of view there are no objections against a first use in humans and the risks connected to the clinical study are medically justifiable in relation to the likely therapeutic benefit of the drug, the clinical trial may take place under the requirements of the legal system in the country in which the trial is carried out.

Clinical investigations

Need for and requirements of clinical trials

The potential to exactly describe the desired effects as well as the undesired side effects of a newly discovered substance in animal experiments has always led to the question of whether clinical trials are necessary at all. Today everybody agrees that this question can only be answered with a definite "Yes". This clear commitment to clinical trials results from the fact that data received from animal experiments – especially with regard to quantitative values – may not be transferred to humans, especially sick persons, without further information. Prediction of the pharmacokinetics and drug effects in humans from animal data greatly facilitates phase I studies, but it is obvious that such predictions cannot be made with absolute reliability.

There are essentially three reasons for this:

• there are differences among individual animal species in their reactions to drugs, as well as between animals and humans;
• the considerable differences that are apparent in many cases in terms of absorption, distribution, metabolism, and excretion of drugs between animals and humans prove that the essential degree of safety in the use of a new drug may only be reached if these parameters are also examined in humans;
• many human diseases do not occur in animals and are not sufficiently initiated on an experimental basis. Two striking examples are the pain of cardiac oxygen deficiency occurring in angina pectoris and the whole range of psychotic illnesses. Although experimental methods have been developed to determine the effects of specific substances in these settings, the final proof of a substance's efficacy in the last analysis must be obtained in actual patients.

For these reasons, the clinical trial in healthy volunteers and ill patients is essential to rational drug efficacy determination. However, before the actual clinical study is started, all preclinical results are again carefully checked by a team of experts.

The scientific clinician will want to understand the results of in vivo and in vitro experiments and dose-concentration-response investigations examining the mechanisms and effects of the intended pharmacodynamic target, of tests of other functional actions, and of studies of acute and subacute/subchronic and genetic toxicity. These actions will have to be considered in relation to the potential exposure of humans and the reversibility and treatment of predictable adverse reactions.

Transfer of a candidate compound from the laboratory and animal test environment to trials in human subjects is a highly critical stage in drug development, and it is justified only if the preclinical investigations in pharmacology, pharmacokinetics, and toxicology suggest that the new substance is safe and superior to drugs and therapeutic regimens already on the market. In the case of a positive risk-benefit evaluation, the dose for first use in humans has to be determined.

Clinicopharmacologic investigations

In drug research, clinical pharmacology is the connecting link between preclinical and clinical research. Clinical pharmacology produces the necessary basis for the clinical trial of a new substance in patients with the target indication(s). During the clinical phase of drug development, clinical pharmacology concentrates on all aspects of use of the drug in humans employing the methods and knowledge of such associated disciplines as natural and clinical science.

In particular, the following clinicopharmacologic questions need to be answered during the investigation:

• how is the substance tolerated?
• what effect does the substance have on the healthy versus the ill human being?
• on what mechanisms are these effects based?
• what are the pharmacokinetic characteristics of the drug under physiologic and pathologic conditions?
• what factors influence the kinetic and dynamic properties of the drug?
• what undesired side effects will be seen, and how can one cope with them?

Today, the clinical study of a new drug in humans generally is divided into four phases and is carried out in three groups of volunteers and patients so as to keep the risk as small as possible (Tab. 8.1). The first investigation in humans – called a *phase I study* – generally is carried out in voluntarily recruited, usually healthy male subjects. This phase requires especially accurate planning and equally accurate observation during the course of the study. For this reason, many consider this phase to be the safest step of the entire drug investigation. However, during phase I studies with new substances, unforeseen effects (e.g., allergic reactions) may arise. Therefore, it is essential to carry out clinicopharmacologic studies only in units with suitable emergency equipment and with a staff that is experienced in emergency medicine. Volunteers must receive regular checkups before and during the clinical trial, as well as for a sufficient length of time after the last administration of the drug. To ensure that the volunteer has not taken any other substances before or during the current study, a careful drug anamnesis and a urinalysis for drugs and narcotics are performed. If possible, volunteers should receive yearly checkups, even if they have not participated in a study in the meantime. In exceptional cases, mainly where the use of a new drug in healthy volunteers is not advisable (e.g., cytostatics), first use of the new substance should be tested in voluntary patients.

The aim of investigations during phase I is to study the tolerability of the new substance in humans, to describe the behavior of the compound in the human organism (pharmacokinetics), and, if possible, to deliver first indications on the pharmacodynamic effect of the new substance in humans. Furthermore, undesired effects should be registered at the earliest possible stage, and clinically relevant drug interactions should be clarified.

To receive reliable answers to all these important questions during clinicopharmacologic studies, a close cooperation with biometry is necessary during the planning and evaluation of each individual study. Before each study begins, a suitable study design (e.g., open trial, crossover, single or double blind, group comparison, etc.) must be developed, a sample size for the main targets to be examined must be estimated, and a suitable evaluation method must be determined. During the study, the randomization, inclusion and exclusion criteria, type and time points of measurements, and completeness of the list of findings must be ensured. Before the actual study is started, the study protocol must be inspected by an independent review board (IRB) or an independent ethical committee (IEC), which in Germany is connected to the regional medical council or the universities.

All clinical investigations must be carried out in accordance with the declaration of the World Medical Association of Helsinki (1964) and its modified forms of Tokyo (1975), Venice (1983), Hong Kong (1989), and, the latest, Somerset West (1996). They specify that "…concern for the interests of the subject must always prevail over the interests of science and society". However, it must be emphasized that these recommendations are only guidelines for physicians all over the world; they do not relieve physicians of the ethical or legal requirements of the jurisdictions in which they work.

Safety and tolerability To select the dosage with which a human investigation is to be started is one of the most difficult tasks of the clinical pharmacologist. In general, investigations start with doses of 1/5 to 1/10 the dosage known to be effective from animal investigations or 1/50 to 1/100 the toxicologic "no effect" dose, respectively. Sometimes the first dose chosen is even lower. If these

first dosages are well tolerated by the first volunteers, then the dose is increased gradually by a factor of 2 to 3 under the same investigational conditions up to a range where a therapeutic effect is expected. An increase in dosage above this range up to the occurrence of the first undesired side effects in healthy volunteers (the so-called maximum tolerated dose, MTD) is not generally accepted from a clinicopharmacologic point of view. For this, the risk-benefit relation must be estimated for every case. On the one hand, the entire probable therapeutic dose range should be measured during phase I investigations so as to give optimal treatment to patients with the target indication(s) as long as the safety of the healthy volunteer is ensured. On the other hand, a new molecule may appear to be well tolerated in phase I trials at very large multiples of a pharmacologically effective dose. However, clinical trials at too high a dose may attribute an unacceptable safety profile to an otherwise good drug. I think that the concept of "maximum tolerated dose" is a flawed one and that the early inclusion of a voluntary patient in phase I studies to demonstrate the minimum maximally effective dose is an acceptable compromise.

Since most drugs must be administered repeatedly, multiple-dose administration must be investigated. After each study, the group of responsible physicians discusses the results and decides on further procedures. In this way, the reactions of each volunteer can be analyzed on the basis of measured values in blood and urine, in terms of the electrocardiogram, and in light of blood pressure mon-

---

Table 8.1 Features of phases I to IV of clinical drug development

Phase I
Aims: (1) Tolerability; (2) pharmacokinetics; (3) pharmacodynamics; (4) interactions with other drugs; (5) undesired effects.
Results: (1) First tolerability assessment; (2) basic pharmacokinetics after single dose and under steady-state conditions known; (3) data on pharmacologic effect (if available by noninvasive methods) known; (4) determination of the first dose in patients and the dosing interval; (5) first data on the frequency of undesired effects known; (6) decision on continuation of clinical investigation

Phase II (first use in patients; therapeutic exploratory studies)
Aims: (1) Pharmacodynamics; (2) efficacy; (3) dose-finding (minimal, optimal and maximal well tolerated effective dose); (4) relative tolerability; (5) special pharmacokinetics.
Results: (1) Dose range and dosing interval known; (2) extensive pharmacodynamics known; (3) extensive pharmacokinetics known; (4) first estimate on tolerability in patients; (5) decision on continuation of clinical investigation

Phase III (wide-ranging clinical investigation; therapeutic confirmation studies)
Aims: (1) Confirm efficacy and tolerability in larger numbers of patients - of different ages and sex - in different countries - of different races - of different life-styles + eating habits; (2) type and frequency of adverse drug events; (3) treatment of patients with impaired liver or kidney function and of geriatric patients; (4) long-term clinical trial - tolerance development - general tolerability - interactions with other drugs - information about side effects; (5) comparison with established treatment methods; (6) long-term efficacy in chronic diseases
Results: (1) Indications and contraindications known; (2) dose- and concentration-response-relationship demonstrated; (3) type, duration, and frequency of side-effects known; (4) safety profile established; (5) clinically relevant interactions known (6) comparability or superiority to standard therapy demonstrated; (7) application for registration of the substance accomplished

Phase IV (after approval/registration)
Aims: (1) Recording and assessment of rare adverse drug events; (2) further information about the efficacy and tolerability profile; (3) studies in certain patient populations, e.g., different races, children, etc.; (4) long-term field studies to assess the influence of the treatment on morbidity and mortality (intervention studies); (5) further information about drug interaction.
Results: (1) Secured knowledge on the value of the new drug regarding efficacy and tolerability (drug safety); (2) knowledge of the influence on morbidity and mortality; (3) possible discovery of new indications

itoring before the next step of the investigation. Only under these conditions may the tolerability and safety of a substance be judged correctly, which is required prior to the start of phase II. During these tolerability studies, parallel investigations are started on chronic animal toxicity.

Pharmacokinetic investigations The aim of pharmacokinetic investigations of a new drug in humans is to determine the behavior of the compound within the human organism, i.e., a clarification of questions regarding absorption, bioavailability, distribution, metabolism, and excretion. If a new substance is administered to a human being for the first time during phase I, the pharmacokineticist measures the concentration in plasma and compares it with the results of preclinical pharmacokinetic investigations. With the aid of these findings, data related to efficacy, tolerability, and toxicology are easier to transfer from animals to humans. In the process of clinical development, differences between individuals are evaluated and the influence of illnesses and concomitant medication is described. By correlating efficacy and concentration curves, pharmacokineticists contribute to finding the best drug form, the right dosage, and the optimal dosing scheme. Since drugs are developed today for an international market, pharmacokineticists are able to deliver valuable information by describing common interests as well as differences between different cultures and races. In contrast with preclinical pharmacokinetics, in clinical pharmacology only a limited number of volunteers and patients may be recruited to investigate pharmacokinetic parameters. Therefore, clinical pharmacology has developed mathematical procedures that allow one to describe the most important kinetic parameters on the basis of relatively few data in plasma and urine, as well as in other body fluids and tissues, if necessary and justifiable. These procedures permit pharmacokineticists to make statements, for example, on the rate and extent of absorption, residence time of the drug in the organism, and the primary routes of elimination.

If the drug is destined for chronic administration, investigations also must be carried out after multiple administrations. Results must reveal if and to what extent pharmacokinetic target parameters change until the "steady-state condition" is reached. Studies on absolute and relative bioavailability must provide information on the rate at which and extent to which the effective substance reaches the systemic circulation or the target organ after the final galenic drug formulation has been developed. A possible influence of food intake on pharmacokinetics also should be evaluated at an early stage. One of the requirements for pharmacokinetic investigations in humans is the availability of a selective, precise analytical method. As a result of continuing advances in methodology, it may already be possible to determine the presence of most substances in human blood or urine after the administration of very small doses. In many cases it is possible to determine the kinetics of the most important metabolites by using nonradioactive products. Otherwise,

an investigation with radioactively labeled material must be performed in phase II after proof of efficacy has been achieved.

The aim of pharmacokinetic studies during phase I in healthy volunteers is to receive first-hand information about dose, dosing interval, and optimal route and form of administration and to identify risk groups. Further investigations on tolerability and pharmacokinetics of a new drug, e.g., in elderly volunteers or in patients with liver and kidney failure, should only be carried out after the first signs of efficacy in patients with the target indication(s) have been collected during phase II. This also applies to investigations of interactions with other substances. These types of investigations should be performed only in healthy volunteers and patients and should be of proven clinical relevance, i.e., that interactions with other drugs are expected on the basis of their pharmacokinetic and pharmacodynamic properties.

Pharmacodynamic investigations Besides gathering data on tolerability and pharmacokinetics, the aim of phase I investigations must be to determine the pharmacodynamic effects of the new substance on healthy volunteers, i.e., the clinicopharmacologic effects, which are similar to the experimental findings in animals but not comparable as far as therapeutic efficacy is concerned. Efficacy is always connected to a therapeutic goal and may only be determined in patients with the target indication(s).

In order to measure pharmacodynamic effects in healthy volunteers, sensitive, noninvasive methods are needed. In addition, these methods must be safe and reproducible, and they must deliver findings that are comparable with the results of invasive methods. They are designed to show correlations between plasma concentration, dosage, and pharmacodynamic effect so as to determine a dose range suitable for therapeutic use and provide information on the time of maximal effect, the duration of effect, and the decline of that effect. Furthermore, the influence on essential or vitally important organs or organ systems after therapeutic dosages must be examined, and if possible, the working mechanism must be explained. During recent years, very sensitive, noninvasive methods have been developed that have gained an increasing significance for the evaluation of drug effects in clinical pharmacology. These methods mainly evaluate the cardiovascular system (e.g., ergometry, echocardiography, Doppler sonography, and venous occlusion plethysmography), the respiratory system (e.g., spirography, ergospirometry, whole-body plethysmography, and interruption methods including provocation tests or blood-gas and respiratory-gas analyses), the gastrointestinal system (e.g., esophageal manometry, pH-metry, H_2 breath test, and abdominal ultrasonography), and the central nervous system (e.g., electroencephalography with evoked potentials, psychometric tests, pain stimulating tests, electromyography, pupillometry, transcranial Doppler sonography, and visual scales). Which of these methods is finally included into the study protocol besides the biochemical investigations depends on the working spectrum of the new substance as well as the criteria chosen for the surveillance of the physiologic factors.

Result of clinicopharmacologic investigations After the first clinicopharmacologic profile of the new drug has been established by investigations of tolerability, pharmacokinetics, and pharmacologic effects in healthy volunteers during phase I and a decision has been made to continue the clinical trial, the aim is now to answer the important question of the therapeutic efficacy in patients with the target indication(s). The more thorough the studies carried out during phase I, the earlier a decision can be made on continuation or discontinuation of further development, thus avoiding additional risks and costs. However, this does not automatically stop all clinicopharmacologic investigations. Transition to further phases of clinical study is gradual. Besides investigations of tolerability and pharmacokinetics in subpopulations, patients with liver and kidney failure, as well as patients with additional illnesses and concomitant drug intake, are examined. The aim is to establish concentration- and dose-effect correlations with the help of the treating physician in patients with the target indication(s). The purpose of these so-called dose-finding studies is to establish the dosages and, if concentration-response relations are measurable, the concentrations at which minimal, mean, and maximal effects can be achieved or undesired side effects may occur. The aim of these key studies in drug development is to make sure that each patient is treated with the dose that is optimal for him/her.

Phases II to IV of clinical drug investigations

The next phase of clinical trials consists of small-scale studies for additional safety and clinical pharmacology, as well as preliminary efficacy studies in patients (phase II studies, i.e., therapeutic exploratory studies). To begin with, the first signs for efficacy, dose finding, and relative tolerability in patients with the target indication(s) are collected during phase IIa in a pilot study in one or two hospitals before this knowledge is ensured and completed during phase IIb by recruiting a larger number of patients. If during phase II of the clinical investigation it was clearly demonstrated that the substance under investigation works for one or the other of the target indications, which doses are necessary, and which side effects are expected, these results must be manifested during phase III in a larger number of patients (several hundred to several thousand) under practical hospital conditions or with general practitioners (phase III studies, i.e., therapeutic confirmation studies). These results are then carefully collected. They provide information on indications and contraindications; dose- and concentration-response relationships; type, duration, and frequency of side effects; long-term tolerability and rare side effects; clinically relevant interactions; and comparability with or superiority to standard therapy. They are the basis for all licensing applications at the responsible health authorities. After the licensing number has been presented, the new drug is launched. However, the launch of a drug is by far not the end of the surveillance and test phase. Only by critical, long-term control is the position of a new drug within the entire spectrum of drugs determined.

Phase IV of the clinical investigation (i.e., therapeutic use) involves recognition and evaluation of extremely rare side effects that appear only after the drug is administered to many people of different genetic, cultural, and social origins; confirmation of long-term tolerability and quantification of therapeutic risk; scientific confirmation of the therapeutic concept, as well as differentiation between other therapeutic measures during treatment of the same illness; and discovery of new indications. Phase IV studies also include costly intervention trials that are directed not only toward demonstrating the drug's specific therapeutic effect in a desired area but also toward elucidating the drug's overall positive effect on morbidity and mortality. A number of countries request that so-called empiric reports be presented at certain time intervals after registration has taken place on the basis of data received during phase IV. In rare situations, it may be necessary to change the indications on the basis of these investigations during phase IV.

Owing to the increasing costs of clinical development, and given that the traditional approach required considerable resources to estimate therapeutic success and may have resulted in overdosing, the objectives and process of clinical drug development have been changing.

Instead of moving from discovery through development phases in sequential steps, drug development should be streamlined, combining preclinical and early clinical development (phase I and IIa) as an exploratory stage and phase IIb/III as a confirmatory stage. Exploratory development consists of all preclinical and clinical work required to answer all questions related to key failure points and to the likelihood for success at an earlier stage, whereas in the confirmatory stage unequivocal demonstration of effectiveness and safety should be made in a multicenter clinical trial in a large number of patients. The key question is, "How can we show benefit of our NCE without spending the large amounts of money associated with large clinical trials in the confirmatory stage (traditional phase IIb/III)?" or, in other words, "How can we improve the quality of decisions in the exploratory stage of drug development?". At first, due to its fundamental influence on informativeness and efficiency of the drug development process, clinical pharmacology as a link between research and development, must be fully integrated in the discovery evaluation of the new compound and in all phases of drug develoment.

Discovery experiments should be done to critically evaluate the compound and the "killer" experiments should be done as soon as possible avoiding the "ostrich principle". Genomic technology should be used to identify novel, proprietary, disease-related targets and to characterize preclinical test systems. Pharmacogenomics is the study of how a patient's response to a drug is affected by his/her genes. It addresses the question of why different patients respond to the same drug in different ways. In terms of clinical trial patients, to select putatively responsive patient groups for large clinical trials may prevent selecting the wrong patient population and avoid expensive repetition of these trials. More sophisticated clinical pharmacokinetics would answer the question if the drug is present at the disease site for a sufficient time. The integration of pharmacokinetic and pharmacodynamic principles into drug development called "the pharmacokinetic-pharmacodynamic guided approach during phase 0 of drug development" contributes to making drug development more rational and more efficient. One of the major roles of PK/PD data in drug development is to provide information on concentration-effect-relationships and on the variability associated with the effects.

The appropriate use of surrogates and models may be significant in determining drug actions in humans and in assisting in dose selection. Taking respsonsibility for the development and validation of new surrogates and models gives clinical pharmacologists a major opportunity to assume a pivotal role in drug development.

OUTLOOK

Despite considerable success in medical research, most diseases known today are not treated causally but rather only symptomatically. For instance, in the case of heart failure or coronary heart disease, certain complaints of the patient, such as shortness of breath or angina pectoris, may be alleviated or improved by the administration of drugs such as diuretics, cardiac glycosides, angiotensin-converting enzyme (ACE) inhibitors, nitrates, beta-blockers, or calcium antagonists; however, the actual cause of the illness cannot be treated, and symptoms reappear after drug administration is stopped. A therapy that is able to fight the cause of the disease, in the sense that a complete cure is achieved, is available in only approximately 10% of all illnesses. For diseases without a cure so far, such as AIDS, cancer, rheumatism, and Alzheimer's disease, intensive drug research is a must for humanitarian, medical, social, political, and economic reasons.

An analysis of registered, already-marketed drugs during recent years shows that despite enhanced efforts and dramatically rising development costs, the innovative potential of the classic approach to the discovery of new drugs is steadily decreasing. Therefore, and in order to make sure that drug research does not wind up a dead-end street, it is absolutely necessary to develop new, innovative drugs with the help of new technologies such as molecular and cell biology, gene technology or immunology, and combinatorial chemistry and robot-supported substance screening. The most significant scientific scenario that could set the stage for a new burst of innovation is the combination of genomic science and combinatorial chemistry.

Genetic factors participate in the development of many human diseases. Information about genetic disease-causing mechanisms and explanations of their pathophysiology are likely to be significant in the development of new therapies. At present, most drug researchers use databanks containing gene sequences very much like libraries. If they are working on a particular class of receptors, enzymes, or signaling proteins, they can use the library to see what other related structures exist and what their functions might be. If, on the other hand, the function of all or most of the estimated 100,000 genes in the human body were to be known, this information not only would be valuable as a reference, but it could, indeed, become the starting point for a large number of drug discovery programs and could revolutionize drug research. The inevitable conclusion is that a well-balanced further development of gene technology is an important goal for responsible health politics.

However, society also must become aware that good health care has a price. Although current public perceptions often focus on cost rather than value, in some quarters, pharmaceuticals are increasingly being seen as the most cost-effective form of health care.

Suggested readings _____

DiMasi JA, Hansen RW, Graboswki HG, Lasagna L. Cost of innovation in the pharmaceutical industry. J Health Econ 1991;10:107-42.

Drews J. The impact of globalization on pharmaceutical research and development. Drug Inform J 1993;27:1059-64.

Kaitin KJ, Mattisen N, Northington FK, Lasagna L. The drug lag: An update of new drug introductions in the United States and in the United Kingdom, 1977 through 87. Clin Pharmacol Ther 1989;46:121-38.

Kuhlmann J. Wirkung und Wirksamkeit von Arzneimitteln. Arzneimitteltherapie 1988;6:43-50

Lis Y, Walker SR. Novel medicines marketed in the U.K. (1960-1987). Br J Clin Pharmacol 1989;28:333-43.

MacInnes R, Lumley CE, Walker SR. New chemical entity output of the international pharmaceutical industry from 1970 to 1992. Clin Pharmacol Ther 1994;56:339-49.

Roland R. The contribution of clinical pharmacology surrogates and models to drug development: a critical appraisal. Br J Clin Pharmacol 1997;44:219-25.

Tansey IP, Armstrong NA, Walker SR. Trends in pharmaceutical innovation: the introduction of products on the UK Market, 1960-1989. J Pharm Med 1994;4:85-100.

Wurtman RJ, Bettiker RL. The slowing of treatment discovery, 1965-1995. Nature Med 1995;1:1122-5.

Central nervous system

SECTION

2

Central nervous
system

Management of pain

Troels S. Jensen, Ron C. Kupers

Pain can be produced by the application of a noxious or otherwise aversive stimulus. In addition, pain also may result from a disease or from an injury to the peripheral or central nervous system. Apart from treating the underlying disease, it is necessary to relieve patients of their pain.

Our knowledge of the physiologic, biochemical, and molecular mechanisms of pain has increased considerably over the past three decades. This has led to major improvements in the treatment of acute and cancer-related pain. In contrast, progress in the treatment of many chronic pain conditions, in particular neuropathic pain, has been at a slower pace. Today, we are still facing the fact that many patients with chronic pain cannot be treated adequately with the available therapeutic armamentarium. In the pharmacologic treatment of acute pain, aspirin-like and morphine-like drugs still form the keystone of most therapies. In chronic pain conditions, little was known about the underlying physiopathology until recently. Consequently, therapeutic possibilities also remained limited.

DEFINITION AND CHARACTERISTICS OF PAIN

Acute pain and chronic pain

Acute pain results from the activation of nociceptors — a specific group of high-threshold receptors — by a noxious stimulus. After encoding at the nociceptor level, the noxious information is carried to the central nervous system (CNS) by specific populations of afferent nerve fibers, the unmyelinated C fibers and the small myelinated A-delta fibers. Acute pain is associated with a number of autonomic, psychologic, and behavioral responses. At the physiologic level, acute pain induces segmental and suprasegmental reflex responses that help the organism to maintain homeostasis. These include release of glycogen from the liver as an energy source, increased respiration and pulse rate, muscular responses (hypermotility and increased muscle tension), elevation of blood pressure, increased perfusion of high-priority organs (e.g., myocardium, brain, and skeletal muscles), and a concomitant decrease in blood flow to low-priority organs (e.g., gastrointestinal tract and genitourinary tract). These

responses are in proportion to the intensity of the noxious stimulus, and they help the organism to a "fight or flight" type of reaction and later enhance healing.

In contrast, chronic pain is the result of a persistent noxious input to the nervous system resulting in sensitization of central neurons. Alternatively, chronic pain may derive from lesions in the peripheral or central nervous system. Unlike acute pain, chronic pain serves no biologic function; it neither warns the organism against tissue injury nor has a role in the healing process. The autonomic signs that are observed in acute pain are replaced by vegetative signs: sleep disturbances, changes in appetite, reduced libido, irritability, loss of interests, a deterioration in interpersonal relationships, and an increased somatic preoccupation. Many patients with chronic pain deteriorate physically because of disturbances in sleep and appetite and the excessive use of medication.

Clinical pain

From a didactic point of view, pain can be divided into three categories: (1) physiologic pain, (2) inflammatory pain, and (3) neuropathic pain, each having particular characteristics.

Physiologic pain is related to a direct activation of high-threshold heat- and mechanosensitive receptors. The noxious activity is short and self-limited, and within certain limits, there is a linear relationship between stimulus intensity and evoked pain (Fig. 9.1). Physiologic pain is related to an acute activation of afferent pain processing systems and a resulting recruitment of distinct modulatory systems acting at different synaptic relays in the spinal cord and the brain.

Inflammatory pain results from the activation of sensitized and/or silent nociceptors at the site of injury. Inflammatory pain is either provoked or spontaneous, long-lasting, but self-limited. There is a linear relationship between stimulus intensity and pain intensity, but in contrast to the acute nociceptive pain, the stimulus-response curve is shifted to the left. In general, there is a facilitation of afferent noxious inputs to the nervous system, which may give rise to a hyperalgesia with lowering of pain threshold and tenderness (Fig. 9.1).

Classic examples of inflammatory pain are postoperative and posttraumatic pain and arthritis.

Neuropathic pain results from a dysfunction or lesion of the peripheral or the central nervous system. Neuropathic pain can be caused by activity in both low- and high-threshold fibers. This type of pain has a complex stimulus-response curve reflecting both a loss of afferent information and a sensitization of central projecting neurons (Fig. 9.1).

The essential characteristics of neuropathic pain are:
- spontaneous, continuous, and paroxysmal pains;
- allodynia: pain evoked by a nonnoxious stimulus;
- hyperalgesia: increased pain response to noxious stimulus;
- hyperpathia: increased threshold to evoke a sensation and an increased response in the suprathreshold range;
- aftersensations: the persistence of a sensation after cessation of stimulation;
- referred pain: pain in an area distant from the stimulation site;
- wind-up-like pain: increased pain response following repetitive stimulation;
- pain in an area with a sensory deficit.

These phenomena may occur separately or in combination, regardless of the underlying cause. The spontaneous, ongoing pain is usually of a burning character with an overlying unpleasant tingling sensation. Patients also may complain of short (seconds) paroxysmal attacks of sharp, shooting, stabbing, or electric-like pains. The onset of neuropathic pain is often delayed after the causative event, sometimes up to months or even years. Neuropathic pain is often associated with somatosensory deficits, and the distribution of the pain usually encompasses the area of somatosensory dysfunctioning. This holds true for pain of both peripheral and central nervous system origin.

Examples of peripheral neuropathic pain conditions include painful neuropathies, nerve injury pain, postherpetic neuralgia, and postamputation pain. At the spinal level, spinal cord injuries and multiple sclerosis are among the most important types, but certain types of low-back pain also may be due to nerve lesions. At the supraspinal level, the far most common condition is post-stroke pain (formerly termed *thalamic pain*). Although neuropathic pains are less common than the traditional inflammatory and physiologic types of pain, they are important for several reasons: (1) neuropathic pain is in general difficult to diagnose, (2) the mechanisms and treatment of neuropathic pain are distinct, (3) neuropathic pain can persist for years and is a burden for both patients and society, and (4) it is assumed that unrelieved pain in cancer patients is due to unrecognzed neuropathic pain.

PAIN MEASUREMENT

In recent years, important progress has been made in the field of pain measurement. It is now recognized that pain is a complex and multidimensional experience. This has lead to the development of new instruments for pain assessment that take into account these various aspects.

How to measure pain? Unfortunately, there is no "golden standard" for pain measurement.

Outcome measures

In the evaluation of a pharmacologic or nonpharmacologic intervention, therapeutic success is often equated with pain reduction. As a result, many clinicians limit themselves to the measurement of pain and pain relief, thereby overlooking other important aspects of the therapeutic outcome, such as functional improvement or improvement in quality of life.

Pain and pain relief Pain is still often measured only in terms of intensity. However, intensity is just one of the relevant dimensions of the pain sensation. Other dimensions that also should be assessed formally are the pain quality, the temporal profile of the pain, and the affective component. The pain experience has an important sensory component, which can be described in terms of intensity, quality, temporal characteristics, and anatomic distribution.

Pain intensity This is the most frequently assessed dimension of therapeutic outcome. The visual analogue scale (VAS), verbal category scales, and numerical rating scales are used most commonly. An example of a numerical rating scale is the 101-point rating scale, whereby the subject is asked to rate his/her pain by giving a number between 0 (no pain) and 100 (most intense pain). A widely used category scale is the four-point intensity scale (i.e., none, mild, moderate, and severe pain). However, this scale does not have enough levels to accurately

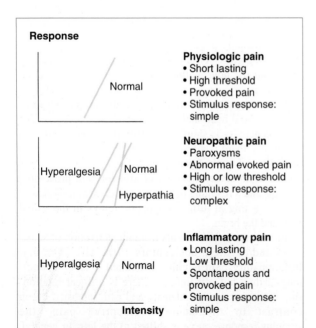

Figure 9.1 The relationship between stimulus intensity and evoked response in three clinical pain conditions: acute (= physiologic) pain, neuropathic pain, and inflammatory pain.

describe treatment effects. Improved category scales with more descriptors are available and should be used instead.

In many clinical pain conditions, pain intensity fluctuates over time. Asking for a mean pain intensity rating leaves the practitioner ignorant about the actual pain levels. In such cases, it may be necessary to rate the percentage of time the pain falls within certain intensity categories. A slightly different approach has been taken in the Brief Pain Inventory (BPI) of Wisconsin, which involves measurement of the pain intensity when it is worst and when it is least and the average pain intensity.

Whereas pain intensity scales focus on the present pain experience, pain relief scores rely on the patient's memory of pain. Since patients tend to overestimate their past pain, the use of pain relief scores may lead to an overestimation of the effects of the treatment, certainly in cases of prolonged follow-up. On the other hand, there is some evidence that pain relief category scales are more sensitive to small reductions in pain.

Pain quality and affect Pain also can be described in qualitative and affective terms. Assessment of pain quality may give important information on the underlying etiology of the pain. There is also evidence that the success of an intervention can be correlated with the qualitative characteristics of the pain. The McGill Pain Questionnaire (MPQ) offers a list of pain quality descriptors. A short form of the MPQ permits an easy and quick estimation of the pain experienced. However, it is not yet clear whether the MPQ can distinguish between different pain categories.

Temporal characteristics of the pain Pain can show different temporal profiles. Pain can be steady (continuous), intermittent, steady and intermittent, or evoked. This can be assessed by simple scales. Since an intervention may exert a differential effect on these components, it is recommended to measure them separately.

Anatomic location of the pain This can be assessed by asking the patient to mark or shade the painful areas on a line drawing. Recently, automated drawing systems have been proposed, and these may be of value for more accurate measurements.

Multiple assessments It is important to distinguish between current pain and usual pain. Usual pain is the average of an individual's report of pain intensity over a specified period of time. The primary outcome variable of interest in a clinical study is a comparison of the average pain experienced before and after the intervention. Single pain intensity ratings offer no reliable measure of average pain because pain reports may change substantially over time. In addition, multiple factors influence pain ratings obtained at a single time point. Therefore, the use of verbal home diaries is advisable. A composite pain intensity score calculated from an average of 12 ratings across 4 days provides a reliable and valid measure of average pain.

Assessment of quality of life and health status An increasing number of clinical trials include measures of quality of life (QoL). These have become an important indicator of treatment "success." Examples of QoL scales that have been validated for chronic pain populations are the Sickness Impact Profile (SIP), the SIP Roland, the West Haven-Yale Multidimensional Pain Inventory, the Nottingham Health Profile, and the SF-36.

Assessment of side effects Side effects can be evaluated by means of a checklist with prespecified events or on the basis of a spontaneous report by the patient. Whereas the checklist may lead to an overreporting of events, the spontaneous report approach may lead to an underestimation of side effects. It is advisable to score each side effect for its severity (i.e., absent, mild, moderate, severe, or very severe).

Determination of "success". A difficult problem in evaluation of the efficacy of a treatment is the definition of the outcome criteria for success. There is a long tradition in using 50% pain reduction as the criterion for success. A valuable alternative to the 50% pain reduction criterion is the use of a total pain relief (TOTPAR) score, which is the area under the curve of pain relief against time. In order to standardize TOTPAR scores, the TOTPAR obtained is divided by the maximal possible TOTPAR score and presented as a %max TOTPAR. Another useful measure is the numbers needed to treat (NNT), which is defined as the number of patients needed to be treated to obtain one patient with more than 50% pain relief. NNT is calculated as 1 divided by the proportion of patients obtaining a certain effect with treatment minus the proportion obtaining the same effect with placebo. A drawback of these success criteria is that they do not take into account patient satisfaction. Patients often balance pain relief against factors such as side effects, expectations, functional improvements, and the cost and benefits of a treatment. In future studies it may be important also to include numbers needed to harm (NNH) values. NNH is the number of patients needed to be treated to find one patient with more than 50% side effects. An effective and useful drug therefore will be one with small NNT and high NNH values, respectively.

Drug therapy

In recent years, our understanding of the mechanisms of clinical pain has increased significantly. In particular, hyperexcitability, an important mechanism for the transition of acute pain to chronic pain, has been elucidated. As a result, many new compounds have been introduced that target this increased excitability.

Analgesia is defined as an abolition of pain in response to a noxious stimulus; in practice, however, there is usually only a partial analgesia. *Analgesics* are defined as drugs that give rise to pain relief without significanlty influencing level of consciousness or other sensory modalities.

From a pharmacologic point of view, analgesics can be

Table 9.1 Antipyretic analgesics

Compound	Bioavailability (oral) (%)	T_{max} (h)	Plasma protein binding (%)	$t_{1/2}$ (h)	Site of action	Antipyretic/anti-inflammatory	Usual daily dose (mg) (adult)
Nonacidic							
Acetaminophen (paracetamol)	75-100	0.5-2	5-50	1,5-2	Spinal cord/nociceptors	+/-	1000-4000
Metamizol	100	1-2	70	7	Spinal cord/nociceptors	+/(-)	500-1000
Acidic							
Acetylsalicylic acid	50-75	2	90	0,25	Nociceptors/CNS	+/+	1000-4000
Diflunisal	75-100	2-3	>98	12	Nociceptors/CNS	+/+	1000
Indomethacin	100	1-2	>90	2-3	Nociceptors/CNS	+/+	50-150
Ibuprofen	75-100	0.5-2	>99	1,5-2,5	Nociceptors/CNS	+/+	900-2400
Ketoprofen	100	1-2	>99	1,5-2,5	Nociceptors/CNS	+/+	150-200
Naproxen	90-100	2-4	>99	12	Nociceptors/CNS	+/+	500-1000
Piroxicam	100	2-3	>99	48	Nociceptors/CNS	+/+	20-40
Phenylbutazone	75-100	2-4	99	72	Nociceptors/CNS	+/+	200-400

divided into (1) antipyretic analgesic drugs, (2) opioid analgesics, (3) sodium channel blockers, (4) antidepressants, (5) NMDA receptor-blocking agents, and (6) other drugs.

ANTIPYRETIC ANALGESICS

These drugs can be subdivided into acidic and nonacidic compounds. Whereas the acidic drugs show anti-inflammatory activity, the nonacidic lack such an activity. Table 9.1 summarizes the pharmacology of various drugs belonging to this class, therapeutic dosages, and side effects.

Arachidonic acid released from membrane phospholipids following tissue injury is transformed via cyclooxygenase and lipoxygenase into prostaglandins and leukotrienes, respectively. Prostaglandins stimulate nociceptors in the region of tissue injury. In addition, prostaglandins also sensitize nociceptors, probably by lowering the threshold for activating polymodal C-nociceptors. The acidic antipyretic drugs have a peripheral site of action. Acetylsalicylic acid (ASA) and other antipyretics inhibit the synthesis of prostaglandins from arachidonic acid by a competitive and noncompetitive interaction with cyclooxygenase. Subsequent studies revealed that cyclooxygenase exists in two isoforms, a constitutive form (COX1) and an inducible form (COX2) that appears after inflammation (see Chap. 44). In addition to a clear peripheral effect, antipyretics also have a central action. Nonsteroidal anti-inflammatory drugs (NSAIDs) also may have an analgesic effect via an action at different brain sites.

The list of existing NSAID drugs is extensive. There is at present no documented difference between different NSAIDs acting as COX1 inhibitors. It remains to be seen whether the new COX2 inhibitors will have a better clinical effect than the existing ones. Antipyretics generally are used for mild to moderate types of pain. Acute and chronic types of pain associated with inflammation of different etiology form an indication for acidic antipyretic drugs. Typical examples are arthritis, posttraumatic pain, postoperative pain, cancer pain, burn injury, myofascial pain, and headache. Indications for nonacidic anti-inflammatory drugs are visceral types of pain with colics, cancer pain in the early phase with mild to moderate pain, headache, and acute types of pain with no signs of inflammation. In general, the time period for analgesic treatment with NSAIDs should be limited to a few weeks or months because of the risk of adverse effects following long-term exposure.

Adverse effects

The major adverse effects of the antipyretic analgesics are allergic reactions and gastrointestinal (GI) disturbances. GI ulcers and bleeding are severe problems occurring with almost all drugs apart from the nonacidic antipyretic analgesics. The reported frequency of GI side effects is up to 30%. The risk increases markedly in the elderly. Other important side effects are allergic manifestations and renal, bone marrow, and liver impairment. Although there are differences among drugs, adverse effects are generally seen after the prolonged use of most NSAIDs.

SPECIFIC ANTIPYRETIC ANALGESIC DRUGS

ASA is a potent inhibitor of cyclooxygenase, exerting both peripheral and central actions. Notwithstanding, its main therapeutic action is a peripheral one with both antipyretic and anti-inflammatory components. The anti-inflammatory effect occurs with doses up to 4 to 6 g per day. It is contraindicated in patients with peptic ulcer or other conditions with increased risk of bleeding.

Among analgesic NSAIDs, diflunisal is a derivative of ASA with a similar mechanism of action. It is readily absorbed from the GI tract. Stable plasma levels are obtained within 4 to 5 days following a diflunisal dose of 0.5 g twice daily. Diflunisal is excreted in a glucuronated form by the kidneys. Other NSAIDs may be used for specific painful conditions such as gout (see Chap. 71).

Acetaminophen (paracetamol) has analgesic and antipyretic effects but no anti-inflammatory effects. Its main action is assumed to be at the level of the dorsal horn. Acetaminophen is readily absorbed from the GI tract and metabolized in the liver. It is excreted by the renal route, and the plasma half-life is 2 to 3 hours. After overdosing with acetaminophen (>8 g), a reactive metabolite is formed that may give rise to hepatic centrilobular necrosis. The hepatic necrosis becomes manifest within 2 to 4 days of ingestion. Consequently, acetaminophen is contraindicated in severe hepatic and renal insufficiency.

OPIOIDS

The use of opium – the juice of the poppy seed (*Papaver somniferum*) – in pain treatment dates back more than 3000 years. There is a long list of natural and synthetic opioids that all have morphine-like properties. Opioids belong to the most powerful analgesics that are used for severe acute and chronic painful conditions, in particular malignant pain (see below).

Chemical structure and classification

Opioids exert their effects by interacting with one or several classes of opioid receptors termed μ (mu), κ (kappa), and ∂ (delta). These receptors bind to both synthetic and naturally occurring opioid peptides. Three distinct families of opioid peptides have been identified: the enkephalins, the endorphins, and the dynorphins. They all bind to G-proteins in the cell membrane, displaying seven transmembrane-spanning loops. Opioids hyperpolarize the cell membrane by increasing an inward-directed K^+ channel and a concurrent inhibition of a voltage-dependent Ca^{2+} channel. While the latter mechanism corresponds to a presynaptic inhibition of afferent transmitter release, the former reflects a postsynaptic activation of K^+ channels. Opioids may produce analgesic effects in the mesencephalic periaqueductal gray matter and reticular formation, the rostroventral medulla, the thalamus, the amygdala, and the cortex. Opioids produce their analgesic action by at least three different mechanisms: (1) recruitment of descending inhibitory systems from brain to the spinal cord, (2) activation of an ascending inhibitory system originating in the brainstem and projecting to thalamus and forebrain, and (3) a local inhibitory effect at the level of either the peripheral nociceptor, the dorsal horn of the spinal cord, or the different relays in the brain and brainstem.

Pharmacokinetics

Following oral administration, opioids are absorbed almost completely. The analgesic effect of orally administered opioids is two- to fourfold less than that seen after a corresponding parenteral administration due to a "first pass" metabolic action in the liver. The more lipid-soluble opioids have a faster onset of action than the water-soluble ones. Because of differences in the intestinal and hepatic metabolism of different opioids, there is a large variability in bioavailability. Opioids are eliminated mainly following hepatic metabolism, and the $t^1/_2$ is generally short. Table 9.2 presents a summary of the pharmacokinetics of different opioids.

Pharmacodynamic effect

The activity of opioids is related to both the affinity and the

---

Table 9.2 Opioid analgesics

Compound	Bioavailability (%)	T_{max} (h)	$t_{1/2}$ (h)	Potency ratio	Duration of action (h)
Codeine	60-70	1-2	15	0.1	6
Tramadol	60-70	1-2	5-6	0.1	6
Dextropropoxyphene	-	1-2	8-24	-	5
Methadone	80-100	0.5-1	15-40	2-4	8
Meperidine (Pethidine)	50-60	2-3	2-5	0.125	3
Pentazocine	20	0.75-1	2-3	0.125-0.25	3
Sufentanil	-	0.25	-	1000	0.5
Buprenorphine (sublingual)	50-60	1-1.5	3	70	6-8
Slow release morphine	-	3-5	-	-	-
Morphine oral	-	1-1.5	1-7	1	4
Morphine parenteral	-	0.5-1	1-7	3	3
Ketobemidone	25-50	1-1.5	2-3	1.5	4
Oxycodone	-	-	-	1	4

(Potency ratio = multiply dose with potency ratio to obtain equivalent dose of morphine.)

efficacy of the specific agent to the receptor. Agents that produce their action by occupation of a small fraction of available receptors have a greater efficacy than agents with a lesser action on the same fraction of opioid receptors. The rank order of the analgesic potency of commonly used opioids is sufentanil > buprenorphine > morphine (Tab. 9.2).

Pain relief

Opioids produce pain relief by their ability to change pain perception without significantly altering other sensory qualities. While opioids have a limited, if any, effect on the pain threshold, their effect on pain tolerance is more distinct. The analgesic effect of opioids is largely attributable to a major effect on the affective component of pain processing and only to a lesser extent on the sensory-discriminative aspect of pain. While pain is still perceived following opioid administration, its unpleasantness is much reduced. It is assumed that long-lasting constant deep pain is more effectively relieved than short-lasting sharp pain. Although the potency of individual opioids differs considerably (Tab. 9.2), the ratio between analgesic and limiting side effects (respiratory depression) appears to be similar across drugs.

Respiratory and cough depression

Opioids exert a depressant effect on the respiratory center in the brainstem by reducing its sensitivity to CO_2. Opioids often also reduce the cough reflex, but there is no simple relation between cough and respiratory depression, suggesting that these effects are mediated by different receptor types. Particular attention should be paid to patients with a reduced ventilatory capacity.

GI effects

Opioids exert a series of effects on GI function, including a reduction in intestinal motility, an increase in intestinal tone, and reduced secretion from pancreatic, biliary, and intestinal glands. This leads to constipation, one of the most disturbing adverse effects associated with the use of opioids.

Urinary effects

Opioids increase the tone of the urinary tract, resulting in urinary retention.

Emetic and miotic effects

Several opioids affect the chemoreceptive center in the medulla. This may cause emesis, the severity of which varies considerably with individual drugs. A miotic effect, due to an action on the cholinergic part of the oculomotor nucleus in the mesencephalon, is seen almost invariably.

Pruritus

Itching is seen with the use of several opioids. It is probably related to a release of skin histamine.

Tolerance and dependency

As a result of repeated opioid administrations, tolerance may develop; the opioid dose has to be increased to obtain the same analgesic action (see Chap. 81). There is also cross-tolerance with other opioid drugs. Besides analgesic tolerance, tolerance also develops to the respiratory depressant and euphoric effects of opioids. Tolerance to the GI effects is rare, implying that constipation persists. Psychological dependency also may develop, which means that the individual has a craving for the drug in order to obtain an euphoric action. This occurs typically among drug addicts and is seen only rarely in chronic pain patients.

Indications

Opioids are used for the treatment of severe acute and cancer-related pain. They are most effective for visceral and deep somatic types of pain. It has been claimed that opioids are not effective for neuropathic pain, but recent studies have shown that certain neuropathic pain conditions such as postherpetic neuralgia and traumatic nerve injury pain do show a clear, albeit limited response to opioids.

Contraindications

Morphine is contraindicated in mild and recurrent nonmalignant pain conditions such as intermittent visceral pain, migraine, and most myofascial disorders. In conditions with respiratory insufficiency, opioids must be used with care. The same holds true for use in patients with increased intracranial pressure because a slight elevation in $PaCO_2$ may further increase pressure.

SPECIFIC OPIOID DRUGS

Morphine Following oral administration, morphine is readily absorbed from the upper part of the intestines. However, the bioavailability of oral morphine is low (35%) due to a large "first pass" metabolism in the liver. Morphine is metabolized to morphine-3-glucuronide and morphine-6-glucuronide by conjugation with glucuronic acid. It is estimated that 65% of administered morphine is converted to these metabolites. While morphine-6-glucuronide is an active metabolite with profound analgesic activity, morphine-3-glucuronide lacks such activity. Long-term morphine treatment increases the bioavailability because of an accumulation of the morphine-6-glucuronide. Morphine-3-glucuronide may have toxic effects, which in part can be responsible for the myoclonus and hyperalgesia seen following high doses of morphine.

After epidural administration, less than 20% of the morphine passes the dura, and the rest is absorbed systemically. Owing to morphine's high water and low fat solubility, the onset of analgesia is slow and the duration correspondingly long (8-10 h).

Fentanyl Fentanyl is a synthetic lipophilic opioid with an analgesic potency that is 100-fold higher than that of morphine. It is mainly used for spinal or transdermal administration. Its action is maximal within 5 minutes, and the duration of action is correspondingly short (<30 min). Owing to its high fat solubility, it can be used for transdermal administration. Fentanyl patches are available commercially. They are indicated for malignant types of pain.

Buprenorphine Buprenorphine is a highly lipophilic mixed opioid agonist/antagonist with an analgesic potency that is 25- to 50-fold higher than that of morphine. It is mainly used for sublingual administration, with a bioavailability of approximately 50%. Its duration of action is 8 to 10 hours.

Methadone Methadone is a synthetic μ-receptor agonist with a complex pharmacokinetic profile. Following oral administration, it is readily absorbed from the intestine with a bioavailability of 80%. Whereas the initial half-life is 12 to 14 hours, this can increase to 24 hours following long-term treatment. There is a risk of accumulation after high single doses administered within a short interval.

Codeine Codeine is a prodrug of morphine. Following oral administration, it is readily absorbed with a bioavailability of 60 to 70%. Approximately 10% of codeine is metabolized into morphine in the liver. Poor CYP2D6 metabolizers (see Chap. 6) may show a reduced metabolic conversion and, consequently, a reduced analgesic effect. On a milligram basis, codeine's analgesic action corresponds to 650 mg ASA, and its duration of action is around 4 hours. The main side effects of codeine are GI, particularly constipation.

Tramadol Tramadol is a synthetic drug with combined μ-receptor agonist and norepinephrine reuptake properties. It is readily absorbed from the GI tract. It undergoes polymorphic CYP2D6-mediated transformation to an active metabolite; poor metabolizers are therefore almost insensitive to the analgesic effect. Tramadol is mainly used for moderately intense pain, both of the nociceptive and neuropathic types.

Naloxone Naloxone is an opioid antagonist with affinity to μ, κ, and σ receptors. Although animal studies show that small doses of naloxone may have a slight analgesic effect, this is without clinical relevance. Naloxone is used mainly to treat opioid overdosing phenomena. It is administered parenterally, usually intravenously, in a dose of 0.4 to 0.8 mg, and within a few minutes it antagonizes all opioid actions associated with μ-receptor stimulation (see Chaps. 80 and 81). Naloxone's action is short-lasting, with a plasma half-life of 1 hour. This may necessitate repeated administrations.

Opioids combined with other drugs Several combinations of weak opioids with other analgesics exist (e.g., antipyretic analgesics with codeine). One of the most commonly used preparations contains 500 mg ASA and 10 mg codeine. However, there is no clear evidence for a higher efficacy of this preparation than for ASA alone. In contrast, 500 mg acetaminophen combined with 25 mg codeine has been shown to be more effective than either drug administered alone.

SODIUM CHANNEL BLOCKERS

In the normal primary afferent neuron, where somatic inputs are translated into appropriate firing patterns, the encoding region is located at the very end of the peripheral axon. Na^+ is important in this process. However, this capacity is absent over the rest of the axon. Even when strong stimuli are applied, the midnerve portion of afferent axons is incapable of generating sustained action potentials. In contrast to normal axons, the midpart of chronically injured afferents develops foci of ectopic activity. This results in spontaneous firing and in abnormal responses to a wide range of externally applied stimuli. Microneurographic recordings in humans have shown that the activity induced

Table 9.3 Sodium channel blockers

Compound	Mechanisms of action	Pain condition	Start dose (mg/day)	Usual daily dose (mg)	Side effects
Carbamazepine	Sodium channel block	Trigeminal neuralgia Diabetic neuropathy Poststroke pain	150	600-900	Dizziness, sedation, rash
Oxcarbazepine	Sodium channel block	Trigeminal neuralgia	300	1200-1600	Dizziness, sedation, rash, low plasma Na^+
Phenytoin	Sodium channel block	Trigeminal neuralgia Diabetic neuropathy	100	250-350	Sedation, dizziness, ataxia
Mexiletine	Sodium channel block	Diabetic neuropathy	100	400-600	Nausea, vomiting, dizziness
Lamotrigine	Sodium channel block Inhibition of glutamate release	Diabetic neuralgia	25	100-200	Sedation, rash

at the ectopic neural pacemaker site is at the basis of the observed paresthesia and pain. The abnormal ectopic firing is produced by an accumulation of Na+ channels at places where myelin is stripped from large-diameter axons, in the neuroma end bulb and in unmyelinated axon sprouts in the neuroma. Administration of the Na+ channel blockers tetrodotoxin (TTX) or lidocaine at the level of the neuroma can suppress ectopic firing.

Sodium channel blockers are mainly of two types: tetrodotoxin-sensitive (TTXs) and tetrodotoxin-resistant (TTXr) ones. These channels are present in the CNS and in sensory nerves, respectively. The preceding data provide a rationale for the beneficial effect of Na+ channel blockers such as local anesthetics and carbamazepine on neuropathic pain. A numbers of drugs are known to exert a blocking effect on the TTXr channels. This list includes carbamazepine, oxcarbazepine, phenytoin, lidocaine, mexiletine, and lamotrigine (see Chap. 10). These drugs have all been used in neuropathic pain conditions (Tab. 9.3). Early support for an analgesic effect of carbamazepine in neuropathic pain comes from studies showing that carbamazepine inhibits the spontaneous activity in experimental neuromas.

More recently, it was reported that carbamazepine significantly reduces spontaneous activity and evoked responses (to both noxious and innocuous stimuli) of dorsal horn neurons. However, only in a limited number of chronic pain conditions is the preceding basic evidence matched by similar evidence from controlled clinical trials. Carbamazepine has been shown to have an analgesic effect in patients with trigeminal neuralgia, but there is at present no evidence that carbamazepine has an effect on other types of face pain. Carbamazepine and phenytoin are also effective in the treatment of pain resulting from diabetic neuropathy. Apart from these drugs, there is only limited, if any, evidence for an analgesic effect of sodium channel blockers or other anticonvulsants in neuropathic and other types of chronic pain. Nevertheless, these drugs are used widely in chronic pain conditions. For example, valproate is often used for many conditions of so-called neuropathic pain. Lamotrigine is a sodium channel blocker with an additional weak glutamate

reducing capacity. Lamotrigine titrated to a dose of 100 mg bid can be used effectively as an add-on therapy in patients with trigeminal neuralgia.

Several new drugs whose action depends partially or completely on a sodium channel blocking effect are currently under investigation. Systemic treatment with local anesthetics such as lidocaine has been introduced within the last decade. Controlled trials have documented that systemically administered lidocaine in a dose of 5 mg/kg intravenously for 30 to 60 minutes has an analgesic effect. This effect occurs at a plasma concentration above 1 to 3 µg/kg. Continuous monitoring of blood pressure and electrocardiogram is necessary. Lidocaine is particularly effective in hyperalgesia associated with neuropathic pain, but its mechanism of action is not known in detail. In many peripheral neuropathic pain conditions, sodium channels are upregulated, and new channels are expressed in the periphery and in dorsal root ganglion (DRG) cells. DRG neurons expressing sodium channels are 10-fold more susceptible to lidocaine than the peripheral nerve terminals. Besides its sodium channel-blocking capacity, lidocaine probably also affects secondary-transmission neurons, and it has been suggested that it can block long-term potentiation by interfering with secondary messenger systems. Controlled trials have shown that the analgesic effect of lidocaine may outlast lidocaine plasma levels for days or even weeks.

ANTIDEPRESSANTS

Antidepressants are among the most widely used drugs for chronic pain conditions. They are indicated mainly for neuropathic pain conditions. Antidepressants have been divided into tricyclic antidepressants (TCAs), tetracyclic antidepressants (TTCAs), serotonin reuptake inhibitors (SSRIs), and noncyclic antidepressants. The most widely studied drugs are the TCAs, for which there is ample evidence that they exert potent analgesic effects in certain chronic pain conditions.

Pharmacokinetics and dosing

The pharmacokinetics of these drugs are described in Chapter 13.

Table 9.4 Mechanisms of action of TCAs

Compound	Monoamine reuptake inhibition		Receptor block				
	5-HT	NE	Musc. cholinergic	α-adrenergic	H₁-histaminergic	NMDA	Sodium channel
Tricyclic antidepressants							
Imipramine	+	+	+	+	+	(+)	+
Amitriptyline	+	+	+	+	+	+	+
Clomipramine	+	+	+	+	+	NA	
Desipramine	-	+	+	+	(+)	NA	+
Nortriptyline	-	+	+	+	(+)	NA	+

(NA = not assessed.)

The TCAs imipramine, clomipramine, and amitriptyline are powerful 5-hydroxytryptamine (5-HT, serotonin) reuptable blockers. Since their metabolites also block the reuptake of norepinephrine (NE), these drugs are considered balanced reuptake blockers of both 5-HT and NE. Desipramine and nortriptyline, on the other hand, have a selective effect on NE reuptake. In addition to their reuptake activity, TCAs also exert an inhibitory effect on α-adrenergic, histaminergic, and cholinergic receptors, and they have a membrane-stabilizing effect, probably due to their Na^+ channel blocking action. Finally, a weak NMDA receptor-blocking effect has been demonstrated recently for some of these drugs. Table 9.4 present an overview of the pharmacodynamic activity of the various antidepressants used.

TCAs have a specific analgesic effect that can be separated from their well-known antidepressant action. The onset of the analgesia is faster and requires a lower plasma concentration, and pain is relieved equally well in depressed and nondepressed patients.

Indications for the TCAs

Consistent with the multitude of actions of TCAs, these drugs differ markedly in their activity in patients with chronic pain, in particular neuropathic pain. About 60% of patients do get some pain relief from TCAs, but only rarely is complete pain relief obtained. Controlled trials have documented an analgesic effect of TCAs for the following conditions: painful diabetic neuropathy, postherpetic neuralgia, posttraumatic nerve injury pain, central poststroke pain, chronic tension-type headache, migraine (prophylaxis), and chronic pain of unknown etiology.

Side effects

TCAs are associated with a long list of side effects, which can be attributed to their interaction with several receptor systems. Approximately 25% of enrolled patients in controlled trials drop out because of side effects. Elderly patients usually experience more severe side effects. Side effects of TCA include anticholinergic: dry mouth, accommodation difficulty, palpitation, micturition problems; antihistaminergic: sedation; α-adrenergic blockade: hypotension, dizziness, nausea; and sodium channel blockade: heart conduction disturbances, negative inotropic effect.

EXCITATORY AMINO ACID ANTAGONISTS

Excitatory amino acids (EAAs) such as L-glutamate and L-aspartate are major excitatory transmitters in the spinal dorsal horn. They play an important role in nociceptive processing under normal and pathologic conditions. A large proportion of primary afferent fibers contains glutamate and aspartate. The vast majority of substance P–containing C fibers also contains glutamate.

At least three different classes of receptors are activated following the release of EAAs: the *N*-methyl-D-aspartate (NMDA) receptor, the non-NMDA (AMPA) receptor, and a metabotropic glutamate (mGlu) receptor. AMPA and the NMDA receptor are ionotropic receptors. Whereas the AMPA and mGlu receptors are associated with fast excitatory postsynaptic potentials, the NMDA receptor seems to amplify the depolarization response. The ionotropic AMPA and NMDA receptors operate ionophores that allow the passage of Na^+ and Ca^{2+} through the NMDA channel and smaller cations through the AMPA channel.

The NMDA receptor and its associated channel may be modulated at distinct points. Under physiologic conditions, the NMDA channel is blocked in a voltage-dependent fashion by the binding of Mg^{2+} inside the ion channel. The Mg^{2+} block can be removed by lowering the cell membrane voltage. Thus, NMDA-associated channel activation requires a ligand binding and a change in membrane voltage. Repetitive C-fiber activity induces not only glutamate release but also the release of excitatory neuropeptides such as substance P that produce a depolarization that removes the Mg^{2+} block. Furthermore, glycine, acting at a strychnine-insensitive site, is necessary as a coactivator at the NMDA receptor. Following activation of the NMDA channel, a cascade of events takes place leading to the entry of Ca^{2+} into the cell, a change in membrane potential, and finally, hyperexcitability.

Hyperexcitability is the biologic cornermarker of all types of chronic pain. There is evidence that the NMDA receptor is the key pharmacologic site for modulating this hyperexcitability. Studies have shown that this wind-up effect can be blocked by NMDA receptor antagonists. In animal models of peripheral mononeuropathic pain, NMDA antagonists are effective in reducing signs of pain, even when they are administered weeks after nerve injury. NMDA receptors are also involved in inflammatory and ischemic pain, as well as in tactile allodynia.

The observation that the NMDA receptors play a significant role in hyperexcitability and in pain states associated with sustained afferent noxious input has led to the development of an entire series of drugs with NMDA receptor antagonistic properties. The NMDA receptor activity can be modulated in at least three different ways by inhibiting glutamate release (e.g., by adenosine A1 activation or by lamotrigine), blocking NMDA receptor activity (e.g., by ketamine, dextrorphan, or memantine; see below), and blocking substances following NMDA activation (blockade of NO and other mediators).

Ketamine is a dissociative anesthetic that binds to the phencyclidine site of the voltage-gated NMDA receptor channel, thereby producing a noncompetitive inhibition of the channel. Ketamine in subanesthetic doses, from 0.125 to 0.5 mg/kg iv, relieves certain forms of postoperative and chronic neuropathic pain. A limiting factor of ketamine use is its psychomimetic side effects such as dizziness, floating sensations, illusions, and time-altered bodily perceptions. At present, there is not enough information to warrant long-term oral treatment with ketamine. Other channel blockers have been introduced that have an affinity for the phenyclidine site inside the ion channel. Dextrorphan,

Table 9.5 Other analgesic compounds

Compound	Mechanisms of action	Pain condition	Start dose	Usual daily dose	Side effects
Baclofen	GABA(B) receptor agonist	Trigeminal neuralgia	5 mg t.i.d. po	10-20 mg t.i.d.	Sedation
Gabapentin	Ca^{2+} channel bloker	Diabetic neuropathy Postherpetic neuralgia	400 mg t.i.d. po	2400-3000 mg	None
Topical capsaicin	Depletion of substance P	Diabetic neuropathy	0.075% cream topical	Slight local pain	
Clonidine	α_2-Adrenergic agonist	Postoperative pain Neuropathic pain	150 µg epidurally or inthrathecally	Same	Hypotension

memantine, and amantadine are examples of such weak channel blockers. Dextrorphan is a metabolite of the antitussive agent dextrometorphan. In some but not all studies, this substance was able to block neuropathic pain.

Animal studies have further drawn attention to the therapeutic potential of combining NMDA antagonists with other drugs. A typical example is the combination of low doses of opioids with NMDA antagonists. Low to moderate doses of opioids delay but do not prevent wind-up. NMDA antagonists, in turn, do not affect the initial response of the dorsal horn neuron to afferent input, but they prevent the occurrence of wind-up. In contrast, the combination of low doses of opioids with low doses NMDA antagonists does inhibit nociceptive responses. Another example of a potentially interesting therapeutic approach is the combination of NMDA receptor antagonists with local anesthetics. Since local anesthetics block voltage-sensitive Na^+ channels, their combination with NMDA antagonists may abolish NMDA-mediated wind-up (Tab. 9.5).

PRINCIPLES OF PAIN TREATMENT

An appropriate and rational pain treatment plan depends on a thorough analysis of the patient's pain: etiology, temporal profile (i.e., acute/chronic), localization (i.e., intensity and quality), signs of inflammation, signs of neuropathic pain, psychosocial factors, and functional status including sleep.

Acute pain

In acute pain conditions with a well-defined noxious stimulus and signs of inflammation, antipyretic agents are recommended when the pain is mild; stronger types of pain require treatment with antipyretics combined with mild opioids such as tramadol. In postoperative conditions and in instances of insufficient pain relief, stronger opioids must be used. The risk for the development of dependence is insignificant, and tolerance is not an issue in acute pain conditions.

Chronic pain

Malignant pain Pain due to cancer is seen in 70 to 90% of the patients with advanced cancers. In 75% of patients with cancer pain, the pain is due to an invasion of tissue by the tumor. In 30 to 35% of patients, pain is musculoskeletal; in 20%, pain is a result of the drug treatment. In less than 10 to 20% of patients, the cause of the pain can not be found. In cancer pain, the pain can be either nociceptive, inflammatory, or neuropathic. Pain treatment starts with antipyretic drugs such as ASA or acetaminophen in sufficiently high doses, followed by weak and strong opioids according the World Health Organization (WHO) ladder principle, in which pain treatment and drug dose are intensified in a stepwise fashion as the disease and pain progress. When chronic opioid treatment is considered, treatment should be based on a slow-release preparation with a fast-acting as-needed opioid administration to adjust doses in the phase where pain treatment has not been stabilized yet. It is always important to include laxatives when opioid treatment is started. When cancer pain is associated with neuropathic types of pain, TCAs, sodium channel blockers, or gabapentin can be added (see Tab. 9.5). In cancer pain associated with metastatic involvement of bone and in patients with incident pains, radiotherapy can provide sufficient pain relief.

Nonmalignant pain A thorough pain analysis is essential in this category of patients. In chronic nonmalignant pain, opioids should not be used or should be used only with great care to avoid the risks associated with long-term treatment: physical dependence, psychologic dependence, and tolerance. This holds true particularly for the remitting types of pain such as viscereal pain and headache. Pharmacologic treatment usually should be limited to antipyretic analgesics and nonopioid analgesics. The character of the latter depends on the pain type in question. NSAIDs may be used for their central actions but not for their anti-inflammatory effects because inflammation is seen rarely in chronic pain.

In neuropathic types of pain, a long list of drugs is available. Often, several types of drug combinations will have to be tried out. It is important to test the effect of different drugs in a sufficient dose and for a sufficient period of time.

Although, as a rule, sodium channel blockers are used for conditions with a paroxysmal component and TCAs for pain conditions with hyperalgesia, at present there are no data available that permit such a selection of drugs entirely on the basis of mechanisms encountered. Opioids have been shown to have an effect on some forms of neuropathic pain but should be used with great care.

New areas of drug development

Adenosine is an endogenous substance with actions in both the spinal cord and the brain and is available as an antiarrhythmic agent (see Chap. 24). Adenosine is believed to exert an antinociceptive effect at the spinal dorsal horn level. Adenosine modulates the nociceptive threshold in various types of experimentally induced pain. Manipulations that increase the amount of available adenosine levels in the dorsal horn, e.g., by adenosine kinase and adenosine deaminase inhibitors, produce analgesia and also enhance opioid-induced antinociception. Intrathecal administration of a selective adenosine A1 agonist reduces levels of substance P in the cerebrospinal fluid. In behavioral studies it was found that intrathecal administration of an adenosine receptor agonist dose-dependently abolishes tactile allodynia in rats with partial nerve injury. Studies in humans have shown that iv adenosine may relieve experimentally induced ischemic pain and increase the cutaneous heat-pain threshold. Recent reports show that systemic adenosine infusions may relieve neuropathic pain and allodynia.

Nicotinic cholinergic agents Following the early demonstration of an antinociceptive activity of nicotine, a number of analgesic derivatives were tested. Epibatidine, an alkaloid isolated from Ecuadorean frog skin, also binds to nicotinic acetylcholine (ACh) receptors. Animal studies show that epibatidine has a powerful analgesic action, but with severe adverse effects Compounds more selective for neuronal than for neuromuscular nicotinic acetylcholine receptors has been developed recently. A promising new potent neuronal nicotinic receptor ligand (ABT-594) is 100 times more potent than morphine. It has a broad spectrum of antinociceptive activity. ABT-594 selectively reduced neuronal activity produced by noxious mechanical and thermal stimuli but not by innocuous stimuli. Clinical studies on this compound are ongoing.

GABA This major inhibitory neurotransmitter is believed to be responsible for more than 40% of all the neuronal inhibitory actions that take place in the nervous system. Three main classes of γ-aminobutyric acid (GABA) receptors have been described: GABA(A) receptors, GABA(B) receptors, and the recently discovered GABA(C) receptor. GABA(A) and GABA(C) are both ligand-gated chloride (Cl) channels. On activation, an increase in membrane Cl conductance occurs. In contrast, GABA(B) receptors are GTP-binding protein-coupled receptors linked to membrane Ca^{2+} and K^+ channels. GABA-containing axon terminals are found both pre- and postsynaptically on primary afferent terminals. In the spinal cord, the highest concentration of GABA is found in dorsal horn interneurons. In the superficial laminae of the dorsal horn, GABA is often colocalized with glycine.

GABA is released in response to noxious stimuli. Both GABA(A) and GABA(B) receptor agonists produce analgesic effects. Whereas GABA(A)-mediated antinociception is more important at supraspinal sites, GABA(B)-mediated antinociception takes place at both spinal and supraspinal sites. Baclofen is a GABA(B) receptor agonist with both spinal and supraspinal sites of action. Monoamines are involved in baclofen's analgesic action at the supraspinal level. In contrast, at the spinal level, baclofen probably acts by directly inhibiting the release of excitatory neurotransmitters, such as glutamate, CGRP, and substance P, from primary afferent fibers. Intrathecal administration of the GABA(A) receptor antagonist bicuculline produces tactile allodynia in the rat. Although there is overwhelming experimental evidence for the involvement of the GABA system in pain processing, particularly neuropathic pain, there are only limited indications that the GABA-ergic system plays a role in clinical pain states. However, it has been shown that baclofen at a dose of 10 mg three times daily is effective in trigeminal neuralgia.

Nitric oxide synthase (NOS) inhibitors Nitric oxide (NO) is a diffusible gas that acts as a neurotransmitter. By generating NO, neurotransmitters such as glutamate, substance P, bradykinin, and ACE activate guanylate cyclase and elevate cGMP intracellular levels. NO is involved in nociceptive processing, and it plays an important role in the development and maintenance of hyperalgesia. Increased NO synthase levels occur in the dorsal root ganglion and in the dorsal horn after peripheral nerve injury, chronic arthritis, and capsaicin and formalin injections in the rat hind paw. Chronic administration of the NOS inhibitor L-NAME directly to the site of nerve injury can abolish thermal hyperalgesia. Allodynia was blocked temporarily when L-NAME was injected intrathecally. NOS inhibitors also block the NMDA-induced release of NO from the rat spinal cord. Clinical application of these drugs must await future development.

Calcium channel blockers Voltage-sensitive calcium channels (VSCCs) regulate the influx of calcium (Ca^{2+}) into the neuron and gain control over neuronal excitability (see Chaps. 23 and 24). Several types of VSCCs are involved in nociceptive processing. L-type VSCC blockers potentiate and prolong the antinociceptive action of opioids. The selective P-type VSCC blockers produce an analgesic effect in both acute pain tests and the formalin test, while N-type VSCC blockers produce their analgesic effects in animal models of acute, tonic, and neuropathic pain. There is at present only limited clinical evidence for a role of Ca^{2+} blockers in pain treatment. However, the L-type Ca^{2+} antagonist verapamil has a prophylactic effect in the treatment of chronic paroxysmatic hemicrania, also known as *cluster headache*.

Gabapentin is a newer antiepileptic that probably acts on a subclass of Ca^{2+} channels (see Chap. 10). Despite its structural similarity to GABA, gabapentin is without any action on the GABA-ergic system. Gabapentin has an analgesic effect in inflammatory and neuropathic pain models but is without effect on normal nociceptive responses. Gabapentin's potential role in the treatment of neuropathic pain is further supported by recent studies showing that it reverses both cold and mechanical allodynia in neuropathic rats. Two controlled clinical trials in postherpetic neuralgia and painful diabetic neuropathy have demonstrated that gabapentin at a dose up to 3600 mg is superior to placebo. Gabapentin does not interact with sodium channel blockers such as phenytoin and carbamazepine. The T_{max} following oral administration is 2 to 3 hours, and the elimination half-life is 5 to 7 hours. The side effects of gabapentin are few, but peripheral edema has been described following gabapentin administration.

Neurokinin receptor antagonists Following noxious stimulation of C fibers, the tachykinins substance P (SP) and neurokinin A (NKA) are released in the spinal dorsal horn. They act mainly on the NK1 and NK2 receptors, densely concentrated in dorsal horn laminae I and II. In the human CNS, NK1 receptors predominate and play an important role in nociceptive processing. SP displays a high affinity for the NK1 receptor. NK2 receptors play a major role in acute nociceptive pain, whereas NK1 antagonists only produce minor effects. In conditions of inflammation and hyperalgesia, the NK1 receptors become more important. Several NK1 and NK2 receptor antagonists have been developed and tested in animals. The results of these studies are inconsistent, but so far there are no obvious effect of these drugs in clinical pain conditions.

α_2-Receptor agonists Under normal circumstances, sympathetic stimulation does not provoke a pain sensation, but pain after peripheral nerve injury sometimes shows an abnormal responsiveness to sympathetic stimulation. Units from injured nerves are excited directly by sympathetic stimulation, and this effect can be mimicked by intraarterial injections of small amounts of norepinephrine. In contrast, sympathetic stimulation has no effect on uninjured nerves. Newly developed animal models of neuropathic pain produce a sympathetically mediated pain that is reduced after sympathectomy. Spinal administration of α_2 agonists, e.g., clonidine, reverses allodynia in these animals. These drugs reduce sympathetic outflow by a direct action on preganglionic neurons, and they potentiate morphine analgesia.

Suggested readings _____

ASHBURN MA, STAATS PS. Management of chronic pain. Lancet 1999;353:1865-9.

BESSON JM. The neurobiology of pain. Lancet 1999; 353:1610-5.

COOK RJ, SACKETT DL. The number needed to treat: a clinically useful measure of treatment effect. Br Med J 1995;310:452-4.

DRAY A, URBAN L, DICKENSON A. Pharmacology of chronic pain. Trends Pharmacol Sci 1994;15:190-7.

HARDMAN JG, LIMBIRD LE, MOLINOFF P.B, et al. Goodman and Gilman's The pharmacological basis of therapeutics, 9th ed. New York: Pergamon Press, 1996.

FELSBY S, NIELSEN J, ARENDT-NIELSEN L, JENSEN TS. NMDA receptor blockade in chronic neuropathic pain: a comparison of ketamine and magnesium chloride. Pain 1996;64:283-91.

JENSEN TS. Opioids in the brain: supraspinal mechanisms in pain control. Acta Anaesthesiol Scand 1997;41:123-32.

JENSEN TS, TURNER JA, WIESENFELD-HALLIN Z. Progress in pain research and management, vol 8. Seattle: IASP Press, 1997.

MAX MB, LYNCH SA, MUIR J, et al. Effects of desipramine, amitriptyline and fluoxetine on pain in diabetic neuropathy. N Eng J Med 1992;326:1250-6.

MCQUAY HJ, MOORE RA. An evidence-based resource for pain relief. Oxford: Oxford University Press, 1998.

PORTENOY RK, LESAGE P. Management of cancer pain. Lancet 1999;353:1695-700.

YAKSH TL, AL-RODHAN NRF, JENSEN TS. Sites of action of opiates in production of analgesia. In: Progress in Brain Research, vol 77. Amsterdam: Elsevier Science, 1988, pp 371-94.

YAKSH TL. Anesthesia: biological foundations, 1st ed. Philadelphia: W. B. Saunders, 1997.

10

Epilepsy

Emilio Perucca

Epilepsy is the most common serious brain disorder. Worldwide, it affects about 40 million people, and 100 million will have been affected at some time in their life. Epilepsy accounts for 1% of the world's burden of disease, the same as breast cancer in women and lung cancer in men.

If inadequately treated, epilepsy can have serious medical consequences, including an increased risk for mood disorders, physical injuries, and sudden unexpected death. Of even greater importance are its social, cultural, and legal stigmas; people with epilepsy may suffer more from ignorance, prejudice, and discrimination than from the actual manifestations of the disease. This situation is even more regrettable when one considers that epilepsy is fully treatable in up to 80% of affected patients, and yet, between 70 and 90% of the over 30 million affected people who live in developing countries receive no treatment.

Epilepsy represents an important burden not only in human suffering but also in terms of costs to society. Using a model based on incidence and prognosis, the total treatment cost per patient with epilepsy in the United States has been estimated tentatively at $ 4272 for patients in remission compared with $ 138,602 for patients with severe refractory epilepsy. In this model, indirect costs account for 62% of the total, whereas drug treatment cost amount to 34 to 52% of direct costs.

In most studies in Europe and the United States, antiepileptic drugs account for about 20% of direct medical health care expenditures, but this proportion is increasing steadily with the introduction of new drugs. In a cohort study of patients assessed at 8 years after diagnosis in the United Kingdom, the newer agents vigabatrin and lamotrigine accounted for more than 60% of antiepileptic drug costs, although only 5% of patients were receiving these drugs. It is no surprise, therefore, that cost is a factor limiting the prescription of some drugs, especially in developing countries.

Disease presentation

Epilepsy is characterized by recurrence of seizures, defined as the manifestation of paroxysmal and disordered neuronal discharges in the brain. Seizures can vary widely in their clinical presentation, depending on site, extent, and mode of propagation of the paroxysmal discharge. Seizures can be either partial or generalized (Tab. 10.1). *Partial seizures* are those in which the first clinical and electroencephalographic (EEG) signs indicate an initial activation of a neuronal system limited to part of a cerebral hemisphere. If consciousness is not impaired, the seizure is called *simple partial*, whereas in the presence of impairment of consciousness the event takes the form of a *complex partial seizure*. If the focal discharge propagates to both hemispheres, it will evolve into a *secondarily generalized seizure*, which may be *tonic-clonic* or, more rarely, *clonic* or *tonic*. Seizures that are generalized at the onset without clinical or electrophysiologic evidence for a focal origin are defined as *primarily generalized*. These seizures, which involve both hemispheres simultaneously, may be convulsive or non-

Table 10.1 A simplified classification of seizures based on the proposals of the Commission on Classification of the International League against Epilepsy

Partial seizures (without impairment of consciousness)
Simple partial seizures
With motor symptoms
With somatosensory or special sensory symptom
With automatic symptoms or signs
With psychic symptoms
Complex partial seizures (with impairment of consciousness)
Simple partial onset followed by impairment of consciousness
With impairment of consciousness at onset
Partial seizures evolving to secondarily generalized seizures
Simple partial seizures evolving to generalized seizures
Complex partial seizures evolving to generalized seizures

Generalized seizures (convulsive or nonconvulsive)
Absence seizures
Typical absence seizures
Atypical absence seizures
Myoclonic seizures/myoclonic jerks
Clonic seizures
Tonic seizures
Tonic-clonic seizures
Atonic (astatic) seizures

Unclassified seizures (includes all seizures unclassifiable because of inadequate data and some which defy classification in the preceding categories, e.g., infantile spasms)

Table 10.2 Simplified classification of epileptic syndromes based on the proposals of the Commission on Classification of the International League against Epilepsy

Localization-related (partial) epilepsies
Idiopathic with age-related onset. Examples: epilepsy with centrotemporal spikes, epilepsy with occipital spikes
Symptomatic or cryptogenic

Generalized epilepsies
Idiopathic (age-related onset). Examples: benign neonatal convulsions, grand mal seizures on awakening, juvenile myoclonic epilepsy
Cryptogenic or symptomatic (age-related onset). Examples: West's syndrome (infantile spasms), Lennox-Gastaut syndrome
Symptomatic (includes many pathologic conditions complicated by epileptic seizures)

Epilepsies undetermined, whether partial or generalized
With both partial and generalized seizures. Examples: neonatal seizures, continuous spike-wave during sleep, Landau-Klefner syndrome
Without clear features allowing to determine whether seizures are partial or generalized. Example: tonic-clonic seizures in which the clinical and EEG features do not allow to determine whether seizures are primarily and secondarily generalized

Special syndromes
Examples: febrile convulsions, other situation-related seizures, Kojewnikow's syndrome

---

convulsive and include absence, tonic-clonic, myoclonic, clonic, tonic, and atonic seizures. The term *status epilepticus* is used to indicate a situation when seizure activity is so prolonged or so frequently repeated as to create a fixed and long-lasting condition. Especially when seizures are convulsive, status epilepticus represents a life-threatening condition requiring emergency treatment.

Classification of the disease (i.e., syndromic classification) is at least as important as classification of the symptom (i.e., seizure classification). As shown in Table 10.2, epileptic syndromes are also differentiated into partial, generalized, or undetermined depending on the presence or lack of evidence for a focal or generalized onset of the epileptic discharge. The syndromic classification also incorporates etiologic information, and a distinction is made between *idiopathic* (when there is no known etiology other than a genetic predisposition), *symptomatic* (when there is an identified abnormality that triggers the seizures), and *cryptogenic* forms (when the clinical picture suggests a symptomatic form, but the abnormality causing the seizures is not identified).

Treatment

Treatments of general use in the disease

The modern treatment of epilepsy started in 1867 with the introduction of bromide, the first effective anticonvulsant.

The use of bromides, however, declined sharply with the introduction of safer and more efficacious agents, namely, phenobarbital, phenytoin, primidone, ethosuximide, carbamazepine, benzodiazepines, and sodium valproate. These compounds, all of which became available before the late 1960s, are often referred to as the "established" or "conventional" antiepileptic drugs and still represent the mainstay of antiepileptic therapy worldwide. Starting in the late 1980s, though, a new wave of drugs has reached the marketing stage, including vigabatrin, oxcarbazepine, lamotrigine, gabapentin, topiramate, tiagabine, zonisamide, and felbamate. In general, the new antiepileptic drugs are reserved for the treatment of patients refractory to the older agents, but evidence is starting to accumulate that the new medications with selective mechanisms of action may be valuable as first-line management of specific epilepsy syndromes. When drugs are used correctly, about 70 to 80% of patients will achieve complete freedom from seizures without unacceptable side effects.

Nonpharmacologic treatment

Nonpharmacologic approaches, including epilepsy surgery, are also available, but most of them are restricted to patients who fail to respond to drug therapy.

Behavioral treatment

Modification of behavior may be sufficient to prevent seizures, one example being the avoidance of trigger stimuli in reflex epilepsies. Precautions that may be useful in patients with photosensitive epilepsy include viewing television from an appropriate distance or obliquely, covering one eye, viewing in good ambient light to reduce contrast, using polarized glasses, and avoiding flickering lights, such as those used in discotheques. Other behavioral approaches that may be used in different types of epilepsy include desensitization, relaxation, biofeedback techniques, aversive therapies, and positive reinforcement.

Modification of behavior and/or life-style also may improve seizure control in drug-treated patients. Factors that may precipitate seizures include excessive intake of alcohol, sleep deprivation, and stressful or irregular lifestyles.

Dietary manipulation

Among dietary manipulations used to improve seizure control, application of the ketogenic diet in children is by far the most widely used. The diet is rich in fat and low in carbohydrates and proteins, resulting in ketosis and acidosis. Although the mechanism by which a ketotic state may prevent seizures is unclear, it has been suggested that the diet may have a valuable role in drug-refractory epilepsy, particularly in children with myoclonic and akinetic seizures. Advocates of the diet recommend implementation under strict supervision by a dietitian, preferably after a period of hospitalization to ensure adequate metabolic responses. Despite continuing favorable reports, the efficacy of the diet has not been evaluated in large-scale, well-conducted controlled trials, and concerns exist about potential long-term side effects.

Vagus nerve stimulation

Experimental and clinical studies indicate that stimulation of afferent vagal fibers can suppress or prevent seizure activity. This has led to the development of a commercial device, similar to a pacemaker, that is implanted in the chest and attached to the left vagus nerve by a stimulating lead. The stimulator is programmed to deliver regular pulses of stimuli for 24 hours a day, and it also may be activated "on demand" by the patient with an external magnet. Studies showing a reduction in seizure frequency (but very rarely complete seizure control) have been conducted mostly in patients with refractory partial epilepsy, but relatively promising results also have been reported in patients with generalized seizures. This treatment is reserved for patients unresponsive to drugs, but additional studies are needed to determine its precise indications and overall clinical impact.

Surgical treatment

Although brain surgery as a treatment for epilepsy has been practiced since the birth of medicine, it is only in the last few decades that impressive advances have been made. Candidates for surgery are patients in whom seizures (1) are not adequately controlled by drugs, (2) interfere significantly with quality of life, and (3) are triggered or mediated by anatomic substrates that can be identified and treated successfully by surgery without unacceptable sequelae. Examples include temporal lobe epilepsy with hippocampal sclerosis; limbic and neocortical epilepsies due to restricted, easily resectable lesions; certain childhood epilepsies amenable to hemispherectomy, such as Sturge-Weber syndrome or Rasmussen's encephalitis; and some catastrophic generalized symptomatic epilepsies.

Drug therapy

If exception is made for the treatment of ongoing seizures and status epilepticus, antiepileptic drugs are prescribed prophylactically to prevent the recurrence of seizures. In animal models, some antiepileptic drugs also exhibit antiepileptogenic activity, in that they are effective in antagonizing the process that leads to establishment of an increased susceptibility to seizures. If this effect also occurs in humans, early drug treatment would be expected to have a favorable impact on the course of the disease. However, in most forms of epilepsy there is no evidence that this is the case.

Drug treatment should be considered only after a correct diagnosis has been made. Although this sounds obvious, differentiation between epileptic and nonepileptic attacks (e.g., psychogenic seizures, syncopal episodes) is not always easy. All efforts should be made to identify correctly the type(s) of seizure(s) and the precise syndrome because these are important in determining drug selection, in deciding the duration of treatment, and in formulating a long-term prognosis.

A single ictal episode may not be sufficient to establish a diagnosis, and usually it does not warrant institution of treatment. In fact, a large proportion of patients who have a single, unprovoked tonic-clonic seizure will not have a recurrence if they remain untreated. Although prescription of antiepileptic drugs after a first seizure does reduce the risk of relapse, indiscriminate application of this practice is unwarranted because it will expose to the adverse effects of treatment many patients who will not have further seizures anyway. Treatment after a first seizure may be justified in patients known to be at particularly high risk for seizure recurrence, such as those with interictal epileptiform EEG abnormalities and those with an identified brain abnormality thought to be responsible for the seizure.

Pharmacologic treatment is usually indicated when

Table 10.3 A classification of antiepileptic drugs based on their probable spectrum of activity against different seizure types

All seizures and syndromes	All seizures except absences	Partial and generalized tonic-clonic seizures	Absence seizures
Valproic acid	Phenobarbital	Carbamazepine[1]	Ethosuximide
Lamotrigine[2]	Primidone	Phenytoin[a]	
Benzodiazepines[3]		Vigabatrin[1,4]	
Topiramate[5]		Oxcarbazepine[1]	
Zonisamide[5]		Gabapentin	
Felbamate[5]		Tiagabine	

[1]Carbamazepine, phenytoin, vigabatrin, tiagabine oxcarbazepine, and possibly gabapentin may exacerbate myoclonic and absence seizures (and possibly other generalized seizure types).
[2]Lamotrigine has been reported to aggravate severe myoclonic epilepsy.
[3]Benzodiazepines occasionally may exacerbate tonic seizures, especially in patients with Lennox-Gastaut syndrome.
[4]Vigabatrin is also effective against infantile spasms.
[5]Evidence of efficacy against some generalized seizure types is preliminary.

two or more seizures have occurred. The decision to start treatment, however, should be taken after consultation with the patient or family and should take into consideration a multitude of factors such as the age of the patient, his or her social background, the need to hold a driver's license or to work under hazardous conditions, etc. Situations in which treatment may be witheld even after repeated ictal episodes include a very low frequency of seizures, particularly when these occur during sleep and do not disturb the patient's life, and some reflex epilepsies that can be managed by avoiding exposure to the triggering stimulus. As a general rule, uncomplicated febrile seizures also should not receive continuous pharmacologic prophylaxis. Some benign idiopathic partial epilepsies of childhood, especially rolandic epilepsy, also may not need to be treated.

Antiepileptic drugs are prescribed sometimes in patients who never had a seizure but are considered at risk for epilepsy, most notably after severe head trauma or brain surgery. If exception is made for the short-term use of iv phenytoin to reduce the frequency of early seizures after supratentorial surgery, these treatments are rarely justified.

Long-term treatment

The treatment of epilepsy should involve initially prescription of a single drug. Monotherapy has many advantages, including easier individualization of therapy, a lower risk of toxicity, avoidance of adverse drug interactions, and improved patient compliance. Up to 80% of patients with newly diagnosed epilepsy achieve complete seizure control with a single drug. Selection of the drug depends on the characteristics of the patient, the drug's efficacy spectrum, the drug's side-effect profile, and additional factors.

Since the efficacy of individual antiepileptic drugs varies in relation to seizure type (Tab. 10.3), the seizure pattern is the most important factor in drug selection. Drug choice is also facilitated by syndromic diagnosis, because some drugs may aggravate certain seizure types in specific syndromes. For example, carbamazepine is effective against tonic-clonic seizures but may aggravate myoclonic manifestations and absences. Since all these seizures may coexist in juvenile myoclonic epilepsy, use of carbamazepine in these patients may precipitate myoclonic jerks and absences even when these were not present before treatment. Three possible therapeutic approaches are summarized below.

The seizure-oriented approach According to this approach, drug choice is determined primarily by seizure type and syndromic form. In most European countries, carbamazepine is usually preferred for partial seizures (with or without secondary generalization), whereas valproic acid is generally preferred in patients with primarily generalized seizures and in those with mixed seizure types.

The popularity of carbamazepine in partial seizures derives from its high efficacy, good tolerability, and relative ease of use, including the possibility of twice-daily dosing (especially with controlled-release formulations). Phenytoin is as effective as carbamazepine and is still a popular first-line drug, especially in North America, but its use is complicated by saturation kinetics and cosmetic side effects (e.g., gingival hyperplasia, coarsening of facial features, and hirsutism). Valproic acid is also similarly effective to carbamazepine, but its long-term side effects, especially weight gain, tremor, and teratogenicity, are of concern to some practitioners. Oxcarbazepine gained acceptance in some countries as an alternative to carbamazepine because of its lower allergenic potential and reduced susceptibility to drug interactions. Phenobarbital and primidone, on the other hand, are rarely chosen as first-line drugs in partial seizures because they are possibly less effective and have definitely more prominent side effects.

Valproic acid is regarded as the first-line drug in most forms of generalized epilepsy. Many generalized epilepsies are characterized by mixed seizure patterns (e.g., tonic-clonic, myoclonic, and absence seizures), and valproic acid has the advantage of being effective in all seizure types. Ethosuximide is a valuable alternative in patients with absence seizures but, unlike valproic acid, is ineffective in preventing tonic-clonic seizures that may occur in some of these patients. Likewise, carbamazepine and phenytoin may be valuable in controlling primarily generalized tonic-clonic seizures, but they may aggravate (or precipitate) other generalized seizure types. Barbiturates have a broader spectrum of activity, but they may aggravate absence seizures, and their tolerability profile is inferior to that of valproic acid.

Some special syndromes require different approaches. Most notably, infantile spasms (e.g., West syndrome) are usually managed initially with corticotrophin, steroids, or vigabatrin.

The broad-spectrum approach Since valproic acid is active against all seizure types irrespectively of syndromic form, it has been suggested as a first-line drug in all patients. This approach has some justification because a precise characterization of seizure types is not always easy in a patient with newly diagnosed epilepsy, and early definition of a syndromic form is even more difficult. For example, the initial manifestations of juvenile myoclonic epilepsy may be restricted to a few tonic-clonic seizures, and administration of a narrow-spectrum drug such as carbamazepine in these patients may precipitate other seizure types such as myoclonic jerks and absences. Administration of valproic acid to all patients will avoid this problem and will ensure complete seizure control in the majority; patients not responding adequately to this strategy could then be referred to a specialist for further assessment.

A disadvantage of this approach is that it underemphasizes the need for a precise diagnostic workup. A correct syndromic diagnosis early in the course of the disease is of utmost importance in establishing the required duration of treatment. If this information has not been obtained before effective treatment is instituted, long-term clinical management may be jeopardized.

The low-budget approach   In 28 countries that contain 40% of the world population, the per capita annual gross national product is barely sufficient to cover a year's supply of carbamazepine or valproic acid for one or two patients. Only phenobarbital, phenytoin, and ethosuximide may be available at prices affordable by the general population. Cost of pharmaceuticals is undergoing close scrutiny even in affluent societies, and the price of new antiepileptic drugs is cited as a major reason for reserving their use to patients unresponsive to older compounds.

Optimization of dosage and dosing schedule   Dosage requirements vary greatly from one patient to another as a result of interindividual differences in pharmacokinetics and pharmacodynamics. Therefore, dose individualization is as important as drug selection.

When response has to be achieved rapidly (e.g., in status epilepticus or serial seizures), effective serum drug concentrations can be produced with a loading dose. In most situations, however, this approach is undesirable because it carries the risk of severe side effects, and it is common practice to start treatment with a small dosage and to increase it gradually up to a target maintenance level. The rate of titration depends on the characteristics of the drug. Some agents, such as phenytoin and gabapentin, can be titrated up over relatively few days, whereas others, such as primidone, lamotrigine, and topiramate, may require a longer escalation period to mini-

mize potential intolerance. The target maintenance dosage, in turn, varies depending on age, body weight, type of epilepsy, associated disease, preexisting drug treatment, and other variables. For example, idiopathic epilepsies tend to respond to lower dosages compared with most symptomatic or cryptogenic forms. Conversely, patients with a high seizure frequency before starting therapy, multiple seizure types, or associated neurologic handicaps are expected to need higher dosages.

The need for dosage adjustment should be evaluated regularly, taking into consideration clinical response and pharmacokinetic features. For long-half-life drugs such as phenytoin and phenobarbital, it may take weeks for the serum concentration to stabilize following a dosage change, and this should be taken into account when evaluating response. Monitoring serum drug concentrations may provide supportive information, but it should not be regarded as a substitute for clinical judgment. Some patients may respond optimally at concentrations below the lower limit of the usually quoted "tharapeutic range," whereas others may tolerate and indeed require concentrations in excess of this range. In particular, no patient can be considered drug resistant unless seizures persist at the maximal tolerated dosage (within an acceptable range), irrespective of serum drug concentrations.

Patients must be informed about the risks of abrupt interruption of therapy, with special reference to withdrawal seizures and status epilepticus. Compliance should be facilitated by using the simplest possible dosing schedule. A qd or bid schedule is acceptable and feasible with

Table 10.4 Ranges of maintenance oral dosages and optimal serum concentrations of the main antiepileptic drugs

| | Maintenance dosage[1] | | Optimal serum concentrations |
	Adults	Children	
Carbamazepine	400-2400 mg/d	5-40 mg/kg/d	17-47 µmol/l
Clobazam	10-40 mg/d	0.5-1 mg/kg/d	NA[2]
Clonazepam	1-20 mg/d	0.01-0.2 mg/kg/d	NA[2]
Ethosuximide	500-1500 mg/d	15-40 mg/kg/d	280-700 µmol/l
Felbamate	1200-3600 mg/d	15-45 mg/kg/d	NA[2]
Gabapentin	1200-4800 mg/d	Insufficient data	NA[2]
Lamotrigine	75-700 mg/d	1.5-15 mg/kg/d	NA[2]
Nitrazepam	—	0.25-3 mg/kg/d	NA[2]
Oxcarbazepine	600-3000 mg/d	10-30 mg/kg/d	NA[2]
Phenobarbital	50-200 mg/d	2-5 mg/kg/d	40-170 µmol/l
Phenytoin	150-450 mg/d	5-9 mg/kg/d	40-80 µmol/l
Primidone	500-1500 mg/d	5-25 mg/kg/d	23-70 µmol/l[3]
Tiagabine	20-60 mg/d	Insufficient data	NA[2]
Topiramate	200-600 mg/d	5-15 mg/kg/d	NA[2]
Valproic acid	500-3000 mg/d	10-60 mg/kg/d	350-700 µmol/l
Vigabatrin	1500-3000 mg/d	30-100 mg/kg/d	NA[2]

(Dosages may not correspond to those approved by regulatory authorities and should be considered indicative. Some patients require dosages and serum concentrations outside the indicated ranges.)
[1]Starting dosage is usually lower than maintenance dosage.
[2]Not applicable. Optimal serum concentrations not yet defined or monitoring of serum concentrations not indicated.
[3]It is usually sufficient to measure the metabolite phenobarbital.

most antiepileptic drugs. Some drugs have a short half-life, and more frequent administrations may be required to avoid intermittent side effects associated with excessive fluctuations in blood levels, especially in patients receiving high dosages. For carbamazepine and valproic acid, controlled-release formulations are available.

Evaluation of response and serum drug level monitoring

Evaluation of response should be based primarily on seizure counts and careful assessment of side effects. EEG recordings are usually of limited value in determining the need for dosage adjustments. The EEG, however, may be useful in monitoring clinical response in patients with absence seizures (whose manifestations have a well-defined EEG correlate) and in those with frequent subclinical epileptiform EEG discharges associated with cognitive impairment. Evaluation of EEG findings also may be useful in determining the risk of seizure recurrence in patients undergoing discontinuation of therapy.

As mentioned earlier, the monitoring of serum drug concentrations (i.e., therapeutic drug monitoring) may provide additional information in determining the need for dosage adjustments. Since the amount of drug in serum is in equilibrium with the drug concentration in the brain, therapeutic and toxic effects of many drugs correlate better with blood concentrations than with the prescribed daily dose. If all patients showed an optimal response at a fixed concentration, individualization of dosage based on serum drug level monitoring would be very simple. Unfortunately, this not the case, owing to the wide interpatient variability in serum level at which an optimal response is achieved.

Factors responsible for the variability in optimal serum drug concentrations include variation in drug binding to serum proteins, confounding effects produced by active metabolites or concomitant drugs, time-related changes in pharmacologic response, and differences in the type and severity of the disease. For example, patients with primarily generalized tonic-clonic seizures and a low pretreatment seizure frequency may be controlled at concentrations lower than those required in patients with symptomatic epilepsy and multiple seizure types or a high frequency of seizures at baseline. Therefore, the concept of "therapeutic ranges" of serum drug concentrations (Tab. 10.4) should be interpreted flexibly, realizing that some patients achieve optimal responses at concentrations outside these ranges. Achievement of seizure control at low concentrations is so common that it has led to the suggestion that the lower limit of the therapeutic range should be disregarded. The variability in optimal concentrations, however, does not necessarily reduce the value of serum level monitoring. In fact, it is often possible to identify the drug concentration at which the best response is achieved in an individual patient. This "individualized" concentration will be useful in evaluating subsequent alterations in response that may occur in the same patient.

In practice, the value of therapeutic drug monitoring is

greatest for phenytoin, which shows saturable pharmacokinetics and a relatively strong correlation between serum level and response. Monitoring serum concentrations also may be useful for ethosuximide and carbamazepine, although the dosage of these drugs may be individualized on clinical grounds. For phenobarbital, development of tolerance to the sedative effects results in a large variation in the levels at which toxicity occurs. For valproic acid, the correlation between serum drug levels and response is also variable. If these shortcomings are understood, a number of situations can be identified in which measurement of drug concentrations may prove particularly useful. These include (1) failure to obtain an adequate therapeutic response despite administration of high dosages (knowledge of the blood level may help in identifying the source of unsatisfactory response, such as unusual pharmacokinetics or poor compliance); (2) confirmation of suspected drug toxicity (some adverse effects such as incoordination, exacerbation of seizure frequency, or mental symptoms may be ascribed to underlying or associated diseases, and detection of a serum drug level in the toxic range facilitates differential diagnosis); (3) optimization of dosage for drugs showing dose-dependent kinetics or optimization of dosage in conditions associated with altered or variable pharmacokinetics, such as pediatric or old age, pregnancy, hepatic impairment, and renal failure (interpretation of serum levels in some of these conditions, however, should be cautious due to the possibility of changes in drug binding to serum proteins); (4) detection of pharmacokinetic drug interactions (changes in serum drug levels after addition or withdrawal of another drug can be identified readily and, if appropriate, dosage can be adjusted prior to the occurrence of adverse consequences); (5) detection of pharmaceutical inequivalence; (6) management of drug overdose, and (7) confirmatory diagnosis of poor compliance.

For a meaningful use of therapeutic drug monitoring, samples must be collected and assayed correctly. Measurements are taken usually at steady state, i.e., at least 5 half-lives after the last dose change. Interpretation of data should take into account the interval elapsed between drug intake and sampling. For long-half-life drugs, such as phenobarbital, drug level fluctuations during a dosing interval are negligible and time of sampling is relatively unimportant. For other drugs, a morning sample before intake of the first daily dose usually provides an estimate of the trough concentration. With agents such as carbamazepine and valproic acid, a second sample at the time of peak may be useful in assessing the possibility of excessively high concentrations associated with intermittent adverse effects.

Management of patients refractory to initial treatment

Although up to 80% of patients are expected to achieve freedom from seizures on the initially prescribed drug, response rate varies with syndromic form, and idiopathic epilepsies usually respond much better than symptomatic epilepsies. In patients who fail to respond to the initial drug, two approaches may be followed. One involves substituting the initial drug with another; in general, substitution is carried out gradually, with the dosage of the initial drug being tapered off while that of the alternative agent is increased. The other approach involves adding the alternative drug and mantaining the patient on combination therapy. Since up to 30 to 40% of patients with partial and/or generalized tonic-clonic seizures, unresponsive to initial treatment achieve seizure freedom on an alternative monotherapy, most physicians correctly prefer to substitute a second drug rather than exposing the patients to the more prominent side effects associated with combination therapy. There are, however, patients who do better on a drug combination, and the actual strategy may vary depending on individual factors.

The probability of achieving seizure freedom decreases with increasing number of drugs to which a patient has been unsuccessfully exposed, and in many patients who are unresponsive to various drugs and drug combinations, optimal management rests on the compromise between the desire to minimize seizure frequency and the need to avoid intolerable side effects.

The role of the new antiepileptic drugs

Several new antiepileptic drugs have been licensed over the last 10 years. As clinical experience increases and results of new studies become available, information on their risk-benefit profile undergoes continuous refinement. At the time of registration, new drugs usually were indicated as add-on treatment in patients refractory to established agents. For many of these compounds, trials in newly diagnosed epilepsy were subsequently completed, leading to the finding that new drugs are not more efficacious than older agents when given as initial therapy. Although in most studies there has been a trend toward better tolerability compared with older agents, the trial design often favored the new drug. Clinical experience with the new drugs is also limited, raising concern that serious side effects may have been undetected, especially in high-risk subpopulations of patients. Concern about safety was rekindled by the discovery of aplastic anemia and hepatotoxicity among patients exposed to felbamate and more recently by reports of an unexpectedly high frequency (1:50 to 1:300) of serious skin reactions in children exposed to lamotrigine. In light of the preceding considerations, new antiepileptic drugs are usually reserved for patients who have failed on at least one of the established primary drugs. One condition in which first-line use of a new drug may be justified is West syndrome (i.e., infantile spasms), particularly if associated with tuberous sclerosis, in which vigabatrin appears to be remarkably effective.

Drug interactions in epilepsy

Since antiepileptic drugs are usually given for a long time and sometimes in combination, the risk of adverse interactions is considerable (see Chap. 6). Among pharmacokinetic interactions, the most common involve displacement from plasma protein binding sites and interference with drug metabolism. Protein-binding interactions, one example being the displacement of phenytoin by valproic acid, are of limited significance because the displaced drug is rapidly eliminated and/or distributed into a large extravas-cular space; however, such interactions need to be taken into account when interpreting plasma drug levels in clinical practice. In fact, in the presence of a protein-binding interaction, the total concentration of the displaced agent will underestimate the amount of free, pharmacologically active drug, and therapeutic and toxic effects may occur at unusually low total concentrations.

Among metabolic drug interactions, many involve enzyme induction. By inducing some families of cytochrome P450 isoenzymes (especially CYP2B, -3A, -3C, and -2E and glucuronyltransferases), phenytoin, carbamazepine, and barbiturates stimulate the metabolism and increase dosage requirements of other compounds that are substrates of these enzymes. These may include other anticonvulsants or medications used for unrelated conditions (Tab. 10.5). Although the newer antiepileptic drugs are less likely to cause enzyme induction, stimulation of enzyme isoforms responsible for the metabolism of oral steroid contraceptives has been reported with oxcarbazepine, topiramate, and felbamate. To minimize the risk of contraceptive failure, patients taking anticonvulsants interacting with the pill should receive a preparation with a high estrogen component (e.g., 50 μg ethinyl estradiol).

Interactions mediated by enzyme inhibition are equally important. Anticonvulsants acting as enzyme inhibitors include valproic acid and felbamate; by this mechanism, valproic acid increases plasma levels of phenobarbital and lamotrigine, whereas felbamate increases the plasma lev-

---

Table 10.5 Examples of drugs whose metabolism is accelerated by enzyme-inducing antiepileptic drugs (e.g., carbamazepine, phenytoin, phenobarbital, and primidone)

Benzodiazepines	Methsuximide
Beta blockers (some)	Metronidazole
Carbamazepine	Metyrapone
Chloramphenicol	Mexiletine
Chlorpromazine	Mianserin
Clozapine	Neuromuscular
Corticosteroids	blocking agents
Coumarin anticoagulants	Oral steroid contraceptives*
Cyclosporine	Paroxetine
Digitoxin	Pethidine
Dihydropyridine calcium	Primidone
antagonists	Quinine
Disopyramide	Quinidine
Doxycycline	Theophylline
Ethosuximide	Thioridazine
Felbamate	Thyroxine
Fentanyl	Tiagabine
Flunarizine	Topiramate
Griseofulvin	Tricyclic antidepressants
Haloperidol	Valproic acid
Ketoconazole	Vitamin D
Lamotrigine	Zonisamide
Methadone	

*The metabolism of oral steroid contraceptives is also stimulated by oxcarbazepine, topiramate, and felbamate.

els of phenobarbital, phenytoin, carbamazepine, 10,11-epoxide, and valproic acid. Drugs prescribed for unrelated conditions may inhibit the metabolism of anticonvulsants, examples being the elevation of plasma carbamazepine levels by macrolide antibiotics, cimetidine, verapamil, diltiazem, and propoxyphene.

Pharmacodynamic interactions may play a role in the high prevalence of adverse effects in patients receiving excessive polytherapy, even when dosage and plasma levels of individual drugs are in the low range. Pharmacodynamic interactions, however, also could be beneficial, one example being the favorable therapeutic index of the combination of valproic acid and ethosuximide in patients with atypical absence seizures refractory to either agent given alone. A possible therapeutic synergism also has been suggested for the combination of lamotrigine and valproic acid.

Duration of treatment

Since some epilepsies have a benign course and enter permanent remission, the possibility of withdrawing treatment should be considered. There are no fixed rules on whether and when drug discontinuation should be attempted, and the decision should be made individually. It is essential that the decision to stop or continue treatment be made after extensive discussion with the patient, who should be informed about the risk of relapse and the fact that in the event of seizure recurrence control is almost always achieved following reintroduction of therapy. In some benign childhood epilepsies it is usual to attempt withdrawal of therapy after approximately 2 years of remission, whereas in adults the time frame may range from 2 to 5 years. Treatment should never be stopped abruptly because this carries a high risk of withdrawal seizures and status epilepticus. If a decision to stop treatment is reached, this should be done gradually, usually over at least 6 months.

Among factors predictive of seizure relapse the most important is clearly the syndromic form. Since many age-related idiopathic epilepsies of childhood show a high remission rate, relapse is less likely in children than in adults. The risk of remaining seizure-free after drug withdrawal in a pooled population of children with different seizure types is 70 to 80%, but lower risks are observed in specific syndromes such as childhood absence epilepsy and benign idiopathic partial epilepsy with centrotemporal spikes (rolandic epilepsy). In adults, the proportion of patients remaining seizure-free at 2 years after drug discontinuation is about 60%, compared with about 80% among patients who continue on treatment. Juvenile myoclonic epilepsy is one syndrome in which relapse after drug withdrawal is almost constant, and discontinuation of treatment should be discouraged.

Febrile seizures

Febrile seizures occur in 3 to 5% of children under 5 years of age and are usually associated with a body temperature in excess of 38° C. Although continuous prophylaxis with valproic acid and phenobarbital may reduce the risk of recurrence, administration of these drugs to children who present with uncomplicated febrile seizures has no effect on long-term prognosis, and the side effects outweigh any possible benefit. For this reason, continuous pharmacologic prophylaxis is generally not indicated.

In most patients in whom there are sound reasons to minimize recurrences, the best approach is intermittent prophylaxis with rectal diazepam (0.3-0.5 mg/kg, using the parenteral solution or especially designed rectal capsules) at the time a febrile episode is detected.

Epilepsy in pregnancy

Administration of antiepileptic drugs during the first trimester of pregnancy is associated with an approximate 6% risk of fetal malformations, compared with a 2-3% risk in an unexposed population. No drug-specific abnormalities have been recorded, except for neural tube defects, particularly spina bifida, after exposure to valproic acid (1-2% risk) and, to a lesser extent, carbamazepine. Most available information relates to established drugs, and there are no sufficient data for the new agents.

Since risk increases with dosage and number of drugs, treatment should be optimized before pregnancy by prescribing a single agent at the lowest possible dosage, divided into at least two or three daily administrations. In most situations, any fetal anomalies are likely to have occurred already by the time pregnancy is diagnosed, and changes in treatment during gestation are unwarranted because worsening of seizure control could do greater harm than the drugs themselves. Should seizures deteriorate during pregnancy, appropriate dosage adjustments are indicated. Folate (4 mg per day) before conception and for the first 12 gestational weeks is effective in reducing the risk of neural tube defects in children whose siblings had such a defect, but its value in preventing the teratogenicity of anticonvulsants is unknown, and some authors recommend lower folate dosages in epileptic women who are not taking valproate and/or carbamazepine and have no history of neural tube defects in previous pregnancies. Newborns of mothers treated with established antiepileptic drugs are at risk of developing a serious internal hemorrhage during the first 24 hours of life. This can be prevented by prophylaxis with vitamin K given to the mother during the last month of gestation and parenterally to the newborn at the time of birth.

Status epilepticus

Status epilepticus, i.e., prolonged or recurrent seizure activity without recovery of function between seizures, encompasses a wide variety of conditions, depending on electroclinical characteristics and the context in which seizures are observed. Convulsive status epilepticus involves a high risk of permanent neuronal damage and mortality, and it requires aggressive emergency treatment. Management should include general supportive measures, assessment and treatment of underlying causes (including, if appropriate, correction of hypoglycemia and potential thiamine deficiency), and parenteral administration of antiepileptic drugs. In general, there are two therapeutic stages: the administration of drugs aimed at stopping seizure activity and the use of drugs to depress cerebral activity and thus ictal activity (general anesthesia). Many protocols have been proposed. One approach in adult patients involves treating early status with lorazepam (4 mg) or, alternatively, diazepam (10 mg) iv repeated after 10 minutes if necessary. Established status epilepticus may be treated with phenytoin (15-18 mg/kg iv at 50 mg/min, with lorazepam if not already given) and/or phenobarbital (10 mg/kg iv at 100 mg/min). In patients refractory to earlier treatments, general anaesthesia is instituted with concomitant EEG monitoring and continued for 12 to 24 hours after the last electrographic or clinical seizure.

The drugs used to treat complex partial status are simi-

Table 10.6 Pharmacokinetic parameters of the major antiepileptic drugs in adults

	Bioavailability (oral) (%)	Plasma protein binding (%)	Distribution volume (l/kg)	$t_{1/2}$ (h)	Main routes of elimination	Major active metabolites
Carbamazepine	≥75	75	1.2	5-26[a,b]	Oxidation	10,11-epoxide
Clobazam	≥90	90	1.2	10-50[a]	Oxidation	N-desmethyl-clobazam
Clonazepam	≥80	85	3.0[d]	20-50[a]	Nitroreduction and acetylation	No
Ethosuximide	≥90	0	0.7	30-60[a]	Oxidation	No
Felbamate	≥80	30	0.8	10-25[a]	Renal excretion and oxidation	No
Gabapentin	≥35[c]	<5	0.8[d]	5-7	Renal excretion	No
Lamotrigine	≥95	55	1.2[d]	8-30[a] 30-90[e]	Glucuronidation	No
Nitrazepam	≥70	85	2.0[d]	20-50[a]	Nitroreduction and oxidation	No
Oxcarbazepine[f]	—	40	—	10-25[a]	Glucuronidation	MHD
Phenytoin	≥80	90	0.8[d]	10-20[g]	Oxidation	No
Phenobarbital	≥80	55	0.6[d]	75-125	Renal excretion, N-glucosidation, and oxidation	No
Primidone	≥90	10	0.7[d]	4-22[a]	Renal excretion and oxidation	Phenobarbital
Tiagabine	≥90	96	1.2[d]	2-13[a]	Oxidation	No
Topiramate	≥80	13	0.7	10-30[a]	Renal excretion and oxidation	No
Valproic acid	≥95	90	0.2	5-20[a]	Glucuronidation and oxidation	No
Vigabatrin[i]	≥60	0	0.8	5-8	Renal excretion	No
Zonisamide	≥50	50	1.5	25-70[a]	Glucuronidation, acetylation, and oxidation	No

[a]Shortest values within this range are found in enzyme-induced patients.
[b]Values in chronically treated patients (elimination is slower after single doses).
[c]Bioavailability decreases with increasing dosages (see text).
[d]Vd calculated after intravenous administration.
[e]Patients comedicated with valproic acid.
[f]Oxcarbazepine is a prodrug for its monohydroxyderivative (MHD). Indicated parameters refer to MHD.
[g]Half-life after single small doses. Half-life lengthens (up to 30-100 h) with increasing serum concentration.
[h]Binding decreases with increasing concentrations.
[i]Vigabatrin is a racemic mixture of 2 enantiomers that show similar pharmacokinetics.

lar to those used for convulsive status. Intravenous diazepam and/or phenytoin may be effective, but there are situations in which oral administration may be feasible. Recent evidence that complex partial status also can cause neuronal damage may influence ongoing controversy about the need for aggressive treatment in these patients. Absence status, on the other hand, is not considered to cause neuronal damage, and its treatment usually involves an iv benzodiazepine.

Drug classes

CARBAMAZEPINE

Carbamazepine was introduced in the treatment of epilepsy in 1963. Its primary mode of action involves blockade of voltage-dependent sodium channels. Carbamazepine is available in different oral dosage forms, which include syrups and conventional and sustained-release formulations. In adults, carbamazepine may be started at 200 mg daily and increased to 400 to 800 mg per day over a period of 7 to 10 days (see Tab. 10.4). The drug is usually administered in two to four daily doses, with a twice-daily schedule being particularly appropriate with controlled-release formulations.

Carbamazepine is usually considered as the drug of choice for partial seizures (with or without secondary generalization), and it also may be used to treat primarily generalized tonic-clonic seizures not complicated by other seizure types.

Pharmacokinetics (Tab. 10.6)

Carbamazepine is metabolized by CYP3A and, to a lesser extent, CYP2C8, CYP1A2, and glucuronyltransferases, whereas its active 10,11-epoxide metabolite (CBZ-E) is inactivated by hydrolases. Compared with adults, children metabolize carbamazepine at a faster rate and require larger dosages on a body weight basis.

After a dosage increment, the increase in serum carbamazepine concentrations may be smaller than expected due to dose-dependent autoinduction. Optimal serum concentrations are usually 17 to 47 µmol/l (4-11 µg/ml), but some patients require levels outside this range.

Side effects

The most common side effects include dizziness, fatigue, diplopia, headache, somnolence, and incoordination. These may occur transiently at initial exposure or intermittently in relation to fluctuation in serum drug concentration, and they can be managed by reducing the dosage, by dividing it into more frequent administrations, or by switching to a sustained-release form. Dyskinesias, dystonias, tremor, and psychiatric disturbances are observed less commonly. Non-central nervous system (non-CNS) side effects include gastrointestinal symptoms, hyponatremia, water retention, hyposexuality, menstrual irregu-

larities, vitamin D deficiency, and heart conduction disturbances (especially in the elderly). Allergic or idiosyncratic effects range from a mild skin rash (5-15%) to serious reactions. Exposure to carbamazepine during pregnancy has been associated with an increased risk of fetal malformations, including neural tube defects, and neonatal hemorrhage.

Contraindications

Carbamazepine may exacerbate absence, atonic, or myoclonic seizures in generalized epilepsies, particularly in patients showing bursts of diffuse and bilaterally synchronous spike-and-wave activity in their EEGs. Because of this, it is contraindicated in juvenile myoclonic epilepsy and progressive myoclonic epilepsy. Carbamazepine is also contraindicated in patients with acute intermittent porphyria and should be used cautiously in patients with cardiac conduction defects.

Interactions

Phenobarbital, primidone, and phenytoin reduce serum carbamazepine concentrations by stimulating its metabolism. Conversely, an increase in carbamazepine levels may be caused by macrolide antibiotics, isoniazid, metronidazol, certain antidepressants, verapamil, diltiazem, cimetidine, danazol, and propoxyphene. Valproic acid, valpromide, valnoctamide, felbamate, and progabide may increase serum CBZ-E.

Because it is an enzyme inducer, carbamazepine reduces the serum concentration of valproic acid, clonazepam, ethosuximide, lamotrigine, topiramate, tiagabine, and many other drugs, including tricyclic antidepressants, neuroleptics, oral steroid contraceptives, glucocorticoids, oral anticoagulants, cyclosporine, theophylline, and certain chemotherapeutic and cardiovascular drugs.

VALPROIC ACID

Valproic acid was introduced into clinical practice in 1967. Its multifactorial mode of action includes enhancement of gamma-aminobutyric acid (GABA)-mediated inhibition, blockade of voltage-activated sodium channels, and inhibition of gamma-hydroxybutyrate release. Valproic acid is the active principle common to several chemical forms, including the acid itself, sodium valproate, magnesium valproate, calcium valproate, divalproex sodium, and the amide derivative valpromide. Liquid and solid oral dosage forms are available, including regular-release, enteric-coated, and sustained-release forms. An iv formulation is also available. In adults, the starting dosage may be 400 to 500 mg per day, increased to 600 to 1000 mg per day after 4 to 5 days (Tab. 10.4). The drug is usually given bid or tid daily, but once-daily dosing may be feasible in some patients.

Valproic acid is effective against all seizure types and is considered the drug of choice in most generalized epilepsies, especially those associated with multiple seizure types. Valproic acid is also a possible alternative to carbamazepine or phenytoin in patients with partial seizures.

Pharmacokinetics (Tab. 10.6)

Although valproic acid has a high bioavailability, absorption may be delayed for several hours when enteric-coated tablets are taken with food. Sustained-release formulations are also available. Elimination is partly by conjugation with glucuronic acid and partly by oxidation. Children metabolize the drug at a faster rate than adults.

The increment in total valproic acid concentration may be less than expected from the increment in dosage because binding to plasma proteins decreases at high dosages. However, the relation between free drug concentration and dosage is approximately linear. Serum valproic acid concentrations are poorly correlated with therapeutic effects, and the proposed optimal range (350-700 μmol/l or 50-100 μg/ml) should be interpreted flexibly.

Side effects

Side effects may include nausea, vomiting, dyspepsia, neurologic symptoms (e.g., tremor, fatigue, sedation, dizziness, headache, stupor), and hair loss. Weight gain may be troublesome during chronic use. Less common adverse effects include hyperammonemia (possibly associated with encephalopathy), thrombocytopenia, coagulation disorders, hyperandrogenism and an increased incidence of polycystic ovaries, and potentially fatal hepatotoxicity and pancreatitis. The risk of liver toxicity ranges from 1 in 600 among children less than 2 years of age on polytherapy, to 1 in 50 000 in the population at large. Maternal exposure to valproic acid is associated with a 1 to 2% risk of fetal spina bifida and other neural tube defects.

Contraindications

Because of the risk of hepatotoxicity, valproic acid should be used cautiously in patients younger than 2 years of age. The drug is contraindicated in patients (particularly children) with metabolic defects potentially associated with Reye-like symptoms and in patients with a history of liver disease and pancreatitis. Consideration of the risk-benefit ratio is recommended in women of childbearing potential.

Interactions

Serum valproic acid levels are decreased by carbamazepine, phenytoin, and barbiturates and increased by felbamate, isoniazid, and possibly fluoxetine and chlorpromazine. Diazepam, salicylic acid, phenylbutazone, and naproxen may displace valproic acid from plasma proteins. By acting as a metabolic inhibitor, valproic acid may increase the serum concentration of phenobarbital, lamotrigine, carbamazepine-10,11-epoxide, lorazepam, nimodipine, and zidovudine.

PHENYTOIN

Phenytoin was discovered in 1947 and introduced rapidly into clinical practice. Like carbamazepine, it exerts its antiepileptic effect primarily by blocking voltage-dependent sodium channels. Phenytoin is available in liquid (syrups) and solid oral dosage forms. Parenteral formulations for im and iv use are also available. A phenytoin prodrug (fosphenytoin) with improved tolerability due to avoidance of an irritant solvent has been developed for both im and iv use. In adults, a reasonable starting oral dosage is 100 mg daily, increased to 200 to 250 mg per day over 5 to 10 days. Further adjustments can be based on clinical response and serum drug level monitoring (Tab. 10.4). Phenytoin is usually given qd or bid daily.

Phenytoin is as effective as carbamazepine in the treatment of partial seizures (with or without secondary generalization) and primarily generalized tonic-clonic seizures. In these conditions, it represents a valuable alternative to carbamazepine. Intravenous phenytoin has an important place in the management of convulsive status epilepticus.

Pharmacokinetics (Tab. 10.6)

Phenytoin is usually well absorbed when taken orally, although there may be differences between formulations. Since im absorption is slow and erratic and may cause muscle damage, patients unable to take the drug orally should be treated preferably by slow iv infusion. Alternatively, fosphenytoin may be used.

Phenytoin is metabolized extensively by cytochromes CYP2C9 and CYP2C19 to inactive metabolites. The elimination rate decreases with increasing dosage owing to saturation of metabolic enzymes. Children metabolize phenytoin at a faster rate than adults and require larger doses than adults.

Owing to phenytoin's saturable metabolism, serum levels are nonlinearly related to dose. At serum concentrations near or above the lower limit of the optimal range (40-80 μmol/l or 10-20 μg/ml), dose adjustments should be cautious because small increments in dosage can result in a disproportionately large increase in serum drug levels.

Side effects

The most common side effects include dizziness, tremor, ataxia, dysarthria, diplopia, nystagmus, and cognitive dysfunction. Other side effects include headache, dyskinesias, dystonias, and an encephalopathy associated with psychomotor slowing, psychiatric disturbances, stupor, and even coma. Side effects during chronic treatment may include hirsutism, coarsening of facial features, Dupuytren's contracture, gum hyperplasia (reduced with good oral hygiene), acne, peripheral neuropathy, hyposexuality, folate and vitamin D deficiency, and depression of cellular and humoral immunity. Hypotension and cardiac dysrhythmias may occur, particularly after intravenous dosing. Ischemic and inflammatory changes of the hand may occur after iv dosing. Maternal exposure to phenytoin is associated with an increased risk of birth defects and neonatal hemorrhage.

Contraindications

Like carbamazepine, phenytoin may exacerbate some generalized seizures in patients with generalized epilepsies, and it is contraindicated in juvenile myoclonic epilepsy and progressive myoclonic epilepsy. The drug is also contraindicated in uncompensated diabetic mellitus and in acute intermittent porphyria; caution is required in patients with impaired glucose tolerance. Because of its cosmetic side effects, phenytoin should not be used as a first-line agent in children and females.

Interactions

Drugs that may decrease serum phenytoin levels include antacids, some nasogastric feeding formulas, some antineoplastic drugs, sucralfate, and vigabatrin. Phenytoin is displaced from plasma proteins by valproic acid, phenylbutazone, salicylates, amiodarone, tolbutamide, diazoxide, and various sulfonamides. An increase in serum phenytoin levels and possible phenytoin toxicity may be caused by felbamate, phenylbutazone, methsuximide, topiramate, sulthiame, progabide, viloxazine, trazodone, omeprazole, ticlopidine, isoniazid, chloramphenicol, some sulfonamides, miconazole, fluconazole, cimetidine, amiodarone, diltiazem, bishydroxycoumarin, and disulfiram. Because it is an enzyme inducer, phenytoin may reduce the serum concentrations of various drugs, causing the same interactions described earlier for carbamazepine. Phenytoin, however, also may cause an increase in serum phenobarbital levels.

PHENOBARBITAL

Used clinically since 1912, phenobarbital is the grandfather of existing anticonvulsants, but it is certainly not obsolete. Its effects are probably mediated mainly by enhancement of GABAergic inhibition. Phenobarbital is available as liquid and solid oral dosage forms and also as parenteral formulations for iv or im use. In adults, treatment may be started with 30 to 50 mg at bedtime, to be increased to 60 to 100 mg at bedtime after 10 to 15 days if clinically indicated (Tab. 10.4).

Phenobarbital is effective in the management of all seizure types except absence seizures, which may be exacerbated. Although it is similarly effective to other primary drugs, it is seldom used as first-line treatment in developed countries because of its inferior tolerability. Intravenous phenobarbital still has a place in the management of convulsive status epilepticus.

Pharmacokinetics (Tab. 10.6)

Phenobarbital is eliminated partly by renal excretion (10-55% of an oral dose) and partly by N-glucosylation and oxidation. The latter is mediated by CYP2C9 and, to a lesser extent, CYP2C19 and CYP2E1. Elimination may be impaired in premature newborns, but in infants and children it is usually faster than in adults.

Serum phenobarbital levels show an approximate linear relationship with dosage. The commonly quoted therapeutic range is 10 to 40 µg/ml (40-170 µmol/l), but patients receiving chronic treatment may tolerate levels causing severe toxicity in acutely exposed subjects.

Side effects

Phenobarbital tends to cause sedation and mental slowing in adults and hyperkinesia, irritability, and cognitive dysfunction in children. Other possible effects include dizziness, dysarthria, incoordination, and psychiatric disorders. Withdrawal manifestations such as anxiety, tremor, confusion, seizures, and status epilepticus may occur when the dosage is reduced too rapidly. Patients treated chronically with phenobarbital may develop various fibrosing disorders, some of which are reversible on drug discontinuation. These include reflex sympathetic dystrophy, shoulder-hand syndrome, frozen shoulder, and Dupuytren's contracture. Other side effects may include in hyposexuality, vitamin D and folate deficiency, and various hypersensitivity reactions. Maternal exposure may be associated with an increased risk of birth defects and neonatal hemorrhage.

Contraindications

Phenobarbital is contraindicated in acute intermittent porphyria and hypersensitivity to barbiturates and structurally related drugs.

Interactions

Serum phenobarbital levels are increased by valproic acid, felbamate, phenytoin, methsuximide, acetazolamide, propoxyphene, chloramphenicol, and quinine. Because it is an enzyme inducer, phenobarbital may reduce the serum concentration of various drugs, causing the same interactions described earlier for carbamazepine.

OTHER BARBITURATE DERIVATIVES

Primidone Primidone is a deoxybarbiturate available only for oral use. It is readily absorbed, negligibly bound to plasma proteins, and eliminated with a half-life of 4 to 22 hours. Although approximately 50% of the dose is excreted unchanged in urine, a significant proportion is converted to phenobarbital that accumulates in serum at clinically effective concentrations. Most of the therapeutic and toxic effects are mediated by phenobarbital, and it is unclear whether there is a significant contribution from the parent drug and from the other weakly active metabolite PEMA.

Primidone should be started with a low dose (e.g., 62.5 mg per day in adults) to avoid manifestations of acute intolerance (e.g., nausea, malaise, headache, dizziness) and increased gradually (Tab. 10.4) over a period of about 3 weeks. It is usually given bid or tid. Its indications, side effects, and interaction potential are mostly overlapping with those of phenobarbital. Methsuximide, clonazepam, isoniazid, and nicotinamide may increase the serum levels of unchanged primidone, presumably by inhibiting its metabolism.

Methylphenobarbital   Methylphenobarbital (mephobarbital), a methylated derivative of phenobarbital, is a racemic mixture of two enantiomers. The *R*-enantiomer is rapidly cleared by CYP2C19-mediated hydroxylation, whereas the *S*-enantiomer is demethylated slowly to phenobarbital, which is largely responsible for the clinical effect. In patients with genetically determined CYP2C19 deficiency (2-5% of Caucasians and 20% of Japanese), hydroxylation is impaired, and the *R*-enantiomer is also converted to phenobarbital, resulting in potentially toxic concentrations. Indications, side effects, and interaction potential of methylphenobarbital are similar to those of phenobarbital.

ETHOSUXIMIDE

Ethosuximide was introduced in 1958 and remains the most widely used succinimide. Its activity is mediated by inhibition of T-type calcium channels in thalamic neurons. Ethosuximide is available as a syrup and as capsules. In adults, treatment may be started with 250 mg per day, which may be increased to 500 to 750 mg per day over a period of 1 to 2 weeks (Tab. 10.4). It is usually administered twice daily.

Ethosuximide is indicated for the treatment of absence seizures, where it is as effective as valproic acid.

Pharmacokinetics (Tab. 10.6)

Ethosuximide is oxidized by CYP3A isozymes to inactive metabolites, elimination being faster in children and in patients comedicated with enzyme inducers. Most patients achieve a good response at concentrations of 280 to 700 μmol/l (40-100 μg/ml).

Side effects

The most common side effects include nausea, vomiting, abdominal discomfort, sedation, behavioral disturbances, anorexia, headache, and hiccups. Skin rashes and, more rarely, other hypersensitivity reactions may be observed.

Contraindications

Ethosuximide is contraindicated in patients with known hypersensitivity reactions to succinimides. Caution is required in patients with a history of behavioral disorders and in those with acute intermittent porphyria.

Interactions

Serum ethosuximide levels are decreased by enzyme-inducing anticonvulsants such as carbamazepine, phenytoin, and barbiturates. Ethosuximide itself appears to be devoid of enzyme-inducing activity. A combination of valproic acid and ethosuximide may be effective in absence seizures refractory to either agent given alone.

METHSUXIMIDE

Compared with ethosuximide, methsuximide may have a broader spectrum of activity, being putatively effective against absence seizures and partial seizures, but adequate, controlled trials are lacking. Its effects are mediated mostly by the *N*-desmethyl metabolite, which accumulates in serum at concentrations 700 times higher than those of the parent drug. Methsuximide is used rarely today, being prescribed occasionally in the management of refractory epilepsies. Side effects include drowsiness, confusion, dizziness, incoordination, headache, mood and personality changes, hiccups, visual disturbances, anorexia, nausea, vomiting, and thirst. Methsuximide may increase the serum concentrations of phenytoin, phenobarbital, and other drugs.

BENZODIAZEPINES

Benzodiazepines were first used in the management of epilepsy in 1965. Their action involves enhancement of GABAergic inhibition through modulation of the GABA-benzodiazepine receptor complex (see Chaps. 13 and 82).

Benzodiazepines are available in different dosage forms for oral, rectal, im, and iv use. Oral maintenance dosages for clobazam, clonazepam, and nitrazepam are summarized in Table 10.4.

The main value of benzodiazepines in epilepsy is in the iv treatment of status epilepticus or serial seizures (see section on Status Epilepticus for dosing information). Lorazepam may be preferred, but diazepam, clonazepam, and midazolam are also used. Diazepam by rectal or oral route is also used to abort recurring seizures, and the rectal route is indicated for intermittent prophylaxis against recurrence of febrile convulsions.

Benzodiazepines are effective against all seizure types, but their value for maintenance oral treatment is limited by side effects, the common (though not invariable) loss of therapeutic effect during prolonged use, and the problem of withdrawal seizures on discontinuation. The most commonly used benzodiazepine for oral treatment is clobazam, which is relatively less sedating and may produce remarkable responses in some patients with refractory partial and generalized epilepsies.

Pharmacokinetics

The pharmacokinetics of clobazam, clonazepam, and nitrazepam are summarized in Table 10.6.

Side effects

The most significant side effects after iv dosing may include sedation, respiratory depression, hypotension, and phlebitis. Rarely, iv benzodiazepines may precipitate tonic seizures in patients with Lennox-Gastaut syndrome. During chronic treatment, benzodiazepines may cause drowsiness, ataxia, cognitive dysfunction, dizziness, visual disturbances, depression, and in children, hyperkinesia, behavioral disorders, and hypersalivation.

Interactions

The clearance of most benzodiazepines is accelerated by phenytoin, carbamazepine, and barbiturates. Intake of benzodiazepines with other CNS depressants, including alcohol, may result in pharmacodynamic potentiation of adverse CNS effects.

LAMOTRIGINE

Lamotrigine was licensed in the early 1990s and is now available in over 70 countries worldwide. Its primary action consists in blockade of voltage-dependent sodium channels, but additional mechanisms cannot be excluded. Lamotrigine is available as tablets. To minimize the risk of hypersensitivity reactions, the dosage should be escalated slowly. In adults taking enzyme inducers, treatment may be started with 25-50 mg per day and increased to 100 to 300 mg per day over 3 to 8 weeks. In adults on valproic acid, the initial dose should be 25 mg on alternate days for 2 weeks, 25 mg per day for 2 weeks, and then 50 mg per day, possibly increased to 100 mg per day, after 1-2 weeks. Maintenance dosages range from 75 to 700 mg per day in adults and 1.5 to 15 mg/kg per day in children (Tab. 10.4); the lowest dosages are used in patients comedicated with valproic acid and the highest in those taking enzyme-inducing anticonvulsants. Lamotrigine is usually given twice daily, but once-daily dosing is feasible in monotherapy or in combination with valproic acid.

Lamotrigine is effective against partial and generalized seizures. In placebo-controlled add-on trials in refractory partial seizures, about 20% of patients (after subtraction of the placebo response) showed a greater than 50% reduction in seizure frequency on lamotrigine. The drug, however, seems to be especially valuable in generalized epilepsies. Its main use is in the management of patients refractory to established drugs.

Lamotrigine shows linear pharmacokinetics, and its elimination is markedly affected by the type of comedication (Tab. 10.6). Children metabolize lamotrigine at a faster rate compared with adults.

The most common side effects are skin rashes (and, rarely, other hypersensitivity reactions), headache, nausea and vomiting, diplopia, dizziness, ataxia, tremor, and sedation. Skin rashes, which may be serious, are reduced by low dose escalation. The estimated incidence of lamotrigine-induced Stevens-Johnson syndrome is 1 in 1000 in adults and 1 in 50 to 1 in 300 in children. Lamotrigine should be used cautiously in patients with a history of serious hypersensitivity reactions. Caution is required in patients with severe myoclonic epilepsy, which may be aggravated by lamotrigine. A favorable synergistic interaction with valproic acid has been reported in patients refractory to either agent given alone.

VIGABATRIN

Vigabatrin, available for routine use since 1989, was designed as an irreversible, enzyme-activated suicide inhibitor of GABA transaminase. Through blockade of this enzyme, vigabatrin inhibits the degradation of GABA, resulting in increased brain GABA levels and enhanced GABAergic transmission. Vigabatrin is available as tablets and as a water-soluble dispersion for oral use. The starting dosage in adults is usually 500 mg per day, which can be increased to 1500 to 2000 mg per day over 1 to 3 weeks. Maintenance dosages up to 3000 mg per day may be used (Tab. 10.4). Vigabatrin is usually given bid, but once-daily dosing is feasible.

Vigabatrin is effective in the management of partial seizures, with or without secondary generalization, and infantile spasms (i.e., West syndrome). In placebo-controlled add-on trials in refractory partial seizures, about 35% of patients showed a greater than 50% reduction in seizure frequency. The main use of vigabatrin is in the add-on treatment of patients refractory to other drugs, but first-line use has been advocated in infants with spasms, especially those associated with tuberous sclerosis.

Vigabatrin exhibits linear pharmacokinetics. Because of its irreversible mode of action, the duration of effect is much longer than its short serum half-life (Tab. 10.6).

Adverse effects may include sedation, dizziness, headache, depression, and behavioral disturbances, including psychosis. During chronic treatment, weight gain may be troublesome. At present, use of vigabatrin is greatly restricted following the recent discovery of potentially irreversible concentric bilateral constriction of the visual fields in over one third of chronically treated patients.

Vigabatrin may aggravate myoclonic and absence seizures in patients with generalized epilepsies. Vigabatrin should be avoided or used with caution in patients with a history of behavioral disturbances or severe depression. Elderly patients and patients with impaired renal function should receive lower dosages.

Vigabatrin may cause a modest and inconsistent reduction in the serum levels of phenytoin.

GABAPENTIN

The GABA analogue gabapentin was introduced in the early 1990s. Its mode of action involves enhancement of GABAergic transmission, possibly through increased brain GABA synthesis, but other actions have been hypothesized. Gabapentin is available as capsules for oral use. In adults, it can be started at 300 mg per day and increased to 900 to 1800 mg per day over 5 to 10 days. Higher doses may be used if appropriate (Tab. 10.4). Gabapentin is usually given three times daily.

Gabapentin is effective against partial seizures, with or without secondary generalization. In placebo-controlled add-on trials in refractory partial seizures, about 15% of patients showed a greater than 50% reduction in seizure frequency, but better results appear to be obtained at dosages higher than those used in early trials. Absorption may aggravate myoclonic seizures.

The drug is absorbed through a saturable mechanism in the gut, and its bioavailabilty decreases from about 60% at low dosages to around 30% above 2400 mg per day (Tab. 10.6); as a result, serum drug concentrations increase less than proportionally with increasing dosages.

Side effects may include sedation, dizziness, ataxia, fatigue, headache, tremor, and weight gain. Behavioral disturbances may occur, especially in mentally retarded children. Caution is required in patients with impaired renal function, who may require lower dosages. No major interactions have been described.

TOPIRAMATE

Topiramate, initially licensed in 1995, has a multifactorial mode of action, including blockade of voltage-dependent sodium channels, antagonism of excitatory amino acids at AMPA receptor sites, and enhancement of GABAergic transmission. It also inhibits carbonic anhydrase. Topiramate is available as tablets and as a special formulation for oral use. In adults, treatment may be initiated with 25 mg per day and increased slowly over several weeks according to clinical response. In difficult-to-treat epilepsies, optimal adult maintenance dosages are usually in the range of 200 to 400 mg per day in two divided doses (see Tab. 10.4).

Topiramate is effective against partial seizures and generalized tonic-clonic seizures, but there is suggestive evidence of efficacy also in other seizure types. The effectiveness against absence seizures is, however, uncertain. In placebo-controlled add-on trials in refractory partial seizures, about 35% of patients showed a greater than 50% reduction in seizure frequency. Topiramate is currently indicated for patients refractory to established drugs.

The drug is is cleared mainly by renal excretion (Tab. 10.6), but in patients taking enzyme inducers, metabolism contributes importantly to elimination. Children eliminate topiramate at a faster rate than adults.

The most common side effects are dizziness, fatigue, diplopia, nystagmus, sedation, confusion, mental slowing, ataxia, anorexia, impaired concentration, paresthesias, agitation, headache, and weight loss. Owing to inhibition of carbonic anhydrase, a 1.5% incidence of symptomatic nephrolithiasis has been reported. Topiramate is teratogenic in animal models, but the clinical relevance of this finding has not been established. Topiramate should not be used or should be used with extreme caution in conditions where inhibition of carbonic anhydrase is undesirable, such as metabolic or respiratory acidosis and a history of nephrolithiasis.

Serum topiramate levels are decreased by enzyme-inducing anticonvulsants such as carbamazepine, phenytoin, and barbiturates. Topiramate may decrease the efficacy of the contraceptive pill by inducing its metabolism.

Pheytoin levels are increased inconsistently by topiramate.

OXCARBAZEPINE

Oxcarbazepine, the 10-keto analogue of carbamazepine, was licensed in the late 1980s. Its primary mode of action involves inhibition of voltage-dependent sodium channels, similarly to carbamazepine. Oxcarbazepine is available as tablets for oral use, but a parenteral form of the active metabolite monohydroxycarbazepine (MHD) is under development. In adults, treatment may be started at 150 to 300 mg per day, to be increased by 150 mg every second day to 600 to 1200 mg per day. For further dosing information, see Table 10.4.

Oxcarbazepine is effective against partial seizures and generalized tonic-clonic seizures, and it may be used as an alternative to carbamazepine.

Oxcarbazepine is converted rapidly to MHD, for which it is considered to be a prodrug (Tab. 10.6). Side effects include sedation, dizziness, headache, diplopia, nausea, and ataxia. Compared with carbamazepine, oxcarbazepine less commonly causes a skin rash, whereas hyponatremia (usually asymptomatic) is more common. Contraindications are similar to those listed for carbamazepine.

Interactions are far less common with oxcarbazepine than with carbamazepine. The serum concentration of the active metabolite MHD may be reduced moderately by enzyme-inducing anticonvulsants. Oxcarbazepine may decrease the efficacy of the contraceptive pill by inducing its metabolism.

TIAGABINE

Tiagabine, licensed in 1997, is a nipecotic acid derivative that acts by enhancing GABAergic transmission through inhibition of GABA reuptake. It is available only as tablets for oral use. In adults comedicated with other anticonvulsants, treatment may be started with 7.5 to 15 mg per day and increased gradually to 30 mg per day over 2 to 3 weeks. Optimal maintenance dosage is 30 to 60 mg per day, usually in two or three divided doses given at meal times (Tab. 10.4).

Tiagabine is effective in the management of partial seizures, with or without secondary generalization. Its main use is as an add-on medication in patients refractory to established drugs.

Tiagabine is is eliminated by CYP3A-mediated oxidation, a reaction that is accelerated in patients taking enzyme-inducing anticonvulsants (Tab. 10.6).

Side effects include dizziness, headache, tremor, impaired concentration, sedation, fatigue, nausea, diarrhea, behavioral disturbances, depressed mood, and emotional lability. Caution is required in patients with hepatic impairment. Precipitation or aggravation of myoclonic and nonconvulsive seizures has been reported.

Serum tiagabine levels are decreased by enzyme-inducing anticonvulsants such as carbamazepine, phenytoin, and barbiturates.

LESS COMMONLY USED DRUGS

Felbamate Felbamate was licensed in the United States in 1993, but use was curtailed drastically following reports of aplastic anemia and fatal liver toxicity. Its mode of action involves antagonism of NMDA-mediated responses at the glycine regulatory site, blockade of voltage-dependent sodium channels, and enhanced GABAergic transmission. It is rapidly absorbed, is 30% bound to plasma proteins, and eliminated partly by renal excretion and partly by metabolism with a half-life of 15 to 23 hours. Felbamate is effective against partial seizures, generalized tonic-clonic seizures, and probably other seizure types. In a controlled trial, it has been found to be effective in reducing drop attacks associated with Lennox-Gastaut syndrome. It is currently used in patients who failed on other drugs, and in some countries the only approved indication is the management of refractory Lennox-Gastaut syndrome under monitoring of hematologic and liver function. Dosing information is given in Table 10.4. Side effects include anorexia, nausea, vomiting, sedation, headache, weight loss, dizziness, diplopia, insomnia, and hypersensitivity reactions. The incidence of aplastic anemia is estimated at 1 in 2000 to 3000 and that of fatal liver damage 1 in 24 000 to 30 000. Felbamate increases the plasma levels of phenobarbital, phenytoin, carbamazepine-10,11-epoxide, and valproic acid, and it reduces the serum levels of oral steroid contraceptives.

Zonisamide Zonisamide was developed in the 1980s in Japan, where it is now licensed. Its mode of action may involve inhibition of voltage-dependent sodium channels, T-type calcium channels, and carbonic anhydrase. It is absorbed rapidly, is less than 50% protein bound, and is eliminated partly by renal excretion and partly by metabolism with a half-life of about 60 hours. Shorter half-lives (about 30 hours) are observed in patients taking enzyme-inducing anticonvulsants. Zonisamide is effective against partial seizures and probably various generalized seizure types. Promising results have been reported in progressive myoclonic epilepsy. Maintenance dosage is usually 200 to 600 mg per day in adults and 4 to 10 mg/kg per day in children, given as one or two daily doses. Side effects include somnolence, ataxia, anorexia, confusion, mental slowing, nervousness, fatigue, dizziness, headache, behavioral disturbances, gastrointestinal symptoms, weight loss, and skin rashes. Nephrolithiasis has been described in initial studies in the United States, but it does not appear to have been a problem in Japan.

Acetazolamide (see Chap. 17) Acetazolamide is a carbonic anhydrase inhibitor that is absorbed rapidly, is over 90% bound to plasma proteins, and is eliminated unchanged in urine. Its distribution half-life is about 2 hours, whereas elimination half-life is 12 to 15 hours. The efficacy of acetazolamide in epilepsy has not undergone adequate, controlled evaluation, but the drug is considered to be of value against various seizure types and especially against absence seizures. Dosage usually ranges between 3 and 20 mg/kg per day. Since efficacy may be limited by development of tolerance, acetazolamide has been proposed for intermittent use, especially in conditions such as catamenial epilepsy. Possible adverse effects include sedation, fatigue, depression, paresthesias, sexual dysfunction, anorexia, weight loss, dysgeusia, hypokalemia, nephrolithiasis, skin rashes, and other hypersensitivity reactions. Acetazolamide should be used cautiously and at lower dosages in the elderly and wherever inhibition of carbonic anhydrase is undesired. Acetazolamide may decrease the serum levels of primidone and increase those of carbamazepine. Potentiation of acetazolamide toxicity by salicylates may occur.

New areas of drug development

The newer generation of antiepileptic drugs has been a welcome addition to the therapeutic armamentarium, but it has reduced only modestly the problem of drug-resistant epilepsy. Therefore, the search for safer and/or more effective anticonvulsants continues. A number of agents, including levetiracetam, remacemide, and losigamone, are currently in advanced clinical development and may become available in the near future. Ongoing mechanistic development of novel drugs is aimed at enhancing inhibition, particularly GABAergic transmission, at reducing excitation through antagonism of excitatory transmitters or ion channel modulation, and at testing the implications of neuroprotective effects with respect to prevention of epileptogenesis. Other lines of development stem from progress in our understanding of the pathogenesis of epilepsy. Genetics in particular is making fast advances, and gene therapy might become a treatment option in the future. Despite all this, experience has taught us that serendipity still plays an important part in therapeutic breakthroughs.

One of the greatest challenges in current epileptology is the development of diagnostic tools that may be used to predict response to individual drugs and rationalize drug choice. For example, higher response rates with GABAergic drugs might be achieved if their use was restricted to individuals whose seizures were caused by documented defects in GABAergic transmission. Development of imaging techniques such as magnetic resonance spectroscopy holds promises in this direction, and the management of epilepsy might become less empirical in the years to come.

BEGHI E, PERUCCA E. The management of epilepsy in the 1990s: Acquisitions, uncertainties, and perspectives for future research. Drugs 1995;49:680-94.

BRODIE MJ, DICHTER MA. Established antiepileptic drugs. N Engl J Med 1996;334:168-75.

BRODIE MJ, TREIMAN DM. Modern management of epilepsy. Bailleres Clin Neurol. Vol 5. London: Baillières-Tindall, 1996.

DE SILVA M, MACARDLE B, MCGOWAN M, et al. Randomised comparative monotherapy trial of phenobarbitone, phenytoin, carbamazepine, or sodium valproate acid for newly diagnosed childhood epilepsy. Lancet 1996;347:709-13.

HELLER AJ, CHESTERMAN P, ELWES RDC, et al. Phenobarbitone, phenytoin, carbamazepine, or sodium valproate for newly diagnosed adult epilepsy: a randomized comparative monotherapy trial. J Neurol Neurosurg Psychiatry 1995;58:44-50.

LEVY RH, MATTSON RH, MELDRUM B. Antiepileptic Drugs, 4th ed. New York: Raven Press, 1995.

MATTSON RH, CRAMER JA, COLLINS JF, AND THE DEPARTMENT OF VETERAN AFFAIRS EPILEPSY COOPERATIVE STUDY NO. 264 GROUP. A comparison of valproic acid with carbamazepine for the treatment of complex partial seizures and secondarily generalized tonic-clonic seizures in adults. N Engl J Med 1992;327:765-71.

PERUCCA E. Clinical implications of hepatic microsomal enzyme induction by antiepileptic drugs. Pharmacol Ther 1987;33:139-44.

PERUCCA E. The new generation of antiepileptic drugs: Advantages and disadvantages. Br J Clin Pharmacol 1996;42:531-43.

PERUCCA E, GRAM L, AVANZINI G, DULAC O. Antiepileptic drugs as a cause of worsening seizures. Epilepsia 1999;39:5-17.

RICHENS A, PERUCCA E. Clinical pharmacology and medical treatment. In: Laidlaw J, Richens A, Chadwick D, eds. A Textbook of epilepsy. Edinburgh: Churchill-Livingstone, 1993:495-559.

RICHENS A, DAVIDSON DLW, CARTLIDGE NEF, EASTER DJ. A multicentre comparative trial of sodium valproate and carbamazepine in adult onset epilepsy. J Neurol Neurosurg Psychiatry 1994;57:682-87.

SHORVON S. Antiepileptic drug monotherapy versus polytherapy: Economic aspects. Epilepsia 1997;38(suppl 5):S17-S20.

SHORVON S, DREIFUSS F, FISH D, THOMAS D. The Treatment of Epilepsy. Oxford: Blackwell Science, 1996.

VERITY CM, HOSKING G, EASTER DJ. A multicentre comparative trial of sodium valproate and carbamazepine in paediatric epilepsy. Dev Med Child Neurol 1995;37:907-1108.

11

Extrapyramidal disorders

Gilles Fenelon, François Le Doze, Gilles-Louis Defer

Extrapyramidal disorders include such classic common and debilitating diseases as Parkinson's disease (PD), Huntington's disease (HD), and a number of parkinsonian syndromes (Tab. 11.1). Although the clinical neuropathologic and pathophysiologic aspects of these disorders are distinct, all induce abnormalities in the control of movement and are responsible for substantial medical and social problems.

Table 11.1 Classification of parkinsonian syndromes

I - Parkinson's disease
  Idiopathic
  Inherited
  Juvenile parkinsonisn

II - Secondary parkinsonism
  A. Iatrogenic: neuroleptics, α-methyldopa, lithium, diazoxide, flunarizine, cinnarizine
  B. Toxic: manganese poisoning, mercury poisoning, carbon monoxide poisoning, carbon disulfide poisoning, cyanide poisoning, ethanol, N-methyl-4 phenyl 1, 2, 3, 6, tetrahydropyridine (MPTP)
  C. Metabolic: hypoparathyroidism, hepatocerebral degeneration, Gaucher's disease
  D. Encephalitis letargica
  E. Vascular
  F. Brain tumor
  G. Trauma
    Punch-drunk syndrome
  H. Hydrocephalus

III - Parkinsonism with other symptoms
  A. Sporadic disorders
    1. Progressive supranuclear palsy
    2. Multi system atrophy including striatonigral degeneration
    3. Parkinson-ALS dementia
    4. Corticobasal degeneration
    5. Alzheimer's disease with parkinsonism
    6. Dementia with Lewy body
  B. Inherited
    1. Huntington's disease
    2. Wilson's disease
    3. Hallervorden-Spatz disease
    4. Neuroacanthocytosis
    5. Spinocerebellar atrophy

During the last decades, these prototypical neurodegenerative diseases have both benefited from important scientific discoveries concerning pathophysiologic mechanisms. Especially for PD, the relationship between the dopaminergic denervation of the striatum (caudate and putamen), major symptoms, and dysfunction of the striatopallidothalamocortical circuitry through a direct and an indirect pathway has been clearly demonstrated. For HD, there was, on the one hand, identification of the responsible gene abnormality (chromosome 4), i.e., a repeated string of a trinucleotide (CAG), the length of which seems to determine the age of onset (anticipation phenomenon), and, on the other hand, a better understanding of the mechanisms of the cellular energetic failure observed in this disease.

In parallel with these major advances in determining the pathophysiologic mechanisms of these diseases, a number of new therapeutic approaches have widened available options for the management of most extrapyramidal disorders. This was particularly true for PD, where new drugs and new therapeutic strategies including surgical procedures were developed.

EXTRAPYRAMIDAL DISORDERS AND PARKINSON'S DISEASE

The term *extrapyramidal motor disease* was first used by Wilson to qualify progressive lenticular degeneration and shaking palsy (i.e., Parkinson's disease). He wished to attract attention to the fact that, in these diseases, pyramidal tracts remained intact. However, attempts to describe an "extrapyramidal" motor system on anatomic and physiologic ground have failed, and the term *extrapyramidal syndrome* remains fuzzy because it does not refer to any precise set of movement disorders. It is now used either as a synonym for *parkinsonian syndrome* or as an equivalent of *movement disorders.* In this section, focus will be on Parkinson's disease.

Pathophysiology

Parkinson's disease may be defined as the combination of

a clinical syndrome (parkinsonism) and a distinctive pathology consisting of cell loss affecting mainly the melanized dopaminergic neurons of the Substantia Nigra, with typical inclusions in the remaining neurons, the Lewy bodies. This cell death is of unknown origin. Its main neurochemical consequence is a severe dopamine deficit in the striatum, which induces a disinhibition of the subthalamopallidal structures. These changes lead to defective frontal cortical motor control (and defective brainstem motor activity), resulting in akinesia. However, the exact consequences on the function of the basal ganglia circuitry are still being debated. Moreover, the pathophysiology of some components of parkinsonism (tremor and postural disturbances) is still poorly understood.

Diagnosis

The first step in the diagnosis of PD is to identify parkinsonism. Parkinsonism consists of a combination of akinesia, rigidity, tremor, and postural disturbances. Akinesia itself is a symptom complex that includes slowness of movement (bradykinesia) with progressive fatiguing when the movement is repetitive, poverty of movement (e.g., amimia, loss of arm swing), reduction of amplitude, and difficulties initiating movement. Rigidity (typically "lead pipe") is usually associated with akinesia. The characteristic tremor is a 3- to 5-Hz rest tremor, often intermittent, and initially absent in about 30% of the patients. Once the characteristic features of parkinsonism are recognized, it should be established whether this is due to PD, the most common cause of parkinsonism, or some other disorder. The clinical diagnostic criteria formulated by the United Kingdom Parkinson's Disease Society Brain Bank are used commonly (Tab. 11.2). It should be emphasized that no final diagnostic test is available and that, even when strict clinical criteria are applied, neuropathologic series have shown that more than 15% of patients are labeled erroneously as having PD during life. False-positive cases are mainly due to progressive supranuclear palsy and multiple system atrophy.

Evolution

Treatment with levo-dopa (L-dopa) always leads to major clinical improvement. However, in most cases, the "L-dopa honeymoon" only lasts a few years, to be followed by long-term motor complications: fluctuations, dyskinesias, and axial motor disorders. Cognitive and neuropsychiatric problems also may occur. Schematically, younger patients are at higher risk of developing early fluctuations and dyskinesias, whereas older patients are more at risk of suffering axial motor disorders and cognitive impairment. In general, PD patients vary considerably in their responses to antiparkinsonian drugs

With the passage of time, an increasing proportion of patients undergo fluctuations of their response to L-dopa. End-of-dose deteriorations or wearing-off effects are the

---

Table 11.2 U.K. Parkinson's Disease Society Brain Bank: clinical diagnostic criteria for Parkinson's disease

Step 1 - Diagnosis of parkinsonism
Bradykinesia and at least one of the following: muscular rigidity, rest tremor, postural instability (not caused by primary visual, vestibular, cerebellar, or propioceptive dysfunction)

Step 2 - Exclusion criteria for Parkinson's disease
Neuroleptic treatment at onset of symptoms
Other possible cause (e.g., history of encephalitis, repeated head injury, or repeated strokes; presence of cerebral tumor or communicating hydrocephalus)
Additional neurologic signs, such as cerebellar signs, Babinski sign, early severe autonomic involvement, supranuclear gaze palsy, oculogyric crises, early severe dementia
Lack of response to large doses of levodopa (if malabsorption excluded)

Step 3 - Supportive prospective positive criteria for Parkinson's disease (Three or more required for diagnosis of definite Parkinson's disease)
Unilateral onset
Rest tremor present
Progressive disorder
Persistent asymmetry affecting side of onset most
Excellent response (70-100%) to L-dopa
Severe L-dopa-induced chorea
L-Dopa response for 5 years or more
Clinical course of 10 years or more

---

earliest fluctuations, developing after a couple of years. The patient begins to experience a loss of effect at the end of dosing periods. These fluctuations therefore are predictable and clearly related to the L-dopa intake schedule. Later in the treatment, motor fluctuations become more abrupt and random, the patient switching rapidly from one state to another (on-off phenomenon). Other types of fluctuations include failure of the patient to respond to one dose of L-dopa (often in the afternoon) or a delayed response after the first dose in the morning (delayed on). Nonmotor phenomena are often associated with motor fluctuations, and they include anxiety, depression, sensory symptoms, and symptoms of autonomic dysfunction. The pathophysiology of fluctuations is debated; peripheral pharmacokinetic, central pharmacokinetic, and central pharmacodynamic factors may play a part.

Dyskinesias are another long-term complication of dopatherapy and represent a major burden of the disease. The term refers to abnormal involuntary movements that generally appear or predominate on the most affected side. Usually they occur with fluctuations and may be described on the basis of the symptoms (e.g., ballistic, choreic, dystonic, etc.) and the location (e.g., face, limbs, or trunk). L-dopa-induced dyskinesias may be divided into three main types. *Peak-dose dyskinesias* are the most common type. They typically appear in the middle of a dosing period and usually take the form of choreic movements. However, a combination of chorea and dystonia may occur. *Diphasic dyskinesias* appear at the beginning or the end of a dosing period. They predominantly involve the lower limbs and are more severe (but of shorter duration) than peak-dose dyskinesias. Finally, *painful dystonic cramps* may occur in the "off" state, particularly in the early morning. Several studies were aimed at risk factors and showed a greater prevalence of male patients and more frequent occurrence of motor fluctuations and dyskinesias in the young-onset group with longer duration of PD and L-dopa treatment, higher L-dopa dosage, and multiple combined therapies.

In one study of 811 L-dopa-responsive patients, predictable "offs" were noted in 20% in the first 5 years and in 58% after 15 years. Unpredictable or sudden offs and early morning dystonia were less common. Disease duration was associated with greater percentages of patients with off periods or dyskinesias (up to 70% after 15 years), although patients with 6 to 15 years of disease duration saw relatively little increase in the frequency of these complications. A minority of patients (approximately 30%) with disease duration higher than 10 years did not experience off periods or dyskinesia.

In PD, parkinsonism remains dopa-sensitive throughout the course of the disease. However, in older patients, some motor disturbances may respond poorly to treatment, such as difficulties in gait, postural stability, swallowing, and speech disorders. These "axial" disorders are often associated with cognitive changes and are thought to depend on nondopaminergic mechanisms (at least in part), especially impaired serotoninergic transmission secondary to inhibition or downregulation of aromatic amino acid decarboxylase.

Nonmotor disorders are constant in the course of PD. Sensory disturbances, sleep disorders, and dysautonomia are common. Dysautonomic disturbances include orthostatic hypotension, constipation, urinary problems, impotence, sweating episodes, and seborrhea. Cognitive changes may be mild or severe (dementia). The exact prevalence of mild cognitive impairment is unknown. It does not interfere with daily life and is revealed by neuropsychologic assessment. These mild cognitive changes mainly consist of impairment in visuospatial tasks, memory, and executive functions. Dementia affects 20 to 40% of patients with PD. The same impairments are observed, to a higher degree, with frequent hallucinations and delusions. Typically, aphasia, apraxia, and agnosia are not present, thus creating a different picture than in Alzheimer's disease. Dementia preferentially affects older patients. Relations with the severity of motor dysfunction are still a matter of debate. Psychiatric aspects are also important to consider. Most patients experience some degree of anxiety, sometimes as panic attacks aligned with the off periods. Depression is also common. Population studies have shown that major depressive disorders have a low prevalence (under 8%), whereas depressive symptoms are present in as many as 45% of the patients. The respective parts of organic and psychosocial factors in the pathogenesis of depression in the course of PD are not clearly established. Finally, hallucinations, mainly visual, may develop in as many as 25% of the patients. The precise role of treatment is difficult to assess because nearly all patients are treated. The main risk factor for visual hallucinations is the presence of cognitive deficits.

An important issue is to determine whether treatments (mainly dopatherapy) increase the life expectancy of parkin-

sonian patients. In the pre-L-dopa era, the mortality ratio (ratio of observed to expected deaths) was 2.9 and 1.6 in the two main available studies. Since L-dopa has been used, mortality was first said to decrease significantly. However, recent prospective case-control studies have shown that parkinsonian patients still have a greater than twofold increased risk of mortality. Thus, it is difficult to draw a definite conclusion on the effects of L-dopa on mortality.

Finally, few studies have evaluated the burden of PD on society, family, and the individual. A cross-sectional, descriptive study of 109 patients assessed income, health status, health-related costs, and household activities. The total per capita societal burden was approximately $ 6000 per year. The direct costs of the disease reflect a small portion of the burden. The hidden costs, in the form of lost wages, informal care, and changing roles, are substantial.

Treatment

Drug therapy

Charcot was probably the first to inaugurate the pharmacologic treatment for PD using anticholinergic agents such as atropine. Until the middle of the twentieth century this was the only treatment, but at that time, new anticholinergic synthetic compounds became available that produced fewer undesirable effects owing to better brain access.

In 1959, dramatic improvements in the understanding of the neurobiology of PD underlined the lack of neostriatal dopamine in the pathophysiology of the main features. Thus, dopaminergic treatment was initiated in the 1960s, based on the administration of L-dopa, soon associated with peripheral dopa decarboxylase inhibitor in order to enhance its bioavailability. More recently, dopaminergic agonists such as apomorphine, ergolines (e.g., bromocriptine, pergolide, and lisuride), as well as nonergoline compounds (e.g., ropinirole, pramipexole, and talipexole) were developed to replace or to synergize with the effects of L-dopa. New compounds such as COMT inhibitors (catechol-*O*-methyltransferase inhibitor) are now available. They prevent the formation of 3-*O*-methyldopa from L-dopa. This metabolite competes with L-dopa to penetrate the blood-brain barrier and may be at the origin of psychic side effects.

Future developments in pharmacologic treatment may be based on an etiopathologic approach through the use of neurotrophic factors (e.g., nerve growth factor, brain-derived neurotrophic factor, and ciliary neurotrophic factor) to counteract neuronal death.

Drug classes

LEVO-DOPA

L-Dopa is active after transformation into dopamine by a dopa decarboxylase. In the central nervous system (CNS), action is mediated through the activation of postsynaptic receptors, mainly D1 and D2. D1 receptors are positively coupled with cAMP, whereas D2 are not. Autoreceptors, probably D2, are implicated in the feedback regulation of presynaptic dopamine release (Tab. 11.3).

Pharmacokinetics

L-Dopa is rapidly absorbed, mainly at the ileal level. *Tmax* is between 30 and 120 minutes, and elimination half-life range from 1 to 3 hours. About 1% of an oral dose enters the brain, owing to extensive metabolism, first into the intestinal wall (dopadecarboxylase and monoamine oxidase metabolize 90% of the dose), thereafter in the blood and peripheral tissues (dopadecarboxylated and catechol-O-methyltransferase metabolize 9% of the dose). It si decarboxylated into dopamine of which only 10% reaches the brain, while the remaining peripheral fraction is responsible or cardiovascular and gastrointestinal effects. Further metabolic products include homovanillic acid, 3, 4 hydroxyphenylacetic acid and 3-0-methyldopa. Levodopa metabolites are rapidly eliminated by the kidney: 80% in 24 hours, while biliary elimination is negligible. Levodopa is excreted into breast milk. In order to ameliorate L-dopa access to the brain, some of these metabolic steps can be counteracted by specific compounds. Benserazide (BS) and carbidopa (CB) are now constantly used in conjunction with L-dopa to increase its half-life by inhibiting peripheral decarboxylation. BS is associated with L-dopa in a ratio of 4:1 (12.5 mg

---

Table 11.3 Major antiparkinsonian drugs

I - L-Dopa + enzyme inhibitor
Levo dopa + dopa-decarboxylase inhibitor
Levo dopa + benserazide
Levo dopa + carbidopa

Catechol-*O*-methyltransferase (COMT) inhibitors
Entacapone
Nitecapone
Tolcapone

Monoamide oxidase inhibitors B
Selegiline
Lazabemide

II - Synthetic anticholinergics
Trihexyphenidyl
Biperiden
Scopolamine
Tropatepine
Benztropine

III - Dopamine receptor agonists
Apomorphine
Ergolines
Bromocriptine
Pergolide
Lisuride
Cabergoline
Terguride

Nonergolines
Piribedil
Ropinirole
Pramipexole
Talipexole

Others
Amantadine

Table 11.4 Major antiparkinsonian drugs: principal pharmacokinetic data

Compound	Absorption (%)	T_{max} (h)	Distribution volume (l/kg)	Biotransformations	Metabolites	Excretion	$t_{1/2}$ (h)	Initial daily dose	Daily maintenance dose
Benserazide	70	1	NA	NA	Yes	60% kidney 40% biliary	0,5	12.5 mg/50 mg of L-dopa	50 to 300 mg
Bromocriptine	30-40	0.5 to 2	1 to 3.4	Liver	Numerous; mainly 2-bromo-lysergic acid and 2-bromo-isolysergic acid	Biliary	3-48	1.25 mg x 2	3,75 to 40 mg
Carbidopa	40-70	0.5 to 5	NA	Liver	Glucuronides	Kidney	2-3	10 mg for 1 00 mg L-dopa	20 to 110 mg
L-dopa	41±6	0.5 to 2	NA	Decarboxylation Methylation	Dopamine Dihydroxy-3,4-phenylacetic 3-O-methylopa Monovanillic acid	Kidney, feces, air, milk	1-3	(+ carbidopa or benserazide) 25 to 100 mg 2 to 3 times	200 to 1100 mg
Lisuride	≈100	1.25±1	2.5	Liver (first pass effect	Numerous; mainly keto-2-hydroxy-3-lisuride	Kidney, biliary	2-3	0.1 mg bid	2-4 mg
Pergolide	NA	1 to 2	NA	Liver	No β-glucuronide	50% kidney 50% biliary	27	0.05 mg	2 to 4 mg
Ropinirole	36-57	1.5	6.7	Liver	CYP1A2	Kidney	6	0.25 mg x 3	9 to 20 mg

(NA= not available.)

(Continued)

Table 11.4 (Continued)

Compound	Absorption (%)	T_{max} (h)	Distribution volume (l/kg)	Biotransfor-mations	Metabolites	Excretion	$t_{1/2}$ (h)	Initial daily dose	Daily maintenance dose
Cabergoline	45	0.5 to 4	NA	Liver	NA	Kidney	63-68	1 mg/day	3 to 7 mg
Piribedil	NA	1	–	–	–	–	–	–	50 mg x 2
Pramipexole	NA	1.3	High/NA	Marginal (10%)	Unidentified	Kidney	8-12	1.5 mg	1.5 to 4.5 mg
Entacapone	30-45	1	181	Liver	β-glucuronide	Kidney	0.5	–	200 mg/L-Dopa intake
Selegiline	2	0.5 to 2	5	Liver (first pass effect ++)	5 metabolites (L-amphetamine)	Kidney-biliary depending on the metabolite	2.5 to 21	5 mg x 2	2.5 to 10 mg
Apomorphine	Complete (subcutaneous)	–	–	–	–	–	–	–	20 µg/kg (sc)
Amantadine	NA	1 to 4	6	Marginal (10%)	Unidentified	Kidney	9 to 34	100 mg x 2	200 mg or 300-400 mg*
Trihexyphenidyl	60	1.3	NA	Liver	Hydroxylation	Kidney	3.3 to 4	2 mg	2 to 5 mg

(NA = not available.)
*In case of dyskinesias.

BS for 50 mg L-dopa). For CB, the ratio is 10:1 (10 mg CB for 100 mg L-dopa). During therapeutic use, CB and BS do not cross the blood-brain barrier. These two coumpounds are metabolized. CB's half-life after oral administration is around 3 hours. L-Dopa metabolites are eliminated rapidly by the kidney: 80% in 24 hours. Biliary elimination is negligible. L-dopa is eliminated in the milk (Tab. 11.4).

Interactions

Coadministration with sympathomimetic amines may result in increased blood pressure secondary to a synergistic action on α- and β-adrenergic peripheral receptors. Monoamine oxidase inhibitors A (MAOI-A) associated with L-dopa could induce rapid and uncontrolled variations in blood pressure. The use of type B MAOIs specific for dopamine (e.g., selegiline) may prevent this kind of side effect.

For the same reason, tricyclic antidepressants (TCAs) should be prescribed cautiously. The association of L-dopa with serotonin uptake inhibitors is dangerous because of the occurrence of a possibly fatal serotoninergic syndrome. Because of their pharmacodynamic antagonist actions on L-dopa and dopaminergic drugs in general, neuroleptics should be avoided. Some authors advocate their use at low dosage to treat dyskinesias or psychic disturbances. Pyridoxine, a dopa decarboxylase coenzyme, weakens the efficacy of L-dopa. Orthostatic hypotension can be observed when L-dopa is administered with sympatholytic antihypertensive drugs (see "Side effects").

Therapeutic use

L-Dopa remains the most effective treatment for parkinsonian motor disability. Classically, it is also considered that an initial positive response to this treatment is a "cornerstone" of the diagnostic criteria. Besides its clear clinical efficacy, side effects of L-dopa generally are milder that those of dopamine agonists, particularly in the elderly. The potential efficacy of controlled-release (CR) L-dopa has been demonstrated in terms of quality of life and "on period" time in fluctuating PD patients. More interesting is the fact that an early administration of CR L-dopa in nonfluctuating patients can reduce future motor fluctuations. A recent 5-year study comparing CR L-dopa with standard L-dopa first administered to nonfluctuating PD patients found no difference in terms of reaching the primary endpoint (motor fluctuations) between the two treatment groups, although activities of daily living subscores on the Unified Parkinson's Disease Rating Scale (UPDRS) were better in the CR L-dopa group. These results need further confirmation, however.

Use of L-dopa in parkinsonian patients is mostly related to the experience of the clinician. Typically, first L-dopa administration is initiated at low dose combined with a peripheral decarboxylase inhibitor twice or three times daily. Thereafter, total dose and the number of drug administrations per day are adapted to the motor response of the patient.

Pathophysiologic issues

The pharmacologic mechanisms of motor fluctuations are

not fully understood but can be separated into three groups: (1) central pharmacokinetics, or delivery of dopamine from presynaptic to postsynaptic receptors, (2) peripheral pharmacokinetics, or delivery of L-dopa from an exogenous source to the brain, and (3) pharmacodynamics, or alterations in the interactions between dopamine and striatal receptors. Changes in central pharmacokinetics caused by diminished presynaptic dopamine storage capacity probably account for early end-of-dose "wearing off." As patients lose further storage capacity, peripheral kinetics may play an important role in the fluctuation of response, i.e., from erratic gastric emptying or variables that change gut-to-blood and blood-brain barrier transport. Finally, erratic motor responses (e.g., the "on-off" phenomenon) in advanced PD may be caused in part by alterations at the striatal dopamine receptor. Aromatic L-amino acid decarboxylase (AAAD) is the second enzyme in the sequence leading to the synthesis of catecholamines and serotonin, and it is the rate-limiting enzyme for the synthesis of the trace amines. The "on-off" phenomenon, where there are fluctuations between "off" periods of marked akinesia over several hours with "on" periods of improved motility also may be related to oscillating or poorly modulated AAAD activity and conversion of L-dopa to DA.

Pathophysiology of dyskinesias is not fully understood, but peak-dose dyskinesia appear to arise mainly as a consequence of postsynaptic alterations that follow exposure to nonphysiologic intrasynaptic dopamine changes in patients who have lost the buffering afforded by dopaminergic terminals. In a 3-year clinical and pharmacokinetic follow-up study, a dissociation of the kinetic-dynamic relationship of L-dopa motor and dyskinesia effects was found, possibly reflecting different cerebral handling of exogenous L-dopa-derived dopamine with disease progression. There is a continuum between the first dyskinesias and those observed during the period of maximal clinical improvement. These dyskinesias also can appear in the reverse order, as if there were an "oscillator" determining a sequence of alternating patterns, and electrophysiologic recordings showed irregular bursting patterns of discharges in the motor thalamus. Nondopaminergic mechanisms have been claimed, and a positron emission tomographic (PET) study pointed to an altered opioid transmission as part of the pathophysiology of L-dopa-induced dyskinesias. Comparison of 2- and 21-hour L-dopa infusions indicated that the duration of response after discontinuing the longer infusions was briefer than after discontinuing the short infusion, suggesting the development of tolerance. Moreover, dyskinesia severity was greater during long infusions.

Generally speaking, it seems that dopaminergic denervation is required, since no dyskinesia is observed in patients treated with L-dopa and devoid of PD. The nature of the dopaminergic receptor implicated in the mediation of the effect may be relevant. Bromocriptine, a weak D1 antagonist and a powerful D2 agonist, rarely produces dyskinesias. D1 receptor activation could be critical in this respect.

DOPAMINE RECEPTOR AGONISTS

Major characteristics of this class of drugs are (1) no need for biotransformation by degenerating neurons, particularly in advanced stages of the disease, (2) much longer duration of action than L-dopa, (3) direct receptor activation with the possibility to target some subpopulations of dopaminergic neurons (D2 receptors with ropinirole), and (4) absence of oxidative metabolism, reducing the risk of neurotoxicity.

Dopamine receptors were divided initially in two categories: D1 and D2. Other classes (D3, D4, and D5) have been now identified. The D1 receptor family includes not only D1 (called D1A) but also D5 (called D1B). The stimulation of one of these receptors results in an increase in intracellular cAMP. At the intracellular level, D2 stimulation inhibits the formation of cAMP. Because of the different receptors, dopamine has variable effects on the extrapyramidal system. Agonist occupancy of the D1 receptor activates the "direct" loop, which has an inhibitory effect on the internal part of the globus pallidus (Gpi), whereas occupancy of the D2 receptor activates the "indirect" loop, which has an inhibitory effect on the external part of the globus pallidus (Gpe). D2 stimulation is less effective in inducing motor effects than combined D2 and D1 stimulation. This can be expected based on the physiologic functioning of the cortical-basal ganglia loops, where both direct and indirect loops work in parallel. Regarding their capacity to stimulate D1 versus D2 receptors, the actions of the different agonist compounds vary (Tab. 11.5). They also differ with respect to their duration of action. Cabergoline has a very long duration of action, up to 48 hours. Bromocriptine and pergolide have durations of action between 3 and 8 hours, respectively, and apomorphine, the most potent D1/D2 agonist, has the shortest duration of action, between 1 and 2 hours (see Tab. 11.4).

Therapeutic use

There is general agreement that dopamine agonists are very useful in the treatment of parkinsonian patients in all stages of the disease. However, and classically within the dose ranging where they are used, their clinical efficacy is considered to be slightly lower than that of L-dopa. Progressive reduction of therapeutic efficacy over time seems to be the main drawback. However, their use is associated with a low risk of motor fluctuations or the occurrence of abnormal

Table 11.5 Receptor activity of dopamine agonists

Compound	D1	D2
Apomorphine	+	+++
Lisuride	0	++
Bromocriptine	-	++
Pergolide	+	++
Ropinirole	0	+++

+ = agonism; ++ = strong agonism; +++ = very strong agonism; – = antagonism; 0= no effect.

movements. Significant side effects include nausea, postural hypotension, sleepiness, delusions, and hallucinations. Thus, dopamine agonists should be administered progressively in combination with peripheral antivomiting therapy (domperidone) to reduce the risk of GI side effects.

Since many dopamine agonists are available around the world (e.g., bromocriptine, lisuride, piribedil, pergolide, cabergoline, pramipexole, ropinirole), the choice of one drug depends directly of the country market, available clinical studies, and the clinician's own experience. Bromocriptine, pergolide, and lisuride are similar semisynthetic ergoline derivatives with full D2 agonist activity. The pharmacologic activity of bromocriptine depends on the presence of dopamine at the synaptic level. Lisuride can be used both orally and subcutaneously. However, use is limited by the occurrence of dyskinesias and neuropsychiatric side effects. Pergolide has a short half-life but a more prolonged clinical effect (around 5-6 h). In different clinical trials it demonstrated similar efficacy and side effects as bromocriptine. Its theoretical advantage is based on D1 and D2 receptor agonist activity and perhaps a better therapeutic index. A low dose should be used for the first administration because of the classic risk of postural hypotension. Cabergoline is a long-acting D2 dopamine agonist with a long duration of action. This is a theoretical advantage in reducing motor fluctuations, and several studies have reported good efficacy of this compound in patients with severe fluctuations.

Ropinirole is a new potent nonergoline D2 agonist that is active peripherally and centrally. Ropinirole has a powerful dose-dependent activity, comparable with L-dopa, and it is effective as an adjunct to L-dopa in patients with or without motor fluctuations. Safety data were collected from 1364 patients involved in different therapeutic trials with ropinirole. The major side effects observed were nausea, somnolence, edema, abdominal pain, vomiting, dyspepsia, and hallucinations (mean daily dose 8.7 mg). When used as adjunctive therapy with L-dopa (mean daily dose 8.2 mg), the major side effects were dyskinesia, nausea, hallucinations, and confusion. Most side effects decreased over time despite progressive increases in dose, except for the hallucinations. No significant changes in cardiovascular and biologic parameters were observed.

Originally introduced as adjunctive therapy to L-dopa in patients with a fluctuating or deteriorating responses to L-dopa, dopamine agonists are now increasingly proposed as an early treatment alone or in combination with L-dopa. The 6-month interim reports of two studies using ropinirole as an early treatment of PD have been published recently. The first compared ropinirole and L-dopa, the second compared ropinirole and bromocriptine, taking into account if the patient received selegiline or not. In the first study (ropinirole versus L-dopa), the percentage of improvement using the motor part III of the UPDRS was significantly higher for L-dopa (44%) versus ropinirole (32%), but with no significant difference in the proportion of responders (defined as an improvement of at least 30% in the UPDRS score). In the second study, ropinirole was better than bromocriptine (improvement in UPDRS score and proportion of responders) only in the group of patients without selegiline. In the group with selegiline,

the therapeutic effect was similar. The reasons behind this apparent augmentation of the effect of bromocriptine by selegiline remains to be elucidated. There was no interaction between treatment and the selegiline stratum in the study comparing ropinirole and L-dopa.

A special place may be given to apomorphine, available in some countries. It is the most powerful dopamine agonist administered by sc injection or by constant sc infusion using a pump device. After sc injection, motor effect is generally obtained in less than 15 minutes. However, since it is a powerful emetic drug, GI side effects should be prevented by regular administration of domperidone. Other side effects include postural hypotension, sedation, and cutaneous induration at the site of injection. This therapy is reserved especially for treatment of "off periods" in patients with severe motor fluctuations. In this selected population, no clinically significant tolerance or loss of therapeutic effect was seen during long treatment periods. In a group of 71 patients with 1 to 5 years of follow-up, the use of apomorphine (continuous waking-hours infusion or repeated intermittent injections) led to a mean reduction in daily "off period" time by about 50%. Moreover, the incidence of neuropsychiatric toxicity remained low. However, the therapeutic effect is progressively marred by an increase in "on phase" dyskinesias and L-dopa-resistant disability.

MUSCARINIC RECEPTOR ANTAGONISTS

Muscarinic receptor antagonists were used widely before the discovery of L-dopa. Although their mechanism of action is unclear, they appear to act in the neostriatum on intrinsic cholinergic innervation. Antiparkinsonian effects are modest on akinesia and hypertonia, but the antitremor activity is remarkable. These agents generally are used to complement dopaminergic therapy. Several drugs of this class are used for this indication, including biperiden, tropatepine, benztropine mesylate, and trihexyphenidyl.

Diphenhydramine is classically included in this group despite the fact that it is an antihistamine drug but with central anticholinergic properties. Trihexyphenidyl is the prototype of this group and the most used drug. It has the same pharmacodynamic properties as atropine of central and peripheral competitive muscarinic antagonism. Its pharmacokinetics are characterized by rapid and complete absorption. In fact, 72 hours after intake, 56% is excreted as hydroxylated metabolite. Classic therapeutic oral doses range from 2 to 15 mg per day (see Table 11.4) for trihexyphenidyl, from 0.5 to 6 mg per day for benztropine, from 2 to 8 mg per day for biperiden, and from 75 to 400 mg per day for diphenhydramine.

Adverse effects of these agents result directly from their anticholinergic properties: mental confusion and sedation. They should be used with caution in patients with narrow-angle glaucoma. They also may produce constipation, urinary retention, diminished salivation, and tachycardia. Any other drug with anticholinergic activity, e.g., antispasmodics or TCAs, can potentiate these side effects. Moreover, their use is clearly associated with worsening cognitive function, particularly in the elderly.

In addition, sudden discontinuation should be avoided because of the possibility of cholinergic crises. Tachycardia, mydriasis, agitation, delusions, and possibly coma characterize intoxication.

AMANTADINE

This old antiviral drug, used in the prevention of influenza, is a weak antiparkinsonian agent generally used as an adjunctive therapy. It is well absorbed from the GI tract and has a long duration of action with a half-life of 15 hours in normal controls. Amantadine is mainly excreted unchanged in the urine and may accumulate in patients with renal dysfunction, especially the elderly. Today, although it is generally well tolerated, it is used less than a few years ago. Its mechanism of action in PD is unclear. However, recent advances in explicating the role of glutamate in basal ganglia neurotransmission may support its potential use in the treatment of dyskinesias. Amantadine administered in a double-blind, placebo-controlled, crossover study in 18 patients over 3 weeks reduced the severity of L-dopa-induced dyskinesias by 60% compared with placebo without altering the antiparkinsonian effect of L-dopa. The usual dose is 100 mg bid up to 400 mg per day in the treatment of dyskinesias. Amantadine favors the occurrence of psychic disturbances when coadministered with anticholinergic drugs. In addition, acute psychiatric complications following amantadine withdrawal have been described recently.

SELEGILINE

This drug, a monoamine oxidase B inhibitor (MAOI-B), has a mild antiparkinsonian effect. It enhances the effect of dopamine by inhibiting one of the two main catabolic enzymes of the mediator. Selegiline has a weak bioavailability but crosses the blood-brain barrier. It is highly bound to plasma proteins and intensively metabolized by the liver. Clinically, the drug will increase, in combination, the therapeutic effect of L-dopa, and it has been used mainly as adjunctive therapy to reduce motor fluctuations later on in the course of the disease. The usual therapeutic dose is 5 to 10 mg per day. At the end of the 1980s it was suggested that in untreated patients, selegiline could slow the progression of the disease and delay the need to introduce L-dopa therapy. At that time it was argued that this clinical observation could be related to a true "neuroprotective" effect. This question was heavily debated until it was demonstrated that the potential neuroprotective effect seen during the DATATOP study was not apparent on longer follow-up. Moreover, a study from the United Kingdom suggested that, in combination with L-dopa, the use of selegiline may be associated with a significant increase in mortality after 5 years of treatment. This study has received many criticisms, especially concerning death data collection and statistical analysis. Thus, clinical guidelines for the best therapeutic use of selegiline are difficult to establish, but this drug may be considered as a weak antiparkinsonian agent useful as adjunctive therapy.

CATECHOL-*O*-METHYLTRANSFERASE (COMT) INHIBITORS

New and selective compounds that inhibit COMT have been developed. COMT catalyses the transfer of a methyl group to a catechol substrate that inactivates L-dopa in particular, as well as norepinephrine and dopamine. In PD, COMT inhibitors prevent the degradation of L-dopa in peripheral tissues and enhance its brain bioavailability. Such an L-dopa–sparing effect allows reduction of the L-dopa dose. These agents offer an adjunctive therapy in unstable patients on L-dopa therapy, especially those with end-of-dose fluctuations. In such patients, the clinical benefit results in a diminution of the "off period" and an increase in the "on period." Two COMT inhibitors are available: tolcapone and entacapone. They differ by their mechanism of COMT inhibition: peripheral for entacapone and peripheral and central for tolcapone. The two have quite similar half-lives of about 2 hours. Entacapone 200 mg should be prescribed with every L-dopa dose; tolcapone is prescribed in a fixed dose: 100 or 200 mg three times daily.

Some drug interactions may occur because of the catechol structure of several adrenergic compounds. COMT inhibitors can potentiate some drugs, such as bronchodilators, isoprenaline, dopamine agonists (apomorphine, dobutamine), antihypertensive drugs (methyldopa), and the β blocker nadolol. COMT inhibitors appear to be well tolerated. Some minor GI problems (diarrhea) can be expected, in addition to the symptoms of L-dopa overdosage. However, severe hepatitis due to tolcapone has just been reported, leading to the withdrawal of the drug from the market in some European countries.

Side effects of L-dopa and dopaminergic drugs (dyskinesias and motor fluctuations excluded)

In recent years, the question of a possible toxicity of L-dopa on dopaminergic neurons has been hotly debated. In actuality, this question probably will be resolved by a properly designed clinical trial. Today, however, there are no data confirming the toxicity of L-dopa, and there are arguments to suggest that L-dopa may increase survival in PD patients, even if this is related simply to delayed disability. Nausea and orthostatic hypotension are due to the peripheral effects of dopamine. Nausea is induced by stimulation of D2 receptors located in the brainstem chemoreceptive trigger zone outside the blood-brain barrier. It may be counteracted by the use of domperidone, which antagonizes the same receptors and has no effect on the CNS. Orthostatic hypotension can be treated by

Table 11.6 Side effects associated with the use of antiparkinsonian drugs

I. Dopamine mediated
  A. *CNS*
    1. Neurologic
      • Dyskinesia
        Peak-dose dyskinesia
        Diphasic dyskinesia
        "Off" dystonia
      • On-off/phenomenon
      • Waning
    2. Psychic
      • Confusion
      • Delusion
      • Depression, anxiety
    3. Neuroendocrine
      • Amenorrhea
  B. *Peripheral*
    1. Abdominal
      • Diarrhea
      • Anorexia, nausea, vomiting
    2. Cardiovascular
      • Orthostatic hypotension
      • Hypertension
      • Supraventricular arrhythmia
    3. Sweating
II. Mediated by other mechanisms
  A. *Anticholinergic*
    • Glaucoma
    • Urinary retention
    • Confusion
  B. *Unknown mechanism*
    • Inflammatory fibrotic syndromes (ergolines)

fludrocortisone therapy or dietary salt supplementation, if necessary (Tab. 11.6).

Dopaminergic drugs can produce hallucinations probably secondary to the stimulation of mesolimbic dopaminergic receptors. A serotoninergic mechanism also can be suspected, since atypical neuroleptics can reverse, at least partially, these side effects. Previously confused or demented patients should be given dopaminergic drugs very cautiously.

The ergoline-derived dopaminergic agonists share with the antimigraine agents ergotamine and methysergide a potential to induce inflammatory-fibrotic syndromes, particularly pleuropulmonary disorders. The incidence of such complications is thought to be around 2 to 6%. Recovery after drug discontinuation does not always occur.

Aging appears to be a risk factor for psychic disturbances inducible by L-dopa and dopaminergic and anticholinergic drugs. In older patients, the association of these compounds should be evaluated. In patients with diminished renal function, amantadine, ropinirole, and L-dopa can accumulate. Therefore, the dose and regimen should be adapted.

Principles of treatment

After reviewing the available drugs to treat PD, the question is how one should initiate the treatment. In other words, when, with which drug(s), and how antiparkinsonian therapy should be started?

Treatment generally is initiated when clinical diagnostic criteria of PD have been established and there is some degree of functional impairment, whatever the underlying symptoms. In all cases, this decision is mainly subjective, depending on the age of the patient, the duration and features of the symptoms, and the nature of the functional impairment. As indicated earlier, the clinical experience of the neurologist is crucial, but therapeutic strategies may be planned on the basis of the patient's age and cognitive status. Elderly patients (>60 years of age) are more prone to develop adverse effects, especially neuropsychiatric, with dopamine agonists and anticholinergic drugs. However, in the elderly, the issue of L-dopa toxicity may be less important. Therefore, in elderly patients, one may administer L-dopa alone early on with a progressive increase in dose (e.g., from 50 mg L-dopa plus 12.5 mg benzerazide tid up to the dose that controls the symptoms) or, if necessary, in combination with another drug according to the main symptomatology. Younger patients (<60 years of age) in whom there are no cognitive disturbances and work activity is still possible will have this disease for many years and will be more likely to develop motor complications with long-term L-dopa treatment. In such patients, the early use of dopamine agonists has been suggested in the last few years, and recent studies demonstrate that early administration of dopamine agonists is sufficient to control the disease in most patients for 1 to 3 years. Therefore, with the exception of patients who have contraindications or who cannot tolerate dopamine agonists, these drugs should be considered for initial therapy. Thereafter, a combination with low doses of L-dopa could easily be proposed to delay the occurrence of motor complications.

When patients have complex refractory oscillations and/or dyskinesias, they may benefit from continuous dopaminergic stimulation with enteral infusions of L-dopa or subcutaneous infusions of apomorphine. However, when pharmacologic strategies are not efficient and the patient has a severe handicap, surgical strategies may be considered (see below).

New treatments for PD

New drugs and new therapeutic strategies have already been developed to increase treatment capacity for PD patients. Among the pharmacologic strategies are the drug pramipexole, which is a selective nonergoline dopamine agonist that acts on D2 and preferentially on D3 dopamine receptors; cocaine derivatives; a blocker of dopamine transport used for brain imaging and reported to protect against neuroleptic parkinsonism; and glutamate antagonists, if they are sufficiently safe for human use.

In recent years, a large and new development of surgical stategies has occurred. In western countries these include lesioning techniques, especially into the pallidum, but more interestingly, chronic electrical stimulation of the thalamus for tremor, of the pallidum for dyskinesias, and of the subthalamic nucleus for all the parkinsonian symptoms. This last surgical procedure seems very promising in that the main symptoms of the disease are improved from 60 to 80% in almost all operated patients, leading to a major reduction in the use of antiparkinsonian drugs in these patients. Ten years after the first report of clinical improvement in PD, brain tissue transplantation remains experimental. Human allografts of mesencephalic embryonic neurons provide clinically significant improvement in most PD symptoms, and these changes are correlated with striatal dopaminergic reinnervation documented by PET or anatomic examination. To achieve optimal results, ventral mesencephalic cells from at least three fetuses are needed per striatum. Tissue availability is the major drawback to the development of this technique, and this explains why there is active preclinical research on xenografts and progenitor cells.

Gene therapy using viral vectors encoding for tyrosine hydroxylase or neurotrophic factors and encapsulated cells secreted from biopolymer capsules are other promising strategies for direct brain therapy in PD.

OTHER EXTRAPYRAMIDAL DISORDERS

Other degenerative parkinsonian syndromes

In these syndromes, additional neurologic symptoms are present at some point in the course of the disease, and the response of parkinsonism to L-dopa is poor or transient. The diagnosis may be easy when patients present with a full-blown clinical picture. However, these conditions may mimic PD at their onset, but even when early atypical signs are present, a precise diagnosis may be difficult within the first years of evolution.

Multiple system atrophy (MSA)

Multiple system atrophy is characterized pathologically by cell loss, gliosis, and characteristic oligodendroglial cytoplasmic inclusions in the nigral, striatal, and olivopontocerebellar areas. This disease includes clinicopathologic syndromes previously reported as independent entities, e.g., olivopontocerebellar atrophy (sporadic type), striatonigral degeneration, and Shy-Drager syndrome. Multiple system atrophy commonly begins in the 50s. Parkinsonism occurs in 90% of the patients, with a combination of cerebellar, pyramidal, and/or autonomic signs and symptoms. Some degree of autonomic deficit is almost invariably present, and it is responsible for impotence, incontinence, and postural hypotension. Characteristic features also include severe dysarthria, dysphagia, stridor, and antecollis. T2-weighted magnetic resonance images (MRIs) may show putaminal hypointensity or a slit hyperintensity of the lateral margin of the lenticular nucleus.

The response to L-dopa is good initially in about 25% of patients. Even in the absence of short-duration motor response, L-dopa may induce predominantly dystonic dyskinesias that often affect the face and neck more than the limbs. In some patients, orthostatic hypotension is severe and requires a pharmacologic intervention. Many drugs have been used in the treatment of neurogenic orthostatic hypotension. The most potent appears to be fludrocortisone, a mineralocorticoid with little glucocorticoid effect, and midodrine, an α_1-adrenoreceptor agonist. These drugs may be used in combination.

Progressive supranuclear palsy (Steele-Richardson-Olszewski disease)

Progressive supranuclear palsy (PSP) is characterized by cell loss and neurofibrillary tangles predominating in the substantia nigra, the pallidum, the subthalamic nucleus, and the upper brainstem. Major clinical features are a supranuclear gaze palsy, predominantly vertical, postural instability with early falls, akinesia and rigidity (axial and proximal more than distal), and cognitive changes of the frontal type. Other features include pyramidal signs, dysphagia and dysarthria, and abormal neck posture (typically in extension). The most characteristic features, such as impairment of voluntary downgaze, may occur late in the course of the disease. Median survival is 6 to 7 years. A midbrain atrophy is apparent on MRI in about half of the patients.

Pharmacologic treatment of PSP has so far been disappointing. It first should be emphasized that PSP is characterized by a unique combination of clinical features and that, at present, no clinical rating scale has been validated to assess this disease. The parkinsonian signs of PSP initially may respond to L-dopa or other dopaminergic agents, but this improvement is not sustained. L-dopa-induced dyskinesias seem to be rare.

Chorea: Huntington's disease

Huntington's disease (HD) is an autosomal dominantly inherited neurodegenerative disorder with a prevalence of about 10 in 100 000 persons in the European population. The main neuropathologic change is a preferential loss of medium spiny neurons in the striatum, but other areas, including deep layers of the cerebral cortex, are involved as disease progresses. HD is characterized by three major symptoms: involuntary movements, changes in behavior and personality, and cognitive impairment. Involuntary movements progress insidiously to chorea, which consists of irregular, unpredictable, brief movements affecting various parts of the body in a continuous, random sequence. Later in the disease, postural stability deteriorates, and other neurologic features may develop, including dysarthria, dystonia, oculomotor disturbances, and in some instances, rigidity. Cognitive changes ultimately lead to dementia. Behavioral problems include early irritability and depression. Symptoms usually appear in midlife and lead to increasing debilitation and death within 10 to 20 years. A juvenile form occurs in about 10% of patients, who commonly presents with a rigid-akinetic syndrome, seizures, and a rapid dementing process. The genetic defect has been located on the short arm of chromosome 4. It involves the expansion of a trinucleotide repeat (CAG) encoding glutamines in the gene coding for huntingtin, a protein the function of which remains unknown.

Symptomatic treatment may provide benefit. Neuroleptics have been used extensively because they improve the chorea and may ameliorate behavioral changes. However, neuroleptics do not improve the progressive dementia, and routine use of these agents has been questioned because they may induce or aggravate mental and motor dysfunctions. Therefore, neuroleptics should be used transiently and at the lowest efficacious dose. Tetrabenazine, a synthetic benzoquinoline that depletes presynaptic storage of monoamines and blocks postsynaptic dopamine receptors, is the most useful drug to control hyperkinetic movement disorders in these patients. Improvement is observed in more than 80% of the patients taking the drug over several months. The usual dosage starts at 25 mg per day, with mean therapeutic dose close to 100 mg per day. Dosage should be titrated in each patient to achieve optimal response. Main side effects include drowsiness, fatigue, parkinsonism, and insomnia. In patients with HD, anxiety and depression may require specific pharmacologic treatment.

To date, no specific treatment has been shown to slow the rate of clinical progression of HD. Negative results of controlled studies have been reported with baclofen, tocopherol (vitamin E), and idebenone. However, in the trial using tocopherol, post-hoc analysis revealed a therapeutic effect on neurologic symptoms for patients early in the course of the disorder.

Dystonia

Dystonia refers to a syndrome of involuntary and sustained muscle contractions usually producing abnormal postures and/or repetitive movements of the affected body part. Mechanisms are poorly understood. The classifications distinguish dystonia according to distribution and cause. Dystonia may be focal (e.g., writer's cramp, torticollis, blepharospasm), segmental (contiguous body regions, e.g., face and neck), multifocal (noncontiguous body regions), or generalized (affecting both legs and at least one other body region). Primary dystonia includes a variety of conditions with no signs of structural abnormality in the CNS; when generalized, it is synonymous with idiopathic torsion dystonia. Secondary dystonias have been described in a long list of conditions, some of which are associated with a hereditary neurologic syndrome (e.g., L-dopa–responsive dystonia associated with a biopterin-deficient state, Wilson's disease), while others

are due to a known toxic or lesional cause (e.g., perinatal brain injury, stroke, drugs). Most lesions responsible for symptomatic dystonia involve the basal ganglia or the thalamus. In a small number of cases, a specific treatment may be instituted (e.g., in Wilson's disease or in L-dopa-responsive dystonia). However, in most instances, only symptomatic treatments can be attempted.

Focal and segmental dystonia may benefit from intramuscular injections of botulinum toxin type A. Botulinum toxin induces an irreversible presynaptic inhibition of acetylcholine release. The resulting muscle weakness is temporary as new neuromuscular junctions develop, and the injections have to be repeated every 3 to 4 months. Maximal weakness usually takes about 1 week to appear. Two types of A toxin are available, Botox® and Dysport®. There is no dose standardization between the two preparations, and it has been calculated that 67 units of Botox® is clinically equivalent to 200 units of Dysport® (i.e., a ratio of 1:3). General guidelines for botulinum toxin therapy include (Botox® value) mean concentration, 5 units/0.1 ml; maximum dose per injection site, 50 units; maximum dose per visit, 400 units; and reinjection no sooner than 3 months. Best results have been obtained so far for blepharospasm and hemifacial spasm, with excellent results in 90% of the patients. Botulinum toxin, in association with physiotherapy, is also the most effective treatment for idiopathic cervical dystonia (spasmodic torticollis); about 75% of patients show improvement. The main side effect is a reversible local paresis due to diffusion of the toxin. With repeated injections, up to 10% of the patients develop resistance to therapy, probably related to the development of blocking antibodies. In such patients, other serotypes of botulinum toxin may be used.

Other medical syptomatic treatments have been used in the various types of dystonias with a limited efficacy in most cases. The most widely used drugs include anticholinergics, dopamine agonists, dopamine antagonists, baclofen, and benzodiazepines. When medical treatment has failed to improve a generalized dystonia, a surgical procedure may be considered. Thalamotomy has been used for a long time. However, it has been suggested recently that unilateral or bilateral pallidotomy or, better, chronic electrical stimulation of the pallidum may have some advantages over thalamotomy.

Acknowledgments

We warmly thank Prof. P. Cesaro for his technical assistance and critical reading of the manuscript.

*Suggested readings*_____

ADLER CH, SETHI KD, HAUSER RA, et al. Ropinirole for the treatment of early Parkinson's disease. Neurology 1997;49:393-9.

BRESSMAN SB. Dystonia. Curr Opin Neurol 1998;11:363-72.

CONTIN M, RIVA R, MARTINELLI P, et al. Relationship between levodopa concentration, dyskinesias, and motor effect in parkinsonian patients: a 3-year follow-up study. Clin Neuropharmacol 1997;20:409-18.

DIAMOND SG, MARKHAM CH, HOEHN MM, et al. Multi-center study of Parkinson's mortality with early versus later dopa treatment. Ann Neurol 1987;22:8-12.

FRANKEL JP, LEES AJ, KEMPSTER PA, et al. Subcutanaeous apomorphine in the treatment of Parkinson's disease. J Neurol Neurosurg Psychiatry 1994;53:96-101.

GOETZ C. New lessons from old drugs: amantadine and Parkinson's disease. Neurology 1998;50:1211-2.

HUGHES AJ. Drug treatment of Parkinson's disease in the 1990s. Drugs 1997;63:195-205.

LANGTRY HD, CLISSOLD SP. Pergolide: a review of its pharmacological properties and therapeutic potential in Parkinson's disease. Drugs 1990;39:491-506.

LEES AJ. Comparison of therapeutic effects and mortality data of levodopa and L-dopa combined with selegiline in patients with early, mild Parkinson's disease: Parkinson's Disease Research Group of the United Kingdom. Br Med J 1995;311:1602-7.

MONTASTRUC JL, RASCOL O, SENARD JM, RASCOL A. A randomized controlled study comparing bromocriptine to which levodopa was later added, with levodopa alone in previously untreated patients with Parkinson's disease: a five-year follow-up. J Neurol Neurosurg Psychiatry 1994;57:1034-8.

PAHWA R, LYONS K, MCGUIRE D. et al. Comparison of standard carbidopa-levodopa and sustained-release carbidopa-levodopa in Parkinson's disease: pharmacokinetic and quality-of-life measure. Mov Disord 1997;12:677-81.

PARKINSON STUDY GROUP. Impact of deprenyl and tocopherol treatment on Parkinson's disease in DATATOP subjects not requiring levodopa. Ann Neurol 1996;39:29-36.

PARKINSON STUDY GROUP. Safety and efficacy of pramipexole in early Parkinson disease: a randomized dose-ranging study. JAMA 1997;278:125-30.

RINNE UK, BRACCO F, CHOUZA C, et al. Cabergoline in the treatment of early Parkinson's disease: results of the first year of treatment in a double-blind comparison of cabergoline and levodopa. Neurology 1997;48:363-8.

VAAMONDE J, LUQUIN MR, OBESO JA. Subcutaneous lisuride infusion in Parkinson's disease: response to chronic administration in 34 patients. Brain 1991;114:601-14.

CHAPTER

12

Dementia

Shibley Rahman, Barbara J. Sahakian

The term *dementia* traditionally has been applied to a progressive syndrome that consists of acquired circumscribed cognitive impairments of intellectual function occurring within a setting of clear consciousness. Modern definitions are more specific. The *Diagnostic and Statistic Manual of Mental Disorders,* fourth edition (DSM-IV), requires the development of multiple cognitive deficits including memory impairment and at least one of the following disturbances: aphasia, apraxia, agnosia, or a disturbance in executive functioning. This must represent a decline from a previously higher level of functioning. A diagnosis of a dementia should not be made if the cognitive deficits occur exclusively during the course of a delirium; however, a dementia and a delirium may both be diagnosed if the dementia is present at times when the delirium is not present.

The major dementias are neurodegenerative in type. This chapter focuses predominantly on dementia of the Alzheimer type the most common cause of dementia in the elderly, accounting for approximately 60 to 80% of cases. We shall consider the options which currently exist for slowing further decline in patients with this form of dementia. Other important forms of dementia also will be discussed briefly, including those which are potentially treatable and those which are related to other disorders (Tab. 12.1).

Disease presentation

The correct clinical diagnosis of dementia depends, as in other medical disorders, on an accurate history and physical examination, as well as on appropriate clinical investigations. In making a clinical diagnosis, the most important element is a clear history (preferably from someone close to the patient). The mode of onset and progression are important. A gradual onset may imply degeneration or a structural cause, whereas an abrupt onset or stepwise progression may suggest a cerebrovascular origin. In addition, it is useful to inquire about the occurrence of any head injury, exposure to toxins, a complete drug history, social history (including degree of alcohol consumption), nutritional changes, and any other diseases (such as diabetes, ischemic heart disease, or malignancy). The complaint of a headache or a focal neurologic deficit may indicate the possibility of a cerebral tumor, e.g., metastasis,

frontal meningioma, or glioma. A family history of neurologic illnesses is important and may identify inherited conditions such as Huntington's disease or Wilson's disease.

The differential diagnosis includes delirium and depression, both of which need to be excluded. If cognitive changes develop over a very short period of time, the diagnosis is likely to be delirium, not dementia. Delirium is an acute state of fluctuating awareness that develops over hours or days and is caused by medical conditions such as liver or kidney failure, urinary tract infection, or hypoglycemia and is reversible. Examination during a lucid interval may show a relative preservation of intellectual faculties. Dementia also can be extremely difficult to differentiate from depression in the elderly. Usually there

Table 12.1 Forms of dementia and their causes

Type of dementia	Examples of specific causes
Potentially treatable disorders that may present as dementia	Chronic subdural hematoma Cerebral tumor Normal-pressure hydrocephalus Alcohol-related dementia Vitamin deficiencies Endocrine disorders Inflammatory and infective disorders Disorders leading to anoxia Toxins Drugs
Dementias unrelated to other disorders	Dementia of the Alzheimer type Diffuse Lewy body disease Frontotemporal dementias
Dementias related to other disorders	Multiple sclerosis Motor neurone disease Huntington's disease Parkinson's disease Parkinsonian syndromes Paraneoplastic dementia Down syndrome Acquired immune-deficiency syndrome (AIDS) Prion diseases

Table 12.2 Aspects of examinations useful to identify abnormalites in the nervous system

Abnormalities	Possible pathology
Vision	Visual field defects may be due to parietal or occipital cortical lobe dysfunction. Abnormal gaze responses may be a manifestation of subcortical pathology
Olfaction	Olfactory function may be altered in frontal lobe syndromes, such as due to head trauma or a subfrontal meningioma
Speech	A pseudobulbar palsy may be seen in multi-infarct states, as well as in pathologies where the brainstem is affected, e.g., in Wilson's disease or Steele-Richardson-Olszewski syndrome
Dyspraxic gait	As in Huntington's disease, this may indicate communicating hydrocephalus
Asymmetric long tract signs	These may be suggestive of cerebrovascular disease
Chorea	As in Huntington's disease, this may be seen when the patient is relaxed in bed or walking, when minor twitches of the fingers and toes become apparent
Gait	Examination of gait can be extremely revealing. Classically, the bent posture and shuffling gait of Parkinson's disease compares with the ramrod stance of progressive supranuclear palsy
Papilledema	This implies that cognitive changes may be due to a space-occupying lesion (such as a cerebral tumor)

is remission in depression, whereas dementia is progressive, with a more abrupt onset; moreover, patients with depression are often slow to answer mental status testing. Psychomotor retardation and insomnia with early morning waking also are commonly present in depression.

Examination should identify any other abnormalities in the nervous systems apart from dementia and the possible etiology of the cognitive impairment. General examination should include a search for endocrine disorders, malignancy, and vasculitic disorders, as well as an assessment of vascular status. Some other useful aspects of the examination are shown in Table 12.2.

In addition to a full clinical history and physical examination, basic investigations of a patient with suspected dementia should be carried out to exclude other conditions in the differential diagnosis, as well as to identify a potentially treatable cause of dementia. Possible investigations are summarized in Table 12.3.

Cognitive neuropsychologic assessment is extremely useful; it has become increasingly acknowledged that, in specialist's hands, it may actually surpass many other procedures as a diagnostic tool. Neuroimaging, together with an informative history and cognitive neuropsychologic examination, constitutes a beneficial approach. In the clinical diagnosis of dementia of the Alzheimer type (DAT), magnetic resonance imaging (MRI) helps to improve the diagnostic accuracy, and recently, new MRI-based techniques for performing volumetric measurement of cortical and subcortical structures have been developed. In recent years, new information has been provided about dementias through the use of such techniques as functional MRI (fMRI), MR spectroscopy (MRS), and MR spectroscopic imaging. Furthermore, perfusion imaging with single-photon emission computed tomography (SPECT) is becoming an important clinical tool ancillary to neuropsychologic testing. In addition, combining these techniques with computed tomography (CT) may even serve to yield a high sensitivity and specificity in diagnosis.

DEMENTIA OF THE ALZHEIMER TYPE (DAT)

The development of effective strategies for the management of DAT represents a central challenge to research in psychopharmacology. The disease is thought to affect approximately 5% of persons over age 65 years and 11% of the population between 80 and 85 years of age (24%

Table 12.3 Outline of possible investigations

Complete blood count (?anemia), erythrocyte sedimentation rate (?underlying malignancy or vasculitic disorder)

Vitamin B$_{12}$, folate

Renal, liver, and thyroid function tests

Serum calcium

Serum free or total copper (?Wilson's disease)

Serology for syphilis

Chest X-ray (e.g., neoplasm of bronchus, secondary deposits), ECG

Serology for HIV (particularly younger patients)

CT or MRI scan

Cognitive neuropsychologic assessment

Toxicology (selected patients)

EEG (?Creutzfeld-Jacob disease, ?subacute sclerosing panencephalitis)

CSF (selected patients)

(Lumbar puncture may cause coning in the presence of a space-occupying lesion or subdural hematoma.)

older than age 85). The Alzheimer's Disease Society estimates that there are now approximately 650 000 people with dementia living in the United Kingdom, of whom 400 000 have DAT. Enormous international scientific efforts are being directed at increasing as much as possible our understanding of the pathogenesis of this disease, with the eventual goal of developing beneficial therapy. As life expectancy increases, the number of patients with DAT is likely to increase, with a massive impact on family, financial, and social responsibilities for the provision of adequate dementia care.

Neuropathology

In DAT, the brain is shrunken, with enlarged ventricles and widened sulci. There is shrinkage of the dendritic tree and increased gliosis and cell loss. The two major neuropathologic hallmarks of DAT throughout the cortical and subcortical gray matter are extracellular senile plaques, the principal component of which is the beta-amyloid (Aβ) peptide, and intraneuronal neurofibrillary tangles, composed of aggregated tau protein in the form of paired helical filaments (PHFs).

Neurogenetics

Dementia of the Alzheimer type represents a heterogeneous syndrome with different genotypes and phenotypes. Most cases are thought to be sporadic without a strong family history. However, genetically defined pedigrees with an early age at onset (under 65 years of age) and a clear autosomal pattern of inheritance of DAT have been recognized. Three separate loci have now been identified at which mutations are associated with the early-onset form of DAT, and marked allelic variability has been found at these loci. The first locus found was the amyloid precursor protein (APP) gene on chromosome 21; three different point mutations at APP 717 and a double mutation at APP 670-671 cosegregate with familial DAT, with ages at onset from 43 to 56 years. APP mutation families are, however, rare.

Most cases of early-onset familial DAT are instead accounted for by a genetic locus, mapped by linkage studies to the long arm of chromosome 14. This locus causes the most aggressive form of familial DAT, with ages at onset as early as 30 years. A novel gene on chromosome 14, presenilin 1, recently has been identified in which mutations are pathogenic for familial DAT. Mutations in a further novel gene, presenilin 2, encoded on chromosome 1, are also associated with early-onset autosomal dominant DAT. In addition, the role of apolipoprotein E (apoE) in the pathogenesis of DAT recently has become clearer. Human apoE is a polymorphic protein with three common alleles, apo ε2, apo ε3, and apo ε4, with a critical role in the modulation of cholesterol and phospholipid transport between cells of different types (see also Chap. 69). Apo ε4 is considered to be associated with sporadic and late-onset familial DAT.

Cholinergic deficits

In the light of much supporting subsequent evidence, the cholinergic hypothesis of geriatric memory dysfunction has generated considerable interest in the functions of the central cholinergic systems and the neuropathologic substrates of DAT. The extent of cholinergic abnormalities correlates with mental state scores obtained from patients with DAT shortly before their death. This finding, together with the observation that systemic administration of the muscarinic acetylcholine receptor antagonist scopolamine to normal volunteers has been found to reproduce many of the deficits in memory, attention, visuospatial functions, and language seen in DAT, lends much weight to the validity of the hypothesis. Patients with DAT perform worse on cholinergic-sensitive tests compared with cholinergic-insensitive tests, suggesting that cholinergic depletion may be responsible for the cognitive deficits seen in early stages of the disease.

The earliest and most consistent post-mortem neurochemical abnormalities in the brains of DAT victims are found in the basal forebrain cholinergic system. The synaptic loss, neuronal atrophy, and degeneration of cholinergic nuclei in the basal forebrain may be associated with reduced cholinergic activity in the hippocampus and a cortical loss of choline acetyltransferase, an enzyme that produces acetylcholine in the neurones. Early involvement of medial temporal structures, including the hippocampal formation and entorhinal cortex, is consistent with the impairment in episodic memory, whereas the semantic memory loss reflects spread to the lateral temporal neocortex.

Neurones of the nucleus basalis of Meynert and cortical cholinergic axons are severely depleted in DAT. A substantial literature indicates a consistent loss of basal forebrain cholinergic neurones in DAT, ranging from 30 to 90%. The loss of cortical cholinergic neurones is usually most severe (up to 85%) in the inferotemporal, midtemporal, and entorhinal cortex and amygdala; less severe (40-70%) in the prefrontal, parietal, and hippocampal complex; and light (4-30%) in the primary visual, motor, and anterior cingulate cortex. Further evidence in favor of the cholinergic deficit hypothesis in DAT comes from the findings of a significant negative correlation between cortical ChAT activity and severity of dementia, whereas cortical levels of other neurotransmitters, e.g., norepinephrine, do not correlate with dementia severity.

Clinical findings

There is a clear consensus that sensory and motor functions are relatively resistant to the pathology of DAT (although a hypokinetic hypertonic motor syndrome may ensue in the final stages). It is, therefore, clear that the disease is characterized primarily by cognitive disability. The neuropsychologic deficits that have been reported are of considerable importance if we are to understand properly the underlying neuropathology.

The presenting problem in patients with DAT is most often expressed in new learning and memory, clinically usually forgetfulness of a minor degree, which may be difficult to distinguish from the effects of normal ageing. The most profound impact is on episodic memory, usually with both verbal and nonverbal material affected. Although the majority of DAT patients show the classic anterograde amnesia, some DAT patients show relatively specific evidence of short-term memory deficits in either or both the verbal and visual modalities. Retrograde memory loss has a temporally graded pattern, with sparing of more distant memories. Working memory, as judged by digit span, is generally normal early on in the disease.

Declarative memory, assessed in tests of delayed matching to sample (DMTS), and associative memory, assessed in tests of paired-associates learning, are particularly sensitive indicators of cognitive symptomatology in early DAT. Semantic memory can be affected early in the course of DAT, but there is considerable variability in the extent of impairment early in the course of the disease. Identification of famous faces may be impaired, which may be correlated with deficits in general semantic memory. A number of recent studies suggest that attentional impairments represent the first nonmnemonic deficits in DAT. Patients in the very early stages of DAT may show a reduced control of the spatial focus of attention, which contributes to deficits in spatial memory, reading, spelling, confrontation naming, and letter cancellation.

Language is typically normal on informal assessment. Visuospatial functioning is good on simple bedside assessment, but deficits may be apparent on formal assessment, which manifest as an inability to copy diagrams. In contrast with patients with frontal dementias, patients with DAT generally have well-preserved personality and do not show marked behavioral disturbance in the mild stages of the disease.

Later in the disease, impaired memory and attention result in marked temporal disorientation. Impairment in working memory is found. Distractibility and executive dysfunction occur that may reflect disconnection of corticocortical tracts. Breakdown of semantic memory leads to word-finding difficulties, diminished vocabulary, semantic paraphasic errors in spontaneous conversation, poor naming ability, reduced generation of exemplars on category fluency testing, and a loss of general knowledge. Marked visuospatial deficits are usually apparent, manifest as an inability of patients to find their way around when driving or to judge distances.

Neuropsychiatric phenomena in patients with DAT are well documented. Patients with DAT may express personality and behavioral changes, e.g., indifference, agitation, and combativeness. Social behavior may decline, and there may be self-care neglect; some patients maintain a good external appearance despite quite profound cognitive impairment. Other common neuropsychiatric symptoms include delusions (most commonly those of theft and suspicion hallucinations (visual > auditory > gustatory > olfactory > haptic), neurovegetative dysfunction (manifest as disorders of sleep, specifically poor sleep, nocturnal arousal, reduced slow-wave sleep, and disturbed

circadian rhythmicity), eating disorders, and troublesome behavior (e.g., restlessness, wandering, anger, and aggression). The mood of patients can vary; it may be predominantly depressed, euphoric, flattened, or labile. Symptoms of depression are recognizable; therefore, it is important that the depression be treated clinically. There also may be effects of the patients' symptoms on their caregivers, such as aggressive behavior, sleep disturbances, and nighttime wandering.

Clinical rating scales

Clinical rating scales are useful for identifying global cognitive impairment and the severity of dementia. Traditionally, they have been considered to be useful screening tests because they are quick and easy to administer.

The Mini Mental State Examination (MMSE) is easy to administer, measures relevant areas of cognition, is available in multiple languages, and has available longitudinal data. It shows good test-retest and interrater reliability. Its major disadvantages are that it does not cover all domains of cognitive functioning; it is insufficiently sensitive for the early detection of dementia, and it is relatively insensitive to change. It also may be subject to considerable bias from sociodemographic variability in subjects.

The Alzheimer Disease Assessment Scale (ADAS) is another attempt to measure specifically gross cognitive deficits considered to be characteristic of patients with DAT, and this test measures the severity of dysfunction in both cognitive and noncognitive domains. The cognitive part (ADAS-cog) has 11 items and a maximum score of 70 and measures memory, language, and praxis. A score of 70 means that the patient is profoundly demented, and a score of 0 means that the patient made no errors at all. This part, therefore, provides broad coverage of cognitive functioning and frequently is used as an outcome measure. The noncognitive part of the scale consists of 10 items and includes measures of mood state and behavioral changes (ADAS-noncog). However, members of the International Working Group on the Harmonization of Dementia Drug Guidelines were recently critical of the ADAS-cog.

The Clinician Global Impression of Change (CGIC) and the Clinician Interview-Based Impression of Change (CIBIC) are scales that measure improvement or worsening in condition since the last assessment. The CGIC is completed by the attending physician, who is supposed to be blind to the results of neuropsychologic testing and without input from relatives or caregivers. An important criticism is that, at present, a number of CGIC scales have not been validated but are nevertheless being employed in clinical trials. The main themes considered in the CIBIC are functional independence, social appropriateness, and mental clarity.

Most recently, computerized neuropsychologic testing batteries have been receiving much attention from investigators in the field of dementia. In particular, the Cambridge Neuropsychological Test Automated Battery (CANTAB) has been employed successfully in the study of a number of neuropsychiatric disorders and has been standardized in a large sample of volunteer subjects. CANTAB is also particularly of use in psychopharmacologic studies. The tests are comprehensive in terms of the range of cognitive functions that they assess, including the domains of attention, visual learning and memory, and working memory and planning. In particular, two CANTAB subtests, paired-associates learning and delayed matching to sample, have been found to be sensitive to early DAT. Scores on these subtests have correctly classified 88% of patients labeled as questionable dementia at initial assessment who subsequently were been found to have probable DAT (pDAT).

Diagnosis

The definitive diagnosis of DAT requires demonstration of characteristic histopathologic features in brain tissue postmortem. In the vast majority of cases, the diagnosis of DAT is made on clinical grounds alone. The report of the NINCDS-ADRDA Work Group on Alzheimer's disease documents now well-established criteria for probable DAT that have been found to produce good interrater agreement in their application. The criteria for the clinical diagnosis of probable DAT include dementia established by clinical examination and documented by the Mini Mental Test, Blessed Dementia Scale, or a similar examination and confirmed by neuropsychologic tests; deficits in two or more areas of cognition; progressive worsening of memory and other cognitive functions; no disturbance of consciousness; onset between the ages of 40 and 90 years, most often after age 65; and absence of systemic disorders or other brain diseases that in and of themselves could account for the progressive deficits in memory and cognition. The diagnosis is supported by progressive deterioration of specific cognitive functions such as language (aphasia), motor skills (apraxia), and perception (agnosia); impaired activities of daily living and altered patterns of behavior; family history of similar disorders, particularly if confirmed neuropathologically; and laboratory results of normal lumbar puncture, normal pattern or nonspecific changes in the electroencephalogram (EEG), and evidence of cerebral atrophy on CT with progression documented by serial observation. From the viewpoint of starting patients on drug therapy, an important criterion is that the dementia syndrome should have been present for at least 6 months.

Treatment

Treatments of general use in the disease

Management is aimed at helping both the patient and the caregiver. Ideally, patients should be in familiar surroundings with support from home visits by health professionals or from attendance at day units. Help at home may include home helpers, incontinence laundry services, and Meals on Wheels. Certain deficits may be corrected so as to provide real benefit, e.g., adequate eyeglasses, hearing aids, etc. As the patient's condition deteriorates, he/she may be admitted to the hospital or into long-stay units. The management of patients is both pharmacologic and nonpharmacologic. Caregivers as well as the patients themselves deserve much attention. It is essential that people with dementia and their caregivers be made aware of as many services and support agencies as possible. This includes financial allowances, legal powers, and support agencies.

Nonpharmacologic treatment

The medical profession is well positioned to assist DAT patients (in the early stages) by encouraging realistic expectations about the disease and possible therapy. Relatives should be involved and supported, and practical help in the home may be arranged. If home care fails, residential or hospital care should be arranged. Treatment of depression and behavioral problems in the patient (e.g., night- and daytime restlessness) may be achieved by means of psychologic treatment or medication. Above all, patients should be given the highest standards of courtesy, privacy, and dignity.

Drug therapy

Therapy is aimed at tackling the symptoms of the disease through enhancing the function of the cholinergic system. An overview is provided in Table 12.4.

Before drug prescription, a detailed assessment of the disease should be completed. An important criterion is that a dementia syndrome be present for at least 6 months. The MMSE may be used as a possible method for monitoring disease progression. Currently, approved evidence of efficacy of treatments is limited to mild to moderate DAT. This is in keeping with the concept that pharmacotherapy aimed at boosting neurotransmitter functioning will no longer be effective when the neural network involved is no longer viable.

Table 12.4 Therapy aimed at tackling the symptoms of the disease

Type of drug and rationale	Examples
Enhanced acetylcholine release	Lecithin 4-AP (4-aminopyridine)
Cholinergic agonists aimed at improving the tonic muscarinic stimulation	Nicotine Arecoline RS86 Oxytremorine Bethanecol
Cholinesterase inhibitors expected to delay the synaptic degradation of ACh, thereby prolonging the postsynaptic stimulation by inhibiting one or more enzymes responsible for its hydrolysis	Donepezil Tacrine Physostygmine Velnacrine maleate (HP029)

Since dementia is a progressive condition, a major concern is the point at which treatment should be stopped. While some patients improve very significantly, no further deterioration – albeit temporary – or even a slowing of deterioration might be viewed as a favorable outcome. Early criteria for stopping treatment could include poor tolerance and compliance, deterioration after 3 to 6 months of therapy, or an accelerating deterioration. Drug-free periods could be useful in the evaluation of response; rapid deterioration during a 6-week drug-free "holiday" would indicate that continued treatment might be appropriate.

Treatment of concomitant disorders in patients with DAT

Incidental physical illness may cause a superimposed delirium resulting in a sudden deterioration in cognitive function from which the patient may not recover fully. Delirium is a common complication of chronic dementia, often occurring with even minor medical illnesses such as influenza. Nocturnal delirium may be aggravated by hypnotics and helped by caffeine taken as a strong cup of coffee or tea. The use of antidepressants for people with dementia and concomitant depression is essential. The rationale for the use of antipsychotic drugs in DAT has been based on phenomenologic similarities between delusions and hallucinations and other disruptive behaviors and the symptoms occurring in patients with schizophrenia.

Drug classes

ENHANCING ACETYLCHOLINE RELEASE

The rate of acetylcholine release is related to the rate of acetylcholine synthesis, and the rate of acetylcholine synthesis is related to the rate of choline uptake into cholinergic neurones.

Lecithin The studies using lecithin or different choline salts have failed to support the notion that lecithin has a therapeutic impact on DAT symptoms; so far, no delaying effects on the progression of the disease have been demonstrated successfully. A possible explanation for this is that under normal conditions, the system of choline uptake may be saturated, and an increase in the availability of extracellular choline does not increase the synthesis or release of acetylcholine.

4-Aminopyridine 4-Aminopyridine (4-AP) is a compound derived from pyridine that acts as a cholinomimetic. It blocks K^+ channels in axonal terminals, prolonging the action potential. More Ca^{2+} can move into the cell, leading to enhanced release of acetylcholine. In one study investigating the cognitive and behavioral effects of 4-AP in patients with DAT, no significant difference was found in assessment using ADAS.

CHOLINERGIC AGONISTS

Administration of cholinergic agonists has been shown to have beneficial effects on memory and learning tasks in animals with experimentally induced hypocholinergic states. In humans, relative preservation of postsynaptic M1 sites in DAT has been reported. However, none of the muscarinic agonists have conclusively shown much clinical benefit to patients. Future directions in the development of successful cholinergic agonists may include manipulation of subtypes of muscarinic and nicotinic receptors that are most likely to enhance cognitive function without significant adverse effects.

Nicotine The interest in nicotine is considerable. There is evidence for a significant loss of nicotinic receptors in the cerebral cortex and the parahippocampal gyrus in DAT, as measured both at post-mortem examination and through functional neuroimaging studies (e.g., using [^{11}C]nicotine). Nicotine administration increases the release of acetylcholine by presynaptic nicotinic autoreceptors and has been shown to improve cognitive performance in several species.

Several clinical studies have addressed the acute effects of nicotine given subcutaneously. For example, the effects of subcutaneous nicotine, at doses of 0.4, 0.6 and 0.8 mg, on attention, information processing, and short-term memory in DAT have been investigated in one study that involved computerized neuropsychologic tests from the CANTAB battery. Nicotine administration resulted in a highly significant and dose-dependent improvement in accuracy and speed of responding on the rapid visual information processing (RVIP) task of sustained attention. Further, nicotine significantly improved performance of patients during the attentional phase of a delayed-response matching-to-location-order task in a dose-dependent manner but failed to produce any improvement in the memory phase. Nicotine may assist DAT patients by optimizing attentional processes, which may assist in everyday activities such as following television programs, conversational ability, etc. This could constitute a real benefit for patients in terms of improved relationships with family members and caregivers.

Nicotine is the principal alkaloid in tobacco smoke and can cross the blood-brain barrier easily. Because of the large number of carcinogens also found in tobacco smoke, and also as a consequence of the need to find a more pliable method of administration than smoking or injection, trials have been designed to address whether nicotine in the form of dermal plasters (currently available for smoking cessation) may be beneficial in patients with DAT. The effects of nicotine on cognition in the form of dermal plasters has been examined recently in a placebo-controlled, double-blind study. Most of the patients tolerated the highest doses of 21 mg nicotine per 24 hours, but some received 14 mg per 24 hours. It was found that short-term memory improved significantly after 4 weeks of treatment, on both nicotine and placebo, therefore indicating that nicotine applied in the form of dermal plasters may not be of any significance in the treatment of memory deficits in patients with DAT. However, it is clear that further trials are needed in the future to characterize fully the potential benefits of the use of nicotine.

Arecoline, RS 86, bethanecol   The effects of the muscarinic agonists – arecoline (a mixed muscarine and nicotine agonist), RS 86 (an investigational long-acting agonist) and bethanecol (an agonist with well-known activity on urinary retention) – generally have been shown to be minimal on major DAT symptoms.

CHOLINESTERASE (ChE) INHIBITORS

Two cholinesterase inhibitors had been up to now approved for the treatment of mild to moderate DAT: (1) donepezil (both in Europe and the United States) and (2) tacrine (in the United States only). However, other strategies for therapeutic intervention exist, and examples of drugs shall be discussed.

Donepezil is a piperidine-based derivative that is chemically distinct from the other ChE inhibitors and has been developed specifically for the treatment of DAT. The indications for use of donepezil hydrochloride are the symptomatic treatment of mild to moderate DAT. Donepezil may slow the rate of cognitive and noncognitive deterioration in about 40% of patients with DAT. It has no effect in patients with other causes of confusion or dementia. Mortality is unaffected.

Donepezil is a highly selective, potent, reversible, noncompetitive inhibitor of acetylcholinesterase according to in vitro data. In vivo, donepezil inhibits acetylcholinesterase activity in human erythrocytes and increases extracellular acetylcholine levels in the cerebral cortex and hippocampus of the rat. It has a longer duration of action than either physostigmine or tacrine. Therefore, it is postulated to augment cholinergic function in the CNS, thereby providing therapeutic benefit. The surrogate marker has been evaluated in several human pharmacokinetic and pharmacodynamic trials and in controlled clinical trials. Three trials of donepezil have been published in full.

The first randomized, controlled trial was conducted to examine the efficacy and safety of donepezil in patients with DAT and appeared to have some promising results. The trial, a preliminary dose-ranging study, was randomized and double-blind for 12 weeks, followed by a 2-week single-blind open-label washout. It compared donepezil at three doses (1, 3, and 5 mg) with placebo. Improvements in ADAS-cog were statistically significantly greater with donepezil (5 mg per day) than with placebo. A statistically significant correlation between plasma concentrations of donepezil and AChE inhibition was demonstrated. The correlations between plasma drug concentrations and ADAS-cog score ($p = 0.014$), MMSE score ($p = 0.023$), and patient quality of life scores, assessed by the patient ($p = 0.037$), also were statistically significant, as was the correlation between AChE inhibition and change in ADAS-cog ($p = 0.008$). The incidence of treatment-emergent adverse effects with all three dosages of donepezil was comparable with that observed with placebo.

However, it is important to note that the drug failed to

influence day-to-day functioning or quality-of-life (QoL) measures. The authors of the trial noted that the QoL-P and QoL-C scores showed extensive intersubject variability with no statistical evidence of improvement over placebo and suggested that the caregivers may not be useful informants.

The changes in the ADAS-cog score appear to be dose-related; in the randomized, controlled trials with donepezil, a greater change in ADAS-cog score has been observed consistently with the higher 10-mg-per-day dose than with the 5-mg-per-day dose (Tab. 12.5). Table 12.5 shows the change in ADAS-cog varies and is on the order of a few points, but it is not clear what a change of this magnitude means in terms of everyday function and of real clinical benefit.

Of the two further published trials, one was a phase III randomized, double-blind, placebo-controlled trial conducted to evaluate further the efficacy and safety of donepezil at dosage levels of 5-and-10-mg-per-day versus placebo in patients with mild to moderate DAT. Patients were randomly assigned to treatment with placebo, 5-mg-per-day donepezil, or 10-mg-per-day donepezil for 24 weeks, followed by a 6-week single-blind placebo washout. Donepezil was found to be well tolerated, with few patients having significant side effects. Analysis of liver function tests demonstrated that the incidence of treatment-emergent abnormal laboratory values for patients with 5-or-10-mg-per-day donepezil did not differ statistically from placebo. The 10-mg-per-day donepezil group, compared with placebo, showed the greatest change in mean ADAS-cog score versus placebo, and the authors considered the possibility that an even higher dosage of donepezil might further improve cognitive symptoms, although the 10-mg-per-day dose produced rates of inhibition of AChE on the upper asymptote of the enzyme inhibition curve. The other trial was an interim analysis (at 98 weeks) of a U.S. multicenter open-label extension study. Donepezil produced improvements in performance on the ADAS-cog test that remained superior to baseline for 38 weeks. Another clinical rating scale, the Clinical Dementia Rating Sum of the Boxes, likewise showed improvement, with scores maintained near baseline values for 26 weeks. Donepezil was again well tolerated, with no evidence of hepatotoxicity.

The results concerning donepezil on the whole, therefore appear promising. However, there is currently no information available that may help to predict which patients may benefit most. Studies are required to identify responders from nonresponders on the basis of objective neuropsychologic tests.

Tacrine has been shown to increase presynaptic ACh release through blocking slow K^+ channels and is also thought to increase postsynaptic monoaminergic stimulation by interfering with norepinephrine and serotonin uptake. These latter characteristics occur at concentrations higher than those required to achieve acetylcholinesterase inhibition and, therefore, probably do not contribute to the drug's clinical effects. It is a cholinomimetic agent whose major advantage over physostigmine appears to be a longer half-life and better bioavailability.

Tacrine has been shown to be successful in alleviating some of the cognitive symptomatology in DAT, as measured by improvements in subjective clinical rating scales, with manageable side effects. The conclusion that tacrine is an effective treatment for DAT derives principally from two adequate and well-controlled clinical investigations that evaluated the effects of drug in patients with mild to moderate DAT, assessed using NINCDS criteria. In the 12-week study, patients were randomized to sequences that provided a comparison between placebo and 20-40 and 80-mg-per-day by the end of the study. Statistically significant drug-placebo differences were detected on both the ADAS-cog and the Clinician's Global Impression of Change (CGIC) tests. In the 30-week study, statistically significant drug-placebo differences also were seen on these two principal outcome measures.

The acute effects of tacrine on cognition in a group of patients meeting criteria for probable DAT showed a statistically significant benefit on the five-choice task, where improvements were seen in both speed and accuracy of performance. The pattern of results with the CANTAB battery were supported by an improvement on the concentration/distractibility subscore of the Rosen Alzheimer's Disease Noncognitive scale. Beneficial effects on attentional function in patients with DAT do not rule out a role for ascending cholinergic neurones in learning and memory. The time course of the changes in cognitive function on treatment with tacrine also has been investigated. Cognitive improvement has been found to occur during the first 2 weeks, reaching a maximum at 1 month, and maintained during the rest of the 3-month treatment period.

DONEPEZIL

Dosage and pharmaceutical forms

Treatment is initiated at 5 mg qd. Donepezil should be taken orally, in the evening, just prior to retiring. The 5 mg qd dose should be maintained for at least 1 month to allow the earliest clinical responses to treatment to be assessed and to allow steady-state concentrations of donepezil hydrochloride to be achieved. Following a 1-month clinical assessment of treatment at 5 mg qd, the dose can be increased to 10 mg qd. The maximum recommended daily dose is 10 mg. Doses greater than 10 mg qd have not been studied in clinical trials (Tab. 12.5).

With discontinuation of treatment, a gradual abatement of the beneficial effects is seen. There is no evidence of a rebound effect after abrupt discontinuation of therapy. A similar dose schedule can be followed for patients with renal or mild to moderate hepatic impairment because clearance of donepezil hydrochloride is not affected by these conditions.

Pharmacodynamics and pharmacokinetics

Donepezil hydrochloride is a specific and reversible inhibitor of acetylcholinesterase, the predominant cholinesterase in the brain. Administration of single daily doses of 5-or-10 mg produces steady-state inhibition of acetylcholinesterase activity (measured in erythrocyte membranes) of 63.3 and 77.3%. The inhibition of acetylcholinesterase in red blood cells by donepezil hydrochloride has been shown to correspond closely to the effects in the cerebral cortex. In addition, a significant correlation has been demonstrated between plasma levels of donepezil hydrochloride, AChE inhibition, and change in ADAS-cog score.

Oral administration of donepezil produces predictable plasma concentrations, with maximal values achieved approximately 3 to 4 hours after dose administration. The terminal disposition half-life is approximately 70 hours; thus, administration of multiple single daily doses results in a gradual approach to steady state. Approximate steady state is achieved within 3 weeks of initiation of therapy. Food does not affect the absorption of donepezil hydrochloride. Donepezil hydrochloride is approximately 95% bound to human plasma proteins.

Donepezil hydrochloride is both excreted in the urine intact and metabolized by the cytochrome P450 system to multiple metabolites, not all of which have been identified. Following administration of a single 5-mg dose of ^{14}C-labeled donepezil hydrochloride, plasma radioactivity (expressed as a percent of the administered dose) was present primarily as intact donepezil hydrochloride (30%), 6-O-desmethyl donepezil (11%), donepezil-cis-N-oxide (9%), 5-O-desmethyl donepezil (7%), and the glucuronide conjugate of 5-O-desmethyl donepezil (3%).

Table 12.5 Randomized double-blind studies using donepezil in patients with mild to moderate DAT

Trial	Protocol	Mean change from baseline ΔADAS-cog		
		for placebo	for 5 mg donepezil	for 10 mg donepezil
A	12 weeks + 2 weeks placebo washout	+ 0.7	− 2.5	Not given
B	12 weeks + 3 weeks placebo washout	+ 0.36	− 2.08	− 2.71
C	24 weeks + 6 weeks placebo washout	+ 1.82	− 0.67	− 1.06

Approximately 57% of the total administered radioactivity was recovered from the urine, and 14.5% was recovered from the feces, suggesting biotransformation and urinary excretion as the primary routes of elimination.

Side effects

Cholinesterase inhibitors may have vagotonic effects on heart rate (e.g., bradycardia). The potential for this action may be particularly important to patients with sick sinus syndrome or other supraventricular conduction abnormalities, such as sinoatrial or atrioventricular block. Theoretically, cholinomimetics may cause bladder outflow obstruction, although this was not observed in clinical trials of donepezil.

The most common adverse effects (incidence greater than 5% and twice the frequency of placebo) were diarrhea, muscle cramps, fatigue, nausea, vomiting, and insomnia. Other common adverse effects (incidence greater than 5% and greater than placebo) are headache, pain, common cold, abdominal disturbance, and dizziness. Rare cases of syncope, bradycardia, sinoatrial block, and atrioventricular block were observed. No notable abnormalities in laboratory values were observed, except for minor increases in serum concentrations of muscle creatine kinase. Care should be taken when prescribing to patients with a history of ulcers or asthma.

Interactions and overdose

The clinical experience with donepezil is presently limited. The prescribing physician should be aware of the possibility of new, as yet unknown interactions with donepezil. Donepezil hydrochloride and/or any of its metabolites do not inhibit the metabolism of theophylline, warfarin, cimetidine, or digoxin in humans. The metabolism of donepezil hydrochloride is not affected by concurrent administration of digoxin or cimetidine. In vitro studies have shown that the cytochrome P450 isoenzymes 3A4 and to a minor extent 2D6 are involved in the metabolism of donepezil. Drug interaction studies performed in vitro show that ketoconazole and quinidine, inhibitors of CYP3A4 and -2D6, respectively, inhibit donepezil metabolism. Therefore, these and other CYP3A4 inhibitors, such as itraconazole and erythromycin, and CYP2D6 inhibitors, such as fluoxetine, could inhibit the metabolism of donepezil. In a study of healthy volunteers, ketoconazole increased mean donepezil concentrations by about 30%. Enzyme inducers, such as rifampicin, phenytoin, carbamazepine, and alcohol, may reduce the levels of donepezil.

Overdosage with cholinesterase inhibitors can result in cholinergic crisis, characterized by severe nausea, vomiting, salivation, sweating, bradycardia, hypotension, respiratory depression, collapse, and convulsions. Increasing muscle weakness is a possibility and may result in death if respiratory muscles are involved. General supportive measures should be utilized. Tertiary anticholinergics such as atropine may be used as an antidote for donepezil overdosage. Intravenous atropine sulfate titrated to effect is recommended: an initial dose of 1.0 and 2.0 mg iv, with subsequent doses based on clinical response.

TACRINE

Dosage and pharmaceutical forms

Tacrine hydrochloride is supplied as capsules containing 10, 20, 30, or 40 mg. The initial dosage is 40 mg per day (10 mg qid). This dose should be maintained for a minimum of 6 weeks with every-other-week monitoring of transaminase levels. It is important that the dose should not be increased during this period because of the potential for delayed onset of transaminase elevations. Following 6 weeks of treatment at 40 mg per day, the dose should then be increased to 80 mg per day (20 mg qid), providing that there are no significant transaminase elevations, and the patient is tolerating treatment. Patients should be titrated to higher doses (120 and 160 mg per day in divided doses on a qid schedule) at 6-week intervals on the basis of tolerance. Serum ALT/SPGT should be monitored every other week for at least the first 16 weeks following initiation of treatment, after which monitoring may be decreased to monthly for every 2 months and every 3 months thereafter. For patients who develop ALT/SPGT elevations greater than two times the upper limit of normal, the dose and monitoring regimen should be modified. Because of the elevation of liver transaminases, monitoring of liver function tests is mandatory.

Pharmacodynamics and pharmacokinetics

Tacrine is rapidly absorbed after oral administration; maximal plasma concentrations occur within 1 to 2 hours. The rate and extent of tacrine absorption following administration of tacrine capsules and solution are virtually indistinguishable. Absolute bioavailability is approximately 17%. Food reduces tacrine bioavailability by approximately 30 to 40%. However, there is no food effect if tacrine is administered at least an hour before meals.

The mean distribution of tacrine is approximately 349 liters. Tacrine is about 55% bound to plasma proteins. The extent and degree of the distribution of tacrine within various body compartments have not been studied systematically. Tacrine is extensively metabolized by the cytochrome P450 system to multiple metabolites, not all of which have been identified. The most important metabolite is velnacrine, the 1-hydroxy metabolite, an active but weaker in vitro AChE inhibitor than tacrine. Studies using human liver preparations demonstrated that CYPIA2 is the principal isoenzyme involved in tacrine metabolism.

Side effects

Tacrine is likely to exaggerate succinylcholine-type muscle relaxation during anesthesia. Because of its cholinomimetic action, it may have vagotonic effects (e.g., bradycardia), which may be particularly important to patients with conduction abnormalities, bradyarrhythmias, or a sick sinus syndrome. Tacrine should be prescribed with care in patients with current evidence or history of abnormal liver function, indicated by significant abnormalities in serum transaminase (ALT/SPGT, AST/SPGOT), bilirubin, and gamma-glutamyl transpeptidase levels. Tacrine also may cause bladder outflow obstruction, and in addition, because of its cholinomimetic action, it should be prescribed with care to patients with a history of ulcers or asthma.

The most common adverse effects associated are elevated transaminases, ataxia, and (in a dose-dependent manner) nausea and/or vomiting, diarrhea, dyspepsia, myalgia, and anorexia.

Interactions and overdose

Tacrine is eliminated primarily by hepatic metabolism via cytochrome P450 drug-metabolizing enzymes. Drug-drug interactions may occur when tacrine is given concurrently with agents such as theophylline that undergo extensive metabolism via CYP1A2. Tacrine administration may thereby double the elimination half-life and plasma concentrations of theophylline. Cimetidine increases the C_{max} and area under the curve (AUC) of tacrine by approximately 54 and 64%, respectively. Because of its mechanism of action, tacrine also has the potential to interfere with the activity of anticholinergic medications (including amitriptyline, to a lesser extent other tricyclic antidepressants, and some neuroleptic agents). A synergistic effect is expected when tacrine is given concurrently with succinylcholine, cholinesterase inhibitors, or cholinergic agonists such as bethanecol.

As in any case of overdose, general supportive measures should be used (see Donepezil).

Pharmacoeconomics

The pharmacoeconomic effectiveness of the new cholinesterase inhibitors remains to be determined using a cost-benefit analysis that would need a number of considerations and assumptions. Donepezil in the United Kingdom costs about £ 1000 per patient per year. There is a theoretical limit to the beneficial effects through loss of cholinergic neurones and a pragmatic limit to treatment based on the therapeutic indications for donepezil (i.e., the progression to severe dementia). It is also important to consider that the function of other neurotransmitter pathways (e.g., catecholaminergic, serotonergic, and peptidergic) becomes compromised later on in the natural history of DAT, and, therefore, arguably, drugs that selectively target the cholinergic system may not have an underlying rationale in advanced disease.

It is generally recognized that patients with DAT usually deteriorate to an end stage requiring full nursing care. The most widely quoted estimates of average survival are between 5 and 8 years. The length of survival is highly variable, but recent data indicate that it is strongly associated with dementia severity, as assessed using the MMSE. The mean survival from symptom onset was found to be 9.3 years. The results from stud-

Table 12.6 MMSE and length of survival	
MMSE SCORE	**Mean survival time (years)**
<13	4.9
13 to 18	6.5
19-23	9.8
>23	10.3

ies such as these potentially may be of some practical use in predicting, to some extent, the likely cost of treatment (Tab. 12.6).

A complete analysis of cost-effectiveness also must include the potential improvement in the quality of life for patients and caregivers. A possible association between the other acetylcholinesterase inhibitor, tacrine, and the likelihood of nursing home placement or death in patients with DAT has been evaluated in a 30-week randomized, double-blind, placebo-controlled, parallel-group clinical trial with 663 patients, after which patients were treated openly and followed up for a minimum of 2 years. Patients who remained on tacrine and who were receiving doses more than 80 mg per day or more than 120 mg per day were less likely to have entered a nursing home than patients on lower doses.

OTHER CHOLINESTERASE INHIBITORS

Physostygmine Physostigmine is a natural alkaloid that is absorbed in the gastrointestinal tract, subcutaneous tissue, and mucous membranes. Physostigmine administration was an early attempt at acetylcholinesterase inhibition treatment for DAT, but unfortunately, it failed to produce any lasting improvement in many DAT patients. Both intravenous and oral administration of the drug resulted in short-lasting, modest improvements on neuropsychologic tests of learning, memory, and attention, but the results were of little clinical significance. This could be the result of a number of factors such as administration of subtherapeutic doses, poor absorption from the gastrointestinal tract, highly individual variability in metabolic rates, fluctuation in CNS availability because of the short half-life, or poor blood-brain barrier penetrability. Recent pharmacologic advances have led to the development of controlled-release preparations of physostigmine that produce sustained blood levels for several hours after ingestion. The results of a large multicenter trial of such a preparation are awaiting analysis, but preliminary results appear positive.

Velnacrine maleate Velnacrine is a tetrahydroaminoacridine derivative that inhibits true cholinesterase and pseudocholinesterase. The drug reverses scopolamine- or lesion-induced memory impairments in rodents. A double-blind, placebo-controlled, enriched population design consisting of a 7-week dose-ranging phase followed by a 6-week dose-replication phase demonstrated modest clinical improvement in a subset of patients with DAT. A high incidence of liver toxicity was observed with this agent associated with elevated serum levels of hepatic enzymes in clinical trials.

New areas of drug development

In the near future, it is worth noting that other cholinesterase inhibitors are likely to be developed fully (e.g., metrifonate, rivastigmine, NXX-066, galanthamine). Metrifonate and rivastigmine recently were reported as being safe and well-tolerated (with no hepatotoxic adverse effects) that enhance cognitive, global, and behavioral function in patients diagnosed with mild to moderate DAT. Drugs that boost levels of acetylcholine are also being investigated currently, among them SB-202026, AF-102B, and ABT-418.

Ultimately, the goal of current drug development research is not only to halt the progress of DAT but also to discover ways in which to restore neuronal activity via neurotropins and to prevent neuronal loss. Cholinergic agents may have direct neuroprotective effects as well as symptomatic effects. It has been postulated that nicotine administration in the form of smoking may reduce the risk of developing DAT. The inverse relation between smoking history and DAT appears to be supported by epidemiologic evidence and may be strongly modified by the presence of the apolipoprotein $\varepsilon4$ allele as well as by a family history of dementia.

Neurotrophins are also being considered for their neuroprotective effects. In vitro, embryonic rat septal neurones produce more intracellular acetylcholine in the presence of nerve growth factor (NGF) than in its absence. NGF may slow down the degeneration of cells in DAT. Recently, using PET neuroimaging, after treating DAT patients with moderate dementia with NGF, increases in cortical blood flow and nicotinic receptors were detected.

Molecules with antioxidative properties (e.g., vitamin E, melatonin, and selegiline) are currently under investigation as treatment for DAT. Vitamin E has been found to slow nerve cell damage and death in animal models and cell culture as a result of its antioxidant effects. In a recent double-blind, randomized, placebo-controlled trial, patients with moderate DAT received either the selective monoamine oxidase inhibitor selegiline (10 mg per day), vitamin E (2000 IU per day), both selegiline and vitamin E, or placebo for 2 years. The primary outcome was the time to the occurrence of any of the following: death, institutionalization, loss of the ability to perform basic activities of daily living, or severe dementia. There were significant delays in the time to the primary outcome for the patients treated with selegiline, vitamin E, or combination as compared with the placebo group. Therefore, the authors concluded that in patients with moderately severe impairment from DAT, treatment with selegiline or vitamin E slows the progression of disease. However, it may be worth bearing in mind that there was no improvement in cog-

nitive decline during the 2-year study period.

Much attention recently has turned to ampakines. Information on the involvement of glutamate receptors in the formation of memory has led to the development of a specific type of glutamate-receptor upregulation. These compounds, called *ampakines,* have been found to reduce memory impairment in middle-aged rats. A positive modulator of AMPA-type glutamate receptors has been found to improve delayed recall in aged humans. Elderly subjects (65 to 76 years of age) were tested for recall of nonsense syllables prior to and after oral administration of CX516 [1-(quinoxalin-6 carbonyl)piperidine], a centrally active drug that enhances currents mediated by AMPA-type glutamate receptors. A significant and positive drug effect was found for delayed (5 min) recall at 75 min after treatment; average scores for the highest-dose group were more than two-fold greater than for the placebo group.

Other cognitive enhancers Nootropic drugs, or cognitive enhancers, are being developed to improve cognitive function, particularly age-related memory impairments. Some drugs may have some effect in rats, e.g., endorphins and certain neuropeptides; however, few drugs have so far been shown to improve consistently and substantially impaired or normal memory in humans over long periods.

POTENTIALLY TREATABLE DISORDERS THAT MAY PRESENT AS DEMENTIA

There are a small number of conditions that give rise to dementia and may be potentially treatable. Some of these are summarized in Table 12.7.

Vascular dementias

This is a term for dementias that are associated with cerebrovascular disease. There is no treatment as yet to reverse the effects of vascular dementia; however, prevention, slowing the progression of a new infarct, and symptomatic treatment of cognitive and neurologic deficits are all aims of management. The use of antioxidants such as vitamin C, vitamin E, beta-carotene, gingko-biloba extract may minimize damage due to new strokes.

Multi-infarct dementia (MID) traditionally has been considered to be the second most common dementia in Europe and the United States and accounts for 15 to 30% of all cases of dementia. It is the most common kind of vascular dementia and is more common in men and in people with a high risk of cardiovascular problems. The onset is usually relatively acute, and the progression is stepwise as a number of minor infarcts cause damage to the cortex. Progressive damage leads to a decline in mental abilities, with the site and extent of infarcts determining cognitive effects. Typical features

Table 12.7 Clinical conditions giving rise to dementia

Chronic subdural hematoma
A blood clot leading to pressure on the brain, often as a result of head injury. It commonly occurs in individuals prone to recurrent head trauma (alcoholics, the elderly, epileptics). Treatment is surgical evacuation; recurrence occurs in about 10-40% of cases

Cerebral tumor
Patients with subfrontal meningiomas present with an insidious change in personality or other features of the frontal lobe syndrome. May be treatable through surgery, radiotherapy, or chemotherapy, according to the type of tumor

Normal-pressure hydrocephalus
This disorder is relatively rare but important because of its potential reversibility by surgical treatment with a ventriculoperitoneal shunt. It may be idiopathic or due to subarachnoid hemorrhage, head injury, or meningitis. The ventricles dilate, but the pressure within them is only intermittently high. The classic presentation is a triad of cognitive impairment, gait disturbance, and incontinence

Alcohol-related dementia
This accounts for about 10% of cases. Heavy alcohol use can lead to brain damage directly and indirectly due to vitamin deficiencies (especially Korsakoff's syndrome, an amnesic syndrome associated with alcohol abuse and thiamine deficiency)

Some alcoholics may develop dementia due to demyelination of the corpus callosum and other areas of the cerebral white matter (the Marchiafava-Bignami syndrome)

Toxins
Manganese, lead, aluminium, and mercury may produce some degree of intellectual impairment

Drugs (e.g., hypnotics, tranquilizers, neuroleptics, barbiturates)

Note also that immunosuppressants may permit the development of opportunistic CNS infections

Vitamin deficiencies
Main examples include vitamin B_{12}, folate, and thiamine (B_1) deficiency. Such deficiencies can be identified by blood tests, and appropriate supplements given

Endocrine disorders
Hormone deficiencies, especially hypothyroidism, can lead to symptoms of slowing, apathy, and poor memory. Severe hypothyroidism also can result in a "myxedema madness," characterized by a psychotic state with hallucinations and paranoia

Thyrotoxicosis may cause behavioral disturbance, resembling an anxiety state; in the elderly, it may present as an apathetic form with psychomotor slowing

Chronic hypocalcemia and recurrent hypoglycemia may result in dementia, sometimes accompanied by ataxia and involuntary movements. Treatment is by hormone replacement. Hypercalcemia may result in reversible neuropsychiatric disturbance

Inflammatory and infective disorders
Conditions such as systemic lupus erythematosus (SLE) and infections such as neurosyphilis ("general paralysis of the insane") (now rare) may affect the brain as well as other organs. Both conditions respond to treatment

Progressive multifocal leukoencephalopathy is caused by the JC papova virus, which causes in the presence of chronic disturbed immunity, widespread cortical and subcortical neurologic and cognitive abnormalities. Visual disturbance due to occipital involvement is more evident than in other dementias. The course of the disease is still most often rapidly progressive and fatal, but several patients with prolonged survival and even remission have been reported. Various antiviral therapies have been tried

Anoxic disorders
If the brain receives insufficient oxygen, for example, after cardiac or respiratory failure, or following carbon monoxide poisoning, symptoms of dementia may result. These are not usually reversible

include emotional incontinence, nocturnal confusion, relative preservation of personality, depression, focal neurologic symptoms and signs, and somatic complaints.

Risk factors include older age, male gender, hypertension, hyperlipidemia, diabetes mellitus, atrial fibrillation, congestive heart failure, carotid bruit, cigarette smoking, and alcohol abuse. The evidence of cerebrovascular disease and the resulting ischemic lesion should be confirmed by neuroimaging techniques, including cerebral angiography; the absence of cerebrovascular lesions detectable by CT or MRI is strong evidence against a vascular etiology. Hypertension should be treated with appropriate antihypertensive

agents. Also, any coexisting conditions that predispose to emboli formation (e.g., cardiac arrhythmias, valvular disease) should be treated appropriately. Daily low-dose enterically coated aspirin is indicated because of its antithrombotic effects provided that the risk falls and intracerebral hemorrhage does not contraindicate its use.

Head injury

Head injury is often neglected as a cause of dementia. The frontal and temporal lobes are particularly at risk from nonpenetrating injury causing multiple contusions and shearing lesions. The length of retrograde amnesia and posttraumatic amnesia may indicate its extent. The vulnerability of the frontal lobes is reflected by personality change in the development of a frontal lobe syndrome. There may be difficulties with planning and problem solving, with loss of fluency and an inability to change rapidly from one task to another, and reduction in powers of concentration. This is associated with emotional blunting, loss of insight, or apathetic mood. Alcohol or other substance abuse may be present. Dementia also may occur as a result of recurrent trauma as in boxing, resulting in the characteristic picture of dementia pugilistica (dementia, personality change, progressive ataxia, extrapyramidal features, and dysarthria). It is important to note that the prevalence of DAT is increased in individuals with a history of head trauma.

Wilson's disease (hepatolenticular degeneration)

Wilson's disease is a rare inborn error of copper metabolism, inherited as an autosomal recessive trait mapped to chromosome 13q. There is a defect in the excretion of ceruloplasmin, the copper-binding protein, from the hepatocyte. This is associated with copper deposition in various organs, most importantly the liver and the brain. The disease presents in childhood or young adulthood with either neurologic or hepatic manifestations but may be delayed in onset as late as age 50. Kayser-Fleischer rings in the eye due to copper deposition on Descemet's membrane are characteristic. Neurologic changes may be subtle, such as a progressive decline in mental function (e.g., defects in memory and visuospatial skills), or more obvious, such as a tremor, dysarthria, dysphagia, involuntary movements, akinesia, and rigidity with dystonia, leading to contractures or immobility. A number of psychiatric aspects also have been described, including at least four symptom clusters (most commonly, affective and behavioral/personality, and less commonly, schizophrenia-like and cognitive).

Liver tests often vary, but in the fulminant presentation there is a low serum alkaline phosphatase level. The total copper content in serum may be reduced, in proportion to the reduction of ceruloplasmin, although free serum copper content may be increased, as may be the urinary excretion of copper.

Copper chelation reverses many of the complications and prevents progression. D-Penicillamine is highly effective for copper chelation. Patients and relatives must be warned that the introduction of treatment is associated with a deterioration in neurologic function that is not always reversible. It is not clear why this occurs. All the relatives of a patient must be screened so that specific treatment can be started early. The prognosis is excellent if treatment is instituted before the development of irreversible organ damage. The usual dosage is 1.5 to 2 g per day in divided doses before food, with a maximum of 2 g daily for 1 year (maintenance 0.75-1 g per day); in the elderly, 20 mg/kg per day is given in divided doses.

DEMENTIAS UNRELATED TO OTHER DISORDERS

Frontotemporal dementias

Frontotemporal dementias (FTD) are distinct from the clinical syndromes of frontotemporal dementia resulting in the dementia of the Alzheimer type (DAT), Creutzfeldt-Jacob disease, subcortical vascular disease, and Huntington's disease, as well as in the affective and schizophreniform psychoses. Frontotemporal dementia is the prototypical behavioral disorder, usually with onset before age 65, that arises from frontotemporal cerebral atrophy. Behaviorally, clinical features may have an insidious onset and include an early loss of personal and social awareness; early loss of insight into the disorder; early signs of disinhibition, mental rigidity, and inflexibility; stereotyped and perseverative behavior; distractibility; and impulsivity. There also may be affective symptoms (e.g., depression, anxiety, delusions, emotional apathy, or amimia) or disorders of speech (e.g., progressive reduction of speech, stereotypy, echolalia and perseveration, and late mutism).

Important neurologic signs that may be found at a relatively early stage include early primitive reflexes and incontinence; later signs include akinesia, rigidity, and tremor. Supportive features in the diagnosis of frontotemporal dementia are bulbar palsy, muscular weakness, wasting, and fasciculations (found in motor neurone disease). By using a combination of an informant history, neuropsychology, and neuroimaging, it should be possible to distinguish between FTD and DAT.

There are currently no pharmacologic treatments widely used. However, recent reports of an improvement in executive function in patients with FTD following increased noradrenergic activity produced by the beta$_2$ antagonist idazoxan suggest a promising approach to the development of new treatments. Idazoxan, at doses of 20, 40, 60, or 80 mg, was found to produce dose-dependent improvements in three patients with FTD, particularly on tests of planning, sustained attention, verbal fluency, and episodic memory. Furthermore, since decreased serotonin receptor binding has been reported in the frontal lobes, temporal lobes, and hypothalamus in autopsy-proven FTD cases, the idea has emerged recently that many of the behavioral symptoms may respond to serotonergic agents. In a recent study, benefits were seen in at least half the patients using fluoxetine (20 mg per day), sertraline (50-125 mg per day), or paroxetine (20 mg per day) (see Chap.13). In this context, it is interesting to note that idazoxan also may have a potent and specific agonistic effect on 5HT1A autoreceptors modulating brain serotonin synthesis in vivo.

Diffuse Lewy bodies disease

A significant number of people diagnosed with dementia are found to have tiny spherical eosinophilic inclusion bodies (Lewy bodies) in brainstem nuclei and throughout the cerebral cortex, which may contribute to the death of brain cells. There is disagreement about whether diffuse Lewy body disease is a distinct illness or a variant of Alzheimer's or Parkinson's disease. The dementia often has a mild and insidious onset and may show marked fluctuation on a day-to-day basis. Features include memory loss, personality changes (e.g., apathy, emotional blunting, disengagement), behavioral disturbances (e.g., agitation, mental wandering), delusions (often of a paranoid nature), depression, neurovegetative dysfunction (e.g., insomnia, nightmares, disturbed sleep), extreme confusion, hallucinations, falls and syncope, and motor features of Parkinson's disease. Results using the CANTAB matching-to-sample task indicate that short-term mnemonic processes, mediated by temporal lobe structures, may be severely affected in patients with dementia with Lewy bodies (DLB). There is currently no treatment. However, given that in DLB neocortical choline acetyltransferase levels are considered to be consistently low, therapeutic trials of cholinesterase inhibitors may prove to be promising, since recently it has been reported that two Lewy body patients with extremely low cholinergic activity were found to respond to tacrine.

DEMENTIAS RELATED TO OTHER DISORDERS

Dementia may be related to other disorders that are currently untreatable.

Huntington's disease

This is a rare, dominantly inherited disease that leads to degeneration of nerve cells in certain parts of the brain. Huntington's disease (HD) is caused by the expansion of an unstable trinucleotide repeat sequence, with consequences of cerebral atrophy, reduced gamma-aminobutyric acid (GABA) and glutamic acid decarboxylase, and a reduction in size of the caudate nucleus bilaterally. Molecular diagnosis can now be performed by a simple polymerase chain reaction (PCR)-based assay. Therefore, genetic counseling is vital, but bearing in mind that suicide occurs both in patients with HD and in those at risk. The disease usually appears between the ages of 30 and 50 years, with early symptoms including forgetfulness, clumsiness, depression, and irrational behavior. Cognitively, patients with early HD have been found to have a wide range of cognitive impairments encompassing both visuospatial memory and executive functions, a pattern distinct from those seen in other basal ganglia disorders.

Dementia eventually occurs in the majority of patients that is judged to be the direct pathophysiologic consequence of HD. Patients with HD are significantly worse than patients with DAT matched for dementia severity on tests of pattern and spatial recognition, simultaneous matching to sample, and visuospatial paired associates and other tests sensitive to frontal lobe function. There is no treatment yet to halt the progress of the disease, but some of the psychiatric and behavioral symptoms may be alleviated by drugs.

Parkinson's disease

Parkinson's disease (see Chap. 10) is a disorder characterized by a considerable loss of striatal dopamine content proportional to the loss of substantia nigra neurones. Clinically, characteristic features are tremor, rigidity, postural abnormalities, and akinesia. There also may be marked cognitive deficits in planning and attentional set-shifting. Dementia has been reported to occur in approximately 20 to 60% of individuals with Parkinson's disease. The dementia is judged to be the direct pathophysiologic consequence of Parkinson's disease and is characterized by cognitive and motor slowing, executive dysfunction, and impairment in memory retrieval.

Human immunodeficiency virus (HIV) and the acquired immune-deficiency syndrome (AIDS)

HIV affects the brain in a number of ways, and about 8 to 16% of people with AIDS develop HIV-related dementia (HIV-D) in the later stages of the illness. Symptoms can include apathy, vagueness, confusion, difficulty in concentrating, forgetfulness, withdrawal, and flattened emotions. However, aspects of the person's original personality may remain intact to the end. There may be a mixed cognitive picture with impairments in tests of executive function (in the CANTAB attentional-shifting test), supporting the hypothesis that frontostriatal dysfunction occurs in individuals infected with HIV-1 prior even to the expression of clinical symptoms. AIDS dementia complex is characterized by personality change, psychomotor slowing, and poor concentration. Zidovudine (AZT) is the most thoroughly investigated medication, with patients developing HIV dementia less frequently and showing improvement on neuropsychologic and CNS evaluations; sustained response lasts 6 months to 1 year, and optimal response is achieved at higher, but less tolerated, dosages. The future management of HIV-D may involve multiple agents as more data become available regarding combination therapy (see Chap. 40).

Prion diseases

Human transmissible spongiform encephalopathies such as Creutzfeldt-Jakob disease (CJD) have been transmitted to primates and to other animals through cell-free injections of infected brain tissue. The principal clinical features of prion diseases are the insidious onset (often accounting for the misdiagnosis of DAT), a dementia (usually progressive, but may be rapid in natural history) with or without ataxia, neuropsychiatric changes, a characteristic EEG (not in the case of new-variant CJD) showing periodic spike complexes, and characteristic neuropathologic features (e.g., spongiform change, neuronal loss, gliosis, and amyloid plaque formation).

CJD is a rapidly progressive dementia, often resulting in death within months of presentation. The cognitive features of this condition include severe memory impairment and aphasia; some patients also develop cortical blindness. Myoclonus is present in about 80% of patients. Most cases appear sporadically, striking about one person in a million over the age of 60. However, 5 to 10% of CJD cases occur in a familial context, showing an autosomal dominant pattern of inheritance. Recently, many cases of CJD have been identified in the United Kingdom with a new neuropathologic profile. This *new-variant CJD* is unusual because of particular features: the young age of the patients, clinical findings, and the absence of EEG changes typical for CJD. The observation that there are particular strain characteristics, which may resemble those of bovine spongiform encephalopathy (BSE) transmitted to mice, domestic cats, and macaque, appears to be consistent with the notion that cattle infected with BSE may be the source of the new disease.

The agent that causes the disease has been characterized and is resistant to inactivation by ultraviolet radiation, formalin, heat, and enzymes that denature nucleic acids. The term *prion* has been coined to describe this small proteinaceous infectious particle. Abnormal forms of the prion protein (a ubiquitous protein of unknown function) cause these neurodegenerative diseases. The disease occurs when the normal cellular prion protein undergoes a conformational change to the abnormal form. Prion diseases occur in several mammalian species. Scrapie affects sheep, and bovine spongiform encephalopathy (BSE) occurs primarily in cows. Other prion diseases, affecting humans, include kuru, a disease associated with cannibalism in the Fore linguistic group of Papua New Guinea natives, and Gerstmann-Sträussler-Scheinker syndrome, classically regarded as a chronic cerebellar ataxia, with dementia occurring later in a more prolonged clinical course. Also, a further rare prion disease has been discovered more recently (fatal familial insomnia), which is characterized by disturbances of the autonomic nervous system, severe insomnia, and dementia; nine extended families have so far been identified.

Acknowledgements

SR was funded by an MRC Research Studentship. Preparation of the manuscript was funded by an MRC LINK grant (G9705363) to BJSCPIJ.

Suggested readings

BRAAK H, GRIFFING K, BRAAK E. Neuroanatomy of Alzheimer's disease: a review article. Alzheimers Res 1997;3:235-47.

EAGGER SA, LEVY R, SAHAKIAN BJ. Tacrine in Alzheimer's disease. Lancet 1991;337:989-92.

FOWLER KS, SALING MM, CONWAY EL, et al. Computerized neuropsychological tests in the early detection of dementia: prospective findings. J Int Neuropsychol Soc 1997;3:139-46.

HODGES JR, PATTERSON K. Is semantic memory consistently impaired early in the course of Alzheimer's disease? Neuroanatomical and diagnostic implications. Neuropsychologia 1995;33:441-59.

JELLINGER K. Morphology of Alzheimer's disease and related disorders. In: Maurer K, Riederer P, Beckmann H (eds). Alzheimer's disease: epidemiology, neuropathology, neurochemistry, and clinics. Wien: Springer, 1990:61-77.

KONNO S, STIRLING MEYER J, TERAYAMA Y, et al. Classification, diagnosis and treatment of vascular dementia. Drugs Aging 1997;5:361-73.

MCKHANN G, DRACHMAN D, FOLSTEIN M, et al. Clinical diagnosis of Alzheimer's disease: report of the NINCDS-ADRDA work group under the auspices of the Department of Health and Human Services Task Force on Alzheimer's Disease. Neurology 1984;34:939-44.

MCKEITH IG. Dementia with Lewy bodies. In: Holmes C, Howard R (eds). Advances in old age psychiatry: chromosomes to community care. London: Wrightson Biomedical Publishing, 1997;52-63.

ORRELL MW, SAHAKIAN BJ. Dementia of frontal type. Psychol Med 1991;21:553-56.

PATTERSON CJ, GAUTHIER S, BERGMAN H, et al. Canadian Consensus Conference on Dementia: a physician's guide to using the recommendations. CMAJ 1999;160:1738-42.

PERRY EK, MORRIS CM, COURT JA, et al. Alteration in nicotine binding sites in Parkinson's disease, Lewy body dementia and Alzheimer's disease: possible index of early neuropathology. Neuroscience 1995;64:385-95.

POIRIER J, DELISLE MC, QUIRION R, et al. Apolipoprotein e4 allele as a predictor of cholinergic deficits and treatment outcome in Alzheimer's disease. Proc Natl Acad Sci USA 1995;92:122-60.

ROSLER M, ANAND R, CICIN-SAIN A, et al. Efficacy and safety of rivastigmine in patients with Alzheimer's disease: international randomised controlled trial. BMJ, 1999;318:633-8.

SAHAKIAN BJ, JONES G, LEVY R, et al. The effects of nicotine on attention, information processing and short-term memory in patients with dementia of the Alzheimer type. Br J Psychiatry 1989;154:797-800.

SAHAKIAN BJ, OWEN AM, MORANT NJ, et al. Further analysis of the cognitive effects of tetrahydroaminoacridine (THA) in Alzheimer's disease: assessment of attentional and mnemonic function using CANTAB. Psychopharmacology (Berl) 1993;110:395-401.

Anxiety and depression

Svein G. Dahl, Lars F. Gram

ANXIETY

Anxiety is an nonspecific symptom that may indicate many different conditions ranging from various somatic illnesses and drug dependence to natural reactions to the events of life. Anxiety is also a common component of most psychiatric disorders and, more infrequently, a disease in itself. Genuine anxiety disorders, without symptoms of depression or psychosis, include phobias, panic disorder, and generalized anxiety disorder. Panic attacks can occur on their own but are most common in phobic situations. The major manifestations of anxiety are:

- verbal complaints from the patient;
- somatic and autonomic effects (e.g., restlessness, agitation, tachycardia, sweating, weeping, and gastrointestinal disorders);
- interference with normal productive activities.

The current treatment of anxiety disorders is based primarily on the use of benzodiazepines, which act as agonists on cortical γ-aminobutyric acid A, GABA(A), receptors. Their anxiolytic effects have a short onset of action, depending mainly on the rate of absorption and distribution to the brain. Despite their potent anxiolytic action, the long-term risk: benefit ratio of benzodiazepines remains controversial.

The azapirones (i.e., buspirone and analogues) represent a different class of anxiolytic drugs, which act as agonists or partial agonists on serotonin 5-HT 1A receptors. The anxiolytic effect of buspirone, which has little tendency to induce sedation or dependence, gradually develops over a period of up to 2 to 3 weeks.

Certain antidepressant drugs are also used for the specialized treatment of anxiety disorders. The tricyclic antidepressant clomipramine has a documented therapeutic effect in panic disorders.

Since anxiety is a subjective human phenomenon, closely related to appropriate fear, the distinction between a normal and a pathologic state of anxiety sometimes may be difficult. It is important, therefore, to make a careful evaluation of the patient. When no treatable primary condition is found despite a thorough evaluation, or one is found and properly dealt with, it may be desirable to initiate treatment to relieve the symptoms of anxiety and restore the patient to a normal affect. In such situations, anxiolytic drugs may be used appropriately, although providing no curative treatment.

With a few exceptions, anxiolytic drugs have a dependence-inducing liability and should only be used short term or intermittently. Excessive medication may prove counterproductive in suppressing the patient's own coping mechanisms.

Drug classes

Several different dosage forms of benzodiazepines are available, especially in the case of diazepam, still the most widely used analogue. Intravenous injections may be used for the treatment of acute conditions such as prolonged epileptic discharge (status epilepticus) and acute agitation. Available dosage forms and recommended doses are given in Table 13.1.

BENZODIAZEPINES

A number of different benzodiazepine derivatives currently are used for the treatment of anxiety. These include alprazolam, chlordiazepoxide, chlorazepate, diazepam, halazepam, lorazepam, medazepam, oxazepam, and prazepam. Like other benzodiazepine derivatives, promoted as sedative-hypnotic drugs, those recommended for treatment of anxiety have a common pharmacologic profile and the following major effects: reduction of anxiety, sedation and induction of sleep, anticonvulsant action, and reduction of muscle tone.

Clonazepam and two other benzodiazepines commonly used as anxiolytics, diazepam and chlorazepate, are also used as anticonvulsants. In addition, benzodiazepines are used for preoperative sedation, treatment of acute symptoms related to alcohol withdrawal, and as muscle relaxants in chronic muscle spasm and spasticity.

The anxiolytic, sedative, anticonvulsive, and muscle-

Table 13.1 Dosage forms and recommended doses of antianxiety drugs

Nonproprietary name	Dosage forms[1]	Usual oral dose[2] (mg/d)	Maximum oral dose[2] (mg/d)
Benzodiazepines			
Alprazolam	O, SR	0.75-1.5	4
Chlordiazepoxide	O, I	15-40	100
Chlorazepate	O, SR	10-30	60
Diazepam	O, SR, SU, L, I	5-15	40
Halazepam	O	60-120	160
Lorazepam	O, I	2-4	10
Medazepam	O	4-8	16
Oxazepam	O	20-60	150
Prazepam	O, L	10-30	60
Azapirones			
Buspirone	O	15-30	45 (60)

[1]O = oral solid rapid release; SR = oral sustained release; L = oral liquid; I = injection; SU = suppositories.
[2]Total daily doses for treatment of anxiety in adults, assumed to be divided into two or more portions. Smaller maximal doses are recommended for elderly patients.

relaxant effects of benzodiazepines all seem to be mediated by a similar molecular mechanism involving agonist interaction with the GABA(A) receptor. This receptor is believed to be a pentameric, ligand-gated ion channel that opens by binding of a GABA molecule to the receptor's γ subunit. Binding of a benzodiazepine molecule to an α subunit of the receptor increases GABA-induced Cl-ion conductance through the intrinsic channel.

The first benzodiazepine drug, chlordiazepoxide, was synthesized in 1955 by Leo Sternbach and colleagues. Rearrangement of a six-membered quinazoline ring by chemical reaction with a primary amine led, quite unexpectedly, to formation of a seven-membered 1,4-benzodiazepine-4-oxide. The compound was supposed to be inactive, but its pharmacologic activity was examined 2 years later. It was then discovered that it had sedative, muscle-relaxant, and anticonvulsant activity in animals superior to that of meprobamate, no effect on the autonomic nervous system, and generally a low toxicity. Clinical trials confirmed that the compound had antianxiety and anticonvulsant effects in humans, and it was introduced to the market in 1960, only $2^{1}/_{2}$ years after the start of the pharmacologic studies.

Diazepam, synthesized in 1959, had a similar pharmacologic profile but was 3 to 10 times more potent than chlordiazepoxide in animal tests. It was marketed near the end of 1963 and has since become one of the most widely used drugs in the western world.

Pharmacokinetics

Absorption and distribution Benzodiazepines are lipophilic compounds that easily traverse biologic membranes. They are usually absorbed rapidly and quite completely (80-100%) after oral administration, with peak plasma concentrations occurring within 1 to $1^{1}/_{2}$ hours. Peak concentrations in the brain are attained almost simultaneously. Intramuscular injection may result in slower absorption than oral administration, possibly because the drug is taken up by the surrounding muscular tissue.

Diazepam and other lipophilic benzodiazepines are distributed rapidly to highly perfused tissues including the brain, with a rapid onset of psychotropic effects. They are then redistributed to less well perfused tissues, resulting in a significant fall in brain concentrations. This may result in a relatively brief duration of action after single doses, despite their long elimination half-lives. Excessive peak concentrations in the brain may cause an undesirable degrees of sedation. Diazepam and other benzodiazepines with relatively long half-lives therefore should be given in two to three daily doses for the treatment of daytime anxiety.

Lorazepam and oxazepam are less lipophilic than most other benzodiazepines and more slowly absorbed. This results in a somewhat slower onset of action, which has been suggested to reduce their abuse potential due to less of a "kick" after oral doses.

Elimination rates and steady-state levels As for antidepressant and antipsychotic drugs, benzodiazepines were used for several years before sufficiently sensitive assay methods permitted measurement of their plasma levels in humans after therapeutic doses. When such methods were developed in the early 1970s, it was found that most of the benzodiazepines used for the treatment of anxiety or sleep disturbances had elimination half-lives on the order of 24 hours or longer and that pharmacologically active metabolites often had longer half-lives than the

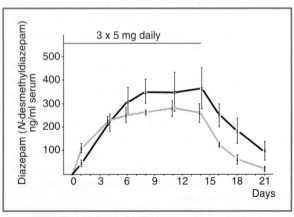

Figure 13.1 Serum concentrations of diazepam (*blue line*) and *N*-desmethyl diazepam (*black line*) after oral administration of diazepam, 15 mg per day, for 2 weeks. (From Hillestad L, Hansen T, Melson H. Diazepam metabolism in normal man. II. Serum concentration and clinical effect after oral administration and cumulation. Clin Pharmacol Ther 1974;16:485-9.)

parent drug. It became evident that these long elimina-
tions half-lives may lead to accumulation of one or more
active compounds in the body for several days and in some
cases for weeks during continued treatment. This is illustrated in Figure 13.1, which shows the accumulation of
diazepam and its active metabolite *N*-desmethyldiazepam
during 2 weeks of treatment with diazepam. Due to its
longer half-life, the metabolite, which only attains relatively low levels after the first dose, continues to accumulate
over a longer period of time and finally reaches higher
steady-state plasma levels than the parent drug.

The half-lives of the benzodiazepines used most frequently as anxiolytics are summarized in Table 13.2.

There are large variations in elimination half-life
between individual drugs. The ranges indicated in Table
13.2 do not include extreme values sometimes observed
in elderly patients or in patients with reduced hepatic
function.

Metabolism

Most benzodiazepine drugs are highly lipophilic compounds that are extensively metabolized before being
excreted into urine. This is illustrated in Figure 13.2,

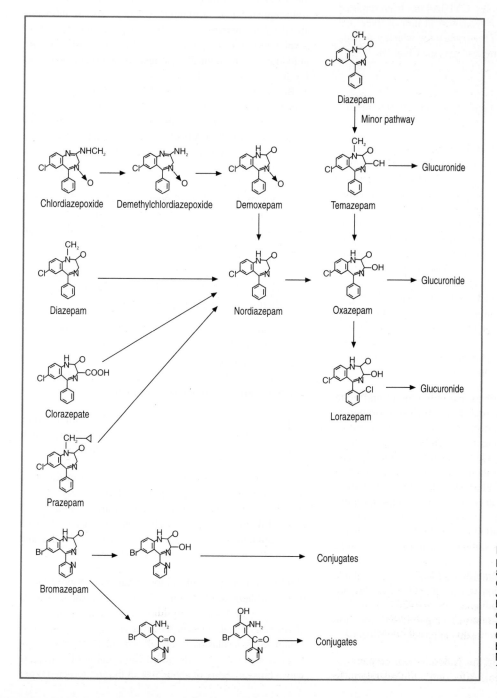

Figure 13.2 Metabolic
pathways of benzodi-
azepines used as anxiolytic
drugs.(From Kaplan SA,
Jack ML. Metabolism of the
benzodiazepines: pharma-
cokinetic and pharmacody-
namic considerations. In:
Costa E (ed). Molecular
biology to clinical practice.
New York: Raven Press,
1983;173-99.)

which also shows that *N*-desmethyldiazepam (nordiazepam) and oxazepam, both used as anxiolytic drugs, are formed as active metabolites from several other benzodiazepines.

Different subfamilies of hepatic cytochrome P450 (CYP) are involved in the metabolism of different benzodiazepines. Therefore, the potential for interaction with any other specific drug differs among different drugs within the benzodiazepine series. Different CYP enzymes also may be involved in different metabolic pathways for one and the same benzodiazepine.

In general, CYP3A4 and CYP2C19 seem to play the most important metabolic roles. CYP3A4 has been reported to be the most abundant CYP enzyme in human liver, and CYP2C19 is one of the CYP enzymes for which a genetic polymorphism has been demonstrated (see Chap. 3).

Properties

Properties of the most commonly used benzodiazepines are reported here.

Alprazolam Alprazolam is a benzodiazepine of high potency that has attained widespread use in the treatment of anxiety and panic disorders. It is rapidly absorbed after oral administration, with peak plasma levels occurring within 0.5 to 2 hours, and it has a bioavailability in the order of 90%. Less than 0.1% of the absorbed dose is excreted unchanged in the urine. Alprazolam is metabolized by CYP3A4, and concurrent administration of erythromycin may significantly increase its elimination half-life, which otherwise is about 10 to 20 hours. Alprazolam has several metabolites, but these do not seem to contribute to the clinical effects. The main metabolite, α-hydroxyalprazolam, which has a half-life similar to that of alprazolam, is less pharmacologically active than the parent compound and does not attain appreciable plasma concentrations. It is conjugated to glucuronides before excretion into the urine.

Chlordiazepoxide Chlordiazepoxide is rapidly and quite completely absorbed after oral doses, but its absorption is slow and erratic after im injection. Therefore, oral administration or iv injections should be used when rapid effects are needed. Chlordiazepoxide has a smaller volume of distribution in the body and therefore attains higher plasma concentrations than most other benzodiazepines after similar doses. It is metabolized to *N*-desmethylchlordiazepoxide, demoxepam, and *N*-desmethyldiazepam, as indicated in Table 13.2. These metabolites are all pharmacologically active and have half-lives similar to or longer than that of the parent compound.

The hydrochloride of chlordiazepoxide is water soluble but unstable both in solution and when exposed to ultraviolet light, under which conditions isomerization to an inactive derivative occurs. Solutions for parenteral injection therefore must be prepared freshly and used immediately.

Chlorazepate is a prodrug for *N*-desmethyldiazepam (i.e., nordiazepam, nordazepam). After oral administration, the drug is decarboxylated to *N*-desmethyldiazepam in the stomach, and peak plasma levels of *N*-desmethyldiazepam are attained in about 1 hour.

Diazepam Diazepam is the most widely studied benzodiazepine, which reflects its widespread use. It is relatively lipid soluble and water insoluble. Oral absorption is rapid and fairly complete (80-100%), with peak plasma levels occurring within 1^1/$_2$ hour. Like chlordiazepoxide, its absorption is slow and erratic after im injection.

Diazepam is almost completely metabolized before excretion into the urine, with *N*-desmethyldiazepam as the major active metabolite. As indicated in Table 13.2, this metabolite generally has a longer elimination half-life than the parent drug. Although the elimination half-lives of benzodiazepines show substantial variations among individuals, the ratio between the half-lives of diazepam and *N*-desmethyldiazepam appears to be relatively constant within individuals, and about 50% longer for the metabolite than for the parent drug.

Both CYP2C19 and CYP3A4 are involved in the *N*-demethylation of diazepam, whereas CYP3A4 is the major enzyme involved in the hydroxylation of diazepam. Poor metabolizers of the CYP2C19 genotype had two to three times longer elimination half-lives of diazepam and *N*-desmethyldiazepam than extensive metabolizers in a Chinese population. It has been suggested that the higher frequency of the CYP2C19 poor metabolizer (PM) phenotype in Oriental (15-20%) than in Caucasian populations (2-5%) may be a reason for the generally lower dosages of diazepam used in Orientals.

Halazepam As indicated in Table 13.2, halazepam is partly metabolized to *N*-desmethyldiazepam and is, accordingly, classified as a long-acting benzodiazepine.

Lorazepam Lorazepam is less lipophilic and more slowly absorbed than diazepam, with peak plasma levels occurring after 2 to 4 hours. It is eliminated mainly by hepatic glucuronidation with a half-life of 8 to 25 hours and is excreted into the urine as conjugated metabolites.

Medazepam As shown in Table 13.2, medazepam has three active metabolites with relatively long half-lives, which may contribute to the duration of its effects in humans.

Oxazepam Oxazepam resembles lorazepam in that it is less lipophilic than diazepam and relatively slowly absorbed, with peak plasma levels occurring after 2 to 3 hours. Like lorazepam, it is eliminated mainly by hepatic glucuronidation and renal excretion of glucuronides and has an elimination half-life of 6 to 20 hours.

Prazepam Prazepam, like chlorazepate, is a prodrug for *N*-desmethyldiazepam but differs from chlorazepate in that the conversion to *N*-desmethyldiazepam occurs mainly as a "first-pass" metabolism in the liver and is slower and less complete. Peak plasma levels of *N*-desmethyldiazepam are reached 4 to 6 hours after oral administration of prazepam, with a bioavailability of about 50% of the administered dose.

Indications

Indications for benzodiazepines include generalized and episodic anxiety and states of phobias, restlessness, tension, and aggression. Benzodiazepines also may be used to treat anxiety related to serious or painful somatic conditions and for treatment of delirium tremens. Alprazolam may be used to suppress predictable and spontaneous panic attacks. It has been maintained that diazepam, lorazepam, and clonazepam also may be capable of suppressing panic attacks when given in sufficiently high doses.

Because of the likelihood of benzodiazepines to induce dependence, treatment with them generally should be as brief as possible and normally should not exceed 8 to 12 weeks. Longer treatment requires precise and repeated evaluations of the patient.

Age-related pharmacokinetic and pharmacodynamic changes may increase the effects of benzodiazepines in elderly patients (see Chap. 89), and prescribing benzodiazepines for the elderly demands special care. Owing to a lower hepatic metabolic clearance, elderly patients may show cumulative toxicity to usual adult dosages, especially for agents such as diazepam, chlordiazepoxide, and prazepam, which are metabolized in the liver by oxidative phase I reactions and have active metabolites with longer half-lives than the parent drug. The elimination of oxazepam and lorazepam, which occurs mainly by hepatic glucuronidation and renal excretion of metabolites, seems to be less affected by age-related physiologic changes. Dosage of benzodiazepines in the elderly generally should be started at 25 to 50% of the usual adult dose range.

Side effects

The main side effects of benzodiazepines are drowsiness, confusion, memory disturbances, and impaired motoric coordination, which may impair job performance and driving skills. The long elimination half-lives of many benzodiazepines may produce substantial after-day impairment (see also Chap. 82).

Although their tendency to produce dependence and withdrawal symptoms is much weaker than for other CNS-depressant drugs such as the barbiturates, it is well recognized that benzodiazepines have a liability to cause physical and psychologic dependence. Patients obtaining dramatic relief of anxiety from benzodiazepines may be reluctant to discontinue use of the drug because abrupt withdrawal after continued use over a long period may cause rebound anxiety, insomnia, sweating, tremor, dizziness, and irritability.

Contraindications

Severe respiratory insufficiency, sleep apnea, pronounced hepatic insufficiency, and known hypersensitivity to benzodiazepines are absolute contraindications. Benzodiazepines should not be prescribed for patients with myasthenia. Since they are excreted in breast milk, benzodiazepines should not be used more than sporadically in nursing mothers. On repeated administration to the nursing mother, the drug may accumulate in the infant, resulting in sedation and general central nervous system (CNS) depression and, in some cases, in a paradoxical reaction with agitation. Even a low concentration of benzodiazepine in the blood may enhance the depressant effects of alcohol, and the combination should be avoided. Due to their CNS depressant activity, benzodiazepines should not be used in combination with car driving or handling of heavy machinery.

Overdose

Benzodiazepines are part of an increasing, worldwide addiction problem. They are used alone or as a part of multidrug abuse to induce euphoria, potentiate opioid actions, or soften the "crash" after the "high" from cocaine or amphetamine abuse. This is reflected in a substantial number of combined opiate-benzodiazepine intoxications (see Chap. 82).

Table 13.2 Elimination of benzodiazepine drugs

Nonproprietary name, active metabolite	Elimination half-life (h)
Alprazolam	9-16
α-Hydroxyalprazolam[1]	15[2]
Chlordiazepoxide	5-15
N-Desmethylchlordiazepoxide	16
N-Desmethyldiazepam	30-100
Demoxepam	14-46
Oxazepam	6-20
Chlorazepate[3]	–
N-Desmethyldiazepam	30-100
Diazepam	20-50
N-Desmethyldiazepam[4]	30-100
Oxazepam	6-20
Halazepam	35
N-Desmethyldiazepam	30-100
Lorazepam[5]	8-25
Medazepam	2-3
N-Desmethylmedazepam	25-85
Diazepam	20-50
N-Desmethyldiazepam	30-100
Oxazepam[6]	6-20
Prazepam[7]	0.5-2
N-Desmethyldiazepam	30-100
Oxazepam	6-20

[1]Only weak biologic activity, probably no clinical effect.
[2]Reported half-life may reflect formation rather than elimination rate of the metabolite.
[3]Prodrug for N-desmethyldiazepam.
[4]About 50% longer than $t_{1/2}$ of parent compound in the same individual.
[5]Hepatic conjugation to inactive glucuronide.
[6]Hepatic conjugation to inactive glucuronide.
[7]Prodrug for N-desmethyldiazepam.

Benzodiazepines generally have relatively low toxicity and less effect on cardiovascular and respiratory function than other sedative-hypnotic drugs. Fatalities due to benzodiazepine overdose alone are uncommon but may occur in the young, the old, the frail, and those with existing respiratory pathology. Severe intoxication resulting from combined overdose of benzodiazepines and other CNS-depressant drugs is often seen in hospital emergency units. Intoxications of benzodiazepines combined with alcohol, opioids, antipsychotic drugs, or antidepressant drugs may produce respiratory collapse and can be fatal.

The specific, competitive benzodiazepine receptor antagonist flumazenil may be used as an antidote in the treatment of acute benzodiazepine intoxication. Flumazenil acts quickly and effectively when administered intravenously, but its action lasts only for about 2 hours.

AZAPIRONES (BUSPIRONE)

Buspirone, together with gepirone and ipsapirone, belongs to the azapirone class of compounds, potent agonists at pre- and postsynaptic 5-HT1A receptors in the brain. Buspirone alleviates both psychic and somatic symptoms of anxiety with a gradual onset of effects, usually within 1 to 2 weeks of treatment. Longer treatment, from 2 to 4 weeks, sometimes may be required before full symptom relief occurs. Buspirone also may have a certain antidepressant effect, independent of its anxiolytic activity.

The exact mechanism of the anxiolytic action of buspirone is not known. Its pharmacologic profile indicates that the main action is on 5-HT1A receptors, both presynaptically in the dorsal raphe as a full agonist and postsynaptically in the hippocampus as a partial agonist.

Pharmacokinetics and metabolism

Buspirone is absorbed rapidly but has a very low bioavailability, about 4%, due to extensive "first-pass" metabolism. As is often the case for drugs with pronounced first-pass metabolism, its bioavailability shows considerable interindividual variation. Concomitant food intake may lead to twice as high a bioavailability as in fasted subjects.

The elimination half-life of buspirone in healthy volunteers ranges from 2 to 11 hours. It is almost completely metabolized before excretion in urine, and at least 12 different metabolites are formed in humans. The main metabolic pathways are hydroxylation and *N*-dealkylation. The dealkylated metabolite had only a weak activity in an animal model of anxiety. Patients with cirrhosis may have significantly longer elimination half-lives of buspirone than patients with normal hepatic function, and substantial inter- and intraindividual variations in half-life and area under plasma drug level curves.

Side effects

The main side effects of buspirone are dizziness, nausea, headache, nervousness, and dry mouth, quite different from those of the benzodiazepines. Buspirone does not cause sedation or motor incoordination, has little effect on cognition, has no respiratory depressant effects, and has no pronounced withdrawal effect on discontinuation of treatment.

Unlike the benzodiazepines, buspirone is rarely associated with dependence or abuse. It therefore may be preferable to benzodiazepines in patients with a history of substance abuse or a likelihood of developing dependency. The lack of cognitive-impairing effects may be an advantage over benzodiazepines in the treatment of elderly patients.

DEPRESSION

Major depression is a serious illness that can cause considerable pain, functional impairment, and even death. In the western world, it is assumed to affect from 5 to 10% of the population. In most countries, the majority of patients identified as having a depression are treated in the primary care setting. It has been maintained, however, that many cases go unrecognized and that those which are identified frequently are inadequately treated. Major depression is a syndrome that includes depressed mood, unrealistically lowered self-esteem, sleep disturbances (often delayed/early wakening), decreased appetite with weight loss, retardation with decreased psychic and motor activity and often a sense of fatigue, decreased motivation, decreased interest, decreased sex drive, and decreased concentration and attention. The patient should have most of these signs and symptoms to qualify for the diagnosis of major depression.

The precise causes of affective disorders remain elusive. However, all antidepressant drugs appear to increase biogenic amine levels at synaptic nerve terminals in the brain, although by different molecular mechanisms of action. These and other observations indicate that depression is caused by a functional deficit of monoamine neurotransmitters at certain sites in the brain, whereas mania results from a functional excess.

For many years, the tricyclic antidepressants (TCAs) and monoamine oxidase (MAO) inhibitors, together with the tetracyclic antidepressant mianserin, were the available drugs for the treatment of depression, in addition to lithium for the treatment of acute mania and prophylaxis in bipolar affective disorders. Over the last decade, this situation has evolved with the introduction of selective serotonin reuptake inhibitors (SSRIs), combined serotonin and norepinephrine reuptake inhibitors (SNRIs), and reversible and more specific MAO inhibitors. The physician therefore may choose between several different pharmacologic approaches in the treatment of a depressed patient.

While the therapeutic profile is somewhat different between the different antidepressant drugs and drug classes, they all have in common a gradual onset of therapeutic effect, which is fully developed after 3 to 10 weeks of treatment.

Treatment

A physician faced with a patient who may have a depressive syndrome must do a differential diagnosis to confirm the depressive illness or to establish that the symptoms are not due to other causes. These may include substance abuse or dependence, other drug therapy, occult malignancies, or other pathophysiologic or etiologic reasons. Different causes of a depressive episode may require different treatments.

Before starting treatment, the depressive episode should be classified as mild, moderate, serious without psychotic symptoms, or serious with psychotic symptoms. Both the therapeutic potential and side-effect profile of the available therapeutic drugs must be taken into account in the choice of treatment. When treatment has been initiated, it is important that before concluding that the patient does not respond to treatment with a certain antidepressant drug, the physician should ascertain that the patient has taken the prescribed drug and has been treated with the right dose and for a sufficiently long period.

The onset of the antidepressant effect is gradual, and it usually takes 2 to 4 weeks to obtain optimal symptom relief. Different features of the depressive illness may respond at different rates. Initially, the treatment may produce a certain psychostimulant effect before the desired effect on depressive mood occurs. The sedative effect of certain antidepressants comes during the initial days of treatment and then gradually weakens as tolerance to this effect develops.

Drug classes

As indicated in Table 13.3, antidepressant drugs usually are administered orally, as immediate-release tablet formulations. Some slow-release formulations are available for once-a-day administration, usually in the evening, but conventional tablets are also often administered in single daily doses. Intramuscular injection or intravenous infusion is sometimes used for a limited period at the beginning of treatment. As for anxiolytic drugs, recommended antidepressant drug dosages in elderly patients are lower than usual adult dosages.

TRICYCLIC ANTIDEPRESSANTS (TCAs)

The first tricyclic antidepressant (TCA), imipramine, was discovered in 1956 when the drug, which has a molecular structure resembling that of chlorpromazine, was tried in the treatment of a wide range of psychiatric patients by R. Kuhn. Imipramine and analogues, together with the then newly discovered antipsychotic drugs, proved valuable both as new therapeutic agents and as research tools to study the neurobiologic pathologies associated with psychiatric diseases. About 4500 articles on imipramine were

Table 13.3 Dosage forms and recommended doses of antidepressant drugs

Nonproprietary name	Dosage forms[1]	Usual oral dose[2] (mg/d)
TCAs		
Amitriptyline	O	75-200
Nortriptyline	O	25-150
Imipramine	O	75-300
Desipramine	O	75-200
Doxepin	O	Initially 50, increase gradually to 200-250
Clomipramine	O, I	50-150
Dosulepin	O	50-150
SSRIs		
Citalopram	O	20-60
Fluoxetine	O, L	20-60
Fluvoxamine	O	100-200
Paroxetine	O, I	20-50
Sertraline	O	50-200
SNRI		
Venlafaxine	O	75-375
Milnacipran	O	50-200
MAOI		
Moclobemide	O	300-600
Other		
Mianserin	O	30-90
Maprotiline	O, I	50-100

[1]O=oral solid rapid release; L=oral liquid; I=injection.
[2]Total daily doses for treatment in adults, assumed to be divided into two or more portions. Smaller maximal doses are recommended for elderly patients.

published during the 10 years following its discovery, and more than 40 years after its discovery, it is still used as a major antidepressant drug in many countries and serves as a model compound. The characteristics of the most widely used TCAs are reported here.

Amitriptyline has relatively strong sedative and anticholinergic effects and therefore may be less suited for treatment of elderly patients. It is often used to treat depression with agitation or anxiety. Nortriptyline is the major metabolite of amitriptyline. Weak sedative, anticholinergic effects and less tendency to cause orthostatic hypotension make it more suitable than other TCAs for treatment of elderly patients. Imipramine has medium-strong sedative and anxiolytic effects in addition to its antidepressant activity. Desipramine has relatively weak sedative properties and is the TCA with the relatively strongest adrenergic

Oral absorption of TCAs is rapid and complete, but the systemic availability is reduced due to "first-pass" metabolism in the liver, which varies from 25 to 75% among patients. The TCAs are extensively distributed into the tissues and have volumes of distribution ranging from 500 to 2500 liters depending on the drug and the patient.

The major metabolites formed by first-pass metabolism of amitriptyline (AMI), clomipramine (CMI), and imipramine (IMI), are the corresponding *N*-demethylated secondary amines (nortriptyline, desmethyl CMI, and desipramine) (Tab. 13.4). These metabolites are pharmacologically active, reach steady-state plasma levels of the same magnitude as those of the parent drug, and contribute to therapeutic and side effects. Ring hydroxylated metabolites, some of which are pharmacologically active, are also formed by first-pass metabolism. These metabolites are conjugated to glucuronides in the liver and excreted in the urine, and they do not appear to contribute significantly to the therapeutic or side effects. The polymorphic CYP enzyme CYP2D6 plays an important role in the oxidative metabolism of TCAs. If hepatic metabolism of TCAs is reduced, this may result in toxic drug levels after repeated therapeutic doses. This may be especially important in the CYP2D6 poor metabolizer (PM) phenotype, which represents about 7% of Caucasian populations.

The elimination half-lives of the TCAs are usually in the range of 1 to 3 days, and steady-state drug levels in plasma are reached after 1 to 3 weeks of treatment. Desmethyl CMI has a longer elimination half-life and requires 2 to 4 weeks to reach steady-state levels in plasma.

Patients who are CYP2D6 PMs (see Chap. 3) have longer elimination half-lives, and the time to reach steady state is prolonged correspondingly. It is important to be aware of the time required before the plasma levels of a certain TCA stabilize at a steady-state level in the individual patient. Excessive plasma levels of TCAs, often seen with standard doses given to patients who are CYP2D6 PMs, are associated with an increased risk of side effects and adverse reactions. In the relatively rare case of ultra-rapid metabolism (UM), higher doses than usual are required to achieve therapeutic blood levels.

The absorbed TCA dose is virtually completely excreted as metabolites in the urine. For imipramine and, in particular, clomipramine, pronounced dose-dependent kinetics at therapeutic doses is well documented.

Activity of metabolites The metabolites formed by *N*-demethylation – AMI nortriptyline and IMI desipramine – are also used as antidepressant drugs per se. All these compounds inhibit the reuptake of norepinephrine and serotonin at synaptic nerve terminals, but the tertiary amines (AMI, CMI, and IMI) are more potent serotonin reuptake inhibitors and less potent norepinephrine reuptake inhibitors than their *N*-demethylated analogues. CMI is the most potent serotonin reuptake inhibitor among the TCAs. AMI and IMI generally have stronger sedative and anticholinergic effects than their *N*-demethylated analogues.

Serum (plasma) concentration monitoring For several of the TCAs, the serum or plasma concentration in

Table 13.4 Elimination of antidepressant drugs

Nonproprietary name, active metabolite	Elimination half-life (h)	Comments
TCAs		
Amitriptyline	10-60	Active metabolite: nortriptyline
Nortriptyline	15-90	
Imipramine	10-30	Active metabolite: desipramine
Desipramine	15-50	
Doxepin	10-25	
Clomipramine	10-40	Nonlinear kinetics
N-Desmethyl-clomipramine	20-50	Active metabolite
Dosulepin	20-60	
SSRIs		
Citalopram	20-40	
Fluoxetine	2-7 days	Nonlinear kinetics
N-Desmethyl-fluoxetine	4-15 days	Active metabolite
Fluvoxamine	20-30	Nonlinear kinetics
Paroxetine	20-40	Nonlinear kinetics
Sertraline	20-30	
SNRIs		
Venlafaxine	5-10	
O-Desmethyl-venlafaxine	10-20	Active metabolite
Milnacipran	5-15	
MAO inhibitors		
Moclobemide	2-6	
Other		
Mianserin	10-20	
Maprotiline	40-45	

effect. Clomipramine is a more potent inhibitor of serotonin reuptake than other TCAs, whereas the primary metabolite, desmethylclomipramine, is a potent inhibitor of both norepinephrine and serotonin reuptake. Doxepin has relatively strong sedative, anxiolytic and anticholinergic effects compared with other TCAs. Dosulepin has relatively strong anticholinergic effects. It has active metabolites with longer elimination half-lives than the parent compound.

patients has been studied systematically in relation to antidepressant effect, side effects, and toxicity. Recommended concentration ranges thus have been defined, forming the basis for drug level monitoring as practiced in particular in hospital settings in several countries. The upper concentration limit has been defined by lack of antidepressant effect for nortriptyline and risk of toxicity (CNS, cardiovascular) for the other TCAs.

Side effects and adverse reactions

The TCAs have, in addition to inhibition of serotonin and norepinephrine reuptake, antagonist action on postsynaptic central and peripheral α-adrenergic, muscarinic, cholinergic, histamine H$_1$, and serotonin 5-HT2 receptors as well as a quinidine-like effect on the cardiac conductance system. These effects explain many of the dose-dependent side effects and adverse reactions that may be an important reason for noncompliance:

- *CNS:* somnolence, tiredness, and difficulty in concentrating. TCAs may produce a state of confusion that may be potentially harmful, especially in elderly patients. Sedative effects of TCAs sometimes may be helpful when difficulty in sleeping is part of the depression symptoms. Restlessness and sleep disturbances are less frequent side effects;
- *peripheral anticholinergic:* dry mouth, accommodation paresis, constipation, urinary retention (especially in elderly male patients), and sweating;
- *cardiovascular:* postural hypotension, probably due to peripheral α$_1$-adrenergic receptor antagonism, may be a problem, particularly in the elderly (nortriptyline is less problematic in this context). Tachycardia and electrocardiographic changes are sometimes observed, and arrhythmias are seen more rarely. Patients attaining abnormally high plasma drugs levels on normal therapeutic doses due to impaired hepatic function or PM genetic polymorphism are especially at risk;

Other side effects include weight gain, reduced sexual drive, and various cutaneous reactions. There is generally a linear relationship between plasma/serum drug levels and the tendency to produce anticholinergic, cardiovascular, and other side effects by treatment with TCAs.

Indications

The primary indications for TCAs are major depression, panic attack (clomipramine), phobic and obsessional states (clomipramine), and neuropathic pain (diabetic, etc.)

Contraindications

The contraindications of TCA therapy are recent myocardial infarction (<6 months), heart failure, narrow-angle glaucoma, micturition problems related to benign prostatic hypertrophy, treatment with a nonspecific MAO inhibitor within the last 2 weeks, and known hypersensitivity to the drug.

Interactions

Tricyclic antidepressants are to a large extent metabolized by CYP2D6, and drugs that are potent inhibitors of this enzyme (e.g., paroxetine, fluoxetine, moclobemide, haloperidol, thioridazine, perphenazine and other neuroleptics, quinidine, and some other antiarrhythmics) may cause elevated plasma/serum levels of TCAs and signs of relative overdose such as confusion in the elderly. Combination of a TCA with a classic irreversible MAO inhibitor may cause severe cardiovascular and CNS toxicity, and combination of clomipramine with an SSRI or moclobemide has been reported to cause severe cases of serotonin syndrome.

Overdose

Ingestion of a dose of about 1000 mg of any TCA (40 tablets of 25 mg) will have serious consequences, and absorption of about 2000 mg may be fatal. The clinical manifestations are coma – often induced from 2 to 6 hours after ingestion – convulsions, respiratory depression, hypotension, cardiac arrhythmias, and hyperthermia. A suspected TCA intoxication requires immediate admission to an emergency care unit.

SELECTIVE SEROTONIN REUPTAKE INHIBITORS (SSRIs)

Like the TCAs, the SSRIs revert depressed mood in depressed patients but do not have mood-elevating effects in normal individuals. There appears to be little difference in antidepressant efficacy among the different SSRIs and in their adverse-effect profiles. Their overall antidepressant efficacies are similar with regard to both induction of response and maintenance of that response over a 1-year follow-up. Their gradual onset of action is similar to that of the TCAs. It has been suggested that TCAs are more effective than SSRIs in hospitalized patients, in particular in those with the melancholic/endogenous type of depression. Some patients appear not to respond to any type of antidepressant drug therapy.

Their major advantages over the TCAs, which may justify their higher price, are a lower toxicity in overdose and generally fewer side effects. It therefore may be easier to complete a treatment with SSRIs than with TCAs, in particular in milder depressions and in elderly depressed patients.

Some of the SSRIs are more prone than the TCAs to inhibit certain hepatic cytochrome P450 enzymes and thus interact with the metabolism of other drugs.

Pharmacokinetics and metabolism

The absorption of oral doses of SSRIs is generally quite complete with a varying but moderate degree of "first-pass" metabolism. Elimination occurs by hepatic metabolism, but renal excretion is significant for some SSRIs (e.g., citalopram). As shown in Table 13.4, the various SSRIs have different elimination rates, the longest of which is for fluoxetine. The elimination half-lives of paroxetine, fluvoxamine, and fluoxetine increase from single to multiple dosing due to saturation of enzymatic metabolic processes. This leads to disproportionately higher steady-state drug levels.

Fluoxetine, N-desmethylfluoxetine, paroxetine, and N-desmethylcitalopram are substrates of the polymorphic enzyme CYP2D6, and three of these (i.e., fluoxetine, N-desmethylfluoxetine, and paroxetine) are also strong inhibitors of CYP2D6. Citalopram is a substrate for CYP2C19, and fluvoxamine is a strong inhibitor of CYP1A2. The inhibitory properties of some of the SSRIs may cause reduced metabolism and increased concentrations of other drugs that are metabolized by these enzymes.

The main kinetic properties of the most commonly used SSRIs are summarized in the following. Citalopram is a racemic mixture of two enantiomers, the S form being more active than the R form. It is well absorbed, has a systemic availability of about 80%, and is metabolized in the liver by CYP2C19 and CYP2D6. Its main metabolite, N-desmethylcitalopram, has only a weak pharmacologic effect (both S and R forms). The elimination appears to be linear, with an elimination half-life of 30 to 40 hours, and steady-state concentrations are reached after 1 to 2 weeks. A smaller fraction of the elimination is renal, and the elimination half-lives are longer in the elderly.

Fluoxetine is a racemic mixture of S- and R-enantiomers of about equal potency. An active metabolite, N-desmethylfluoxetine (S and R forms), has similar potency (serotonin reuptake inhibition). Fluoxetine has nonlinear kinetics, and its elimination half-life increases from about 2 days after single doses to 6 days after repeated dosing. An increase in daily dose therefore leads to disproportionately higher drug concentrations in the body. The elimination half-life of the metabolite ranges from 5 to 15 days, and it may take several weeks to reach steady-state plasma levels after the start of the treatment and to decline from plateau levels to zero on discontinuation.

Fluvoxamine is eliminated mainly by metabolism; none of the formed metabolites has significant potency as a serotonin reuptake inhibitor. Elimination appears to be dose dependent, half-lives of 20 to 25 hours have been reported, and steady-state levels are achieved within 1 to 2 weeks.

Paroxetine is mainly eliminated by metabolism. None of the formed metabolites has significant serotonin reuptake inhibitory effects. Paroxetine is eliminated by metabolism, at low doses/single doses mainly via CYP2D6 (90%) but at multiple dosing, only 50% due to saturation of CYP2D6. Likewise, the elimination half-life is about 20 hours after a single dose and longer after multiple dosing, with about 2 weeks to reach steady state. In contrast to the other SSRIs, paroxetine has some potency as an inhibitor of muscarinic acetylcholine receptors.

Sertraline is eliminated mainly by metabolism; the primary metabolite, desmethylsertraline, is considerably less potent as a serotonin reuptake inhibitor but is eliminated considerably slower than the parent compound. Sertraline is metabolized only to a limited extent via CYP2D6. The kinetics appear to be linear, with elimination half-lives of 20 to 25 hours and about 1 week is required to achieve steady state.

Side effects and adverse reactions

The most frequently reported side effect of SSRIs is nausea, which may occur in up to 20 to 30% of the patients, but usually wears off after 1 to 2 weeks of treatment. Diarrhea is also relatively frequent. Other side effects include headache, sweating, tremor, somnolence, and insomnia. Sexual dysfunction, with reduced libido, anorgasmia, or delayed ejaculation, seems to have been underreported and may occur in up to 30% of patients. Sedation is less pronounced than for the TCAs, with some differences within the group, paroxetine apparently being the most sedative. More rarely, severe hyponatremia and extrapyramidal symptoms have been reported, in particular in elderly patients. Very rarely, cardiac conductance disturbances (e.g., bradycardia, tachycardia) have been reported. On abrupt withdrawal, some patients may experience anxiety, restlessness, headache, etc. A "serotonergic syndrome" with disturbed consciousness, tremor, agitation, etc. has been seen when SSRIs are combined with an MAO inhibitor.

Indications

The primary indications for SSRIs are major depression, panic disorder, obsessive-compulsive disorder, and eating disorders (e.g., bulimia).

Contraindications

Contraindications to SSRIs are treatment with a nonspecific MAO inhibitor within the last 2 weeks, age below 15 years (due to a lack of clinical data for this age group), and known hypersensitivity to the drug.

Interactions

Fluoxetine/norfluoxetine and paroxetine are potent inhibitors of CYP2D6 and thus may cause increased blood levels and toxic symptoms of other drugs metabolized by this enzyme, e.g., confusion in amitriptyline-treated patients. Owing to the very long half-life of norfluoxetine, the interaction may persist for 1 to 3 weeks after discontinuation of fluoxetine.

Fluvoxamine is a potent inhibitor of CYP1A2, and interactions with caffeine, theophylline, and clozapine have been reported. SSRIs combined with MAO inhibitors, including the reversible MAO type A selective inhibitor moclobemide, have been reported to cause a serotonergic syndrome.

Overdose

The acute toxicity of SSRIs is generally lower than that of the TCAs. Despite this, cases of fatal overdoses of SSRIs have been reported, and care should be taken in prescription of SSRIs to suicidal patients. In particular, combined overdose with MAO inhibitors or TCAs may be problematic. Symptoms of overdose are nausea, ocular accommodation paresis, and excitation.

COMBINED SEROTONIN AND NOREPINEPHRINE REUPTAKE INHIBITORS

Like the TCAs, this class of antidepressant drugs inhibits neuronal reuptake of both norepinephrine and serotonin but is devoid of receptor-blocking effects and thus has fewer adverse effects than the TCAs.

Venlafaxine has four active compounds in vivo; *R*- and *S*-venlafaxine and *R*- and *S*-*O*-desmethylvenlafaxine. All four compounds have both serotonin and norepinephrine reuptake inhibitory properties, although with somewhat different relative potencies. It is likely that the serotonergic effect is dominant at low doses and that the adrenergic effect is added at higher doses. Venlafaxine is metabolized via CYP2D6 and CYP3A4, and the elimination half-lives (nonenantioselective) of the parent compound and primary metabolite (*O*-desmethyl) appear to be fairly short, 6 to 12 hours. The side effects resemble those of SSRIs, but at higher doses, adrenergic effects such as hypertension may be seen.

Milnacipran is available as the active racemic *Z*-isomers. It has reuptake inhibitory effects that, compared with venlafaxine, are relatively more potent on norepinephrine than on serotonin reuptake. Elimination takes place both by metabolism and by renal excretion, with elimination half-lives of around 6 to 12 hours, but expectedly longer in the elderly and in patients with impaired renal function. Side effects are SSRI-like plus adrenergic effects such as tachycardia and dysuria.

MONOAMINE OXIDASE (MAO) INHIBITORS

The old irreversible MAO inhibitors were efficacious antidepressants, but they were prone to produce serious side effects, especially in combination with other drugs or with the intake of various foodstuffs rich in tyramine. Some of them also had a certain hepatotoxicity. They have therefore been withdrawn from the market or are used only in selected patients. New MAO inhibitors (e.g., moclobemide), which are reversible and specific inhibitors of type A monoamine oxidase, have efficacy similar to the older MAO inhibitors but do not produce potentially dangerous side effects in combination with the intake of tyramine-rich food.

Moclobemide is well absorbed after oral administration, with a bioavailability of 60% after single doses and 80% after multiple doses due to saturable "first-pass" metabolism, and has a relatively short elimination half-life (Tab. 13.4). Moclobemide has no sedative effects and generally is well tolerated. The most frequent side effects are nausea and other gastrointestinal disturbances, insomnia, and vertigo. Agitation and restlessness may occur. Tablets should be taken after a meal in order to avoid gastrointestinal side effects. Moclobemide inhibits CYP2D6 and may cause a severe serotonergic syndrome when combined with an SSRI or clomipramine.

OTHER ANTIDEPRESSANTS

A number of other antidepressants cannot be assigned to any of the preceding major groups. As for the TCAs, SSRIs, and MAO inhibitors, the extent of their use is highly variable among various countries.

Amoxapine is structurally and pharmacodynamically related to the TCAs but has weak anticholinergic effects and, in addition, a significant dopamine antagonistic effect. This may explain its neuroleptic-like effects in patients, such as extrapyramidal symptoms and elevated serum prolactin levels.

Mianserin appears to act mainly by antagonism on presynaptic α_2-adrenergic receptors in the brain. It has a pronounced "first-pass" metabolism, and it is likely that metabolites may contribute to its effects. It has a certain sedative effect and is frequently used in elderly patients because of its relatively low tendency to produce anticholinergic and cardiovascular side effects.

Mirtazapine acts via antagonism at central α_2-adrenergic auto- and heteroreceptors; it also acts as an antagonist on postsynaptic serotonin 5-HT2 and 5-HT3 receptors. Its most frequent side effects are somnolence and constipation.

Maprotiline is a tetracyclic antidepressant that has a pharmacologic profile similar to those of the TCAs nortriptyline and desipramine. It has an elimination half-life of more than 40 hours and therefore requires more than 1 week of treatment before steady-state drug levels are attained. It is eliminated by hepatic metabolism and renal excretion of metabolites.

Nefazodone has inhibitory effects on serotonin and norepinephrine as well as postsynaptic antagonistic effects on serotonin receptors. CYP3A4 is involved in its metabolism; it has an elimination half-life of 5 to 10 hours.

Trazodone has a complex mechanism of action including inhibition of serotonin reuptake and an antagonist effect on postsynaptic serotonin receptors. CYP2D6 is involved in its metabolism. It has a relatively strong sedative effect but with little after-day effects due to its short elimination half-life.

Reboxetine, available in racemic form, is a selective norepinephrine reuptake inhibitor that has been introduced recently as an antidepressant.

Lithium

Lithium is effectively used in psychotic excitation and in bipolar disorders. Its unique pharmacological properties are solely dependent from the lithium ion, Li^+. Today lithium is primarily used for its antimanic effects.

The exact mode of action of Li^+ in the brain is uncertain. Li^+, at relatively elevated concentrations, can reduce the cellular content of phosphatidyl inositides, abundant second messengers in brain (particularly inositol trisphosphate, IP_3), thus possibly reducing sensitivity of neurons to neurotransmitters. Recent data suggest an enhancing effect of Li^+ on the affinity of membrane associated protein kinases.

Lithium is mainly used prophylactically in bipolar and unipolar manic-depressive illnesses, even if its use has been slightly reduced following the availability of the novel second generation antipsychotic medications. It can attenuate both manic and depressive episodes and can be used therapeutically in mania. Long term clinical data indicate the maintenance of therapeutic efficacy of Li$^+$ overal several decades.

Lithium, under the form of salt, is generally well absorbed with a T_{max} around 4-5 h (longer after slow release formulations) and a biphasic elimination $t_{1/2}$, ranging between 8 and 45 h. Li$^+$ is non protein bound and is eliminated by the kidney. Li$^+$ needs monitoring in plasma and concentrations can be assessed by atomic emission spectrophotometry (sensitivity > 0.15 mmol/l). Therapeutic levels range from 0.75 to 1.25 mmol/l, although a lower range of 0.5-0.8 mmol/l has been proposed. Trough concentrations, ie pre-dose levels should be preferentially assessed. There is as yet an unclear relationship between concentration and therapeutic efficacy. Levels should be primarily evaluated to prevent toxicity.

Li$^+$ is provided in a variety of formulations, the prevaling salt is carbonate, but in Europe also citrate, acetate and glutamate are available. Both tablet and liquid formulations contain between 250 and 940 mg of Li$^+$ salt per dose (5-10 ml for syrups), corresponding to between 5.4 and 10 mmol Li$^+$. Preference is given to sustained-release formulations, allowing more prolonged absorption and stabler serum levels.

Treatment of acute mania should be started with a dose around 30 mmol daily, corresponding to approximately 1,200 mg of one of the major available salts. The dosage should be adjusted based on the Li$^+$ levels and renal function tests. During prophylaxis, a titration from a low dose of 3-4 mmol bid should be started, until a steady state is reached, after approximately one week. Li$^+$ treatment should not be stopped abruptly because of the risk of rebound psychiatric symptoms. Li$^+$ is generally given in association with a major antidepressant for the treatment of depression, or a neuroleptic in the treatment of mania (see Chap. 14). Combination with lithium should be tested in all patients with an inadequate response to antidepressants.

Side effects of Li$^+$ range from kidney disorders with disturbed electrolyte balance, particularly in patients on a low dietary Na$^+$ intake (in case this is suspected, Li$^+$ should be stopped until an adequate rehydratation is achieved). Potentially lethal side effects may occur after intoxication. Li$^+$ concentrations >1.5 mmol/l indicate risk of impending poisoning; features of poisoning (impaired consciousness, tremor, dysarthria) occur at > 2.5 mmol/l; concentrations > 3.5 mmol/l are potentially life threatening. Hemodialysis should be instituted, eventually accompanied by iv Na$^+$ loading and forced diuresis. In mild poisoning, withdrawal of lithium and correction of electrolyte balance are usually sufficient.

Suggested readings

ANDERSSON T, MINERS JO, VERONESE ME, BIRKETT DJ. Diazepam metabolism by human liver microsomes is mediated by both *S*-mephenytoin hydroxylase and CYP3A isoforms. Br J Clin Pharmacol 1994;38:131-7.

BALDESSARINI RJ. TONDO L. DOES lithium treatment still work? Evidence of stable responses over three decades. Archives of General Psychiatry 57:187-90, 2000.

DALEN P, DAHL ML, RUIZ ML, et al. 10-Hydroxylation of nortriptyline in white persons with 0, 1, 2, 3, and 13 functional CYP2D6 genes. Clin Pharmacol Ther 1998;63:444-52.

FULTON B, BROGDEN RN. Buspirone: an updated review of its clinical pharmacology and therapeutic applications. CNS Drugs 1997;7:68-88.

GRAM LF. Fluoxetine (review). N Engl J Med 1994;331:1354-61.

GRIFFITHS RR, WEERTS EM. Benzodiazepine self-administration in humans and laboratory animals: implications for problems of long-term use and abuse. Psychopharmacology 1997; 134:1-37.

HILLESTAD L, HANSEN T, MELSOM H. Diazepam metabolism in normal man. II. Serum concentration and clinical effect after oral administration and cumulation. Clin Pharmacol Ther 1974;16:485-9.

HOLLIDAY SM, BENFIELD P. Venlafaxine: a review of its pharmacolgy and therapeutic potential in depression. Drugs 1995;49:280-94.

KAPLAN SA, JACK ML. Metabolism of the benzodiazepines: pharmacokinetic and pharmacodynamic considerations. In: Costa E, ed. Molecular biology to clinical practice. New York: Raven Press, 1983:173-99.

KASPER S. The place of milnacipran in the treatment of depression. Hum Psychopharmacol 1997;12:S315-41.

ONO S, HATANAKA T, MIYAZAWA S, et al. Human liver microsomal diazepam metabolism using cDNA-expressed cytochrome P450s: role of CYP2B6, 2C19 and the 3A subfamily. Xenobiotica 1996;26:1155-66.

OZDEMIR V, FOURIE J, BUSTO U, NARANJO CA. Pharmacokinetic changes in the elderly: do they contribute to drug abuse and dependence? Clin Pharmacokinet 1996;31:372-85.

PRESKORN SH. Clinically relevant pharmacology of selective serotonin reuptake inhibitors: An overview with emphasis on pharmacokinetics and effects on oxidative drug metabolism. Clin Pharmacokinet 1997;32(suppl 1):1-21.

VON MOLTKE LL, GREENBLATT DJ, SHADER RI. Clinical pharmacokinetics of antidepressants in the elderly: therapeutic implications. Clin Pharmacokinet 1993;24:141-60.

WILDE MI, PLOSKER GL, BENFIELD P. Fluvoxamine. An updated review of its pharmacology and therapeutic use in depressive illness. Drugs 1993; 46:895-924.

YASUI N, OTANI K, KANEKO S, et al. A kinetic and dynamic study of oral alprazolam with and without erythromycin in humans: In vivo evidence for the involvement of CYP3A4 in alprazolam metabolism. Clin Pharmacol Ther 1996;59:514-9.

Psychosis

Göran C. Sedvall

Psychosis and *madness* are terms that can be defined as human states or conditions where a subject's experience of reality is distorted in the absence of gross changes in consciousness. This experiential change, in turn, leads to signs and symptoms that are communicated to or observed by people around the afflicted individual. Thus, delusions, hallucinations, altered speech, and psychomotor behavior, as well as inadequate affective changes, represent the symptoms seen most often in patients in psychotic states. Anecdotal evidence from the arts and literature bear witness to how such alterations in behavior have been common throughout human history.

Scientific description and medical classification of psychotic states occurred during the second half of the nineteenth century in European psychiatry. It was recognized early on that psychotic disturbances can be secondary to gross brain damage resulting from trauma, tumor, or bleeding. Secondary transient psychotic behavior also may result from pharmacologic or toxic actions on the brain by psychotomimetic drugs such as amphetamine, marijuana, and lysergic acid diethylamide (LSD) or by alcohol. However, in most patients evidencing psychotic states, no such gross brain damage or intoxication can be found, and, accordingly, these states have been defined as primary psychotic disorders. Psychotic depression (melancholia), age-related dementia as described by Alois Alzheimer, and paranoid psychotic states were described in the scientific literature as case reports around 1850. The current classification of primary psychotic disorders only became available in the last decades of the twentieth century.

The prevalence, incidence, and epidemiology of psychotic disorders can now be determined with high reliability as a result of the development of generally accepted diagnostic conventions where genetic and environmental mechanisms interact and contribute as risk and protective factors for the disorders. From clinical experience, it is also likely that there are many mixed forms of psychoses that do not easily fit into the different classification systems.

At present, psychotic disorders are classified with high reliability on the basis of such generally accepted diagnostic conventions as the *Diagnostic and Statistical Manual,* 4th Edition (DSM-IV), and the *International Classification of Diseases,* 10th Edition (ICD-10). However, the true nature and specific causative factors for the development of psychoses in an individual patient are still far from clearly understood. Thus, for most psychotic disorders, there are still no biologic or medical diagnostic measures. This is a great problem for the clinician both when it comes to arriving at a reasonable diagnosis and when it comes to making the right choice of treatment for individual patients. Major international surveys concerning the occurrence, distribution, and natural history of the various forms of psychosis have made it clear that from a quantitative standpoint, they represent major health problems in all human societies. Also with regard to the human suffering produced, alleviation of symptoms remains as a major challenge to the medical community. Globally, many millions of people are afflicted by psychotic disorders that make them more or less unable to support themselves so as to achieve an adequate quality of life, placing a heavy burden on their families and society. In 1990, the World Health Organization (WHO) ranked the top 10 causes of human disability. Among these causes, depression, bipolar psychotic disorders, schizophrenia, and dementia were all included, a fact that illustrates the true dimension of the medical problem of psychotic disorders to the community.

Clinical findings

Schizophrenia, bipolar affective disorder, and dementia represent three major classes of psychotic disorders according to the internationally accepted diagnostic classification systems, i.e., DSM-IV and ICD-10. Psychotic symptoms in patients belonging in these diagnostic categories respond to every one of the antipsychotic drugs irrespective of the primary diagnosis. Therefore, the clinical features and natural cause of each one of these groups of conditions will be described below. The primary forms addressed in this chapter are schizophrenia and related disorders.

Schizophrenia

The typical form of schizophrenia afflicts a previously healthy individual in his/her early adulthood (20-30 years). Typical symptoms include auditory hallucinations (usually in the form of commentary voices), delusions of a bizarre nature, and affective outbursts that appear with increasing intensity over weeks or months. Aberrations in the thought process leading to concentration difficulties and specific changes in formal thought and speech are also common. These symptoms, generally classified as *positive* symptoms, are often found in parallel with social isolation, passivity, and loss of initiative, features referred to as *negative* symptoms. In different patients, the mixture of symptoms can vary substantially. Thus, paranoid, disorganized, or catatonic forms of schizophrenia with distinct changes in motor behavior can be distinguished. In addition, the time course for the development of the symptoms may vary considerably.

If untreated, most patients follow a chronic course with exacerbations and a constellation of marked symptoms in the early phases alternating with periods of lower symptom frequency and intensity. The lifetime risk for developing schizophrenia is about 1% in most societies. The general prognosis is poor, with most patients showing early deterioration and a course with more or less intensive periods of positive symptoms and chronic development of negative symptoms that dominate as the patients grow older. The risk is similar in women and men, but men tend to fall ill about 5 years earlier than women. In women, the prognosis generally tends to be somewhat better than in men. A number of chromosomal regions have linked to schizophrenia. Polygenic mechanisms are most likely. About 10% of schizophrenic patients commit suicide. Family, twin, and adoption studies indicate that up to 70% of the causative factors are related to hereditary genetic mechanisms, but a substantial fraction of the variants also appear to depend on environmental factors. A number of chromosomal regions have been linked to schizophrenia. Polygenic mechanisms are most likely. About 30% of patients show evidence of expanded cerebrospinal spaces, particularly within the ventricular system.

Affective psychosis

Although changes in mood, energy, and speed of psychomotor performance represent the primary features of affective disorders, it is not uncommon that psychotic symptoms also predominate in such patients. Thus, severe delusions with paranoid, nihilistic, and/or somatic dimensions may occur. Auditory hallucinations with depressive content also occur. In so-called schizoaffective conditions, a mixture of schizophrenic and affective symptoms are seen. In the DSM-IV and ICD-10, affective disorders are divided into unipolar and bipolar types. Patients with unipolar depressions are liable to recurrent attacks of depressive disorder, whereas those with bipolar disorder are liable to attacks of depression interspersed with episodes of mania. Unipolar manias do exist but are very rare.

The current classification depends predominantly on the clinical phenomena, symptoms, cause, and outcome. The great success of such biologic treatments as drugs and electroconvulsive therapy (ECT) have provided support for biologic theories of etiology and pathophysiology of these disorders and downgraded psychologic theories. Epidemiologic, adoption, and twin studies indicate that genetic mechanisms are of great importance. Several chromosomal regions have been linked to these disorders, some of which seem to increase the risk, but evidence for genes with a protective action also has been presented recently.

The lifetime probability of suffering a mood disorder is estimated to be about 2% for men and about twice that for women. Twice as many women as men suffer from unipolar depression, and about the same holds true for schizoaffective disorder. For bipolar disorder, the ratio is about 3:2. Affective illness is not only common but also serious. About 15% of patients with a depressive illness commit suicide. Of those who made an unsuccessful attempt, about 10% eventually will kill themselves. Patients with unipolar depressions have a higher rate of suicide than other affective disorder patients. The age of onset for bipolar disorder is about 45 years, and for schizoaffective disorder it is 25 to 30 years. General aspects of drug treatment for depression are described in Chapter 13.

Dementia

Psychotic symptoms are not infrequent in age-related disorders involving a decline in cognitive function and memory. The DSM-IV distinguishes several types of dementia. The major forms are Alzheimer's dementia and vascular dementia. Alzheimer's dementia with deterioration of memory for recent episodes is seen in early and late forms. In vascular dementia, besides the disturbance in memory, focal neurologic signs are also present. Alzheimer's dementias have typical histopathologic features in the brain as disclosed at autopsy. These are represented by senile plaques and fibrillary tangles. So far, four distinct genes have been implicated in the pathophysiology of dementia. Together these genes can only account for at most a few percent of patients. However, it has been estimated that these genes may account for up to 20% of patients with dementia developing before age 60. The largest number of patients seen so far constitute a group with cryptogenetic etiology. Patients with various forms of dementia often present with such psychotic manifestations as delusions and hallucinations. Practically all cases of dementia show a progressively deteriorating course. General aspects of drug treatment of dementia are described in Chapter 12.

Treatment

Psychotic symptoms represent severe risk factors for patients and their ability to adjust to personal, interpersonal, and social demands. For the patient with psychotic symptoms and a distorted apprehension of reality, confrontations with other people in the surroundings often lead to affective reactions, such as aggression, depression, and/or paranoid ideation. It is necessary, therefore, either to motivate the patient to begin active drug treatment as soon as possible and/or to seclude or in other ways protect the patient from destructive behavior because of his psychotic experiences.

Since the early 1950s, antipsychotic drugs, so-called neuroleptics, have been in general use for the treatment of psychotic symptoms predominantly in schizophrenia. In Western countries, most schizophrenic patients receive long-term treatment with these drugs. Patients with affective disorders and psychotic symptoms sometimes receive combination therapy with antidepressant drugs and neuroleptics. Manic patients receive neuroleptic treatment often in combination with lithium therapy or anticonvulsants. Many patients with senile psychotic symptoms are treated with low doses of neuroleptic drugs. There are no absolute contraindications to the use of antipsychotic drugs. Many patients dislike such treatment because of difficulty in accepting the negative subjective experience of the dampening effect of the drug and other side effects or poor therapeutic response. Therefore, poor drug compliance is a common problem in the management of many psychotic patients.

Despite such problems, treatment of psychotic patients with neuroleptic drugs has had a dramatic effect on the organization of health care for psychotic patients. This holds true especially for schizophrenic patients, who in most cases benefit markedly from treatment with neuroleptics, which simplify their social adjustment, making institutional care less necessary. Thus, the introduction of antipsychotic drugs during the 1950s probably represents one major reason for the marked reduction in the number of mental institutions and psychiatric beds in most western countries during the last half of the twentieth century. Many schizophrenic patients can now be treated on an outpatient basis with less severe manifestations of psychotic symptoms. This, in turn, has placed greater demands on outpatient and community treatment centers for such patients. Still, drug treatment of psychosis varies with regard to practice in many countries. Therefore, a further development of principles, rules, and recommendations for antipsychotic drug treatment is pertinent to the field of clinical pharmacology.

Nonpharmacologic treatment

Every psychotic patient is in a vulnerable position because of his idiosyncratic reaction to the florid symptoms that often causes anxiety, suspiciousness, and difficulties in communicating in an appropriate manner with nearby people. In many cases, the patient lacks insight into his own situation, and questions and suggestions from other people can be especially disturbing and provocative to the patient. Therefore, it is extremely important in the early stages of treatment to approach the psychotic patient in a respectful, nonprovocative manner. Confrontations should be avoided if at all possible because of the danger to the patient himself and the surroundings. Thus, every measure should be taken to avoid provoking anxiety in the patient during the first phase of treatment. It is most important for the physician to create a relationship with the patient based on confidence. This also holds true for relationships with family members, who are usually highly engaged in the patient's situation. In this way, it is possible to explain to the patient and family the importance of accepting the true nature of the psychotic symptoms so as to gain insight into and to understand the importance of beginning drug treatment at an early stage. Most patients can undergo outpatient treatment. However, in some patients with florid symptoms, inpatient care is necessary so that the patient can be observed carefully to avoid aggression and behavior that can be damaging to others or to the patient himself. In many instances, compulsory treatment in a closed ward is necessary in the early phase of the psychosis.

Many psychotic patients who show behavioral changes and mental confusion, disorganization, and marked manic or depressive reactions benefit from electroconvulsive therapy (ECT). Unilateral or bilateral electroconvulsive therapy given as a series of 4 to 10 treatments (one every second day) can dramatically reduce and sometimes eliminate such symptoms. Patients should be admitted to a psychiatric unit to allow adequate medical monitoring of the treatment and to avoid problems with the retrograde amnesia that usually follows such a treatment series for a few weeks. The problem with ECT is that in the absence of additional neuroleptic drug treatment, the effect is usually only temporary, which necessitates repeated ECT therapy series.

Drug therapy

Drugs of first choice

Since the introduction of chlorpromazine in 1953, more than 50 neuroleptic drugs have been developed and shown to have an antipsychotic efficacy. All the antipsychotic drugs developed so far have antagonistic effects on certain aspects of dopamine signalling in the brain. Thus, they all share an antagonistic affinity for D2-like dopamine receptors. In addition, most of them have other pharmacologic receptor effects (Tab. 14.1) that may explain individual differences in their clinical action profile. Thus, in addition to their antipsychotic action, they have different degrees of tendency to induce extrapyramidal side effects, prolactin elevation, weight gain, and cardiovascular effects, as well as a potential for toxic effects on stem cells in the bone marrow. None of the drugs developed so far seems to have a clear superiority with regard to optimal effects on all these aspects. Moreover, different patients may show a differential response when treated with one or the other of these drugs. The drugs also have different pharmacokinetic properties, some of which may be advantageous when selecting a specific drug for a specific patient. The cost of treatment is also a factor that may be taken into consideration.

It is also important to keep in mind that patients with different symptom profiles may show a differential response to various antipsychotic drugs. Sex and age factors also should be taken into consideration. The drugs of first choice listed below therefore represent the net outcome of personal considerations of the author in terms of the weighting aspects summarized earlier. There is also a growing awareness that the results of well-designed controlled studies, i.e., evidence-based medicine, may not always reflect outcome in the practical clinical situation.

Treatment of positive psychotic symptoms Haloperidol, olanzapine, and risperidone are drugs for which a substantial clinical documentation has verified useful effects against positive psychotic symptoms. For agitated patients and those refusing voluntary treatment, the availability of injectable haloperidol preparations is an advantage. In addition, for the elderly psychotic patient, haloperidol and olanzapine, drugs with a low tendency to induce autonomic side effects, should be recommended as first choice. However, it should be kept in mind that haloperidol, belonging to the series of classic, typical antipsychotics, has a significant liability to induce extrapyramidal side effects at doses above 4 mg per day. Long-term treatment with higher doses may be related to an increased risk for the side effect tardive dyskinesia.

For treatment of the average young schizophrenic patient, the drug of choice should be determined by the relative dominance of the following three symptom categories: (1) positive symptoms, (2) negative symptoms, and (3) anxiety and agitation.

Optimal doses of haloperidol, olanzapine, and risperidone vary considerably in the individual patient. Thus, oral doses for haloperidol typically vary between 2 and 8 mg per day; for olanzapine, 5 and 15 mg per day; and for risperidone, 4 and 12 mg per day. This dose preferably can be given as a single administration before the patient goes to bed.

There is currently no causal treatment for schizophrenia. Accordingly, the antipsychotic drugs available today represent a symptomatic treatment that has to be maintained in order to suppress symptoms. Usually, the appearance of antipsychotic effects after administration of an antipsychotic drug takes 2 to 3 weeks to develop. Further improvement and stabilization of the condition are often obtained during the following 2 months of continuous treatment.

After withdrawal of antipsychotic drug treatment, there is also usually a rather long delay before symptoms reappear. About 80% of schizophrenic patients relapse if neuroleptic treatment is withdrawn. The relapse rate is low during the first 3 to 4 weeks after withdrawal, but most patients relapse within a year. For most schizophrenic patients, antipsychotic drug treatment should continue for at least a year after the first psychotic episode. In many patients, treatment is required lifelong. The decision to withdraw an antipsychotic drug from a schizophrenic patient is a difficult one and should involve consideration of the risk of a relapse. This risk can be estimated from the number and frequency of previous episodes.

Treatment of negative psychotic symptoms Antipsychotic drug treatment usually has a good effect on positive schizophrenic symptoms, which makes it possible for the patient to avoid hospitalization and to initiate social rehabilitation. Unfortunately, the effect of antipsychotic drugs on aspects of negative symptomology is often less satisfactory, which makes it difficult or impossible for patients to return to their premorbid level of functioning with regard to work and social interactions.

For patients with a preponderance of negative symptoms, olanzapine and amisulpride may be first-choice alternatives. For both these drugs, systematic comparative studies against haloperidol using several doses indicate that they have a significantly better effect on aspects of negative symptomology versus the reference drug. For olanzapine, there is also evidence that in schizophrenic patients depressive symptoms may show a significantly

Table 14.1 Receptor affinities of some typical and atypical antipsychotics (Ki values in nM)

Compound	Receptor subtypes							
	D1	D2	5-HT2A	α_1	α_2	H_1	M_1	5-HT2/D2
Haloperidol	15	0.8	28	7.3	1400	550	570	35
Clozapine	268	78	11	48	37	23	228	7.9
Risperidone	851	3.1	0.16	2	7.54	5	NK	5
Olanzapine	31	11	5	19	228	7	1.9	2.2
Quetiapine	1243*	329*	148*	90*	270*	30*	NA	2.2
Amisulpride	>1000	1.3	1867	>1000	800	>1000	>1000	

Ki => 10.000 nM; NA = not active; NK = not known.
*IC$_{50}$

better outcome as compared with treatment with a classic reference drug such as haloperidol. For amisulpride, it is interesting that low doses (50-100 mg) appear to be optimal for negative symptomatology, whereas higher doses (on the order of 300-600 mg) seem to give the optimal response for positive schizophrenic symptoms.

Treatment of anxiety and agitation Anxious and aggressive schizophrenic patients preferably are treated with haloperidol, for which injectable preparations are available.

Drugs of second choice

In the acute phase of a psychotic episode, many schizophrenic patients experience severe anxiety and agitation and may be very aggressive. For such patients, benzodiazepines are often valuable to counteract these symptoms during the latency phase before the antipsychotic action of the neuroleptic agent appears. Many psychotic patients with affective symptoms both of manic and depressive type also can achieve a good benefit from lithium treatment added to the neuroleptic maintenance treatment (see Chap. 13).

Resistance to conventional neuroleptic treatment About 30% of schizophrenic patients have a poor response to conventional neuroleptic drugs such as haloperidol. For such patients, clozapine or some of the more recently developed atypical antipsychotic drugs such as olanzapine and risperidone may be useful. About 30 to 60% of patients resistant to conventional neuroleptic drugs have a relatively good response to clozapine, with an improvement particularly with regard to negative symptoms and delusions.

As mentioned previously, the main benefit of neuroleptic drug therapy appears to be the reduction of positive psychotic symptoms. This, in turn, leads to a reduced need for inpatient treatment. The cost of schizophrenia to society has been estimated in many western countries. In financial terms, the costs for treatment and services to patients (direct costs) can be separated from the costs presented by loss of productivity by patients and caregivers (indirect costs). Western countries allocate about 2% of the national health budgets to the treatment of schizophrenia. Hospitalization and residential care are the two major contributors to direct costs. Drug costs are relatively small and account for less than 4% of the direct costs of schizophrenia. In a 1994 study from the United Kingdom, the annual indirect costs incurred through productivity loss by patients were estimated to be at least four times higher than the direct costs estimated in the same study (Tab. 14.2).

Several pharmacoeconomic studies with different antipsychotic drugs have demonstrated the pharmacoeconomic benefit from antipsychotic drug treatment. Thus, the effect of drug treatment on the demand for inpatient care and better social adjustment markedly reduces direct as well as indirect costs in relation to the direct cost of drug treatment.

Table 14.2 Distribution of costs

Institutional/residential care	74%
Day care	14%
Community-based support	4%
Hospital outpatient care	3%
Depot injection clinics	2%
Other drug treatment	3%

Drug classes

Delay and Deniker introduced chlorpromazine, the prototype of current antipsychotic drugs, as a new treatment modality for psychiatric patients in 1953. At about the same time, the alkaloid reserpine was isolated from the plant *Rauwolfia serpentina*. Both of these drugs were shown to produce antipsychotic actions in manic and schizophrenic patients in the absence of general sedation. On the basis of the effects of these drugs, Delay and Deniker in 1957 defined the term *neuroleptic* to characterize compounds that
- have an antipsychotic effect;
- reduce psychomotor activity;
- produce extrapyramidal symptoms (EPSs) or side effects as in parkinsonism.

The *syndrome neuroleptique,* considered by French workers to be produced by such drugs, has since then been used as synonym for *antipsychotic.* The term *neuroleptic* is not very appropriate because these drugs reorganize and in many patients activate behavior.

The introduction of chlorpromazine into psychiatry undoubtedly constitutes a major therapeutic discovery in modern times. Although compounds of a similar structure had been known for about 100 years at that time, French workers focused interest on their therapeutic potential. Carpentier worked out a method to synthesize phenothiazines, among them chlorpromazine. The general pharmacologic properties of this class of compounds were known, and the compounds were used as antihistamines, hypnotics, sedatives, and antiemetics, as well as in the so-called artificial hibernation advocated by Henry Laborit. The psychiatrist Jean Delay and his coworkers undertook clinical studies with several of these compounds. They clearly systematically outlined for the first time the possibility of using chlorpromazine in the treatment of psychiatric disorders. In their first publication in 1952, they wrote: "in 90% of the treated patients we have been obtaining therapeutic and biological results; 8 patients in a state of exhilaration of the maniacal type were completely cured in a shorter time than required by shock therapy." The term *chemical lobotomy,* to define the mental state of certain patients, does not seem warranted; patients were not euphoric but rather were aware of the favorable effects of treatment, and there was no hyperactivity, mental confusion, or sphincter disturbance.

These first publications on chlorpromazine were soon

followed by a number of open and, later during the 1960s, controlled clinical studies in schizophrenic patients where the effect could be verified and dose recommendations for clinical practice could be presented.

Chemical drug classes

A number of distinct chemicals shown to have antipsychotic properties have been developed over the past 50 years. They are all useful to treat schizophrenia and other psychoses. They are all antipsychotic in general rather than antischizophrenic in particular.

Phenothiazine derivatives A number of phenothiazine derivatives with substituents on the nitrogen in the central ring have antipsychotic properties. These, in contrast to conventional antihistamines, having a two-carbon substitution separating the two nitrogen functions, have a three-carbon substitution. These compounds can be subdivided into those with an aliphatic piperazine or piperidine moiety in the side chain. Aliphatic and piperidine derivatives tend to have a low relative potency with regard to antipsychotic action but have a relatively strong tendency to produce sedation. Piperazine derivatives have a high potency as antipsychotics and also a high liability to produce extrapyramidal side effects. These drugs, on the other hand, have relatively low general sedative properties. Major phenothiazines in clinical use, besides chlorpromazine are mesoridazine, thioridazine, acetophenazine, fluphenazine, and perphenazine. Long-acting formulations (see below) are available for fluphenazine and perphenazine. These compounds are becoming of lesser use these days, with the exception of the long-acting fluphenazine formulations.

Thioxanthene derivatives These compounds represent variants of the phenothiazine structure. The nitrogen in the central ring has been substituted with a carbon. Substitutions with structures similar to those indicated above for the phenothiazines can be added to this carbon. These molecules are characterized by a more rigid configuration of the side chain in relation to the phenothiazine skeleton. Aliphatic and aromatic substitutions have in general similar properties as those for the corresponding phenothiazine derivatives. Major thioxanthene derivatives include chlorprothixene and thiothixene, both of which presently are relatively restricted in use.

Butyrophenones In order to develop compounds with a less complex chemical structure than the phenothiazines, Janssen and colleagues used the aliphatic three-carbon chain as prototype for synthesizing organic chemicals with antipsychotic properties. The prototype butyrophenone, haloperidol, a relatively simple compound, showed properties similar to those of the conventional neuroleptics with a strong antipsychotic action but also a fairly strong tendency to produce extrapyramidal symptoms (EPS). Sedation and autonomic side effects were shown to be less prominent than for chlorpromazine. Haloperidol later became the prototype for developing butyrophenones with different clinical profiles that could be used not only as antipsychotics but also as general anesthetics (e.g., neuroleptic analgesia) as well as in several neurologic conditions such as Huntington's chorea. Haloperidol is available also as a decanoate formulation for depot injections (see below).

Systematic animal models were developed for studying the behavioral effects of antipsychotic drugs. Structure-activity relationships could be defined for a great number of chemical agents designed with the butyrophenone skeleton as a base. This development led to antipsychotic compounds with modified structure-activity relationships, such as pimozide and risperidone.

Substituted benzamides Most antipsychotic drugs were shown early on to have strong antiemetic properties. Besides the butyrophenones, substituted benzamides were shown to exhibit antiemetic as well as antipsychotic properties. Sulpride was the prototype compound. It was used initially to treat gastrointestinal conditions, but later it was also shown to have effects on psychiatric conditions. Sulpride, tiapride, and recently, amisulpride have been shown to exhibit several of the properties of classic antipsychotic drugs.

Clozapine In the search for antipsychotic and antidepressant drugs using chemical modifications of the phenothiazine skeleton, clozapine was developed. By the late 1960s, this drug was shown to have unique properties. It differed markedly from the classic antipsychotic drugs in exhibiting an antipsychotic action but lacking most of the classic extrapyramidal symptoms. The subsequent demonstration that clozapine had a good therapeutic action in many patients previously shown to be resistant to classic neuroleptics brought a lot of attention to the unique properties of this compound. The subsequent demonstration, however, that clozapine may be associated with an increased risk of agranulocytosis (1% of treated patients) encouraged the development of agents with a similar activity profile but less risk, such as olanzapine and quetiapine.

Mechanism of action

As early as the first part of the 1960s, the antipsychotic drugs reserpine, chlorpromazine, and haloperidol were already known to induce profound effects on monoaminergic mechanisms in the brain. Reserpine depleted storage amine pools of these transmitters. Receptors for the monoaminergic transmitters dopamine, norepinephrine, and serotonin were shown to be blocked by drugs such as chlorpromazine and haloperidol, but not the phenothiazine antihistamines. The recent development of molecular genetic methods to identify monoaminergic receptors has shown a marked diversity with many receptor subtypes. Pharmacologic studies have demonstrated that most of the classic antipsychotic drugs have high antagonistic affinities for predominantly the D2 class of dopamine receptors (Tab. 14.1). Extensive animal experimentation indicates that a high D2 antagonistic affinity is related to a high propensity to produce extrapyramidal symptoms and to induce a strong prolactin elevation in plasma, related to blockade of the inhibitory D2 receptors in the pituitary.

Several of the antipsychotic drugs also have a high antagonistic affinity for serotonin (5-HT) 2A receptors (Tab. 14.1). Clozapine in particular and all the more recently developed so-called atypical antipsychotic drugs, such as olanzapine, risperidone, and quetiapine, have high affinities for 5-HT 2A receptors in addition to a relatively high affinity for D2-like dopamine receptors. In fact, many of the newer atypical antipsychotics have been developed on the basis of animal experiments indicating that the addition of a high 5-HT 2A antagonistic affinity may be related to a reduced liability of D2-like antagonists to produce extrapyramidal symptoms.

Using the techniques of positron emission tomography (PET) and single-photon-emission tomography (SPECT), the receptor actions of antipsychotic drugs suggested by animal pharmacologic experiments have been verified and extended by direct clinical experiments in schizophrenic patients and healthy volunteers treated with these drugs. Thus, it has been shown in patients that clinical doses of these drugs induce a significant occupancy of D2 dopamine receptors (see Fig. 14.1 in Color Atlas) and in some cases also 5-HT 2A receptors in the living brain (see Fig. 14.2 in Color Atlas). It also has been possible to

demonstrate significant relationships between the degree of occupancy of these receptors, particularly the D2 dopamine receptors in the basal ganglia, and the various clinical action profiles of these drugs. Occupancy levels above 80 to 90% are related to a high propensity for extrapyramidal symptoms. Brain imaging data also indicate that a low occupancy of D2 dopamine receptors in the basal ganglia may be related to amelioration of negative symptomology in schizophrenic patients. Antipsychotic doses of clozapine induce a lower degree of D2 occupancy than conventional doses of classic neuroleptics. A higher occupancy level after classic neuroleptic administration is related to a therapeutic effect with regard to positive symptomology. So far, PET scan experiments are unclear with regard to the role of 5-HT 2A receptor occupancy in the brain. Drugs such as clozapine, olanzapine, and risperidone produce a more than 90% occupancy of cortical 5-HT 2A receptors at therapeutic doses. This high occupancy may explain the relatively low propensity for extrapyramidal symptoms of drugs showing this property. However, further experimentation of this type is required to verify this assumption.

Table 14.3 Daily doses, kinetic parameters, and cytochrome P450 handling of major classic and atypical antipsychotic agents[1]

	Standard dose mg (tablet, ampoule)	Daily dose range (mg)	Bioavailability (%)	$t_{1/2}$ (h)	Active metabolites	P450s involved
Classic						
Amisulpride	50 100 im	50-300 200-800	45	11-16	No	<5% metabolized
Chlorpromazine	100	100-2000	32	21	Yes	2D6, 1A2
Fluphenazine decanoate im	2 25	2-40 (every 2 weeks)	50	16 6-10 days	Yes Yes	2D6?
Perphenazine enanthate im	10 100	10-60 (2-4 weeks)	30-40	10 8-10 days	Yes	2D6?
Haloperidol decanoate im	2 50-150	1-100 (4 weeks)	40-60	9-67 10-12 days	Yes	2D6, 3A4
Pimozide	6	2-20	20	53	No	3A4
Atypical						
Clozapine	15	25-300	50	12	No	1A2, 2D6
Olanzapine	15	5-20	60	34	No	1A2, 2D6, 2C9
Risperidone	6	2-16	60-70	2-4 EM 17-22 PM	Yes	2D6
Quetiapine	150	50-750	10	6-7	No	3A4

[1]Agents available in most countries were selected.
EM-CYP2D6= extensive metabolizers; PM-CYP2D6= poor metabolizers (see Chap. 3).

Pharmacokinetics

All available antipsychotic drugs undergo extensive metabolism in the liver and other tissues. Most antipsychotics undergo degradation under the influence of several of the isoenzymes related to the cytochrome P450 system. In particular, isoenzyme CYP2D6 is involved in the metabolism of most neuroleptics, but CYP1A3 and CYP2C19 also influence the metabolism of olanzapine. Very recently, pimozide metabolism has been found to be regulated by CYP3A4, and serious adverse events have been associated with the concomitant use of macrolide antibiotics (see Chap. 6); a similar risk, to a minor extent, may be present with quetiapine. Sertindole, a very promising imidazoline derivative, was withdrawn from clinical use recently because of an increased risk of arrhythmias, most likely related to a metabolic interaction. Hydroxylation, oxidation, and conjugation convert the relatively lipid-soluble antipsychotics into more hydrophilic molecules that can be excreted easily (Tab. 14.3).

There are marked interindividual differences in the rate of degradation of all the antipsychotics. Thus, at steady-state administration of these drugs, there are 10- to 20-fold variations in plasma concentrations among individuals. Consequently, it has been difficult to date to define plasma concentration–effect relationships for most antipsychotics. The most extensively examined neuroleptic in this regard is haloperidol. For this drug, plasma concentrations on the order of about 1 ng/ml appear to be related to a clear antipsychotic effect. However, for several antipsychotics in addition to haloperidol, e.g., amisulpride, clozapine, and olanzapine, it has been possible to demonstrate curvilinear relationships between plasma concentrations of the drug at steady state and occupancy level of D2 dopamine receptors in the brain, as measured by PET scan (Fig. 14.3). So far plasma concentration monitoring of neuroleptics has not been applied extensively in clinical psychiatry. However,

the frequent occurrence of CYP2D6 poor metabolizer status among patients treated with antipsychotic medications and the significant impact this may have on the use of some of the newer agents, such as risperidone (Tab. 14.3), has encouraged defining the metabolizer status of patients by one of the recently available gene chip technologies prior to use of these agents (see Chap. 3).

Most antipsychotic drugs are given orally once or several times per day. Steady-state concentrations in plasma usually are obtained within about a week. Because of the failure to demonstrate clear-cut relationships between plasma concentrations and therapeutic effect, plasma monitoring of antipsychotic drug treatment has gained little popularity in practice. Dose adjustment for individual patients therefore usually is based on clinical response of the patient within the first 4 weeks of treatment with a fixed dose. In the absence of an adequate response, the dose is increased by 50 to 100%, and treatment is continued for another 2 to 4 weeks. Patients who do not respond to conventional doses of neuroleptics are often treated with a markedly higher dose or are changed to another type of neuroleptic.

This behavior can be questioned on the basis of studies that have examined the relationship between clinical response and receptor occupancy of D2 receptors in the brain in patients treated with various types of antipsychotics in different doses. Patients treated with chemically distinct types of conventional neuroleptics have similar values for D2 receptor occupancy, as determined by PET scan. Relatively low doses on the order of 4 to 12 mg of haloperidol induce a more than 80% occupancy of the D2 receptors. Detailed dose-response curves for clinical effects have only been established for a few neuroleptics such as chlorpromazine, haloperidol, and sertindole in single studies.

Drug interactions

Metabolism mainly by CYP2D6-regulated pathway makes major antipsychotics quite liable to interactions with concomitantly given drugs affecting this metabolic pathway. This is particularly clear for major selective

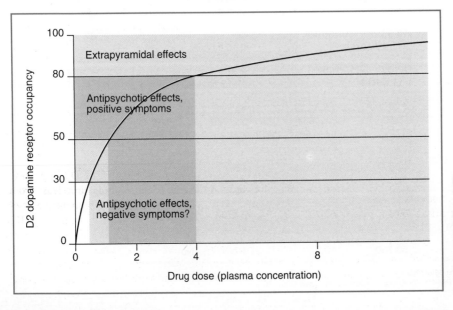

Figure 14.3 Relationship between dose or drug concentration of antipsychotic drug and D2 dopamine receptor occupancy in the brain as measured by PET scan. Note thresholds for occupancy level inducing EPSs, therapeutic effects on positive aspects of schizophrenic symptoms, as well as negative aspects of schizophrenic symptoms.

serotonin reuptake inhibitors (SSRIs) (see Chap. 13) that are all substrates of the same metabolic pathway. Both fluoxetine and fluvoxamine are also potent antagonists of the CYP2D6 enzyme system and thus may markedly increase steady-state blood levels of concomitantly given antipsychotics that are substrates of this pathway. A similar antagonism may be exerted by antiarrhythmic drugs such as quinidine. The case of pimozide (a CYP3A4 substrate) was described earlier.

Intermittent treatment Most patients receive continuous neuroleptic treatment. However, in order to reduce the risk for tardive dyskinesia and other side effects, intermittent treatment has been examined. One study compared continuous with intermittent treatment. The patients who received intermittent treatment were given significantly less drug and exhibited significantly fewer side effects as compared with patients receiving continuous treatment. However, the relapse frequency was considerably higher than for those receiving continuous treatment. There was no difference between the two groups with regard to social function and/or risk for tardive dyskinesia. Therefore, most clinicians do not recommend intermittent treatment.

Injectable depot preparations Haloperidol and several antipsychotics with the piperazine substitution can be esterified with long-chain fatty acid molecules. Injectable depot preparations of such esters so far are available only for typical antipsychotics such as fluphenazine, perphenazine, and haloperidol. These preparations have the advantage of an improved biologic availability and also make it possible to guarantee that the patient is really receiving the drug in case of poor compliance. Depot treatment is an invasive therapy with a slight risk for tissue damage at the injection site. Many patients accept the treatment, but many others consider the regular injections troublesome and in some cases humiliating. Systematic dose-response studies indicate that doses above 25 mg of fluphenazine decanoate every second week or 25 mg of haloperidol decanoate every month result in a reduced frequency of relapses.

Side effects

Antipsychotic drugs cause a number of side effects that often represent a major problem for patients and cause poor compliance. In some cases, side effects also may be dangerous.

Effects on the central nervous system Sedation is the most common side effect at the beginning of treatment. In anxious patients, this side effect is often considered to be a therapeutic component. For many patients, sedation also can be advantageous in improving sleep. Usually, there is tolerance for the sedative effect after a few weeks of treatment. Sedation is particularly marked for antipsychotics with strong antagonism at histamine H1 and catecholamine α1 receptors. However, selective D2 receptor antagonists also may produce sedation that can be reduced by administering the antipsychotic once a day at bedtime.

Extrapyramidal side effects (EPSs), such as tremor, dystonia, akathisia, and muscle rigidity, are common when antipsychotic agents are administered in high doses (Fig.14.3). These effects are considered to be related to blockade of D2 dopamine receptors, particularly in the nigrostriatal system. These side effects can occur during treatment with all antipsychotics but are very uncommon during treatment with clozapine. They are particularly common during treatment with typical antipsychotics with a high potency such as haloperidol. Acute extrapyramidal side effects can be treated rapidly with anticholinergics. When such symptoms occur, dosage preferably should be reduced. Continuous treatment with anticholinergics is usually not indicated.

Tardive dyskinesia (TD) can develop during long-term treatment with neuroleptics and is characterized by stereotypical movements within the orofacial area. These movements often take the form of repeated chewing movements, grimaces, smacking, licking, and blowing mouth movements and tongue or labial movements. Stereotypes can occur in most parts of the body. Stereotypical dyskinetic movements also can vary with dystonic movements within the muscles of the head and the neck. The occurrence of dyskinetic movements was reported in schizophrenic patients before the availability of antipsychotic drugs. However, their occurrence was considerably more common after the advent of neuroleptic treatment. It has been estimated that about 5% of schizophrenic patients develop TD for every year of continued medication. Usually, TD develops during treatment with neuroleptics, but it also may occur after their withdrawal. Advanced age, high neuroleptic dose, and the development of extrapyramidal side effects early during previous treatment, previous brain damage, and female sex are factors that may increase the risk for TD. Clozapine and other atypical antipsychotics with a low tendency for acute extrapyramidal side effects may have a reduced liability to cause TD. The pathogenic mechanisms of TD are still unclear. Withdrawal of neuroleptic treatment can cause substantial improvement. However, this may not be possible in patients with a severe psychosis. Clozapine has been used to treat TD often with satisfactory effects.

Many antipsychotics lower the threshold for epileptic seizures. Low-potency antipsychotics and particularly clozapine have a relatively high liability for causing this side effect. Anticholinergic side effects include dry mouth, disturbed accommodation, disturbed micturition, and bowel obstruction. All antipsychotic drugs tend to exert endocrine effects by increasing the level of prolactin in serum. This is related to blockade of D2 dopamine receptors that mediate inhibition of prolactin release from the pituitary. This effect is particularly pronounced after substituted benzamides and antipsychotics with a high D2 dopamine receptor affinity. The prolactin release may cause galactorrhea, breast swelling, and amenorrhea in women. In men, impotence and gynecomastia may be induced. These effects seem to be less apparent with some of the newer atypical antipsychotics such as olanzapine.

Many antipsychotics cause slight alterations in liver function tests. These side effects are seldom alarming, especially today when antipsychotic drug doses have been reduced.

Hematologic side effects Agranulocytosis, a potentially lethal side effect, occurs in about 0.5% of patients receiving atypical antipsychotics and in about 1% of patients receiving clozapine. Blood counts should be monitored weekly at the beginning of therapy and monthly thereafter. Agranulocytosis is usually reversible if treatment is interrupted immediately.

Neuroleptic malignant syndrome (NMS) This is a rare but potentially lethal complication of antipsychotic treatment. It is a more or less rapidly appearing idiosyncratic reaction with muscular rigidity and autonomic instability with tachycardia, hypo- or hypertension, and sudden blood pressure swings. Hypothermia, sweating, and temperature elevations above 41°C are common. The patient can develop stupor, delirium, and fluctuating consciousness. Early diagnosis and intervention are important to prevent mortality, estimated to be about 20%. The neuroleptic treatment should be interrupted immediately, and the patient should be admitted to a medical emergency unit for intensive care. Patients are often treated with bromocriptine, facilitating dopaminergic signaling (see Chap. 11), and most patients recover within a few days.

Fetal and neonatal risks Most antipsychotic drugs pass the placental barrier, and drug concentrations in the fetus are of the same order as in the mother. Many of the antipsychotic drugs also can be found in breast milk. Animal experiments indicate that antipsychotic drug treatment of pregnant rats causes a delayed development of psychomotor activity in their newborns. These effects are rapidly reversible after drug withdrawal. Although there is no statistical evidence for mutagenic or teratogenic effects of antipsychotic drugs, their use in pregnant women is therefore not recommended unless the patient's clinical condition strongly motivates such treatment. After delivery, breast-feeding is usually not recommended for children of mothers receiving antipsychotic drug treatment.

Side effects of antipsychotic drugs due to reduced drug metabolism and elimination may be related to drug accumulation in patients with liver and kidney damage. In such patients and in older patients, doses should be kept low to avoid drug accumulation and the appearance of side effects.

Indications

An impressive number of controlled comparisons have been made of chemically different categories of antipsychotic drugs versus placebo and/or reference drugs under double-blind conditions. Such studies have demonstrated beyond doubt the significant therapeutic effects of these drugs on positive aspects of schizophrenic symptomlogy and psychotic behavior in patients with manic and schizoaffective disorders, as well as in patients with psychosis of old age. For some of the recently developed atypical antipsychotics, such as clozapine, olanzapine, risperidone, and amisulpride, there is also some evidence for a better effect against negative aspects of schizophrenic symptomatology as compared with conventional doses of classic neuroleptics such as haloperidol.

Contraindications and therapy of overdose

There are no absolute contraindications for antipsychotic drug treatment. As mentioned earlier, previous occurrence of NMS should be a relative contraindication. However, many patients with this condition who responded well after antipsychotic drug withdrawal could be treated later with such drugs with a good therapeutic effect without recurrence of the NMS.

Antipsychotic drugs have a relatively low toxicity, in that vital functions are not severely affected even by high drug concentrations. Overdose treatment should be based on conservative measures, since the drugs are fairly rapidly metabolized and excreted if vital functions are maintained.

New areas of drugs development

Although classic and atypical neuroleptic drugs have a specific place in the treatment of most psychotic patients, the fact that these drugs represent a symptomatic treatment necessitates the development of more causal remedies. Since the etiology and pathophysiology of most psychotic reactions are still obscure, drug development in this field has so far been extensively dependent on animal models (see Chap. 16). Most currently available antipsychotics were developed using pharmacologic models of schizophrenia, where stimulation of dopamine release by such drugs as amphetamine was considered a model of the pathophysiology. This view has come under increased criticism in recent years.

More recently, alterations in serotonergic, glutamatergic, and GABAergic signaling have been the focus of attempts to find new treatments. Thus, antagonists of 5-HT 2A receptors, agonists of 5-HT 1A receptors, and glutamatergic agonists have been proposed as potential antipsychotic drugs. However, so far, compounds with selectivity for each one of these mechanisms have not demonstrated a clear-cut antipsychotic effect in schizophrenic patients.

It seems logical that tracing molecular genetic mechanisms that participate in increasing or reducing the risk for schizophrenic and other psychotic disorders may be a more rational approach to finding the brain systems that should be targeted to develop a more causal treatment for these disorders. The development of the human brain project is a rational strategy to obtain such measures.

Current principles for antipsychotic drug treatment for individual patients are based on the assumption that patients are identical with regard to drug targets in the brain, as well as drug metabolism and kinetics in the body, as is more or less the case in a strain of inbred rats.

It is now well appreciated that the receptor targets of antipsychotic drugs are encoded by functionally polymorphic genes that create a marked individual variability with regard to receptor functions in the brain. Similarly, polymorphism within the cytochrome P450 systems responsible for the metabolic breakdown of most antipsychotic agents may result in more than 10-fold individual variations in the rate of drug metabolism. The develop-

ment of chip and array methodologies for determining individual polymorphisms in such genes will in the near future give important information that will be used to further optimize individual treatment with the drugs that are already available.

Suggested readings _____

BROWN CS, MARKOWITZ JS, MOORE TR, PARKER NG. Atypical antipsychotics. II. Adverse effects, drug interactions, and costs. Ann Pharmacother 1999;33:210-7.

CAMPBELL M, YOUNG PI, BATEMAN DN, et al. The use of atypical antipsychotics in the management of schizophrenia. Br J Clin Pharmacol 1999;47:13-22.

DAVIES JM. Maintenance therapy and the natural course of schizophrenia. J Clin Psychiatry 1985;46:18-21.

DELAY JP, DENIKER O. Characteristiques psychophysiologiques des medicaments neuroleptiques. In: Garattini J, Ghetti V, eds. The psychotropic drugs. Amsterdam: Elsevier, 1957:485-501.

HALL H, HALLDIN C, JERNING E, et al. Autoradiographic comparison of [125I]epidepride and [125I]NCQ 298 binding to human brain extrastriated dopamine receptors. Nucl Med Biol 1997;24:389-93.

JANSSEN PAJ. The evolution of the butyrophenones, haloperidol, and trifluperidol, from meperidine-like 4-phenylpiperidines. Int Rev Neurobiol 1965;8:221-63.

JIBSON MD, TANDON R. New atypical antipsychotic medications. J Psychiatr Res 1998;215:215-28.

MARKOWITZ JS, BROWN CS, MOORE TR. Atypical antipsychotics. I. Pharmacology, pharmacokinetics, and efficacy. Ann Pharmacother 1999;33:73-85.

NYBERG A, NAKASHIMA Y, NORDSTROM A-L, et al. Positron emission tomography of in vivo binding characteristics of atypical antipsychotic drugs. Br J Psychiatry 1996;168:40-4.

SEDVALL G, FARDE L. Chemical brain anatomy in schizophrenia. Lancet 1995;346:743-9.

TRAN PV, TOLLEFSON GD, SANGER TM, et al. Olanzapine versus haloperidol in the treatment of schizoaffective disorder: acute and long-term therapy. Br J Psychiatry 1999;174:15-22.

15

Insomnia

Cesare R. Sirtori

Insomnia is a common symptom; it may be defined as a disturbance or perceived disturbance of the usual sleep pattern of an individual that has troublesome consequences. The consequences may include daytime fatigue and drowsiness, irritability, anxiety, depression, and somatic complaints. Insomnia tends to increase with age and is more prevalent among women. Recent estimates indicate that there is a 10% prevalence of chronic insomnia in the adult population of the United States with an associated annual cost of $90 to $107 billion. Estimates of the incidence of insomnia range from 16.6% in the French adult population to 27.7% in Japanese industrial workers. In a large epidemiologic study in the elderly, 22% of people aged 70 and older reported mild insomnia, and 27% reported moderate to severe insomnia, with women complaining more frequently. In fact, 35% of women versus 13% of men complained of moderate to severe insomnia in the same age group. A rare but important cause of insomnia is the fatal familial insomnia syndrome, recently linked to a prion disease (see Chap. 12) and characterized by early impairment of attention and vigilance, deficits of memory and of temporal ordering of events, and a progressive dreamlike state with features of a confusional state. At neuropathologic examination, there is prominent neuronal loss involving the anterior ventral and mediodorsal thalamic nuclei, with additional cerebral cortical involvement.

People who are divorced, widowed, or separated report having insomnia more often than married people; lower socioeconomic status is also a correlate of insomnia. Insomnia can vary over time but tends to be persistent or recurrent in both clinical and community samples. Persistent insomnia is both a risk factor for and a precursor of mood disorders; an effective treatment of insomnia may represent an opportunity to prevent major depression. Chronic insomnia is also associated with an increased risk of automobile accidents, alcohol consumption, and daytime sleepiness.

Normal sleep physiology

Normal sleep consists of two phases, *rapid eye movement* (REM) *sleep* and *non-REM sleep.* Non-REM sleep is subdivided into four stages. Stage 1 sleep, the lightest stage of sleep, is very brief. Stage 2 sleep is a light stage of sleep comprising up to 50% of total sleep time. Stages 3 and 4, collectively called *slow-wave sleep* or *delta sleep,* are characterized by a deep, restorative sleep. They have a rejuvenating function, and a decrease in these stages is associated with poor sleep quality. REM sleep (about 20% of total sleep time) is associated with high levels of neuronal activity and dreaming. REM rebound occurs on abrupt discontinuation of agents that suppress REM sleep (i.e., barbiturates, some benzodiazepines, tricyclic antidepressants), resulting in vivid and frightening dreams in some individuals.

Sleep involves cycling (approximately four to six cycles per night) between the non-REM and REM stages. Delta sleep dominates early in the night, but as the night progresses, REM periods become longer and more prevalent.

Clinical findings

Patients with insomnia have problems that may include an unrefreshing or nonrestorative sleep as well as the inability to fall asleep (taking more than 30 minutes to fall asleep) or difficulty in maintaining sleep. The duration of insomnia has important diagnostic implications. Transient insomnia, lasting only a few days, is often a result of acute stress, medical illness, "jet lag," or self-medication. Insomnia lasting longer than 3 weeks is considered chronic and usually has different causes. This differential diagnosis is crucial in evaluating secondary problems, including the use and misuse of alcohol and drugs (both a cause and an effect of insomnia) and obsessive concern about the inability to sleep.

The diagnosis of chronic primary insomnia requires difficulty in initiating or maintaining sleep or the presence of nonrestorative sleep for at least 1 month. This may cause marked impairment in social, occupational, or other important areas of functioning. Such a disturbance must not be due to another sleep disorder, a mental disorder, a medical condition, or the use of a drug. A diagnosis of exclusion must be reached after more specific medical and psychiatric diagnoses have been ruled out. The cause of chronic insomnia, whenever possible, should be established before embarking on a long-term approach to management.

The main symptom(s) – insomnia, excessive sleepiness, or disturbed behavior during sleep – should be established first. Possible causes may include concurrent medical conditions or their treatment; use of substances such as caffeine, nicotine, or alcohol; psychiatric disorders such as mood or anxiety disorders; acute or chronic stress (e.g., bereavement); disordered circadian rhythms (e.g., "jet lag," shift work, or advanced or delayed sleep-phase syndrome); sleep-disordered breathing (heralded by snoring or obesity); nocturnal myoclonus, sometimes associated with restlessness of the legs at the beginning of sleep; events such as panic attacks or recurrent nightmares; excessive worrying about not sleeping; and behavior destructive to sleep, including an irregular schedule or the habit of lying in bed ruminating.

The patient, whenever possible, should complete a 2-week diary indicating usual bedtime and time of arising, timing and quantity of meals, use of alcohol, exercise, medications, and description of duration and quality of sleep. If the patient has a bed partner, it is also important to ask whether the patient snores loudly, behaves abnormally during sleep (e.g., has episodes of confusion or combativeness), or is excessively sleepy during the day. Physicians should refer patients suspected of having sleep-disordered breathing for an evaluation that includes electroencephalography (EEG) sleep staging and simultaneous electrocardiography (ECG) and monitoring of respiration and limb movements. The American Sleep Disorders Association also recommends referring a patient if chronic insomnia persists after behavioral and pharmacologic intervention (as described below) or if the sleep symptom is not adequately explained by the type or degree of medical illness or medications. Objective evaluation of insomnia may require sleep laboratory studies by using polysomnography, which includes data recorded from the EEG, electro-oculogram, chin electromyogram, and respiratory monitor.

Sleep parameters commonly measured in sleep studies include sleep latency, the percentage of time spent in each sleep stage, the number of night awakenings, and sleep efficiency (ratio of total sleep time to total time spent in bed). In addition, polysomnography measures physiologic variables such as respiratory effort and airflow, oxygen saturation, leg movements, and heart rate during sleep. These data aid in the detection of such sleep disorders as periodic limb movement disorder (PLMD) or sleep apnea. Polysomnography allows classification of dyssomnias, comprising disorders of initiating or maintaining sleep (insomnias) or excessive sleepiness (hypersomnia).

Dyssomnias may be further divided into *extrinsic* and *intrinsic* sleep disorders. Extrinsic insomnia is attributed to external factors such as inadequate sleep hygiene, drug or alcohol dependency, or situational stress. Intrinsic insomnia develops from causes within the body and includes psychophysiologic insomnia, idiopathic insomnia, obstructive sleep apnea, restless legs syndrome, and periodic limb movement disorder.

Treatment

The primary goals are to remove or mitigate eventual underlying problems associated with insomnia, to prevent progression from transient to chronic insomnia, and to improve the patient's quality of life. Achieving these goals involves educational, behavioral, and often pharmacologic intervention.

Educational and behavioral interventions Patients should be educated about the kinds of behavior that disrupt sleep (stimulus control) and should be instructed in how to stabilize sleep-wake schedules (temporal control). Patients should be told to go to bed only when they are sleepy and to use the bedroom only for sleep and sex and not for reading, watching television, eating, or working. If patients are unable to sleep after 15 to 20 minutes in bed, they should get out of bed and go to another room. They should read with a dim light and avoid watching television, which radiates full-spectrum bright light and has an arousing effect; they should return to bed only when sleepy. The aim is to reestablish the psychologic connection between the bedroom and sleeping rather than the bedroom and insomnia. Patients should get out of bed at the same time each morning regardless of how much they have slept. This stabilizes the sleep-wake schedule (temporal control) and enhances sleep efficiency (the percentage of time in bed spent sleeping). Daytime napping should be minimized or avoided in order to increase the drive to sleep at night.

Another helpful behavioral intervention consists of curtailing the amount of time spent in bed to the actual amount of time spent sleeping. This sleep-restriction therapy was shown to be effective in a randomized clinical trial with elderly subjects. With this method, a slight sleep debt accrues, thus increasing the patient's ability to fall asleep and to stay asleep. The time allowed in bed is increased incrementally, as long as a desired sleep efficiency is maintained. If a patient with chronic insomnia sleeps 5.5 hours nightly, the time in bed is limited to 5.5 to 6.0 hours. The patient then adds approximately 15 minutes per week to the start of each night's time in bed, rising at the same time every morning, as long as at least 85% of the time in bed is spent sleeping. Finally, paradoxical intention should be mentioned; in this the patient is instructed not to fall asleep, with the expectation that efforts to avoid sleep will in fact induce it.

More specialized approaches involve relaxation therapies, such as progressive muscular relaxation and biofeedback, to reduce arousal. Relaxation techniques are a group of behavioral therapeutic approaches that differ widely in their philosophic bases as well as in their methodologies and techniques. The primary objective is the achievement of nondirected relaxation rather than direct achievement of a specific therapeutic goal. The techniques all share two basic components: (1) repetitive focus on a word, sound, prayer, phrase, body sensation, or muscular activity, and (2) the adoption of a passive attitude toward intruding thoughts and a return to the focus. Relaxation techniques also may be used in stress management (as self-regulatory techniques) and have been divided into deep and brief methods.

Deep methods of relaxation include autogenic training, meditation, and progressive muscle relaxation. Autogenic training consists of imagining a peaceful environment and comforting bodily sensations. Basic focusing techniques are used: heaviness and warmth in the limbs, cardiac regulation, centering on breathing, warmth in the upper abdomen, and coolness in the forehead. Meditation is a self-directed practice for relaxing the body and calming the mind. Meditation generally does not involve suggestion, autosuggestion, or trance. The goal of mindfulness meditation is development of a nonjudgmental awareness of bodily sensations and mental activities occurring in the present moment. Concentration meditation trains the person to passively attend to a bodily process, a word, and/or a stimulus. Transcendental meditation focuses on a "suitable" sound or thought (the mantra) without attempting to actually concentrate on the sound or thought. There are also many movement meditations, such as yoga and the walking meditation of Zen Buddhism. Progressive muscle relaxation focuses on reducing muscle tone in major muscle groups. Each of 15 major muscle groups is tensed and then relaxed in sequence.

Brief methods of relaxation include self-control relaxation, paced respiration, and deep breathing and generally require less time to acquire or practice, often representing abbreviated forms of a corresponding deep method. Autogenic training may be abbreviated and converted to a self-control format. Paced respiration teaches patients to maintain slow breathing when anxiety threatens. Deep breathing involves taking several deep breaths, holding them for 5 seconds, and then exhaling slowly.

Drug therapy

Rational pharmacotherapy for insomnia, especially chronic insomnia, in both adult and geriatric patients should use the lowest effective dose, use intermittent dosing (two to four times weekly), and prescribe medications for short-term use (regular use for no more than 3 to 4 weeks). Medications should be discontinued gradually, and the physician and patient should be alert for rebound insomnia following discontinuation. Drugs with shorter elimination half-lives are generally preferred so as to minimize daytime sedation. Alcohol is minimally effective in inducing sleep, may further impair the quality of sleep, and adversely affects performance the next day. A review of controlled medication studies (with a total of close to 10 000 patients) and controlled behavioral-intervention studies (more than 1000 patients) indicates that subjective symptoms and objective signs of chronic insomnia respond to short-term behavioral and pharmacologic intervention. Both types of interventions can reduce the amount of time it takes to fall

Table 15.1 Dosages and pharmacokinetic characteristics of major benzodiazepines used for insomnia

	Time to onset of action (min)	$t_{1/2}$ (h)	Active metabolite(s)	Usual therapeutic dose (mg/day)
Short acting				
Midazolam	20-40	1.7-4	No	7.5-15 oral 0.01 mg/kg iv infusion 3-6 im
Triazolam	15-30	1.5-5	No	0.125
Intermediate-acting				
Estazolam	15-30	8-24	No	0.5-2
Flunitrazepam	60-120	16-26	No	0.5-2
Lorazepam	15-40	8-24	No	0.5-2
Lormetazepam	20-40	8-24	No	0.5-2
Loprazolam	30-60	12-16	Yes	1-2
	45-60	3-25	No	7.5-30
Long-acting				
Clorazepate	30-60	6-8[1] 48-96[2]	Yes	3.75-15
Flurazepam	30-50	9-101[3]	Yes	15-30
Nitrazepam	15-40	24-40	No	5-10
Quazepam	20-45	15-40[1]	Yes	7.5-15

[1] Parent compound.
[2] Active metabolites.
[3] Active metabolites (the parent drug is essentially undetectable).

asleep by 15 to 30 minutes as compared with pretreatment times and the number of awakenings by one to three per night. Pharmacologic agents appear to act more reliably in the short run, and behavioral interventions appear to produce more sustained effects, but no direct comparisons with respect to long-term efficacy are available (Tab. 15.1). Controlled trials clearly indicate that benzodiazepines, zopiclone, antidepressants, and melatonin (only one controlled trial) are effective pharmacologic agents. Stimulus control, sleep restriction, relaxation strategies, and cognitive-behavioral therapy are effective behavioral interventions for short-term management.

Double-blind trials in elderly patients give scientific support for the short-term efficacy (up to 3 weeks) of zolpidem and triazolam in the elderly, as well as temazepam, flurazepam, and quazepam, but not for chloral hydrate. The latter generally is not available in Europe and may well be obsolete by now.

Benzodiazepines

Benzodiazepines remain the mainstay of therapy because of their proven efficacy and relative safety. Benzodiazepines (BDZs) bind to the γ-aminobutyric acid (GABA) receptor, a multimolecular complex comprised of five protein subunits that form a chloride ion channel in the cell membrane (see also Chap. 13). Binding of GABA causes a conformational change that opens the channel, allowing a rapid influx of Cl into the cell and thereby hyperpolarizing the membrane. GABA binding at these receptors is influenced by a number of drugs – including benzodiazepines, barbiturates, neurosteroids, β-carbolines, and alcohol – that have specific binding sites at the GABA(A) receptor complex. Central benzodiazepine-receptor agonists exert a positive allosteric effect that results in an increased affinity of GABA for its binding site, thus potentiating GABAergic transmission.

Major pharmacokinetic features of the benzodiazepines are reported in Table 15.1. These drugs may be divided into short-acting (<6 h), intermediate-acting (6-24 h), and long-acting (>24 h) agents. Short-acting drugs, e.g., triazolam and midazolam (most frequently used for parenteral treatment associated with general anesthetics), may have less respiratory depressant effects as opposed to other benzodiazepines. In the case of triazolam, doses greater than 0.25 mg are not recommended because of increased central nervous system (CNS) adverse effects. Short-acting benzodiazepines may lead to tolerance within 1 to 2 weeks of use as opposed to longer-acting agents.

Intermediate-acting benzodiazepines, e.g., estazolam, flunitrazepam, lorazepam, lormetazepam, loprazolam, and temazepam, are generally well tolerated but may have carryover effects in the elderly. Hangover may become more marked with increasing doses. Finally, long-acting agents, e.g., clorazepate, flurazepam, nitrazepam, and quazepam, are less likely to induce tolerance, thus retaining efficacy for longer periods of time. However, these agents should be avoided in the elderly because of increased risk of falls and hip fractures.

Benzodiazepines increase stage 2 sleep, thus accounting for the increased sleeping time. They have a capacity to reduce the percentage of REM sleep, and withdrawal tends, at least temporarily, to reduce total sleep time (Tab. 15.2).

Toxicity and interaction Benzodiazepines are remarkably well tolerated. Major side effects are reported in Chapter 83. Clinically significant interactions may occur with short-acting benzodiazepines handled by CYP3A4.

Table15.2 Adverse effects of major benzodiazepines and nonbenzodiazepines hypnotics

Drug or drug class	Hangover effects	Rebound insomnia	Time to development of tolerance	Dependence/ abuse potential	Comments
Benzodiazepines					
Short-acting	0	+++	+++	++	May have less respiratory depressant effects versus other benzodiazepines; gradual tapering may reduce rebound
Intermediate-acting	+/++	++/+++	++/+++	++	Hangover effects may become more marked with increasing doses
Long-acting	+++	0	+	++	Avoid in elderly
Zolpidem	+	0	+	+	
Zopiclone	++	++	++	+	Doses > 7.5 mg may cause more adverse effects without increasing efficacy

Such may be the case for triazolam and midazolam, whose metabolic fate may be affected significantly by CYP3A4 inhibitors, e.g., azole antifungals (see Chap. 6). In this case, subjects may be prone to prolonged sleepiness, with consequent danger in driving and other activities requiring attention.

Nonbenzodiazepine sleep-inducing agents

Identification of the central benzodiazepine receptor subtypes (BZ1/BZ2), while still disputed, has indicated that more selective agents than currently available benzodiazepines may be sought. BZ1 receptors occur in brain areas involved in sedation, whereas BZ2 receptors are highly concentrated in areas responsible for cognition, memory, and psychomotor functioning. While benzodiazepines act nonselectively on the two BZ receptor subtypes, newer, more selective agents should have similar hypnotic activity but reduced unwanted CNS adverse effects. Two new agents, zolpidem and zopiclone, currently in wide use were developed based on the concept of receptor selectivity. Another agent, zaleplon, developed with a similar strategy, has just become available in many countries.

Zolpidem This is the first nonbenzodiazepine that selectively binds to the BZ1 receptor. This specificity may account for this agent's minimal anticonvulsant, myorelaxant, and anxiolytic properties. Zolpidem shows a reduced potential for tolerance and abuse. It has a rapid onset of action and a short elimination half-life, ranging from 1.5 to 2.4 hours. It has demonstrated similar improvements in sleep latency and total sleep time compared with benzodiazepines. However, unlike benzodiazepines, which tend to decrease REM and delta sleep, zolpidem does not seem to adversely alter physiologic sleep architecture.

Comparative clinical trials have shown similar effects of zolpidem and triazolam on impairing memory and psychomotor functioning. Maximum impairments were seen approximately 1.5 hours after dosing, i.e., near the time of the estimated peak plasma concentrations for both drugs. Few studies have evaluated rebound effects of zolpidem based on a night-by-night analysis using polysomnographic techniques. Rebound insomnia, i.e., a worsening of sleep below baseline levels, does not appear to occur after discontinuation of zolpidem. The claim that zolpidem is associated with less abuse liability than benzodiazepines remains to be proven. Although clinical trials did not point to any clear evidence of abuse, there have been case reports of chronic abuse, tolerance, and withdrawal symptoms. Individuals with a history of addiction to drugs or alcohol should be monitored carefully while receiving zolpidem.

Zolpidem is biotransformed to inactive metabolites by the CYP3A4 system. However, metabolic handling appears to be minimally affected by potent CYP3A4 antagonists, i.e., itraconazole. The drug therefore can be administered safely in the presence of CYP3A4 inhibitors. Similar lack of interactions has been noted with caffeine or fluoxetine. In contrast, rifampin, like other metabolic inducers, markedly lowers the plasma concentrations, activity, and side effects of zolpidem.

Zolpidem's adverse effects are dose-related, occurring more frequently with 20 mg or more. In a large series of over 1000 patients, the most common adverse effects after 5 to 50 mg of zolpidem were drowsiness (5%), dizziness (5%), headache (3%), and gastrointestinal distress (4%). Between 1 and 2% of the patients also experienced memory disturbances, nightmares, confusion, depression, hangover effects, falls, and asthenia. Recently, there have been several published case reports of unusual CNS adverse effects, such as psychotic symptoms, sensory distortions, and sleepwalking, that may be linked to zolpidem. Otherwise, the next day cognitive functioning and performance are not affected with nighttime zolpidem use, as predicted by its short half-life.

Zopiclone Zopiclone is a non-benzodiazepine that binds to a site close to but not directly corresponding to the benzodiazepine-binding site on the GABA receptor. BZ receptor subtype selectivity is disputed. Zopiclone is short- to intermediate-acting, with a half-life ranging from 3.5 to 6.5 hours and no active metabolites. Compared with benzodiazepines, zopiclone has demonstrated similar improvements in sleep. However, nighttime administration of zopiclone may cause hangover the next morning and impair psychomotor performance similar to that seen with temazepam and nitrazepam. Zopiclone 7.5 mg causes memory impairment up to 2 hours after administration, but there are no morning-after effects. Rebound insomnia is reported when the drug is discontinued. Symptoms of anxiety, decreased sleep duration and sleep quality, and increased sleep latency have been observed on the second day of zopiclone withdrawal after 3 weeks of drug use.

The usual dose for the treatment of short-term insomnia is 7.5 mg taken 30 to 60 minutes before retiring; an initial dose of 3.75 mg is recommended in the elderly and in patients with liver impairment. Zopiclone is a substrate of the CYP3A4 system, and blood levels are moderately, clinically insignificantly raised by azole antifungals. Conversely, rifampin markedly reduces both plasma concentrations and clinical activity.

Although the drug has a low abuse potential, there have been reports of dependence and withdrawal reactions in patients with a history of substance abuse. Most common adverse effects are otherwise mainly of a subjective nature and not different from those of major benzodiazepines. Zopiclone does not appear to offer significant advantages over benzodiazepines in terms of efficacy or adverse effects. The choice of the drug should be based on the clinician's preference and cost considerations.

Other drug classes and OTC products

Low doses of sedating antidepressants such as amitriptyline or trazodone (see Chap. 13) have been used to treat insomnia. Trazodone 50 to 100 mg has been used successfully in patients experiencing insomnia induced by tricyclic antidepressant therapy and in depressed insomniacs. Other agents, e.g., nefazodone and paroxetine, may alleviate sleep disturbances accompanying depression and may have fewer side effects than benzodiazepines and zolpidem, with the advantage of a low risk of overdose. Controlled evaluation of serotonin reuptake inhibitors and other newer antidepressants in the treatment of chronic primary insomnia is lacking. It is possible that use of a low-dose antidepressant (e.g., 10 mg paroxetine per day) would both improve sleep and help prevent depression in chronic insomnia.

A number of over-the-counter (OTC) agents are available, particularly in the United States and less in Europe, for the treatment of insomnia. Two antihistamines (see Chap. 78), i.e., diphenhydramine and doxylamine, are particularly indicated for promoting sleep. These agents unfortunately cause daytime sedation, psychomotor impairment, and anticholinergic adverse effects.

Other nonprescribed medications include valerian and melatonin, widely used as mild hypnotics. Valerian is a herbal product consisting of the underground parts of the plant *Valeriana officinalis*. It is still widely used all over the world, although the responsible components have as yet to be identified. Apparently, volatile oils and valepotriates show hypnotic efficacy. The mechanism seems to be related to the interaction of unknown constituents with the central GABA(A) receptors. Controlled trials with valerian have shown a mild hypnotic activity in the absence of rebound insomnia.

Melatonin is a pineal hormone involved in the regulation of circadian rhythms and in the initiation of sleep. Participation of melatonin in the regulation of sleep-wake cycles in circadian-based sleep disorders such as "jet lag" and delayed sleep phase syndrome is fairly well documented. Less clearly established is the activity of melatonin on sleep, although a trend toward improved subjective sleep has been noted. Melatonin, in available formulations, has a very short half-life (20-50 min), thus not leading to hangover effects in patients. However, there is a question as to the most proper dose, timing of administration (2 h before bedtime or immediately before bedtime), and the possibility that sleepiness may occur erratically during the daytime.

Melatonin, in the form of tablets and capsules and in doses ranging between 0.3 and 10 mg, is widely available, although not regulated (it is still a "dietary supplement" essentially everywhere). Melatonin may be considered for elderly patients with insomnia starting with doses of 1 to 2 mg of a sustained-release formulation. Recent data indicate the potential for melatonin to facilitate the discontinuation of benzodiazepines.

Since the introduction of chlordiazepoxide 30 years ago, all clinical drug trials have addressed only short-term interventions (lasting several days to several weeks) and their immediate responses; there are no data from randomized clinical trials of the ability of interventions to produce sustained effects for more than 35 days. Questions remain unanswered about the long-term efficacy of medications in a disorder that is typically chronic and relapsing. This deficiency, along with the risk of physical dependence, has led the US Food and Drug Administration to establish guidelines that discourage the use of benzodiazepine hypnotics for more than 4 weeks. Although chronic primary insomnia defies easy diagnosis and treatment, clinicians should recognize the importance of determining the cause of insomnia, while bearing in mind that it may have multiple causes in the same patient. Chronic insomnia is often a relapsing disorder, and more data are needed about preventive strategies and the long-term efficacy of both behavioral and pharmacologic approaches. Sleep-restriction therapy and selected antidepressant medications may be promising candidates for studies of long-term efficacy.

Suggested readings

BOOTZIN RR, PERLIS ML. Nonpharmacologic treatments of insomnia. J Clin Psychiatry 1992;53(suppl 6):37-41.

GARFINKEL D, ZISAPEL N, WEINSTEIN J, LANDON M, Facilitation of benzodiazepine discontinuation by melatonin. Arch Intern Med 1999; 159:2456-60.

GENTILI A, EDINGER JD. Sleep disorders in older people. Aging Clin Exp Res 1999;11:137-41.

GILLIN JC, BYERLEY WF. The diagnosis and management of insomnia. N Engl J Med 1990;322:239-48.

GREENBLATT DJ. Pharmacology of benzodiazepine hypnotics. J Clin Psychiatry 1992;53:7-13.

LUPOLOVER R, BALLMER U, HELCL J, et al. Efficacy and safety of midazolam and oxazepam in insomnias. Br J Clin Pharmacol 1983;16:139S-43S.

KUPFER DJ, REYNOLDS CF III. Management of insomnia. N Engl J Med 1997;336:341-6.

MENDELSON WB. Long-term follow-up of chronic insomnia. Sleep 1995;18:698-701.

MORIN CM, CULBERT JP, SCHWARTZ SM. Nonpharmacological interventions for insomnia: a meta-analysis of treatment efficacy. Am J Psychiatry 1994;151:1172-80.

NIH TECHNOLOGY ASSESSMENT PANEL. Integration of behavioral and relaxation approaches to the treatment of chronic pain and insomnia. JAMA 1996;276:313-8.

RACAGNI G, MASOTTO C, STEARDO L. Pharmacology of anxiolytic drugs. Seattle: Hogrefe & Huber, 1997.

REITE M, BUYSSE D, REYNOLDS C, MENDELSON W. The use of polysomnography in the evaluation of insomnia. Sleep 1995;18:58-70.

VGONTZAS AN, KALES A. Sleep and its disorders. Annu Rev Med 1999;50:387-400.

WAGNER J, WAGNER ML, HENING WA. Beyond benzodiazepines: alternative pharmacologic agents for the treatment of insomnia. Ann Pharmacother 1998;32:680-90.

ZAVALA F. Benzodiazepines: anxiety and immunity. Pharmacol Ther 1997;75:199-216.

CHAPTER 16

New areas of drug development

Francesco Clementi

The human brain is a formidably complex apparatus that lies at the very basis of the life of each individual and community of individuals. It consists of more than one hundred billion cells, each of which establishes contacts and relationships with thousands of others by means of about two million miles of axons and around one million billion synapses. This complex machinery allows us to be aware of and respond to the environment, as well as communicate with other individuals. The brain is ultimately responsible for the coordinated life of all our organs and, in particular, for the complex processes going on in our minds, such as memory, learning, attention, recognition, feelings, and behavior. Brain diseases are affecting a growing number of patients and lead to enormous costs for society (Fig. 16.1), particularly in the case of diseases such as Alzheimer's disease (AD), drug addiction, and mood disorders. The difficult task of neuroscientists and pharmacologists is to try to unravel the complexity of this structure, understand how it works, and attempt to develop appropriate therapies.

In recent years, a real scientific revolution has taken place in this field, originating from the fortunate merging of the techniques and cultural approaches of molecular science and engineering. As a result of this cross-fertilization, our understanding of the diagnostic and clinical aspects of brain diseases has greatly improved, and this also has had a remarkable effect on our knowledge of human psychology and behavior.

However, our therapeutic approaches have remained those which have led to the greatest benefit in terms of the number of patients positively affected and the quality of cure. The new benefits come mainly from better use of known drugs or minor modifications of older regimens, trying to improve selectivity and ensure more favorable pharmacokinetics, but the overall results in the case of major central nervous system (CNS) pathologies are still disappointing. There is therefore an impelling urgency to find new therapeutic approaches based on the new possibilities offered by recent progress that has been made in our understanding of brain function and the pathogenesis

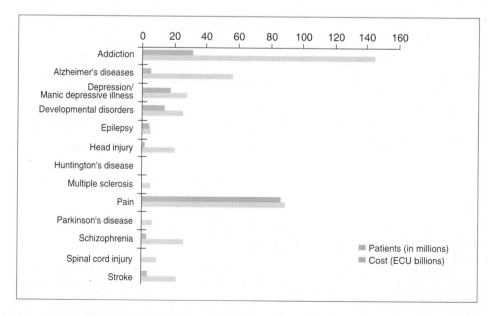

Figure 16.1 Sources for numbers: the Dana Alliance for Brain Initiatives, Washington, New York, USA 1997.

of brain disease. This is important not only in terms of reaching new and safer therapeutic goals but also because a long-standing failure to find new active drugs will alienate patients and physicians from drug-based approaches and lead them toward adopting less valid forms of therapy that are more dangerous for patient health.

In this chapter I shall try to indicate what I believe to be the most promising innovations that could lead to significant improvements in pharmacologic therapy of brain diseases.

Noninvasive brain imaging

The technical improvement that has contributed most to progress in the human neurosciences is the recent explosive development of noninvasive imaging techniques such as magnetic resonance imaging (MRI), positron-emission tomography (PET), single-proton-emission computed tomography (SPECT), and magnetoencephalography. These techniques make it possible to assess the properties of brain tissues and obtain information across scales ranging from system to molecular levels with a high degree of temporal and spatial resolution.

In living humans, it has been possible to associate the activation of specific brain areas with specific mental functions in a number of cases; various neurotransmitters have been localized and their activity monitored during the course of specific brain functions or diseases; for example, a decrease in the number of dopaminergic and neuronal nicotinic receptors in selective brain areas has been clearly shown in Parkinson and AD patients, respectively, and these in vivo neurochemical data have been found to correlate with disease severity.

The combination of these techniques with new molecular and cellular approaches will have a significant impact on our understanding of how the human brain works and the pathogenesis of brain diseases. From a pharmacologic point of view, it can be expected that in the future it will be possible to map a drug in specific brain areas so as to see what brain structures it is affecting and to follow the drug's tissue kinetics in such a way as to evaluate whether or not its effects change in relation to a particular brain activity or disease, and all this safely in living humans. It, thus, finally will be possible to bridge the gap between the data obtained in experimental animals and that obtained in humans.

However, the routine use of these techniques in pharmacologic investigations will greatly depend on the availability of safe and specifically labeled drugs or chemicals and a decrease in the costs of brain imaging. Both these goals will require a lot of effort before they can be reached.

Animal models

One of the main problems affecting pharmacologic research into brain diseases is the ability to find appropriate animal models for in vivo testing of the drugs that have positive effects on relevant targets in vitro or for studying the basic mechanisms of brain diseases. In par-

ticular, the known animal models of human anxiety, depression, and psychosis are not sufficiently reliable predictors of drug activity in humans, although they mimic some of the major neurochemical modifications occurring in patient brains. Any improvement in this field would be of enormous benefit to CNS pharmacology.

A possible breakthrough should come from genetic and molecular biology techniques. The genetic basis of common psychiatric diseases (such as schizophrenia, depression, and anxiety) has been increasingly clarified, and there is a great hope that these investigations will lead to further success. The genetic dissection of behavioral traits of mood is also under active investigation in both humans and animals. In particular, rodents are very useful in trait analysis, and some models of genetically based depression and anxiety have been proposed for validation in terms of drug response, quantitative evaluations, and neurochemical modifications. Degenerative diseases such as AD and Parkinson's disease are also awaiting the development of appropriate models for studying new drugs. It has been found recently that transgenic mice expressing high amyloid and presenilin levels have some of the basic morphologic and behavioral alterations that are present in the brains of AD patients, thus suggesting that a model for Alzheimer's disease is feasible

Brain development

A number of the genes that regulate organization in space (e.g., the frontocaudal organization of brain structures) and time (e.g., when a particular gene has to be switched on and/or off) have been discovered and cloned. In particular, two families of homeobox genes that control anterior head and rostral brain development (*Emx* and *Otx* genes) have been studied carefully. It has been found recently that the human counterpart of *Emx*2 is mutated in schizoencephaly (a congenital disease in which defects of cortex development are associated with deep clefts in the cerebral hemispheres) and that a correlation exists between this gene mutation and the malformations and clinical signs. In such cases in which a gene defect clearly lies at the origin of the disease, it is possible to foresee the use of gene therapy. Many mice carrying homeobox gene mutations have brain malformations that are similar to those found in some human diseases. A typical example is the *Otx*1 null mutant, which contains multiple abnormalities affecting various areas of the cerebral cortex, hippocampus, mesencephalon, and cerebellum and also causes epileptic seizures. Epilepsy is a phenotypically and genotypically heterogeneous disorder, in some cases of which a genetic component has been described. It is possible that the *Otx*1 null mouse may provide a starting point for similar studies in humans.

Genetics and molecular biology in brain pathologies

The fact that genetics, as well as molecular and cell biology, now makes it possible to target the genes involved in genetic diseases, manipulate cells, and insert or delete genes and gene products in cells and tissues in vivo promises to revolutionize not only the experimental approach to brain diseases but also everyday clinical practice. Three scenarios can be envisioned as possible paradigms of such interventions:

1. *Gene therapy.* A number of genes have been found to be connected with severe brain diseases such as AD and Parkinson's disease, amyotrophic lateral sclerosis, and some forms of epilepsy. Furthermore, great progress has been made in dissecting the genetic basis of mood disorders, such as schizophrenia in particular, and this has led to a better understanding of their pathogenesis. In addition, the possibility of knocking out or inserting genes in animals and neuronal cells has allowed the creation of animal models of brain diseases that, in turn, will greatly contribute to the study of possible preventive and therapeutic strategies, as will the increasing feasibility of making an early diagnosis of gene-related diseases. Finally, studies designed to investigate the use of a gene therapy in multiple-gene diseases certainly will soon produce results that can be applied also to many of the brain diseases. Intensive research is now under way to find appropriate vectors to transfer genes to tissue in vivo, an approach that will open up a series of possible applications of gene therapy in brain diseases associated with a specific gene target or the deletion of a specific protein.

2. *Neural transplantation.* It is possible to transplant cells delivering particular molecules that can have beneficial effects on the brain. Myoblasts producing tyrosine hydroxylase and neuron-like cells secreting dopamine or NGF have been used experimentally to ameliorate experimental animal models of Parkinson's and other degenerative diseases, and transplants of dopamine-producing human embryonic cells already have been carried out in some patients with Parkinson's disease with positive preliminary results.

A number of brain diseases, such as tumors or multiple sclerosis, could benefit from local modulation of the immune response or the sustained local release of toxic agents. The transplantation of engineered microglia or astrocytes that release appropriate cytokines or toxic agents could become feasible in the future.

3. *Antisense oligonucleotides.* Another approach is the use of antisense oligonucleotides to inhibit the expression of a selected gene product. Although a number of difficulties have been encountered (e.g., a lack of selectivity, difficult pharmacokinetics, unpredictable results), this could be an interesting possibility in some cases. It has been found that in some degenerative diseases (such as Huntington's disease, a dominant inherited degeneration of caudate and putamen cells), expanded trinucleotide repeats are inserted in particular genes that seem to be of pathogenetic relevance. In such cases, a strategy based on antisense oligonucleotides could be very useful.

However, all these approaches raise a number of ethical issues and questions concerning the safety of such interventions in humans. Preclinical research in this field therefore needs to be particularly thorough and precise, and the discussion of any clinical applications also should involve nontechnical physicians and even philosophers and specialists in the field of ethics.

Signal transduction

This is the classic field in which pharmacologic therapy has obtained the most promising results. This is hardly surprising for a number of reasons. First, given that signal transduction lies at the basis of cell-cell communication, interfering with even one step of this complex process can be expected to have a considerable impact on brain function. Second, since the first steps that activate the transduction machinery are unique in many cases (e.g., neurotransmitter receptors, ion channels), it is possible to develop specific drugs that induce a selective pharmacologic effect by interacting with a specific target. Third, as a result of the contributions made by molecular and cell biology, pharmacology has advanced greatly in recent years. Finally, the fortunate coincidence of technical innovations in the fields of neurochemistry, anatomy, in vivo imaging, and pharmaceutical chemistry has made it possible to bridge the gap between molecular biology and in vivo normal and pathologic situations and, thus, has given us a greater general understanding of brain function.

Some of the new possibilities for a pharmacologic intervention include the fact that a large number of receptor subtypes have been discovered and cloned in all the receptor families and, thus, has made it possible to clarify their role in the cell-cell dialogue. Furthermore, regulatory substances and their receptors, which are known to be peripherally active in the case of nonneuronal functions, have been found to have profound effects on the brain (e.g., cytokines and adhesion molecules). The field of ion channels has expanded enormously in terms of both new members and new pharmacologically active molecules, such as the recently discovered voltage-operated Ca^{2+} channels responsible for the regulation of neurotransmitter release. The number of known neurotransmitter transporters has increased, thus offering new pharmacologic targets. The life of synapses has been elucidated in detail only recently, and its different steps can now be investigated as targets of drugs and toxic agents.

Selective or nonselective drugs?

Before describing some of these possibilities, I would like to discuss a more general question that has emerged as our knowledge of the brain has increased: are the drugs that are active on selective and specific targets better or more useful than relatively unselective drugs? The logical answer would appear to be yes. After all, a greater understanding of the functions of the different molecular components involved in neuronal machinery should lead to the possibility of developing drugs that selectively interact with them, and so it is logical to expect an increase in the selectivity of the therapeutic intervention and a decrease in unwanted side effects. Unfortunately, this is not always the case. We can take the example of the inhibitors of neurotransmitter transporters, which are extremely useful drugs in depression; we now have selective drugs that can block dopamine or serotonin or catecholamine uptake, but their clinical usefulness has not been found to be any better than that of the older nonselective drugs. A second example is given by the neuroleptics. Since the discovery of the classic antipsychotic drugs more than 30 years ago, there has not been any dramatic innovation in the drug-based therapy of psychosis, despite our increased knowledge of the structure and signal transduction of dopamine receptors. The development of selective dopamine D2 or D1 receptor antagonists or selective serotonin antagonists gave rise to some hope, but the greatest recent breakthrough in the treatment of psychosis came from clozapine, a typical "dirty" compound that acts on various different neuroreceptors.

Therefore, although it is logical to think that a clean therapeutic intervention requires drugs that are as target-selective as possible, our existing knowledge of the main brain functions and diseases is not so advanced as to allow us to recognize precisely what target may be relevant or to understand the complex interplay among the possible targets. In some diseases, drugs with a composite effect therefore are probably more useful at the moment because they can act simultaneously on several targets and thus partially compensate for our lack of knowledge of a particular brain function or disease.

Nevertheless, a better knowledge of the structure and function of a possible pharmacologic target does greatly improve the possibility of drug development, as can be seen in the case of neuronal nicotinic receptors.

Neuronal nicotinic receptors

Until recently, nicotinic receptors were neglected because they were thought to be confined mainly to the autonomic ganglia and were likely to play a very minor role in the CNS. However, the recent discovery that they are present in the brain, that they constitute a family made up of numerous subtypes whose different pharmacologic and functional properties depend on their subunit composition, that different subtypes are present in brain in selected discrete areas, and that these molecules may play important roles in major brain diseases (such as Alzheimer's disease, schizophrenia, drug addiction, and Tourette's syndrome) has given rise to an enormous interest in these receptors as possible drug targets. For example, the $\alpha4\beta2$ subtype, which is widespread in the CNS, seems to be involved in pain control, nicotine addiction, and probably memory and attention; the $\alpha7$ receptor, which is mainly present in interneurons and presynaptic terminal, controls the activities of other neurotransmitters, and the $\alpha3\beta4$ subtype is mainly responsible for sympathetic and parasympathetic ganglionic transmission. New and promising nicotinic drugs have been found recently: epibatidine and its derivatives stimulate $\alpha4\beta2$ receptors and have a very strong and long-lasting analgesic activity; the $\alpha7$ receptor-activating drugs now in preclinical study seem to be useful in enhancing cognitive functions in AD patients, whereas the overall stimulation of all the nicotinic receptor subtypes produced by cholinesterase inhibitors has not been found to offer any

dramatic benefit. The recent finding that the $\alpha7$ gene map is very close to a locus controlling a sensory gating disturbance in schizophrenics opens up a possible new pharmacologic approach to the therapy of this pathology.

Adhesion molecules

A number of the molecules responsible for cell-cell recognition have been identified and their functional mechanisms clarified, thus improving our understanding of the selective innervation underlying neuronal circuits. Furthermore, several of these adhesion molecules are essential for the regulation of immune cell responses and the migration of inflammatory cells in inflamed tissues. Traumatic injuries of the brain and spinal cord, which are becoming increasingly more frequent among young people and for which no drug-based therapy is available, probably will benefit from the pharmacologic control of these molecules by helping the growth, regeneration, and homing of axons and by decreasing the inflammatory response. Some experimental approaches have been found recently that can block or stimulate individual adhesion molecules; if these drugs prove to be effective in in vivo models, it is possible that they could find an application in the treatment of human brain injuries. A very preliminary indication of this is the fact that steroids (which are known to modulate adhesion molecules) have a mild activity on spinal cord injuries.

Cytokines

It has been shown that cytokine cell messengers influence brain responses, as well as the response to an aggressive environment, thus finally allowing an understanding of the brain function that modulates stress and defensive responses. However, the study of these molecules at the CNS level is still in its infancy, and a lot of apparently contradictory results have been reported, depending on their concentration at the site of action and the copresence of similar molecules. In addition to being important molecules for the regulation of CNS inflammatory responses, cytokines also can act as neuromodulators and mediators of neurodegeneration and repair. However, their action, receptors, and transduction mechanisms in the CNS are still to be discovered, and so any attempt to intervene in these processes pharmacologically is still very preliminary. A greater understanding of the function of their signal transduction in the brain is important not only for discovering new drugs that are active on the CNS but also for limiting the brain effects of new cytokine-based drugs that are useful for treating inflammation.

Life of synapses

The recent elucidation of the fine details of synapse function has led to the discovery of new targets for pharmacologic intervention. In particular, the molecular machinery of the fusion of synaptic vesicles leading to the release of neurotransmitters has been clearly described, and there is now an open possibility of modulating neurotransmitter release by means of drugs that selectively interact with these molecules. The finding that a number of potent bacterial neurotoxins, i.e., clostridial toxins and in particular tetanus and botulinum toxins, are active through this pathway strongly suggests that a selective pharmacologic approach is feasible. The dramatic effect of botulinum toxins in the treatment of muscle spasticity is an example of the impact that this approach would have if it were possible to find selective targets in the brain synapses, such as inhibition of the release of a specific neurotransmitter.

Use of Ca^{2+} channel blockers in brain diseases so far has been restricted mainly to neurodegenerative diseases and has had very limited success. However, the recent molecular and biophysical description of different ion channels, particularly the recognition of N, L, P/Q, R, and T voltage-operated Ca^{2+} channel subtypes, their relevance in controlling neurotransmitter release, their specific localization in neurons and synapses, especially in perisynaptic and active zone domains, and the discovery of drugs that selectively block or enhance the activity of only one channel subtype, suggests their possible future therapeutic use as neuroprotective agents, modulators of neurotransmitter secretion in mood control, or antiepileptic agents.

As discussed previously, the cloning of a number of neurotransmitter receptor subtypes and the finding of some new neurotransmitter transporters in synaptic plasma membrane and vesicles, as well as the definition of their function at a molecular level, increases the chances of finding more selective drugs capable of interfering with neurotransmitter uptake. However, this pathway has been investigated extensively over recent years, and although the results have been significant, they have not been innovative. We do not expect any great improvements in the pharmacotherapy of mood disease or psychoses from this classic approach.

A multifactorial approach in degenerative diseases

Degenerative diseases have been investigated extensively, and although we are still far from the conclusion of the story, we have gained some insights that have already given rise to therapeutic indications.
There is a general consensus that the greatest therapeutic success in degenerative diseases will come from a concerted attack against multiple targets. Alzheimer's disease offers a paradigmatic example of this multifaceted therapeutic approach. Recent studies have indicated that the disease has various causes and risk factors, the most important of which are β-amyloid deposition in the brain (which plays a significant pathogenetic role), presenilins (which greatly contribute to explaining the early-onset cases), and the apolipoprotein E4 allele (which is associated with an increased risk for the common late-onset familial forms).

Future pharmacologic interventions in this complex disease therefore also should be multifactorial. The possible targets are (1) the secretase enzymes that cleave the amyloid protein precursors, with the aim of increasing the activity of α-secretase (which cleaves the amyloid precursors at the physiologic level) and decreasing the activity

of β- and γ-secretases that give rise to pathologic peptides, (2) the deposition of amyloid, looking for drugs that can decrease the secretion of fibrillar aggregates, (3) microglia and astrocytes, finding drugs that can interfere with the production of cytokines and inflammatory agents, (4) neurodegeneration (the final target of the different noxae produced in Alzheimer's disease), against which systemic or local neuroprotective agents could be extremely important at least in decreasing neuronal loss, and (5) cognitive functions, since the loss of neurons and synapses leads to impaired cognitive function that could be ameliorated by means of drugs capable of stimulating the function of the remaining synapses. The currently used cholinergic, nicotinic and muscarinic drugs are an indication of this type of treatment.

All these targets are very important, but some are still elusive (e.g., the structure of the secretases is not known, and their function has only just been discovered, and the deposition of fibrillar aggregates is a process that is still not understood). Others have been studied more closely as possible drug targets in the case of neurodegeneration, inflammatory reactions, or cognitive functions, but although these are interesting and promising, the clinical results are still very meager.

Given that any therapeutic approach to these targets certainly will be more efficacious the earlier it is administered, the early diagnosis of these diseases is a compelling need. Great innovations are expected in this field as a result of molecular and genetic studies, another consideration that underlines the close correlation between therapeutic efficacy and progress in other fields of medicine.

This brief description of a possible future trend in the pharmacologic treatment of AD patients gives only a partial idea of what is likely to be the complex and multifaceted approach to other degenerative diseases.

Neuronal death

The final common target of degenerative diseases and ischemic insults is neuronal death, and we now have to answer the question of whether it is possible to control it. One of the main causes of neuronal death is a sustained increase of the intracellular concentration of calcium, which can be caused by an increased influx through ligand and/or voltage-gated calcium channels, a reduction in the residual Ca^{2+} by mitochondria or the endoplasmic reticulum, or a decreased Ca^{2+} outflow due to an impaired ion transporter or ion pump. Enormous efforts have been made to find drugs that are capable of decreasing Ca^{2+} influx and therefore could prevent neuronal death. However, although blockers of voltage-operated Ca^{2+} channels and glutamate ionotropic receptors are extremely potent in in vitro models of hypoxia and neuronal degeneration, they have been shown to have very minor effects in in vivo models of brain damage and preliminary clinical trials.

It has been discovered very recently that cyclosporine A and FK506, two major immunosuppressants, can be active in vivo as neuroprotectors against increases in intracellular Ca^{2+} concentrations. This probably occurs as a result of the regulation of IP3 receptors (molecules that control the release of Ca^{2+} from the endoplasmic reticulum) obtained by the binding of cyclosporine A and FK506 to the immunophilin-IP3 complex receptor. This is an interesting approach that complements that of interfering with Ca^{2+} influx.

It has been observed recently that drugs capable of regulating nitric oxide (NO) synthesis also can regulate apoptosis. Finally, it has been claimed that a number of cytokines are neuroprotective factors. However, although these findings are quite interesting and potentially open up new ways of controlling neuronal death, they are still very preliminary, because the results often have been obtained in cultures and therefore are still very far from becoming a possible clinical application.

Drug addiction

This field is of great relevance not only because of its social, economic, and health implications but also because the mechanism of action of pain-controlling drugs is very similar to that of drugs of abuse. The mechanism of drug addiction has been partially elucidated very recently at the molecular level and placed in its correct anatomic and physiologic context. The central role of the activation of the mesolimbic dopamine system (particularly the locus ceruleus) in the main types of drug addiction (i.e., opiates, cocaine, and nicotine) suggests that a common mechanism may underlie this highly complex and very important behavior. It is also possible that the reinforcement, dependence, and tolerance associated with drugs are not just part of a general adaptive supracellular process involving a large number of neuronal circuits and psychologic modifications but are also sustained by cell changes at the level of single neurons. This implies that a perturbation of intracellular events (such as second-messenger pathways), together with modifications in the ion permeability of the plasma membrane, may induce chronic cell changes by means of the activation or suppression of transcription factors. It is possible that new agonist and antagonist molecules may be capable of interfering with the modified pathways (particularly with protein kinases and transcription factors) and thus can offer alternative approaches to controlling drug addiction and open new perspectives for the treatment of both physical and moral pain, as well as for the control of un-rewarding behavior.

Conclusion

Although very general, this brief description of some of the most significant innovations in basic neuroscience has given some idea of the developments that are likely to take place in the future drug-based therapies of brain diseases. Supported by an improvement in our basic understanding of brain function, the progress that is currently being made in the clinical field will allow an earlier and more certain diagnosis. Even more important, these two aspects will indicate with more precision the cellular or functional defects that underlie the pathogenesis of the diseases and further encourage the development of new drugs and exploration of the clinical application of those which are already known. The recent advances made in the fields of experimental and clinical psychology, as well as in the behavioral sciences, also will reinforce the correct application of drugs affecting the human brain and the discovery of possible new therapeutic pathways.

The treatment of brain diseases is certainly one of the most complex tasks that physicians have to face, and this treatment needs to be conducted using all the instruments that we have. Drugs may be the most important, but they are by no means the only approach.

Suggested readings

BENNETT CF. Antisense oligonucleotides: is the glass half full or half empty? Biochem Pharmacol 1988;55:9-19.

BONCINELLI E. Homeobox genes and disease. Curr Opin Gen Dev 1997;7:331-7.

DUMAN RS, HENINGER GR, NESTLER EJ. A molecular and cellular theory of depression. Arch Gen Psychiatry 1997;54:397-605.

FINK DJ, DE LUCA NA, GOINS WF, GLORIOSO JC. Gene transfer to neurons using herpes simplex virus–based vectors. Annu Rev Neurosci 1997;19:265-87.

GOTTI C, FORNASARI D, CLEMENTI F. Human neuronal nicotinic receptors. Progr Neurobiol. 1997;53:199-237.

HENRICKS PAJ, NIJKAMP FP. Pharmacological modulation of cell adhesion molecules. Eur J Pharmacol 1998;344:1-13.

LINDVALL O. Neural transplantation. A hope for patients with Parkinson's disease. Neuroreport 1997;8:III-X.

NESTLER EC. Molecular mechanisms of opiate and cocaine addiction. Curr Opin Neurobiol 1997;7:713-9.

POST RM. Molecular biology of behavior. Arch Gen Psychiatry 1997;54:607-8.

ROTHWELL NJ, HOPKINS SJ. Cytokines and the nervous system: II. Actions and mechanism of action. TINS 1995;18:130-6.

SAMBUNARIS A, HESSELINK JK, PINDER R, et al. Development of new antidepressants. J Clin Psychol 1997;58:40-51.

SMALL GW, RABINS PV, BARRY PP, et al. Diagnosis and treatment of Alzheimer disease and related disorders. JAMA 1997;278:1363-71.

SNYDER SH, SABATINI DM, LAI MM, et al. Neural actions of immunophilin ligands. TIPS 1998;19:21-5.

VERMA IM, SOMIA N. Gene therapy: promises, problems and prospects. Nature 1997;389:239-42.

VOLKOW ND, ROSEN B, FARDE L. Imaging the living human brain: Magnetic resonance imaging and positron emission tomography. Proc Natl Acad Sci USA 1997;94:2787-8.

Kidneys and sexual function, urinary tract

Diuresis and diuretics

G. Dennis Johnston

Conditions that are associated with salt and water retention are common clinical problems. Important examples include congestive heart failure, nephrotic syndrome, chronic liver disease, and renal failure. Diuretics increase sodium and water excretion and therefore are used widely to treat these conditions. In addition, diuretics have been used successfully as antihypertensive agents for 40 years. This action cannot be related easily to effects on sodium and water balance, since very low doses of thiazide diuretics effectively lower blood pressure without activating the renin-angiotensin system, and loop diuretics, which are more effective as diuretic agents, are usually less effective as antihypertensive agents. Diuretics may exert their antihypertensive effects by dilating peripheral resistance vessels or attenuating the vascular responsiveness to endogenous pressor hormones.

Before the introduction of effective synthetic diuretics, attempts to reduce edema in various parts of the body depended on the removal of blood, sweat, or urine. Leeches and scalpels were used to remove blood, whereas herbs were concocted to increase sweating and/or urine flow. The most effective herbal agents to act as diuretics were the xanthine alkaloids present in tea, cocoa, and coffee, but even the most effective of these, aminophylline, does not compare with presently available diuretics.

Soon after the introduction of sulfanilamide, an early antimicrobial sulfonamide, it was observed that very large doses produced an alkaline diuresis. This was attributed to its inhibitory effects on the tubular enzyme carbonic anhydrase, promoting sodium and water loss and retention of hydrogen ions. Sulfanilamide proved too toxic to use as a diuretic, and a number of potent heterocyclic sulfonamides were synthesized that were more water soluble and did not crystallize in the renal tubules. Of these, acetazolamide was the most effective, being 330 times more potent as an inhibitor of carbonic anhydrase than sulfanilamide. It was later discovered that if an amino group was attached to the phenyl ring of this group of compounds, the effect on carbonic anhydrase was reduced, but the overall diuretic effect was maintained. The addition of formic acid to produce the *N*-formyl analogue resulted in an unplanned ring closure to form a ben-

zothiadazine derivative. This was the prototype for the thiazide diuretics from which hydrochlorothiazide, chlorothiazide, and hydroflumethiazide were derived. The loop diuretics furosemide, bumetanide, and piretanide were later produced by replacing the second acidic group of the sulfonamide derivative dichlophenamide with a carboxyl group. Ethacrynic acid, on the other hand, was discovered as a result of attempts to synthesize mercury-free inhibitors of dehydrogenases after the mercurial diuretics mersalyl and merbaphen had been developed. Chlorine and methyl substitutions to the phenyl ring increased the diuretic potency, and eventually ethacrynic acid was synthesized.

Pharmacoeconomic considerations and the clinical use of diuretic therapy

With a few notable exceptions, diuretics are among the most cost-effective drugs in clinical medicine. In the United Kingdom, thiazide diuretics are available for as little as half of one pence or one US cent per day. Indeed, the cheapest available diuretic, bendroflumethiazide, has been shown consistently to reduce stroke and cardiovascular events in hypertensive patients. No equivalent outcome data are available for indapamide, which is 30 times more expensive, for angiotensin converting enzyme inhibitors, or alpha-adrenoceptor antagonists. Low-dose thiazide diuretics remain the most cost-effective treatment for hypertensive patients and should be given in preference to other antihypertensive drugs unless there are well-defined contraindications. Potassium supplements or potassium-sparing diuretics increase the long-term costs and are rarely necessary. The most expensive combinations contain spironolactone, a drug that has no useful role in the treatment of essential hypertension and has a number of unpleasant adverse effects.

It is much more difficult to assess the cost-effectiveness of diuretic therapy in patients with congestive heart failure or other edematous states. There are no placebo-controlled outcome trials, but there is a wealth of clinical evidence to show major symptomatic improvement, especially in congestive heart failure. It seems reasonable to infer that the small cost of long-term diuretic therapy is more than balanced by the reductions in hospital admissions. Potassium-sparing diuretics are required more frequently in heart failure than in hypertension.

There are three basic approaches to the treatment of conditions associated with fluid retention: correction of the underlying disease, sodium restriction, and diuretic therapy. It is unusual for any measure to have a major impact on the underlying disease, other than organ transplants. Compliance with sodium restriction is often a problem, so diuretic use remains the cornerstone for the treatment of congestive heart failure, ascites, chronic renal failure, and nephrotic syndrome. In congestive heart failure, diuretics reduce pulmonary edema and venous congestion, particularly when combined with angiotensin converting enzyme inhibitors. Periodic administration of diuretics to patients with hepatic cirrhosis and ascites can eliminate the need for repeated paracenteses or at least increase the interval between paracenteses. In the nephrotic syndrome, responses to diuretics are often disappointing, and large doses tend to be required in chronic real failure.

The type of diuretic chosen, the route of administration, and the speed of fluid mobilization depend critically on the clinical situation. Acute left ventricular failure requires iv loop diuretics, whereas mild pulmonary edema and venous congestion associated with chronic heart failure are best treated with an oral loop diuretic and the dose adjusted to achieve the optimal result. In other situations, edema does not pose an immediate health risk. In such situations, appearance and discomfort may be the main reasons for diuretic therapy, and partial removal of edema fluid is all that is required using a regimen that produces minimal fluid and electrolyte disturbance. Overdiuresis can result in reduced extracellular plasma volume, leading to hypotension, malaise, and asthenia. Finally, diuretics are useful in lowering blood pressure by mechanisms that do not involve the removal of edema fluid.

HYPERTENSION

Thiazide diuretics remain the drugs of first choice in the treatment of hypertension because their use is supported by a wealth of evidence from randomized clinical trials. Loop diuretics are usually less effective than thiazides when used as monotherapy except in patients with severe renal impairment. They combine effectively with angiotensin-converting enzyme (ACE) inhibitors and other vasodilator drugs in resistant hypertension. Potassium-sparing diuretics are also rarely effective as monotherapy and are used principally to prevent hypokalemia caused by loop and thiazide diuretics. Thiazide diuretics are as effective as other antihypertensive agents for lowering systemic blood pressure. They have a flat dose-response relationship, and there is usually little advantage in increasing the dose above 2.5 mg bendroflumethiazide or 25 mg hydrochlorothiazide. Much lower doses than previously are now used to lower blood pressure. For example, a large number of patients received 10 mg bendroflumethiazide in the Medical Research Council Hypertension Study undertaken in the early eighties (see Chap. 23).

The use of these lower doses has been shown to minimize their adverse metabolic effects. An overview of all long-term outcome trials has demonstrated that treatment regimens based principally on thiazide diuretics and β blockers result in a 38% reduction in stroke and a 16% reduction in coronary events. With the possible exception of dihydropyridine calcium antagonists, there are no outcome data with newer antihypertensive drugs. Thiazides are particularly efficacious in elderly patients because they effectively lower systolic and diastolic blood pressure and appear to have greater coronary protection than in younger patients. Women also tolerate diuretics particularly well because two important adverse effects – gout and impotence – are seen almost exclusively in men. Diuretics have greater efficacy in black patients and are clearly the drugs of first choice when heart failure is also present.

HEART FAILURE

Diuretics remain the principal treatment of the salt and water retention associated with heart failure. In acute heart failure, iv loop diuretics lead to a rapid improvement in symptoms and signs and are required for all patients with severe dyspnea. Initially, in mild heart failure, thiazide diuretics may be sufficient, but for most patients with moderate to severe heart failure, loop diuretics are required. These agents have steep dose-response relationships, and increasing the dose is associated with increased diuretic activity. Since the introduction of ACE inhibitors, however, it is rarely necessary to exceed daily doses of 80 mg furosemide or 2 mg bumetanide. The most effective way to increase diuretic activity is to use combinations of diuretics. Loop diuretics can be usefully combined with potassium-sparing thiazide and thiazide-like diuretics. The potassium-sparing diuretics have the advantage of ameliorating the loss of potassium produced by loop and thiazide diuretics, although this has become less of a problem since the introduction of angiotensin converting enzyme inhibitors.

For patients with increasing edema despite standard diuretic therapy, switching to the iv route can increase the response, possibly due to increased bioavailability and vasodilator activity. There is also evidence that continuous infusions of loop diuretics are more effective than the equivalent doses given as iv boluses. Alternative strategies include strict bed rest and short-term support with inotropic agents. Metolazone is a thiazide-like diuretic that is particularly effective when combined with loop diuretics. Short courses are preferred because of the high risk of hypokalemia, but a small number of outpatients with severe congestive heart failure may require long-term administration. A dose of 2.5 mg on alternate days or twice a week is often all that is required, along with careful monitoring of the electrolytes and creatinine level. Fluid and salt restriction are often forgotten and always should be part of an overall treatment program.

Diuretic resistance refers to a condition in which the edema has become refractory to the action of a diuretic. This may be due to reduced drug delivery or to impaired responsiveness at the renal tubule. Possible approaches include strict bed rest, reduced fluid intake, continuous infusions of loop diuretic, and the addition of metolazone to the loop diuretic.

OTHER EDEMATOUS CONDITIONS

Nephrotic syndrome

Patients with nephrotic syndrome present special problems with fluid volume management. The majority have reduced plasma volume in association with reduced oncotic pressure. In these patients, diuretics may cause further reductions in plasma volume, which can reduce the glomerular filtration rate and blood pressure. Most of the remaining patients have salt and water retention, resulting in expanded plasma volume and hypertension despite reduced oncotic pressure. In these situations, diuretics may be useful in controlling the volume-dependent component of hypertension and reducing the contribution elevated blood pressure may make to the underlying renal disease. Loop diuretics are usually the drugs of first choice because they are more effective when glomerular filtration is reduced. Potassium-sparing diuretics tend to cause excessive potassium retention in patients with renal impairment and usually are contraindicated.

Renal failure

Although renal disease is occasionally associated with salt wasting, most patients exhibit salt and water retention. In severe renal failure, diuretics are usually of little value because there is insufficient glomerular filtration to sustain a significant diuresis. However, most patients with less severe renal impairment can be treated satisfactorily with loop diuretics, especially if heart failure is also present. Certain types of renal disease, especially diabetic nephropathy, are associated with hyperkalemia at a relatively early stage of the disease. In these situations, loop diuretics can be used to reduce the severity of the hyperkalemia.

Hepatic cirrhosis

Hepatic cirrhosis is associated with edema and ascites accompanied by portal hypertension and reduced plasma oncotic pressure. Plasma aldosterone concentrations usually are elevated in response to the reduction in effective circulating volume. When edema and ascites are severe, diuretic therapy can be useful in reducing salt and water retention. However, a large percentage of these patients are resistant to loop diuretics partly because of the high aldosterone concentrations and partly because of decreased secretion of the drugs into tubular fluid. Spironolactone and other potassium-retaining diuretics are often effective because of the potassium-wasting and sodium-retaining effects of high levels of aldosterone. The combination of loop diuretics and spironolactone therefore can be useful. Over vigorous diuresis can cause hypokalemia, metabolic alkalosis, and major

reductions in intravascular fluid volume. Hepatorenal syndrome and hepatic encephalopathy also have been described.

Idiopathic edema

This condition consists of intermittent episodes of salt and water retention in the absence of any recognized underlying pathology. In general, diuretic therapy tends to make the condition worse, and long-term salt restriction is the preferred option.

Acute mountain sickness

Headache, nausea, weakness, and dizziness can occur when travelers rapidly ascend to over 3000 m. In severe cases, cerebral and pulmonary edema can develop. By reducing the production and pH of cerebrospinal fluid, acetazolamide can reduce the severity of the condition if taken 24 hours before the ascent.

OTHER CONDITIONS NOT ASSOCIATED WITH EDEMA

Glaucoma

Inhibition of carbonic anhydrase decreases the formation of aqueous humor and reduces intraocular pressure. Acetazolamide or dorzolamide are therefore of value in acute and chronic glaucoma.

Renal calculi

Thiazide diuretics are probably of benefit in the treatment of renal stones that are associated with hypercalciuria. They enhance calcium reabsorption in the distal convoluted tubule and reduce the amount of calcium excreted in the urine. Salt intake must be reduced because excessive dietary sodium intake can reverse the effect on calcium excretion. Clearly, the dietary intake of calcium also should be reduced.

Hypercalcemia

Loop diuretics can be used in combination with other drugs to reduce the serum calcium level in patients with severe hypercalcemia.

Diabetes insipidus

Thiazide diuretics can reduce polyuria and polydipsia in patients who are not responsive to antidiuretic hormone. The beneficial effect seems to be related to a reduction in plasma volume with a resulting decline in glomerular filtration, enhanced proximal tubular reabsorption of salt and water, and decreased delivery of fluid to the diluting segments. The overall effect is a reduction in urine flow, especially if combined with sodium restriction.

Drug classes

Most clinically effective diuretics exert their effects on specific membrane transport proteins at the luminal surface of the renal tubular epithelial cells. Examples include loop diuretics, thiazide diuretics, and non-aldosterone-dependent potassium-sparing diuretics. Others exert an osmotic effect that prevents water reabsorption in the water-permeable segments of the nephron (e.g., mannitol), inhibit carbonic anhydrase (e.g., acetazolamide), or interfere with hormone receptors in renal epithelial cells (e.g., spironolactone) (Tab. 17.1). For each diuretic there is a principal site of action at a single anatomic segment within the nephron (Fig. 17.1).

CARBONIC ANHYDRASE INHIBITORS

Carbonic anhydrase is present at several sites within the nephron and in the red blood cells of the renal circulation. The enzyme, however, is most plentiful in the luminal membrane of the proximal tubule (Fig. 17.1), where it catalyzes the dehydration of carbonic acid, a critical step in the reabsorption of bicarbonate. Acetazolamide, the most commonly used carbonic anhydrase inhibitor (dorzolamide, a newer inhibitor, is used only in the treatment of glaucoma), blocks sodium bicarbonate reabsorption, causing sodium bicarbonate diuresis and a reduction in the body stores of bicarbonate. Some bicarbonate can be absorbed at other sites within the nephron by carbonic anhydrase-independent mechanisms. The effect of full doses of acetazolamide results in approximately 45% inhibition of the total renal bicarbonate reabsorption.

Pharmacokinetics

Acetazolamide, the only carbonic anhydrase inhibitor in wide clinical use, is well absorbed after oral administration. An increase in urinary pH is observed within 30 minutes of drug administration and reaches a maximum at 2 hours. The effect lasts for about 12 hours, and the elimination half-life is between 6 and 9 hours. Excretion is almost entirely by tubular secretion in the proximal tubule, and the dose thus should be reduced in patients with renal impairment.

Side effects

Most adverse effects of carbonic anhydrase inhibitors relate to an exaggeration of their biochemical actions. Adverse effects therefore include a metabolic acidosis due to a reduction in bicarbonate stores and renal stones due to increased urinary concentrations of calcium and phosphate in an alkaline urine. Hypokalemia also can occur as a result of increased bicarbonate in tubular fluid. The neg-

---

Table 17.1 Dosage and formulation of diuretics

	Dose (mg)	Potency	Formulation
Carbonic anhydrase inhibitors			
Acetazolamide	250-1000 mg	—	Oral, iv
Thiazide diuretics			
Bendroflumethiazide	2.5-5 mg	10*	Oral
Chlorthalidone	12.5-100 mg	1	Oral
Cyclopenthiazide	250-500 mg	100*	Oral
Hydrochlorothiazide	12.5-50 mg	1	Oral
Indapamide	1.25-2.5 mg	20*	Oral
Metolazone	1.25-5 mg	2*	Oral
Loop diuretics			
Furosemide	20-2000 mg	1	Oral, iv
Bumetanide	1-5 mg	40†	Oral, iv
Ethacrynic acid	50-100 mg	0.7†	iv
Torasemide	2.5-40 mg	3†	Oral
Piretanide	6 mg	5†	Oral
Potassium-sparing diuretics			
Amiloride	10-20 mg	1	Oral
Triamterene	75-150 mg	0.3‡	Oral
Spironolactone	100-400 mg	0.1‡	Oral

*Relative to hydrochlorothiazide.
†Relative to furosemide.
‡Relative to amiloride.

ative electrical potential increases, and more potassium is excreted in the urine. Other adverse effects include drowsiness and paresthesias, especially if large doses are used and/or renal impairment is present. Hypersensitivity reactions, fever, rashes, bone marrow suppression, and interstitial nephritis have all been reported.

Acetazolamide should be avoided in hepatic cirrhosis. Alkalinization of the urine will decrease urinary trapping and excretion of ammonium ions. This may contribute to the development of hepatic encephalopathy. Since these drugs induce sodium and potassium loss, they are contraindicated in patients with low sodium or potassium levels.

THIAZIDE DIURETICS

These chemically related compounds inhibit sodium and chloride reabsorption from the luminal side of epithelial cells in the distal convoluted tubule. There is also a small effect on the proximal tubule, but this is probably of little clinical significance (Fig. 17.1). The transport system inhibited by thiazide diuretics has not been characterized accurately, although there is evidence that it is an electrically neutral sodium chloride cotransporter system that is distinct from that present in the thick ascending loop of Henle. There is also an active reabsorptive process for calcium ions in the distal convoluted tubule that is modulated by parathormone. Thiazides increase calcium reabsorption and can cause hypercalcemia or unmask hypercalcemia due to metastatic or nonmetastatic carcinoma, hyperparathyroidism, and sarcoidosis.

Pharmacokinetics

The pharmacokinetic parameters for the most commonly used thiazide diuretics are listed in Table 17.2. Most are well absorbed when given orally but have variable rates of metabolism and renal elimination. The prototype, chlorothiazide, is less lipid-soluble than most other members of the group, and larger doses are required. Chlorthalidone is absorbed slowly and has a longer duration of action, which increase the risk of hypokalemia. Indapamide is excreted primarily in the bile, although enough is excreted by the kidney to exert its diuretic effect on the distal convoluted tubule. Thiazide diuretics are related to the sulfonamides, which are organic acids. They are therefore secreted by the organic acid secretory system and compete to a greater or lesser degree with uric acid secretion. Since they must gain access to the tubular lumen to produce their diuretic activity, drugs such as probenecid can decrease the diuretic response by competing for transport into the proximal tubule. Plasma albumin binding varies considerably among thiazide diuretics and determines the fraction of the drug that undergoes glomerular filtration.

Side effects and interactions

The disadvantages of thiazide diuretics relate mainly to their adverse biochemical effects. Almost all these effects are dose-dependent and can be avoided or minimized by keeping the dose low. Adverse effects that have caused most concern include hypokalemia, hypomagnesemia, hyperuricemia, hyperlipidemia, and glucose intolerance.

Reduced body stores of potassium are due to increased urinary excretion related to increased flow in the renal tubules and activation of the renin-angiotensin-aldosterone system due to decreased plasma volume. Potassium loss is compensated in part by the kidney dur-

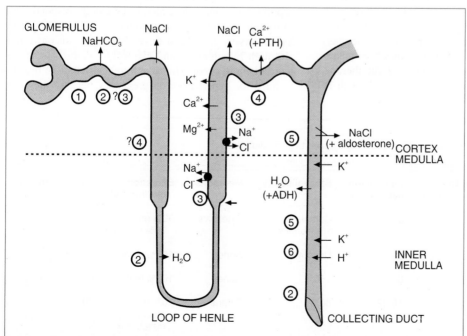

Figure 17.1 Main anatomic sites of action of diuretics: (1) acetazolamide; (2) osmotic diuretics; (3) loop diuretics; (4) thiazide diuretics; (5) potassium-sparing diuretics (PTH= parathormone; ADH= antidiuretic hormone).

ing chronic therapy. The frequency and severity of hypokalemia relate to the dose, the duration of the diuretic activity, the dietary intake of potassium and sodium, and the age of the patient.

The importance of diuretic-induced hypokalemia has caused considerable debate over the last decade. Interest has centered on the association between hypokalemia, ventricular dysrhythmias, and sudden death. The general view is that small reductions in the serum potassium level do not constitute a risk in treated hypertensive patients but that larger decreases do represent a significant risk of sudden death. In addition, hypokalemia increases the risk of toxicity in patients receiving digitalis glycosides and can induce ventricular dysrhythmias in patients with an acute myocardial infarction and those receiving drugs that prolong the QT interval on the electrocardiograph. A relationship between dose and severity of hypokalemia has been demonstrated for most thiazide diuretics that is not paralleled by effects on blood pressure.

There is a considerable amount of literature detailing the adverse effects of thiazide diuretics on plasma lipids. These effects include an elevation of total cholesterol, triglycerides, and low-density lipoprotein cholesterol with little effect on high-density lipoprotein cholesterol. The mechanism is unknown, although the changes have been correlated with hypokalemia and impaired glucose tolerance. It has been suggested that these changes could negate the beneficial effects on blood pressure produced by thiazide diuretics. Recent outcome studies in elderly patients using low doses of thiazides have not confirmed this hypothesis, and the expected beneficial effects on stroke and cardiovascular events are achieved with minimal biochemical derangement.

Diabetes, worsening of diabetic control, insulin resistance, and rarely, hyperosmolar nonketotic diabetic coma have all been described in patients receiving high doses of thiazide diuretics. Most evidence has been obtained in hypertensive patients who develop impaired glucose tolerance or overt diabetes mellitus. Not all studies have reported worsening of glucose tolerance with chronic therapy, however. Although impairment has been described with 10

mg bendroflumethiazide, this has not been demonstrated with the 2.5-mg dose, and a relationship between dose and fasting blood glucose level has been shown for bendroflumethiazide, chlorthalidone, and hydrochlorothiazide in hypertensive patients. In addition, although conventional doses of thiazide diuretics increase insulin resistance, 1.25 mg bendroflumethiazide, a dose that was equally effective in lowering blood pressure, had no effect on insulin resistance. Thiazide diuretics have been associated with an increased incidence of diabetic nephropathy, however, and a higher motality than in those diabetic patients not receiving these drugs. In general, higher doses of diuretics are best avoided in diabetic patients.

Many of the problems relating to hypokalemia could be due to reduced levels of magnesium. Hypomagnesemia, however, is rare with presently recommended doses or when thiazide diuretics are combined with potassium-sparing diuretics.

Elevations of the serum urate concentrations commonly occur with thiazide diuretics and may precipitate gout in up to 5% of treated patients. Although an elevated uric acid level is a marker that often coexists with other cardiovascular risk factors, there is no evidence that it represents an independent risk factor. In the short term, increases are dose-related for chlorthalidone, hydrochlorothiazide, and cyclopenthiazide, but after 1 year or more of treatment, the urate levels tend to be lower.

Impotence, lethargy, photosensitivity, and dizziness also have been described with thiazide diuretics, usually at higher doses. Fever, chills, blood dyscrasisa, pancreatitis, necrotizing vasculitis, acute interstitial nephritis, and noncardiogenic pulmonary edema have been observed rarely.

Thiazides are best avoided in patients with hyponatremia, hypokalemia, diabetes, and hyperuricemia, although problems tend to develop when higher doses are used. Clearly, hypersensitivity to sulfonamides is a contraindication. As with acetazolamide, thiazides can worsen hepatic encephalopathy and precipitate coma in susceptible individuals. In general, the elderly respond well to diuretic therapy, and the greatest outcome benefit in hypertension has been described in these patients, although hypotension and electrolyte disturbances are more likely to occur. Thiazide diuretics cannot be recommended for hypertension in pregnancy because they can

Table 17.2 The pharmacokinetic values for the commonly used thiazide diuretics

Compound	Time to peak effect (h)	Elimination half-life (h)	Bioavailability	Metabolism	Excretion	Plasma protein binding (%)
Bendroflumethiazide	2	3	Complete absorption	Extensive	30% renal, 70% nonrenal	90
Chlorthalidone	4	54	Unknown	None	100% renal	90
Hydrochlorothiazide	4	6	~60%	None	100% renal	60
Indapamide	4	10-22	80%	Extensive	70% renal, mostly as metabolites	70

cause relative hypoperfusion of the placenta. Use of thiazide diuretics during the first trimester may cause an increased risk of congenital defects and hypoglycemia, thrombocytopenia, and electrolyte disturbances in the newborn. There are a few reports that thiazide diuretics may delay labor due to direct smooth muscle effects. Diuretics are not secreted in large enough amounts into breast milk to produce pharmacologic effects apart from thrombocytopenia. They can suppress lactation, however, and should be avoided.

Clinically relevant interactions with thiazide diuretics include hypotension when combined with angiotensin converting enzyme inhibitors; hypokalemia with corticosteroids, laxatives, acetazolamide, and other drugs that reduce the serum potassium level; and arrhythmias with cardiac glycosides and drugs such as quinidine that prolong the QT interval on the electrocardiograph. Thiazide diuretics also may attenuate the effect of hypoglycemic and uricosuric agents and predispose to lithium toxicity by reducing lithium clearance by the kidney. Nonsteroidal anti-inflammatory agents may reduce their antihypertensive and diuretic effects.

LOOP DIURETICS

Loop diuretics selectively reduce sodium and chloride reabsorption by inhibiting the coupled $Na^+,K^+,2Cl^-$ transport system in the thick ascending limb of the loop of Henle (Fig. 17.1). Since this segment of the renal tubule has a large absorptive capacity and diuresis is not limited by the development of acidosis, these drugs are the most effective diuretic agents available.

Pharmacokinetics

The pharmacokinetic values for the most commonly used loop diuretics are listed in Table 17.3. All are rapidly absorbed from the gastrointestinal tract with oral bioavailability ranging from 50 to 90%. They are extensively bound to plasma proteins so that delivery to the renal tubules by glomerular filtration is limited. However, they are efficiently secreted by the organic transport system in the proximal tubule and therefore can produce their effects on the thick ascending loop of Henle. Diuretic response is very rapid and effective after intravenous administration and usually lasts 2 to 4 hours. Diuretic activity correlates positively with concentrations in the renal tubule. Indomethacin and probenecid reduce tubular secretion and hence diuretic activity. Metabolites of ethacrynic acid and furosemide have been identified, but it is unclear whether they have any diuretic activity. Torsemide has a longer elimination half-life and duration of action than furosemide or bumetanide.

Side effects and interactions

Loop diuretics overall cause fewer metabolic problems than thiazide diuretics at equivalent dosages. In addition to the

Table 17.3 The pharmacokinetic parameters for the commonly used loop and potassium-sparing diuretics

Compound	Time to peak effect	Elimination half-life (h)	Bioavailability (%)	Metabolism	Excretion	Plasma protein binding (%)
Loop diuretics						
Bumetanide	1 h oral, <5 min iv	$1\frac{1}{2}$	90	Five metabolites	Renal including metabolites	95
Ethacrynic acid	1-2 h oral, <5 min iv	1	80	Conjugation in liver	Renal including metabolites	>90
Furosemide	1-2 h oral, <5 min iv	1	60	Partial to glucuronide	Renal including metabolites	95
Potassium-sparing diuretics						
Amiloride	3-4 h	6-9	50	None	100% renal	<10
Triamterene	6-8 h	2	50	Extensive to active and inactive metabolite	100% renal	50
Spironolactone	1-3 days	13-24 (canrenoate)	90	80% conversion to active metabolites	Mostly renal, some biliary	>90

well-described electrolyte changes, hyperlipidemia, pancreatitis, and allergic reactions also have been described. The risk of eighth-nerve damage occurs most commonly with ethacrynic acid and least commonly with bumetanide and is seen principally in patients with renal impairment who receive high doses.

Most of the contraindications to the use of loop diuretics are the same as those for thiazides. They are therefore best avoided in patients with liver failure, hypokalemia, hyponatremia, and volume depletion, as well as those receiving lithium In general, loop diuretics have less impact on hypoglycemic and uricosuric drugs than thiazide diuretics. The elderly respond well to loop diuretics, although the risk of hypovolemia and hypotension is greater and urinary retention can be a problem in those with prostatic hypertropy. Safety has not been clearly established in pregnancy, but there is no evidence that loop diuretics reduce amniotic fluid volume or cause thrombocytopenia in the neonate. There are also no reported adverse events with loop diuretics during breast feeding. Interactions with lithium, nonsteroidal anti-inflammatory drugs, ACE inhibitors, corticosteroids, digitalis, quinidine, and uricosuric and hypoglycemic drugs are largely the same as with thiazide diuretics. In addition, there is evidence that ethacrynic acid increases the risk of bleeding in patients receiving warfarin, and furosemide increases the risk of theophylline toxicity in patients with obstructive airways disease. Loop diuretics do increase the nephrotoxicity of the aminoglycoside antibiotics.

POTASSIUM-SPARING DIURETICS

Potassium-sparing diuretics produce effects that are opposite to those of the hormone aldosterone. Spironolactone acts by directly antagonizing the mineralocorticoid receptors, whereas triamterene and amiloride inhibit sodium transport through ion channels in the luminal membrane (Fig. 17.2). All three drugs reduce sodium absorption in the collecting tubules and ducts. Spironolactone prevents sodium reabsorption by decreasing the activity of aldosterone on the sodium-potassium exchanger. It binds to the cytoplasmic mineralocorticoid receptors and prevents translocation of the receptor complex to the nucleus in the target cells. In contrast, triamterene and amiloride do not antagonize the aldosterone receptor but reduce the entry of sodium through the sodium-selective ion channels in the apical membrane of the collecting tubule. Since potassium secretion is coupled with sodium entry in this region of the tubule, potassium retention results.

Pharmacokinetics

Since spironolactone is a synthetic steroid that is a competitive antagonist of aldosterone, its onset and duration of effect are related to the kinetics of aldosterone on the target tissue. Spironolactone is relatively well absorbed (60-70%) and extensively metabolized, undergoes

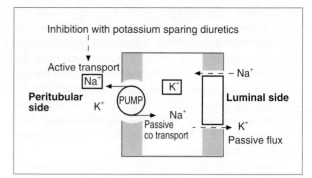

Figure 17.2 The mechanism of action of potassium-sparing diuretics.

enterohepatic recirculation, and is highly protein bound. The elimination half-life of the parent compound is approximately 1.4 days, but its major active metabolite, canrenone, has a much longer half-life of approximately 16.5 hours, which prolongs its clinical effect.

The pharmacokinetic values of triamterene and amiloride are listed in Table 17.3. Triamterene is extensively metabolized to the active metabolite that is excreted in the urine. Its activity is comparable with that of the parent compound. Toxic effects are increased in liver and renal disease. In contrast, amiloride is not metabolized and is largely excreted in urine. All three drugs need to be used with caution in patients with renal failure because of the risk of hyperkalemia.

Side effects

Hyperkalemia is the most common adverse effect of triamterene, amiloride, and spironolactone. Hyponatremia is also relatively common in elderly patients, especially in those with hypothyroidism and poor diet. Nausea, flatulence, and skin rashes also have been described, especially with amiloride. Spironolactone has a high incidence of impotence and gynecomastia in men.

The principal contraindication to the use of potassium-sparing diuretics is the presence of significant hyperkalemia, particularly if there is renal impairment. This effect tends to be more marked in elderly patients. There is no clear evidence that triamterene, amiloride, or spironolactone cause fetal abnormalities, and although excreted in breast milk, all three drugs are probably safe during lactation. Clinically important interactions are mostly with drugs that tend to increase the serum potassium level such as ACE inhibitors, β-blockers, potassium supplements, beta-adrenoceptor antagonists, and nonsteroidal anti-inflammatory drugs. Like other diuretics, lithium clearance can be reduced, and the risk of digoxin toxicity is increased. Aspirin also has been shown to reduce the effectiveness of spironolactone as a diuretic.

OSMOTIC DIURETICS

The proximal tubule and descending limb of the loop of Henle are freely permeable to water. An osmotic diuretic that is not transported promotes water retention in these segments and causes a water diuresis. The resulting increase in urine flow decreases the period the tubular fluid is in contact with the tubular epithelium, and total sodium reabsorption is reduced. Overall, more water than salt is lost, however, and hypernatremia can occur.

Suggested readings

BEERMAN B, GRIND M. Clinical pharmacokinetics of some newer diuretics. Clin Pharmacokinet 1987;13:254-66.

BRATER D. Pharmacodynamic considerations in the use of diuretics. Annu Rev Pharmacol Toxicol 1983;23:45-62.

BRATER D. Clinical pharmacology of loop diuretics. Drugs 1991;41:14-22.

CODY RJ, KUDO SH, PICKWORTH KK. Diuretic treatment for the sodium retention of congestive heart failure. Arch Intern Med 1994;154:1905-14.

COLLINS R, PETO R, MACMAHON S, et al. Blood pressure, stroke and coronary heart disease. Short-term reductions in blood pressure: overview of randomised drug trials in their epidemiological context. Lancet 1990;335:827-38.

JOHNSTON GD. Direct cardiovascular effects of diuretics. In: Puschett JB, Greenberg A, eds. Diuretics: chemistry, pharmacology and clinical applications. New York: Elsevier, 1984:438-46.

JOHNSTON GD. Selecting appropriate antihypertensive drug dosages. Drugs 1994;47:567-75.

LANT A. Diuretics: Clinical pharmacology and therapeutic use, part I. Drugs 1985;29:57-87.

LANT A. Diuretics: clinical pharmacology and therapeutic use, part II. Drugs 1985;29:162-88.

MORRISON RT. Edema and principles of diuretic use. Med Clin North Am 1997;81:689-704.

ROSE BD. Diuretics. Kidney Int 1991;39:336-52.

Siscovick DS, Raghunathan TE, Psaty BM, et al. Diuretic therapy for hypertension and the risk of primary cardiac arrest. N Engl J Med 1994;330:1852-7.

WALMA EP, HOES AW, VAN DOOREN C, et al. Withdrawal of long-term diuretic medication in elderly patients: a double blind randomised trial. Br Med J 1997;315:464-8.

WARD A, HEEL RC. Bumetanide, a review of its pharmacodynamic and pharmacokinetic properties and therapeutic use. Drugs 1984;28:426-64.

Prostate disease

Luc V. M. Baert, Hein Van Poppel, Zbigniew Petrovich

Prostate disease is a very common disorder with a variable natural history that affects middle-aged and older men. It can be divided into benign and malignant prostate disease, each mandating a different therapeutic approach.

BENIGN PROSTATIC HYPERPLASIA

The incidence of clinical benign prostatic hyperplasia (BPH) increases with age. A 40-year-old man who lives to be 80 years old has a 78% chance of developing BPH and a 29% chance of undergoing surgery for BPH. Surgery is the only proven treatment modality in the management of patients with BPH. Transurethral resection of the prostate (TURP), which constitutes 90% of surgical treatment for this disease, brings major and rapid improvement in the frequently distressing signs and symptoms of BPH in about 80% of patients. The facts that surgical complications affect one in five patients treated, that a substantial proportion of severely symptomatic patients are poor surgical risks, and that a group of patients exists who require treatment but refuse surgical therapy lead to an urgent need to continue to search for alternative treatments. Such alternative treatments consist of the following modalities: (1) endoprostheses, (2) balloon dilatation, (3) laser therapy, (4) transrectal or transurethral hyperthermia, (5) transurethral thermotherapy, and (6) treatment with pharmacologic agents.

Prostatism defines the symptoms of the clinical phase of BPH. The symptoms of prostatism are either obstructive or irritative. Obstructive symptoms include (1) decreased force of the urinary stream, (2) decreased caliber of the urinary stream, (3) hesitancy, (4) intermittency, (5) terminal dribbling, and (6) urinary retention. Irritative symptoms include (1) nocturia, (2) frequency, (3) urgency, and in extreme cases (4) urge incontinence. These symptoms are not specific for BPH and can be seen in several other conditions such as carcinoma of the prostate, urinary tract infection (UTI), neurogenic bladder, and urethral stricture.

The symptoms and treatment of BPH are intimately associated with the pathophysiology of prostatic growth. Testis-mediated growth is the result of testosterone conversion by the prostate to dihydrotestosterone (DHT) through actions of the enzyme 5α-reductase. DHT is known to inhibit programmed cell death (apoptosis) in the prostate. Prostate growth occurs with aging because of increased sensitivity to DHT or because DHT production is accelerated. Prostate growth increases bladder outlet resistance through mechanical and functional effects. As the prostate grows, there appears to be increased sensitivity to the neurotransmitters that regulate bladder and urethral function. There is evidence in both dogs and humans that chronic bladder obstruction can change the response of the bladder dome or detrusor to exogenous norepinephrine from a α-adrenoceptor-mediated relaxation to an α-adrenoceptor-mediated contraction.

Treatment

Nonpharmacologic treatment

Prostatectomy is presently the most effective and only proven treatment modality in the management of BPH. Bothersome symptoms of prostatism represent the primary surgical indication in 90% of patients undergoing TURP in the United States. In clinical practice, the diagnosis of BPH and the indications for therapeutic intervention do not depend on histopathologic findings, as the term *benign protatic hyperplasia* may suggest, but on the presence of a collection of nonspecific complaints of prostatism quantified as the *symptom score* and the presence of objective signs such as decreased flow rate, increased postvoiding residual volume, and increased volume of the prostate, along with evidence of difficulty in micturition.

About 80% of patients achieve satisfactory resolution of their symptoms following TURP. Transurethral resection of the prostate is accepted as the primary method of relieving the symptoms of BPH, whereas about 10% of BPH patients, primarily those with larger (>50 g) glands, are treated with open prostatectomy. Hyperthermia of the prostate has been used in the management of BPH for the past 20 years. The fundamental task of prostate microwave hyperthermia is to selectively increase the temperature of the target volume up to 44°C for approximately 1 hour. Initially, hyperthermia of the prostate for BPH was limited to transrectal hyperthermia (TRHT), now infrequently used because of its limited ability to heat the periurethral region of the prostate and limited clinical efficacy.

Transurethral hyperthermia (TUHT) was developed in 1985, and the first clinical study was completed in 1988. Multiple laboratory and phase I and II clinical trials have demonstrated the presence of histologic lesions in the periurethral prostate and have shown objective and subjective improvements in more than 70% of treated patients. TUHT was found to be effective in patients presenting with retention and relatively (30%) ineffective in patients with predominant median lobe hyperplasia.

Transurethral thermotherapy (intraprostatic temperature between 46 and 60 °C) is another microwave heating modality. At such high temperatures, a single 1-hour session has been shown to induce thermocoagulation of BPH tissue. Thermotherapy should be distinguished from hyperthermia in that its goal is to create an irreversible tissue lesion that has a favorable effect on the irritative and obstructive symptoms of BPH.

Drug therapy

In comparing surgery with the alternative treatment modalities, it is appropriate to consider not only treatment efficacy but also its tolerance by patients and the cost of the different types of treatments. Approximately 15% of men undergoing TURP have a relapse and will require reintervention within 8 years. Nonsurgical treatment alternatives are of even greater importance in this group of patients with recurrent disease. The optimal patient for medical therapy has yet to be defined. Many pharmacologic agents have been used in the management of symptomatic BPH patients, with the α-adrenergic blockers being used most frequently. Histologically, the prostate is composed of epithelium, smooth muscle, connective tissue, and glandular lumen. In BPH tissue, the ratio of stroma to epithelium is approximately 5:1. Stromal hyperplasia generally is irreversible; hence this component of BPH may not be influenced hormonally. An important stromal component is smooth muscle. Several studies confirm the presence of smooth muscle as a significant histologic component in BPH tissue.

Drug classes

ALPHA BLOCKERS

The rationale for α-adrenergic blockade in the treatment of symptomatic BPH was based initially on demonstration in rat prostate of smooth muscle contractility in response to the adrenergic agonist norepinephrine. Similar observations in the human prostate pointed to the clinical usefulness of α-adrenergic blockade in symptomatic BPH patients. The next step was demonstration that the contractility of the human prostate is mediated by the α_1-adrenoceptors and that these receptors are concentrated in the bladder base and prostate but not in the bladder body. Alpha$_1$-antagonists could relax the muscle tone of the bladder outlet and prostatic urethra without inhibiting bladder contractility, mak-

Table 18.1 Pharmacologic effects of alpha activation (the contraction of smooth muscle involved in sphincter activity mediated by alpha activation is an important factor in obstruction voiding)

Target organ	α_1	α_2
Vessels	Constriction	Constriction
Bronchi	Constriction	–
Digestive system muscle	Relaxation	–
Digestive system sphincter	Contraction	–
Uterus	Contraction	–
Bladder detrusor	–	–
Bladder sphincter	Contraction	–
Reproductive system	Ejaculation	–
Iris-m.dil.pupillae	Mydriasis	–
Heart	–	–
Skeletal muscle	–	–
Liver	Glycogenolysis	–
Fatty tissue	–	–
Kidney	↓renin secretion	–
Pancreas	↓insulin secretion	–
Neuro-effector junction	–	↓norepinephrine release, →↓blood pressure
Central nervous system	Excitation	Sedation, ↓outflow to orthosympatic system, →↓blood pressure

ing these drugs useful in the treatment of BPH.

Alpha-adrenoceptors, which are transmembrane glycoproteins on the surfaces of specific cells, bind molecules such as norepinephrine and result in the formation of second messengers that modify cell activity. There are two main types, α_1 and α_2 adrenoreceptors (Tab. 18.1). α_1 adrenoreceptors are situated postjunctionally, whereas α_2 adrenoreceptors are prejunctional, regulating neurotransmitter release. Activating α_1 adrenoreceptors leads to a higher concentration of its second messenger, IP-3, whereas activating α_2 adrenoreceptors leads to a lower concentration of its second messenger, cyclic AMP, which has a negative feedback effect on norepinephrine release. Recent studies have led to subdivision of the α_1 adrenoceptors into three subtypes (α_{1a}, α_{1b}, and α_{1d}), and all three receptors have a high affinity for prazosin (α_{1H}). Following the cloning of multiple α_1 adrenoceptors, the contractile response in human prostate has been assigned to the α_{1a}-adrenoceptor subtype, represented in prostate stroma. Many agents have been used in clinical studies. The early studies were performed with nonselective α blockers (Tab. 18.2) such as phenoxybenzamine, an irreversible antagonist. Symptomatic improvement was seen

Table 18.2 Affinity of antagonists on adrenergic receptor subtypes

Antagonist	α_1	α_2	β_1	β_2
Phentolamine	+	+++	-	-
Phenoxybenzamine	+++	+++	-	-
Prazosin	+++	+	-	-
Indoramin	+++	+	-	-

in 18 of 27 BPH patients treated with phenoxybenzamine over a period of 7 days. Clinical use of phenoxybenzamine is now limited because of proven carcinogenicity in rodents.

Prazosin Prazosin, a highly selective α_1 antagonist without subtype selectivity (Tab. 18.3), has long been used clinically as an antihypertensive agent. Several clinical trials with prazosin found a significant reduction in residual urine volume and an increase in urine flow rate, whereas symptomatic improvement was observed in 77% of BPH patients treated. Some investigators found a significant improvement in obstructive symptoms but a minimal effect on irritative symptoms, in contrast to phenoxybenzamine. Prazosin doses used in these studies were low (2-4 mg/day), and the beneficial effect appeared to be dose-related. The treatment side-effect profile of prazosin was superior to that of phenoxybenzamine. Despite these favorable reports, prazosin was not widely accepted in urologic practice. Other limiting factors in the use of prazosin are the requirement for dose titration to prevent cardiovascular side effects such as dizziness and syncope and the relatively short duration of action, which requires two to three daily doses.

Terazosin Terazosin is a structural analogue of prazosin, differing only in the replacement of a furan substituent with tetrahydrofuran. Like prazosin, it has no α_1 subtype selectivity. Terazosin has a longer duration of action, allowing for once-daily administration. Sustained efficacy over 2 years has been demonstrated. As a result of

side effects of terazosin therapy, most commonly consisting of dizziness, asthenia, and light-headedness, 5% of patients withdrew from a phase III clinical trial. Dosages of terazosin employed (20 mg/day) were not well tolerated. A plateau of therapeutic efficacy, however, has not yet been attained at doses of 10 mg per day.

Doxazosin Doxazosin is also a structural analogue of prazosin. It has no subtype selectivity, and it has the longest plasma half-life of the α_1 antagonists used in the treatment of BPH. The longer plasma half-life may result in improved treatment tolerance. Several clinical trials have demonstrated treatment efficacy both in terms of symptom score reduction and an increase in urine flow rate. Despite the use of dose titration, dizziness was still the most commonly observed side effect, seen in up to 24% of patients.

Alfusozin Alfuzosin is another structural analogue of prazosin without subtype selectivity. The efficacy of alfuzosin has been demonstrated in several clinical trials. Long-term beneficial effects of therapy have been confirmed. Cardiovascular side effects are less common than those seen with prazosin, and dose titration is not required. A three-times-daily schedule generally is used because of the short duration of action of alfuzosin. A recent trial with a sustained-release formulation of alfuzosin showed good results with an incidence of side effects similar to that of placebo obtained on twice-daily alfuzosin administration.

Bunasozin Bunazosin, another structural analogue of prazosin, has been shown to be an effective agent in BPH. Studies in hypertensive patients would suggest less orthostatic effect than other prazosin analogues, without the need for dose titration.

Indoramin The design of new α_1 antagonists for BPH has concentrated on agents producing preferential blockade of urogenital vis-à-vis vascular α_1 adrenoceptors, based either on selectivity for the α_{1a}-adrenoceptor subtype or on functional uroselectivity in animal models. The

Table 18.3 Major kinetic parameters and peceptor affinity of currently available α_1 selective antagonists

Compound	$t_{1/2}$ (h)	Daily intakes	α_{1a} subtype selectivity	Need of titration	Affinity for α_{1a} subtype (-pKi)
Alfuzosin	5	3-2	No	No	7.0±0.2
Doxazosin	20	2-4	No	Yes	8.2±0.68
Indoramin	ND	ND	Yes	No	?
Prazosin	Short	2-3	No	Yes	8.6±0.19
Tamsulosin	10	6	Yes	No	9.2±0.56
Terazosin	12	1	No	Yes	6.9±0.12

(Adapted from Kirby RS, Pool JL. Alpha adrenoceptor blockade in the treatment of benign prostatic hyperplasia. Br J Urol 1997;80:521-32.)

main goal at the present time is to reduce the side effects of therapy. On the other hand, nonselective α blockers are preferable in hypertensive patients with BPH. Indoramin is structurally unrelated to prazosin and has selectivity for the α_{1a}-adrenoceptor subtype. The reported affinity ratio of α_{1a} to α_{1b} ranges from a low of 3- to 4-fold to a high of 10-fold. The efficacy of indoramin in patients with BPH with both objective and subjective improvement has been clearly demonstrated. There appears to be no associated decrease in blood pressure, and titration of the dose is not needed because of the lack of orthostatic hypotension. Otherwise, sedation is a commonly observed side effect of indoramin therapy. Indoramin is the leading α_1 antagonist for the treatment of BPH in the United Kingdom. Whether the moderate α_{1a} subtype selectivity is responsible for its initial clinical advantage has yet to be demonstrated.

Tamsulosin Tamsulosin is structurally unrelated to prazosin and shows a moderate degree (13-15-fold) of selectivity for the human α_{1a} versus α_{1b} adrenoceptor. However, it has an equal affinity for the α_{1a} and α_{1d} adrenoceptor. Dose titration is not required. Side effects of the vascular type were not observed in clinical trials. Results of recent large-scale trials confirm the efficacy of tamsulosin. Clinical effects of tamsulosin appear to result from selectivity for the α_{1a}-adrenoceptor subtype or possibly the α_{1L} subtype.

The question remains: How effective is α blockade? Patients who had completed a clinical trial with prazosin and subsequently underwent surgery confirmed the well-known observation that surgery produced a greater improvement in both symptom score and urinary flow rates. While surgery remains superior to therapy with pharmacologic agents, advantage is gained at the cost of lost work time and a greater probability of treatment-related complications.

ANDROGEN SUPPRESSORS

The rationale for androgen suppression therapy is to reduce the size of the adenoma, reducing outlet resistance and improving the symptoms of prostatism. Prostate volume reduction induced by androgen suppression is well known, especially when treating prostatic malignancy. The development and maintenance of BPH require an intact hypothalamus-pituitary-testes-prostate axis. Agents acting by androgen inhibition have their primary effect on the glandular epithelium. Epithelial hyperplasia is usually reversible. Medical castration using several different agents such as gonadotropin-releasing hormone (GnRH) agonists, synthetic antiandrogens, progestational hormones, nonsteroidal antiandrogens, and 5α-reductase inhibitors may at times lead to morbidity greater than the symptoms of BPH. Consequently, the number of well-studied drugs in this category is rather limited.

Finasteride The most extensively studied drug is the 5α-reductase inhibitor finasteride. Finasteride, a neutral 4-aza

steroid, is a selective competitive inhibitor of the type II isoform of 5α-reductase, the most important of the two NADPH-dependent isoenzymes in the human prostate. The mechanism of testosterone reduction involves the formation of a binary complex between the enzyme and NADPH, followed by the formation of a ternary complex with testosterone. The half-life of finasteride is 4.7 to 7.1 hours. The drug undergoes extensive hepatic metabolism through oxidation. Serum dihydrotestosterone (DHT) levels are not lowered to castration levels because of the action of type I 5α-reductase, but nevertheless, finasteride lowers the DHT concentration in prostatic tissue by more than 85%. This drug has no androgenic, estrogenic, or gestagenic properties and has no affinity for the androgen receptor. It needs to be administered for at least 6 to 12 months (5 mg/day). The most important effect of finasteride is in reducing prostate size by 19 to 23%. The average improvement in symptom score is small, with only 1.3 to 1.8 points on the symptom score over placebo. For an average patient, a difference in symptom score of this magnitude would be imperceptible. Furthermore, the use of finasteride does not protect against acute retention.

Efficacy limitations of finasteride have caused investigators to realize that the importance of DHT in BPH may have been overestimated. Nevertheless, a 2-year Scandinavian finasteride study demonstrated worsening of maximum flow rate in the placebo group but improvement in the finasteride group. The mean difference in urinary flow rates between finasteride and placebo groups was only 1.9 ml/s. Prostate volume increased by 12% in the placebo group, whereas it decreased by 19% in the finasteride group.

How does one determine which patients will respond best to which type of therapy, and how does one predict the treatment outcome? Since the onset of improvement with α blockers is rapid (within 1 to 3 weeks), it may be appropriate to give men with symptoms of BPH a trial of α blockade. If the patient does not respond within 3 to 4 months, alternative therapy should be considered. Patients with a history of orthostatic hypotension should not be treated with α blockers. The treatment outcome for patients with α blockade therapy possibly could be predicted by sampling prostate tissue with needle biopsies, with more smooth muscle content predicting better results. As for finasteride, men with small prostates would be expected to have a small improvement only, whereas those with large glands (volumes > 40 cc) are more likely to have a greater benefit. Empiric drug trials still seem to be the best way to differentiate responders to a specific therapy from nonresponders. Nevertheless, it has been reported that patients with a high pretreatment prostate-specific antigen (PSA) level responded well to antiandrogen therapy, whereas those with a low PSA level responded better to α blockade.

Another therapeutic approach to the treatment of BPH, commonly referred to as *phytotherapy,* encompasses a variety of plant extracts. Although this approach has been used for many years, objective evidence for its efficacy has been limited. Several different mechanisms of action have been proposed for these drugs, but the biochemical mechanisms and pathways remain unclear. Some of these agents are in wide use and probably are effective, e.g., *Serenoa repens, Echinacea,* and *Sabal* extracts.

CARCINOMA OF THE PROSTATE

Carcinoma of the prostate constitutes a major and escalating international health problem. The risk of developing a clinically significant prostate cancer during a lifetime is about 10%, and approximately 25% of men with prostate cancer die of the disease. Currently, 9% of all cases are thought to have a genetic basis. Prostate carcinoma expands peripherally through the capsule, favoring passage through the perineural spaces that perforate the capsule only at the upper-outer corner and the apex. Unlike most other forms of cancer, not every prostate cancer constitutes a serious threat to life, and thus not every one necessarily warrants treatment. Many elderly men die "with" rather than "of" prostate cancer.

Bladder outflow obstruction can lead to secondary problems such as recurrent urinary tract infections (UTIs), resulting in frequency, dysuria, and hematuria. Urinary stasis can cause formation of bladder stones, predisposing the patient to recurrent urinary sepsis. Irritation of the bladder trigone by stones may result in suprapubic pain, stranguria, and hematuria. Hematuria may be associated with dysuria due to malignant infiltration of the prostatic urethral urothelium. At least one-quarter of men with prostate cancer at presentation also will have bone metastases detectable by isotopic bone scan. Sudden onset of progressive low back pain is a cardinal symptom. Metastatic disease within the vertebral bodies is common, and compression of the spinal cord causing neurologic symptoms may occur in 1 to 12% of patients. The main diagnostic tools include (1) digital rectal examination (DRE), (2) transrectal ultrasonography (TRUS), and (3) determination of the PSA level in serum.

Several clinical parameters need to be considered when evaluating PSA levels. A definite elevation of PSA is also possible with nonmalignant prostatic diseases. Enlarged glands with BPH account for most borderline elevations of PSA. An antigen level above 10 ng/ml is most unlikely to be due to BPH alone, and further evaluation is indicated. Injury to normal prostate tissue can raise the PSA level for several days. Prostatitis can elevate the PSA level over the short term, as can a prostatic infarction. Initial PSA level at the time of diagnosis is an important parameter to estimate the extent of the prostate tumor. A PSA level of 10 ng/ml or more is frequently associated with a more advanced tumor stage. As long as the PSA level is less than 20 ng/ml, tumor metastasis is unlikely. Adequate staging is very important to define the most efficient form of therapy in an individual patient.

Routine examinations are DRE, TRUS, and TRUS-guided biopsies, leading to a histologic staging using the Gleason grading system. This is a five-step grading system, and the two most prominent grades are added together to give the so-called Gleason score. To exclude lymph node metastases, a computed tomographic (CT) scan of the pelvis is performed. The TNM classification of 1997 is also used commonly in prostate carcinoma.

Treatment

Treatments of general use in the disease

In men with localized prostate cancer and a life expectancy of 10 years or more, the goal is to eradicate the disease. Watchful waiting can be advocated in patients with a shorter life expectancy and low-stage and low-grade tumors but is not acceptable in younger men at higher risk of tumor progression. Because prostate cancer is an androgen-dependent tumor, primary hormonal treatment may be given in patients with clinically localized prostate cancer when they are not suitable candidates for more aggressive treatment. Complete eradication of localized prostate cancer can be achieved either by radical prostatectomy or by radiation therapy.

Radical prostatectomy is used widely today only in men in whom it is likely that the malignancy is completely removable by surgery, affording cure (T1 or T2 disease with low- to moderate-grade pathology). Radiation therapy provides an alternative, definitive treatment approach to localized prostate carcinoma. Locally extensive prostate cancer (T3) is seen in about 40% of all clinically diagnosed tumors, and management remains controversial. Radical prostatectomy, radiation therapy, radiation therapy in combination with hormonal treatment, and primary hormonal treatment are the options most frequently discussed. T3a cancer is defined as having extracapsular extension, whereas in T3b cancer the seminal vesicles are also invaded. In extracapsular tumors, radical prostatectomy often will not succeed in achieving complete tumor excision.

Hormonal therapy before prostatectomy (so-called neoadjuvant) has not been shown to be effective in decreasing the risk of positive surgical margins or to prolong the time to PSA progress in T3c prostate cancer. Various therapeutic shedules can be used in neoadjuvant hormonal therapy: high-dose monotherapy with cyproterone acetate (CPA), a combination of goserelin acetate or leuprorelin acetate with CPA or flutamide, or flutamide monotherapy (products and doses; see below). Radiation therapy also has been used for T3 cancers in the hope of cure. Nearly 90% of these patients have rising serum PSA levels within 10 years of therapy. Recent studies have shown that the combination of radiotherapy and hormonal treatment yields better local control and also improves survival when performed for T3 tumors.

Patients with a preoperative diagnosis of lymph node involvement usually are not considered to be good candidates for radical surgery. Mostly they will be treated by hormonal manipulation. Despite the trend to earlier diagnosis, many patients (up to 33%) still present with either bony and/or soft tissue metastases. Other develop disseminated disease despite the best curative endeavors employed at a stage when the disease was still localized. Hormonal therapy has played a growing role in the treatment of prostate cancer. The basis of hormonal therapy is androgen deprivation, which can be achieved through the inhibition of either androgen production or androgen action. Two pathways have been recognized for the production of androgens in the mammalian body, one in the testis and one in the adrenal cortex (5% of total activity) from androstenedione and dehydroepiandrosterone.

Drug therapy

Bilateral subcapsular orchiectomy, resulting in a 95% reduction in circulating testosterone down to a level of 10 to 50 ng/100 ml within 24 hours, is the most cost-effective and compliant method of androgen deprivation. Estrogen preparations, such as diethylstilbestrol (DES), are very inexpensive but have well-documented complications, such as gynecomastia, impotence, a change in the distribution of body fat, peripheral edema, and cardiovascular complications, that are clearly dose-dependent. Because of these complications, daily doses were reduced to 3 mg. Doses of 1 mg did not suppress the testosterone levels reliably into the castrate range. Gynecomastia can be prevented by superficial radiation of the breast tissue at a dose up to 15 Gy before therapy.

Drug classes

ANTIANDROGENS

Nilutamide, flutamide, bicalutamide Antiandrogens block the action of androgens at the target cells. They may be divided into two types: steroidal with progestational effects and nonsteroidal with only an antiandrogen effect and no other endocrine properties. Testosterone production is not affected. The three pure antiandrogens currently used (nilutamide, flutamide, and bicalutamide) are associated with a rise in serum testosterone and luteinizing hormone (LH) levels resulting from the inhibition of feedback at the hypothalamic-pituitary level. Nilutamide has a half-life of about 40 hours, allowing once-daily administration of 300 mg. Its side effects include hot flushes, nausea, visual disturbances, alcohol intolerance, and rarely, interstitial pneumonia. Flutamide (250 mg tid) has a shorter half-life (5 to 6 hours). Most treated patients retain libido and sexual potency, due to the rise in testosterone level. It is approved for the use only in combination with a GnRH agonist. Gynecomastia, nausea, vomiting, diarrhea, and infrequently, liver dysfunction are the possible side effects. Bicalutamide, with a half-life of 7 to 10 days, appears to elevate serum testosterone levels like flutamide. However, its long half-life enables maintenance of high serum concentrations and allows once-daily dosing (150 mg). The most important complications are breast tenderness (30%), gynecomastia (25%), and hot flushes (8%).

Cyproterone Cyproterone acetate, a steroidal antiandrogen, also has progestational properties, inhibiting

testosterone production. It produces a potent androgen withdrawal effect through its central and peripheral modes of action. The central effect of progestational activity causes partial suppression of pituitary gonadotropins. Side effects are impotence in all patients, fatigue, weakness, headache, gynecomastia, and some cardiovascular toxicity.

DECAPEPTIDE LUTEINIZING HORMONE–RELEASING HORMONE (LHRH) AGONISTS

The administration of decapeptide LHRH agonists (goserelin acetate, 3.6 mg; buserelin acetate, 5.5 mg; leuprorelin acetate, 3.75 mg; and triptorelin acetate, 3.75 mg) causes an initial stimulation of LH and follicle-stimulating hormone (FSH) production with a rise in the serum testosterone level to 140 to 170% of basal levels. Within 2 weeks, however, they cause a suppression of testosterone – by making the pituitary resistant to stimulation by endogenous LHRH – similar to surgical castration. Adrenal testosterone, since it is controlled by adrenocorticotropic hormone (ACTH), is unaffected.

LHRH agonists cannot be given orally because they would be destroyed by peptic digestion. They are available as monthly copolymer and depot suspension formulations to be injected either subcutaneously or intramuscularly. A new long-acting 10.8-mg depot formulation of goserelin has been developed and is effective when used on a 3-monthly basis. The principal side effect is the potential "tumor flare" accompanying the initial rise in testosterone concentration. This can be avoided by the concomitant use of antiandrogens or estrogens during the first 4 weeks. The advantage of LHRH analogues is that they avoid the trauma of orchiectomy and the side effects of estrogen therapy (e.g., gynecomastia, increased platelet adhesiveness).

DRUGS USED FOR TOTAL ANDROGEN DEPRIVATION

Total androgen deprivation is defined as the withdrawal of testicular and adrenal androgens. After medical or surgical therapy, adrenal androgens are responsible for maintaining intraprostatic DHT levels, continuing to stimulate androgen-sensitive cells. Possible therapeutic schedules include a combination of leuprorelin or goserelin acetate or bilateral orchiectomy with either flutamide or nilutamide or bicalutamide. The best results of total androgen blockade are observed in a subgroup of patients with metastatic prostate cancer, namely, the ones with good prognostic factors. Other methods to achieve total androgen blockade involve the use of aminoglutethimide and ketoconazole.

Aminoglutethimide Aminoglutethimide (week 1: 125 mg bid; week 2: 250 mg bid; week 3: 250 mg tid; and afterwards: 250 mg qid) blocks the conversion of cholesterol into pregnenolone, a precursor of adrenal androgens. This effect is accomplished by binding to the cytochrome P-450 moiety of enzyme complexes. Replacement glucocorticoids must be given to avoid cortisol insufficiency and to prevent the reflex rise in ACTH that would overcome the chemical blockade.

Ketoconazole Ketoconazole, a synthetic antifungal imidazole dioxalane, is a potent inhibitor of cytochrome P-450 and, at higher dose (400 mg tid), of C17–20 lyase in the adrenals, thus reducing adrenal androgen production. Plasma glucocorticoids and mineralocorticoids are not affected. Side effects at this high dose are common (e.g., gastrointestinal and hepatic toxicity).

Estramustine Estramustine phosphate, a combination of nitrogen mustard linked to a phosphorylated estradiol, is rapidly dephosphorylated in the body to estramustine and estromustine. About 10% of these metabolites are hydrolyzed to estradiol and estrone, which depress testosterone levels. Cytotoxicity is due mainly to its ability to bind to and disassemble microtubule-associated proteins (MAPs), which are essential to microtubule stability and the cell cycle. Mitotic arrest and cell death are the result. Estramustine accumulates preferentially in the prostate. At a dose of 560 mg per day it elicits complete androgen ablation.

OTHER THERAPIES

Due to clonal selection of androgen-independent cell lines, every advanced prostate cancer treated by androgen ablation eventually may escape from the growth-restraining effects of low androgen levels. For those patients treated initially by monotherapy, the addition of an antiandrogen would seem appropriate. However, this has disappointingly little, if any, beneficial effect. Patients who have been managed with maximal androgen blockade may benefit from cessation of the antiandrogen. This "antiandrogen withdrawal syndrome" is unexplained but could be the result of an agonist effect of the antiandrogen on mutated androgen receptors in tumor cells. PSA declines by 50 to 80% and remains low for about 5 months. Estramustine can be used in combination with vinblastine, a *Vinca* alkaloid that inhibits microtubule formation. PSA decreases by 60% or more, and major pain relief occures in 42% of patients. Another combination is oral estramustine (15 mg/kg/day) and oral etoposide (50 mg/m^2/day) for 21 days, repeating the cycle every 28 days, resulting in significant effect in patients with hormone-refractory carcinoma.

Chemotherapy is of very little value when used on prostate cancers that are refractory to hormonal therapy. The use of such cytotoxic agents in elderly patients carries a great risk for side effects and impairment of renal and hepatic function. Mitomycin C, doxorubicin, and cisplatin have response rates of 20%. Nevertheless, epirubicin (100 mg/m^2 intravenously every 3 weeks) has a response rate of 32%. Side effects are hematologic toxicity, nausea, vomiting, mucositis, and alopecia. There is evidence that some patients with painful bony metastases from prostate cancer may benefit from treatment with bisphosphonates (see Chap. 46). The only side effect is gastrointestinal discomfort when patients continue oral therapy. Use of the β-emitting isotope strontium-89 chloride (150 mBq; slow injection into a fast-running intravenous line) could produce some improvement in pain control in patients with bony metastases. Side effects are thrombocytopenia (dose related, reaching usually 5 to 7 weeks after treatment) and other hematologic signs of toxicity. Care should be taken in patients with renal insufficiency, since the drug is excreted through the kidneys. If the first injection is not beneficial, the second probably will be no more effective. In 80% of responders, the effects last 3 months or longer, after which a further dose may be required, when hematology allows.

Based on laboratory data and published results of numerous clinical trials, it is apparent that major effort is needed to develop new treatment strategies in the management of prostate disease. The number of prostate patients is expected to increase progressively with the increase in the average age of men. This alone should stimulate an interest to develop new pharmologic treatments that are more effective and less toxic than the presently available medications.

Acknowledgments

We would like to express our gratitude to Bjorn Verlinde, MD, Kelly De Keersmaecker, MD, and Filip Ameye, MD for their generous cooperation. We would also like to thank Dr. Paul Tuytens, K.U. Leuven for his help.

Suggested readings

CHAPPLE CR, NOBLE JG, et al. Comparative study of selective α$_1$-adrenoceptor blockade versus surgery in the treatment of prostatic obstruction. Br J Urol 1993;72:822-5.

CHODAK GW. LHRH agonists for the treatment of advanced prostate carcinoma. Urology:1989;33:42-4.

DANESHGARI F, CRAWFORD ED. Endocrine therapy of advanced carcinoma of the prostate. Cancer 1993;71:1089-97.

FREEMAN JA, LIESKOVSKY G, GROSSFELD G, et al. Adjuvant radiation, hormone and chemotherapy in pathological stage D1 adenocarcinoma of the prostate. Urology 1994;44:719-25.

GOETHUYS H, BAERT L, VAN POPPEL H, et al. Treatment of metastatic carcinoma of the prostate. Am J Clin Oncol (CCT) 1997;20:40-5.

HIEBLE JP, RUFFOLO RR JR. The use of alpha-adrenoceptor antagonists in the pharmalogical management of benign prostatic hypertrophy: an overview. Pharmacol Res 1996;33:145-60.

KIRBY RS, POOL JL. Alpha adrenoceptor blockade in the treatment of benign prostatic hyperplasia: past, present and future. Br J Urol 1997;80:521-32.

LABRIE F, DUPONT A, BELANGER A, et al. Combination therapy

with flutamide and castration in advanced prostate cancer: Marked improvement in response and survival. J Steroid Biochem 1985;23:833-41.

LEPOR H, WILLIFORD WO, et al. The efficacy of terazosin, finasteride, or both in benign prostatic hyperplasia. N Engl J Med 1996;335:533-39.

PETROVICH Z, AMEYE F, BAERT L, et al. New trends in the treatment of benign prostatic hyperplasia and carcinoma of the prostate. Am J Clin Oncol 1993;16:187-200.

PETROVICH Z, BAERT L, MALCOLM A, et al. Adenocarcinoma of the prostate: Innovations in management. Am J Clin Oncol 1997;20:111-19.

SHAPIRO E, HARTANO V, et al. The response to alpha blockade in benign prostatic hyperplasia is related to the percent area density of prostate smooth muscle. Prostate 1992;21:297-307.

TAMMELA T. Benign prostatic hyperplasia: practical treatment guidelines. Drugs Aging 1997;10:349-66.

YAGODA A, PETRYLAK D. Cytotoxic chemotherapy for advanced hormone-resistant prostate cancer. Cancer 1993;71:1098-109.

19

Urinary retention and incontinence

Walter Artibani, Francesco Pesce

Normal vesicourethral function involves a *storage phase,* usually lasting several hours, in which urine accumulates in the bladder and a *voiding phase,* lasting less than a minute, in which the bladder is completely emptied. Pressure in the system is always maintained in a low range. During the filling phase, this can occur only in the absence of either involuntary phasic detrusor contractions (detrusor overactivity) or gradual intravesical pressure increments due to a diminished bladder compliance. The normal filling detrusor pressure usually does not exceed 10 to 12 cmH$_2$O at the maximum bladder capacity (500 ml in adults). Low pressure ranges are also maintained during micturition (0-30 cmH$_2$O in females, 25-45 cmH$_2$O in males), provided no anatomic or functional bladder outlet obstruction exists. Causes of anatomic outflow obstruction include bladder neck contracture, benign prostatic hypertrophy (BPH) or prostatic carcinoma, and urethral strictures. Functional types of obstruction include a lack of coordination between detrusor contraction and the relaxation of the smooth or striated urethral sphincter (detrusor-sphincter dyssynergia).

In the normal adult, the entire micturition cycle is under voluntary cerebral control and is regulated by a pontine mesencephalic reticular formation center. All three branches of the nervous system, i.e., parasympathetic, sympathetic, and somatic, are involved. The hypogastric nerves convey the efferent sympathetic fibers to the bladder and urethra. The preganglionic sympathetic neurons are located in the intermediolateral nuclei of the thoracolumbar region (T10-L2 segments) of the spinal cord. There, the axons form the paravertebral (sympathetic) chain ganglia and then the inferior mesenteric ganglion, which sends both preganglionic and postganglionic fibers through the hypogastric nerves to the pelvic plexus and the urogenital organs. The role of the sympathetic supply to the bladder dome is essentially inhibitory of parasympathetic activity during the filling phase, thus enabling accumulation of urine at low pressure and continence. In males, the sympathetic supply to bladder base and bladder outlet plays an important role by increasing the resting tone of these structures during ejaculation, thus pre-

venting the reflux of semen to the bladder (retrograde ejaculation).

The parasympathetic motor supply to the pelvic organs arises from the parasympathetic nucleus in the intermediolateral column of the spinal cord (S2-4). The preganglionic fibers travel through the anterior roots and the pelvic nerves, carrying efferent parasympathetic transmission to both the pelvic plexus and other ganglia in proximity to the bladder, and the wall of the urethra and other pelvic organs, from which postganglionic parasympathetic fibers innervate the smooth musculature of the viscera. Cholinergic neuromuscular transmission is the predominant mechanism responsible for bladder contraction, leading to an intravesical pressure rise and subsequent voiding. A nonadrenergic, noncholinergic (NANC) type of transmission is also known to be involved. The amount of intravesical pressure exerted by a detrusor contraction during voiding is greatly dependent on the grade of simultaneous relaxation of the striated musculature of the pelvic floor and external urethral sphincter (rhabdosphincter). The motor supply of these structures comes from the pudendal nerves (somatic), the motor neurons of which are located in Onuf's nucleus in the ventral horns of the sacral spinal cord (S2-4).

It is likely that sympathetic fibers also play a role in motor innervation of the external urethral sphincter. Both pelvic and, to a lesser extent, hypogastric nerves conduct afferent stimuli from the bladder and urethra to the spinal cord, via the dorsal root ganglia at the sacral and toracholumbar levels, respectively. Sensation from the perineum and genitalia are conveyed by the pudendal nerves to the sacral cord.

Neuroreceptors for the main neuromuscular transmitters are present throughout the lower urinary tract. Cholinergic and α-adrenergic receptors predominate in the bladder body, and β-adrenergic receptors predominate in the bladder base, bladder neck, prostatic urethra, prostate, and to a lesser extent, the external urethral sphincter. The alpha receptors have been subdivided into α$_1$ receptors (postsynaptic), including four undertype receptors (α$_{1A}$, α$_{1B}$, α$_{1C}$, and α$_{1L}$), and α$_2$ receptors (presynaptic). Two subtypes of β-adrenergic receptors have been identified: the β_1 receptors (postsynaptic) and the β_2 receptors (both presynaptic and postsynaptic).

The cholinergic receptors are divided into muscarinic and nicotinic. In the past 10 years, two subtypes of muscarinic receptors, named M1 and M2, have been recognized. The first are located mainly within the central nervous system. The second are found predominantly in the viscera. More recently, M3 receptors also have been found in the detrusor.

Besides acetylcholine and norepinephrine, several other substances, among them prostaglandins, vasoactive intestinal protein (VIP), and somatostatin, have been localized in the vesicourethral area, but their role as neurotransmitters has yet to be elucidated. A precise knowledge of the type, location, and function of vesicourethral neuroreceptors is crucial in order to pharmacologically manipulate lower urinary tract function.

VESICOURETHRAL DYSFUNCTION

Urinary retention and incontinence are the main dysfunctional disorders of the lower urinary tract. They represent a failure in the voiding and storage phases of the micturition cycle, respectively. Not infrequently, the simultaneous combination of the two conditions constitutes a true therapeutic challenge for the clinician.

Urinary retention

An impairment of the voiding phase may be due to a primarily inefficient detrusor contraction (detrusor underactivity), or it may be secondary to bladder outlet obstruction (BOO). Detrusor contractility may be impaired (or completely lacking) as a consequence of neurogenic, myogenic, or psychogenic conditions, or it may be induced pharmacologically. Neurogenic causes include diseases affecting the sacral cord, the cauda equina, or peripheral vesicourethral innervation. Myogenic detrusor underactivity is a common finding in the elderly as a consequence of the aging process. It also may be secondary to chronic BOO (decompensated detrusor). Psychogenic (or psychosomatic) impairment of detrusor contractility usually leads to complete acontractility and total urinary retention. The involuntary psychogenic inhibition of the detrusor is mainly mediated by a hyperactive pelvic floor musculature, which prevents the detrusor contraction from being triggered.

Pharmacologic inhibition of voluntary detrusor contractility, usually by means of anticholinergic agents, may be pursued intentionally in order to treat a hyperreflexic neurogenic voiding dysfunction, in combination with intermittent catheterization. More frequently, this is a side effect of drugs used for other purposes (antidepressants, antiparkinsonians, antiepileptics, etc.). Eventually, bladder emptying becomes incomplete, leading to the presence of residual urine that is prone to become infected. The anatomic capacity of the bladder tends to increase, but its functional capacity decreases because the filling phase begins with a bladder that is already partially filled. Bladder compliance may decrease, causing a progressive pressurization in the system during filling and leading, in the most severe instances, to upper urinary tract dilatation and deterioration (chronic urinary retention and obstructive uropathy). Depending on the concomitant presence of detrusor instability (i.e., the presence of involuntary, uninhibited detrusor contractions during the filling phase), urinary urge incontinence may coexist. This combination of detrusor dysfunction (underactivity and instability), quite common in the elderly population, is rather unsuitable for pharmacologic manipulation, since all the drugs used for decreasing involuntary detrusor hyperactivity also depress the voluntary detrusor contractility, aggravating bladder retention.

Urinary retention also may be secondary to organic or functional BOO, i.e., an impediment to urinary flow located at the level of the bladder neck (internal or smooth muscle urethral sphincter), prostatic urethra, or external (striated muscle) urethral sphincter. Table 19.1 enumerates various causes of BOO, the most commonly being benign prostatic hypertrophy (BPH).

Urinary incontinence

Urinary incontinence may be due to an overactive bladder (urge incontinence or detrusor incontinence) or to a weak and/or hypermobile sphincter mechanism (stress incontinence or urethral incontinence). In females, incompetence of the sphincter mechanism may be caused by direct damage (induced by surgery, trauma, or neuropathy) or indirect damage (such as that following several periurethral surgical procedures). Urethral hypermobility is secondary

---

Table 19.1 Causes of bladder outlet obstruction (BOO)

Organic
  Benign prostatic hypertrophy
  Prostatic carcinoma
  Marion's disease
  Bladder neck contracture following:
    TURP
    Open prostatectomy
    Radical prostatectomy
    Neobladder-urethral anastomosis

Functional
  Neurogenic
  Detrusor-external sphincter dyssynergia (DESD)
  Nonneurogenic
  Detrusor-bladder neck dyssynergia (BND)
  Detrusor-perineal floor incoordination (Hinman's syndrome)

Note: Marion's disease, described in 1927, is a congenital hypertrophy of bladder neck musculature. After the initial hypothesis of Turner-Warwick, its occurrence is today considered extremely rare or even questioned, in favor of a functional etiology (bladder neck dyssynergia). Hinman's syndrome, also called *nonneurogenic neurogenic bladder,* is a nonneurogenic incoordination between detrusor contraction and relaxation of the pelvic floor during voluntary voiding.

to defective support of the pelvic floor musculature and organs, usually following previous pregnancies. In males, urinary stress incontinence is essentially due to intrinsic sphincter deficiency either on a neurogenic basis or, more frequently, following direct damage in the course of prostatic surgery or as a result of pelvic trauma.

The overactive bladder is defined by the cystometric finding of phasic "unhibited" detrusor contractions during the filling phase while the patient is attempting to "hold the urine", i.e., to inhibit the micturition reflex. If this urodynamic diagnosis is made in a patient with a known neurologic disease, the condition should be termed *detrusor hyperreflexia.* Otherwise, *detrusor instability* is the recommended terminology. Since urge and stress incontinence reflect totally different pathophysiologic conditions, their possible means of management are also completely different and are discussed separately.

Treatment

URINARY RETENTION DUE TO DETRUSOR UNDERACTIVTY (DU)

DU may be the result of pharmacologic treatment for other diseases with drugs known to exert a depressing effect on the detrusor, such as tricyclic antidepressants, antiparkinsonians, and so forth. In this case, the efforts of the urologist, together with the specialist treating the other disease should be aimed primarily at substituting or reducing the dosage of the medication responsible for DU.

All other instances in which DU is caused by neurogenic, myogenic, and psychogenic factors are currently treated predominantly by nonpharmacologic measures, since the great majority of drugs employed in the past to induce or enhance the voiding reflex have not been demonstrated to be effective in clinical practice or in the more recent literature.

Nonpharmacologic treatment

Intermittent catheterization (IC) can be used when bladder emptying is completely or partially impeded by DU. Intermittent bladder drainage is carried out by the patient or a caregiver with a small catheter at time intervals calculated not to exceed the bladder capacity at each evacuation. If the patient's oral intake is maintained at reasonable levels (1-1.5 l/d), IC can be applied as many as 4 to 5 times daily. The procedure is generally easy and safe.

IC has become the method of choice in treating the vast majority of neurogenic voiding dysfunctions, and patients with nonneurogenic DU as well can, in some instances, benefit from this minimally invasive method. In neuropathic patients in particular, in whom the experience is more extensive, IC has dramatically decreased the occurrence of all complications related to indwelling catheterization, including urinary tract infections (UTIs), bladder stones, urethral diverticula and fistulas, upper urinary tract deterioration, and bladder carcinoma.

Neuromodulation by chronic direct stimulation of the sacral roots (usually S3, monolaterally) by means of an implantable electrical stimulator is now a viable method for treating some forms of functional retention. The main indication for this kind of treatment, popularized by Tanagho and Schmidt under the term *neuromodulation,* is urinary retention due to an involuntary hyperactivity of the pelvic floor muscles, usually on a psychogenic basis, resulting in the inhibition of the micturition reflex.

Drug therapy

Cholinergic agonists such as bethanechol chloride and carbachol, are acetylcholine-like agents used orally or given by sc injection to patients with detrusor underactivity, especially those with postoperative and postpartum retention. Dosages of approximately 5 to 10 mg sc every 4 to 6 hours or 50 mg po up to four times a day (im injection is very painful and should be avoided) have not provided satisfactory results. Probably bethanechol only causes an increase in the tension of the smooth detrusor muscle, but it does not induce a physiologic micturition reflex. These drugs today are very seldom indicated. Side effects include flushing, increased sweating and salivation, nausea, vomiting, abdominal pain, diarrhea, and bronchospasm.

Anticholinesterases, particularly distigmine bromide, a widely used drug for its long-lasting action and its supposed relative selectiveness for the bladder, have not provided any statistically significant effect on the resumption of voiding after prostatectomy. Such drugs are not useful in cases of neurogenic detrusor areflexia.

Prostaglandins have been tested, based on the hypothesis that they may act as exciting neurotransmitters capable of maintaining tone and detrusor contractility. PGE_2 seems to cause a clear reduction in the tone of the smooth urethral muscle, whereas $PGF_{2\alpha}$ increases it. However, controlled clinical studies have not supported this hypothesis, and these medications are rarely used in current clinical practice.

Opioid antagonists exercise a stimulating effect on the detrusor reflex. They have proved controversial results, and because of the impracticability of administering such narcotic agents, they are not used in current clinical practice.

URINARY RETENTION DUE TO BOO

Most patients with complete or significant chronic incomplete urinary retention with abundant postvoiding residual urine secondary to bladder outlet obstruction (BOO) are managed by nonpharmacologic means. If the cause of urinary retention is functional BOO of neurogenic origin, the treatment of choice is conservative, by means of IC (see above), usually associated with anticholinergic medication to treat the concomitant detrusor hyperreflexia. When this is not possible, an endoscopic treatment may be indicated in male patients, in the form of a transurethral sphincterotomy and/or bladder neck incision. If a sphincterotomy is performed, the resolution of urinary retention and the decrease in intravesical pressures, detrimental to the upper urinary tract, are achieved at the cost of urinary incontinence. The procedure can lead to such complications as severe hemorrhage, crisis of autonomic dysreflexia, and impotence.

In cases of organic BOO, mainly due to benign prostatic hypertrophy (BPH), many surgical, endoscopic, or mini-invasive procedures are available. The "gold standard" is still represented by transurethral resection of the prostate or open prostatectomy. Transurethral incision of prostate for glands smaller than 30 g, laser prostatectomy, transurethral thermotherapy, transurethral needle ablation, and high-intensity focused ultrasound are all alternative treatments under evaluation. In general, they are less invasive (and therefore less prone to complications), but they are also less effective than the traditional methods. (see Chap. 18) Their role in the patient unfit for more standard surgery or unwilling to undergo more invasive treatment has to be elucidated.

Phytotherapy

Before the development of 5α-reductase inhibitors and α-adrenoreceptor blockers, various phytotherapeutic agents (plant extracts) were used. The most widely used phytotherapeutic agents are *Serenoa repens* (320 mg daily) and *Pygeum africanum* (200 mg daily). Their exact mechanism of action has not been elucidated completely, and they likely act at several different levels. The nonphytotherapeutic agent mepartricin has been isolated from a Streptomyces strain. The usual oral dose is 40 mg per day. Both phytotherapeutic agents and mepartricin are well tolerated and have no significant side effects.

α-Adrenoreceptor blockers and 5α-reductase inhibitors are described in Chapter 18.

OVERACTIVE BLADDER

Nonpharmacologic treatment

Overactive bladder and its symptoms are treated primarily by means of pharmacologic manipulation, mainly with drugs with anticholinergic activity. However, there are some instances when drugs are ineffective, not toler-

---

Table 19.2 Nonpharmacologic treatment modalities of overactive bladder

Functional electrical stimulation (FES) of the pelvic floor
Acupuncture
Neuromodulation (permanent sacral nerve stimulation)
Posterior sacral rhizotomy + sacral anterior root stimulation
Bladder augmentation (enterocystoplasty) + bladder neck closure and continent vesicostomy
Bladder autoaugmentation (detrusorectomy)

---

ated, or contraindicated. In these circumstances, several other treatments are available to help the patients suffering from the most severe symptoms, such as urinary incontinence (Tab. 19.2). These treatments include noninvasive modalities such as functional electrical stimulation of the pelvic floor and acupuncture or surgical interventions aimed at either denervating the bladder or augmenting its capacity by incorporating a segment of the gastrointestinal tract. A description of the mechanisms of action, clinical results, and side effects of these modalities is beyond the scope of this review. Nonpharmacologic treatments should be provided only by specialists in voiding dysfunction, following a careful urodynamic evaluation.

Drug therapy

The pharmacologic manipulation of the lower urinary tract for the management of bladder overactivity is usually quite effective and represents the most successful application of uropharmacology. Medical treatment is the first-line option for this condition, in conjunction with behavioral modifications. Nonmedical (rehabilitative or surgical) therapies are also available, should the drugs be ineffective or poorly tolerated in a specific patient.

Several drugs exist, working at different levels and with various mechanisms of action. The largest group of these drugs acts by decreasing detrusor contractility. This can affect voluntary detrusor contractility as well, thereby creating or exacerbating bladder retention, especially if BOO or detrusor underactivity coexists. A thorough urodynamic evaluation is recommended before beginning such a pharmacologic treatment, especially in patients at risk for retention, such as males, the elderly, and neurogenic patients.

Drugs acting by reducing detrusor contractility

Several drugs are potentially useful and have been employed clinically in this regard. Almost all of them

---

Table 19.3 Drugs decreasing bladder overactivity and their usual dosages

Pure anticholinergic agents
Propantheline (15-60 mg tid to qid po)
Trospium chloride (20 mg bid po)
Tolterodine (2 mg bid po)
Smooth muscle relaxants with anticholinergic activity
Oxybutynin chloride (7.5-15 mg tid po or 5 mg in 30 ml of water intravesically)
Dicyclomine hydrochloride (20 mg tid po)
Flavoxate (100-200 mg tid po)
Calcium antagonists with anticholinergic activity
Propiverine hydrochloride (10-15 mg bid or tid po)
Tricyclic antidepressants with anticholinergic activity
Imipramine hydrochloride (25 mg once to qid po)
Doxepin (25 mg once to qid po)
Desipramine (25 mg once to qid po)
Nortriptyline (25 mg once to qid po)

have in common an anticholinergic (antimuscarinic) effect. In some cases this is the only mechanism of action, whereas in others this action is coupled with other actions. A list of various drugs that act by reducing detrusor contractility, schematically divided by mechanism, is provided in Table 19.3.

Anticholinergic drugs

Since detrusor contraction is induced mainly by stimulation of post-ganglionic parasympathetic cholinergic (muscarinic) receptors in the detrusor wall by acetylcholine (Ach), cholinergic blocking can cause a reduction in detrusor contraction. In patients with detrusor overactivity, this results in an increase in the threshold and a decrease in the amplitude of uninhibited contractions and a corresponding increase in bladder functional capacity. The associated "storage" symptoms such as frequency, urgency, and urge incontinence are therefore improved or cured.

Anticholinergic agents, along with smooth muscle relaxants and tricyclic antidepressants with anticholinergic properties, are not selective for the bladder but are equally effective on many other organs. Several side effects must be expected, including the following: xerostomia (dry mouth), blurred vision due to impairment of visual accommodation, constipation, tachycardia (due to vagal blockage), xerophthalmia, nausea, urinary retention, and cognitive deficits. Strict contraindications to the use of anticholinergic agents are narrow-angle glaucoma and BOO (because of a risk of total bladder retention).

Specific recommendations for patients on chronic antimuscarinic agents are (1) limitation of exposure to high-temperature environments for a prolonged time and (2) reduction in dosage in the elderly population. These drugs reduce perspiration, limiting the exchange of heat between the body and the external environment. Furthermore, the sensitivity to anticholinergic side effects increases with age, particularly in relation to the central nervous system, such as memory impairment, drowsiness, and confusion. As a general rule, an individual titration of drug dosage is advisable for a maximum therapeutic effect with minimal side effects.

Propantheline bromide This quaternary ammonium derivative was the first pure anticholinergic drug used for the treatment of bladder overactivity. The usual dosage is 15 to 60 mg po every 6 to 8 hours. At its lowest dosage, this medication has been shown to reduce the symptoms by about 15% over placebo. Side effects were found in 50% of the patients, with discontinuation in approximately 20%.

Oxybutynin chloride This medication has a strong muscle-relaxant activity, as well as anticholinergic and local anesthetic actions. It is currently the most widely used drug in the treatment of detrusor overactivity and probably the most effective. At an oral dose of 15 mg per day, this agent reduces "storage" symptoms in more than 85% of patients. The incidence of side effects is as high as 68% of the patients, dry mouth being the most common. Both efficacy and incidence of side effects are dose-related, as

is the case for all the anticholinergic agents. The usual oral dose for chronic therapy is 7.5 to 15 mg tid.

To reduce adverse effects, an alternative route of administration is used, namely, intravesical instillation of oxybutynin dissolved in normal saline or distilled water. This has been shown to be an effective means of managing overactive bladder, especially detrusor hyperreflexia of neurogenic origin in patients already using IC. In this way, many patients can obtain similar beneficial effects without suffering from the anticholinergic side effects usually associated with oral administration of oxybutynin. A possible explanation is that the intravesical instillation of the drug may prevent the formation of a hepatic metabolite, N-desethyl-oxybutynin, responsible for the occurrence of the side effects. Symptomatic improvement has been demonstrated in 55 to 90% of the studied population. The main reason for discontinuing therapy is the inconvenience of the route of administration, which requires a preliminary preparation of the compound and the insertion of a transurethral catheter. The usual dose is one 5-mg tablet dissolved in 30 ml of sterile water (normal saline or distilled water) bid or tid. The drug is left in the bladder until the next catheterization or an episode of incontinence takes place.

Trospium chloride This is another quaternary ammonium derivative with antimuscarinic properties, and it has documented efficacy on detrusor hyperreflexia similar to that exerted by oxybutynin but with less severe side effects. The oral dose employed is 20 mg bid.

Propiverine hydrochloride This is a benzylic derivative with muscle-relaxant and mild antimuscarinic effects. It has a documented favorable effect on detrusor hyperreflexia and a reasonable adverse-effect profile. The usual oral dose is 10 to 15 mg bid or tid.

Dicyclomine hydrochloride This has both antimuscarinic and muscle-relaxant activities. The scarce data in the literature indicate its efficacy in the treatment of urinary urge incontinence compared with placebo. No published data on the side effects are available, and the worldwide published clinical experience is limited. The usual oral dose is 10 to 20 mg tid.

Flavoxate hydrochloride The results of recent studies on the efficacy of this widely used muscle relaxant (and very weak antimuscarinic) for the treatment of detrusor overactivity are controversial. In the clinical practice, the side effects of this agent are limited, and it may be tested in patients in whom antimuscarinic adverse effects are to be avoided. The common oral dose is 100 to 200 mg tid or qid.

Tricyclic antidepressants (TCAs) The compounds belonging to this category have a strong anticholinergic effect and are potentially useful in increasing the storage function of the bladder in selected patients.

This anticholinergic effect is both central and peripheral. This group of drugs has other pharmacologic actions as well (see Chaps. 9 and 13). They also increase bladder outlet resistance, probably due to blockade of norepinephrine reuptake and the consequent increased α-adrenergic effect at the level of bladder base and proximal urethra. TCAs may be particularly useful in clinical conditions where an overactive bladder and urethral sphincter weakness coexist, such as some forms of female mixed incontinence and postprostatectomy incontinence. A mean increase in maximum urethral pressure of 30 cmH$_2$O has been demonstrated during therapy with imipramine.

Another pharmacologic effect of TCAs is sedation secondary to an antihistaminic action. This has to be taken into account when these drugs are prescribed for detrusor overactivity, and patients must be warned against sleepiness in case they drive or operate hazardous machinery. The half-life of this group of drugs is quite long, and this is particularly true in the elderly, who must take TCA agents at greater intervals.

The most widely used compound in this group for the treatment of overactive bladder is imipramine, which has been employed successfully in the management of primary nocturnal enuresis at a single dose of 25 mg at bedtime. The usual dose for the control of overactive bladder symptoms is 25 mg tid or qid in adults. Other TCAs used for overactive bladder include doxepin, desipramine, and nortriptyline.

Besides the usual anticholinergic side effects, many other adverse effects have been described (see Chap. 13), among which is delayed ejaculation. For this reason, these agents are currently used for the management of premature ejaculation. The following two points must be carefully taken into account when prescribing TCAs. They are contraindicated in people concomitantly treated with monoamine oxidase (MAO) inhibitors (because of the risk of severe central nervous system toxicity, such as hyperpyrexia, seizures, and coma), and discontinuation of therapy should be gradual.

Being relatively inexpensive compared with classic anticholinergic agents and muscle relaxants, TCAs are often the only possible treatment for overactive bladder in developing countries.

Tolterodine tartrate This is a selective competitive muscarinic receptor antagonist developed for the pharmacologic manipulation of detrusor overactivity and related symptoms, and it has only recently been released (Tab. 19.4). In vitro and in vivo studies evaluating its efficacy in comparison with oxybutynin have shown that tolterodine has the same efficacy as oxybutynin in reducing the symptoms of detrusor overactivity. In fact, the symptomatic improvement obtained by tolterodine 1 mg bid, tolterodine 2 mg bid, and oxybutynin were similar and statistically higher than placebo. In particular, the incontinence episodes per 24 hours were reduced in each active treatment group by a mean of 40 to 60% of baseline. Although these data, based on the findings of micturition charts, seemed to demonstrate a similar positive effect of the two dosages of tolterodine, the urodynamic data failed to show an advantage of the smaller dosage (1

mg) over placebo. Therefore, the higher dosage (2 mg bid) of tolterodine is preferable.

The tolterodine 2-mg group showed a much lower incidence of side effects than the oxybutynin group. Dry mouth was reported in 40% of patients taking the full dosage of tolterodine, compared with 80% of patients taking oxybutynin. Only 8% of patients in the tolterodine 2-mg group withdrew from the study because of side effects (a percentage not too different from the 5% withdrawal incidence in the placebo group), compared with 20% in the oxybutynin group. The pharmacologic explanation for the higher tolerability of tolterodine can be found in the results of preliminary in vitro studies demonstrating that tolterodine has eight times less potency than oxybutynin at the salivary muscarinic receptors, whereas the two drugs show the same potency in antagonizing bladder muscarinic receptors.

Drugs acting by reducing detrusor sensitivity

This is a recent and promising field of research. The two drugs that have so far been tested are capsaicin and, less extensively, resiniferatoxin. They are still under evaluation, and their clinical application for the treatment of overactive bladder, outside research conditions, is not yet approved.

Capsaicin is a derivative of hot red pepper that has the botanical name *capsicum.* The pungent compound, when applied to sensitive tissues (skin, mucosa, etc.), has an initial algogenic effect, followed soon after by an anti-inflammatory and analgesic effect that is therapeutically useful. Capsaicin is employed as a cream in the topical treatment of the painful lesions of herpes zoster. Clinical studies have shown that the intravesical instillation of a solution of 1 to 2 m*M*/l of capsaicin in alcohol is helpful in reducing bladder overactivity of neurogenic origin (mainly multiple sclerosis and spinal cord injury). Its mechanism of action is aimed selectively at the vanilloid receptors of the bladder wall, thus desensitizing the unmyelinated afferent C-fibers by an initial emptying of the stores of peptides such as substance P, various neurokinins, etc. In normal conditions, e.g., when the C-fibers conducting painful sensation are not affected by the neurotoxin capsaicin, the release of these tachykinins causes bladder contraction. There is evidence that the voiding reflex, which in the intact animal is mediated by the afferent myelinated α fibers, in spinal cord-injured (SCI) animals is mediated by the C-fibers sensitive to capsaicin. The effect of capsaicin instillation on bladder overactivity is transient, normally lasting 2 to 7 months. However, the treatment is safe and can be

Table 19.4 Main anticholinergic drugs: major kinetic parameters

	Bioavailability (%)	Volume of distribution (l/kg)	T$_{max}$ (h)	t$_{1/2}$ (h)
Oxybutynin	6	–	–	2-3
Tolterodine	17-65	0.9-1.6	0.7-1.0	2-3

repeated. The only side effect reported is a brief and tolerable suprapubic burning sensation.

Resiniferatoxin, another neurotoxin affecting C-fibers, is approximately 1000 times more potent than capsaicin. The few studies conducted to date have shown that this drug, when instilled in the bladder of SCI patients at a concentration of 50 to 100 n*M,* exerted a positive effect without the transient suprapubic burning sensation caused by capsaicin. The beneficial effects lasted at least 3 months. Further placebo-controlled studies are needed to confirm the role of this very promising therapy.

URETHRAL INSUFFICIENCY (URINARY STRESS INCONTINENCE)

Pharmacotherapy of this disorder traditionally has been directed at stimulating the α-adrenergic receptors of the proximal urethra. Therefore, α-adrenergic agonists, such as phenylpropanolamine, have been employed since the 1970s, mainly in the conservative treatment of female stress incontinence.

Phenylpropanolamine hydrochloride, when used in stress incontinence leads to a partial subjective improvement of incontinence but in almost no case a complete relief. The usual oral dose is 25 to 100 mg bid. Side effects include nausea, anxiety, agitation, insomnia, sweating, and hypertension. This agent should be used with caution in patients with hypertension or cardiac disease.

Imipramine, besides its anticholinergic effect, also causes an increased outlet resistance by an enhanced adrenergic effect secondary to inhibition of norepinephrine reuptake. This double action may be useful in some patients presenting with both bladder overactivity and urethral sphincter deficiency, as is some cases of postprostatectomy and female stress incontinence. The usual oral dose is 25 mg tid or qid.

Estrogen therapy is aimed at increasing urethral coaptation in postmenopausal women. Conjugated estrogens (e.g., estriol, estrone) can be taken either by mouth or vaginally. The usual dose is 0.3 to 1.25 mg per day po and 2.5 to 10 mg per day by vaginal administration. Some studies have confirmed at least a limited positive effect in postmenopausal women. Estrogen therapy is contraindicated in patients with cancer of the breast or uterus.

Several nonpharmacologic treatments have been

Table 19.5 Nonpharmacologic treatment options for urinary stress incontinence

Pelvic floor rehabilitation
Biofeedback
Suburothelial injection of:
  Teflon
  Fat
  Collagen (Contigen)
  Silicone (Macroplastique)
Vaginal needle suspension (Pereyra-Raz procedure)
Abdominal colposuspensions (Marshall-Marchetti, Burch)
Pubovaginal sling procedures with:
  Rectus fascia
  Fascia lata
  Alloplastic material

described, and they are usually much more effective in treating urinary stress incontinence than pharmacotherapy (Tab. 19.5).

Pelvic floor exercises, with or without biofeedback techniques, are a noninvasive method with a reasonably positive effect and are recommended by many authors as the first-line treatment in patients with mild to moderate female stress incontinence. Less impressive results have been described in postprostatectomy incontinence. Such exercises are not useful at all in patients with a complete neurogenic lesion.

Suburothelial injection of bulking agents in the urethral sphincter area is currently considered the second option, in consideration of the relatively minimal invasiveness and acceptable results. The most suitable indication is considered the intrinsic sphincter deficiency (ISD) in both females and males. Teflon and fat have been abandoned recently, and extensive research is underway to find even more effective and practical bulking material.

If a more invasive approach is to be considered, a thorough videourodynamic evaluation, including measurement of the Valsalva leak-point pressure, is strongly recommended. Among the classic surgical operations for female patients, recent studies have shown a limited success in the long run (5 years and longer) of vaginal needle suspensions. The transabdominal approach is preferred. For the most severe cases or for postprostatectomy incontinence, implantation of an artificial sphincter is a viable option.

Suggested readings _____

Brynne N, Stahl MMS, Hallen B, et al. Pharmacokinetics and pharmacodynamics of tolterodine in man: a new drug for the treatment of urinary bladder overactivity. Int J Clin Pharmacol Ther 1997;35:287-95.

Bultitude ML, Hills NH, Shuttleworth K. Clinical and experimental studies on the action of prostaglandins and their synthesis inhibitors on detrusor muscle in vitro and in vivo. Br J Urol 1976;48:631-7.

Christensen H, Haltby N, Jorn AF, et al. Cholinergic block-

ade as a model of the cognitive deficits in Alzheimer's disease. Brain 1992;115:1681-99.

Clinical Practice Guideline Update. Urinary incontinence in adults: Acute and chronic management. AHCPR publication no 96-0682. Rockville, MD, Agency for Health Care Policy and Research, Public Health Service, U.S. Department of Health and Human Services, March 1996.

Delaere K, Thomas C, Moonen T, Debruyne F. The value of prostaglandin E$_2$ and F$_{2a}$ in women with abnormalities of bladder emptying. Br J Urol 1981;53:306.-9

Douchamps J, Derenne F, Stockis A, et al. The pharmacokinetics of oxybutynin in man. Eur J Clin Pharmacol 1988;35:515-20.

FEINBERG M. The problems of anticholinergic adverse effects in older patients. Drugs Aging 1993;4:335-48.

LAPIDES J, DIOKNO A, SILBER S, LOWE B. Clean intermittent self-catheterisation in the treatment of urinary tract disease. J Urol 1972;107:458-16.

MADERSBACHER H, STOHRER M, RICHTER R, et al. Trospium chloride versus oxybutynin: A randomized, double-blind, multicentre trial in the treatment of detrusor hyperreflexia. Br J Urol 1995;75:452-6.

SCHMIDT RA. Implantable neuroprosthetics in urology. Urodynamica 1992;1:29-33.

STANTON SL. Diseases of the urinary system: drugs acting on the bladder and urethra. Br Med J 1978;1607-8.

THOR KB, ROPPOLO JR, DE GROAT WC. Naloxone induced micturition in unanesthetized paraplegic cats. J Urol 1983;129:202-5.

THUROFF JW, BUNKE B, EBNER A, et al. Randomized, double-blind, multicenter trial on treatment of frequency, urgency, and urge incontinence related to detrusor overactivity: oxybutynin versus propantheline versus placebo. J Urol 1991;145:813.

VAPNEK JM, SCHMIDT RA. Restoration of voiding in chronic urinary retention using the neuroprosthesis. World J Urol 1991;9:142.

WEESE DL, ROSKAMP DA, LEACH GE, ZIMMERN PE. Intravesical oxybutynin chloride: experience with 42 patients. Urology 1993;41:527-30.

WEIN AJ. Neuromuscular dysfunction of the lower urinary tract and treatment. In: Walsh, Retik, Vaughan, Wein, eds. Campbell's Urology, 7th ed. Philadelphia: WB Saunders, 1997;953-1006.

Male impotence

Richard Sachse

Impotence is the failure to achieve erection, ejaculation, or both and comprises a variety of symptoms such as loss of libido, failure of erection, premature ejaculation, ejaculatory failure, and the inability to achieve orgasm. This chapter focuses on erectile dysfunction, defined by the U.S. National Institutes of Health Consensus Development Conference as "the inability to achieve or to maintain an erection sufficient for satisfactory sexual performance." According to the Massachusetts Male Aging Study, the prevalence of erectile dysfunction of any degree is 40% among 40-year-old men and 70% among 70-year-old men.

ERECTILE DYSFUCTION

Physiology and pathophysiology Penile erection is triggered by two main mechanisms: local sensory stimulation of the genital organs (reflexogenic erection) and via stimuli emanating from the brain (psychogenic erection). Whereas reflexogenic erections are mediated by a spinal reflex pathway, psychogenic erection is regulated by supraspinal centers including the thalamus and the limbic system. Probably reflexogenic and psychogenic mechanisms act synergistically.

Erection is a neurovascular phenomenon, regulated by complex neurophysiologic mechanisms that cause relaxation of the smooth muscle tone in penile blood vessels and sinusoids. This leads to a decrease in peripheral resistance and dilatation of the sinusoids, allowing increased blood flow into the corporal sinusoids through the internal pudendal and cavernosal arteries. Blood is stored in the expanding sinusoidal system, and the venous outflow is reduced by compression of the subtunical venules.

Etiologic factors for erectile disorders may be characterized as psychogenic or organic, but they derive most commonly from problems in both areas. Psychogenic stimuli not only can cause erection but also are able to inhibit the erectile response. Reflexogenic erections and activation of the parasympathetic dilator nerves to the penis may be inhibited by messages from the brain to the sacral cord. Also, an increase in penile smooth muscle tone, opposing the smooth muscle relaxation required for erection, may be caused by excessive sympathetic outflow or elevated blood catecholamine levels. Common psychogenic causes of erectile dysfunction are anxiety, depressive states, disinterest in the sexual partner, conflicts over sexual preference, etc.

Organic diseases causing erectile dysfunction are numerous. Impotence is more strongly associated with age than with any other variable. However, aging itself may not cause erectile dysfunction but rather raises the probability of suffering from organic diseases causing erectile dysfunction. The most common organic factor in men over 50 years of age is atherosclerosis. Since the cavernous arteries as well as the coronary arteries are end arteries without collateral circulation, they are therefore affected by the same risk factors as those relevant for coronary heart disease such as hypertension, smoking, and hyperlipidemia.

Diagnosis To work out the etiology of erectile dysfunction in each particular patient is inevitable for the selection of appropriate therapy. Medical and sexual history can be useful in evaluation of risk factors, associated diseases, and drug consumption. A slowly progressive loss of erectile function associated with the absence of nocturnal erections is suggestive of an organic origin, whereas a rapid onset of erectile dysfunction associated with maintained nocturnal erections is often due to psychogenic factors. Physical examination can reveal penile diseases or signs of hypogonadism, and where necessary, specific laboratory testing should be performed and endocrinopathies should be ruled out. Often included in the evaluation of erectile dysfunction is assessment of the maximal erectile capacity with the help of a pharmacoerection test, a pharmacopenile duplex ultrasonograph, and the testing of the nocturnal penile tumescence and rigidity.

Treatment

Therapy of erectile dysfunction has evolved tremendously since the 1960s, when it was thought that 90% of erectile dysfunction was of psychogenic origin. During the late 1970s, penile implants represented the only alternative to arterial bypass surgery or surgery for venoocclusive dysfunction, which frequently had disappointing long-term

Table 20.1 Drugs for intracavernosal pharmacotherapy

Drug	Main pharmacologic effect
Papaverine	Nonselective inhibition of phosphodiesterases
Phentolamine	α-Receptor antagonism
Prostaglandin E$_1$ (alprostadil)	Adenylate cyclase activation
Moxisylyte	α-Receptor antagonism
Linsidomine	Nitric oxide donation
Forskolin	Adenylate cyclase activation
Vasoactive intestinal peptide	Adenylate cyclase activation
Calcitonin gene-related peptide	Direct corporal smooth muscle relaxation

results. The 1980s were characterized by less invasive therapies, and the pioneering work of Virag and Brindley led to the introduction of intracavernous injection of vasoactive agents. In addition, nowadays a number of alternative forms of therapy are available or under development, including topical or intraurethral pharmacotherapy as well as oral drug therapy.

Intracavernosal pharmacotherapy

Intracavernosal application of vasoactive agents not only has revolutionized the diagnosis of erectile dysfunction by providing a better insight into penile hemodynamics, physiology of erection, and pathophysiology of erectile dysfunction but also has been the cornerstone for the pharmacologic treatment of erectile dysfunction. The intracavernosal application of vasoactive agents is capable of locally altering penile blood flow and inducing an erection despite neurologic diseases or alterations in penile arterial blood flow. It allows high concentrations of the pharmacologically active substance at the end organ without severe systemic side effects. Ideally, the lowest dose for induction of a rigid erection is determined individually to avoid side effects. A summary of intracavernosal drugs is provided in Table 20.1.

Papaverine Papaverine is an opium alkaloid (benzylisoquinoline) derived from *Papaver somniferum* that has a direct myotonolytic effect on smooth muscle cells, exerted by a nonselective inhibition of cyclic nucleotide phosphodiesterases. The resulting intracellular accumulation of the second messengers cyclic adenosine monophosphate (cAMP) and cyclic guanosine monophosphate (cGMP) leads to an activation of protein kinases, which causes phosphorylation of membrane proteins and a decrease in intracellular levels of free calcium, thus promoting corporal smooth muscle relaxation and in turn increasing blood flow into the cavernosal spaces.

Since 1982, a substantial amount of data on patients receiving papaverine monotherapy has been published. Patients with psychogenic or organic erectile dysfunction have excellent response rates on intracavernosal administration of 16 to 120 mg papaverine, with sufficient erections being achieved in 60 to 93%. Complications after intracavernosal papaverine injection are priapism in 7.1%; corporal nodules, indurations, and fibrosis in 5.7%; pain in 4.0%; hematoma at the injection site in 11.4%; and elevated liver enzymes in 1.6%. Other systemic side effects are peripheral vasodilation, hypotension, and reflex tachycardia.

The intracavernous concentration of papaverine after local administration of 80 mg shows a steady decrease and represents, after 60 minutes, still about 15% of the concentration at 5 minutes after administration. In the peripheral circulation, papaverine concentrations are at the detection limit before intracavernosal injection and were still small but significantly elevated 30 and 60 minutes after injection. Papaverine is not metabolized locally but excreted via the liver. It is released slowly from the corpora cavernosa, leading to a slight but measurable elevation of peripheral concentrations. In patients with a clinically significant venous or cavernous insufficiency, this elevation of peripheral papaverine concentrations may explain systemic side effects such as mild hypotension or liver enzyme elevation. In patients without venoocclusive dysfunction, the relatively high local concentrations may be maintained, which could explain the relatively high rate of priapism.

Phentolamine Phentolamine is a competitive α_1- and α_2-adrenoceptor antagonist and a direct smooth muscle relaxant. The intracavernous injection of phentolamine provokes arterial dilatation but has no effect on venous return without a significant rise in intracorporal pressure. Monotherapy with phentolamine does not produce sufficiently rigid erections. Therefore, phentolamine is used in combination with other agents. The combination of papaverine and phentolamine results in a significantly better erectile response with a lower incidence of prolonged erections, the most severe side effect of papaverine monotherapy. This combination roughly equals the efficacy of prostaglandin E$_1$. The combination of phentolamine, papaverine, and prostaglandin E$_1$ can be regarded as the most effective intracavernosal pharmacotherapy available today.

The plasma half-life of phentolamine is approximately 30 minutes. It is almost completely metabolized by the liver before excretion, with less than 10% excreted unchanged renally. Systemic side effects include hypotension, reflex tachycardia, and nasal congestion.

Prostaglandin E$_1$ (Alprostadil) Prostaglandin E$_1$ (PGE$_1$) is a naturally occurring prostaglandin. By activating adenylate cyclase, it enhances cAMP formation, which in turn causes relaxation of corporal smooth muscle cells by stimulating the intracellular reuptake of calcium. It is a potent relaxant of the corporal smooth muscles, spongiosum, and cavernous artery. In the venous system it leads to constriction of the vascular wall with a decrease in outflow.

Alprostadil, a synthetic prostaglandin, analogous to the naturally occurring PGE_1, is officially approved for the intracavernosal treatment of erectile dysfunction in most countries. After injection, it produces dose-dependent erections in the clinically recommended dose range from 5 to 60 µg. The best response can be observed in patients with neurogenic erectile dysfunction, whereas higher doses are required in patients with mixed vasculogenic erectile dysfunction. Response rates are higher than 70%, with satisfaction rates higher than 85% in patients and their partners. Complications after intracavernosal alprostadil injection are remarkably lower than after papaverin: priapism in 0.36%; corporal nodules, indurations, and fibrosis in 0.8%; pain in 7.2%; and hematoma at the injection site in 6.6%. About 50% of patients experience penile pain as the main side effect after injection, but only in 11% of the injections. The only significant systemic side effect is hypotension, and this is observed only after high-dose injections. In summary, alprostadil, despite a relatively high incidence of penile pain, has a very good safety profile with a low incidence of such serious adverse events as priapism and fibrosis.

The kinetics of intracavernous PGE_1 is very rapid, the 60-minute value representing only 4% of the concentration at 5 minutes after injection of 20 µg. No increase in systemic PGE_1 concentration could be observed. The major initially circulating, biologically inactive metabolite, 15-keto-13,14-dihydro-prostaglandin E_1, has an intracavernous concentration 60 minutes after injection of 40% compared with the 5-minute value. Peripheral measurement of the metabolite shows a significant increase after 30 minutes about doubling basal concentrations, followed by a decrease back to basal levels. Due to the rapid metabolism during passage in the lung and the short peripheral half-life of only 30 seconds, PGE_1 cannot be found in the periphery, in contrast to the metabolite, with a half-life of 8 minutes. The local metabolism into a biologically inactive substance can explain the low rate of priapism and the very low risk of systemic side effects.

Moxisylyte Moxisylyte is a competitive norepinephrine antagonist that acts on postsynaptic α_1 receptors. The inhibition of the constant adrenergic tone leads to relaxation of corporal smooth muscle cells. In vitro, moxisylyte is less potent than phentolamine. Moxisylyte is approved for the intracavernosal treatment of erectile dysfunction in a few countries.

Moxisylyte proved clearly less active than papaverine in inducing rigid erections in patients with erectile dysfunction. In a comparative study, moxisylyte proved to be significantly less efficacious than PGE_1 (50% versus 71%). Conversely, the incidence of prolonged erections including priapism and of pain was clearly lower. Fibrotic lesions were observed equally in both treatment groups. Despite the better tolerance compared with PGE_1, its discontinuation rate was significantly higher, suggesting a lower satisfaction due to the lower efficacy. Treatment with moxisylyte may be considered in patients with hypersensitivity to the injections and in those with significant pain following PGE_1 injection.

After intracavernosal or intravenous administration of 10 mg moxisylyte, unchanged moxisylyte is not detectable in plasma. The first step in biotransformation of moxisylyte, deacetylation by the cholinesterase into the active metabolite deacetylmoxisylyte (DAM), is very rapid, with a plasma half-life of moxisylyte of approximately 1 minute. The $t_{1/2}$ values for unconjugated DAM after intracavernosal and intravenous administration were 1.04 and 1.02 hours, respectively, with mean residence times (MRTs) of 1.37 and 1.12 hours, respectively. A tourniquet placed before intracavernosal injection increases the MRT of unconjugated DAM up to 1.68 hours (~25%) and also seems to increase efficacy.

Combinations of intracavernosal drugs The use of combinations of vasoactive drugs for intracavernosal injection therapy was introduced to take advantage of the combination of drugs that rely on different mechanisms of action. Not only would this produce a pharmacologic synergism enhancing the overall therapeutic effect, but it also would reduce the side effects by lowering the dose of each compound. In addition, combination therapy may save costs by reducing the doses of the relevant compounds. Historically, the first drug combination included papaverine and phentolamine, which was as effective as monotherapy with alprostadil but has a lower incidence of pain and a higher risk of priapism and local fibrotic complications. The combination of alprostadil and phentolamine was shown to be effective with a similar complication rate as alprostadil monotherapy. A triple combination of 7.6 mg papaverine, 0.25 mg phentolamine, and 2.5 µg alprostadil was found to be as effective as 20 µg alprostadil with a low incidence of penile pain. Combinations including moxisylyte have not as yet been reported.

Other agents The nitric oxide donor linsidomine was shown to be less effective than PGE_1 monotherapy and papaverine-phentolamine combination therapy. Its excellent safety profile and low cost make linsidomine a possible alternative that still has to be investigated. Forskolin increases the activity of alprostadil in vitro and in vivo without significant systemic side effects. Experience with forskolin is still limited, but it appears that forskolin might find its place as an additional component in already established drug combinations. The vasoactive intestinal peptide (VIP) has been shown to induce erections in combination with phentolamine. When administered alone, however, it only produces a weak erectile response. The calcitonin gene-related peptide (CGRP) in combination with alprostadil is able to induce erections in patients not responding to the combination of papaverine and phentolamine. To date, there is only limited experience.

In conclusion, intracavernous pharmacotherapy is one of the cornerstones of medical treatment of erectile dysfunction. Despite the good response rates, dropout rates during therapy are very high-up to 40 to 50% in long-term follow-up, in most cases due to a lack of efficacy or due to "needle phobia". To overcome this problem, suitable patients should be better selected for this therapy, a proper dose

Table 20.2 Drugs for topical or transurethral pharmacotherapy

Drug	Main pharmacologic effect
Prostaglandin E$_1$ (MUSE)	Adenylate cyclase activation
Prazosin	α_1-Receptor antagonism
Prostaglandin E$_2$ (dinoprostone)	Adenylate cyclase activation
Nitroglycerin	Nitric oxide donation
Minoxidil	Potassium channel opening
Papaverine	Nonselective inhibition of phosphodiesterases

titration should be performed before initiating the therapy, and dose adjustment should be done after a certain time.

Topical and transurethral pharmacotherapy

In order to offer less invasive treatment options, researchers always attempt to develop alternative delivery systems. A couple of different vasoactive agents have been tested for topical administration. However, drug absorption through the skin remains the major block to reaching adequate drug concentrations in the corpora cavernosa. Only drug administration in the urethral mucosa seems to be an effective route for administration of vasocative agents for absorption and transfer to the erectile bodies of the corpora cavernosa and the corpus spongiosum (Tab. 20.2).

Prostaglandin E₁ (Alprostadil, MUSE) Alprostadil also is officially approved for transurethral therapy of erectile dysfunction in many countries. Alprostadil is delivered to the distal urethra by a proprietary drug-delivery system (MUSE, Medicated Urethral System for Erection) followed by massage of the distal shaft. Twenty percent of the medication is absorbed into the corpus cavernosum, whereas 80% is absorbed into the systemic circulation. As discussed earlier, alprostadil undergoes rapid lung metabolism and has a half-life of 30 seconds in the periphery.

In a double-blind, placebo-controlled study of 1511 men suffering from chronic erectile dysfunction from various organic causes, intraurethral alprostadil in doses from 125 to 1000 µg resulted in 65.9% of the patients having sufficient erections. These were randomly assigned to the different treatments for 3 months at home. About 65% of the patients receiving alprostadil reported having sexual intercourse at home at least once as compared with 19% in the placebo group. Seven of 10 administrations of the drug were followed by intercourse. The most frequent adverse event was penile pain, reported after 10.8% of alprostadil administrations and by 32.7% of the men, but only 2.4% of the men discontinued the study because of it. There were no cases of priapism or fibrosis. Hypotension was observed during the clinical testing in

3.3%, its frequency increasing with dose. Newer data indicate that systemic side effects such as dizziness, sweating, and hypotension occur in 5.8% after transurethral administration of 1000 µg alprostadil. As compared with intracavernosal administration of alprostadil, intraurethral administration requires much higher doses and is clearly less effective but has relatively few adverse effects.

Other topical treatments Prazosin, an α_1-receptor antagonist, can improve the efficacy of intraurethral alprostadil when they are given together intraurethrally. The efficacy rate was comparable with that of intracavernous administration of alprostadil. However, experience with this combination is limited. PGE$_2$, an oxytocic agent with vasodilatory effects similar to those of PGE$_1$, gave in a pilot study a positive response in 70% of men. Thirty percent had full penile tumescence after intraurethral administration of 800 µg PGE$_2$ cream. Nitroglycerin, a nitric oxide donor, has been administered topically to the penis. It commonly results in mild increases in tumescence but seldom in rigidity sufficient for intercourse. Side effects include severe headache and hypotension. The vasodilator minoxidil was shown to be more effective in a direct comparison than nitroglycerin after topical administration. Other studies found the drug not to be effective. Papaverine was tested for transdermal administration. Full erections were present in only 15% of the patients but also were present with placebo. Topical administration of papaverine seems to augment reflex erections in selected patients.

In summary, transurethral therapy with alprostadil is a suitable alternative for patients with erectile dysfunction of psychogenic, neurogenic, or mild vasculogenic etiology. The systemic side effects are mild, and there are no risks of significant cardiovascular reactions.

Oral pharmacotherapy

Oral agents for the treatment of erectile dysfunction have been used since the era of the alchemists, with many of the agents used being nothing better than placebo. Still, oral therapy seems to be the ultimate goal for restoring potency (Tab. 20.3). Only the scientifically and seriously tested substances are discussed. The discussion of hormonal therapy

Table 20.3 Drugs for oral pharmacotherapy

Drug	Main pharmacologic effect
Yohimbine	Centrally acting α_2-receptor antagonism
Trazodone	Centrally acting serotonin antagonism
Apomorphine	Centrally acting dopamine agonism
Phentolamine	α-Receptor antagonism
Sildenafil	Phosphodiesterase 5 inhibition
L-Arginine	Nitric oxide precursor
Korean red ginseng	?
Naltrexone	Opioid receptor antagonism
Pentoxifylline	Hemorrheologic effect

is also omitted, since therapy with testosterone or bromocriptine should remain restricted to those patients with hypogonadism or prolactinoma, respectively.

Yohimbine Yohimbine is an indole alkaloid obtained from the bark of the yohimbine tree. It is an extensively studied mainly centrally acting α_2-adrenoceptor antagonist that is thought to increase the central sympathetic drive, which in turn facilitates stimulated erections. Yohimbine 5 mg tid or 15 mg bid is generally well tolerated, but some patients experience anxiety, nausea, palpitations, dizziness, nervousness, insomnia, and headache. The outcome data for yohimbine in impotence clearly indicate a therapy with marginal efficacy. Yohimbine does not appear to be effective for organic erectile dysfunction and should not be recommended for the standard patient.

Trazodone Trazodone, a triazolopyridine derivative, is a centrally acting antidepressant (see Chap. 13) that inhibits serotonin reuptake. In addition, it is thought to exert an α-adrenergic blocking function, thus interfering with the sympathetic control of penile detumescence. Trazodone is administered empirically in patients with erectile dysfunction in oral doses from 50 to 200 mg per day. In earlier studies, response rates of up to 60% were reported. In patients with psychogenic erectile dysfunction, a combination therapy of trazodone and yohimbine had a response rate of 71% as compared with 18% with placebo. However, in a more recent double-blind, placebo-controlled study, no erectogenic effect of trazodone could be demonstrated in patients with erectile dysfunction not selected on the basis of etiology.

Apomorphine Apomorphine, synthesized from morphine in the nineteenth century, has been used as an emetic, sedative, and aphrodisiac. Apomorphine is structurally similar to dopamine and was shown to have potent activity on D_1 and D_2 dopamine receptors. In earlier studies with sc, po, or sublingual delivery, the drug may have been effective on erection but was associated with unacceptable side effects such as nausea, vomiting, yawning, and drowsiness. A modified form of apomorphine was shown to induce erections in 8 of 12 patients with psychogenic erectile dysfunction after sublingual administration of 3- or 4-mg tablets and absorption through the oral mucosa. Clinical development of apomorphine has recently been stopped due to excess risk of hypotension.

Phentolamine Phentolamine has been used for a long time in intracavernous pharmacotherapy (see above). Systemic administration may exert an erectogenic effect both by a central effect and by a direct effect on the corpora cavernosa. Phentolamine was shown to be effective after 50-mg oral administration, with 11 of 16 patients being able to penetrate and to ejaculate after 1.5 hours. After buccal administration of 20 mg, 21 of 69 patients could produce erection sufficient for intercourse. Later studies gave more ambiguous results. In a recent randomized, double-blind, placebo-controlled study, a beneficial effect of oral doses of phentolamine of 20, 40, and 60 mg (up to 50% of treated patients) was observed in too small a clinical sample to reach statistical significance. The drug is still under development.

Sildenafil Sildenafil is a potent and competitive inhibitor of cGMP-specific phosphodiesterase 5 (PDE5). It was officially approved for the oral treatment of erectile dysfunction in 1998. During sexual stimulation, penile nonadrenergic-noncholinergic nerves, as well as endothelial cells of penile blood vessels and of the corpora cavernosa, release nitric oxide (NO), which mediates vasodilation of the penile vascular resistance bed. Nitric oxide diffuses into the smooth muscle of the blood vessels and corporal smooth muscle and activates guanylate cyclase. The activated guanylate cyclase then converts guanosine triphosphate to the active second messenger cGMP, which results in a decrease in intracellular calcium and promotes smooth muscle relaxation. Inhibition of PDE5, the predominant isozyme metabolizing cGMP in the corpus caverrosum, leads to accumulation of cGMP and therefore augments the natural response on sexual stimulation.

Sildenafil was shown to enhance the induced NO-dependent relaxation of human corpora cavernosa in vitro but did not relax unstimulated tissue. Sildenafil inhibits the PDE5 with a geometric mean IC_{50} of 3.5 nM. IC_{50} values for the isozymes PDE2, PDE3, and PDE4 were more than 1000 times greater than that for PDE5, the IC_{50} for PDE1 are approximately 80-fold greater, and the IC_{50} for PDE6 are approximately 9-fold greater. Preclinical data revealed no special hazard based on conventional studies of safety, pharmacology, repeated-dose toxicity, genotoxicity, carcinogenicity, and toxicity to reproduction.

Since sildenafil demonstrates affinity on PDE6, which is present in the retinal photoreceptors and is involved in phototransduction, visual function tests were performed in humans after receiving therapeutic doses of sildenafil. Mild and transient differences in the Farnsworth-Munsell color discrimination test could be observed 1 hour after oral administration of 100 mg sildenafil.

Due to its vasodilatory effect, mild and transient decreases in blood pressure with a mean maximum of 8.4 mm Hg systolic were observed in healthy subjects after a single oral dose of 100 mg sildenafil, but no significant electrocardiographic changes were seen. No effect on sperm motility or morphology after single oral doses of 100 mg sildenafil was demonstrated.

In patients in the fasted state, sildenafil is rapidly absorbed, reaching maximal plasma concentrations 0.5 to 2 hours (median 60 minutes) after oral administration. The mean absolute oral bioavailability is 41% (range 25-63%). Area under the curve (AUC) and C_{max} increase in proportion with dose in the recommended oral dose range of 25 to 100 mg. When sildenafil is taken with food, the rate of absorption is reduced, with a mean delay in T_{max} of 60 minutes and a mean reduction in C_{max} of 29%. Approximately 96% of sildenafil and its major circulating *N*-desmethyl metabolite is bound to plasma proteins. The mean steady-state volume of distribution (V_{ss}) is 105 liters.

Sildenafil is extensively metabolized predominantly by the CYP3A4 (major route) and CYP2C9 (minor route) hepatic microsomal isoenzymes. The major *N*-desmethyl metabolite occurs in plasma concentrations that are 40% of those of unchanged sildenafil and has an in vitro potency of 50% compared with sildenafil. Sildenafil as well as its main metabolites are excreted mainly by the biliary route. Total-body clearance of sildenafil is 41 l/h, and the terminal half life 3 to 5 hours.

Severe renal diseases may raise the AUC of sildenafil and its main metabolite levels up to about 90% compared with young, healthy subjects. The pharmacokinetic behavior is not significantly altered in patients with mild to moderate renal insufficiency after receiving oral doses of 50 mg. However, in patients with severe renal insufficiency (creatinine clearance < 30 ml/min), the AUC and C_{max} of sildenafil increased significantly by 100 and 88%, respectively. In patients with mild to moderate liver cirrhoses (Child-Pugh A and B), the AUC and C_{max} of sildenafil increased significantly by 84 and 47%, respectively.

The single-dose AUC and C_{max} for sildenafil increased about 50% when coadministered with the nonspecific CYP3A4 inhibitor cimetidine (800 mg). Coadministration of 100 mg sildenafil with the specific CYP3A4 inhibitor erythromycin raised both the AUC and C_{max} for sildenafil by 2.6- and 2.1-fold, respectively. Coadministration of the CYP2C9 inhibitors tolbutamide and warfarin revealed neither pharmacokinetic nor dynamic interactions. The bioavailability of sildenafil was not affected by single doses of antacid. Coadministration of alcohol did not result in a pharmacokinetic or pharmacodynamic interaction. Population pharmacokinetic analysis did not reveal clinically relevant interactions with CYP3A4 inducers, CYP2D6 inhibitors, diuretics, calcium channel blockers, beta-blockers, angiotensin-converting enzyme (ACE) inhibitors, or angiotensin II antagonists.

In an early randomized, double-blind, crossover pilot study, 12 patients with erectile dysfunction of no established organic cause undergoing visual sexual stimulation and subsequent penile plethysmography had significantly longer erections after taking sildenafil as compared with placebo. The median time of onset of erection after taking sildenafil was 25 minutes. In a further randomized, placebo-controlled clinical trial in 532 men aged 24 to 87 years with erectile dysfunction, increasing doses of sildenafil were associated with greater efficacy, with 56, 77, and 84% of patients taking 25, 50, and 100 mg, respectively, reporting improved erections compared with 25% of those taking placebo. In another placebo-controlled study in 329 patients with organic, psychogenic, and mixed erectile dysfunction, improved erections were reported by 74% of patients receiving 25 to 100 mg sildenafil versus 16% for placebo. In this study, the mean number of successful attempts at sexual intercourse per month was 5.9 for patients receiving sildenafil as compared with 1.5 for those receiving placebo. Sixty-five percent of all attempts were successful for all patients receiving sildenafil versus 20% for patients receiving placebo. Improved erections also were reported by 50 and 52% of diabetic patients with erectile dysfunction treated with 25 and 50 mg of sildenafil, respectively, compared with 10% of those receiving placebo. In a small study in patients with erectile dysfunction

after radical prostatectomy, 12 of 15 patients who had undergone bilateral nerve-sparing procedures had a positive response to sildenafil. None of the 3 patients who had undergone a unilateral nerve-sparing procedure responded, nor did any of the 10 patients who had undergone a non-nerve-sparing procedure.

In healthy subjects, sildenafil augmented the hypotensive effect of glyceryl trinitrate but had no discernible effect on blood pressure alone. In patients with stable angina taking isosorbide mononitrate or glyceryl trinitrate, sildenafil substantially decreased blood pressure for more than 6 hours and increased heart rate for about 2 to 3 hours, often to the point of being symptomatic. These results are consistent with the known effect of sildenafil on the NO/cGMP pathway. Therefore, coadministraton with nitric oxide donors or nitrates in any form is contraindicated.

The safety of sildenafil has not been tested in patients with severe hepatic impairment, hypotension of less than 90/50 mm Hg, recent history of stroke or myocardial infarction, and known hereditary degenerative retinal disorders such as retinitis pigmentosa. Therefore, the use of sildenafil is contraindicated in these patients until further information is available.

Safety and tolerability data of oral sildenafil in the treatment of erectile dysfunction have been evaluated in 4274 patients (2722 sildenafil, 1552 placebo; age range 19-87 years) who received double-blind treatment over a period of up to 6 months and in 2199 patients who received long-term, open-label sildenafil for up to 1 year. The rate of discontinuation due to adverse events was similar for patients treated with sildenafil (2.5%) and placebo (2.3%). Treatment-related adverse events occurred in 37.2% of sildenafil-treated patients and 9.6% of placebo-treated patients. The most frequent adverse events were headache (16% sildenafil, 4% placebo), flushing (10% sildenafil, 1% placebo), and dyspepsia (7% sildenafil, 2% placebo). Abnormal vision was observed in 6.5% of patients receiving sildenafil versus 0.4% receiving placebo. There were no reports of priapism, which, however, was reported in postmarketing surveillance. Finally, there were no significant differences in the overall incidence of adverse events for patients taking sildenafil with or without concomitant medications, the overall adverse events incidence being higher in patients on CYP3A4 inhibitors than in subjects on no medications (76.0 versus 62.7%).

Other oral agents Korean red ginseng, L-arginine, naltrexone, and pentoxifylline have been tested in small studies suggesting that they may play a role in the treatment of erectile dysfunction. However, these studies have not yet been followed up.

In conclusion, oral therapy is the most convenient therapy with the best patient compliance. The approval of the first oral PDE5 inhibitor sildenafil revolutionized the treatment of erectile dysfunction. Until the approval of sildenafil, no effective oral medication for patients with erectile dysfunction was available. However, since sildenafil is not efficacious in all patients, and since for a large number of patients it is not suitable due to its side effects and interaction profile, other forms of therapy still play an important role in the treatment of erectile dysfunction.

AHLEN VAN H, PESKAR BA, STICHT G, HERTFELDER H-J. Pharmacokinetics of vasoactive substances administered into the human corpus cavernosum. J Urol 1994;151:1227-30.

BALLARD SA, GINGELL CJ, TANG K, et al. Effects of sildenafil on the relaxation of human corpus cavernosum tissue in vitro and on the activities of cyclic nucleotide phosphodiesterase isozymes. J Urol 1998;159:2164-71.

BECHARA A, CASABE A, CHELIZ G, et al. Prostaglandin E_1 versus mixture of prostaglandin E_1, papaverine and phentolamine in nonresponders to high papaverine plus phentolamines doses. J Urol 1996;155:924-25.

BOOLELL M, GEPI-ATTEE S, GINGELL JC, ALLEN MJ. Sildenafil, a novel effective oral therapy for male erectile dysfunction. Br J Urol 1996;78:257-1.

BRINDLEY GS: CAVERNOSAL ALPHA BLOCKADE. A new method for investigating and treating erectile impotence. Br J Psychiatry 1983;143:312-37.

BUVAT J, LEMAIRE A, HERBAUT-BUVAT M. Intracavernous pharmacotherapy: comparison of moxisylyte and prostaglandin E_1. Int J Impot Res 1996;8:41-6.

FELDMAN HA, GOLDSTEIN I, HATZICHRISTOU DG, et al. Impotence and its medical and psychological correlates: results of Massachusetts male aging study. J Urol 1994;151:54-61.

GOLDSTEIN I, LUE TF, PADMA-NATHAN H, et al. Oral sildenafil in the treatment of erectile dysfunction. N Engl J Med 1998;338:1397-1404.

LINET OI, OGRINC FG. Efficacy and safety of intracavernosal alprostadil in men with erectile dysfunction. N Engl J Med 1996;334:873-7.

MARQUER C, BRESSOLLE F. MOXISYLYTE. A review of its pharmacodynamic and pharmacokinetic properties, and its therapeutic use in impotence. Fundam Clin Pharmacol 1998;12:377-87.

MONTAGUE DK, BARADA JH, BELKER AM, et al. Clinical guidelines panel on erectile dysfunction: summary report on the treatment of organic erectile dysfunction. The American Urological Association. J Urol 1996;156:2007-11.

NATIONAL INSTITUTES OF HEALTH. Consensus Development Conference Statement on Impotence. Bethesda, Md., National Institutes of Health, 1992.

PADMA-NATHAN H, HELLSTROM WJG, KAISER FE, et al. Treatment of men with erectile dysfunction with transurethral alprostadil. N Engl J Med 1997;336:1-7.

PORST H. The rationale for prostaglandin E_1 in erectile failure: a survey of worldwide experience. J Urol 1996;155:802-15.

VIRAG R. Intracavernous injection of papaverine for erectile failure (letter). Lancet 1982;2:938.

21

Kidney disease and drug elimination

Cesare R. Sirtori

Drug elimination may take place by parallel routes, and the relative importance of each route is related to the solubility of the excreted molecule. All water-soluble drugs are excreted, partially or totally by the renal route. Lipophilic drugs are transformed metabolically into more water-soluble metabolites that are easily excreted by the kidney. Nonmetabolized lipid-soluble drugs are instead mainly excreted by other routes, e.g., the biliary route, whereas volatile drugs are preferentially excreted by the lungs.

Renal elimination may be the only pathway of excretion for highly water-soluble molecules such as aminoglycoside antibiotics. At the other extreme, highly lipophilic molecules are eliminated in minimal percentage by this route.

FUNCTIONAL BASIS OF THE RENAL ELIMINATION OF DRUGS

Excretion of drugs is tightly integrated into the main renal function, which is regulation of the composition and volume of extracellular fluids within optimal limits. This is controlled by two basic processes: (1) glomerular filtration, which separates large amounts of fluids from plasma, and (2) tubular transport (secretion and reabsorption) of electrolytes and other solutes. In the course of evolution, the kidneys have refined this function to a high degree of efficiency, thus reaching a filtering capacity of renal glomeruli 100-fold higher than that of muscle capillaries. Tubular transport, in particular at the proximal convoluted tubule, is far superior to the transport capacity of any other structure with a similar activity.

About 20% of plasma circulating in the kidneys is filtered. This constitutes approximately 50 times the volume of extracellular fluids (about 17 liters in an adult). The volume of preurine produced by glomerular ultrafiltration in the 24 h is thus approximately 170 liters. Only 1% of the ultrafiltrate is excreted into the urine, whereas 99% is reabsorbed with differential processes in the different segments of the nephron (65% in the proximal tubule and a further 15% along the descending branch of the loop of Henle, thus allowing only the remaining 20% to reach the distal tubule). The distal convoluted tubule and the collecting duct are responsible, in equal parts, for the hormone-regulated reab-

sorption of the residual volume of filtrate that is not excreted. The function of the tubules is thus reabsorption not only of water but also of all substances that are essential for the electrolyte and metabolic balance of the body (electrolytes, glucose, amino acids, vitamins, etc.).

Processes responsible for the excretion of drugs do not significantly differ from those for endogenous substrates. Drugs and water-soluble metabolites are filtered into the preurine; in the tubular lumen, they may either diffuse passively, according to a concentration gradient, into the extravascular parenchymal spaces or may be selectively reabsorbed, even against gradient, by the same tubular systems responsible for the transfer of endogenous metabolites from the lumen to blood vessels. Finally, some drugs also may be secreted into urine through active transport processes from the vascular pole to the lumen by tubular cells.

The principles regulating transfer of drugs at the renal level, based on physicochemical and general biochemical laws, do not differ to a significant extent from those operating in other biologic structures responsible for drug absorption and distribution. Variables such as molecular size, water and lipid solubility, and pK_a, dictating ionic dissociation as a function of hydrogen concentrations, affinity for tubular transport systems, and plasma protein binding, are all of essential importance.

Glomerular filtration and tubular reabsorption/secretion

Glomerular filtration depends on the pressure gradient across the filtering membrane. Different types of pressure are integrated, thus determining the effective filtration pressure (P_{eff}). The hydrostatic pressure of capillary glomeruli (P_{cap}) is partially counterbalanced by the colloido-osmotic pressure of capillary blood (P_{onc}) and the hydrostatic pressure in Bowman's capsule (P_{bow}):

$$P_{eff} = P_{cap} - P_{onc} - P_{bow} \qquad (21.1)$$

P_{cap} (about 50 mm Hg) is higher than that of capillaries in all other body areas, making glomerular filtration very efficient. P_{eff}, on the other hand, is kept constant, even when systemic blood pressure varies widely (between 80 and 200 mm Hg), because resistance in afferent arterioles is regulated as a function of blood pressure (thus in some cases contributing also to the maintenance of elevated pressure).

When applied on the filtering surface (S), P_{eff} is characterized by a specific hydraulic conductance (C_{hy}) that determines the filtered volume in time units, i.e., the velocity of glomerular filtration, generally expressed as glomerular filtration rate (GFR):

$$GFR = S \times C_{hy} \times P_{eff} \qquad (21.2)$$

where the $S \times C_{hy}$ product defines the filtration coefficient K_f.

GFR is about 170 liters/24 h, i.e., 120 to 130 ml/min, corresponding to about one-fifth of renal plasma flow (RPF). GFR fluctuates during the 24 h, following a circadian rhythm, increasing during the day by about 30% above the mean values and decreasing at night to a minimum 30% lower than the mean daily values. Disease and drug treatment may drastically affect these values.

Tubular reabsorption occurs predominantly in the proximal tubule, where up to 65% of water and NaCl are reabsorbed, whereas other molecules, e.g., drugs and endogenous metabolites, are reabsorbed at percentages that vary as a function of physicochemical characteristics. The fraction reabsorbed in the proximal tubule is constant and independent of GFR.

Drug reabsorption occurs at different percentages as a consequence of the different physicochemical factors regulating drug diffusion. The area of absorption is very ample, particularly in the proximal tubule, because of the brush-border structure, which increases surface contact of the luminal poles of tubular cells about 40-fold. Paracellular diffusion, on the other hand, is difficult because of the tight junctions between the lateral membranes of tubular cells. Along the nephron, drug concentrations in the tubular lumen may vary significantly, particularly because the reabsorption of drugs may be proportionally different from that of water. The initial concentration gradient between the lumen and surrounding capillaries may increase, thus varying the rate of reabsorption in the different sections of the tubule. Drug concentration in the ultrafiltrate may reach toxic levels for renal cells and cause irreversible damage. It also may exceed saturation levels, with consequent precipitation or crystal formation, e.g., in the case of drugs of low water solubility, such as the old sulfonamides used in protozoan disease. Precipitation also may be favored by certain urinary pH values. Molecules with a high lipid/water partition coefficient diffuse from preurine to peritubular capillaries. Overall, there is a minimal diffusion across the tubular membrane and very little reabsorption of water-soluble drugs. Drug ionization is also an important regulatory factor, since lipid-soluble molecules may diffuse back only in the undissociated form. The pH of the filtrate may move the ratio between the dissociated and undissociated forms of a drug, favoring or antagonizing reabsorption and delaying or accelerating excretion. This phenom-

enon occurs when the drug's pK_a and urinary pH differ by no more than 1 pH/pK_a unit; otherwise, changes are insignificant. Urinary acidification, reaching a maximum in the distal tubule and the collecting duct, facilitates net reabsorption and reduces excretion of weak acids such as salicylates and barbiturates, while reducing, in contrast, the reabsorption and facilitating excretion of weak bases such as alkaloids. An opposite effect is seen with urinary alkalinization.

In addition to passive diffusion, renal tubules can selectively transport metabolites such as glucose, amino acids, phosphates, sulfates, and bicarbonate through active reabsorption. These are saturable mechanisms, each displaying a threshold value. Most typical is glucose, with a renal threshold of around 2 g/liter, above which glucose may appear in urine.

Transport systems for the active reabsorption of endogenous metabolites are quite specific, and only in limited cases do they apply to drugs or metabolites. Small polypeptides are only partly reabsorbed by the various systems of amino acid transport; in most cases, proteins or filtered peptides are first hydrolyzed to amino acids by enzymes in the brush border of tubular cells.

The most efficient and specific reabsorption system is that for anions, operating in the reabsorption of uric acid and other anions, which takes place in the luminal membranes of the proximal tubules. Acidic drugs, such as probenecid, which are an efficient substrate for this transport system, by competing with uric acid, inhibit reabsorption and induce uricosuria (see Chap. 71). It should be noted that the active reabsorption system for anions is analogous to that for the tubular secretion of acidic substances, although transport in tubular cells appears to be less specific. As a consequence, most weak acids are secreted by renal tubules and not reabsorbed, whereas only a limited number of molecules such as uric acid, with a high affinity for reabsorption transporters, are retained and reenter the circulation.

Some macromolecules can bind receptor sites on the brush border and stimulate endocytosis-exocytosis. The best example is aminoglycoside antibiotics, for which endocytosis results in vacuolar and lysosomal accumulation with ensuing cell damage, enzyme release, and tubular cell necrosis. A renal protein receptor for aminoglycosides has been described recently. This very large molecule (megalin, GP 330), a polymer of cellular low-density lipoprotein (LDL) receptors, had been identified originally as the antigen for Heymann's nephritis, a rat model of membrane glomerulonephritis. Elucidation of the binding of aminoglycosides to megalin may allow the design of better-tolerated aminoglycosides (Fig. 21.1).

Tubular secretion is the transport of a substance in luminal fluid against a concentration gradient. It uses energy (provided by an Na pump in the basolateral membrane) and is blocked by enzyme inhibitors. The mechanism of active secretion of anions and cations, only partly clarified, is relatively nonspecific but saturable. In the case of saturable mechanisms, renal excretion of the substance increases only as a proportion of the GFR.

The best characterized tubular secretion system is that of anions, mainly controlling tubular secretion of uric and

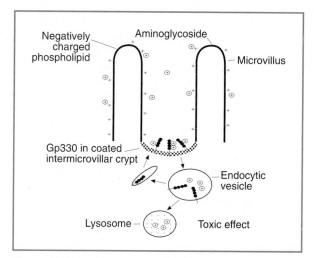

Figure 21.1 Possible model for the interaction of aminoglycoside antibiotics with the renal proximal tubular epithelium. Aminoglycosides concentrate in the intravillar space by binding to negatively charged phospholipids on cell surfaces and are subsequently delivered to negatively charged Gp330/megalin in the intravillar crypts. This leads to uptake and accumulation of the drug in lysosomes, where the polybasic molecules may exert their toxic effects on the cells.

oxalic acids. Optimal transport takes place for a substrate with two negative charges separated by 0.6 to 0.7 nm and a hydrophobic chain of a length of 0.8 to 1 mm, although the system can accommodate various types of organic anions. Many different exogenous organic acids have affinity for the anion transporters for uric acid and are secreted by the same tubular system. Best known examples are penicillin and other β-lactams, sulfonamides, salicylates (see Chap. 7), barbiturates, and diuretics such as furosemide, thiazides, and acetazolamide. The same system favors elimination of water-soluble drug metabolites and conjugates of glucuronic acid, sulfuric acid, or glycine.

Saturability of the system leads to competition between acidic substrates of both exogenous and endogenous origin. Penicillin secretion, when competitively reduced by probenecid and pyrazinamide, may increase uricemia by competing with the tubular secretion of uric acid. Salicylates at low doses inhibit urate secretion, whereas at high doses they reduce uricosuria by competing with tubular reabsorption (see Chap. 71).

Basic substances, such as catecholamines, serotonin, histamine, thiamine, and creatinine, are secreted by the cation system, different from that of anions but similarly energy-dependent and stereospecific. The major feature of transported substances is the presence of positively charged -NH₂ groups at physiologic pH. Through this route, natural and synthetic alkaloids, including atropine, hexamethonium, meperidine, morphine, and neostigmine, are secreted. The anatomic location of this second secretory system is similar to that for anions; it is saturable and may compete with drugs or endogenous substrates, whereas it is insensitive to acidic substances.

Recently, a ubiquitous mechanism for drug transport has found an unexpected role in the renal control of toxic substance accumulation. The P-glycoprotein system, originally detected as a membrane transport controller, confers mul-

tidrug resistance to cancer cells by active cellular extrusion of a wide range of drugs. Of the two types of human P-glycoprotein (Pgp), type I MDR1Pgp, is also responsible for the renal excretion of xenobiotics, peptides, steroids, and phospholipids and also is a regulator of swelling-activated Cl channels. The *MDR1* gene and protein are expressed in mesangial, proximal tubule, thick loop of Henle, and collecting duct cells, where Pgp-mediated transport occurs. Exposure of kidney cells to more than one Pgp substrate may result in competition and increased toxicity, as is the case for cyclosporine A (CsA), tacrolimus, digoxin, ivermectin, and dexamethasone. Antagonism to Pgp may lead to a considerably enhanced toxicity of CsA, whereas, conversely, knock-out of Pgp reduces the elimination of both CsA and digoxin. The role of Pgp in the active transport of steroid hormones, antibiotics, and calcium channel blockers explains its potential responsibility for the renal toxicity of cationic xenobiotics and metabolites. The reduced elimination of CsA following administration of calcium channel blockers, e.g., verapamil, is generally attributed to CYP3A4 inhibition (see Chap. 6). Experimental data show, however, that competition for Pgp also may contribute to the observed kinetic changes.

Evaluation of the renal excretion of drugs

Rate of drug elimination into the urine varies as a function of the amount of drug in the body at that moment (X_t) according to a proportionality factor (k_e) known as the *renal elimination constant:*

$$dX_u = k_e \times X_t \, dt \tag{21.3}$$

This equation may be simplified by using, instead of instantaneous velocity, the mean velocity in a time interval t calculated according to the concentration of drug in the urine (U) multiplied by the volume produced in that time interval (V_u/t). Since the total amount of drug in the body at time t is given by the concentration (C_t) times the apparent volume of distribution (V_d), Eq. (21.3) becomes

$$UV_u/t = k_e \times V_d \times C_t \tag{21.4}$$

The rate of renal excretion depends on plasma concentrations according to a proportionality factor, represented by the product of the renal elimination constant k_e and the volume of distribution V_d, i.e., by the renal clearance (CL_R). The general definition of CL_R is the rate of renal excretion normalized by the drug concentration in plasma, i.e., converting Eq. (21.4) to

$$(UV_u/t)/C_t = k_e \times V_d \tag{21.5}$$

Equation (21.5) can be applied directly and allows estimation of CL_R for endogenous and exogenous substances. The drug concentration measured in an aliquot of collected urine is multiplied by the volume of urine excreted in the time t, allowing calculation of the excreted drug. This value is divided by the plasma concentration of the substance at an intermediate time in the interval of urinary collection. When CL_R and the V_d are obtained, the renal elimination constant k_e can be calculated directly:

$$k_e = CL_R/V_d \qquad (21.6)$$

Since the half-life $(t_{1/2})$ of an exponential process is given by $0.693/k$, the $t_{1/2}$ of renal excretion will be

$$t_{1/2}r = 0.693(V_d/CL_R) \qquad (21.7)$$

CL_R thus represents the volume of plasma cleared of a substance by the kidney in a unit of time. If the drug is eliminated exclusively by the kidneys, CL_R correspond to total clearance, and k_e or the $t_{1/2}$ thereof correspond, respectively, to the k_e or elimination $t_{1/2}$ from the body.

CL_R of a drug varies as a function of the mechanism involved. For a drug exclusively eliminated by the renal route without reabsorption, CL_R corresponds to the GFR (i.e., approximately 120 ml/min), whereas if the drug is also eliminated by tubular secretion, CL_R may reach a value approximately equal to that of renal flow (i.e., about 650 ml/min). If, finally, the drug is filtered but not secreted and partly reabsorbed, CL_R may have a value below the GFR (e.g., 30 ml/min).

Since renal extraction has values between 0 and 1, and because renal flow is approximately 650 ml/min, CL_R is between 0 and 650 ml/min. This allows measurement of the CL_R of a substance eliminated in a single passage through the kidneys and rapidly secreted by the renal tubules. This is the case for penicillin and *para*-aminohippuric acid (PAH), both with a CL_R of approximately 650 ml/min in normal subjects. Since the plasma volume is about half the blood volume, renal blood flow is approximately 1300 ml/min, i.e., a value close to 25% of cardiac output.

The filtering capacity of renal glomeruli, approximately one-fifth of total renal flow, can be measured with a substance that is only filtered, without reabsorption or secretion, e.g., inuline. Inuline clearance (CL_{In}) may be used to evaluate glomerular filtration in a single patient. However, this method has been replaced by the simpler evaluation of creatinine clearance (CL_{Cr}). Creatinine is an endogenous muscular metabolite introduced into the circulation at constant velocity and eliminated almost totally by glomerular filtration. If conditions are maintained, creatinine concentration alone may allow an indirect estimation of clearance and, therefore, of glomerular filtering capacity (see below). Such conditions may not be met, for example, in the elderly (see Chap. 89) and in newborns (see Chap. 87).

DRUG KINETICS IN THE COURSE OF RENAL DISEASE

Since drug concentrations in plasma and tissues depend on dose, absorption, V_d, protein binding, and clearance,

renal disease may significantly affect kinetics. In the course of renal disease, gastric pH tends to increase, and the rate/amount of absorption also may decrease as a consequence (e.g., of altered motility/emptying as well as vomiting). In addition, the use of chelating drugs (e.g., aluminum hydroxide, calcium carbonate, or acetate) may lead to the binding of molecules such as iron, aspirin, or the quinolones (see Chap. 6).

Edema and hypotension also may reduce absorption of drugs given by the intramuscular or subcutaneous route. Edema and ascites also increase the V_d and reduce protein binding of drugs because of a concomitant decrease in albumin and retention of compounds competing with protein-binding sites. The final result is a reduction in total plasma concentration, increased V_d, and an increase in the free/bound ratio. An increased free fraction theoretically (may lead to increased pharmacodynamic activity, but this is compensated by metabolism and clearance (see Chap. 6). In renal failure, protein binding of phenytoin, digoxin, furosemide, nonsteroidal anti-inflammatory drugs, penicillin, salicylates, benzodiazepines, propranolol, quinidine, and tricyclic antidepressants is altered. Renal failure also may interfere with the liver metabolic handling of drugs, resulting in some cases in enhanced (e.g., phenytoin, digoxin, and propranolol) or reduced (e.g., quinidine) oxidation. In general, altered drug metabolism in the course of renal failure has limited clinical significance.

Drug excretion in renal failure

Since the renal clearance of a drug (CL_R) depends on glomerular filtration rate (GFR), tubular secretion (T_S), and/or tubular reabsorption (T_R), then

$$CL_R = GFR \times unbound\ drug + T_S - T_R \qquad (21.8)$$

Kinetics in the course of renal insufficiency generally are characterized by an increased elimination $t_{1/2}$. The half-life $t_{1/2} = 0.693k_e$ is determined by the efficiency of elimination k_e, a constant depending on renal (k_R) and metabolic (k_M) clearances. Thus, Eq. (21.6) may be reformulated as

$$k_e = (k_R + k_M)/V_d \qquad (21.9)$$

Knowledge of k_R therefore appears to be essential for an understanding of major kinetic parameters in the course of renal insufficiency.

In multiple-dose schedules, average drug concentrations in plasma at steady state (C_{ss}), assuming that dose and interval of administration τ are constant, are described by the following ratio:

$$C_{ss} = (F \times dose \times t_{1/2})/(\tau \times 0.693 \times V_d) \qquad (21.10)$$

where F is drug bioavailability and τ generally is expressed in hours (see Chap. 2). In renal insufficiency, lengthening of $t_{1/2}$ may lead to increased C_{ss} unless τ is appropriately modified. The best index of change in renal drug handling is provided by calculation of CL_R (see also Eqs. 21.5-21.7):

$$CL_R = UV_u/C_p \qquad (21.11)$$

where U is the urinary concentration (in mg/dl), C_p is the plasma concentration (in mg/dl), and V_u the urinary volume (in ml/min).

In order to avoid urine collection, CL_R may be calculated according to the formula of Cockcroft and Gault, only requiring measurement of serum creatinine S_{Cr}:

$$CL_R \text{ (ml/min)} = [(140 - \text{age, years}) \times \qquad (21.12)$$
$$\times \text{ body weight, kg}]/(72 \times S_{Cr})$$

This needs appropriate correction in the case of reduced muscle mass such as in the elderly or newborns (see Chaps. 87 and 89).

For obese patients, the lean body weight (LBW) should be used. Correction for males (H is height in cm) is

If H > 152.4 cm, LBW (kg) = 50 + (H − 152.4) × 0.89
If H < 152.4 cm, LBW (kg) = 50 − (152.4 − H) × 0.89

For females:

If H > 152.4 cm, LBW (kg) = 45.4 + (H − 152.4) × 0.89
If H < 152.4 cm, LBW (kg) = 45.4 − (152.4 − H) × 0.89

S_{Cr} should not be used or should be used with caution if it is higher than 4 mg/dl and in patients with muscular diseases (e.g., atrophy, cachexia).

In order to calculate doses or intervals of administration τ, a correction factor Q also can be used:

$$Q_r = k_e/k_n \qquad (21.13)$$

where k_e is the elimination constant in a patient with reduced filtration and k_n is the elimination constant in a patient with normal renal function. Variations in dosage

thus can be expressed either as

$$D_r = D_n \times Q_r \qquad (21.14 \text{ a})$$

where D_r is the reduced dose and D_n is the normal dose, or as a change in interval τ

$$\tau_r = \tau_n/Q_r \qquad (21.14 \text{ b})$$

Reduction in dosage and increase in the interval of administration obviously are not the same intervention. When drug effects depend from the rapid attainment of therapeutic concentrations, results may be achieved more easily by giving full doses at longer intervals versus giving reduced doses at normal intervals. Table 21.1 gives examples of dosage or interval modifications as a function of the degree of renal impairment.

A renal failure nomogram can be a simple and useful tool (Fig. 21.2). The left-hand side represents the fraction of renally eliminated drug F_u. On the numeric abscissa, the endogenous CL_{Cr} is given in ml/min/1.73 m². Below this there are two additional scales for the corresponding S_{Cr} (in mg/dl) for males and females (adult age and normal muscular function). The right-hand side ordinate represents the ratio $R = t_{1/2,norm}/t_{1/2,rf}$ (rf = renal failure). Considering elimination of a drug in renal failure, e.g., digoxin, with an F_u of 0.76, a straight line is drawn between 0.76 on the left ordinate and 1.0 on the right ordinate. Assuming CL_{Cr} of 40 ml/min/1.73 m² (or equivalent S_{Cr}), a vertical line is drawn from 40 on the abscissa so as to the intersect with the previously drawn line. From the intersection a parallel to the abscissa is drawn. This gives an R value of 0.49, and by the equation

$$t_{1/2,rf} = t_{1/2,norm}/R \qquad (21.15)$$

since the $t_{1/2,norm}$ for digoxin is 41 h, $t_{1/2,rf} = 41/0.49 = 83.7$ h.

Table 21.1 Examples of dose (% of maximal) or interval modification hours as related to glomerular filtration rate (GFR) for some major antibiotics

Drug	Method	GFR > 50 (ml/min)	GFR 10-50 (ml/min)	GFR <10 (ml/min)	Supplement after dialysis
Ampicillin	I	6	6-12	12-16	Yes
Gentamicin	D	60-90	30-70	20-30	Yes
Netilmicin	D	60-90	30-70	20-30	Yes
Cefotaxime	I	6-8	8-12	12-24	Yes
Cefoxitin	I	8	8-12	24-48	Yes
Erythromycin	D	-	-	-	No
Nalidixic acid	D	100			?
Sulfonamides	I	12	18	24	Yes
Doxycycline	I	12	12-18	18-24	No
Vancomycin	I	24-72	72-240	240	No

Examples:
Ampicillin: method I, change from an interval of 6h for normal GFR to 12-16h for GFR < 10 ml/min.
Gentamicin: method D, change from a dose 60-90% of maximal for normal GFR to 20/30% of maximal for GFR < 10 ml/min.

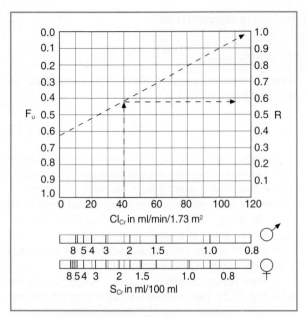

Figure 21.2 Inset nomogram renal failure. The example provided shows estimation of the digoxin elimination half-life in renal failure. Detailed explanations are provided in the text. (CL_{Cr} = creatinine clearance; S_{Cr} = serum creatinine).

Drug excretion during dialysis

Renal failure patients at the terminal stage are treated with a renal substitution therapy, i.e., hemodialysis, hemodiafiltration, hemofiltration, or peritoneal dialysis. All these can remove drugs from the circulation. Therefore, at times, dosage adjustments are necessary.

Dialysis membranes influence removal of drugs as a function of surface area and size of pores. The diameters of pores of cuprophan filters, used in traditional dialysis, are about 0.001 μm, allowing the free passage of molecules with molecular weights (M_r) less than 500.

Diffusion of higher-molecular-weight molecules is difficult and stops for M_r above 1000. Passage through the dialysis membrane is proportional to the blood/dialysis bath concentration gradient, flow of blood and dialysate, and filtering surface area. Protein binding limits drug diffusion, and V_d influences the dialyzable fraction. This is high for drugs with $V_d < 1$ liter/kg, modest for drugs with $V_d = 1$ to 2 liters/kg, and very scarce for drugs with $V_d > 2$ liter/kg.

Hemodialysis, hemodiafiltration, and hemofiltration, using filters with pores of 0.01 μm, allow the best passage of molecules of higher molecular weight. Removal is thus independent of the concentration gradient (diffusion) but occurs for convection, i.e., passage of drug through the membrane together with ultrafiltered water. In the case of peritoneal dialysis, drug removal is very modest, and the limiting factor is the very low flow; the peritoneal membrane also allows passage of drugs in the opposite direction, and this may be important for the antibiotic treatment of peritonitis, which often complicates treatment.

Drug dosage during dialysis follows the rules described for renal insufficiency, considering, however, that drug supplementation is required at the end of dialysis for dialyzable drugs. This can be accomplished by monitoring the amount of drug excreted in the ultrafiltrate. Alternatively, some authors have suggested a correction based on the drug's sieving coefficient (S_c), i.e., the solute's ability to convectively permeate the membrane; S_c values range from 0 (for macromolecules that do not cross the membrane) to 1 (for microsolutes whose transport is not affected by the membrane). The factor p for drug dosage adjustment therefore may be

$$p = Q_x + (UFR \times S_c)/CL \qquad (21.16)$$

where Q_x reflects the remaining elimination capacity of the body (extrarenal elimination), and CL is the clearance in a patient with normal renal function. Coefficients for S_c are provided by different sources. The administered dose D is computed as $D = pD_0$, where D_0 is the dose for otherwise healthy individuals.

Suggested readings

Bressolle F, Kinowski J-M, de la Coussaye JE, et al. Clinical pharmacokinetics during continuous hemofiltration. Clin Pharmacokinet 1994;26:457-71.

del Moral RG, Olmo A, Aguilar M, O'Valle F. P glycoprotein: A new mechanism to control drug-induced nephrotoxicity. Exp Nephrol 1998;6:89-97.

Lam YWF, Banerji S, Hatfield C, Talbert RL. Principles of drug administration in renal insufficiency. Clin Pharmacokinet 1997;32:30-57.

Moestrup SK, Cui S, Vorum H, et al. Evidence that epithelial glycoprotein 330/megalin mediates uptake of polybasic drugs. J Clin Invest 1995;96:1404-13.

Schinkel AH, Wagenaar E, van Deemter L, et al. Absence of the mdr1a P-glycoprotein in mice affects tissue distribution and pharmacokinetics of dexamethasone, digoxin, and cyclosporin A. J Clin Invest 1995;96:1698-705.

Schinkel AH, Mayer U, Wagenaar E, et al. Normal viability and altered pharmacokinetics in mice lacking mdr1-type (drug-transporting) P-glycoproteins. Proc Natl Acad Sci USA 1997;94:4028-33.

Vrhovac B, Sarapa N, Bakran I, et al. Pharmacokinetic changes in patients with oedema. Clin Pharmacokinet 1995;28:405-18.

Cardiovascular
diseases

Drugs used in cardiovascular diseases

Lajos Matos

Cardiovascular diseases accounted for 30% of global mortality in 1998. This death toll is not evenly distributed; cardiovascular disease accounted for 46% of all deaths in developed countries and 25% of all deaths in developing countries. Cardiovascular disease will continue to have a leading role in global mortality in the future as well, and disability-adjusted life years (DALY) loss attributable to cardiovascular disease, which is already high, according to projected estimates for 2020, will have a significant further rise. Thus, we need more and better drugs to address this disease because pharmaceutical therapy is highly cost-effective for both patients and society.

This chapter provides an introduction to the clinical pharmacology of drugs used in cardiovascular disease, presented in alphabetical order.

ADENOSINE

Adenosine is an endogenous nucleoside produced in many tissues and organs. Its effects depend primarily on binding to cell surface receptors. Its mode of action involves enhanced potassium conductance and inhibition of cyclic adensine monophosphate (cAMP)-induced calcium influx. The results are hyperpolarization and suppression of calcium-dependent action potentials. In cardiac electrophysiologic studies, a lengthening of the sinus cycle and a prolongation of the AH interval, followed by partial or complete atrioventricular nodal block, without any effect on the His-Purkinje interval, are observed. Adenosine has minimal vagal effects and no appreciable negative inotropic or hypotensive effect.

Adenosine is not absorbed from the gastrointestinal tract. After iv injection, it is distributed rapidly in the body and crosses the blood-brain barrier. Its half-life is estimated to be less than 10 s; however, because of its fast clearance, no reliable pharmacokinetic data are available.

Adenosine can restore sinus rhythm in about 90% of patients with atrioventricular nodal reentrant tachycardia (AVNRT) and atrioventricular reciprocating tachycardia (AVRT), but it is ineffective in multifocal atrial tachycardia.

Interactions

- Methylxanthines (theophylline, caffeine): competitive antagonism.
- Dipyridamole: inhibits cellular uptake of adenosine.
- Carbamazepine: conduction inhibition can be enhanced.

Administration

Administration is by rapid bolus injection.

ALPHA$_1$ BLOCKERS

Stimulation of α_1 adrenoreceptors at postsynaptic sites leads to vasoconstriction, increases peripheral resistance, and elevates blood pressure. Blockers of these receptors therefore are vasodilators. Selective postsynaptic α_1-adrenoceptor inhibitors decrease peripheral vascular resistance and lead to vasodilatation without inducing reflex tachycardia or reducing cardiac output. In addition, because α_1 blockers leave α_2 receptors practically unaffected, they do not induce endogenous catecholamine release from the sympathetic nerve endings. Alpha$_1$ blockers act favorably in the lipid profile, improve insulin sensitivity, and are equally effective in all age groups. Specific advantages include improvement in urodynamics and symptoms in patients with benign prostatic hyperplasia (BPH).

Interactions

- Diuretics, calcium antagonists, β blockers: concomitant administration may produce a substantial reduction in blood pressure (low initial dosage recommended).
- False-positive laboratory test results may occur in screening for pheochromocytoma (urinary VMA and MHPG metabolites of norepinephrine) in patients treated with prazosin.

Although α_1 blockers are highly bound to plasma proteins (Tab. 22.1), in vitro data in human plasma indicate that they have no effect on protein binding of other drugs (e.g., cardiac glycosides, hypoglycemic agents, antiarrhythmics, and anti-inflammatory drugs).

Side effects

Side effects include first-dose hypotension and pancreatitis (prazosin, doxazosin).

Administration

Administration is by the oral route.

ANGIOTENSIN-CONVERTING ENZYME (ACE) INHIBITORS

In response to different factors, such as sodium depletion and symphathetic stimulation or reduced renal artery pressure, an enzyme (renin) is produced by the kidney cortex. Renin converts angiotensinogen, a circulating glycoprotein, into angiotensin I. This is a biologically inactive form, converted by angiotensin-converting enzyme (ACE) into a highly potent vasoconstrictor, angiotensin II. ACE inhibitors reduce angiotensin II levels and thus prevent vasoconstriction. Both sympathetic activity and norepinephrine release are reduced, whereas vagal activity probably is increased. Sodium excretion and potassium retention are facilitated because aldosterone release is reduced. There is an increased water loss as well because antidiuretic hormone (ADH) secretion is also blocked. ACE inhibitors reduce bradykinin degradation; bradykinin stimulates release of nitric oxide and of other vasodilators. ACE inhibitors also reduce left ventricular mass, partly by decreasing blood pressure and partly by producing a direct antiproliferative effect. Pharmacologic and pharmacokinetic characteristics of ACE inhibitors are given in Table 22.2.

Main indications

- Hypertension and hypertensive heart disease.
- Congestive heart failure.
- Acute myocardial infarction.

Interactions

- Anesthetics: hypotensive effect may be enhanced.
- Antacids: bioavailability may be reduced.
- Diuretics: increased risk of first-dose hypotension.
- Lithium: ACE inhibitors decrease lithium clearance.
- Nonsteroidal anti-inflammatory drugs (NSAIDs): antihypertensive effect of ACE inhibitors reduced.
- Potassium-sparing diuretics or potassium supplements: concomitant administration may lead to hyperkalemia.

Side effects

- Cough: nonproductive, dry cough.
- Hyperkalemia: in most patients an ACE inhibitor-induced decrease in aldosterone secretion triggers a rise in serum potassium levels.
- Renal insufficiency: high-risk patients also would respond with hypotension (see below).
- Angioneurotic edema: could be severe but is rare (0.1 to 0.2%).
- Skin rash: seen in 5 to 10% of patients.
- Dysgeusia: taste alteration or loss, probably caused by zinc binding by the ACE inhibitor.

Table 22.1 Main pharmacodynamic and pharmacokinetic characteristics and recommended dosages of alpha$_1$ blockers for cardiac therapy

	Doxazosin	Prazosin	Terazosin
Onset of action (min)	60-120	>30	15-20
To peak effect (h)	6-7	1-1.5	1-2
Duration of action (h)	16-36	4-6	>18
Plasma half-life (h)	22	3	10-12
Bioavailability (%)	60-70	60-80	80-90
Protein binding (%)	>90	>90	>90
Metabolism	Hepatic	Hepatic	Hepatic
Excretion	Renal (10%)	Bile, feces	Renal (40%)
Pregnancy	No	No	No
Elderly half-life	Longer half-life	Longer half-life	Longer half-life
Impaired liver function	Longer effect	Longer effect	Longer effect
Impaired renal function effect	Minimal effect	Longer half-life	Minimal effect
Effect of food on absorbtion	No effect	No effect	No effect
Daily dose (mg)	1-16	2-20	1-20
Daily dosing frequency	1	2-3	1

Table 22.2 Pharmacologic, pharmacokinetic, and dosing data of ACE inhibitors

	Prodrug	SH group?	Protein binding (%)	Peak effect (h)	Metabolism	Elimination	$t_{1/2}$ (h)	Daily dose (per day)	(mg)
Benazepril	Yes	No	95-97	2	Hepatic	Renal	10-11	1	10-20
Captopril	No	Yes	30	1-2	Hepatic (partially)	Renal	2-3	2-3	25-150
Cilazapril	Yes	No	Unknown	3-7	Hepatic + blood	Renal	3-9	1	1.5-5
Delapril	Yes	No	Unknown	1-2	Hepatic + blood	Renal	1-5	2	15-30
Enalapril	Yes	No	<50	2-4	Hepatic	Renal	6-11	1-2	5-40
Fosinopril	Yes	No	>90	2-4	Hepatic	Renal + hepatic	>24	1	5-40
Lisinopril	No	No	None	4-8	None	Renal	12-13	1	5-40
Moexipril	Yes	No	Moderate	1-2	Hepatic	Renal	2-9	1	7.5-30
Perindopril	Yes	No	20	2-3	Hepatic	Renal	>24	1	2-8
Quinapril	Yes	No	95-97	1-2	Hepatic	Renal	2-3	1-2	5-40
Ramipril	Yes	No	50-60	3-6	Hepatic	Renal	14-30	1	2.5-10
Spirapril	Yes	No	89	4-6	Hepatic	Renal	>12	1	6
Trandolapril	Yes	No	80-94	4-6	Hepatic	Renal	>24	1	1-4

Administration

Administration is by the oral route or iv (enalaprilat).

ANGIOTENSIN II INHIBITORS

There are two main classes of angiotensin II receptors, labeled as AT_1 and AT_2, respectively, and angiotensin II inhibitors act directly at these receptors. Practically all cardiovascular effects of angiotensin II – including vasoconstriction, stimulation of aldosterone, catecholamine release, and cell proliferation – are controlled by AT_1 receptors. The functions of AT_2-binding sites are still unclear (control of cardiac mass?). Drugs acting on AT_1 receptors have no effect on bradykinin metabolism and therefore are more selective than ACE inhibitors. Effects can be summarized as arteriolar vasodilatation, blockade of aldosterone and norepinephrine release, reduction in central sympathetic tone, and blockade of endothelin release. Consequently, blood pressure is reduced, sodium and water reabsorption are decreased, and cerebral autoregulation is improved.

Some AT_1 antagonists act as unchanged molecules on the receptor; others are prodrugs. Some act competitively, whereas others do not. The main characteristics of AT_1 antagonists in clinical practice are shown in Table 22.3. AT_1 antagonists offer a therapeutic alternative to patients unable to tolerate ACE inhibitors because of cough, which is no more frequent on AT_1 antagonists than on placebo.

Main indications

These are identical with those of ACE inhibitors.

Interactions

No significant pharmacokinetic interactions have been found with diuretics, digoxin, warfarin, cimetidine, and phenobarbital.

Administration

Administration is by the oral route.

Table 22.3 Characteristics of AT_1 antagonists in clinical use

Agent	Prodrug	Antagonism	Daily dose (per day)	(mg)
Candesartan cilexetil	Yes	Noncompetitive	1	2-8
Eprosartan	No	Competitive	1	400-1200
Irbesartan	No	Competitive	1	50-100
Losartan	Yes	Noncompetitive	1	25-100
Valsartan	No	Competitive	1	80-160

ANTIARRHYTHMIC AGENTS

A traditional and still widely used classification of antiarrhythmic drugs is based on their effects on cardiac action potential. The main electrophysiologic properties and classification of antiarrhythmics are shown in Table 22.4.

Chapter 24 provides a critical evaluation of the current classification of antiarrhythmic agents.

There are compounds (e.g., adenosine, cardiac glycosides, and magnesium) that produce antiarrhythmic activity by unclassified mechanisms. These are discussed separately (e.g., see Adenosine above). Basic pharmacodynamic and pharmacokinetic characteristics of antiarrhythmic agents are summarized in Table 22.5.

CLASS IA

Disopyramide

Interactions

- Negative inotropic agents (e.g., β blockers): these may further depress myocardial function.
- Agents prolonging the QT interval: arrhythmogenicity may be enhanced.
- Verapamil: constipation may be enhanced.

Side effects

- Hypoglycemia may be seen in diabetes mellitus.
- In BPH, anticholinergic effect of the drug may cause urinary retention.

Administration

Administration is by the oral route.

Procainamide

Interactions

The doses of neuromuscular blocking agents (e.g., succinylcholine) should be reduced because procainamide decreases acetylcholine release.

Side effects

A lupus-like reaction is seen (particularly in slow acetylators).

Administration

Administration is by the oral route or iv.

Quinidine

Interactions

- Decreases digoxin clearance (serum digoxin levels increase).

Table 22.4 Modified Vaughn-Williams classification of antiarrhytmic agents and some of their electrophysiologic effects

Class	Main electrophysiologic properties	Drug	Ventricular fibrillation threshold	Arrhythmogenic action (%)[1]
IA	Inhibition of fast inward sodium current Repolarization lengthened QT interval lengthened	Disopyramide Procainamide Quinidine	Decreased Decreased Decreased	1-6 0-21 1-20
IB	Inhibition of fast inward sodium current QT interval unchanged	Aprindine Lidocaine Mexiletine Phenytoin Tocainide	Increased Increased Increased Increased	 16 1-20 0-8
IC	Inhibition of fast inward sodium current QT interval lengthened	Encainide Flecainide Lorcainide Propafenone	Increased Increased Increased Increased	12-37 4-28 8-24 5-15
II	Beta-blockers: inhibition of β₁-adrenergic receptor mediated effects		Increased	
III	Sodium channel activation, potassium channel blockade QT interval increases	Amiodarone Bretylium Ibutilide	Increased Increased Increased	4-30 4
IV	Calcium antagonists: blocking of slow inward calcium channel	Diltiazem Nifedipine Verapamil	Increased Unchanged Increased	 18

[1]Data from studies reported in the literature.

• Effects of coumarin anticoagulants enhanced.

Side effect

Thrombocytopenia.

Administration

Administration is by the oral route.

CLASS IB

Lidocaine

Interactions

Drugs decreasing liver blood flow (e.g., propranolol) reduce lidocaine clearance.

Administration

Administration is iv.

Table 22.5 Pharmacodynamics and pharmacokinetic characteristics of antiarrhythmic agents

Class	Drug/ administration	Onset of action	Peak of action	Duration of action	$t_{1/2}$	Protein binding (%)	Bioavailability (%)
IA	Disopyramide, po	30-300 min	30-300 min	90-480 min	6-7 h	10-70	50-95
	Procainamide						
	po	5-15 min	60-90 min	4-20 h	3-5 h	15-20	75-95
	iv	<10 s	<10 s	-	-	-	-
	Quinidine, po	60 min	60-300 min	12 h	4-8 h	70-85	80 ± 15
IB	Lidocaine, iv	Immediate	Dose-dependent	10-20 min	1-2 h	60-80	NA
	Mexiletine, po	30-120 min	2-4 h	8-12 h	9-12 h	60-75	80-90
IC	Flecainide, po	60-120 min	60-360 min	24-48 h	12-24 h	40	>90
	Propafenone, po	60 min	60-180 min	8-12 h	8 h	80-90	3-10 dose-dependent
II	See β-blocking agents						
III	Amiodarone						
	po	1-3 wks	Dose-dependent	>50 days	30-110 days	90-96	35-65
	iv	12 h	15-30 days	>50 days	20-47 days	96	22-86
	Ibutilide, iv	Immediate	Immediate	Dose-dependent	2-12 h	40	NA
	Sotalol, po	2-4 h	2-3 h	24 h	7-15 h	Not bound	>90
IV	See Calcium channel blocking agents						

Class	Drug	Metabolism	Excretion	Renal impairment	Hepatic impairment	Elderly
IA	Disopyramide	Hepatic	Renal	Reduce dose	Reduce dose	Reduce dose
	Procainamide	Hepatic unchanged	(50-60%)	Reduce dose	Reduce dose	Reduce dose
	Quinidine	Hepatic/renal (60-85%)	Renal (15-40% unchanged)	Reduce dose	Reduce dose	Reduce dose
IB	Lidocaine	Hepatic	Renal (10% unchanged)	Reduce rate of infusion	Reduce rate of infusion	Reduce dose
	Mexiletine	Hepatic	Mainly biliary	Reduce dose	Reduce dose	Reduce dose
IC	Flecainide	Hepatic	Renal	Reduce dose	Reduce dose	Reduce dose
	Propafenone	Hepatic "metabolites"	Renal + biliary	No effect	Reduce dose	Reduce dose
II	See β-blocking agents					
III	Amiodarone	Hepatic	Mainly biliary	No dose adjustment needed	Reduce dose	Reduce dose
	Ibutilide	Hepatic	Renal	No dose adjustment needed	Reduce dose (?)	Reduce dose (?)
	Sotalol	Not metabolised	Renal (unchanged)	No dose adjustment needed	No dose adjustment needed	Start with low dose
IV	See Calcium channel blocking agents					

Mexiletine

Interactions

Concomitant administration of hepatic enzyme inducers (e.g., phenobarbital or phenytoin) may lower mexiletine levels.

Side effects

In patients with parkinsonism, tremor may be potentiated.

Administration

Administration is by the oral route.

CLASS IC

In the Cardiac Arrhythmia Suppression Trial (CAST, 1989) it was shown that mortality among patients treated with class IC drugs increased more than twofold compared with those treated with placebo. There is indirect evidence that other sodium channel blockers may produce similar effects. Encainide was withdrawn from the market in the United States in 1991 because of the results of the CAST study. At present, the drug is available only through the manufacturer for those patients who received encainide prior to its withdrawal and who cannot be switched to another antiarrhtyhmic agent. It is therefore not reviewed in detail here.

Flecainide

For characteristics, see Table 22.4.

Interactions

Flecainide may increase the propranolol level, and vice versa.

Side effects

- Precipitation or worsening of heart failure;
- visual problems;
- dizziness.

Administration

Administration is by the oral route.

Propafenone

Interactions

Propafenone increases serum digoxin, propranolol, and warfarin levels.

Administration

Administration is by the oral route.

CLASS II

See β-blocking agents.

CLASS III

Amiodarone

Interactions

Blood levels of class IA, IB, and IC antiarrhythmics as well as those of oral anticoagulants, quinidine, and digoxin are increased.

Side effects

See Table 22.6.

Administration

Administration is by the oral route and intravenously.

Table 22.6 Adverse effects of amiodarone therapy

Early events (mainly following intravenous administration)

Cardiovascular
Circulatory collapse, bradycardia, sinus arrest, arrhythmogenicity (relatively rare)

Central nervous system
Flushing, headache, insomnia, hallucinations, dizziness, ataxia, memory disturbances

Gastrointestinal
Bitter taste, nausea, vomiting, constipation

Late events

Pulmonary
Infiltrates and fibrosis (0.07-13%; fatal in up to 3.9%)

Thyroid gland
Hypothyroidism or hyperthyroidism (3-7%)

Ophthalmologic
Corneal deposits, haloes, reduced visual acuity, macular degeneration, optic neuropaty (with complaints, 1.4-6%)

Cardiovascular
Negative chronotropism, sinus arrest, atrioventricular block, torsades des pointes (relatively rare)

Dermatologic
Photosensitivity, permanent grayish-blue discoloration of the skin (10%), rashes

Muscular
Proximal muscle weakness, gastrointestinal nausea, constipation, weight loss

Hepatic
Increase in transaminase levels (10-20%), hepatotoxicity (uncommon, but may be fatal)

Hemopoietic
Thrombocytopenia

Other
Breast pain, gynecomastia, epididymitis, porphyrinogenicity

Ibutilide

Following iv administration, this recently marketed drug restored sinus rhythm in about 50% of patients with atrial flutter and about 30% of patients with atrial fibrillation (for pharmacodynamic and kinetic characteristics, see Tab. 22.5).

Interactions

Coadministration of digoxin, calcium antagonists, or β blockers had no effects on ibutilide kinetics.

Side effects

Side effects include nausea and torsades des pointes (see Tab. 22.4).

Administration

Administration is by iv infusion.

Sotalol

Interactions

Sotalol interacts with catecholamine-depleting drugs (e.g., guanethidine and reserpine) causing an excessive reduction in resting sympathetic tone.

Administration

Administration is orally or by iv infusion.

CLASS IV

See calcium antagonists.

β-ADRENERGIC BLOCKING AGENTS

These drugs are structurally similar to catecholamines and are competitive inhibitors. Two subtypes of β receptors have been identified: β_1 and β_2. Although β_1 receptors are found mainly in the heart and β_2 receptors usually are found in smooth bronchial muscles, in some organs, including the heart, both subtypes are present. β blockers have different affinities for β_1 or β_2 receptors; those having a greated affinity for β_1 receptors are known as *cardioselective*. Selectivity, however, is relative; with higher doses, β_2 activity also becomes evident.

Some β blockers also activate β receptors in the absence of catecholamines, having partial intrinsic sympathomimetic activity (ISA), and therefore are partial agonists. They also differ in their pharmacokinetic characteristics. Those with low lipid solubility (e.g., atenolol and nadolol) are absorbed less readily by the gastrointestinal tract, metabolized to a lesser extent, have low plasma protein binding, and have a longer plasma half-life than do those with high lipid solubility (e.g., alprenolol and propranolol). Characteristics of the different beta-blockers are shown in Tables 22.7 and 22.8, respectively. These two tables also include frequency and average daily doses.

NONSELECTIVE β BLOCKERS WITHOUT ISA

Nadolol, propranolol, sotalol, timolol

The characteristics of nonselective β blockers are reported in Table 22.7.

Table 22.7 Characteristics of nonselective β blockers

	Lipid solubility	Protein binding (%)	Metabolism	Elimination	Onset of action (h)	Peak effect (h)	$t_{1/2}$ (h)	Dosing frequency per day	Daily dose (mg)
Nonselective, without ISA									
Nadolol	No	20-30	–	Renal (metabolites)	1	2-4	20-24	1	40-240
Propranolol	Strong	80-95	Hepatic	Renal	1-2	2-3	3-6	2-4	80-320
Sotalol	No	10	–	Renal	1	2-3	7-15	1-2	160-320
Timolol	Strong	10	Hepatic	Renal	0.5	1-2	3-5	1-3	10-60
Nonselective,	**with ISA**								
Carteolol	Weak	20-30	–	Renal	0.5-1	1-2	6-7	1	10-40
Oxprenolol	Strong	70-80	Hepatic	Renal	1	1	2	2-3	60-480
Penbutolol	Strong	80-98	Hepatic	Renal	0.5-1	1-3	20-25	1	10-20
Pindolol	Moderate	40	Hepatic	Renal	1	1-3	2-5	1-3	15-45

Interactions

- Adrenoreceptor stimulants: hypotensive effect may reverse.
- Class I antiarrhythmics: cardiac depression and bradycardia.
- Calcium antagonists (especially diltiazem and verapamil): additive negative inotropic and chronotropic action and hypotension.
- Disopyramide: additive effect.
- General anesthetics: negative inotropic effect.
- Lidocaine: unwanted lidocaine effects may be exaggerated.
- MAO inhibitors: increased hypotensive effect.
- NSAIDs: antihypertensive effect may be reduced.
- Quinidine: beta-blocking effect may be increased.

Side effects

The following must be considered valid to different degrees for all β blockers:

- in obstructive airways disease, an increase in airway resistance may occur;
- in pheochromocytoma, blood pressure elevation occurs because nonselective β blockade leaves α vasoconstrictor activity unopposed;
- in diabetes, signs of hypoglycemia may be masked.

NONSELECTIVE β BLOCKERS WITH ISA

Carteolol, oxprenolol, penbutolol, and pindolol

See also Table 22.7.

Interactions and side effects

See Nonselective β blockers without ISA.

SELECTIVE β BLOCKERS WITHOUT ISA

Atenolol, betaxolol, bisoprolol, esmolol, and metoprolol

See also Table 22.8.

Interactions

- Epinephrine: there may be sudden hypertension with bradycardia (less likely than with nonselective beta-blockers).
- Class I antiarrhythmics: cardiac depression and bradycardia are seen.
- Digoxin: serum digoxin levels may be elevated.
- General anesthetics: possible myocardial depression.
- Ergotamine: peripheral vasoconstriction could be increased.
- Prazosin: first-dose effect may be potentiated.

SELECTIVE β BLOCKERS WITH ISA

Acebutolol and celiprolol

See also Table 22.8.

Interactions

- Alcohol: central depressant effect is potentiated.
- Amiodarone: negative inotropic effect is potentiated.
- Quinidine: effects of the β blocker may be increased.

Table 22.8 Characteristics of selective β blockers

Selective β blockers	Lipid solubility	Protein binding (%)	Metabolism	Elimination	Onset of action	Peak effect	$t_{1/2}$	Daily dosing	Daily dose
Without ISA									
Atenolol	No	3-10	Minimal	–	1 h	2-4 h	3-6 h	1-2	25-100 mg
Betaxolol	Moderate	50	Extensive	Renal	2 h (+hepatic)	2-8 h	16-22 h	1	10-40 mg
Bisoprolol	Moderate	30	Minimal	Renal	1-3 h	2 h	10-12 h	1	2.5-20
Esmolol[1]	No	55	Extensive	Renal	2 min	2-5 min	9 min	Not for chronic use	25-300 µg/kg/min
Metoprolol	Moderate	12-88	Extensive	Renal	1 h	1-2 h	3-6 h	2-3	50-400 mg
With ISA									
Acebutolol	Weak	10-20	Extensive	Renal (+biliary)	1h	1-4 h	3-10 h	1-2	200-1200 mg
Celiprolol[2]	Weak	25-30	Minimal	Renal (+biliary)	0.5-1 h	2-3 h	5-6 h	1	200-400 mg

[1]iv
[2]ß$_1$ ISA at lower doses; ß$_2$ ISA at higher doses

DUAL-ACTING β BLOCKERS

Some β blockers act as competitive antagonists on both α and β adrenoreceptors. Adding a vasodilator to a β blocker may significantly increase the success rate of hypertension therapy over monotherapy, but it may cause serious side effects. However, molecules with dual action have been developed, and they show few adverse reactions.

Carvedilol

Carvedilol is a β blocker with no ISA that binds to $β_1$ and, to a lesser extent, $α_1$ receptors; α blockade seems to be the primary mechanism responsible for vasodilatation. Carvedilol possesses pronounced antioxidant properties as well and inhibits the aberrant proliferation of vascular smooth muscle cells. It also was found to be effective in the management of congestive heart failure (CHF).

Peak plasma concentrations after oral administration are reached after 1 to 2 hours. Bioavailability is 25%, but in patients with liver impairment, it may be increased up to 80%. Plasma protein binding is 98%. Carvedilol is extensively metabolized by the liver, and because excretion is primarily biliary, 60% of a single dose appears as metabolites in feces. Only about 1% is eliminated in unchanged form through the kidneys. Elimination $t_{1/2}$ is approximately 7 hours.

Interactions

Interactions occur with diltiazem and verapamil, resulting in a potentially additive effect on atrioventricular conduction.

Labetalol

Labetalol has a ratio of 3:1 ratio of β to α antagonism, being a racemic mixture of four isomers (two inactive, one potent α blocker, and one potent selective $β_2$ agonist, respectively). Labetalol is specifically indicated to control blood pressure in severe hypertension, even during pregnancy. Following oral administration, peak plasma levels are reached in 1 to 2 hours, with an absolute bioavailability of 25% because of extensive "first pass" metabolism. Protein binding is 50%. Metabolism is hepatic. Excretion is via the urine and bile.

Side effects

The most common side effect is reversible hepatic and cholestatic jaundice.

Administration

Administration is orally or by iv infusion.

CALCIUM CHANNEL BLOCKERS

Calcium channel blockers (CCBs) inhibit calcium entry into the cells by blocking voltage-dependent calcium channels. In phase 0 of the action potential there is a fast inward sodium current through the so-called fast channels, whereas during phase 2 there is a slow inward calcium current through the slow channels. These slow channels are a hundred times more specific for calcium than for sodium; they are *slow calcium channels*. Two or more slow channels exist: the so-called voltage-dependent calcium channels (VDCs), which are blocked by CCBs, and the receptor-operated calcium channels, which are blocked by β-blocking drugs.

CCBs differ from one another in their chemical structure, selectivity, and specificity. A summary of basic characteristics, including daily dose, is given in Table 22.9.

Archetypes: dihydropyridines, e.g., nifedipine

Interactions

- Beta blockers: may precipitate heart failure.
- Quinidine: serum levels of quinidine may decrease.

Benzothiazepines, diltiazem

Interactions

- Digoxin: serum digoxin levels may be increased.
- Anesthetics: hypotension may be induced.
- Interactions occur between all CCBs and 3A4 substrates (e.g., azole antifungals, statins, macrolides)

Table 22.9 Some characteristics of calcium channel blockers (CCBs)

Agent	To onset of action (h)	$t_{1/2}$ (h)	Daily dose (per day)	(mg)
Archetypes				
Nifedipine[1]	0.5-1	6-11	3-4	20-40
Nifedipine GITS	2	17	1-2	30-40
Diltiazem	0.5-1	4-6	2-3	180-360
Diltiazem SR	2-3	5-7	1-2	180-480
Verapamil	0.5-1	3-12	2-3	120-360
Verapamil SR	0.5-1	4-12	1	240-480
Gallopamil	0.5-1	4-5	2-3	150-200
Later versions				
Felodipine ER	2-5	12-17	1	5-10
Isradipine	20 min	2-6	2	5-10
Nicardipine	30 min	8-9	2-3	60-120
Nimodipine	1	5	3-4	90-160
Nisoldipine	30 min	2-11	1-2	10-40
Nitrendipine	1	8-20	1-2	10-40
Amlodipine	1-2	35-50	1	5-10
Lacidipine	1	8	1	2-8

(ER=extended release; SR=sustained release; GITS=gastrointestinal therapeutic system).
[1]Chewing and swallowing the short-acting formulation: time to onset of action is about 10-20 min.

Phenylalkylamines, verapamil

Interactions

Lithium sensitivity may be increased.

More recent

These are all dihydropyridines, but with more advantageous pharmacologic effects (vascular selectivity) and/or pharmacokinetic action (longer duration) (Tab. 22.9).

CARDIAC GLYCOSIDES AND OTHER POSITIVE INOTROPIC AGENTS

Digitalis glycosides bind to cell membrane–bound potassium ATPase; by inhibiting this enzyme, they allow sodium to enter myocardial cells, from which it is driven out by a sodium-calcium exchange process. Higher intracellular calcium concentrations lead to enhanced myocardial contractility. Digitalis increases the refractory period of the conduction system and has a negative dromotropic effect. There is an increase in vagal tone, resulting in a negative chronotropic effect (also due to the increased inotropy).

Pharmacodynamic and pharmacokinetic characteristics as well as dose recommendations concerning the most frequently used cardiac glycosides – digoxin and digitoxin – are given in Table 22.10.

Interactions

Serum digitalis levels are decreased by antacids, dietary fibers, chemotherapeutic agents, rifampicin, cholestyramine, colestipol, metoclopramide, phenobarbital, and neomycin. Serum digitalis levels are increased by ACE inhibitors, antifungal agents, amiodarone, cyclosporin A, benzodiazepines, NSAIDs, CCBs, erythromycin, disopyramide, quinidine, and tetracyclines.

Side effects

- Gastrointestinal: anorexia, naurea, vomiting.
- Neurologic: apathy, visual disturbances, psychosis.
- Cardiac: various arrhythmias and conduction disturbances.

In case of serious side effects because of overdose, administration of digoxin-specific Fab antibody fragments is the therapy of choice. This approach is effective in both digoxin- and digitoxin-related intoxication, as well as in situations of refractory hyperkalemia. The antibody fragments quickly reduce the ratio of active, unbound glycosides in a few minutes, after which the bound complexes are excreted by the kidneys.

Deslanoside

This deacetyl lanatoside C is usually given iv because reliable clinical results cannot be achieved by oral administration. Its effect occur about 5 to 10 minutes after intravenous injection; full action is exerted after about 2 hours. Half-life is about 33 hours, and the effect persists for 2 to 5 days.

Interactions and side effects

See Digoxin.

Dobutamine

Dobutamine stimulates β_1 receptors and – weakly – β_2 receptors alike. It is administred by iv infusion. Peak action appears in 10 minutes, with a plasma half-life of a few minutes.

Dopamine

Dopamine stimulates sympathetic adrenergic receptors and dopaminergic receptors in the renal, coronary, and cerebrovascular regions, producing vasodilatation.

Dopexamine

Similar to dopamine, dopexamine probably stimulates

Table 22.10 Pharmacodynamic and pharmacokinetic characteristics of digitalis glycosides

	Digoxin	Digitoxin
To onset of action		
po	30-120 min	60-360 min
iv	5-20 min	-
To peak action		
po	1-5 h	8-12 h
iv	1-4 h	-
Plasma half-life	30-48 h	4-6 days
Duration of action	5-6 days	14 days
Protein binding	20%	90%
Metabolism	Slight, hepatic	Hepatic recirculation
Excretion	Renal, 60-70% unchanged	Renal, in the form of metabolites
Dose (daily)		
po loading	0.25 mg bid for 2 days	- 0.05-0.15 mg
po maintenance	0.25 mg qd	
iv	0.75 mg over 5 min then in 2 h intervals 0.25 mg, max 1.5 mg	
Hepatic impairment	No effect	Dose reduction
Renal impairment	Delayed excretion	Dose reduction not required
Elderly	Reduce dose	Reduce dose

dopaminergic (DA_1 and DA_2) receptors and β_2 adrenoceptors. More trials are needed to establish its precise role in cardiovascular therapy.

DIURETICS

Diuretics inhibit tubular electrolyte reabsorbtion. Thiazide-type diuretics inhibit sodium chloride cotransport in the distal renal tubules. Loop diuretics inhibit sodium-potassium-chloride cotransport in the ascending limb of the loop of Henle, with a weak effect in the proximal tubule. Potassium-sparing diuretics have an effect on sodium channels in the distal renal tubule, resulting in a weak natriuretic effect and potassium retention.

All three diuretic groups increase the excretion of sodium. This means that all diuretics can decrease blood pressure in doses not high enough to result in enhanced diuresis. First, plasma volume is decreased; then this volume change is restored, but with a slight fall in peripheral vascular resistance. Characteristics of the three types of diuretics currently used are shown in Table 22.11.

Interactions

- ACE inhibitors or anesthetics: hypotension may worsen.
- ACTH, corticosteroids, laxatives: hypokalemia may worsen.
- Antidiabetic agents: a dose increase may be necessary.
- Digitalis: hypokalemia or hypomagnesemia decrease the threshold of digitalis-induced arrhythmias.
- Drugs prolonging QT intervals: arrhythmias may be induced.
- Lithium clearance is reduced.
- Muscle relaxants: neuromuscular action may be increased.
- NSAIDs: antihypertensive effect of the diuretic may be reduced.

Side effects

Side effects include hypokalemia and hypomagnesemia (except with potassium-sparing agents) and glucose intolerance.

Table 22.11 Characteristics of different types of diuretics

Drug	To onset of action	To peak effect	Plasma half-life	Duration of action	Usual daily dose (mg)
Thiazide-type diuretics					
Bendroflumethiazide	1-2 h	2 h	3 h	12-20 h	2.5-10
Chlorothiazide	1 h	2-3 h	1-2 h	6-12 h	250-2000
Chlorthalidone	1 h	3-4 h	50-55 h	6-12 h	50-200
Cyclopenthiazide	1-2 h	?	?	6-12 h	0.25-1.5
Hydrochlorothiazide	2 h	4 h	5-6 h	6-12 h	25-200
Hydroflumethiazide	1-2 h	3-4 h	5-6 h	6-12 h	50-200
Indapamide	1-2 h	?	10-20 h	18-24 h	2.5
Mefruside	1-2 h	4-12 h	3-12 h	20-24 h	25-50
Methyclothiazide	2 h	4-6 h	?	22-24 h	2.5-10
Metolazone	1 h	2-4 h	6-8 h	24-48 h	5-20
Polythiazide	2 h	5-6 h	24 h	24-48 h	0.5-4
Xipamide	2 h	3-5 h	6-8 h	22-26 h	20-80
Loop diuretics					
Bumetanide					
po	30 min	1-2 h	1-2 h	4-6 h	1-5
iv	2-5 min	15-30 min	1-2 h	2-3 h	1-2
Ethacrynic acid					
po	30 min	1-2 h	30-60 min	6-8 h	25-150
iv	<1 min	30-40 min	30-60 min	2-3 h	50-100
Furosemide					
po	1 h	1-2 h	45-90 min	5-6 h	20-600
iv	<1 min	<1 min	45-90 min	2-3 h	20-40
Piretanide	20-30 min	1-2 h	30-50 min	4-6 h	6-12
Potassium-sparing drugs					
Amiloride	1-2 h	3-4 h	6-9 h	22-24 h	5-20
Spironolactone	Slow	2-4 days	12-24 h	2-3 days	50-400
Triamterene	2-4 h	6-24 h	1-2 h	12-16 h	50-250

NITRATES AND NITRIC OXIDE DONORS

The intact endothelium produces an endogenous factor, *endothelium-derived relaxing factor* (EDRF), which has been identified as nitric oxide or as a related nitrosothiol derivative. Exogenous nitrates enter the vascular wall, where they are converted to nitric oxide.

This process is independent of the intact endothelium; therefore, exogenous nitrates can replace deficient EDRF. Structure-activity studies indicate that all nitrate preparations used clinically are capable of releasing nitric oxide in vascular smooth muscle target issues. On the other hand, they can all induce cross-tolerance when given continuously and in large doses. Therefore, pharmacokinetics govern the choice of drug and mode of treatment when using nitrates. Pharmacokinetic characteristics and usual doses of clinically employed nitrate preparations are given in Table 22.12.

Interactions

- Acetylcholine: effects may be reduced with concomitant administration of nitrates.
- Alcohol: potentiates vasodilatating effects of nitrates.
- Heparin: effects of heparin may be decreased.
- Other vasodilators: efficacy may be potentiated by nitrates.

- Sildenafil: life threatening hypotension may occur.

Side effects

Major acute side effects are generally an exaggerated extension of the therapeutic action: vasodilatation, orthostatic hypotension, tachycardia, and headache. Long-acting preparations provide higher and more even blood levels, which, paradoxically, lead to a loss of efficacy over time (i.e., tolerance). Nitrate tolerance probably is caused by a multifactorial process, including (1) depletion of sulphydryl donors, decreasing intracellular formation of nitric oxide and sulphydryl-containing compounds; (2) reflex vasoconstriction and sodium retention, produced by vasodilatation-induced sympathetic activation; (3) lower hematocrit value, caused by increased intravascular volume and hemodilution, limiting the ability of nitrates to moderate left ventricular filling pressure; and (4) an increase in free radical production by the enothelium during nitrate therapy. Significantly increasing blood nitrate levels, e.g., by sublingual nitrates, could restore the acute effect even in cases of nitrate tolerance. Coadministration of sulphydryl donors (e.g., N-acetylcysteine) was unable to prevent tolerance. Nitrate tolerance can be effectively avoided by nitrate-free intervals (interval dosing) only.

Molsidomine is a prodrug that is converted to 3-morpholino sydnonimine (SIN-1) in the liver, which by a spontaneous ring opening is changed to SIN-1A (N-mor-

Table 22.12 Characteristics and usual dosages of nitrate preparations

Drug	To onset of action	To peak effect	Plasma half-life	Duration of action	Usual daily dose (mg)
Glyceryl trinitrate (GTN)					
Sublingual tablet	<1 min	3-4 min	3-4 min	~30 min	0.3-0.9[1]
Buccal aerosol	<1 min	3-4 min	4-5 min	~30 min	1-2 puffs
Buccal tablet	<1 min	3-4 min	3-5 min	3-5 h	3 x 1-5[3]
Sustained-release tablet	>1 h	60-120 min	4-5 min	8-10 h	2 x 2.6-6.4
Transdermal ointment	15	60 min	~30 min	6-7 h	7.5-30
Patch	30-40 min	120 min	~3 min	>24 h	$0.2\text{-}0.4\ mg/m^2$
iv	<1 min	~2 min	~7 min	[2]	10-200 µg/min
Isosorbide dinitrate (ISDN)					
Sublingual tablet	3-4 min	6-10 min	60 min	120 min	2.5-10
Buccal aerosol	2-3 min	4-6 min	?	30-60 min	1-2 puffs
Chewable tablet	2-3 min	4-5 min	~20 min	60-120 min	5-10
Sustained-release tablet	30 min	60-100 min	4 h	8-10 h	2 x 40-80
iv	<1 min	~2 min	20 min	[2]	2-12 mg/h
Isosorbide mononitrate (ISMN)					
Tablets	20 min	30-40 min	20-30 min	10 h	20-120
Sustained-release tablet	30 min	3-4 h	3-4 h	15-17 h	30-120
Pentaerythrol tetranitrate					
Tablets	30 min	?	10 min	6 h	3 x 30-60

[1]At the onset of an attack or before exercise to prevent pain.
[2]Continuous infusion may lead to tolerance after 24 h.
[3]Higher dose in congestive heart failure (i.e., 3 x 5 mg).

pholino-N-N-nitroso-aminoacetonitrile), the active drug, resulting in the release of NO, the active variety. After oral administration, absorption is almost 100%. Onset of action is in 10 to 15 minutes, and peak plasma level is achieved after 60 minutes. Molsidomine is extensively metabolized, and 90% of the metabolites are excreted by the kidneys. Molsidomine is regarded as an alternative to nitrate interval treatment, especially to bridge the therapeutic gap that seems necessary for effective nitrate use.

Interactions

Antihypertensive agents (e.g., β blockers, CCBs) used concomitantly may add to a hypotensive effect.

Side effects

Side effects include headache, rarely flush, dizziness, hypotension, and palpitations.

Suggested readings

ANTIPLATELET TRIALIST'S COLLABORATION. Collaborative overview of randomized trials of antiplatelet therapy: I. Prevention of death, myocardial infarction, and stroke by prolonged antiplatelet therapy in various categories of patients. Br Med J 1994;308:81-106.

THE CARDIAC ARRHYTHMIA SUPPRESSION TRIAL (CAST) INVESTIGATORS. Preliminary report: effect of encainide and flecainide on mortality in a randomized trial of arrhythmia suppression after myocardial infarction. N Engl J Med 1989;321:406-12.

CLELAND JFG, WALKER A. Is medical treatment for angina the most cost-effective option? Eur Heart J 1997;18(suppl. B):B35-42.

FLAKER GC, BARTOLOZZI J, DAVIS V, et al. Use of a standardized heparin nomogram to achieve therapeutic anticoagulation after thrombolytic therapy in myocardial infarction. Arch Intern Med 1994;154:1492-6.

GRACE AA, CAM AJ. Quinidine. N Engl J Med 1998;338:35-45.

HANSSON L, ZANCHETTI A, CARRUTHERS SG, et al. Effects of intensive blood-pressure lowering and low-dose aspirin in patients with hypertension: Principles results of the Hypertension Optimal Treatment (HOT) randomized trial. Lancet 1998;351:1755-62.

KOREN G, PASTUSZAK A, ITO S. Drugs in pregnancy. N Engl J Med 1998;338:1128-37.

LATINI R, MAGGIONI AP, FLATHER M, et al. ACE inhibitor use in patients with myocardial infarction: summary of evidence from clinical trials. Circulation 1995;92:3132-7.

MURRAY KT. Ibutilide. Circulation 1998;97:493-7.

PARKER JD, PARKER JO. Nitrate therapy for stable angina pectoris. N Engl J Med 1998;338:520-31.

TEO KK, YUSUF S, FURBERG CD. Effects of prophylactic antiarrhythmic drug therapy in acute myocardial infarction: an overview of results from randomized controlled trials. JAMA 1993;270:1589-95.

23

Hypertension

Helge Hohage, Karl Heinz Rahn, Cesare R. Sirtori

Disease presentation

Hypertension (HTN) is defined as an elevation of arterial blood pressure above an arbitrarily defined normal value. This normal value differs according to sex and age; men have higher average pressures than women, and in most populations, older people have higher pressures than younger people. Most candidates for antihypertensive therapy have a systolic pressure (SP) above 140 mmHg, a diastolic pressure (DP) above 90 mmHg, or both. The presence of other risk factors (e.g., smoking, hyperlipidemia, target-organ damage) is also an important determinant in the decision to treat, since the incidence of morbidity and mortality significantly decreases when hypertension is diagnosed early and is treated properly. The prevalence of hypertension varies in different subgroups of the population, but it is estimated that overall approximately 20% of all adults are affected.

About 90% of patients have essential hypertension, and only a small number (<10%) of people with hypertension have identifiable causes, such as renal disease or endocrine tumors; these latter are often managed by surgical means. Most patients diagnosed as hypertensive, however, are simply at the upper end of the normal distribution of blood pressure values for their population group. No single mechanism has been identified to explain the higher blood pressure values in such people, but genetic factors play a role, because blood pressure is strongly influenced by inheritance in a polygenic fashion. This type of hypertension is designated *essential hypertension.* It is noteworthy that essential hypertension occurs four times more frequently among blacks than among whites, and it occurs more often among middle-aged males than among middle-aged females.

Unless rapid in onset and severe, hypertension does not produce noticeable symptoms. However, several cardiovascular diseases are common or more severe in persons with high blood pressure; these include atherosclerosis, coronary artery disease, aortic aneurysm, congestive heart failure, stroke, diabetes (with particular reference to insulin resistance), and renal and retinal disease. The frequency and severity of end-organ damage are increased in smokers and diabetics. The purpose of treating hypertension is to prevent these significant cardiovascular complications.

The choice of therapy for a patient with hypertension depends on a variety of factors: age, sex, race, body build, and lifestyle of the patient; cause of the disease; the presence of other coexisting diseases; rapidity of onset and severity of the hypertension; and the presence or absence of other risk factors and diseases, e.g., smoking, alcohol consumption, obesity, diabetes, hyperlipidemia, and others.

Antihypertensive drugs can be divided into nine classes on the basis of their mechanisms of action. Whenever possible, monotherapy is advisable, but if blood pressure is not controlled by a single drug, additional drugs frequently are administered in a stepwise manner. Many experts believe that a thiazide diuretic or β-blocker should be the first choice for monotherapy, based on the proven ability of these drugs to decrease cardiovascular mortality. Others suggest that ACE inhibitors, calcium channel blockers, and α-blockers are often the best choice for monotherapy. Nevertheless, treatment is initiated with any of four drugs depending on the individual patient: a diuretic, a β-blocker, an ACE inhibitor, or a calcium channel blocker.

Certain subsets of hypertensive patients respond better to one class of drug than another. For example, black patients respond well to diuretics and calcium channel blockers, whereas β-blockers and ACE inhibitors frequently are less effective.

There are also several nonpharmacologic therapies for hypertension. Patients differ in their sensitivity to these techniques, but on average, only modest reductions (5–10 mmHg) in blood pressure can be achieved by these means. Despite the modest effect of nonpharmacologic interventions, when viewed across large populations, specific people may be classified on the basis of their sensitivity to these interventions. For example, a "salt-sensitive" person's blood pressure will decrease rapidly in response to a low-sodium diet. The major advantage of nonpharmacologic therapies is their relative safety and freedom from side effects compared with drug therapy. However, most patients with hypertension require drug treatment to achieve an adequate, sustained blood pressure reduction. Approximately two-thirds of patients require therapy with two or more drugs.

Arterial blood pressure is the product of cardiac output (CO) and total peripheral resistance (TPR). Patients with recent-onset essential hypertension tend to have an elevated CO. Most patients with chronic sustained hypertension have a normal or low CO and a fixed, elevated TPR. Currently available drugs lower blood pressure by decreasing CO,

Table 23.1 Site and mechanism of action of antihypertensive drugs

Drug	Heart	Kidney	Vascular smooth muscle	Central nervous system	Effect
ACE inhibitors, AT$_1$ antagonists		Decrease in blood volume	Relaxation of vascular smooth muscle		↓CO ↓TPR
α-Blockers	Decrease in force and rate of cardiac contraction		Relaxation of vascular smooth muscle		↓CO ↓TPR
β-Blockers	Decrease in force and rate of cardiac contraction	Decrease in blood volume		Decreased sympathetic outflow	↓CO ↓TPR
Calcium channel blockers			Relaxation of vascular smooth muscle		↓TPR
Centrally acting sympatholytics				Decreased sympathetic outflow	↓CO ↓TPR
Diuretics		Decrease in blood volume			↓CO
Vasodilators			Relaxation of vascular smooth muscle		↓CO ↓TPR

(CO = cardiac output; TPR = total peripheral resistance.)

Table 23.2 Physiologic reponses to antihypertensive drugs

Drug	Heart rate	CO	TPR	Plasma volume	Plasma renin activity
ACE inhibitors, AT$_1$ antagonists					
α-Blockers	↓←	↓←	↓	↑←	←
β-Blockers	↓	↓	↑←	←	↓
Calcium channel blockers	↑←	←	↓	←	↑←
Centrally acting sympatholytics	↓	↓	↓	↑←	↓←
Diuretics	↑←	↓	↓	↓	↑
Vasodilators	↑	↑←	↓	↑	↑

TPR, or both (Tab. 23.1). However, CO and TPR are not independent variables; changes in one can indirectly affect the other. Reduction in blood pressure produced by any means may activate one or more physiologic mechanisms that oppose a drug-induced decrease in blood pressure (Tab. 23.2).

Physiologic systems involved in blood pressure regulation

Renin-angiotensin-aldosterone system

The kidney provides for the long-term control of blood pressure by altering blood volume. A decrease in arterial pressure causes a release of the enzyme renin from the kidney into the blood. Renin generates angiotensin I from a circulating substrate, angiotensinogen, that is synthesized in the liver and other tissues. Angiotensin I is converted to angiotensin II by the "converting enzyme," found in the endothelial cell membrane, especially in the lungs. Angiotensin II (ATII), the body's most potent circulating vasoconstrictor, constricts blood vessels, enhances sympathetic nervoaus system activity, and causes renal salt and water retention by direct intrarenal actions and by stimulating the adrenal gland to release the potent mineralocorticoid aldosterone.

Sympathetic nervous system

A decrease in blood pressure activates the baroreflex, producing increases in sympathetic nervous system activity. As a consequence, the force and rate of cardiac contraction are increased, and cardiac filling is enhanced, resulting in an elevated CO. Furthermore, most blood vessels are constricted, leading to an increase in TPR. Finally, mediated by renal sympathetic nerves innervating renal blood vessels and tubules, sodium chloride and water excretion by the kidney is reduced.

Vasopressin system

A decrease in arterial pressure causes a baroreflex-mediated release of vasopressin (antidiuretic hormone), which acts on the renal collecting duct to enhance water retention.

Fluid retention by the kidney

A decrease in arterial pressure causes the kidney to excrete less sodium chloride and water. This results in part from the direct intrarenal hydraulic effect of reduced renal perfusion pressure and in part from the other mechanisms listed earli-

Table 23.3 Randomized, placebo-controlled trials of antihypertensive therapy

		Therapy	N	CHD	Stroke	CHF	Mortality	CVD	Duration (years)
VA-NHLBI[1]	D-high	Treatment	508	8	0	—	2	2	1.5
		Control	504	5	0	—	0	0	
VA-II	D-high	Treatment	186	11	5	0	10	8	3.3
		Control	194	13	20	11	21	19	
HDFP[1]	D-high	Treatment	5485	171	102	—	349	195	5.0
		Control		189	158	—	419	240	
Oslo Study	D-high	Treatment	406	14	0	0	10	7	5.5
		Control	379	10	5	1	9	6	
ANBPS	D-high	Treatment	1721	33	13	3	25	8	4.0
		Control	1706	33	22	3	35	18	
MRC[1]	D-high	Treatment	4297	119	18	—	128	69	4.9
		Control	8654	234	109	—	253	139	
USPHS	D-high	Treatment	193	15	1	0	2	2	7.0
		Control	196	18	6	2	4	4	
HSCSG	D-high	Treatment	233	7	37	0	26	15	3.0
		Control	219	9	42	6	24	19	
EWPHE	D-high	Treatment	416	48	32	19	135	67	4.7
		Control	424	59	48	23	149	93	
MRC-O[1]	D-low	Treatment	1081	48	45	—	134	66	5.8
		Control	2213	159	134	—	315	180	
SHEP	D-low	Treatment	2365	104	103	56	213	90	4.5
		Control	2371	141	159	109	242	112	
SHEP-P	D-low	Treatment	443	15	11	6	32	14	2.8
		Control	108		4	6	2	7	5
MRC-O[1]	β-block	Treatment	1102	80	56	—	167	95	5.8
		Control	2213	159	134	—	315	180	
MRC[1]	β-block	Treatment	4403	103	42	—	120	65	4.9
		Control	8654	234	109	—	253	139	
Coope and Varrender	β-block	Treatment	419	35	20	22	60	37	4.4
		Control	465	38	39	36	69	50	
STOP-H	β-block	Treatment	812	25	29	19	36	17	2.0
		Control	815	28	53	39	63	41	
CAPP	ACE-inh	Treatment	5492	162	189	75	—	76	6.1
		Control[2]	5493	161	148	66	—	95	

[CHD= fatal or nonfatal coronary heart disease; CHF= fatal or nonfatal congestive heart failure; CVD= cardiovascular mortality; D-high= high-dose diuretic therapy; D-low= low-dose diuretic therapy (high-dose diuretic therapy included studies that generally used starting drugs and doses greater than or equal to chlorthalidone 50 mg, hydrochlorothiazide 50 mg, bendroflumethiazide 5 mg, methyclothiazide 5 mg, or trichlormethiazide 2 mg); VA-II= Veterans Administration Cooperative Study Group on Antihypertensive Agents, II; HDFP= Hypertension Detection and Follow-up Program; ANBPS= Australian National Blood Pressure Study; MRC= Medical Research Council; USPHS= U.S. Public Health Service Hospitals; HSCSG= Hypertension-Stroke Cooperative Study Group; EWPHE= European Working Party on High Blood Pressure in the Elderly; MRC-O= Medical Research Council-Older Adults; STOP= Swedish Trial in Old Patients with Hypertension; SHEP= Systolic Hypertension in the Elderly Program; SHEP-P= Systolic Hypertension in the Elderly Program Pilot Study; and CAPP= Captopril Prevention Project.]
[1]No data are available on CHF.
[2]Conventional diuretic/β blocker theraphy.

er. The resulting expansion of extracellular fluid and plasma volumes tends to increase CO and arterial pressure and thus reduce the antihypertensive action of any drug.

Cardiovascular risk factors and effects of antihypertensive therapy

Although the goal of antihypertensive therapy is to reduce end-organ damage associated with chronically elevated blood pressure, the effects of therapy on other cardiovascular risk factors also must be considered. The end-organ damage is not related exclusively to blood pressure level. If an antihypertensive drug effectively lowers blood pressure but increases the influence of other risk factors for cardiovascular disease, the benefit of therapy is reduced accordingly.

Hypertension is considered among the most important cardiovascular risk factors; i.e., it goes together with factors such as hyperlipidemia, cigarette smoking, diabetes, sedentary lifestyle, excess body weight (particularly at the abdominal level), and a number of others. The concepts of *cardiovascular risk factor* and *global cardiovascular risk* are discussed in Chapter 69.

A number of placebo-controlled, randomized long-term studies have assessed the major cardiovascular disease endpoints after treatment with a number of different antihypertensive drugs, in particular diuretics, both high and low doses, and β-adrenergic blockers. A smaller number of studies have evaluated the activity of the newer antihypertensive drug classes, i.e., calcium channel blockers and ACE inhibitors. Although these latter drug classes are now far more widely used than diuretics and β-blockers, the clinical trial evidence in terms of health outcomes is meager.

Cardiovascular event outcomes following long-term diuretic and β-blocker therapy within randomized, controlled trials were analyzed by a meta-analysis. Table 23.3 provides data from 17 trials, i.e., those involving at least 200 patients per treatment group, generally drug versus placebo, as well as from a recent trial (CAPP) comparing an ACE inhibitor with conventional diuretic/β-blocker therapy. Globally, compared with placebo, β-blocker therapy was effective in preventing stroke, with a relative risk (RR) versus placebo of 0.71 and with 95% confidence intervals (CI) of 0.59 to 0.86, as well as in preventing congestive heart failure (RR = 0.58; 95% CI = 0.40-0.84). High-dose diuretic therapy versus placebo reduced the risk of stroke (RR = 0.49; 95% CI = 0.39-0.62) and of congestive heart failure (RR = 0.17; 95% CI = 0.07-0.41). Low-dose diuretic therapy prevented not only stroke (RR = 0.66; 95% CI = 0.55-0.78) but also congestive heart failure (RR = 0.58; 95% CI = 0.44-0.76), coronary disease (RR = 0.72; 95% CI = 0.61-0.85), and total mortality (RR = 0.90; 95% CI = 0.81-0.99). These data, therefore, clearly indicate that both drug classes are effective, and the use of high-dose diuretics poses no particular advantage. The more recent studies, particularly the STOP and SHEP studies, carried out in older patients, show a definite benefit also in this age group and clearly indicate that reduction of, particularly, systolic

blood pressure is most beneficial in elderly patients. Data from the CAPP study would, however, suggest little difference in the efficacy of an ACE inihibitor, with only an apparent disadvantage in stroke risk.

Global evaluation of the active treatment effect on blood pressure in this series of studies showed a net reduction of 6 mmHg diastolic and (with less precision) of 12 mmHg systolic. It also should be noted that in the majority of studies, about 25% of patients randomized to placebo or control groups received active antihypertensive treatment at some stage.

The issue of vigorous versus less vigorous reduction in blood pressure has been of major concern. Some authors have suggested that a too vigorous reduction in blood pressure may be associated with an increased cardiovascular risk, the so-called J-curve concept. In order to assess how far blood pressure should be lowered so as to achieve the greatest benefit, as well as to evaluate whether a too low blood pressure may cause some harm, patients in the very recent Hypertension Optimal Treatment (HOT) randomized trial (18,790 patients from 26 countries aged 50 to 80 years with diastolic blood pressures between 100 and 115 mmHg) were randomly assigned to target diastolic blood pressures. A third of the patients were allocated to each target pressure: <90 <85, and <80 mmHg. Felodipine, a calcium entry blocker (see below) was given as baseline therapy, with the addition of other agents according to a five-step regimen. In addition, half the patients were randomly assigned 75 mg per day of aspirin and the other half a placebo. Although the study did not really succeed in achieving the target blood pressures (the three groups achieved diastolic pressures, respectively, on average of 85.2, 83.2, and 81.1 mmHg), still the study did not indicate any increase in the risk of adverse events in patients with the lowest end of study blood pressure. Actually, the lowest incidence of major cardiovascular events occurred at a mean DP of 82.6 mmHg, and the lowest risk of cardiovascular mortality occurred at 86.5 mmHg. Further reduction below these blood pressures, although not providing any further benefit, was safe. Only in patients with diabetes mellitus did achievement of a blood pressure of less than 80 mmHg, compared with the target group of less than 90 mmHg, result in 51% reduction in major cardiovascular events.

Other cardiovascular risk factors that can be affected by antihypertensive drugs include plasma glucose, potassium, and uric acid concentrations. In particular, insulin resistance is now recognized to be prevalent in patients with hypertension. The resulting high insulin concentration is a risk factor for coronary artery disease. Thus it is noteworthy that thiazides and β-blockers increase insulin resistance, whereas ACE inhibitors and prazosin decrease it. Calcium channel antagonists do not affect insulin resistance. There is interpatient variability in the response of these metabolites to antihypertensive drugs, and so therapeutic generalizations are difficult. Nonetheless, thiazide diuretics appear most likely to cause pressure-independent changes in cardiovascular risk, whereas calcium channel antagonists and ACE inhibitors actually may improve the metabolic risk profile. Nonselective β-adrenergic receptor blockers without intrinsic sympathomimetic activity have been shown to reduce the risk of sudden death during or after myocardial infarction in hypertensive patients. The mechanism is presumed to be a protection against catecholamine-induced ventricular fibrillation.

Drug classes

DIURETICS (see also Chap. 17)

Diuretics are currently recommended as the first-line drug therapy for hypertension. Low-dose diuretic therapy is safe and effective in preventing stroke, myocardial infarction, congestive heart failure, and death. Recent data show that diuretics are superior to β-blockers in older patients. Diuretics reduce fluid volume by inhibiting electrolyte transport in the renal tubules. Various diuretic drugs are used in the therapy of hypertension. The molecular mechanism of the antihypertensive action of diuretics is not known, but receptor proteins for thiazides and "loop" diuretics have now been cloned. Initial administration of a diuretic produces a pronounced increase in urinary water and electrolyte excretion and a reduction in extracellular and plasma volumes. These changes result in a decrease in CO, which is primarily responsible for producing the decrease in arterial pressure. Some investigators suggest that this initial decrease in extracellular water volume is the full explanation for the antihypertensive effect. After several days, the urinary excretion returns to normal, but blood pressure remains reduced. Subsequently, plasma volume and CO also return to, or approximately to, pretreatment values, and the TPR decreases, whereas blood pressure remains lowered. The decline in TPR initially may involve autoregulatory vascular adjustments of various tissues in response to decreased perfusion, but this mechanism would not be expected to remain operative after CO is normalized.

Other possible mechanisms include a decreased vascular reactivity to norepinephrine and other endogenous pressor substances and a decreased "structural" vascular resistance secondary to the removal of sodium chloride and water from blood vessel walls. These changes could result directly from the tissue actions of diuretic drugs or indirectly from the generalized loss of sodium and water from the body. However, the antihypertensive actions of diuretics do not parallel their efficacy in causing fluid loss, except in patients with renal insufficiency.

Finally, some diuretics relax vascular smooth muscle directly, but the vasodilatation produced by most agents in this class occurs only at doses well above the effective diuretic range. An exception is indapamide, which is a vasodilator at normal therapeutic doses, an action probably producing a major portion of its antihypertensive effect.

Use of diuretics in HTN

The therapy of hypertension is the most important use of diuretics. They have long been the mainstay of antihypertensive medications, since they are inexpensive, convenient to administer, and well tolerated. Diuretics are effective in reducing systolic and diastolic blood pressure for extended periods in most patients with mild to moderate essential hypertension. After 3 to 7 days of treatment, the blood pressure stabilizes at a lower level and can be maintained indefinitely by a daily dosage level of the drug that causes lower peripheral resistance without having a major diuretic effect. Many patients can be continued for years on the thiazides alone, although a small percentage will require additional medication. Diuretics are often used as adjuncts to other antihypertensive agents to prevent fluid retention, and they potentiate the hypotensive effect of most other drugs They are more effective in black than in white patients, perhaps because there is a high incidence of low-renin hypertension among blacks. Lower doses of diuretics are required to treat hypertension than to treat edema. Larger doses do not result in a greater blood pressure reduction but in the greater incidence and severity of side effects.

Thiazides are also used in the treatment of mild to moderate congestive heart failure to reduce extracellular volume. If they fail, loop diuretics may be useful.

In addition, thiazides have the unique ability to produce a hyperosmolar urine. Thiazides can substitute for the antidiuretic hormone in the treatment of nephrogenic diabetes insipidus. The urine volume of such individuals may drop from 11 to about 3 liters per day when treated with the drug. Pharmacokinetics, major pharmacodynamics, and toxicologic features of the diuretics most commonly used in hypertension are given in Chapter. 22.

Thiazide diuretics

Thiazide diuretics are effective orally. Most cause a demonstrable diuretic effect within an hour of oral administration, but it takes 1 to 3 weeks to produce a stable reduction in blood pressure and to exhibit a prolonged biologic half-life (40 h). All thiazides are secreted by the renal organic cation transporter. Chlorthalidone is given once a day for the treatment of hypertension. Indapamide is metabolized and excreted by the gastrointestinal tract and the kidneys; it therefore is less likely to accumulate in patients with renal failure and may be useful in their treatment.

Hypokalemia is the most frequent problem encountered with the thiazides and can predispose patients on digitalis to ventricular arrhythmias. Activation of the renin-angiotensin-aldosterone system by the decrease in intravascular volume contributes significantly to urinary K+ losses. The K+ deficiency can be overcome by spironolactone, which interferes with aldosterone action, or by triamterene, which acts to retain K+. Low-sodium diets blunt the potassium depletion caused by thiazide diuretics. There is concern that the hypokalemia frequently associated with diuretic treatment may increase the incidence of sudden cardiac death. The monitoring of serum potassium concentrations and the use of potassium supplements are often recommended in patients receiving diuretics.

Because they decrease the amount of acid excreted by the organic acid secretory system, thiazides increase serum uric acid. Being insoluble, the uric acid deposits in the joints, and a full-blown attack of gout may be seen in individuals predisposed to gouty attacks (see Chap. 71). It is important, therefore, to perform periodic blood tests for uric acid levels.

Volume depletion can cause orthostatic hypotension or light-headedness. In contrast to loop diuretics, the thiazides inhibit the secretion of Ca^{2+}, sometimes leading to elevated levels of Ca^{2+} in the blood.

Thiazides should be used with caution in patients with diabetes mellitus. These patients may become hyperglycemic and have difficulty in maintaining appropriate blood sugar levels. Hypersensitivity reactions such as bone marrow suppression, dermatitis, purpura, acute pancreatitis, necrotizing vasculitis, and interstitial nephritis are very rare. Finally, it should be mentioned that thiazide diuretics are not effective in patients with inadequate kidney function (creatinine clearance less than 50 ml/min).

Loop or high-ceiling diuretics

Bumetanide, furosemide, torsemide, and ethacrynic acid are four diuretics that exert their principal action on the ascending limb of the loop of Henle. Compared with all other classes of diuretics, these drugs have the highest efficacy in mobilizing Na^+ and Cl^- from the body. Ethacrynic acid has a steeper dose-response curve than furosemide; it shows greater side effects than those seen with the other loop diuretics; and is not as widely used. In contrast, bumetanide is much more potent than furosemide.

Loop diuretics are administered orally or parenterally. They are absorbed readily from the gastrointestinal tract, although to variable degrees. Ethacrynic acid, bumetanide, and furosemide are bound extensively to plasma proteins, but they are secreted rapidly by the renal transport system for organic cations. Owing to their short half-lives (1-2 h), the duration of action is relatively brief, 1 to 4 hours.

The loop diuretics act promptly, even among patients who have poor renal function or who have not responded to thiazides or other diuretics. In contrast to thiazides, loop diuretics increase the Ca^{2+} content of urine. The loop diuretics cause decreased renal vascular resistance and increased renal blood flow. They are the drugs of choice for reducing the acute pulmonary edema of congestive heart failure. Because of their rapid onset of action, they are useful in emergency situations, such as acute pulmonary edema, that call for a rapid, intense diuresis. Furthermore, loop diuretics are also useful in treating hypercalcemia because they stimulate tubular Ca^{2+} secretion.

Owing to their high efficacy, loop diuretics can cause a severe and rapid reduction in blood volume, with the possibility of hypotension, shock, and cardiac arrhythmias. Furthermore, the heavy load of Na^+ presented to the collecting tubule results in increased exchange of tubular Na^+ for K^+, with the possibility of inducing hypokalemia. The loss of K^+ from cells in exchange for H^+ leads to hypokalemic alkalosis. Potassium depletion can be averted by use of potassium-sparing diuretics or dietary supplementation with K^+.

Potassium-sparing diuretics

These agents act in the collecting tubule to inhibit Na^+ reabsorption, K^+ secretion, and H^+ secretion. The major use of potassium-sparing agents is in the treatment of hypertension, most often in combination with a thiazide. It is extremely important to closely monitor K levels in patients treated with any K-sparing diuretic. Exogenous potassium supplementation usually is discontinued when potassium-sparing diuretic therapy is instituted.

Spironolactone is a synthetic aldosterone antagonist that competes with aldosterone for intracellular cytoplasmic receptor sites. The spironolactone receptor complex is inactive, and this results in a failure to produce proteins that normally are synthesized in response to aldosterone. These mediator proteins normally stimulate the Na^+-K^+ exchange sites of the collecting tubule. Thus a lack of mediator proteins prevents Na^+ reabsorption and therefore K^+ and H^+ secretion. In contrast to this, triamterene and amiloride block Na^+ transport channels, resulting in a decrease in Na^+-K^+ exchange; they have K^+-sparing diuretic action similar to that of spironolactone. Both triamterene and amiloride frequently are used in combination with other diuretics, usually for their potassium-sparing properties. For example, much like spironolactone, they prevent the K^+ loss that occurs with thiazides and furosemide.

Although spironolactone has a low efficacy in mobilizing Na^+ from the body in comparison with the other drugs, it has the useful property of causing the retention of K^+. Because of this latter action, spironolactone is often given in conjunction with a thiazide or loop diuretic to prevent K^+ excretion that otherwise would occur with these drugs. Spironolactone is the only potassium-sparing diuretic that is routinely used alone to induce net negative salt balance. It is particularly effective in clinical situations associated with secondary hyperaldosteronism (see Chap. 26).

Spironolactone is almost completely (70%) absorbed orally and is strongly bound to proteins. It is rapidly converted during its first passage through the liver to an active metabolite, canrenone. The action of spironolactone is largely due to the effect of canrenone, which has mineralo-corticoid-blocking activity. The potassium salt of canrenoate is a water-soluble substance that can be administered iv. Spironolactone induces hepatic cytochrome P450. Spironolactone is available in capsule forms in daily doses from 25 to 100 mg (higher for drug-resistant edema). A spironolactone cream is available in some countries for the treatment of acne. Fixed-dose combinations, e.g., spironolactone 25 mg and hydrochlorothiazide 25 mg or spironolactone 50 mg and furosemide 20 mg, are also available for the management of edematous conditions. The active metabolite canrenone is also available in an oral daily dose of between 50 and 100 mg.

Triamterene and amiloride generally are given orally. About 50% of the oral dose of each drug is absorbed. Triamterene is about 60% bound to plasma proteins, amiloride to a lesser extent. Both drugs have apparent vol-

Table 23.4 Possible interactions and problems observed with diuretics

Drug	Interaction
ACE inhibitors (ACE I)	Hyperkalemia with potassium-sparing diuretics, first dose hypotensive effect of ACE I
Adrenal steroids	↑ Hypokalemia
Aminoglycosides	↑ Ototoxicity, ↑nephrotoxocity
Antiarrhythmics	↓ Antiarrhythmic effects
Antidiabetics	↓ Antidiabetic effects
Chlorpropamide	Hyponatremia
Corticosteroids	Electrolyte disturbances
Digitalis	↑ Risk of digitalis toxicity
Indomethacin	↓ Antihypertensive effect
Lithium	↓ Lithium clearance
Phenytoin	↓ Diuretic effects of furosemide
Probenecid	↓ Diuretic effects of loop diuretics
Psychotropics	↑ Hypotensive effects
Sotalol and others	↑ Risk of arrhythmias
β-Blockers	↑ Blood glucose, urates, lipids

umes of distribution greater than the body water. Amiloride is not metabolized, but the metabolism of triamterene is extensive. The onset of antihypertensive action occurs in 2 to 3 days, with a plateau of action within 2 to 3 weeks.

Adverse effects and clinical problems

Because spironolactone chemically resembles some of the sex steroids, it does have minimal hormonal activity and may induce gynecomastia in males and menstrual irregularities in women. Because of this, the drug should not be given in high doses on a chronic basis. At low doses, spironolactone can be used chronically with few side effects. Hyperkalemia, nausea, lethargy, and mental confusion can occur. Similar to spironolactone, the most serious side effect of amiloride and triamterene is hyperkalemia (Tab. 23.4).

B-ADRENERGIC RECEPTOR BLOCKERS

Like diuretics, β-blockers (see Chap. 22) are currently recommended as first-line drug therapy for hypertension. The common characteristic of β-blockers is their ability to antagonize competitively the effects of the sympathetic effectors norepinephrine and epinephrine on cardiac β-adrenergic receptors. Compounds that are selective for the β_1-adrenergic receptors are effective antihypertensives; thus one hypothesis is that all drugs in this class exert their effects on blood pressure through β_1-adrenergic receptor blockade.

Numerous explanations have been proposed for the antihypertensive response to β-blockers, but none has been accepted universally. In patients with renin-dependent hypertension (e.g., renovascular hypertension), much of the blood pressure reduction produced by β-blockers is caused by inhibition of renin release secondary to blockade of β_1-adrenergic receptors present on renin-secreting juxtaglomerular cells in the kidney and innervated by sympathetic nerves. Many hypertensive patients with low or normal plasma renin activity, however, also respond to β-blocker therapy. Thus the therapeutic response cannot be predicted on the basis of pretreatment plasma renin values. Furthermore, β-blockers such as pindolol, which have strong intrinsic sympathomimetic agonist activity, decrease blood pressure without affecting plasma renin activity.

Acute and chronic decreases in CO are observed in most studies assessing β-blockers in hypertensive patients, but in some studies CO is reported to return to normal over a period of days to weeks, whereas TPR also declines over the same time. Initially, peripheral vascular resistance tends to rise (probably chiefly a reflex response to the reduced CO, but also because the α-adrenoceptor (vasoconstrictor) effects are no longer partially opposed by β_2-adrenoceptor (dilator) effects, and peripheral flow is reduced. The universal decrease in TPR that follows may be the result of a long-term autoregulatory response to decreased tissue blood flow or to other effects of the drugs. However, some patients exhibit an increase in TPR after β-blockade, which has led to speculation that vascular α-receptors may be activated. For this reason, β-blockers are contraindicated in patients with peripheral vascular disease. An initial decrease in CO therefore may be necessary for the antihypertensive action of β-blockers to occur, but it is not sufficient alone because CO declines similarly in patients whose blood pressure does not decrease in response to β-blockers. Furthermore, β-blockers with intrinsic sympathomimetic activity decrease blood pressure with little or no change in CO.

The sharp decrease in blood pressure hours after β-blockade causes a reflex increase in the plasma catecholamine concentration, which is less than that produced by direct-acting vasodilators. This may reflect an ability of β-blockers to interfere with cardiovascular reflexes or to inhibit release of norepinephrine from sympathetic nerve terminals by blocking a facilitatory prejunctional β_2-adrenergic receptor. However, although not all β-blockers inhibit baroreflexes or sympathetic neurotransmission, all lower blood pressure.

There is some evidence, such as reduced excretion of catecholamines, that β-blockers have a central nervous system (CNS)-mediated sympathoinhibitory effect. Several of these drugs (e.g., propranolol) readily penetrate into the brain, and side effects attributable to perturbation of CNS processes are common with such agents. Studies in experimental animals also have shown that selective administration of β-blockers into the cerebral ventricles lowers blood pressure at doses that are ineffective peripherally. Some drugs in this class, however, do not readily penetrate into the brain after oral administration but still retain antihypertensive efficacy, a finding that opposes a CNS mediated effect. Furthermore, sympathetic neural activity is not reliably reduced by β-blockers at clinically effective doses.

Table 23.5 Pharmacodynamic properties of β-adrenoceptor antagonists

Drug	β₁-Blockade potency ratio (propranolol = 1.0)	Relative β₁ selectivity	Intrinsic sympathomimetic activity	Membrane-stabilizing activity
Acebutolol	0.3	+	+	+
Atenolol	1.0	++	0	0
Betaxolol	1.0	++	0	+
Bisoprolol	10.0	++	0	0
Bucindolol	1.0	0	+	+
Carteolol	10.0	0	+	0
Carvedilol	10.0	0	0	+
Esmolol	0.02	++	0	0
Labetalol	0.3	0	+	0
Metoprolol	1.0	++	0	0
Nadolol	1.0	0	0	0
Oxprenolol	0.5-1.0	0	+	+
Penbutolol	1.0	0	+	0
Pindolol	6.0	0	++	+
Propranolol	1.0	0	0	++
Sotalol	0.3	0	0	0
Timolol	6.0	0	0	0

β-Adrenoceptor selectivity

Some β-adrenoceptor blockers have higher affinity for cardiac β₁-receptors than for cardiac and peripheral β₂-receptors (Tab. 23.5). The ratio of the amount of drug required to block two receptor subtypes is often described as the *selectivity* of the drug. The question is whether the differences between selective and nonselective β-blockers constitute clinical advantages. In theory, there is less likelihood of causing bronchoconstriction, but in practice, none of the available β₁-blockers is sufficiently selective to be used safely in asthma. The main practical use of β₁-selective blockade is in diabetics, where β₂-receptors mediate both the symptoms of hypoglycemia and the counterregulatory metabolic responses that reverse the hypoglycemia.

Some β-blockers also have agonist action; i.e., they are partial agonists. This is sometimes described as *intrinsic sympathomimetic activity* (ISA). These agents cause less of a fall in resting heart rate than do the pure antagonists and may be less effective in severe angina pectoris, in which reduction of heart rate is particularly important. There is also less of a fall in CO, and possibly fewer patients experience unpleasantly cold extremities, although intermittent claudication may be worsened by β-block regardless of whether there is a partial agonist effect. Both classes of drugs can precipitate heart failure, and indeed no important difference is to be expected because patients with heart failure already have high sympathetic drive.

Abrupt withdrawal may be less likely to lead to a rebound effect if there is some partial agonist action, since up-regulation of receptors, as occurs with prolonged receptor blockade, may not have occurred.

β-blockers that act as competitive antagonists at both the β- and α₁-adrenergic receptors include labetalol and carvedilol. Oral labetalol has never gained popularity (a potential unpredictability of effect may be due to the presence of four stereoisomers with different metabolic handling), and the drug is used mainly for hypertensive emergencies; instead, carvedilol is used quite widely, particularly in western Europe. Carvedilol exerts peripheral vasodilatory effects, mediated in part by α₁-antagonism, and has shown significant effectiveness in both hypertension and congestive heart failure (see Chap. 26). This latter activity also has been explained based on the potent antioxidant properties of the compound.

Use of β-blockers in HTN

Beta-blockers are more effective for treating hypertension in white than in black patients and in young patients compared with older ones. β-blockers are particularly effective in younger patients and those with high plasma renin activity. They are useful in treating conditions that may coexist with hypertension, such as supraventricular tachycardias, previous myocardial infarction, angina pectoris, glaucoma, and migraine headache. In addition, β-blockers are used in the treatment of aortic dissection, hepatic portal hypertension, cardiac failure, hyperthyroidism, and pheochromocytoma.

These agents may take several weeks to develop their full effects. A substantial advantage of β-blockade in hypertension is that physiologic stresses such as exercise, upright posture, and high environmental temperature are not accompanied by hypotension, as they are with agents that interfere with α-adrenoceptor-mediated homeostatic mechanisms. With β-blockade these necessary adaptive α-receptor constrictor mechanisms remain intact. The pharmacokinetics, daily doses, and major features of β-blockers used in the treatment of hypertension are given in Chapter 22.

β-blockers are administered orally, with labetalol also

being available for iv use. Lipophilic compounds are almost completely absorbed after oral administration. The antihypertensive effect usually is observed within a few hours. Typically, more than one dose must be given per day, although the long half-life of some drugs and the availability of long-acting preparations have made possible single-dose-per-day administration. For some of the lipid-soluble β-blockers, especially timolol, plasma half-life may not reflect the duration of β-blockade because the drug remains bound to the tissues near the receptor long after therapeutic concentrations of drug have disappeared from the bloodstream. Interestingly, the ocular formulation of timolol may be extensively absorbed systemically, and adverse effects can occur in susceptible patients.

Lipid-soluble agents are metabolized extensively (hydroxylated, conjugated) to water-soluble substances (some of which are active) that can be eliminated by the kidney. They are subject to hepatic "first pass" metabolism after oral administration, especially propranolol (up to 80% metabolized). Plasma concentrations of drugs subject to extensive hepatic first-pass metabolism vary greatly between subjects (up to 20 times) because the process is so much affected by two highly variable factors, speed of absorption and hepatic blood flow, of which the latter is the rate-limiting factor. The bioavailability of propranolol may be increased by the ingestion of food and during long-term administration of the drug.

Water-soluble agents show more predictable plasma concentrations because they are less subject to liver metabolism, being excreted unchanged by the kidney; thus their half-lives are much prolonged in renal failure, e.g., the atenolol half-life is increased from 7 to 24 hours. Water-soluble agents are less widely distributed and may have a lower incidence of effects attributed to penetration of the CNS, e.g., nightmares.

Side effects and clinical problems

Frequently observed side effects of β-blocker therapy include nausea, anorexia, fatigue dizziness, lethargy, insomnia, hallucinations, and bradycardia. It is preferable to use selective β$_1$-antagonists in patients with asthma or diabetes, but any β-blocker should be used with caution. Abrupt cessation of β-blockers has been associated with tachycardia, angina pectoris, myocardial infarction, and hypertension as a result of up-regulation of β-receptors in response to long-term β-blocker therapy. Some β-blockers (particularly those without intrinsic sympathomimetic activity) decrease high-density lipoprotein and increase triglyceride concentrations in blood. Furthermore, β-blockers may decrease libido and sexual potency, which can reduce patient compliance severely. Availability of sildenafil (see Chap. 20) has made this less of a problem. The cold extremities that are characteristic of chronic therapy are probably due chiefly to reduced CO with reduced peripheral blood flow rather than to the blocking of peripheral (β$_2$) dilator receptors, for the effect occurs also with the β$_1$-selective agents. Bronchoconstriction (β$_2$-receptor) occurs as expected, especially in asthmatics (in whom even eyedrops can be fatal). In elderly patients with chronic bronchitis, there may be gradually increasing bronchoconstriction over weeks (even

with eyedrops). Plainly, the risk is greater with nonselective agents, but β$_1$-selective agents are not totally selective and may precipitate asthma.

Patients near congestive heart failure (CHF) need sympathetic drive to provide adequate cardiac output per minute; a drop in heart rate may induce cardiac failure. However, newer studies indicate that cardioselective or nonselective β-blockers without intrinsic activity may prove very useful in the management of patients with CHF (see Chap. 26).

Hypertension may occur whenever block of β-receptors allows preexisting α-effects to be unopposed, e.g., pheochromocytoma. In addition, heart block may be made dangerously worse. Hypoglycemia also may occur, especially with nonselective members, which block β$_2$-receptors, and especially in diabetes and after substantial exercise owing to impairment of the normal sympathetic-mediated homeostatic mechanism for maintaining the blood glucose level; i.e., recovery from iatrogenic hypoglycemia is delayed. However, since α-adrenoceptors are not blocked, hypertension can occur as the sympathetic system discharges in an attempt to reverse the hypoglycemia. In addition, the symptoms of hypoglycemia, insofar as they are mediated by sympathetic mechanisms (anxiety, palpitations), will not occur (although cholinergic sweating will), and the patient may miss the warning symptoms of hypoglycemia and slip into coma. β$_1$-selective drugs are preferred in diabetes.

Overdose, including self-poisoning, causes bradycardia, heart block, hypotension, and low-output cardiac failure that can proceed to cardiogenic shock; death is more likely with agents having membrane-stabilizing action. Bronchoconstriction can be severe, even fatal, in patients subject to any bronchospastic disease; loss of consciousness may occur with lipid-soluble agents that penetrate the CNS. Receptor blockade will outlast the persistence of the drug in the plasma.

Rational treatment of overdose includes the following:
- atropine (1-2 mg iv as one or two bolus doses) to eliminate the unopposed vagal activity that contributes to bradycardia;
- glucagon (5-10 mg iv followed by infusion of 1-10 mg/h) to be used at the outset in severe cases;
- if there is no response, iv injection or infusion of a β-adrenoceptor agonist, e.g., isoprenaline (4 mg/min, increasing at 1- to 3-minute intervals until the heart rate is 50-70 beats/min);
- for bronchoconstriction, albuterol may be used; aminophylline should be given intravenously very slowly to avoid precipitating hypotension.

Interactions

β-blockers exert multiple interactions, pharmacokinetic as well as pharmacodynamic. Agents metabolized in the liver provide higher plasma concentrations when another drug that inhibits hepatic metabolism (e.g., cimetidine) is added. Enzyme inducers enhance the metabolism of this class of β-blockers. β-adrenoceptor blockers themselves reduce hepatic blood flow (fall in CO) and reduce the metabolism of other β-blockers, of lidocaine, and of chlorpromazine.

Most nonsteroidal anti-inflammatory drugs (NSAIDs) attenuate the antihypertensive effect of β-blockers (but not perhaps of atenolol), presumably through inhibition of the formation of renal vasodilator prostaglandins. β-adrenoceptor blockers potentiate the effect of other anti-hypertensives, particularly when an increase in heart rate is part of the homeostatic response (Ca^{2+} blockers and α-adrenoceptor blockers). Combination with verapamil (iv) is hazardous in the presence of atrioventricular nodal or left ventricular dysfunction because the latter has stronger negative inotropic and chronotropic effects than do other calcium channel blockers.

Furthermore, nonselective β-blockers potentiate hypoglycemia of insulin and sulfonylureas. The most important pharmacokinetic/pharmacodynamic interactions are given in Table 23.6.

Cardioselective β-adrenoceptor blocking agents are used in hypertension of pregnancy, including preeclampsia. Both lipid- and water-soluble members enter the fetus and may cause neonatal bradycardia and hypoglycemia. In early pregnancy they appear not to be teratogenic.

CENTRALLY ACTING SYMPATHOLYTICS

Centrally acting sympatholytics can be used alone in the treatment of mild to moderate hypertension that has not responded adequately to treatment with first-line antihypertensives. Sympatholytics are often used in combination with a diuretic. They are believed to decrease blood pressure by causing a reduced sympathetic nerve firing rate; the locus of their action is within the CNS. The reduced sympathetic discharge is functionally selective, because a hypotensive effect is obtained with only minimal impairment of baroreflexes. Drugs in this class include methyldopa, clonidine, moxonidine, rilmenidine, guanfacine, and guanabenz. Reserpine also may act in part by this mechanism.

Clonidine, guanfacine, and guanabenz are relatively selective agonists at α$_2$-adrenergic receptors (i.e., their interaction with α$_1$-adrenergic receptors is minimal, especially in the CNS). In addition, radioligand binding assays have characterized I$_1$-imidazoline sites in the brain stem as the site of action for these agents in the rostral ventrolateral medulla. Drugs such as moxonidine and rilmenidine, still not available in most countries, seem mainly to act by this latter mechanism. Whether blood pressure reduction is due to stimulation of I$_1$-imidazoline sites and/or α$_2$-adrenergic receptors is still a point of discussion.

Nevertheless, these agents readily enter the brain after systemic administration. Findings that (1) blood pressure is lowered in experimental animals by low doses injected directly into the cerebral ventricles, into specific brain regions, or selectively into the arterial blood supply of the brain and that (2) the depressor response to peripherally and centrally administered clonidine or guanabenz can be attenuated by the intracerebral injection of α$_2$-adrenergic receptor antagonists indicate that blood pressure is reduced as a result of an effect of these substances on α$_2$-adrenergic receptors in the CNS. The precise brain site (or sites) where α$_2$-agonists act to lower blood pressure is controversial, but current evidence favors the ventrolateral medulla.

Some studies have shown that the antihypertensive effect of clonidine may involve the release of endogenous opiate peptides. Central-acting sympatholytics are notable for causing less orthostatic hypotension than many other antihypertensive agents do. They also do not impair renal

Table 23.6 Possible pharmacokinetic/pharmacodynamic interactions with β-blockers

Drug	Interaction	Effect
Aluminum hydroxide gel	Decreased absorption of β-blockers	↓Clinical effect of β-blockers
Aminophylline	Mutual inhibition ·	
Ampicillin	Decreased absorption of β-blockers	↓Clinical effect of β-blockers
Calcium	Decreased absorption of β-blockers	↓Clinical effect of β-blockers
Calcium channel blockers	Decreased hepatic clearance of β-blockers	↑Clinical effect of β-blockers
Cimetidine	Decreased hepatic clearance of lipid-soluble β-blockers	↑Clinical effect of β-blockers
Fluvoxamine	Decreased hepatic clearance of propranolol	↑Clinical effect of propanolol
Glucagon	Enhanced clearance of lipid-soluble β-blockers	↓Clinical effect of β-blockers
Hydralazine	Decreased hepatic clearance of lipid-soluble β-blockers	↓Clinical effect of β-blockers
Lidocaine	Decreased hepatic clearance of lidocaine	↑Clinical effect of lidocaine
Phenobarbital	Increased hepatic metabolism of β-blockers	↓Clinical effect of β-blockers
Phenothiazines	Increased phenothiazine and β-blocker blood concentrations	↑Clinical effect of β-blockers
Propafenone	Decreased hepatic clearance of lipid-soluble β-blockers	↑Clinical effect of β-blockers
Quinidine	Decreased hepatic clearance of lipid-soluble β-blockers	↑Clinical effect of β-blockers
Smoking	Enhanced first-pass hepatic degradation	↑Reduced levels of lipid-soluble drugs
Warfarin	Decreased clearance of warfarin	↑Clinical effect of warfarin

function and thus are suitable for hypertensive patients with renal insufficiency.

Clonidine is an imidazoline that acts as an agonist to α_2-adrenoceptors (postsynaptic) in the brain, suppressing sympathetic outflow and reducing blood pressure. At high doses, it also activates peripheral α_2-adrenoceptors (presynaptic receptors) on the adrenergic nerve ending; these mediate negative-feedback suppression of norepinephrine release. Clonidine reduces blood pressure with little postural or exercise drop and would be a drug of first choice were it not for a serious handicap. Abrupt or even gradual withdrawal (e.g., because of forgetfulness, intercurrent illness, need for surgery, etc.) causes a rebound hypertension (in up to 50% of patients) akin to the hypertensive attacks of pheochromocytoma (with high plasma catecholamine concentration). The onset may be rapid (a few hours) or delayed for as long as 2 days; it subsides over 2 to 3 days. Treatment is either to reinstitute clonidine, im if necessary ($t_{1/2}$ = 6 h), or to treat as for pheochromocytoma. Clonidine thus cannot be regarded as a drug of first choice. Recently, in many countries, a transdermal formulation of clonidine, containing 2.5 or 5 mg, to be applied once weekly, has been made available. It can be used safely when drug ingestion is difficult (e.g., postoperatively) or in conditions of mild, unstable hypertension.

Clonidine does not decrease renal blood flow or glomerular filtration rate and therefore is useful in the treatment of hypertension complicated by renal disease. Because it causes sodium and water retention, clonidine usually is administered in combination with a diuretic.

Methyldopa is the drug in this class most commonly employed clinically for reducing blood pressure. Methyldopa (L-isomer) is a prodrug and must be converted in the CNS by dopa decarboxylase and dopamine-hydroxylase to active α-methylnorepinephrine to exert an effect on blood pressure. Because α-methylnorepinephrine is a strong agonist at α_2-adrenergic receptors, it also may act at that site. The related metabolites α-methylepinephrine and α-methyldopamine have been found to have similar actions. As with clonidine, a potential site of action for methyldopa is within the nucleus of the solitary tract. Noradrenergic innervation of the nucleus of the solitary tract provides the neural substrate for the local synthesis and release of α-methylnorepinephrine and related amines. α-Methyldopa reduces total peripheral resistance and decreases blood pressure. CO is not affected, and blood flow to vital organs is not reduced. As with clonidine, renal blood flow is not diminished, and α-methyldopa is of special value in hypertensive patients with renal insufficiency and in pregnant women, in whom long-term successful use has been documented. Methyldopa is available in 250- and 500-mg tablets, to be used in divided doses bid, generally up to 2 g per day.

Pharmacokinetics

The sympatholytic agents are administered orally. Clonidine, guanabenz, and guanfacine have a rapid onset of action (a few hours). Clonidine is well absorbed after oral administration, and the bioavailability is nearly 100%. The peak concentration in plasma and the maximal hypotensive effect are observed 1 to 3 hours after an oral dose. The elimination half-life of the drug ranges from 6 to 24 hours. About half the administered drug can be detected unchanged in the urine. For hypertension, therapy is usually started with oral doses of 0.1 mg twice a day; the maximum dose is 2.4 mg per day.

Methyldopa ($t_{1/2}$ = 1-5 h) is reliably absorbed from the gut and readily enters the CNS. It also takes several hours for methyldopa, a prodrug, to take effect because it must be converted to the active species. Peak concentrations in plasma occur after 2 to 3 hours. The apparent volume of distribution is small (0.4 liter/kg), and it is eliminated with a half-life of about 2 hours. Methyldopa is secreted in the urine primarily as the sulfate conjugate (50-70%) and as the parent drug (25%). The half-life of methyldopa is prolonged in patients with renal failure. Owing to metabolization to the active metabolite, the peak effect of methyldopa is delayed for 6 to 8 hours. The duration of action, even of a single dose, is usually about 24 hours, allowing once- or twice-daily dosage (see Tab. 23.7).

Guanfacine is well absorbed after oral administration and has a large volume of distribution (4-6 liters/kg). About 30% of guanfacine appears unchanged in the urine; the rest is metabolized. The half-life for elimination ranges from 12 to 24 hours. The initial dose is usually 0.5 to 1 mg per day and should be taken at bedtime to minimize problems with somnolence. The dose may be increased in 1-mg increments at intervals of at least several weeks. Doses of 3 mg per day generally are adequate.

Table 23.7 Pharmacokinetic properties of imidazoline receptor agonists

Drug	T_{max} (h)	Bioavailability (%)	Plasma half-life (h)	Protein binding (%)	Volume of distribution (l/kg)
Moxonidine	1	88	2		1.83
Rilmenidine	1.5-2	Not available	8	<10	4.2

Guanabenz has a half-life of 4 to 6 hours and is metabolized extensively in the liver; dosage adjustment may be necessary in patients with hepatic cirrhosis.

Adverse effects and clinical problems

Adverse effects are largely those expected from the mode of action of centrally acting sympatholytics; they include dry mouth, sore or black tongue, sedation (frequent), headache, nightmares, depression, involuntary movements, nausea, flatulence, constipation, dizziness, positive Coombs' test with, occasionally, hemolytic anemia, leukopenia, thrombocytopenia, and hepatitis. These effects occur, to a variable degree, in at least 50% of patients treated with centrally acting sympatholytics. Drug withdrawal may be necessary. Gynecomastia and lactation occur as a result of interference with dopaminergic suppression of prolactin secretion. Any failure of male sexual function is probably secondary to sedation.

Methyldopa produces a positive direct Coombs' test in 20 to 30% of patients and hemolytic anemia in 1%. The incidence of methyldopa-induced hepatitis is unknown, but about 5% of patients will have transient increases in transaminase activities in plasma. Because of its adverse effects, methyldopa is no longer a drug of first choice in routine long-term management of hypertension.

A special problem associated with clonidine (and with other centrally acting α_2-agonists) is a dramatic hypertensive response that occurs in some patients after abrupt withdrawal of therapy. It can be counteracted or prevented with the use of peripherally acting sympatholytic agents. However, clonidine should never be used with a β-adrenoceptor blocker, which exacerbates withdrawal hypertension. Marked bradycardia is observed in some patients. Tricyclic antidepressants antagonize the antihypertensive action and increase the rebound hypertension of abrupt withdrawal.

IMIDAZOLINE AGONISTS (I₁)

Moxonidine and rilmenidine act selectively and have very little central α_2-agonist activity.The only adverse effect consistently associated with these drugs is dry mouth (approximate placebo-corrected incidence is 10%). Sedation is not pronounced. Rebound hypertension is a less important problem with these longer-acting drugs because omission of a single dose will not trigger the rebound. Although there is good evidence for the existence of an imidazoline receptor in the CNS distinct from the α_2-receptor, it is not certain that desired and undesired effects of a drug will be mediated through different receptors. These drugs have as yet limited distribution and also limited experience.

Rilmenidine is almost completely absorbed, and peak plasma concentration are reached in 1.5 to 2 hours. The elimination half-life is about 8 hours, blood pressure reduction being maintained well beyond plasma half-life; 65% of the drug is excreted by the kidneys. The renal clearance is

300 ml/min, with a total clearance of 450 ml/min. In older persons, drug absorption is delayed and the half-life prolonged to 13 hours. Renal insufficiency and renal failure are other situations that alter the pharmacokinetics of rilmendine. In patients with a creatinine clearance of 30 ml/min per 1.73 m, the elimination half-life is prolonged to 29 hours, and in patients with severe renal impaiment, the half-life is prolonged to 42 hours. The drug is poorly dialyzed. Thus patients on hemodialysis do not require an addional dose after a dialysis session. Moxonidine is 89% absorbed orally, and peak plasma concentration occurs after about 1 hour. The half-life is about 2 hours, but as with rilmenidine, the antihypertensive action of moxonidine is longer than would be expected; 90 to 96% of the drug is excreted by the renal route with a renal clearance of 530 ml/min and a total clearance of 830 ml/min. In contrast to rilmenidine, the pharmacokinetics of moxonidine are unchanged in older persons. In patients with renal insufficiency, however, there is a significant increase in in the half-life and C_{max}.

PERIPHERALLY ACTING SYMPATHOLYTICS

Sympatholytics with a peripheral action lower blood pressure by interfering with sympathetic neural control of cardiac and peripheral vascular function through effects produced on the sympathetic neuroeffector junction. Adrenergic neuron-blocking drugs are taken up into adrenergic nerve endings by the active, energy-requiring, saturable amine (norepinephrine) pump mechanism. They accumulate in the norepinephrine storage vesicles, from which they are released in response to nerve impulses. They do not, however, adequately control supine blood pressure and are prone to interact with multiple other drugs affecting adrenergic function.

Guanethidine and guanadrel inhibit the exocytotic release of norepinephrine by a local anesthetic-like action on the nerve terminal. Long-term treatment also results in depletion of transmitter from storage granules in peripheral sympathetic nerves. Guanethidine and guanadrel do not enter the brain. Guanethidine has been used to reduce intraocular pressure and to inhibit thyrotoxic eyelid retraction. Guanadrel and guanethidine are seldom used because of the frequent incidence of severe side effects. These include include fluid retention, dizziness, weakness, retrograde ejaculation, impotence, and diarrhea.

Reserpine is an alkaloid used in medicine since ancient times. It blocks the uptake of dopamine and norepinephrine into storage granules of the sympathetic nerve terminal and subsequently depletes the terminal of neurotransmitter. Thus less transmitter is released during terminal depolarization. Reserpine also acts centrally to decrease sympathetic outflow by an unknown mechanism. This could be related to depletion of norepinephrine or serotonin in the brain. Like guanethidine, reserpine is now seldom used because of the frequent incidence of severe side effects, e.g., sedation, inability to concentrate, psychotic depression, weight gain, and nasal congestion. A number of elderly patients, however, still find benefit from fixed-dose combinations of reserpine (0.25 mg) and a thiazide diuretic (generally chlorthalidone 50 mg).

These act at the postjunctional side of the sympathetic neuroeffector junction. They occupy α_1-adrenergic receptors selectively and block the effects of norepinephrine released from sympathetic nerves. Experimental data indicate that prazosin and other α_1-antagonists such as doxazosin and terazosin also inhibit sympathetic nerve activity through a central mechanism. Alpha-adrenergic blocking agents decrease peripheral vascular resistance and lower arterial blood pressure by causing the relaxation of both arterial and venous smooth muscle. They cause only minimal changes in CO, renal blood flow, and glomerular filtration rate. Therefore, long-term tachycardia and increased renin release do not occur. Prazosin, because of an infrequent but disturbing severe, transient hypotensive effect occuring at the beginning of treatment (first-dose effect), is now seldom used. Newer agents have in fact an improved kinetics, generally allowing single daily doses, and are better tolerated.

Peripheral α_1-adrenergic blockers are used to treat mild to moderate hypertension and are prescribed in combination with β-blockers or diuretics for additive effects. Very recently, doubts have been raised on the effectiveness of doxazosin in preventing CHF in hypertension, compared to chlorthalidone. Concomitant use of a β-blocker may be necessary to blunt the short-term effect of reflex tachycardia.

Doxazosin and terazosin are suitable for once-daily dosing. Terazosin is more soluble in water and has a higher bioavailability (90%). Furthermore, the half-life is approximately 12 hours, with a duration of action of almost 18 hours, allowing administration once daily of doses ranging between 1 and 20 mg. The half-life of doxazosin is approximately 20 hours, and its duration of action may extend to 36 hours. Bioavailability and metabolism are similar to those of prazosin. Usually, single daily doses range from 1 to 16 mg.

Their first-dose effect is less pronounced than in the case of prazosin. Nevertheless, patients should be started at a lower dose than intended for maintenance (detailed pharmacokinetic date are given in Chapter 22). Trimazosin, which is available in a few countries, has a shorter half-life (3 h) and may share some of the unwanted effects of prazosin.

Phentolamine, a nonselective α-adrenoceptor blocker is given iv or im (5-10 mg repeated as necessary) for the treatment of adrenergic hypertensive crises, e.g., pheochromocytoma or MAO inhibitor-sympathomimetic interaction. It has been suggested for the oral treatment of erectile dysfunction (see Chap. 20).

CALCIUM CHANNEL BLOCKING AGENTS

As early as 1964 it was observed that the effects of certain phenylalkylamines such as prenylamine and verapamil on isolated cardiac papillary muscle preparations were indistinguishable from the effects of Ca^{2+} removal. These drugs, like Ca^{2+} depletion, counteract the effects of Ca^{2+} on the cardiac contractile system by inhibiting the influx of Ca^{2+} into cells through specific voltage-dependent Ca^{2+} channels located in cell membranes. Ca^{2+} channels are membrane-spanning, funnel-shaped glycoproteins that function like ion-selective valves. When conformational changes in the channel macromolecule occur, the activation and inactivation "gates" move into and out of an occluding position. This determines opening and closing of the channel pore. Ca^{2+}-binding sites present in the pore ensure the ion selectivity of the channels.

Based on their electrophysiologic and pharmacologic properties, the voltage-dependent Ca^{2+} channels can be divided into different types. The best characterized are the L-type channels (long-lasting, large channels), the T-type channels (transient, tiny channels), and the N-type channels (found in neuronal tissue and resembling neither of the other two in kinetics and inhibitor sensitivity). Only the L-type Ca^{2+} channels are affected by calcium antagonists.

The primary modulator of voltage-dependent Ca^{2+} channels is the membrane potential (voltage). Under resting conditions, when the voltage-dependent Ca^{2+} channels are closed, the membrane potential is -30 to -100 mV (intracellular with reference to extracellular), depending on the cell type. The free intracellular Ca^{2+} concentration ($<10^{-7}$ M) is more than four orders of magnitude lower than the extracellular free Ca^{2+} concentration (1-1.5×10^3 M). This large concentration gradient represents an enormous driving force for Ca^{2+} to enter the cell and can be maintained only by a membrane that is largely impermeable to Ca^{2+} and contains active-transport systems that pump Ca^{2+} extracellularly out of the cytosol. The intact cell membrane fulfills these requirements. On excitation, a rapid depolarization of the cell membrane follows, voltage-dependent Ca^{2+} channels open, and Ca^{2+} enters the cell. Before the next depolarization occurs, Ca^{2+} channels must recover from inactivation and be ready to open from a resting (closed) conformation.

Many chemical compounds are known to inhibit voltage-dependent Ca^{2+} channels, but drugs that have a *primary* effect on Ca^{2+} channels belong to one of the following chemical groups: 1,4-dihydropyridines, phenylalkylamines, and benzothiazepines. The chemical structures of the representative drugs are completely different; hence one may expect that they bind to distinct sites of the L-type Ca^{2+} channel. The interaction of calcium channel modulators with Ca^{2+} channels is complex. Distinct but allosterically interacting receptors exist for the structurally different chemical groups of drugs, such that 1,4-dihydropyridines (nifedipine-like drugs), phenylalkylamines (verapamil-like drugs), and benzothiazepines (diltiazem-like drugs) bind to different binding sites. For example, verapamil inhibits the binding of diltiazem, and diltiazem inhibits verapamil binding. The other agents exhibit similar allosteric interactions. All these receptors are located on the same α_1 subunit of the L-type voltage-dependent Ca^{2+} channels. All excitable tissues contain voltage-dependent Ca^{2+} channels and high-affinity, reversible, and stereospecific binding sites for Ca^{2+} antagonists. However, Ca^{2+} antagonists do not affect every tissue equally. Some tissues rely primarily on exogenous Ca^{2+}

(atrioventricular node) and are more sensitive to these drugs than other tissues (skeletal muscle) that require little or no external Ca^{2+} for function. There are subtypes of voltage-dependent Ca^{2+} channels that show different sensitivities to Ca^{2+} antagonists. Because the distribution of the channel subtypes differs in various tissues, the drug sensitivity of the tissues also varies. In addition, even the L-type Ca^{2+} channels are different in various tissues in terms of their affinities for calcium antagonists. The different pharmacologic properties and pharmacokinetics of the several classes of calcium channel blockers are shown in Tables 23.8 and 23.9, and usual daily doses and time to onset of action are given in Table 22.9.

Clinical use in HTN

Calcium antagonists, encompassing several heterogeneous groups of chemicals, are effective in the treatment of several cardiovascular disorders, particularly angina pectoris, supraventricular tachycardias, and hypertension. For this last indication, calcium channel blockers (CCBs) are recommended when the preferred first-line drugs are contraindicated or ineffective. In hypertensive patients, one retrospective study suggests that use of short-acting CCBs, especially in high doses, is associated with an increased risk of myocardial infarction. CCBs have an intrinsic natriuretic effect; as a consequence, they do not usually require the addition of a diuretic. CCBs are useful in patients who also have asthma, diabetes, angina, and/or peripheral vascular disease. Endothelial dysfunction and platelet activation with thromboxane release may contribute to spasm or alterations in internal mammary artery graft flow during coronary artery surgery (see Chap. 25). An additional field in which CCBs may be used is in patients with kidney failure. They increase renal blood flow and glomerular filtration rate with vasodilatation of afferent as well as efferent arterioles, reducing intraglomerular

pressure. Therefore, they may be useful in diabetic nephropathy, glomerular lesions, microalbuminuria, and proteinuria. In human diabetic nephropathy at least, proteinuria was lowered more effectively by the combination of an ACE inhibitor and a CCB than when either drug was used as monotherapy, despite a similar fall in blood pressure.

Side effects, clinical problems, and toxicity

Most side effects of major CCBs result from excessive vasodilatation or cardiodepression (Tab. 23.10). Generally, side effects such as dizziness, headache, palpitations, and flushing diminish or disappear when the dose is decreased. It may be necessary to discontinue the drug if any of the other side effects occur. Although true withdrawal symptoms are not observed as such, sudden withdrawal of large doses of calcium antagonists can precipitate angina. These drugs have not been observed to cause tachyphylaxis or tolerance.

Side effects occur in approximately 8 to 10% of patients receiving verapamil and may result from excessive vasodilatation and blockade of AV node. During oral administration, the most frequent side effects are constipation, headache, nausea, dizziness, and ankle edema. The edema is not a sign of sodium retention. It is due to a rise in intracapillary pressure as a result of the selective vasodilatation of the precapillary arterioles. This side effect can be attenuated by combining the CCB with a vasodilator that is more potent at relaxing the postcapillary venules. Constipation does not appear to be a problem with either nifedipine or diltiazem. Verapamil may produce its side effects by acting on autonomic receptors. Rare side effects are galactorrhea and reversible hepatic damage. Adverse effects of overdose include hypotension, AV node block, bradycardia, congestive heart failure, and (rarely) ventricular asystole. Verapamil toxicity, like the effects of all calcium antagonists, may be reversed with isoproterenol alone or in combination with calcium gluconate.

Table 23.8 Pharmacologic effects of calcium channel blockers

Drug	Heart rate				Myocardial contractility	Peripheral vasodilatation	Conduction		
	Acute	Chronic	SA node	AV node			Cardiac output	Coronary blood flow	Myocardial O_2 demand
Amlodipine	↑	↑-	-	-	↓	↓↓	↑-	↑	↓
Bepridil	↓	-	↓	↓	V	-	V	↑	↓
Diltiazem	↓	-	↓	↓	↓	↓	V	↑	↓
Felodipine	↑	↑-	-	-	-	↓↓	↑-	↑	↓
Isradipine	↑	↑-	-	-	-	↓↓	↑-	↑	↓
Nicardipine	↑	↑-	-	-	-	↓↓	↑-	↑	↓
Nifedipine	↑	↑-	-	-	↓	↓↓	↑-	↑	↓
Nimodipine	↑	↑-	-	-	-	V	↑-	↑	↓
Nisoldipine	↑	↑-	-	-	-	↓↓	↑-	↑	↓
Verapamil	↑	↓	↓	↓	↓↓	↓	V	↑	↓

Note: ↑ = increase; ↓ = decrease; - = no change; V = variable.

Table 23.9 Pharmacokinetics of calcium channel blockers

Drug	Absorption (%)	Bioavailability (%)	Protein binding (%)	Volume of distribution (liters/kg)	Half-life (h)	Clearance (ml/min/kg)
Diltiazem	>90	35-60	78	5.0	4.1-5.6	15
Verapamil	>90	10-20	90	4.3	4-6 iv / 6-8 po	15
Amlodipine	>90	60-65	>95	21	35-45	7
Felodipine	>95	15-25	>99	10	15.1 + 2.6	12
Isradipine	90-95	17	97	2.9	8.8	10
Nicardipine	>90	~30	>90	0.6	~1 iv	14
Nifedipine	>90	65	90	1.32	~5	500-600
Nimodipine	>90	13	>95	1.7	8-9	19
Nisoldipine	87	5	>99		7-12	

Side effects of nifedipine may occur in 17 to 20% of patients, primarily but not exclusively related to excessive vasodilatation. Headache, dizziness, flushing, ankle edema, hypotension, nasal congestion, and provocation of angina are mitigated by careful dose titration. If this is unsuccessful, it may be necessary to discontinue the drug and substitute another calcium antagonist. In addition to the side effects listed earlier, gum hypertrophy also may occur.

Side effects are rare (2 to 5%) during diltiazem treatment and occur mainly in patients receiving high doses. Headache, flushing, and hypotension may result from excessive vasodilatation, and AV nodal block may result from depression of the AV node.

Before administering calcium antagonists to patients concurrently taking digitalis preparations, two possible drug interactions must be considered. Depression of AV conduction may occur as a result of the combined depressive effects of digitalis and calcium antagonists on the AV node. Digitalis toxicity also may occur if the renal clearance of digoxin is reduced by a calcium antagonist.

The combination of nifedipine with a β-blocker for the treatment of hypertension can be advantageous. Although both drugs directly decrease blood pressure, the reflex effects of nifedipine that increase heart rate and plasma renin activity prevent severe hypotension when the drugs are used in appropriate doses. Although it has no significant effect on AV nodal conduction, nifedipine produces a small negative inotropic effect in the presence of β-blockade. Therefore, this combined therapy is not recommended for patients with impaired ventricular function. In this setting, the combination of verapamil and β-blockers may cause severe hypotension, AV node block, or heart failure. In several studies, diltiazem and β-blockers have been used safely, but again, caution should be observed.

Diltiazem, nicardipine, and verapamil should be used with care in patients treated with immunosuppressive drugs because these drugs raise cyclosporine concentration.

Most widely used CCBs

Verapamil Verapamil was the first selective Ca^{2+} channel blocker available for the treatment of cardiovascular disorders. Like nifedipine, it has both coronary and peripheral vasodilatory effects. It is a more potent negative inotropic agent than nifedipine. The reflex increase in adrenergic tone caused by a sudden decrease in blood pressure mitigates but does not overcome the strong direct negative inotropic and chronotropic effects of verapamil. Because of these prominent cardiodepressant effects, verapamil is generally contraindicated in the treatment of congestive heart failure and should not be used in patients with bradycardia, second- or third-degree heart block, or sick sinus syndrome.

Table 23.10 Clinical problems observed with major calcium channel blockers

Verapamil
(Problems in 8 to 10% of patients)

Cardiodepression
Hypotension
AV node block
Peripheral edema
Headache
Constipation
Vertigo

Nifedipine
(Problems in 17 to 20% of patients)

Hypotension
Headache
Peripheral edema
Vertigo
Fatigue

Diltiazem
(Problems in 2 to 5% of patients)

Hypotension
Peripheral edema
AV node block
Cardiodepression

Nifedipine Nifedipine has a relatively selective effect on arterial resistance vessels. By dilating coronary blood vessels and increasing coronary blood flow, particularly through narrowed coronary arteries (e.g., vasospasm), nifedipine increases oxygen and nutrient supply to the ischemic myocardium. As a result of the dilatation of peripheral arterial resistance vessels, the arterial blood pressure (afterload) decreases. Although the decrease is much more significant in hypertensive patients than in normotensive individuals, any sudden decrease in blood pressure in either can result in a reflex increase in the heart rate and contractility. If the reflex increase in contractility is stronger than the direct negative inotropic effect of nifedipine, the overall result may be a slight increase or no effect, rather than a decrease in contractility. These effects produce a favorable hemodynamic state in patients suffering from angina pectoris and mild congestive heart failure simultaneously. However, there is always the potential for nifedipine to exacerbate incipient heart failure already present because of its direct cardiac negative inotropic action. In contrast to verapamil and diltiazem, which inhibit AV nodal conduction, nifedipine has no significant effect on AV nodal conduction in vivo.

The efficacy of nifedipine in the treatment of mild to moderate hypertension is equivalent to that of β-blockers or diuretics. Although it is effective alone, its use in combination with low doses β-blockers can be particularly efficacious because the reflex increases in heart rate and plasma renin activity produced by nifedipine are attenuated by the β-blocker.

Diltiazem Diltiazem has some pharmacologic effects similar to those of nifedipine but resembles verapamil in its other actions. Like all calcium antagonists, diltiazem increases coronary blood flow and decreases elevated blood pressure. Like verapamil, it inhibits AV nodal conduction, although less effectively than verapamil, and should not be used where there is bradycardia, second- or third-degree heart block, or sick sinus syndrome. Diltiazem is approximately as efficacious as nifedipine in dilating coronary arteries but produces fewer side effects. It is effective in decreasing hypertension and has fewer negative inotropic and chronotropic effects than do the β-adrenergic blocking drugs. Diltiazem is approved by the Food and Drug Administration (FDA) for the treatment of angina pectoris (caused by coronary artery spasm), chronic exercise-induced stable angina, and hypertension.

Other calcium antagonists

Nicardipine is a newer dihydropyridine calcium antagonist that is similar to nifedipine. It increases coronary blood flow in patients with coronary artery disease without causing rnyocardial depression. It also decreases systemic vascular resistance and has a potent antihypertensive effect. At higher doses, nicardipine does have a direct negative inotropic effect on the heart and can lead to worsened heart failure in some patients with severe left ventricular dysfunction. It has little or no effect on the conduction system. Nicardipine shows little interaction with digoxin and warfarin.

Isradipine and *felodipine* are other dihydropyridine antagonists used to treat essential hypertension. Isradipine decreases systemic vascular resistance and has potent antihypertensive effects. A sudden decrease in blood pressure may result in a reflex increase in heart rate. At higher doses, isradipine may have a direct negative inotropic effect on the heart, and caution therefore should be exercised in patients with congestive heart failure who are receiving it, particularly when the drug is used in combination with a β-blocker. Isradipine has no detrimental effects on the conduction system and is indicated for the treatment of hypertension alone or in combination with thiazide diuretics. Isradipine appears to have no significant effect on cyclosporine trough levels, creatinine clearance, or renal plasma flow in hypertensive kidney transplant recipients. Chronic treatment with isradipine may favorably affect the platelet function and fibrinolytic system in essential hypertension in patients with or without other cardiovascular risk factors.

Unlike some other calcium antagonists, *felodipine* has very little effect on cardiac function. It has a relatively long duration of action and in an extended-release formulation is appropriate for the treatment of hypertension with a once-daily dose. A reflex increase in heart rate frequently occurs during the first week of therapy, but this increase attenuates over time. The increase in heart rate is inhibited by β-blocking agents. Felodipine, a CYP3A4 substrate, is markedly affected by compounds metabolized through this route; most notable is the case of grapefruit juice, which may laed to significant side effects when combined with felodipine, e.g., vasodilatation, tachycardia, and possibly circulatory collapse. Felodipine has been used, with very good results, in the primary prevention HOT study (see above).

Amlodipine is a low-clearance dihydropyridine that is effective for the treatment of hypertension and angina with once-daily dosing, resulting in improved patient compliance and a minimal fluctuation in serum drug concentrations. Its good bioavailability (60-65%), slow rate of elimination (half-life = 45 h), and almost total absence of drug interactions give a pharmacokinetic profile not seen with other calcium antagonists. Amlodipine is not suitable for emergency reduction of blood pressure. It is safe, however, in patients with cardiac failure (PRAISE study; see Chap. 26). The safety of amlodipine for the treatment of angina or hypertension in patients with left ventricular hypertension also has been established.

Interestingly, treatment of smooth muscle cells with amlodipine alone and an amlodipine-lovastatin combination ameliorated the atherogenic effect of low-density lipoproteins (LDLs). As compared with amlodipine alone, the combination demonstrated a considerably higher antiatherogenic effect on LDL.

Nimodipine is a second-generation dihydropyridine with apparent selectivity for cerebral blood vessels. It has been approved for the treatment of neurologic complications that occur after subarachnoid hemorrhage. It also has been approved for the treatment of neurologic deficits caused by cerebral vasospasm after subarachnoid hemorrhage resulting from ruptured congenital intracranial aneurysms.

ORALLY ACTIVE DIRECT VASODILATORS

The direct vasodilators hydralazine and minoxidil are used in combination with other drugs for the treatment of severe or resistant hypertension. They lower blood pressure by directly relaxing arterial smooth muscle (Tab. 23.11). They differ from calcium channel blockers by having different presumed cellular mechanisms of action and a greater selectivity for arterial smooth muscles. Calcium channel antagonists do not show selectivity but affect both arterial and venous smooth muscle.

The cellular mechanism by which *hydralazine* causes vascular relaxation is not known but may involve intracellular accumulation of cyclic guanosine monophosphate (cGMP). At the present time, hydralazine has little place in the routine oral therapy of hypertension. It may be used, however, together with nitrates in congestive heart failure (see Chap. 26). Since the compensatory baroreceptor-mediated sympathetic activity causes tachycardia and increased CO, postural hypotension generally is not a problem. Usually, 5 to 20 mg may be given iv over 20 minutes; the maximum effect occurs in 10 to 80 minutes.

Minoxidil appears to cause vascular relaxation by increasing cellular potassium permeability, thus leading to K^+ efflux from the cell, membrane hyperpolarization, and inhibition of stimulated calcium influx through receptor-mediated calcium channels. It is administered orally for the treatment of severe to malignant hypertension that is refractory to other drugs, including hydralazine. The relatively strong renal vasodilator activity of this drug makes it particularly useful in patients with renal insufficiency.

Pharmacokinetics

Hydralazine is well absorbed after oral administration; the bioavailability, however, is low (16% in fast acetylators, 35% in slow acetylators). The acetylated form is inactive. Thus the dose necessary to reduce blood pressure is larger in fast acetylators. The half-life of hydralazine is 1 hour, and the hypotensive effects can last as long as 12 hours. Hydralazine shows hepatic and extrahepatic metabolization. The peak concentration of hydralazine occurs within 30 to 120 minutes of oral administration. Usually, the dose is 25 to 100 mg bid.

After oral administration, minoxidil is well absorbed from the gastrointestinal tract. Peak plasma concentrations are detected about 1 hour after administration; the maximal hypotensive effect, however, occurs later, possibly because of formation of active metabolites. Only 20% of the drug is excreted unchanged in the urine; the main route of elimination is by hepatic metabolism. The glucuronide conjugate of minoxidil is less active but has a longer half-life than minoxidil (3-4 h). The duration of action (24 h) is longer than expected. The initial dose is usually 4 mg, which can be increased to 40 mg qd or bid.

Side effects

Common side effects of hydralazine are headache, flushing, nasal and conjunctival congestion, lacrimation, palpitations, dizziness, fatigue, tachycardia, and vomiting. The incidence and severity of side effects are greater in slow acetylators. With prolonged use of doses above 100 mg, a reversible syndrome of myalgia and arthralgia proceeding to disseminated lupus erythematosus may occur, especially in slow acetylators. The condition is reversible after discontinuation of the drug. As with other drugs that increase the vascular capacity, blood volume increases, thereby reducing the effectiveness of blood pressure reduction. Therefore, a combination therapy with diuretics may be useful.

Reflex tachycardia may be severe in patients treated with minoxodil and may require concomitant use of a β-blocker. An increase in CO also may occur. Minoxidil causes serious sodium and water retention, leading to volume overload, edema, and congestive heart failure. Concomitant administration of a diuretic may be necessary. Additional side effects of minoxidil are palpitations and abnormal hair growth. The last effect may limit compliance in female patients, but it is exploited to treat male-pattern baldness, in which case it is applied topically.

Table 23.11 Mechanism and site of action of vasodilator drugs

Drug	Mechanism	Vessels affected
Nitrates	Direct effect, conversion to NO, increase in cGMP	Venous
Hydralazine	Direct effect, EDRF-dependent formation of NO, increase in cGMP, K^+-channel agonist	Arteriolar
Nitroprusside sodium	Direct effect, conversion to NO, increase in cGMP	Arteriolar and venous
Minoxidil	Direct effect, K^+-channel agonist	Arteriolar

ACE INHIBITORS

Renin, an enzyme produced by the kidney in response to a number of factors including adrenergic activity and sodium depletion, converts the circulating glycoprotein angiotensinogen into the biologically inert decapeptide angiotensin I, which is then changed by the angiotensin-converting enzyme (ACE or kininase II) into the highly potent vasoconstrictor angiotensin II (ATII). The angiotensin-converting enzyme is widely distributed, but its highest activity is in the endothelium of the pulmonary vasculature, probably because of the long length of pulmonary capillaries. Other renin-angiotensin systems are located in the brain, heart, and many other organs, the relevance of which, however, is uncertain. Bradykinin (an endogenous vasodilator occurring in blood vessel walls) is also a substrate for ACE; it is probably a minor contributor to the vasodilator action of ACE inhibitors, except in patients without kidneys or other low-renin causes of hypertension. However, either bradykinin or one of the neurokinin substrates of ACE (such as substance P) may cause cough.

ATII acts on two G-protein–coupled receptors, of which the angiotensin AT1 subtype accounts for all the classic actions of angiotensin. These include also stimulation of aldosterone (sodium-retaining hormone) production by the adrenal cortex.

When the ATII concentration in plasma is relatively high (i.e., approximately 100 pg/ml), the peptide causes direct arterial constriction. Inhibition of ATII formation reduces vasoconstriction, and blood pressure decreases. However, hypertensive patients with lower, or even normal, plasma concentrations of ATII also exhibit a depressor response to ACE inhibition. The mechanism of this effect is less clear. One possibility is that the ACE inhibitors act by blocking

the tissue generation of ATII. ATII also can be produced by intrarenal renin, in which case the peptide exerts an antinatriuretic and antidiuretic effect. Inhibition of intrarenal ATII formation by ACE inhibitors could lower blood pressure by promoting salt and water excretion in a manner similar to that of the diuretic agents. Finally, ACE inhibitors act by inhibiting brain ACE. An increase in intracerebral concentrations of ATII in experimental animals causes an elevation in arterial pressure mediated through activation of the sympathetic nervous system. The ACE inhibitors could reduce the activity of the sympathetic nervous system in a manner similar to that of centrally acting sympatholytic agents.

In addition, ATII stimulates cardiac and vascular smooth muscle cell growth, probably contributing to the progressive amplification of hypertension once the process is initiated. Limited studies to date have shown that the AT_2 receptor subtype is coupled to inhibition of muscle growth or proliferation.

ACE inhihitors reversibly inhibit angiotensin-converting enzyme that cleaves angiotensin I to form the potent vasoconstrictor ATII. These inhibitors also diminish the rate of bradykinin inactivation. They lower blood pressure by reducing peripheral vascular resistance without reflexly increasing CO, heart rate, or contractility. Vasodilatation occurs as a result of the combined effects of lower vasoconstriction caused by diminished levels of ATII and the potent vasodilating effect of increased bradykinin; renal blood flow may increase. By reducing circulating ATII levels, ACE inhibitors also decrease the secretion of aldosterone, resulting in decreased sodium and water retention. The pharmacodynamic effects of ACE inhibitors are summarized in Table 23.12. The presence of an SH group in some ACE inhibitors (see Tab. 22.2) may account for some antioxidant activity.

Use in HTN

Like β-blockers, ACE inhibitors are most effective in hypertensive patients who are white and young. However, when used in combination with a diuretic, the effectiveness of ACE inhibitors is similar in white and black hypertensive patients. ACE inhibitors are also effective in the management of patients with chronic congestive heart failure. ACE inhibitors are now a standard in the care of patients following myocardial infarction, in which they may reverse the vascular remodeling and cardiac hypertrophy of hypertension. Therapy is started 24 hours after the end of the infarction. In addition, ACE inhibitors may become a standard therapy in diabetic patients, in whom beneficial effects on kidney long-term function have been described. There is increasing evidence that the beneficial effects of ACE inhibitors are greater than would be expected from blood pressure reduction alone.

ACE inhibitors are particularly efficacious when the raised blood pressure results from excess renin production (renovascular hypertension). The effect is immediate, and there may be an initial brisk, even serious, drop in blood pressure (first-dose effect) so that therapy is best initiated at bedtime and the patient warned. Patients already taking a diuretic should omit this for a few days before the first

Table 23.12 Hemodynamic and hormonal effects of ACE inhibition in patients with hypertension

Hemodynamic parameter	Hypertension
Blood pressure	↓
Systemic vascular resistance	↓
Heart rate	↔
Stroke volume	↔
Cardiac output	↔
Ejection fraction	↔
Renal blood flow	↔↑
Renal vascular resistance	↔↓
Glomerular filtration rate	↔
Forearm blood flow	↑
Cerebral blood flow	↔↑
Angiotensin II	↓
Angiotensin I	↑
Renin	↑
Aldosterone	↔
Converting-enzyme activity	↓
Kinin levels	↑↔
Plasma norepinephrine	↔
Prostaglandins (urinary)	↑

Table 23.13 Adverse effects and clinical problems in ACE inhibitor therapy

Hypotension
  Hyperkalemia
  Functional renal impairment
  Acute renal failure
  Nephrotic syndrome
  Accumulation in patients with impaired kidney function
Cough
Fever
Skin rash
Angioneurotic edema
Taste disturbances
Hemodialysis-associated anaphylaxis
Hematologic
  Leukopenia
  Anemia
Hepatobiliary
  Cholestasis
  Hepatocellular dysfunction
Teratogenic effects
  Skeletal malformation
  Neonatal renal failure

dose. The antihypertensive effect increases progressively over weeks with continued administration (as with other antihypertensives), and the dose may be increased at intervals of 2 weeks.

ACE inhibitors have a useful vasodilator and diuretic-sparing (but not diuretic-substitute) action in all grades of heart failure (see Chap. 26).

Pharmacokinetics

Kinetic data and daily doses of major ACE inhibitors are summarized in Table 22.2.

Except for captopril and lisinopril, which do not require deesterification after absorption, ACE inhibitors are prodrugs. Captopril is well absorbed from the gastrointestinal tract, and peak plasma concentrations occur within\1 hour. It has the shortest half-life (2-3 h) of all the ACE inhibitors and is partly metabolized and partly excreted unchanged (40%); in renal failure, elimination is reduced, and adverse effects are more common. The bioavailability of captopril (65%) is significantly reduced by food, and captopril should be given 1 hour before meals. The initial dose for the treatment of hypertension is 25 mg, given bid or tid. After 2 weeks, it may be increased to 100 mg per day. In patients with heart failure or on intensive diuretic therapy, 6.25 mg or less may be the initial therapy.

In contrast to captopril, the bioavailability of enalapril is little affected by food. It is rapidly absorbed after oral administration. Peak plasma levels are observed within 3 to 4 hours, with a maximal reduction in blood pressure 4 to 6 hours after ingestion. Since enalapril is a prodrug ($t_{1/2}$ >30 h) that is converted to the active enalaprilat ($t_{1/2}$ = 10 h), the onset of action is slower than with captopril. Responses to enalaprilat given intravenously are apparent in 15 minutes. The duration of action of enalapril, however, is prolonged; it binds more tightly to the converting enzyme and persists

longer in the plasma, allowing an effective treatment with a single daily dose, and some enzyme inhibition is still present at 24 hours. Oral daily doses range from 10 to 40 mg.

In contrast to the ACE inhibitors just mentioned, lisinopril is slowly and incompletely (30%) absorbed. Most of the drug is cleared by the kidney unchanged, with a half-life of about 12 hours. It is noteworthy that short-term treatment (10-12 weeks) causes a significant decrease in CO. For blood pressure reduction, the initial dose is 10 mg per day. To achieve the desired blood pressure reduction, the dosage can be increased to 20 to 40 mg per day.

Other members of this group include benazepril, delapril, perindopril, ramipril, cilazapril, moexipril, spirapril, trandolapril, and quinapril (see Tab. 22.2). Fosinopril is cleared by both the liver and the kidney. Trandolapril and perindopril are among the few ACE inhibitors with a sufficiently long half-life to guarantee high trough/peak plasma ratios on once-daily dosing, but once again, the clinical significance of this is insufficient to recommend any claim of superiority over other drugs in the class.

Side effects

ACE inhibitors are generally very well tolerated. The major side effect is cough, to a varying degree, in 2-10% of treated patients. It may require change to an ATII antagonist. Other adverse effects are listed in table 23.13

ANGIOTENSIN II (ATII) ANTAGONISTS

ATII antagonists block the binding of ATII to the AT_1 subtype angiotensin receptors in blood vessels and other tissues. Most physiologic effects of the peptide are thus inhibited. These agents have antihypertensive actions similar to these of ACE inhibitors but may produce fewer side effects because bradykinin and prostanoid metabolism are not altered. Since they have no effect on bradykinin, they are likely to be even less effective than ACE inhibitors in the absence of renin secretion. Losartan, a nonpeptide, was the first available angiotensin (AT) receptor antagonist. The pharmacologic effects of losartan are similar to those of ACE inhibitors in that losartan produces vasodilatation and blocks aldosterone secretion. Until further experience with these drugs has been gained, their main use is in patients responding to an ACE inhibitor who develop cough. The AT_1 blockers have not yet been introduced for the treatment of cardiac failure; this is likely to be a matter of time. Major clinical characteristics of currently available AT_1 blockers are summarized in Table 22.3.

Pharmacokinetics

Losartan is a highly selective competitive ATII receptor blocker with a noncompetitive active metabolite. The drug is only one-third absorbed after oral dosing (Tab. 23.14), and this is not affected by food. Losartan is highly bound to plasma proteins, and the half-life ranges between 1.3 and 2.2 hours. That of the metabolite is much longer, permitting adequate once-daily doses. Excretion is one-third urinary and two-thirds biliary. Mean plasma clearance after intravenous administration is 8.1 ml/kg per minute, with a renal clearance of 0.92 ml/kg per minute. Whereas renal excretion is only a minor pathway for the unchanged drug, 55% of the active metabolite is excreted renally. Daily doses of 50 to 100 mg have been found to be as efficacious as ACE inhibitors, felodipine, or atenolol in reducing blood pressure. Blood pressure lowering with losartan once or twice daily is evident within 1 week and reaches a maximum after 6 weeks. Dosage adjustment of losartan in the presence of renal insufficiency does not seem mandatory, since the area under the curve (AUC) and half-life do not change. In mild to moderate liver cirrhosis, however, the total clearance of losartan should be decreased by approximately 50%.

The absorption after oral administration of most other angiotensin receptor antagonists is rapid to intermediate (Tab. 23.14). Peak plasma concentrations are achieved withn 1 to 4 hours. Angiotensin receptor antagonists are lipophilic drugs and highly bound to plasma proteins with intermediate values for their terminal volume of distribution. They are mainly metabolized in the liver, generating both active and inactive metabolites, which are further eliminated in the bile or through the kidney. Metabolism involves the cytochrome P450 system as well as UDP-glucuronyltransferases.

Side effects

No significant drug-related adverse effects have been reported, other than those due to excessive hypotension in salt-depleted subjects, and it is certain that losartan does not cause dry cough. Sometimes postural dizziness has been observed. However, fetotoxicity has been reported, and AT_1 antagonists are contraindicated in pregnant women.

Interactions

In vitro data suggest that the transformation of losartan to its metabolite E-3174 is catalyzed by CYP3A4. Thus modulators of this enzyme may influence pharmacokinetics. Pretreatment with cimetidine generated an 18% increase in losartan AUC without affecting the AUC of the metabolite E-3174. The half-life of both was unchanged. In contrast, ketoconazole significantly reduced conversion of losartan to E-3174, thus ultimately leading to a reduction in the hypotensive effect. Induction of cytochromes by pretreatment with phenobarbital decreased both AUCs (losartan and E-3174) by 20%, whereas no significant changes in half-life and renal clearance were detected.

DRUGS FOR HYPERTENSIVE EMERGENCIES

Under some clinical circumstances (Tab. 23.15), blood pressure must be reduced in a rapid but controlled fashion for a relatively short period. Hypertensive emergencies are rare but life-threatening situations (see also Chap. 87). Diastolic blood pressure is either over 150 mmHg (systolic blood pressure > 210 mmHg) in an otherwise healthy person or 130 mmHg in an individual with pre-existing complications. Several of the antihypertensive agents already discussed can be given parenterally for this purpose. Other drugs are used exclusively to rapidly reduce blood pressure, including the direct-acting vasodilators nitroprusside and diazoxide and the α_1-antagonist urapidil.

Nitroprusside (Tab. 23.16) acts by increasing cGMP concentrations in vascular smooth muscle cells and thereby reducing intracellular calcium ion concentrations. It is administered iv and causes prompt vasodilatation with reflex tachycardia. It is capable of reducing blood pressure in all patients, regardless of the cause of hypertension. The drug has little effect outside the vascular system, acting equally on arterial and venous smooth muscle. Nitroprusside is metabolized rapidly and requires continuous infusion. Close monitoring of blood pressure is mandatory.

Diazoxide, although related chemically to the thiazide diuretics, produces direct vasodilatation by an activation

Table 23.14 Pharmacokinetic properties of angiotensin receptor antagonists

Drug	Bioava-ilability	T_{max} (h)	Effects of food	Protein binding (%)	Volume of distribution (liters)	Half-life (h)	Clearance (l/h)	First pass	Active drug	Dose reduction in	
										kidney failure	hepatic failure
Losartan	33	0.25-2	No influence	98	27	1.3-2.2	36	+	No	No	Yes
Ibersartan	60-80	1-2	No influence	90	53-93	11-15	15	No	Yes	No	No
Valsatan	26-39	<2	Reduction of absorption	96	12	5-6	2-7	No	Yes	No	No

of the ATP-dependent K⁺ channel. In contrast to nitroprusside and trimethaphan, which produce equivalent relaxation of arteries and veins, diazoxide is primarily an arterial vasodilator. For patients with coronary insufficiency, diazoxide is administered iv with a β-blocker, which reduces reflex tachycardia. Diazoxide is used in the treatment of hypertensive emergencies, hypertensive encephalopathy, and eclampsia.

Labetalol is both an α- and β-blocker. Labetalol does not cause reflex tachycardia and carries the contraindications of a nonselective β-blocker. It is a racemic mixture; one isomer is a β-adrenoceptor blocker (nonselective), and the other blocks α-adrenoceptors. The β-blockade is 4 to 10 times greater than the α-blockade, varying with dose and route of administration. Labetalol can be useful as a parenterally administered drug in the rare patient who requires emergency blood pressure reduction.

Urapidil is both an α₁-antagonist and a central sympatholytic. Urapidil produces a reduction in peripheral resistance and a fall in diastolic and systolic blood pressure, usually without reflex tachycardia. Changes in glucose or lipid metabolism have not been reported. Urapidil may have a potential role in eclampsia, and its beneficial effects on preload and afterload may be of value in patients with congestive heart failure. It has been used successfully in the to improve myocardial perfusion after coronary stenting.

Pharmacokinetics

Major kinetic parameters of the four drugs most frequently used in hypertensive emergencies are given in Table 23.16. Diazoxide is given rapidly iv (<30 s) at a dose of 1 to 3 mg/kg (maximum 150 mg). The maximum effect occurs within 5 minutes and lasts for at least 4 hours. Additonal injections may be given after 5 to 15 minutes. The duration of action is variable and can be as short as 4 hours or as long as 20 hours. Usually, an infusion may be begun at 0.3 to 1.0 µg/kg per minute, and control of blood pressure is likely to be established at 0.5 to 6.0 µg/kg per minute. Approximately 20 to 50% of the drug is eliminated unchanged by the kidney; the rest is metabolized in the liver.

Nitroprusside is an unstable molecule given by continuous iv infusion; full effects occur in seconds, and recovery takes place within a few minutes of terminating the infu-

Table 23.15 Conditions requiring rapid blood pressure reduction

Acute left ventriculare failure
Aortic dissection
Coronary insufficiency
Hypertensive encephalopathy
Intracranial hemorrhage
Malignant hypertension
Pheochromocytoma
Refractory hypertension of pregnancy

sion. Because the drug decomposes in light, only fresh solutions should be used. Most patients respond to an infusion of 0.5 to 1.5 µg/kg per minute. If an infusion rate of 10 µg/kg per minute does not produce adequate reduction in blood pressure, administration of nitroprusside should be stopped.

Labetalol doses of 50 mg may be given iv over 1 minute with the patient supine and repeated at 5-minute intervals up to a maximum of 200 mg; atropine reverses or prevents severe bradycardia.

Urapidil is is given as a slow iv injection of the hydrochloride in an initial dose equivalent to 25 mg of the base, followed by infusion of 9 to 30 mg per hour.

Side effects and toxicities

The side effects of drugs used for hypertensive emergencies can be significant. The usual side effects of diazoxide are hyperglycemia, tachycardia, and fluid retention. The concurrent use of a nonthiazide diuretic frequently is required. Blood glucose and potassium levels should be monitored carefully. Diazoxide is strongly alkaline, and extravasation should be avoided. Moreover, diazoxide relaxes the uterus.

Side effects of nitroprusside therapy are few. Nitroprusside is metabolized to cyanide ions, which mainly remain in erythrocytes. Sometimes, an infusion of sodium thiosulfate is required to produce thiocyanate, which is less toxic and is eliminated by the kidneys. Measurement of plasma thiocyanate level may be useful in determining

Table 23.16 Pharmacokinetic parameters of drugs used for hypertensive emergencies

Drug	Route of administration	Half-life (h)	Bioavailability (%)	Volume of distribution (l/kg)	Protein binding (%)	Onset of action	Duration (h)	First pass
Nitroglycerin	po	8-9	<1		60	10-20 min	2-3	+
	iv					Immediate		
Nitroprusside	iv					seconds		
Diazoxide	iv	20-60		0.21	94	1-5 min	<4	
Urapidil	iv	4.7 2.7 (iv)	70-80 (po)		80			
Labetalol	iv	4	20	9.4	50			+

whether the patient is suffering from toxicity from prolonged infusions, e.g., hypothyroidism or acute toxic psychosis. Cyanide concentrations should be monitored in patients with liver disease. Other reversible side effects of nitroprusside include nausea, headache, abdominal cramping, and dizziness.

Postural hypotension (characteristic of α-receptor block-

ade) is likely to occur at the outset of therapy with labetolol and if the dose is increased too rapidly. Urapidil is reported to be well tolerated, with adverse effects generally transient and most frequent at the beginning of the therapy. Dizziness, nausea, headache, fatigue, orthostatic hypotension, palpitations, nervousness, itching, and allergic skin reactions have been reported. The drug should be used with care in elderly patients and those with severe hepatic insufficiency, in whom the half-life may be markedly prolonged.

Suggested readings

ALDERMAN CP. Adverse effects of the angiotensin-converting enzyme inhibitors. Ann Pharmacother 1996;30:55.

ALLHAT Officers and Coordinators. Major cardiovascular events in hypertensive patients randomized to doxazosin vs chlorthalidone. JAMA 2000;283:1967-75

BAUER JH, REAMS GP. The angiotensin II type 1 receptor antagonists:a new class of antihypertensive drugs. Arch Intern Med 1995;155:1361-8.

EVANS RR, DiPETTE DJ. New or developing antihypertensive agents. Curr Opin Cardiol 1997;12:382-8.

FOUAD TF. Hemodynamic effects of inhibitors of the renin-angiotensin system. J Hypertens (suppl) 1994;12:S25-9.

GALES MA. Oral antihypertensives for hypertensive urgencies. Ann Pharmacother 1994;28:352-8.

GODFRAIND T. Calcium antagonists and vasodilatation. Pharmacol Ther 1994;64:37-75.

HEAGERTY AM. Functional and structural effects of ACE inhibitors on the cardiovascular system. Cardiology 1991;79 (suppl 1):3-9.

HANSSON L, ZANCHETTI A, CARRUTHERS SG, et al. Effects of intensive blood-pressure lowering and low-dose aspirin in patients with hypertension: principal results of the hpertension optimal treatment (HOT) randomised trial. Lancet 1998;351:1755-62.

HANSSON L, LINDHOLM L, NIKKANEN L, et al. Effect of angiotensin converting enzyme inihibition compared with conventional therapy in cardiovascular morbidity and mortality in hyertension: the Captopril Prevention Project (CAPP) randomized trial. Lancet 1999;353:611-16.

KIRSTEN R, NELSON K, KIRSTEN D, HEINTZ B. Clinical pharmacokinetics of vasodilators, part I. Clin Pharmacokinet 1998;34:457-82.

KIRSTEN R, NELSON K, KIRSTEN D, HEINTZ B. Clinical pharmacokinetics of vasodilators, part II. Clin Pharmacokinet 1998;35:9-36.

PSATY BM, SMITH NL, SISCOVICK DS, et al. Health outcomes associated with antihypertensive therapies used as first-line agents: a systematic review and meta-analysis. JAMA 1997;277:739-45.

RAMSAY LE, UL HAQ, YEO WW, JACKSON PR. Interpretation of prospective trials in hypertension: do treatment guidelines accurately reflect current evidence? J Hypertens 1996;14(suppl 5):S187-94.

SCHACHTER M. New ideas for treating hypertension. J Hum Hypertens 1995;9:663-7.

VAN ZWIETEN PA, PFAFFENDORF M. Similarities and differences between calcium antagonists. pharmacological aspects. J Hypertens 1993;11(suppl):S3-11.

WILSON TW, QUEST DW. Comparative pharmacology of calcium antagonists. Can J Cardiol 1995;11:243-9.

The clinical use of antiarrhythmic drug therapy

Robert J. MacFadyen

Recent times have seen improved understanding of the risks of drug therapy for arrhythmia. Clinical trials have resulted in a reduction in the scope of chronic antiarrhythmic drug therapy, but these treatments remain important in the management of most patients. The aim is to control symptoms or improve prognosis at a drug concentration that produces no major adverse effects. For some drugs, concentration measurements can define antiarrhythmic and proarrhythmic (arrhythmia-provoking) effects as well as adverse effects.

CLASSIFICATION OF ANTIARRHYTHMIC DRUGS

There are two main systems of classification. The simplest system is based on cellular electrophysiology, the *Vaughn-Williams classification*. More recently, an alternative has been developed known as the *Sicilian gambit*. The name relates simply to the site of the inaugural meeting of the working group.

Modified Vaughn-Williams classification

This system is based on the broad effects of antiarrhythmic drugs on electrocardiographic (ECG) intervals with one main electrophysiologic property per agent. Assessment is based on the action potential changes in isolated cardiomyocytes from normal animal tissue. This does not translate well to clinical practice but remains in widespread use (Tab. 24.1).

Class I drugs

These agents affect the voltage-dependent sodium channel, and subdivisions have been added based on the effects of drugs on action potential duration. Class Ia drugs prolong this characteristic, class Ib drugs shorten it, and class Ic drugs have little or no effect. The class was complicated further by a consideration of the binding kinetics of drugs to the sodium channel, which depend on heart rate. Time constants for ion binding are long for class Ia and Ic drugs but short for class Ib drugs.

Class Ia drugs include quinidine, procainamide, and disopyramide. They all possess a similar range of electrophysiologic effects but have varying effects on electrophysiologic intervals. Pharmacokinetic properties affect the onset and duration of drug effect. They possess individual additional properties, e.g., marked anticholinergic effects with quinidine, an active metabolite of procainamide (*N*-acetyl procainamide), and myocardial depressant effects and peripheral vasodilator activity and a proarrhythmic effect with disopyramide.

Class Ib agents include the standard agent used in acute-onset ventricular arrhythmia, lignocaine, with rapid-onset blockade of the sodium channel. Similar agents having this effect include tocainide and mexiletine, which now have restricted use and most often only in combination with class III drugs in specialised circumstances.

Class Ic agents include a variety of compounds with slower onset sodium channel blocking activity, from little used agents such as encainide and lorcainide to more recent, widely studied, and widely used agents such as flecainide and propafenone. Propafenone has significant class II β-blocking activity.

Class II drugs

This class contains drugs blocking the sympathetic nervous system. These agents interact at a number of other sites that contribute to antiarrhythmic effect. The main agents are the β-adrenergic blocking drugs, including non-receptor-selective lipophilic drugs, e.g., propranolol; drugs with high intrinsic sympathomimetic activity, e.g., pindolol; and β_1-selective agents, e.g., metoprolol and atenolol (see Chap. 23). The β_1-specific drug sotalol has multiple activities (see below). Agents in other classes such as amiodarone (class III) and propafenone (class Ic) have β-blocking activity that may be clinically important.

Table 24.1 The modified Vaughn-Williams classification of antiarrhythmic drugs

Class	Examples	Depolarization	Repolarization
Class I	*Membrane-active drugs*		
Ia	Quinidine Procainamide Disopyramide Moricizine	Moderate depression of Na^+ current; intermediate kinetics	Prolonged
Ib	Lidocaine Tocainide Mexiletine Phenytoin	Limited depression of Na^+ current; rapid kinetics	No effect or shortened
Ic	Flecainide Propafenone	Marked depression of Na^+ current; slow kinetics	Minimal effect
Class II	*β-Adrenoceptor blocking drugs* Propranolol Esmolol Acebutolol		
Class III	*Drugs that prolong repolarization* Amiodarone Bretylium tosylate Sotalol Ibutilide		
Class IV	*Ca^{2+} entry-blocking drugs* Verapamil Diltiazem		
	Unclassified in this system Digoxin Adenosine		

Class III drugs

Drugs in this class prolong the repolarization phase of the action potential. The mechanism of action varies, but examples of these agents include sotalol, amiodarone, dofetilide, ibutilide, and bretylium. Whereas ibutilide and dofetilide possess primarily class III effects, amiodarone and, to a degree, sotalol have a wide range of activities; e.g., amiodarone has β-blocking (class II), calcium antagonists (class IV), have class I and class III activities.

Class IV drugs

This class incorporates the calcium channel blocking agents. It includes all calcium channel blocking drugs active on the conducting tissues of the heart (i.e., largely excluding the dihydropyridine agents nifedipine, nicardipine, isradipine, etc.) (see Chap. 23). These agents have vasodilator effects that may contribute to their antiarrhythmic profile by reducing ischemia.

Problems with the Vaughn-Williams classification

Each drug has multiple actions at different concentrations and potentially different effects depending on heart rate, sympathetic activation, and the loading state of the heart. Drugs within one Vaughn-Williams class can share the class effect but achieve this by a variety of mechanisms. Frequently, class III activity on ventricular repolarization is associated with a class I effect. Many such agents have been developed yet failed to progress into clinical use.

Beneficial clinical effects of an antiarrhythmic drug are not always ascribed to their classification. Effectiveness may be related to improved myocardial perfusion in one patient, improved cardiac output in another, or a primary electrophysiologic effect in a third. In most instances, the link between the mechanisms of arrhythmogenesis and clinical effectiveness is unclear.

Functional classification: the Sicilian gambit

In this system, the activity of each drug is classified by its site of action on an individual patient's arrhythmia. All drugs have combined effects and broadly depend on four basic steps of classification: (1) the mechanism for an arrhythmia is defined (Tab. 24.2); (2) the electrophysiologic property is identified whose modification is likely to suppress the arrhythmia; (3) the responsible ion current or receptor mediating that modification is identified, and (4) a drug enacting the desired change is selected and dose titrated (Fig. 24.1).

This may seem complex initially, but the mecha-

DRUG	CHANNELS Na Fast	CHANNELS Na Med	CHANNELS Na Slow	Ca	K	μ	α	β	M₂	P	PUMPS Na-K ATPase	CLINICAL EFFECT Left ventricular function	Sinus rate	Extra cardiac	PR Interval	QRS width	JT interval
Lidocaine	○											→	→	◍			↓
Mexiletine	○											→	→	◍			↓
Tocainide	○											→	→	●			↓
Moricizine	●											↓	→	○		↑	
Procainamide		●			◍							↓	→	●	↑	↑	↑
Disopyramide		●			◍			○				↓	→	◍	↑↓	↑	↑
Quinidine		●			◍		○	○				→	↑	◍	↑↓	↑	↑
Propafenone		●						◍				↓	↓	○	↑	↑	
Flecainide			●	○								↓	→	○	↑	↑	
Encainide			●									↓	→	○	↑	↑	
Bepridil	○			●	◍							?	↓	○			↑
Verapamil	○			●		◍						↓	↓	○	↑		
Diltiazem				◍								↓	↓	○	↑		
Bretylium					●	▨		▨				→	↓	○			↑
Sotalol					●			●				↓	↓	○	↑		↑
Amiodarone	○			○	●	◍		◍				→	↓	○	↑		↑
Alinidine					◍	●						?	↓	●			
Nadolol								●				↓	↓	○	↑		
Propranolol	○							●				↓	↓	○	↑		
Atropine									●			→	↑	◍	↓		
Adenosine										□		?	↓	○	↑		
Digoxin									□		●	↑	↓	●	↑		↓

Figure 24.1 A summary of individual antiarrhythmic drug effects. All drugs should, of course, be understood to have proarrhythmogenic effects under certain conditions, e.g., dilated or failing heart, ischemia, or electrolyte/acid-base imbalance. Drug combinations are subject to pharmacokinetic and pharmacodynamic interactions in many instances. Some of these interactions are clinically useful others range from counterproductive to toxic. Relative potency of block: ○ = Low; ◍ = Moderate; ● = High; □ = Agonist; ▨ = Agonist/Antagonist; A = Activated state blocker; I = Inactivated state blocker.

nisms used are limited and the actions of drugs are well characterised. This system defines the likely clinical response more accurately and includes all available drugs.

Table 24.2 Simple classification of arrhythmogenic mechanisms

Abnormal impulse initiation
Due to automaticity of cardiomyocytes
   From within normal automatic conducting tissue
   From an abnormal decrease in the normal cycle
      of high membrane potential
Due to triggered activity
   Not automatic requiring a depolarization source
      during repolarization phase
Abnormal impulse conduction
Due to reentry circuits
   Set up by an area of slowed conduction and
   unidirectional conduction block causing recirculation
   or circus impulses. These can be sited in SA node,
   atria, AV node, or within the ventricular conducting
   system/ventricular muscle

PRACTICAL ASPECTS OF ANTIARRHYTHMIC DRUG USE

General clinical practice points

The history should define the functional status of the patient, as well as the frequency and sequelae of arrhythmia. Consider the use of stimulants (e.g., ephedrine, amphetamine derivatives, cannabinoids, or thyroid hormone), "recreational" drug use (use urine screening), and excessive intake of alcohol- or caffeine-containing preparations. Some general conditions predispose to arrhythmia (e.g., electrolyte imbalance, adrenergic or thyroid hormone excess). A family history of cardiac illness or sudden death is important.

Minor abnormalities of cardiac rhythm are common in sedentary normal people, athletes, and patients across the range of cardiac diseases. They are not always of significance. Before specific antiarrhythmic treatments are considered, it may be useful to define the presence or absence of cardiac disease by:

Table 24.3 The patient and ECG assessment

Patient assessment
Rhythm assessment
Static 12-lead ECG; rhythm strip; ambulatory study;
  exercise ECG
Patient symptoms
Duration, frequency, aggravating features, relieving
  features
Temporal relationship to rhythm
  Cardiac assessment as necessary
Concomitant disease, ischemic, valve, ventricular
  function
  General cardiac risk factors to be corrected
  Efficacy of treatment to be assessed
Symptoms, rhythm, exercise capacity, outcome
  morbidity/mortality

ECG assessment
All patients should have a 12-lead ECG and rhythm
  strip at rest
Ambulatory ECG recorder can be useful with frequent
  symptoms
Use patient-activated recorders for intermittent
  symptoms

- *echocardiography*: if heart is enlarged or a murmur detected;
- *stress testing* (radionuclide, electrocardiographic, or echocardiographic): if chest pain is evident;
- *exercise study*: to assess functional capacity and observe the relationship of rhythm to exercise (arrythmias disappearing on exercise are rarely significant, whereas those provoked by exercise are usually important).

Arrhythmia can be a cause of symptoms or a secondary response to another illness. Antiarrhythmic drug therapy is considered (1) in those patients who are symptomatic, (2) in those with established heart disease, or (3) in those with a major clinical event (e.g., resuscitated sudden death).

Antiarrhythmic treatment should incorporate an integrated approach to reduce cardiovascular risk factors (e.g., weight reduction, exercise therapy, lipid management, blood pressure control, smoking cessation): (1) control heart failure, (2) correct oxygenation (e.g., lung disease), (3) reduced ischemia (e.g., revascularization), (4) correct valve dysfunction, and (5) correct electrolyte disorders.

Treatment goals should be outlined clearly and include one or several of the following: (1) symptom control, (2) improved exercise capacity, (3) preventing secondary sequelae (e.g., thromboembolism), and rarely, (4) primary prevention of arrhythmia (e.g., asymptomatic congenital prolongation of the QT interval).

Therapeutic drug monitoring

Beneficial and adverse effects of antiarrhythmic drugs both relate to concentration (occasionally to the proportion bound to protein). Almost all these drugs have a narrow therapeutic index (adenosine probably being the

notable exception). Monitoring concentration can be useful for most drugs in attempting to minimize toxicity and proarrhythmic effects. In the case of amiodarone, the key compartment that reflects its efficacy is not clear. The concentration of desethylamiodarone in white blood cells may be useful.

Whereas therapeutic drug monitoring is used frequently in North America to monitor the effectiveness of therapy, using steady-state target ranges for drug concentration, it is not used routinely elsewhere (with the exception of digoxin). There is no need to measure drug concentration routinely unless there is a suspicion of toxicity or failure of compliance despite serious underlying arrhythmia. Parameters of effectiveness are given in Table 24.3.

CLINICAL ASPECTS OF ANTIARRHYTHMIC DRUG USE

Bradyarrhythmia

Significant bradyarrhythmia generally presents with presyncopal/syncopal attacks or exercise intolerance. It is generally degenerative in origin or secondary to ischemic damage. Patients may present with fast palpitations in relation to a tachyarrhythmia following bradyarrhythmia.

Part of the general assessment of bradyarrhythmia is to identify it as a primary or secondary cardiac phenomenon. It is also important to identify tachyarrhythmia occurring after bradyarrhythmia, e.g., paroxysmal atrial fibrillation (a tachyarrhythmia) secondary to sinus node dysfunction.

While drug therapy is used in the emergency management of bradyarrhythmia (see below), it is not applied widely in chronic or paroxysmal bradyarrhythmia. Aminophylline has been examined in sinus node disease, but it is not an adequate substitute for appropriate pacemaker therapy.

Drug treatment of specific bradyarrhythmias

Sinus bradycardia and junctional rhythm

Rate is greater than 60 beats per minute, with a P wave present (i.e., sinus bradycardia). The P wave is inverted or buried within or after the QRS complex in the case of junctional rhythm. Both are common with the onset of inferior infarction or in response to β-blockade. This

---

Table 24.4 Bradyarrhythmia management

Bradyarrhythmia may present as a secondary
  tachyarrhythmia
Only symptomatic bradyarrythmia requires treatment
  unless in the context of myocardial infarction or
  breakthrough tachyarrhythmia
Drug therapy has little role in long-term management
Acute therapy with bolus atropine (max. 3 mg)
  or isoprenaline by infusion can buy time to arrange
  pacemaker therapy

Table 24.5 Digoxin toxicity

Serious overdose is rare but accompanied by hyperkalemia and renal dysfunction, visual and gastrointestinal upset, and arrhythmia

Nondrug treatment:
- hospital admission
- gastric lavage and activated charcoal instillation
- correct electrolytes including magnesium

If symptomatic, then antibody therapy is indicated

Antibody therapy (Digibind = digoxin-specific antibody fragments) may rapidly control rhythm and electrolytes and promote elimination

Atrial arrhythmia needs only atrial pacing unless AV block, when ventricular wire is mandatory (care over induction of incessant ventricular tachycardia during manipulation)

Avoid direct current (dc) countershock unless ventricular fibrillation occurs

should be treated only if it is symptomatic, e.g., hypotension, or if it is associated with ventricular arrhythmia.

First choice: Atropine 0.5 to 1mg iv bolus, which may be repeated if required. Maximum dose in 24 hours is 3 mg. Large doses (>1.8 mg) may give rise to toxicity/mental confusion and urinary retention, particularly in the elderly. Avoid in patients with glaucoma or a history of prostatism.

Atrioventricular block

First-degree atrioventricular (AV) block This is characterised by one P wave per QRS complex but with a PR interval of greater than 200 ms. It is not uncommon after inferior myocardial infarction (MI) and in patients treated with β-blockers. Those on β-blockers alone may have a marginal and acceptable first-degree AV block.

First choice: This requires no drug treatment, but the patient should be observed carefully for signs of progression to more severe forms of AV block. The combination of β-blockers and diltiazem/amlodipine or other nodally active calcium channel blockers may have additive nodal suppressive effects.

Second- and third-degree (complete) AV block Second-degree AV block may be type I (Wenckebach) with progressive lengthening of the PR interval to intermittent block of AV conduction or type 2 with intermittent and unpredictable AV block. Type I is usually asymptomatic and benign, whereas type 2 may be symptomatic and progress to third-degree, or complete, AV block. Therapy is necessary if there are associated symptoms (e.g., hypotension, syncope, cardiac failure, or escape ventricular rhythms).

First choice: Atropine 0.5 to 1 mg should be given intravenously and repeated, if necessary, up to a maximum of 3 mg. Atropine at a total dose of 3 mg intravenously is sufficient to block all vagal tone. There is no benefit to be gained from further drug treatment. If the block is persistent, arrange for hospital admission so that the patient can be paced.

AV block in the context of inferior MI usually resolves within 10 days, and permanent pacing is not normally

necessary. In the context of anterior infarction, the damage is usually more severe, and permanent pacing generally is required. A summary of treatment policies is given in Table 24.4.

Digitalis toxicity

Digoxin toxicity can be associated with many arrhythmias. Death usually results from asystole, ventricular fibrillation, or pump failure. Fatal overdose is associated with advanced age, structural heart disease, male sex, high-grade AV block, and hyperkalemia. Bradyarrhythmia and high-grade AV block are common. Digoxin toxicity can be associated with ventricular bigeminy, multifocal atrial tachycardia (often in conjunction with AV block), or accelerated idioventricular rhythm. Visual symptoms, abdominal pain, nausea, and vomiting accompany all significant overdoses.

Nonpharmacologic treatment Treatment should involve hospital admission, consideration of gastric lavage, and oral treatment with activated charcoal. Digoxin must be discontinued, and the plasma digoxin level and renal function should be checked. In addition, fluid or electrolyte imbalance should be corrected (Tab. 24.5).

First choice: With risk factors for serious toxicity (above), digoxin antibody fragments (Digibind) should be given in line with digoxin concentration and body weight as an urgent therapy [Digibind dose in number of vials (38 mg-fragments) = serum digoxin concentration (ng/ml) × weight (kg)/100]. This is well tolerated and quickly reverses arrhythmias, electrolyte imbalance, and myocardial depression with rapid elimination of the drug.

Second choice: Temporary pacemaker support (caution advised).

Tachyarrhythmias

The impact of a tachyarrhythmia can range from asymptomatic to syncope. The rhythm may be a symptom of primary cardiac disease or secondary to systemic illness. Identification and specific treatment of structural heart disease is an essential part of effective therapy.

Drug treatment of supraventricular and nodal tachycardia

A summary of supraventricular tachycardia management is reported in Table 24.6 Major drugs are discussed in Chapter 22.

Sinus and atrial tachycardia

Generally, these rhythms are well tolerated provided the heart is otherwise normal. When the heart is abnormal (e.g., cardiomyopathy, diffuse or focal coronary ischemia, valvular disease, or hypertrophy) or the propagation rate is very high, then acute cardiac failure or cardiogenic

---

Table 24.6 Supraventricular tachycardia management

Acute therapy (intravenous)
Vagal maneuvers: diagnostic and potentially therapeutic
Adenosine: intravenous escalating dose (3, 6, 9, and 12 mg),
response (2 min)
If unsuccessful, consider bolus intravenous dosing with
verapamil, or flecainide, or disopyramide

Do not use intravenous digoxin
If unsuccessful, consider rate control with intravenous
β-blockade, e.g., atenolol 5 mg over 10 min or esmolol
infusion
If blood pressure is unstable or patient failed treatment,
arrange dc countershock

Chronic therapy (oral)
Sequential trials of monotherapy, monitored by symptoms,
exercise capacity, repetitive ECG recording: β-blockade
(sotalol preferred), or verapamil (never with β-blockade)
Or if structurally normal heart: class I agent:
oral propafenone, or oral flecainide, or oral disopyramide
Or if structurally abnormal heart: amiodarone [caution in
chronic therapy; advise against sun exposure; monitor
baseline and regular TFT (TSH, thyroid peroxidase
antibody if abnormal) and fT3, along with clinical
thyroid status] and diffusion factor (for onset of
asymptomatic pulmonary fibrosis)

Avoid combination treatments unless carefully controlled
Consider definitive electrophysiologic diagnosis and
radiofrequency pathway ablation at an early stage
in resistant cases

---

shock can result. The most common symptomatic presentation is palpitation.

Three basic types exist. The first type is atrial tachycardia due to enhanced automaticity in an atrial focus that can include the sinoatrial node. Here, P waves are visible before the QRS complex but with abnormal P-wave morphology. This is often associated with AV block (consider digoxin toxicity if this is a known treatment). The second type is AV nodal reentry tachycardia. Usually this presents in young adults and is more common in women. No P waves are visible. The third type is AV reentry tachycardia (the tachycardia associated with the Wolff-Parkinson-White syndrome). This also presents in young adults. Inverted P waves may be seen after the QRS complex or in the ST segment, and a pseudo-right bundle-branch block (RBBB) pattern is seen in V_1.

Nonpharmacologic treatment Reversible causes should be treated, e.g., pain, fever, pericarditis, ischemia, and cardiac failure. Carotid sinus massage can be performed. This can be combined with techniques to increase vagal tone such as elevation of the legs with the head-down tilt or immersion of the face in ice-cold water. These manuevers may terminate a reentrant tachycardia and clarify atrial tachycardia (e.g., expose flutter waves). Hemodynamically unstable patients should receive prompt direct current (dc) cardioversion.

Drug therapy
First choice: the first drug treatment is intravenous adenosine in ascending doses of 3, 6, 9, and 12 mg at 2-minute intervals *or* verapamil (5-mg bolus repeated in 10 minutes if required). Digoxin must not be used because it may precipitate uncontrolled atrial fibrillation.

Second choice: in patients in whom the heart is structurally normal or hemodynamic compromise may result from prolonged arrhythmia, a variety of class I agents may be considered as acute iv therapy: (1) flecainide 1.5 mg/kg given in 100 ml of 5% dextrose over 15 minutes, followed by 1.5 mg/kg in 100 ml of 5% dextrose given over the following 1 hour, *or* (2) procainamide at an initial dose of 1 g in 5% dextrose (100 ml) given over 30 minutes, followed by 120 mg in 5% dextrose (100 ml) given over the following 1 hour, *or* (3) disopyramide 2 mg/kg to a maximum of 150 mg over 5 minutes by slow intravenous injection.

If these are unsuccessful, then slowing of AV conduction can be achieved with an iv β-blocker, e.g. 5 mg atenolol, given as a slow intravenous injection over a minimum of 10 minutes, provided that ventricular tachycardia can be ruled out. Alternatively, esmolol, a very short acting ($t_{1/2} = 10$ min) β-blocker can be given by iv infusion (10-150 μg/kg/min) following a loading dose (500 μg/kg) if there is concern over side effects.

Chronic oral treatment Treatment should focus on symptom control, which may be different from the frequency of arrhythmia on ECG monitoring. Symptoms may depend on arrhythmia rate and/or duration and patient sensitivity. Asymptomatic patients or those with infrequent paroxysms responsive to vagal maneuvers may require no drug therapy. Active patients with a normal heart or older patients intolerant of drug therapy with poor symptom control should be considered for a clinical electrophysiologic study to identify and ablate the responsible pathway.

Chronic drug treatment of supraventricular tachycardia is a balance of symptom relief and side effects. Patients should have sequential trials of monotherapy. Holter studies may be used to assess rhythm control in conjunction with symptoms.

Preexcitation syndromes

The Wolff-Parkinson-White syndrome presents with a short PR interval plus QRS complex widening. It represents reentrant tachycardia mediated by an accessory pathway. Most common in young men, it may present as paroxysmal atrial fibrillation but is often an asymptomatic finding. It may require no treatment if asymptomatic and associated with a structurally normal heart and normal exercise stress studies.

When patients present in tachycardia, acute treatment is as above. β-blockade should be avoided, and digoxin therapy is contraindicated. If atrial fibrillation is present and the heart rate is above 200 beats per minute, drug therapy with procainamide, disopyramide, or quinidine is effective but prompt dc cardioversion is preferred.

Table 24.7 Atrial flutter/fibrillation management

Vagal maneuvers and adenosine are diagnostic and potentially therapeutic in some patients

Seek a primary cause and treat this separately (e.g., sepsis, alcohol, ischemia, valve dysfunction, thyroid disease)

Paroxysmal arrhythmia may be a response to sinus node dysfunction best treated by elective atrial pacing

Consider elective cardioversion to restore sinus rhythm

Acute therapy

Consider early dc countershock; immediate in compromised patients, in hospital with recent-onset arrhythmia or deferred elective after establishing anticoagulation (3 weeks) where heart is abnormal or duration is indeterminate

Rate control and chemical cardioversion: where heart is normal, consider intravenous bolus dosing with flecainide, or procainamide, or disopyramide

Do not use intravenous digoxin [may be proarrhythmogenic in prexcitation (Wolff-Parkinson-White) and efficacy is not marked]

Where heart is abnormal (e.g., cardiomegaly, acute pulmonary edema), consider dc countershock if recent onset, or bolus dosing with intravenous amiodarone by a central vein

Chronic therapy

Principle: rate control and low-intensity whole-body anticoagulation

Attempt to minimize therapies by combinations:
- use β-blockade where concurrent ischemia or hypertension (sotalol is preferred with class III effect)
- use calcium channel blocking drugs with peripheral vascular disease
- consider class I drugs: flecainide, procainamide, etc. if normal heart (rare)
- use amiodarone with low dose and appropriate monitoring when other agents fail

Intractable symptoms or recurrent uncontrollable paroxysmal disease can be considered for definitive electrophysiologic investigation and ablation therapy (refer to regional cardiac electrophysiology service)

Amiodarone and sotalol are the agents of choice if chronic therapy is required. Intolerance of the tachycardia or drug side effects should lead to early consideration of electrophysiologic study and catheter-based pathway ablation.

Atrial flutter

Table 24.7 reports a summary of atrial flutter management principles. Characteristic flutter waves in precordial leads V_1 and V_2 or limb lead II may be better seen after carotid sinus massage or diagnostic use of adenosine (see above). Acute-onset atrial rate is typically around 300 beats per minute with 2:1 AV block. A regular, narrow complex (unless a BBB pattern is present) tachycardia of 150 beats per minute should be suspected to be atrial flutter with a 2:1 block irrespective of flutter waves being evident on the ECG.

Nonpharmacologic treatment

Low-energy dc shock (25-100 W) can achieve conversion to sinus rhythm. Anticoagulation to cover cardioversion is probably unnecessary for atrial flutter or short-lived atrial fibrillation (<2 days). Electrical cardioversion is safe in the presence of digoxin within the therapeutic range (1–2 ng/ml) and with a normal serum potassium level. Digoxin excess can lead to the induction of intractable arrhythmia.

Treatment may be as for supraventricular tachycardia (see above). Recurrent atrial flutter should be treated as for atrial fibrillation, i.e., oral amiodarone in low dose after appropriate loading (600 mg daily in divided doses for 1 week, followed by 400 mg daily in divided doses for 1 week, followed by 100-200 mg daily thereafter; check thyroid function and pulmonary diffusion coefficient, and warn regarding sun exposure).

Atrial fibrillation

Table 24.7 reports a summary of atrial fibrillation (AF) management principles. Atrial fibrillation is characterised by no recognisable P waves, fibrillatory waves, and QRS complexes that are irregularly irregular. AF can be transient in acute MI and may need observation only. Other reversible causes include hypertension, valvular heart disease, chronic heart failure, thyrotoxicosis, pneumonia, and major surgery, sepsis, or injury. A cause of AF should always be sought because "lone" AF is rare. AF considerably reduces cardiac output, limits exercise capacity, and is never benign. AF is associated with increasing age but its prevalence is rising above the changes in age distribution of the population. Paroxysmal AF may occur in response to sinus node disease and may be best treated by appropriate pacemaker therapy. The natural history of untreated paroxysmal AF is degeneration to chronic AF.

Observation alone is rarely appropriate with sustained AF, but if the ventricular rate is well controlled and/or a secondary cause is identified (e.g., sepsis), no treatment may be required. A primary cause (e.g., sepsis, thyroid disease, ischemia, valve dysfunction, or hypertension) should be treated if evident.

Restoration of sinus rhythm should be attempted in all patients in whom the left atrium is normal and should be considered in most others. Anticoagulation for 3 weeks followed by electrical cardioversion should be arranged. Anticoagulation should not be discontinued immediately because both the recurrence rate (3 months) and the embolic risk (7 days) extend after restoration of sinus rhythm.

Drug therapy

Digoxin is poorly effective for rate control in ambulant patients but may be useful if there is ventricular dysfunction or significant exercise limitation. When administering digoxin, it is important to check the serum potassium and blood urea and creatinine levels and adjust maintenance (but not loading) dosage. If there is no associated hypotension or acute circulatory failure and no digoxin has been given recently, give 0.5 mg orally and 0.25 mg orally every 6 hours for the first 24 hours, with maintenance treatment thereafter. If for any reason the patient is unable to take the drug by mouth, or if more rapid control is required, digoxin can be given intravenously in a dose of 0.75 to 1.0 mg in a 50-ml infusion of 5% dextrose over 2 or more hours (response will take at least 6 hours). Maintenance doses (0.0625-0.25 mg daily) can be given by infusion over 2 or more hours. If the ventricular response remains rapid, consider adding a β-blocker, verapamil, or amiodarone.

Alternative therapies should be used with great caution, if at all, in heart failure. In the absence of left ventricular dysfunction, class Ic agents are safe and provide more effective rate control with higher reversion to sinus rhythm than digoxin. Flecainide and procainamide have roughly equivalent efficacy and can be administered intravenously (see above). Propafenone is an oral agent with class Ic and β-blocking activity that can sustain sinus rhythm in paroxysmal AF. It may be combined with other agents, but care should be taken with its β-blocking activity in heart failure. Amiodarone has useful class Ic/class II activity iv (300 mg over 2 hours) in attempting "chemical cardioversion." It should not be used as chronic therapy (class III effect) unless other agents are ineffective. While acute toxicity is documented (hepatitis), chronic therapy is associated with a range of hepatic, thyroid, and pulmonary side effects. β-blockade is more effective as a chronic therapy than digoxin and can be useful with additional ischemic heart disease or hypertension. β-blockade can help reduce the symptoms of paroxysmal disease alone or in combination with digoxin. Sotalol (80-160 mg bid) may be the agent of choice combining class II and III effects. Calcium channel blocking drugs can prove useful in AV node control alone or combined with digoxin. They should be avoided altogether if there is significant left ventricular dysfunction and are contraindicated when a β-blocker is already in use.

Ventricular arrhythmias

The management of ventricular arrhythmia by drugs has been reduced in recent years. The presence of ventricular arrhythmia in a patient with heart disease *but preserved ventricular function* does not predict increased cardiac mortality. Ventricular arrhythmia is only rarely seen in a structurally normal heart. Ventricular arrhythmia (as frequent ventricular premature beats or nonsustained ventricular tachycardia) in the presence of impaired ventricular function does predict increased cardiac mortality and sudden death. Unifocal ventricular premature beats disappearing on exercise are benign. Uniform ventricular tachycardia at a rate of less than 150 beats per minute on exercise without evidence of structural heart disease is benign. Neither requires treatment.

All patients with ventricular arrhythmia who are being considered for antiarrhythmic drug therapy must undergo appropriate testing to exclude ongoing ischemia as a cause, ambulatory ECG monitoring to exclude primary bradyarrhythmia, and an assessment of ventricular struc-

ture. Some authorities recommend a signal-averaged ECG to look for late potentials (optional marker if available, interpretation is still a specialist practice). The role of electrophysiologic testing is controversial. Neither susceptibility to reproducible programmed stimulation, the nature of the resulting arrhythmia, nor titrated drug suppression reliably predicts improved outcome.

The treatment of asymptomatic arrhythmia has been reduced substantially. While many drugs achieve suppression of arrhythmia, e.g., the class 1a agents (i.e., quinidine, procainamide, disopyramide, and moricizine), the class 1b agents (i.e., lignocaine, tocainide, phenytoin, and mexilitine), and the class 1c agents (i.e., encainide and flecainide), survival is worse in treated patients with impaired ventricular function. Treatment should be avoided outside specialist practice.

The only agent that may protect from sudden death in impaired ventricular function is amiodarone. This is not a class III effect, since efficacy does not appear to be extended to "pure" class III-acting drugs such as ibutilide and dofetilide and is not shared by sotalol. Amiodarone usage remains proarrhythmogenic (see below) in a minority of patients and is accompanied by significant side effects.

Ectopy and coupled ventricular rhythms/ nonsustained ventricular tachycardia

Multifocal ectopy has a relationship to underlying cardiac disease and mortality but not to sudden cardiac death or serious arrhythmia. Antiarrhythmic treatment is not recommended. The occurrence of coupled ectopy remains an unclear area of management. The frequency of events is important, but the prognostic significance of these events for individual patients is unclear.

Treatment may be considered for patients who have had previous or resuscitated ventricular tachycardia, ventricular fibrillation, or syncope/sudden death (see below). The safest therapy is β-blockade. There is no clear preferred therapy, but large outcome trials are available for metoprolol, timolol, and pindolol.

The position for asymptomatic ventricular tachycardia is similar to that for unifocal or coupled ectopy. This arrhythmia is associated with increased cardiac mortality in impaired ventricular function. Interpretation may be difficult without invasive assessments, but adenosine can be useful in diagnosis. Circulatory impairment, circulatory failure, or secondary ischemia requires prompt dc countershock or overdrive pacing for control.

Intravenous lignocaine (50-200 mg by slow injection) can be useful prior to hospital transfer. Bolus magnesium (1-2 g) by infusion can be used if facilities to support blood pressure are available. If hypokalemia is present, KCl 20 to 30 mmol per hour up to a total of 60 mmol should be given intravenously, and hypomagnesemia should be treated (10 ml 50% magnesium sulfate in 100 ml of 5% dextrose intravenously over 1 h). If ventricular tachycardia is well tolerated and unresponsive to magnesium infusion, lignocaine 50 mg should be given over 2 minutes and repeated to a maximum dose of 200 mg for signs of toxicity (e.g., seizures).

In the context of an acute MI, both primary ventricular tachycardia and ventricular fibrillation (occurring within the first 24 h) do not require a maintenance regimen if cardioversion can be achieved and there is subsequently no ectopy. Care should be exercised if any degree of AV block exists, and prophylactic temporary pacing may be required.

In the absence of cardiac failure, if intravenous lignocaine successfully terminated the arrhythmia, then an infusion may be given as 1 g lignocaine in 500 ml of 5% dextrose (0.2% solution, 2 mg/ml) at 2 mg per minute (60 ml/h) for 2 hours and then 1.5 mg per minute (45 ml/h) for a total of 24 hours

If the preceding regimen fails to suppress the ventricular tachycardia, or if ventricular contractility is impaired, amiodarone should be given as an alternative, not concurrent, therapy. This is administered through a central vein except in an emergency, in which a large-bore cannula in an antecubital fossa vein is acceptable. High-dose intravenous amiodarone is given as follows:

Emergency: 300 mg diluted in 20 ml of 5% dextrose over 5 minutes

Loading dose: 300 mg diluted in 250 ml of 5% dextrose over 1 to 2 hours

Maintenance dose: 15 mg/kg in 500 ml of 5% dextrose over 24 hours (maximal additional dose: 1200 mg)

In infarct-related arrhythmias, long-term oral therapy is not indicated routinely. Monitoring for 24 hours after discontinuation of treatment is required. If significant ventricular arrhythmias occur outside the context of infarction or without an identifiable precipitant, then referral for electrophysiologic investigation should be considered. With significant impairment of left ventricular function, early consideration should be given to the use of an implantable cardioverter defibrillator. Device management is now established as more effective than drug therapy in life threatening arrhythmia. While cost effectiveness has also been defined the total financial impact of implementing such result remains problematic for most healthcare systems around the word. The best interim medical therapy is probably β-blockade and amiodarone (if tolerated).

Ventricular fibrillation and "resuscitated sudden cardiac death"

Resuscitated sudden death involves a variety of arrhythmias but is predominantly associated with ventricular fibrillation. Preceding ventricular tachycardia, sinus arrest, or AV block can be implicated. The majority of patients have underlying coronary artery disease or cardiomyopathy, but approximately 10% have a "primary" arrest with a normal heart. These patients may have a variety of occult cardiac diseases not evident at the time of the event.

Acute ventricular fibrillation arrest requires assisted cardiopulmonary massage until electrical defibrillation can be applied. Protocols are simple and effective, and community education, combined with the increased skills of paramedical personnel and the general public, has increased the numbers of survivors. Underlying disease should be identified and specific treatments given if indicated. As with ventricular tachycardia, device management in the form of an implantable defibrillator may be superior to drugs. Trial data is not yet available in this group.

As with the management of recurrent ventricular tachycardia in the abnormal heart, there is no clear-cut indication for one drug therapy. No agreement exists on the need or benefits of electrophysiologic testing in guiding drug selection.

Drug-induced arrhythmias and proarrhythmic effects of antiarrhythmic drugs

Cardiac arrhythmia can result from the administration of antiarrhythmic or other drugs. In general, bradyarrhythmia results from the predictable responses to agents such as β-blockers, digitalis, and calcium channel blocking drugs. Emergency management is required where there is hemodynamic instability or this is likely and is best achieved by appropriate pacemaker therapy. Offending drug combinations must be suspended. Antiarrhythmic drugs, particularly in combination, should be avoided. The use of temporary (or sometimes permanent) atrial pacing, which can increase the heart rate and shorten the QT interval, should be considered. In an emergency, an isoprenaline infusion may be used to achieve the same aim until pacing is established (2 mg/500 ml of 5% dextrose = 4 μg/ml; run at 2-10 μg/min, 30-150 ml/h) This runs a risk of increasing ischemia and aggravating tachyarrhythmia.

Tachyarrhythmia in response to drug therapy is less predictable and generally more serious. Many agents have intrinsic proarrhythmic effects, particularly in the presence of left ventricular impairment, e.g., class Ia and Ic agents such as flecainide, moricizine, procainamide, tocainide, and mexilitine or class III drugs such as ibutilide, dofetilide, and amiodarone. Identification can be very difficult in patients who generally already have serious arrhythmia prior to treatment. Some drugs may cause specific patterns, e.g., torsades de pointes tachycardia (see below) with amiodarone or sotalol, but this is the exception rather than the rule. Therapeutic drug monitoring may be useful, but proarrhythmia is not reliably predicted by serum concentrations.

Drug-induced torsades de pointes

Torsades de pointes is a polymorphic ventricular tachycardia characterised by twisting of the QRS complex about baseline. It can be mistaken for ventricular fibrillation, but it is usually self-terminating and recurrent. It may be aggravated by antiarrhythmic drugs, and associated, syncope is common. The causes are bradycardia, hypokalemia/hypomagnesemia, antiarrhythmic drugs prolonging the QT interval (e.g., sotalol, amiodarone), tricyclic antidepressants, pimozide, erythromycin, oxybutynin, terfenadine, and congenital long-QT syndrome.

Suggested readings

BAUMANN JL, SCHEON MD, HOON TJ. Practical optimisation of anti-arrhythmic drug therapy using pharmacokinetic principles. Clin Pharmacokinet 1991; 20:151-66.

CARDIAC ARRHYTHMIA SUPPRESSION TRIAL INVESTIGATORS. Preliminary report: effect of encainide and flecainide on mortality in a randomised trial of arrhythmia suppression after myocardial infarction. N Engl J Med 1989;321:406-12.

ECHT DS, LIEBSON PR, MITCHELL LB, et al. Mortality and morbidity in patients receiving encainide, flecainide or placebo: The Cardiac Arrhythmia Suppression Trial. N Engl J Med 1991;324:781-8.

HARRISON DC. The Sicilian gambit: reasons for maintaining the present anti-arrhythmic drug classification. Cardiovascular Res 1992;26:566-7.

KOLATSKY TJ. The Sicilian gambit and anti-arrhythmic drug development. Cardiovascular Res 1992;26:562-5.

LATINI R, MAGGIONI AP, CAVALLI A. Therapeutic monitoring of anti-arrhythmic drug therapy using pharmacokinetic principles. Clin Pharmacokinet 1990;20:151-66.

NATTEL S, TALAJIC M. Recent advances in understanding the pharmacology of amiodarone. Drugs 1988;36:121-31.

PRATT CM, MOYE LA. The cardiac arrhythmia suppression trial: casting suppression in a different light. Circulation 1995; 91:245-7.

ROSEN MR, FOR THE EUROPEAN WORKING GROUP ON ARRHYTHMIAS. The Sicilian gambit: a new approach to the classification of anti-arrhythmic drugs based on their actions on arrhythmogenic mechanisms. Eur Heart J 1991;12:1112-31.

SCHOLZ H. Classification and mechanisms of action of anti-arrhythmic drugs. Fund Clin Pharmacol 1995; 8:385-90.

SCHWARTZ PJ, ZAZA A. The Sicilian gambit revisited: theory and practice. Eur Heart J 1992;13:23-9.

SINGH BN, VAUGHAN-WILLIAMS EM. A fourth class of anti-arrhythmic action? Effect of verapamil on ouabain toxicity, on atrial and ventricular intracellular potentials and on other features of cardiac function. Cardiovasc Res 1994;6:109-19.

VAUGHAN-WILLIAMS EM. The relevance of cellular to clinical electrophysiology in classifying anti-arrhythmic actions. J Cardiovasc Pharmacol 1992;20:S1-7.

ZIPES DP. Treatment of arrhythmias and abnormalities in conduction. In: Willerson JT, ed. Treatment of heart diseases, chap 3. London: Gower Medical, 1992.

Angina and coronary heart disease

James A. de Lemos, Christopher P. Cannon

Over the past few decades, dramatic progress has been made in the management of coronary artery disease. Despite these improvements, however, ischemic heart disease remains the most common cause of death in the industrialized world. As management options have expanded, the complexity of clinical decision-making has increased significantly. New insight into the pathophysiology of the stable and unstable coronary syndromes has highlighted the need to tailor the therapeutic approach based on the underlying pathophysiologic mechanisms.

CORONARY ISCHEMIA

Pathophysiology Coronary atherosclerosis develops silently over decades and is characterized by the formation of lipid-rich plaques that form at vulnerable sites in the coronary circulation. Both traditional (e.g., age, cholesterol, smoking, diabetes, family history, hypertension) and novel (e.g., homocysteine, inflammatory markers) risk factors are critical for the development and progression of atherosclerosis over time. Many atherosclerotic plaques grow slowly and silently and become manifest only when they narrow the lumen of the artery sufficiently to cause limitation of blood flow. In this circumstance, ischemia will occur when myocardial oxygen demand increases, such as during exercise or emotional stress. Other atherosclerotic plaques may change more abruptly, leading to an unstable ischemic pattern, with rest ischemia or infarction. Rupture or erosion of a lipid-rich atherosclerotic plaque exposes the subendothelial plaque components to circulating blood. Platelet adhesion and aggregation at this site lead to the formation of a thrombus, which can cause myocardial ischemia or infarction (Fig. 25.1). The prominent role of platelets, thrombin, and the fibrin clot in the pathophysiology of myocardial ischemia and infarction underlies the principles of antiplatelet, antithrombin, and fibrinolytic therapies.

There is a substantial body of evidence indicating that coronary artery thrombosis plays an important role in the pathogenesis of acute ischemic syndromes. Six sets of observations contribute to this concept: (1) at autopsy, thrombi are usually seen at the site of a ruptured plaque, (2) coronary atherectomy specimens obtained in patients with acute myocardial infarction (MI) or unstable angina demonstrate a high incidence of acute thrombotic lesions, (3) coronary angioscopic observations indicate that thrombus is frequently visualized in patients, (4) coronary arteriography has demonstrated ulceration or irregularities suggesting a ruptured plaque and/or thrombus in 25 to 85% of patients depending on the timing of angiography and the definition of thrombus in each series, (5) markers of platelet activity and fibrin formation are increased, and (6) antithrombotic therapy with aspirin and heparin improves the clinical outcome of patients with acute coronary syndromes. Accordingly, current treatment (and

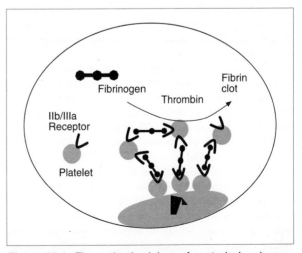

Figure 25.1 The pathophysiology of acute ischemic syndromes. Atherosclerotic plaque rupture leads to platelet adhesion, activation, and subsequent aggregation, which is mediated via the Gp IIb/IIIa receptor. Thrombin is activated on the platelet membrane and catalyzes the conversion of soluble fibrinogen to insoluble fibrin, forming the thrombus characteristic of all the acute coronary syndromes.

ongoing research) is focused on improving antithrombotic therapies for acute ischemic syndromes.

In clinical practice, coronary angiography is employed extensively in patients with acute ischemic syndromes, and thus the morphology of coronary artery lesions can help identify the pathophysiology in certain patients. *Active lesions* tend to be associated with greater than 50% diameter narrowing (or greater than 75% cross-sectional area loss); they are frequently located eccentrically, with an irregular border and intraluminal filling defects that may represent thrombus. Such lesions are more likely to be associated with the pathologic features of plaque rupture, hemorrhage, and superimposed thrombus. These *vulnerable* plaques typically have a thin fibrous cap and a rich lipid core. In addition, activated macrophages frequently are seen at the shoulder of the plaques, which may contribute to plaque rupture. *Nonactive lesions* are more likely to be either symmetric or asymmetric with smooth borders and a broad neck. In addition, intraluminal filling defects are seen rarely. Histologically, these lesions are characterized by less lipid accumulation and inflammatory cell infiltration and an intact fibrous cap. Of the large number of atherosclerotic lesions, most are nonactive; however, multiple factors, including endothelial function, plaque consistency, focal coronary artery tone, and local sheer stress forces, contribute to plaque rupture, formation of platelet-rich thrombi, and resulting unstable angina.

Disease presentation

The spectrum of ischemic heart disease

Ischemic heart disease can be viewed as a spectrum, ranging from stable angina to acute MI and sudden cardiac death (Tab. 25.1). Frequently, the first presentation of ischemic heart disease is stable angina pectoris, which typically is described as a tightness in the chest, a pressure (not a pain) brought on by exertion and relieved by rest. If the pattern of angina is worsening, accelerating, or occurring at rest, it is referred to as *unstable angina.* Some patients with a crescendo pattern of pain will have a prolonged episode and develop some degree of myocardial necrosis, with elevation of cardiac enzymes but no Q-wave development on the electrocardiogram (ECG), referred to as a *non-Q-wave MI.* Other patients will have a prolonged episode of pain (and usually ST-segment elevation on the ECG) and develop a Q-wave MI.

Most clinical presentations of coronary artery disease can be classified into one of these four categories: stable angina, unstable angina, non-Q-wave MI, and Q-wave MI. Recent work, however, has brought to light several other syndromes, falling in between these categories, where clinical presentation and prognosis differ. Indeed, many patients with significant coronary artery disease are completely asymptomatic. In this age of advanced diagnostic testing, coronary stenoses and/or inducible ischemia sometimes can be detected on screening tests. Between patients with stable angina and those with unsta-

Table 25.1 The spectrum of ischemic heart disease

Stable angina
Symptoms of exertional tightness in the chest, a pressure (not a pain) brought on by exertion and relieved by rest. No rest pain

Silent ischemia
Evidence of ischemia in the absence of clinical symptoms such as chest pain. Usually detected by ST-segment depression on a Holter monitor. Present in a subset of patients with stable or unstable angina

Unstable angina
The pattern of angina is worsening, accelerating, and/or occurring at rest. Cardiac enzymes (e.g., CK-MB) are negative. ECG can show ST-segment or T-wave abnormalities

Microinfarction
A syndrome of ischemia intermediate in severity between unstable angina and non-Q-wave MI, with small elevations in CK-MB, troponin T, or other cardiac enzymes, but a normal total CK

Non-Q-wave MI
A similar pattern of accelerating pain at rest, frequently with a prolonged episode. Cardiac enzymes are elevated, CK and CK-MB greater than upper limit of normal. ECG can show ST-segment depression or deep T-wave inversion but does not have Q waves

Q-wave MI
An acute episode of prolonged pain associated with elevated cardiac enzymes and new Q waves (or LBBB) on the ECG. Some MIs can be clinically silent

ST-segment elevation MI
An acute episode of prolonged pain associated with elevated cardiac enzymes, but the initial ECG at presentation demonstrates acute occlusion of a coronary artery. This has also been termed a *reperfusion-eligible MI*

Non-ST-segment elevation MI
An acute episode of prolonged pain associated with elevated cardiac enzymes, but without ST-segment elevation, indicating a probable patent infarct-related artery but severe coronary stenosis. Such MIs usually develop into a non-Q-wave MI

Sudden death
Acute cardiac death, usually out of hospital. Presumed to be due to acute MI and/or ventricular arrhythmia

(MI = myocardial infarction; EGG = electrocardiogram; LBBB = left bundle-branch block.)

ble angina are a high-risk group with clinically stable symptoms yet significant ambulatory ischemia that can be detected by ambulatory Holter monitoring. Similarly, between patients with unstable angina and those with non-Q-wave MI, a patient may have what has been called a *microinfarction;* these patients have either a very small but nondiagnostic elevation of cardiac creatine kinase (CK) or no elevation in CK but elevation of other cardiac proteins such as the cardiac-specific troponins.

In the pre-thrombolytic era, the distinction of Q-wave and non-Q-wave MI was a very useful one, in that patients with non-Q-wave MI usually presented with ST-segment depression or T-wave changes on the ECG, indicative of partial but not complete coronary occlusion, whereas those with Q-wave MI usually presented with ST-segment elevation on the ECG, indicative of an acute coronary occlusion. However, with current aggressive reperfusion therapies, decisions regarding early treatment must be made immediately and cannot wait until the following day to see if Q waves have developed. Thus, a more useful distinction is the dichotomization between ST-segment elevation MI and non-ST-segment elevation MI. At the extreme of the ischemic heart disease spectrum are patients with sudden cardiac death. Many patients have an acute coronary occlusion as the etiology of the catastrophic arrest. However, with aggressive emergency medical personnel who respond rapidly and treat with advanced cardiac life support procedures, more patients are presenting following resuscitated *sudden cardiac death.*

One of the major roles of cardiologists, critical care physicians, emergency physicians, internists, and cardiac nurses is to discriminate ischemic heart disease from other noncardiac diseases. Although the initial concern is cardiac ischemia, only one of seven patients actually will have ischemic heart disease. Conversely, presentations with ischemia take on many nuances that do not always fit the classic descriptions: patients can present with syncope (without chest pain) and be found to be suffering an MI. Following cardiac or noncardiac surgery, pain medication can mask many of the symptoms and alter the pattern of cardiac enzymes used to diagnose infarction. In addition, patients may present with two clinical events – for example, a myocardial infarction and a cerebrovascular accident. Thus, the astute clinician must evaluate the individual patient's presentation carefully to try to identify the underlying clinical syndrome(s) in order to initiate appropriate therapy.

Treatment

The balance between oxygen supply and demand

Coronary ischemia is fundamentally an imbalance between myocardial oxygen supply and demand. Myocardial oxygen supply is determined by the status of the coronary circulation and the ability of red blood cells to deliver oxygen to the myocardium. Myocardial blood flow typically increases in response to heightened demand, via endothelium-dependent smooth muscle relaxation and subsequent vessel dilatation. In the presence of even mild degrees of atherosclerotic damage, however, the ability of the endothelium to promote vessel dilatation is impaired, and myocardial blood flow cannot increase in response to increased demand. When the area of the coronary artery is narrowed by greater than 70 to 80%, maximal blood flow is reduced, and under instances of increased demand, ischemia may develop. As the atherosclerotic plaque grows, blood flow is reduced proportionally, and ischemia becomes more severe. It should be noted, however, that dynamic factors and vessel tone are quite important in determining minute-to-minute coronary

blood flow: Active lesions may have increased vascular tone and greater impairment in blood flow than would be expected for the degree of fixed stenosis in the vessel. In unstable syndromes, plaque rupture can lead to instantaneous cessation of blood flow, with sufficient imbalance between supply and demand of oxygen to cause cellular necrosis. Finally, in the presence of anemia, less oxygen is delivered per unit of blood flow. It is not uncommon for patients with only mild coronary artery disease to develop angina in situations where the hematocrit is significantly decreased.

Myocardial oxygen demand is determined by heart rate, wall stress, and the contractile state of the ventricle. Clinically, oxygen demand is assessed indirectly via measurement of the heart rate and blood pressure. Common causes of increased oxygen demand include physical or emotional stress, uncontrolled tachycardia from arrhythmias such as atrial fibrillation or supraventricular tachycardia, poorly controlled hypertension, and noncardiac illnesses such as infection and thyrotoxicosis. In addition, left ventricular hypertrophy, whether due to hypertension, aortic stenosis, or another cause, is associated with increased oxygen demand.

The primary goal of the management of all the coronary syndromes is to maximize oxygen supply and reduce oxygen demand (Tab. 25.2). Both pharmacologic and nonpharmacologic means are used to improve oxygen supply. The most definitive means of improving coronary blood flow is via revascularization. Both coronary artery

Table 25.2 Agents that increase O_2 supply or reduce O_2 demand

Increase O₂ supply	Decrease O₂ demand
Revascularization	Heart rate
PCI	Beta-blockers
CABG	Ca²⁺ channel blockers
Angiogenic factors	Verapamil
TMR	Diltiazem
	Amiodarone
Medical therapy	
Thrombolytic therapy	Cardiac contractility
Antithrombotic therapy	Beta-blockers
Aspirin	Ca²⁺ channel blockers
Gp IIb/IIIa inhibitors	Verapamil
Heparin	Diltiazem
LMWH	
Coronary vasodilators	Wall stress
Nitrates	Nitrates
Ca²⁺ channel blockers	Beta-blockers
	Ca²⁺ channel blockers
Other	ACE inhibitors
IABP	Other anti-HTN agents
	IABP

(PCI = percutaneous coronary intervention; CABG = coronary artery bypass graft surgery; TMR = transmyocardial laser revascularization; LMWH = low-molecular-weight heparin; HTN = hypertension; IABP = intraaortic balloon pump.)
Note: Treatments listed in *italics* remain experimental at this time.

bypass grafting (CABG) and percutaneous coronary interventions (PCIs) have proven to be extremely effective revascularization techniques in suitable patients. Methods of PCI include percutaneous transluminal coronary angioplasty (PTCA), intracoronary stenting, and a variety of new catheter-based techniques, including direct and rotational atherectomy, suction thrombectomy, and laser ablation of plaque material. Pharmacologic methods to restore blood flow include thrombolytic therapy (for acute MI), antiplatelet therapy (for all forms of coronary artery disease), and antithrombin therapy (for unstable angina and acute MI). In addition, vasodilators such as nitroglycerin and calcium channel antagonists improve oxygen supply by relaxing vascular smooth muscle and effecting coronary vasodilation.

Two exciting new methods are under development for the improvement of myocardial oxygen supply. Genetically engineered vascular endothelial growth factors, such as vascular endothelial growth factor F (VEGF) and basic fibroblast growth factor (bFGF), appear to stimulate new vessel growth and may prove to be a medical alternative to revascularization, particularly in patients unsuitable for standard percutaneous or surgical techniques. Transmyocardial laser revascularization (TMR) is a novel surgical therapy for patients who are not candidates for CABG or PCI. A laser is used to create channels through ischemic myocardium in an epicardial-to-endocardial direction. Initial studies show relief of angina and decreased objective evidence of ischemia in some patients. Interestingly, autopsy studies in animal models demonstrate that the newly created channels close almost immediately after they are created; this suggests that TMR improves ischemia not by creating new "channels" for blood flow but rather by stimulating angiogenesis by some unknown mechanism. Catheter-based techniques for laser revascularization are currently under development as well.

Risk-factor modification

Correction of modifiable risk factors is essential for the treatment of patients with established coronary disease, whether they have stable angina or acute MI (secondary prevention). In addition, modification of risk factors can prevent the development of coronary disease in patients without evident disease (primary prevention). The benefits of aggressive risk-factor modification are profound and are in fact more dramatic than those with any of the expensive treatment strategies described below. In secondary prevention trials, lipid-lowering therapy with hydroxymethylglutaryl (HMG) coenzyme A (CoA) reductase inhibitors has been shown to reduce cardiac mortality by as much as 20 to 30%. As a result of these studies, most patients with coronary disease, including those with total cholesterol and low-density lipoprotein (LDL) cholesterol levels in the so-called normal range, should be treated with lipid-lowering therapy. The only exception are patients with a serum LDL cholesterol of less than 125 mg/dl, in whom the benefits have not yet been clearly defined (see Chap. 69).

Aggressive treatment of hypertension is important not only because hypertension contributes to the progression of underlying atherosclerosis but also because lowering blood pressure reduces oxygen demand and may relieve ischemia. Although there are numerous agents to choose from, the initial agent chosen to treat essential hypertension should be one that has added anti-ischemic properties, such as a beta-blocker or calcium channel antagonist. In patients who have had a Q-wave MI or who have reduced left ventricular function, angiotensin-converting enzyme (ACE) inhibitors have a special role, as will be described below.

Growing clinical evidence supports the role for intensive glucose control in diabetic patients to reduce microvascular complications. Although the benefits in terms of macrovascular complications are not as robust, careful control of diabetes should reduce ischemic complications as well. In addition, because renal failure is such an important contributor to coronary events in diabetic patients, prevention of renal disease will undoubtedly reduce ischemic complications.

Smoking is a particularly frustrating risk factor for practicing physicians and ancillary staff. Although smoking's contribution to coronary artery disease is indisputable, efforts to convince patients to stop smoking are often unsuccessful, and recidivism is high in those few patients who are able to stop.

Male sex and the postmenopausal state in females are risk factors for the development of coronary disease. Estrogen deficiency is associated with unfavorable effects on plasma lipids and endothelial function. A wealth of epidemiologic data supports the role for hormone replacement therapy (HRT) for the prevention of coronary artery disease; to date, however, confirmatory evidence from prospective, randomized trials is lacking. In fact, in the recently reported HERS trial, HRT was not associated with benefit through 4 years of follow-up and was associated with excess thrombotic events in the first year of treatment. Decisions about HRT are complex and require individualization and a multidisciplinary approach to be successful.

Many novel risk factors for coronary disease have been identified, such as fibrinogen, homocysteine, and C reactive protein (CRP); with the exception of homocysteine, however, no reliable treatments for these risk factors have been identified. Modest doses of supplementary folate (amounts included in typical multivitamins) reduce total serum homocysteine levels. Studies are needed to determine whether folate supplementation will reduce coronary artery disease morbidity and mortality.

Therapy for chronic stable angina

Stable angina is characterized by anginal chest pain that occurs with exertion only and is not progressive over time. With the exception of several high-risk subsets of patients that will be described below, stable angina is associated with good long-term survival. Therefore, for most patients with stable angina, the focus of therapy is to improve symptoms and prevent MI (Tab. 25.3). The most important initial management step is to identify and modify cardiac risk factors, as outlined earlier. Further therapy focuses on prevention of MI and optimizing the balance between oxygen supply and demand.

Aspirin Aspirin is the cornerstone of therapy for the prevention of MI in patients with stable angina. Although there are no direct data showing reduction in the incidence of acute MI or death in patients with stable angina, aspirin has been shown to reduce mortality in patients with acute MI, prevent reinfarction in patients with unstable angina, and prevent an initial infarction in healthy male physicians without prevalent coronary artery disease. Although the optimal aspirin dose has not been defined, doses between 81 and 325 mg daily (with enteric coating) are safe and effective, with tolerable side effects.

Nitrates Nitrates have been a mainstay of therapy for patients with symptomatic angina and can be given via intravenous, sublingual, oral, and topical routes (Tab. 25.4). The clinical effects of nitrates are mediated through several distinct mechanisms, including the following: (1) dilatation of large coronary arteries and arterioles leads to redistribution of blood flow from epicardial to endocardial regions. Nitroglycerin provides an exogenous source of nitric oxide (NO) to vascular endothelium, facilitating coronary vasodilation even when damaged endothelium is unable to generate endogenous NO due to coronary artery disease. It is important to emphasize that these coronary vasomotor effects may either increase or decrease collateral flow. (2) Peripheral venodilatation leads to an increase in venous capacitance and a substantial decrease in preload, thus reducing myocardial oxygen demand. Nitrates are consequently of particular value in treating patients with left ventricular (LV) dysfunction and congestive heart failure (CHF). (3) Peripheral arterial dilatation, typically of a modest degree, may decrease afterload. In addition, nitrates have been shown to relieve dynamic coronary constriction, including that induced by exercise. Nitrates also may have an inhibitory effect on platelet aggregation, although the clinical significance of this finding is unclear.

For patients with infrequent anginal episodes, periodic use of sublingual nitroglycerin can effectively ameliorate symptoms and abort anginal attacks. For patients who have predictable angina with certain activities, sublingual nitroglycerin taken immediately before the activity is particularly helpful in preventing symptoms. For patients with more frequent angina or evidence of silent ischemia on ambulatory monitoring, chronic nitrates are indicated. When dosing any form of chronic nitrate preparation, consideration must be given to nitrate tolerance, which develops as early as 24 hours after beginning therapy. To prevent tolerance and the reduction in therapeutic efficacy that accompanies it, a nitrate-free period should be given each day. In general, this should occur when the patient is least likely to develop angina, which is typically while the patient is sleeping. Table 25.4 outlines recommended doses and kinetic features of the most common oral and topical nitrate preparations. Common side effects of all nitrate preparations are headache and flushing. In addition, patients who are volume depleted or who depend on higher intravascular volume to maintain CO (as in the case of critical aortic stenosis) may develop hypotension when given short-acting nitrates. It should be noted that sildenafil, a phosphodiesterase inhibitor used to treat impotence, must not be given with any form of nitrate because the combination can precipitate severe hypotension and even death (see Chap. 20).

Table 25.3 Treatments for coronary artery disease

Primary prevention	Secondary prevention	Stable angina	Unstable angina/NQMI	ST-Segment elevation MI
Statins	**Statins**	**Aspirin**	**Aspirin**	**Thrombolytic therapy**
Anti-HTN rx	**Aspirin**	Beta-blockers	**Heparin**	**Aspirin**
Smoking cessation	**Beta-blockers**	Ca²⁺ antagonists	**LMWH**	**Heparin**
Aspirin	**Clopidogrel**	Nitrates	**Gp IIb/IIIa inhibitors**	Gp IIb/IIIa inhibitors
B vitamins	**Warfarin**	PCI[1]	**Beta-blockers**	**Beta-blockers**
HRT	**Gemfibrozil**	CABG[2]	**Ca²⁺ antagonists**	Ca²⁺ antagonists
Anti-oxidants			Nitrates	Nitrates
			PCI[1]	**ACE inhibitors**
			CABG[2]	PCI[1]
				CABG[2]

(Statins = HMG CoA reductase inhibitors; HTN = hypertension; HRT = hormone replacement therapy; PCI = percutaneous coronary intervention; CABG = coronary artery bypass graft surgery; LMWH = low-molecular-weight heparin.)
Note: Treatments in bold print have been shown to prevent myocardial infarction or reduce mortality. Treatments in normal font either relieve symptoms or decrease ischemia. Treatments in italics are as yet unproven therapies.
[1]PCI has not been shown to reduce mortality, except as primary therapy for ST-segment elevation MI.
[2]CABG reduces mortality only in select patient subsets (see text).

Beta-blockers Adrenergic receptors are present in most organs and have myriad functions. In the cardiovascular system β_1-adrenergic receptors are found in ventricular myocardium and cardiac conduction tissue, whereas β_2 receptors are prominent in the smooth muscle of the peripheral vasculature and the bronchial airways. Both efficacy and side effects of beta blockade can be explained by inhibition of the effects of catecholamines on these target sites. The beneficial effects of β-blockers in patients with angina include β_1-receptor-mediated reduction of heart rate and contractile force, with consequent reduction in myocardial oxygen demand. Beta-blockers have little or no effect on myocardial blood flow; in fact, under certain circumstances, such as cocaine ingestion, β-blockers can increase coronary vasomotor tone and reduce myocardial blood flow. In this setting it is believed that beta blockade allows unopposed β-receptor-mediated coronary vasoconstriction.

Some important adverse effects, on the other hand, are due to blockade of β_2-receptors: β_2-blockade can precipitate claudication in patients with peripheral vascular disease and bronchospasm in patients with asthma or chronic obstructive pulmonary disease. β_1-selective agents in general are preferable in patients with coronary artery disease, since they have fewer extracardiac side effects. Other reported side effects of β-blockers include fatigue, depression, impotence, and reduced peak exercise performance. Beta-blockers have a modest adverse effect on serum lipids, which is probably not significant in light of their other beneficial effects. In patients with diabetes, addition of a β-blocker may make glucose control slightly more difficult, but more important, these agents may supress the autonomic symptoms of hypoglycemia. For this reason, they should be used with extreme caution in patients with diabetes and frequent hypoglycemic episodes. Beta-blockers with intrinsic sympathomimetic activity (ISA) generally should be avoided in patients with coronary artery disease, unless severe bradycardia limits appro-

Table 25.4 Selected characteristics of common nitrate preparations

Preparation	Dose	To onset of action	To peak effect	Plasma half-life	Duration of action	Comments
Nitroglycerin						
Sublingual tablet	0.15-0.9 mg q5min x 3	<1 min	3-4 min	3-4 min	30 min	For acute therapy
Buccal spray	0.4 mg dose; 1-2 puffs q5min x 3	<1 min	3-4 min	3-5 min	30 min	For acute therapy; simple to use
Buccal tablet	1-5 mg tid-qid	<1 min	3-4 min	3-5 min	3-5 h	Do not chew or swallow
Sustained-release tablet	2.5-6.5 mg bid-qid	>1 h	60-120 min	4-5 min	8-10 h	
Intravenous infusion	Start at 10-20 mg/min (as needed to max of 300 mg/min)	<1 min	2 min	7 min	Tolerance develops within 24 h	Titrate to chest pain or blood pressure goal; tolerance develops rapidly
Ointment	0.5-2 in tid-qid	15 min	1 h	3 min	6-7 h	Tolerance develops rapidly
Transdermal patch	0.4-1.2 mg/h; on for 12 h, then off 12 h	30-40 min	2 h	3 min	>24 h	Useful for patients with nocturnal angina
Isosorbide dinitrate						
Sublingual tablet	2.5-10 mg q2-3h	2-4 min	5-10 min	60 min	120 min	For acute use; slower than NTG
Buccal spray	1-3 sprays q2-3h	2-3 min	5 min	15 min	30-60 min	For acute therapy
Oral capsule	10-60 mg bid-tid	20-30 min	30-60 min	30-50 min	Up to 8 h	To prevent tolerance, stagger doses to allow 10-14 h nitrate-free period
Sustained release tablet	40-80 mg qd	30 min	1-3 h	4-5 min	8 h	
Isosorbide-5-mononitrate						
Oral tablet	20-30 mg bid	20 min	30-40 min	3-5 h	10 h	Give doses 7-8 h apart to prevent tolerance
Sustained-release tablet	30-240 mg qd	30 min	3-4 h	3-5 h	15-18 h	

priate dosing of conventional agents. In this circumstance, beta-blockers with ISA can be particularly useful.

Beta-blockers should be a primary component of the pharmacologic regimen for most patients following acute MI or unstable angina, as will be discussed below. In stable angina, they are also extremely effective, although there are no long-term trials showing a mortality benefit in these patients. In general, beta-blockers appear to provide symptom relief comparable with that of nitrates and calcium channel antagonists; certain subsets of patients, however, may derive particular benefit from beta-blockers. These include patients with concomitant atrial or ventricular arrhythmias and patients with compensated LV dysfunction. Chemico-physical properties and detailed kinetic/metabolic characteristics of major β-blockers are given in Tables 22.7 and 22.8. Dose recommendations for a variety of different β-blocker preparations are provided in Table 25.5.

Calcium channel blockers Despite recent concerns in the lay press, calcium channel antagonists remain an impor-

Table 25.5 Clinical characteristics of selected beta-blockers

Preparation	Dose	To onset of action	To peak effect	Plasma half-life	ISA	Metabolism/ of action	Comments
β₁-Selective agents							
Acebutolol	200-600 mg qd-bid	1 h	1-4 h	3-10 h	Yes	Hepatic/ renal	Potent ISA
Atenolol	50-100 mg qd	1 h	2-4 h	6-9 h	No	Renal	Avoid in renal failure
Betaxolol	5-40 mg qd	2 h	2-8 h	12-22 h	No	Hepatic/ renal	Limited experience in CAD
Bisoprolol	2.5-20 mg qd	1-2 h	2-3 h	7-15 h	No	Hepatic/ renal	Limited experience in CAD
Celiprolol	200-400 mg qd	30-60 min	2-3 h	5-6 h	Yes	Renal	Also has vasodilating properties
Esmolol (IV)	5-300 mg/kg/min	2 min	2-5 min	5-9 min	No	Hepatic	Extremely short half-life; very expensive
Metoprololol	po: 25-100 mg bid-qid iv: 2.5-10 mg q4-6h	po: 1 h iv: <5 min	1-2 h	3-6 h	No	Hepatic	Use IV form initially in AMI or unstable angina
Xamoterol	100-200 mg qd-bid	1 h	1-2 h	15-20 h	Yes	Renal	
Nonselective agents							
Alprenolol	100-200 mg tid-qid	30-60 min	1-2 h	3-4 h	Yes	Hepatic/ renal	
Carteolol	10-40 mg qd	30-60 min	1-2 h	6-7 h	Yes	Renal	
Carvedilol	6.25-50 mg bid	30-60 min	60-90 min	6 h	No	Hepatic	Combined beta-blocker and vasodilator used in CHF
Labetalol	po: 100-300 mg bid iv bolus: 20-80 mg iv infusion: 2 mg/min	po: 2 h iv: 5 min	po: 3 h iv: 10 min	6-8 h (po)	No	Hepatic	Combined α₁/β₂-blocker; used for severe HTN or hypertensive emergencies
Nadolol	40-240 mg qd	1 h	2-4 h	20-24 h	No	Renal	
Oxprenolol	80-160 mg bid	1-2 h	2-3 h	2 h	Yes	Hepatic	Sustained release preparation available
Penbutolol	10-20 mg qd	30-60 min	1-3 h	20-25 h	Yes	Hepatic/ renal	
Pindolol	5-20 mg tid	1 h	1-3 h	2-6 h	Yes	Hepatic/ renal	Most potent ISA effect; has some vasodilating properties
Propranolol	20-80 mg qid	1-2 h	2-3 h	3-6 h	No	Hepatic	Sustained-release form available
Sotalol	80-240 mg bid	1 h	2-3 h	7-18 h	No	Renal	Antiarrhythmic drug only
Timolol	10-30 mg bid	30 min	2-3 h	3-5 h	No	Hepatic/ renal	Mainly used for glaucoma

tant class of agents for the treatment of stable angina. They provide symptom relief that is at least comparable with that of beta-blockers and in general have a very favorable side-effect profile. These agents fall into three main groups: dihydropyridines, of which nifedipine is the prototype; benzothiazepines, of which diltiazem is the only member; and phenylalkylamines, of which verapamil is the only member (Tab. 25.6). All these agents block the entry of calcium into cells via voltage-sensitive (L-type) calcium channels. In vascular smooth muscle cells, this causes coronary and peripheral vasodilation. In cardiac tissue, this leads to depression of myocardial contractility, cardiac pacemaker function, and atrioventricular (AV) nodal conduction. The differences between the three classes of calcium channel blockers relate to differences in their primary sites of action.

Dihydropyridine calcium channel antagonists can be viewed as almost pure vasodilators. They dilate resistance vessels in both the peripheral and coronary beds and improve coronary blood flow. Although dihydropyridine-type calcium channel blockers may reduce oxygen demand by reducing blood pressure and wall stress, this is countered by a reflex increase in heart rate, making the overall effect on oxygen demand unpredictable. This factor causes nifedipine alone, for example, to be of little use in treating ischemia. The addition of a β-blocker can block reflex tachycardia, however, and the combination of these two agents can be extremely effective. Short-acting preparations of nifedipine appear to be responsible for most of the problems associated with this class of drugs, and there is no reason to use short-acting nifedipine in contemporary practice. Rapid hemodynamic fluctuations frequently occur, particularly in elderly patients, with potentially serious adverse consequences. Sustained-release preparations, on the other hand, appear to avoid these rapid hemodynamic changes and are safe when used properly. Although long-acting nifedipine preparations are generally well tolerated, peripheral edema and headache can be seen in some patients. These side effects may be somewhat less common with second- and third-generation agents such as amlodipine. Amlodipine causes less reflex tachycardia than other dihydropyridines and usually has a neutral effect on heart rate. This property allows it to be used effectively as monotherapy for the treatment of angina. In addition, amlodipine may be particularly effective in patients with reduced LV function.

Verapamil has the most direct cardiac effects of the calcium channel blockers (Tab. 25.6), and therefore, it has the greatest effect on cardiac conduction and contractility. On

Table 25.6 Characteristics of selected calcium channel antagonists

Preparation	Dose	To onset of action	Plasma half-life	HR	SVR	Comments
Nifedipine						
Sublingual	10-20 mg tid	5-10 min	2-5 h	↑↑	↓↓↓	Should no longer be used
Oral	10-30 mg tid	10-20 min	2-5 h	↑↑	↓↓↓	Should not be used routinely
Sustained release	30-90 mg qd	2 h	2-5 h	↑↑	↓↓↓	Use in combination with β-blocker; use as monotherpy only in patients with bradycardia
Diltiazem						Very favorable side effect profile
Oral	30-90 mg tid	15-30 min	4-6 h	↓	↓↓	
Sustained release	180-480 mg qd	2-3 h	5-10 h	↓	↓↓	
Intravenous	0.25 mg/kg bolus; 0.15 mg/kg/h infusion	<5 min	3-5 h	↓↓	↓↓	Used iv to control supraventricular arrhythmias; expensive
Verapamil						Reduces myocardial contractility more than other agents
Oral	40-120 mg tid	30-60 min	3-12 h	↓↓	↓	
Sustained release	240-480 mg qd	30-60 min	4-12 h	↓↓	↓	
Intravenous	2.5-10 mg bolus; 5-10 mg/h infusion	<5 min	2-7 h	↓↓↓	↓	Useful to control supraventricular arrhythmias; less expensive than iv diltiazem
Newer agents						
Nicardipine						
Oral	20-30 mg tid	20 min	2-4 h	↑	↓↓	Should be combined with β-blocker
Intravenous	10-15 mg/h for 30 min; then 3-5 mg/h	<5 min	1-2 h	↑	↓↓↓	Effective agent to treat hypertensive emergencies
Amlodipine	2.5-10 mg qd	1-2 h	30-50 h	→	↓↓↓	May be particularly effective in patients with LV dysfunction
Felodipine	5-20 mg qd	2 h	9-17 h	↑	↓↓↓	
Isradipine	2.5-10 mg bid	20 min	2-10 h	→	↓↓↓	

(HR= heart rate; SVR= systemic vascular resistence.)

the other hand, it has the least vasodilating action. Verapamil also facilitates ventricular relaxation and thus may be particularly helpful in patients with diastolic dysfunction and angina. Although these effects are qualitatively similar to those of the beta-blockers, the negative inotropic effects of verapamil are more powerful, and verapamil should be avoided in patients with LV dysfunction or conduction disease. The most common side effects seen with verapamil are constipation and headache.

Diltiazem has actions intermediate between verapamil and nifedipine (Tab. 25.6), which explains why adverse effects are very rare with diltiazem. In particular, diltiazem causes less myocardial depression and has less effect on AV nodal conduction than verapamil. Sustained-release preparations of diltiazem, like verapamil, are widely available. These long-acting preparations generally are superior in terms of patient satisfaction and compliance. In patients with atrial arrhythmias, in whom tight control of heart rate is necessary, shorter-acting (or even iv) preparations may be preferable, at least until a stable dose is reached.

The negative inotropic and chronotropic properties of diltiazem and verapamil make these drugs, like β-blockers, effective agents for reducing myocardial oxygen demand. In distinction to β-blockers, however, these two agents are coronary vasodilators and therefore increase myocardial blood flow and oxygen supply as well. For this reason, calcium antagonists are the agents of choice for patients with coronary artery spasm or Prinzmetal's variant angina. For patients with the more typical form of exertional angina, diltiazem and verapamil improve symptoms and prolong exercise duration. Although these drugs can be used safely with nitrates, when they are given in combination with β-blockers, patients must be observed closely for bradycardia because both agents have depressant effects on sinus rate and AV nodal conduction. Finally, in the setting of presumed calcium channel blocker toxicity or overdose, iv calcium carbonate or calcium gluconate should be administered immediately.

Coronary artery bypass grafting for chronic stable angina

Revascularization, by either percutaneous (PTCA, stent, atherectomy, etc.) or surgical technique, provides excellent symptom relief for patients with stable angina. Surgical revascularization with coronary artery bypass grafting (CABG) has been performed for over three decades; more recent refinements in technique include the use of arterial conduits, minimally invasive approaches, and improved myocardial protection. These factors have combined to reduce surgical mortality, reduce perioperative complications and morbidity, and prolong the period of symptom relief following surgery.

Several randomized trials from the 1970s and 1980s compared CABG with medical therapy for patients with stable angina. Although they were performed in an era when both surgical and medical therapy were quite different from what it is today, these studies still provide the best available data to guide decision-making. Overall, symptom relief with CABG is excellent and clearly superior to medical therapy, with approximately 85% of patients reporting either complete relief or significant improvement of angina following surgery. The benefits of bypass surgery wane over time, however, and by 10 years, approximately half of venous conduits have failed. Graft failure is associated with the return of angina in many patients. Long-term survival is similar between CABG and medical therapy, except in certain high-risk groups: patients with left main coronary artery disease (>50%) and patients with LV dysfunction and multivessel coronary artery disease have a significantly lower mortality when treated with CABG compared with medical therapy. In the future, the use of multiple arterial grafts and genetically altered vein grafts should improve long-term surgical results even further.

Percutaneous coronary intervention

The number of percutaneous revascularization procedures performed has grown explosively in recent years despite lack of evidence supporting a reduction in mortality in any subgroup of patients tested to date. Percutaneous transluminal coronary angioplasty (PTCA) by use of a balloon is very effective for relief of angina in patients with coronary artery disease, provided they have suitable lesion characteristics. Patients with one or two discrete coronary stenoses are the most appropriate candidates for PTCA. Initial success rates for PTCA are greater than 90 to 95% in experienced hands. Complications, such as acute closure of the target vessel (usually due to intimal trauma and dissection), have been reduced dramatically with the use of "bail out" intracoronary stenting and the addition of glycoprotein IIb/IIIa receptor inhibitors. In the modern era, emergent CABG for failed PTCA is very rarely required.

Restenosis remains the "Achilles heel" of PTCA, with rates ranging from 30 to 50% after 6 months to 1 year depending on lesion location and morphology and vessel size. Application of an intracoronary stent appears to reduce restenosis rates significantly, and several trials have documented up to 50% reductions in both angiographic restenoses and target lesion revascularization. Unfortunately, many vessels are too small to be stented effectively; restenosis rates in these small vessels are disappointingly high, regardless of whether stents are applied. Furthermore, the pathobiology of in-stent restenosis appears to be different from the typical restenosis after plain balloon angioplasty. After balloon angioplasty, much of the restenotic process appears to be due to adverse vessel"remodeling", a process that can be limited by intracoronary stenting. In-stent restenosis, on the other hand, is a process of cellular proliferation and tissue ingrowth, with the consequence that treatment has proven to be extremely difficult. Therapy is more technically challenging than with post-PTCA restenosis, often requiring tissue ablative techniques such as atherectomy. Although the use of stents emitting either beta or gamma radiation shows promise as a means of halting tissue proliferation and limiting in-stent restenoses, many obstacles, both clinical and regulatory, will need to be overcome before radiation therapy becomes an accepted means of preventing restenoses.

After stent placement, optimal adjuvant therapy includes aspirin and ticlopidine (for 2-4 weeks). Ticlopidine is a thienopyridine antiplatelet agent that appears to inhibit platelet aggregation by 20 to 30%, via blockade of the binding of adenosine diphosphate (ADP) to its platelet receptor. The regimen of ticlopidine (250 mg bid) and aspirin is associated with a lower incidence of stent thrombosis than warfarin-containing regimens. Important side effects of ticlopidine include rare cases of neutropenia and thrombocytopenia that necessitate monitoring the complete blood count (CBC) at least biweekly. Clopidogrel (see below) is a structurally similar agent, apparently is devoid of neutropenic side effects, and can be given once daily. Studies evaluating adjunctive clopidogrel (75 mg/d) following coronary stenting are currently underway.

Choosing between medical therapy, percutaneous coronary intervention, and coronary artery bypass grafting

Several studies comparing angioplasty with medical therapy have been performed in patients with one- or two-vessel coronary artery disease. Mortality and infarction rates are generally similar, but angioplasty does appear to provide somewhat better symptom relief than medical therapy. A recent study with the statin atorvastatin (AVERT study) has shown significant reduction in the need for angioplasty in such patients. Studies comparing multivessel angioplasty with CABG have been performed in carefully selected patients who meet criteria for both procedures. In these selected patients, overall mortality rates are similar, but repeat revascularization is much more common in patients treated initially with angioplasty. Of note is the consistent increase in mortality seen in patients with diabetes mellitus who are treated with multivessel angioplasty instead of surgery.

In summary, patients with left main coronary artery disease or multivessel coronary artery disease and LV dysfunction should in general be treated with CABG. In addition, diabetic patients with multivessel disease appear to benefit from the more complete revascularization that surgery offers. Patients with larger ischemic burdens as assessed by ambulatory ECG monitoring or exercise scintigraphy may benefit from revascularization, either by PCI or by surgery. Most of the remaining patients can be treated initially with medical therapy, unless they prefer more definitive revascularization. In general, β-blockers should be the first agents chosen, with calcium channel blockers as an alternative. The decision between these two agents is often based on associated comorbid medical conditions and the side effects of each agent. In low-risk patients, decisions between medical therapy, PCI, and surgery may depend on patient preference, local expertise, and even cost considerations. Patients who remain symptom-limited despite medical therapy should undergo catheterization with an eye to revascularization if coronary anatomy is suitable. In many of these patients, "culprit" vessel PCI can provide effective and lasting symptom relief.

Therapy for unstable angina and non-Q-wave myocardial infarction

Across the spectrum of myocardial ischemia, the syndromes of unstable angina and non-Q-wave MI (NQMI) are often considered together because of their similar clinical presentation, disease pathophysiology, and clinical management strategies. Patients usually present to the hospital with a worsening pattern or prolonged episode of ischemic pain. The ECG may show ST-segment and T-wave changes (but not ST-segment elevation). On the basis of cardiac enzymes, patients are characterized as having MI or unstable angina.

Within these broad groups of patients, however, several subsets merit further consideration. First, between the traditional categorization of unstable angina and NQMI, a patient may have what has been called a *microinfarction* or *infarctlet*, with a very small but nondiagnostic elevation of cardiac (CK) or no elevation of CK but elevation of other cardiac proteins such as troponin T. In one study, patients with an elevated isoenzyme CK-MB level but with a normal total CK level had a greater than 10 times higher risk of death or reinfarction than patients without CK or CK-MB elevation. Similar observations have been made with cardiac troponin I and cardiac troponin T.

Among patients with acute MI, the traditional dichotomization is between Q-wave and non-Q-wave MI (NQMI). However, in the current era of aggressive treatment, a more relevant dichotomy is made based on the presence or absence of ST-segment elevation, a marker for acute coronary occlusion. In those with ST-segment elevation, immediate reperfusion therapy with thrombolysis (or primary PTCA) is clearly beneficial (see ST-Segment Elevation MI below). In those without ST-segment elevation, however, thrombolysis is not beneficial and may be harmful. For all patients with acute ischemic syndromes (with or without ST-segment elevation), antithrombotic therapy (currently with aspirin and heparin) plays a central role, with the goal of stabilizing or "passivating" the acute coronary lesion. In addition, it is important to control ischemia with β-blockers and nitrates and, if needed, revascularization.

Antithrombotic therapy Antithrombotic therapy plays a major role in the acute treatment and prevention of acute ischemic syndromes. Antithrombotic therapy, if present at the time of plaque rupture (e.g., aspirin) or administered acutely at the time of a clinical event (e.g., aspirin or heparin), can limit the development of thrombosis and lessen the degree of thrombosis and subsequent lesion stenosis, which causes clinical ischemia. Antithrombotic therapy also can prevent the local thrombosis from progressing to a complete occlusion (i.e., MI). Over a period of days to weeks, antithrombotic therapy acts to passivate the lesion and allow endogenous fibrinolysis to dissolve the acute thrombosis and restore the acute lesion to a stable plaque (see also Chap 74).

Several major studies have demonstrated clear beneficial effects of aspirin in patients with acute ischemic syn-

Table 25.7 Glycoprotein IIb/IIIa inhibitors that are in current clinical use

	Abciximab	Tirofiban	Eptifibatide
Dose	Bolus: 0.25 mg/kg Infusion: 0.1 µg/kg/min	Bolus: 0.4 µg/kg/min for 30 min Infusion: 0.1 µg/kg/min	Bolus: 180 µg/kg over 1-2 min Infusion: 2 mg/kg/min
Mechanism of action	Fab-fragment of monoclonal antibody	Nonpeptide	Cyclic heptapeptide
Plasma half-life	10-30 min	2 h	2-3 h
Duration of action	Up to 10 days	4 h	4 h
Indications	Coronary interventions	Unstable angina/ NQMI	Coronary interventions Unstable angina NQMI
Cost	++++	++	++

dromes. These studies found that patients with unstable angina or NQMI treated with aspirin instead of placebo had a 50 to 70% reduction in the risk of death or MI. Consistent positive results from clinical trials support the use of aspirin in all patients with unstable angina or NQMI, unless they have a contraindication.

One study conducted in the mid-1980s showed a 50% reduction in cardiac events through follow-up in patients with unstable angina who were treated with ticlopidine instead of placebo. Note, however, that no benefit was seen within the first 5 to 10 days of therapy. Clopidogrel has not been studied in unstable angina. Thus, ticlopidine (and possibly clopidogrel) are potential alternatives in patients allergic to aspirin.

The development of a class of drugs that inhibit platelet aggregation by binding to the platelet glycoprotein (Gp) IIb/IIIa receptor offers a new promising antithrombotic tool. By preventing the final common pathway of platelet aggregation, fibrinogen-mediated cross-linkage, these agents are much more potent than aspirin and inhibit platelet aggregation in response to all types of stimuli (e.g., thrombin, ADP, collagen, etc.). There are three broad categories of Gp IIb/IIIa inhibitors (Tab. 25.7): (1) the monoclonal antibody to the Gp IIb/IIIa receptor, abciximab, (2) the intravenous peptide and nonpeptide small-molecule inhibitors, such as eptifibatide and tirofiban, and (3) the oral Gp IIb/IIIa inhibitors, such as sibrafiban. Three Gp IIb/IIIa inhibitors are currently approved for use by the U.S. Food and Drug Administration (FDA): abciximab and eptifibatide for use in coronary angioplasty and tirofiban and eptifibatide (Integrilin) for unstable angina/non-ST-segment elevation MI. In addition, several agents are being evaluated as adjuncts to reduced-dose thrombolytic therapy.

Abciximab, the Fab fragment of the monoclonal antibody, binds very tightly to the Gp IIb/IIIa receptor. Thus, the antiplatelet effect lasts much longer than the infusion period. On the other hand, if bleeding occurs, stopping the drug will not reverse the antiplatelet effect immediately; transfusion of platelets, however, will allow the antibodies to redistribute among all the platelets, thereby reducing the level of platelet inhibition.

The peptide and peptidomimetic inhibitors (e.g., tirofiban and eptifibatide) are competitive inhibitors of the Gp IIb/IIIa receptor. Thus, the level of platelet inhibition is directly related to the drug level in the blood. Since both inhibitors have short half-lives, the antiplatelet activity reverses after a few hours when the drug infusion is stopped. On the other hand, for prolonged antiplatelet effect, the drug needs to be given iv for a longer period of time.

The third group of Gp IIb/IIIa receptor inhibitors are the oral agents. These agents are also competitive inhibitors and are usually prodrugs that are absorbed and then converted to active compounds in the blood. The oral agents all have longer half-lives, such that they can be given bid or tid in order to achieve relatively steady levels of Gp IIb/IIIa inhibition. With oral dosing, long-term therapy (i.e., >1 year) is possible. However, the long half-life also means that if bleeding occurs, the drug must be removed from the circulation in order to reduce the antiplatelet effect. This can be accomplished at present acutely by hemodialysis or charcoal hemoperfusion. These agents are currently under development or only available in some countries.

Gp IIb/IIIa inhibition was first shown to be beneficial during high-risk coronary angioplasty, e.g., for patients with acute coronary syndromes, with 25 to 50% reductions in ischemic complications. Significant benefit persisted for up to 3 years. Benefit from administration of Gp IIb/IIIa inhibitors also has been observed when using coronary stents and when performing "primary" and "rescue" PTCA in acute ST-segment elevation MI. Thus, given this broad experience with Gp IIb/IIIa inhibitors in PTCA, especially in high-risk patients with acute coronary syndromes, they have become a new therapeutic standard for coronary intervention.

Two agents, tirofiban and eptifibatide, are currently approved for the treatment of unstable angina and NQMI. Three large phase III trials have been performed with these agents. When used together with aspirin and heparin, they appear to reduce by 10 to 32% the combined incidence of death, MI, and/or recurrent ischemia. As a result of these findings, the use of tirofiban or eptifibatide is becoming standard for high-risk patients with unstable angina and non-ST-segment elevation MI. To date, Gp IIb/IIIa inhibitors have been studied only in concert with unfractionated heparin. Their use with low-molecular-weight heparins (LMWHs) requires further study.

A major concern with the Gp IIb/IIIa inhibitors is the potential for bleeding. Some studies suggested that Gp IIb/IIIa inhibitors are associated with increased bleeding, but careful evaluation has suggested that bleeding is more associated with excessive heparinization and prolongation of the activated partial thromboplastin time (aPTT) than with use of the Gp IIb/IIIa inhibitors per se. Use of lower doses of heparin and careful monitoring of the level of anticoagulation should avoid bleeding complications in patients receiving Gp IIb/IIIa inhibitors.

Thrombocytopenia is the other major side effect of Gp IIb/IIIa inhibition. Platelet counts falling below 100000/mm³ occur in approximately 1 to 2% of patients treated with Gp IIb/IIIa inhibitors, and platelet counts falling to less than 50000/mm³ occur in less than 0.5% of patients. Thrombocytopenia generally occurs on either the first day after beginning therapy or after approximately 2 weeks of therapy. The mechanism by which it occurs is not well understood. Fortunately, it is nearly always reversible, with platelet counts returning to normal after a few days.

Heparin also appears to be beneficial in unstable angina and non-ST-segment elevation MI. The greatest benefit has been observed during the period of therapy, with a rebound in recurrent events after stopping heparin. This rebound may be largely mitigated by the addition of aspirin. A recent and comprehensive meta-analysis showed a 33% reduction in death or MI at 2 to 12 weeks follow-up in patients treated with heparin plus aspirin versus aspirin alone, 7.9% versus 10.4%. Thus, these data support the use of the combination anticoagulant and antiplatelet therapy in acute coronary syndromes.

Unpredictability of the anticoagulant effects of heparin, so-called heparin resistance, is thought to be due to the size variability of the individual heparin molecules and to the neutralization of heparin by circulating plasma factors and by proteins released by activated platelets. Clinically, frequent monitoring of the anticoagulant response using the aPTT is recommended, with adjustments made according to a standardized nomogram (Tab. 25.8), definitely shown to facilitate the attainment of a target aPTT.

The traditional heparin dose used has been a 5000-unit bolus followed by a 1000 unit per hour infusion and then titrated according to the aPTT. The use of weight-adjusted heparin has been suggested as a means of improving aPTT control and patient safety. Weight adjusting the initial heparin bolus and infusion appears both to increase the proportion of patients who reach target aPTT and also to decrease the frequency of a large "overshoot" of the target aPTT, which is commonly seen with standard heparin dosing and has been associated with excess bleeding. Based on available data, the current optimal regimen appears to be weight-adjusted dosing (70 unit/kg bolus and 15 unit/kg per hour infusion), frequent monitoring of aPTT (every 6 hours until the aPTT is in the target range and every 12-24 hours thereafter), and titration of heparin using a standardized nomogram, with a target range of aPTT between 1.5 and 2 times control or between 50 and 70 seconds. Values for the aPTT below this range are associated with an increase in recurrent events, whereas values above this range are associated with excess bleeding.

Complications of heparin therapy are not limited to excess bleeding. Long-term treatment has been associated with osteoporosis, and thrombocytopenia is a potentially very serious complication. Mild dose-related thrombocytopenia is seen frequently and is of little clinical consequence. More severe thrombocytopenia is due to immune-mediated platelet destruction and paradoxically may be accompanied by clinical thrombosis. Severe thrombocytopenia tends to occur later in treatment, after 5 to 7 days of therapy, but may occur earlier in patients previously exposed to heparin. Although the thrombocytopenia almost always resolves after discontinuation of heparin, patients who have thrombotic complications have significant morbidity and mortality. In addition, many patients with heparin associated thrombocytopenia continue to need intravenous anticoagulation. In such patients, argatroban, an experimental antithrombin agent, has been used with success.

A major advance in the use of heparin has been in the development of low-molecular-weight heparins (LMWHs). These drugs are obtained by depolymerization of standard, unfractionated heparin and selection of those fragments with lower molecular weight. LMWHs have a molecular weight of 4000 to 5000 Da, in comparison with unfractionated heparin, which has an average molecular weight that varies from 12,000 to 15,000 Da. As compared with unfractionated heparin, which has nearly equal anti-factor IIa (thrombin) and anti-factor Xa activity, LMWHs have increased ratios of anti-factor Ia to anti-factor Xa activity: either 1:2 (dalteparin) or 1:3 (enoxaparin or nadroparin). LMWHs have several potential advantages over standard, nonfractionated heparin: (1) LMWHs inhibit both factor IIa and factor Xa, thereby inhibiting both thrombin activity and its generation, (2) LMWHs also induce a greater release of tissue factor pathway inhibitor than standard heparin and are not neutralized by platelet factor 4, (3) from a safety perspective, LMWHs do not increase capillary permeability (which may lead to fewer bleeding complications) and most recently have been found to have a lower rate of thrombocytopenia and osteoporosis, and (4) the high bioavailability and repro-

---

Table 25.8 Heparin nomogram using weight-adjusted heparin

aPTT (s)	Repeat heparin bolus	Stop heparin infusion (min)	Rate change (U/kg/h)	Repeat aPTT
<35	70 U/kg	0	+4	6 h
35-45	0	0	+2	6 h
45-70	0	0	0	Next A.M.
71-90	0	0	−2	6 h
>90	0	60	−3	6 h

(Heparin dosing in acute ischemic syndromes: initial bolus of 70 units/kg, followed by an infusion at 15 units/kg/h. The infusion will be adjusted to an aPTT of 45-70 s. Measurement of the aPTT will be done at 6, 12, and 24 h following the initiation of heparin and daily thereafter for each day the patient is on heparin. An aPTT should be measured 6 h after any change in the rate of heparin infusion.)
U= units.

ducible anticoagulant response of LMWHs allow for sc administration without any required monitoring of the coagulation system. This factor alone represents a major clinical improvement over unfractionated heparin.

In two large trials of patients with unstable angina or NQMI, enoxaparin, a LMWH with a 1:3 anti-factor IIa/anti-factor Xa ratio, lowered the incidence of death, MI, or recurrent ischemia by approximately 15% compared with standard unfractionated heparin. In separate trials, no difference was seen when dalteparin, a LMWH with a ratio of 1:2, was compared with unfractionated heparin. These results suggest that (1) enoxaparin appears to represent a modest improvement over standard unfractionated heparin in terms of clinical efficacy, and (2) the LMWH agents cannot be considered interchangeable members of a single class of drugs. At this time, enoxaparin is the only LMWH indicated for the treatment of unstable angina or NQMI. It should be administered with aspirin, a dose of 1 mg/kg sc bid.

Thrombolytic therapy Because thrombolytic therapy is beneficial in the treatment of patients with acute MI presenting with ST-segment elevation, it had been hoped that it also might improve outcome in the other acute coronary syndromes. Unfortunately, however, clinical trials have shown that not only do thrombolytic agents not help in these syndromes, they actually may harm patients. In the TIMI IIIb trial, for example, the incidence of death or MI through 42 days was actually higher in the patients treated with tissue plasminogen activator (tPA) than in control patients (8.8% versus 6.2%, p = 0.05) due to an increase in recurrent MI in patients with unstable angina. Accordingly, routine thrombolytic therapy is not recommended for patients with non-ST-segment elevation MI.

The proposed mechanism for an adverse effect of thrombolysis in unstable angina and non-ST-segment elevation MI is a prothrombotic effects of thrombolytic agents. Thrombolysis is known to activate platelets, increase fibrinopeptide A, and expose clot-bound thrombin, which is enzymatically active and can lead to more clot formation. Because most patients with unstable angina and non-ST-segment elevation MI have a patent culprit artery, these prothrombotic forces can lead to progression of the thrombus to 100% occlusion, thereby creating an ST-segment elevation MI.

Antianginal therapy The same agents described in detail earlier for the treatment of chronic stable angina are used to treat unstable angina and non-ST-segment elevation MI. The following brief discussion will focus on the points unique to this clinical syndrome.

Nitrates are very useful in the acute management of ischemia and should be given sublingually initially if the patient is experiencing ischemic pain. If pain persists after 3 sublingual tablets and initiation of beta blockade, intravenous nitroglycerin is recommended. Topical or oral nitrates can be used if the episode of pain has resolved or can replace iv nitroglycerin if the patient has been pain-free for 24 hours. Since the goal of nitrate therapy is relief of pain, nitrates frequently can be tapered off in the long-

term management of patients, with primary therapy composed primarily of aspirin and beta-blockers.

The use of beta-blockers is recommended in unstable angina. Several placebo-controlled trials have shown benefit in reducing subsequent MI. In addition, in patients with non-Q-wave MI, beta-blockers reduce infarct size, reinfarction, and mortality. Early iv beta blockade appears to provide benefits in both unstable angina and acute MI. Thus, beta blockade is recommended in all patients without contraindications (e.g., bradycardia, AV block, hypotension, pulmonary edema, history of bronchospasm). If ischemia and chest pain are ongoing, early iv beta blockade should be used, followed by oral beta blockade. A reduced ejection fraction is not an absolute contradiction to beta blockade, and indeed, such patients may derive added benefit.

Calcium channel blockers may be used in patients who have persistent or recurrent symptoms but are recommended only after nitrates and beta blockade have been initiated. In patients with contraindications to beta blockade, heart rate control can be accomplished with a calcium channel blocker (e.g., diltiazem or verapamil). No beneficial effect has been observed with calcium channel blockers in reducing mortality in patients with NQMI, and among those with LV dysfunction or CHF, a harmful effect has been observed. Although some studies have suggested a benefit in terms of prevention of recurrent infarction in patients with NQMI and normal LV function, this remains a controversial point, and beta-blockers should be the agents of choice in unstable angina or NQMI.

Angiography and revascularization At present, two general approaches to the use of cardiac catheterization and revascularization in unstable angina/NQMI exist: one involves early cardiac catheterization and revascularization with PCI or bypass surgery as appropriate; the other is a more conservative approach that uses initial medical management with catheterization and revascularization only for recurrent ischemia. There has been considerable debate as to whether an early invasive strategy might be better than a conservative approach. Advocates of the invasive approach note that the definitive management can be accomplished in several days; angiography can identify the 10 to 15% of patients with normal coronary arteries (who could be discharged home), as well as the 5 to 10% of patients with critical left main or severe three-vessel coronary artery disease who benefit from coronary bypass surgery; in the remaining patients who need revascularization, it can be carried out expeditiously, and the patient can return home rapidly.

On the other hand, with a more conservative approach using vigorous medical therapy, particularly in patients who have never previously received antianginal medication, unstable angina may quickly "cool off". If the patient remains symptom-free on medical therapy after beginning to ambulate, he/she may be treated conservatively. Treadmill exercise testing, with or without adjunctive imaging, may help to further define patient management. If the pattern of angina remains unstable or if ECG changes suggest ongoing ischemia, then coronary angiography is warranted.

There has been debate as to whether an early invasive strategy might be better than a conservative approach. Two large trials have prospectively evaluated this question. The TIMI IIIB trial found that both the early invasive and early conservative strategies led to a similar incidence of serious adverse outcomes, and thus both strategies are suitable for patients with these acute ischemic syndromes. However, since nearly two-thirds of patients required catheterization despite aggressive medical treatment, the early invasive arm could be viewed as a more expeditious strategy for unstable angina and non-Q-wave MI.

The recent VANQWISH (VA Non-Q-Wave Infarction Strategies in-Hospital) trial compared invasive and conservative strategies in patients with non-Q-wave MI and found no significant difference in the primary end-point of death or nonfatal MI during a 12- to 44-month follow-up. However, there were significantly more deaths in patients assigned to the invasive compared with the conservative strategy at hospital discharge and at 1 year. Much of the early hazard in the invasive group was explained by a very high (13.4%) perioperative mortality in patients receiving CABG; although this has been a point of criticism, similarly high perioperative mortality rates have been reported in patients with recent MI.

Thus, balancing TIMI IIIB and VANQWISH, one must individualize the approach for the patient population and the success rates of the coronary interventions—both angioplasty and bypass surgery. In a broad group of patients with unstable angina and non-ST-segment elevation MI, in which angioplasty can be carried out in the majority of patients with low complication rates, an invasive strategy may be considered appropriate and more expeditious than an early conservative strategy. In patients with more severe infarction and higher frequency of multivessel disease requiring bypass surgery and/or at hospitals where intervention complication rates are higher, a more conservative approach may be most appropriate. Given the importance of this issue, trials are currently ongoing to reexamine the relative benefits of invasive versus conservative strategies in this patient population in the current era of Gp IIb/IIIa inhibition and coronary stenting.

PTCA versus CABG The indications for surgical revascularization in unstable angina are similar to those for chronic stable angina. CABG is recommended for patients with disease of the left main coronary artery, multivessel disease involving the proximal left anterior descending artery, and multivessel disease and impaired LV function. For other patients, either PTCA or CABG is suitable. PTCA has a lower initial morbidity and mortality than CABG but a higher rate of repeat procedures, whereas CABG is associated with more effective relief from angina. In patients in need of revascularization, the choice should be individualized.

Therapy for ST-segment elevation MI

Transmural MI is caused by complete thrombotic occlusion of an epicardial coronary artery and is associated with ST-segment elevation on the 12-lead ECG. Untreated, transmural necrosis usually develops, and Q waves are seen on the ECG. Primary therapy for ST-segment elevation MI involves the rapid reestablishment of antegrade flow in the occluded infarct-related artery.

Thrombolytic therapy The benefits of thrombolytic therapy for acute ST-segment elevation MI are related to early achievement of infarct-related artery (IRA) patency. Early, successful coronary reperfusion limits infarct size, decreases LV dysfunction, and improves survival. Patients who achieve normal (TIMI grade 3) flow in the IRA 90 minutes after thrombolysis have the lowest mortality (3.6%), patients with slow (TIMI grade 2) antegrade flow have an intermediate mortality of 6.6%, and patients with no flow or only a trickle of flow (TIMI grade 0 or 1 flow) have the highest mortality (9.5%). A patent IRA not only enhances regional myocardial function but also limits LV dilatation and dysfunction and reduces electrical instability after MI.

Time is a critical determinant of the success of any thrombolytic regimen. Patients treated within 1 hour of the onset of chest pain have an almost 50% reduction in mortality if treated with thrombolytics; patients treated after 12 hours do not benefit at all. For each hour earlier that a patient is treated, there is an approximately 1% absolute decrease in mortality, which translates into an additional 10 lives saved per 1000 patients treated.

Thrombolysis has been shown to reduce mortality in numerous placebo-controlled trials. The Fibrinolytic Therapy Trialists' overview of all the large placebo-controlled studies showed a 2.6% absolute reduction in mortality for patients with ST-segment elevation MI treated within the first 12 hours after the onset of symptoms. Patients presenting with left bundle-branch block (LBBB) and a strong clinical history for acute MI also derive a large benefit from thrombolysis. However, as noted earlier, those without ST-segment elevation or LBBB do not benefit from thrombolysis and indeed may be harmed.

All the thrombolytic (fibrinolytic) agents currently available and under investigation are plasminogen activators. They all work enzymatically, directly or indirectly, to convert the single-chain plasminogen molecule to the double-chain plasmin, which has potent intrinsic fibrinolytic activity. Highlights of differences in dosing, pharmacokinetics, recanalization rates, and cost are shown in Table 25.9.

Most of the recent studies indicate that accelerated tPA with intravenous heparin is currently the most effective therapy for achieving early reperfusion and enhanced survival in acute MI, but it is also substantially more expensive and is associated with more intracranial hemorrhage. Reteplase is a new double-bolus agent that appears to have similar efficacy and risk to tPA but may be simpler to administer. When deciding which agent to use, cost-benefit analysis is often performed. The cost-benefit ratio is in favor of tPA compared with streptokinase in patients presenting early after symptom onset with a large area of

Table 25.9 Thrombolytic agents in current clinical use

	Alteplase	Reteplase	Streptokinase	Anistreplase (APSAC)	Urokinase
Fibrin-selective	+++	++	-	-	-
Half-life	5 min	15 min	20 min	70 min	4 min
Dose	15-mg bolus; then 0.75 mg/kg over 30 min; then 0.5 mg/kg over 60 min	Two 10-unit bolus doses given 30 min apart	1.5 million units over 30-60 min	30 units as slow bolus over 5 min	3 million units over 1 h
Adjunctive heparin	Yes	Yes	No	No	No
Possible allergy	No	No	Yes	Yes	No
TIMI 2/3 flow (90 min)	80%	80%	60%	60%	65%
TIMI 3 flow (90 min)	55%	55%	32%	NA	NA
Cost	+++	+++	+	++	+++

(NA = not available.)

injury (e.g., anterior acute MI) and at low risk of intracranial hemorrhage. In groups with smaller potential for survival benefit and a greater risk for intracranial hemorrhage, streptokinase appears to be the agent of choice, particularly in view of the cost. Additional considerations include avoiding reuse of streptokinase or anistreplase for at least 2 years (preferably indefinitely) because of a high prevalence of potentially neutralizing antibody titers and because of the risk for allergic reaction on second exposure to these drugs. Other promising thrombolytic agents under investigation include lanoteplase, TNK-tPA, prourokinase, and staphylokinase.

Thrombolysis is indicated for patients presenting within 12 hours of symptom onset if they have ST-segment elevation (or new LBBB), provided they have no contraindications to thrombolytic therapy (Tab. 25.10). Less clear indications include patients who are older than 75 years of age, those who can be treated only more than 12 to 24 hours after the onset of acute MI, and those who are hypertensive but present with high-risk MI. Patients should not be treated if the time to treatment is greater than 24 hours and their ischemic symptoms have resolved or if they present only with ST-segment depression.

Current thrombolytic regimens achieve patency (TIMI grade 2 or 3 flow) in approximately 80% of patients but complete reperfusion (TIMI grade 3 flow) in only 50 to 60% of patients. For patients who fail thrombolysis, rescue PTCA can be performed; in high-risk patients, particularly those with anterior MI, this appears to improve outcome. Whether patients with partial reperfusion (TIMI grade 2 flow) benefit from rescue PTCA is not yet clear. Even after successful

thrombolysis, a significant 10 to 20% risk of reocclusion is present. Reocclusion and reinfarction are associated with a 2- to 3-fold increase in mortality.

Bleeding is the most common complication of thrombolytic therapy, and major bleeding occurs in 5 to 15% of patients. Intracranial hemorrhage (ICH) is the most devastating bleeding complication of thrombolytic therapy and is associated with very high mortality and almost universal

Table 25.10 Contraindications to thrombolytic therapy

Absolute	Relative
Active internal bleeding	Blood pressure consistently >180/110 mm Hg
History of CNS hemorrhage	History of stroke at any time in past
Stoke of any kind within the last year	Known bleeding diathesis diabetic retinopathy
Recent head trauma or CNS neoplasm	Proliferative diabetic retinopathy
Suspected aortic dissection	Prolonged CPR
Major surgery or trauma within 2 weeks	Prior exposure to SK or APSAK Pregnancy

(CNS = central nervous system; SK = streptokinase; APSAC = anisolylated plasminogen streptokinase activator complex [anistreplase]; CPR = cardiopulmonary resuscitation.)

disability in survivors. In major clinical trials, ICH has occurred in 0.4 to 0.8 % of patients; in clinical practice, where higher-risk patients are treated, rates are likely to be higher.

Primary PCI An alternate method of achieving coronary reperfusion is use of immediate or *primary* PTCA, without concomitant administration of thrombolytic therapy. Initial randomized trials have shown that primary PTCA appears to be more beneficial in reducing death or MI than administration of a thrombolytic agent. In addition, this therapy avoids the risk of ICH seen with thrombolytic therapy. The relative benefits of primary PTCA are greatest in patients at highest risk, including those with cardiogenic shock, right ventricular infarction, large anterior MI, and increased age (due partly to increased ICH rate with thrombolytic therapy). However, as with thrombolysis, rapid time to treatment is critical to success. In addition, operator and institutional experience seem to be vital to realize the full benefit of primary PTCA or stenting. The superb procedural and clinical results seen in single-institution studies have not been replicated in larger trials and registries.

More recent developments include the use of primary stenting for acute MI and the use of Gp IIb/IIIa inhibitors as adjunctive agents. Stenting certainly appears to be safe, even in the thrombus-rich environment of acute MI, but further study is needed to determine whether a strategy of primary stenting is superior to one of primary PTCA with "bailout" stenting. Adjunctive Gp IIb/IIIa inhibitors in primary PTCA appear to be more clearly beneficial. These agents can be administered when the patient arrives in the emergency room, and in addition to facilitating reperfusion, they reduce the incidence of periprocedural complications.

Although primary PTCA and stenting are excellent reperfusion options in dedicated centers that can perform the procedures quickly and expertly, given current logistic and financial constraints, most patients will continue to be treated initially with thrombolytic therapy. Efforts should be made to transfer patients with contraindications to thrombolytic therapy to centers that can perform primary angioplasty. In addition, recent studies have confirmed the safety of immediate PTCA following thrombolytic therapy. Investigations are underway to reexamine the use of combined thrombolytic and interventional strategies to optimize reperfusion and prevent reocclusion.

Aspirin In the setting of acute ST-segment elevation MI, aspirin decreases reocclusion by over 50%, decreases reinfarction by nearly 50%, and reduces morality by 25%, a benefit comparable with that of streptokinase. Following MI, chronic aspirin therapy also reduces subsequent cardiac events, a benefit that now has been observed to persist for up to 4 years of follow-up. Thus, aspirin has had a dramatic effect in reducing adverse clinical events and constitutes primary therapy for all acute coronary syndromes. A dose of 162 to 325 mg daily is currently recommended (see also Chap. 74).

Heparin In acute ST-segment elevation MI, heparin is also an important adjunctive agent to decrease reocclusion following administration of tPA. Although no clear difference in infarct-related artery patency is seen at 90 minutes, there is higher patency between 18 hours and 5 days in patients randomized to receive iv heparin, suggesting that the benefit of heparin is a result of decreased reocclusion rather than enhanced thrombolysis. Further analysis of these studies has demonstrated that patency is greatest in patients who have effective anticoagulation, with an aPTT of greater than 2 times control or greater than 60 seconds, and suggest that a target aPTT between 50 and 70 seconds is optimal. Following streptokinase or anistreplase (APSAC), heparin has not been shown to be of benefit. Therefore, iv heparin may be considered optional in streptokinase- or APSAC-treated patients. Sc heparin has been shown to be of no benefit in preventing reinfarction or death compared with placebo.

Warfarin In secondary prevention trials after MI, anticoagulant therapy with warfarin has been shown to reduce the rate of death and recurrent MI. Warfarin monotherapy appears to be at least as effective as aspirin in the general population, and there are several circumstances in which benefit or potential benefit with warfarin therapy exceeds that of aspirin. First, warfarin is superior to aspirin in prevention of systemic emboli in patients with atrial fibrillation. In addition, beneficial effects in reducing systemic emboli also have been observed in patients after MI with documented LV dysfunction. No significant benefit has been observed with the combinations of warfarin plus aspirin versus monotherapy with either agent alone, and the combination is associated with increased risk for hemorrhage. Thus, warfarin is a suitable alternative to aspirin following MI as monotherapy, but there is no evidence to support a combination regimen of warfarin plus aspirin.

Clopidogrel Clopidogrel, like its sister drug ticlopidine, is a thienopyridine derivative that inhibits platelet aggregation, increases bleeding time, and reduces blood viscosity. The two agents achieve their antiaggregatory action by inhibiting the binding of ADP to its platelet receptors. Clopidogrel has been tested for secondary prevention in patients with either recent MI, stroke, or documented peripheral arterial disease and has been shown to reduce the incidence of MI by approximately 20% compared with aspirin. Based on these findings, the FDA recently approved clopidogrel for secondary prevention of vascular events among patients with symptomatic atherosclerosis, at a dose of 75 mg given orally once per day. Whether clopidogrel provides additive benefit to aspirin is not yet known. Further studies are needed to determine the circumstances under which clopidogrel should be used instead of, or in addition to, aspirin and Gp IIb/IIIa inhibitors. At the present time, the recommendation is to use clopidogrel as secondary prevention in patients who cannot take aspirin and to consider its use in addition to aspirin for patients on aspirin with recurrent cardiac or vascular symptoms.

Beta-blockers The β-blockers were among the first therapeutic interventions designed to limit the size of acute MI.

Studies administering the β-blocker within an appropriate time window following onset of acute MI have definitively demonstrated a mortality benefit associated with β-blocker therapy, both in patients who receive thrombolytic therapy and in those who do not. Much of this benefit is due to a reduction in sudden cardiac death, which appears to result from the prevention of cardiac rupture and ventricular fibrillation. In addition to reducing mortality, prolonged treatment with β-blockers reduces the incidence of nonfatal reinfarction.

It is striking that the long-term mortality benefits of the β-blockers following an index MI (i.e., secondary prevention) extend to most members of this class of agents. There does not seem to be a significant difference between agents with or without cardioselectivity (see Chap. 22). However, the presence of intrinsic sympathomimetic activity reduces the benefit considerably, and these agents should not be used in acute MI. Reduction in heart rate appears to be a critical feature associated with the protective effect of β-blockers. Indeed, there is a significant relationship between the magnitude of heart rate reduction observed on the active agent and the magnitude of reduction in mortality. The magnitude of benefit from long-term use of β-blockers also depends on the patient's risk of mortality associated with the index MI. In clinical trials, those patients with electrical or mechanical complications experienced a much greater relative benefit. The benefits from routine β-blocker use seem to persist as long as the active agent is continued. It is therefore most appropriate in the setting of ST-segment elevation MI to begin with iv β-blocker therapy immediately, followed by oral therapy that is maintained indefinitely in patients who can tolerate it.

The side effects from prolonged β-blocker use generally have been quite minor and are similar to those seen with placebo. In studies that report it, the incidence of heart failure is slightly but significantly higher in patients receiving β-blockers than in patients receiving placebo. However, patients with a history of mild or moderate chronic heart failure (CHF) actually experienced greater benefit from β blockade than did patients without CHF.

Nitrates Early studies demonstrated that nitrates may reduce infarct size and improve regional myocardial function when administered early in the course of acute MI. A meta-analysis of these earlier studies prior to the acute reperfusion era indicated that nitrates reduced the odds of death after acute MI by approximately 35%. More recent trials from the thrombolytic era do not support the routine use of long-term nitrate therapy in patients with uncomplicated acute MI. However, it is reasonable to use iv nitroglycerin for the first 24 to 48 hours in patients with acute MI and recurrent ischemia, CHF, or significant hypertension. It should be continued orally or topically in patients with CHF and large transmural MIs as well. Intravenous administration is recommended in the early stage of acute MI because of its onset of action, ease of titration, and the opportunity for prompt termination in the event of side effects.

Calcium channel blocking agents Studies that have investigated calcium channel blockers, particularly the dihydropyridines, for the early treatment of MI, have found no benefit for these agents. Short-acting nifedipine, in fact, has been found to be detrimental when used without a β–blocker to blunt the reflex sympathetic activity. Nicardipine, a newer-generation dihydropyridine agent, also has been found to nonsignificantly increase mortality and reinfarction.

Verapamil and diltiazem have been given to patients as secondary prevention after stabilization of their index MI. Although these agents appear to have no effect on mortality following acute MI, when given several days to weeks after an uncomplicated MI, they reduce the rate of reinfarction, an effect that seems similar for both agents. Verapamil in particular is detrimental to patients with heart failure or bradyarrhythmias during the first 24 to 48 hours after acute MI.

It should be emphasized that there have not been studies comparing the efficacy of verapamil or diltiazem with that of a beta-blocker. Beta-blockers more consistently reduce both mortality and reinfarction and should be recommended for patients who can tolerate such medication. Verapamil or diltiazem may be a reasonable alternative for patients who cannot tolerate a β-blocker but who can tolerate one of the calcium channel blockers, e.g., patients with severe chronic obstructive pulmonary disease (COPD) or asthma. It should be noted, however, that many patients who cannot tolerate a beta-blocker because of concern of excessive bradycardia or CHF may experience similar complications from diltiazem or verapamil.

Angiotensin-converting enzyme (ACE) inhibitors ACE inhibitors have become a mainstay in the treatment of patients with acute MI because they prevent the deleterious LV chamber remodeling that may occur after MI and because they may prevent the progression of vascular pathology. The LV dysfunction associated with acute MI leads to a perceived reduction in circulating blood volume and blood pressure, which is compensated by an increase in the renin-angiotensin-aldosterone system as well as an increase in sympathetic tone. These effects lead to salt and water retention as well as vasoconstriction, which in turn further dilates the left ventricle and causes progressive LV dysfunction. This vicious cycle can be interrupted by ACE inhibitors, which block the increased renin-angiotensin activity and thereby prevent the progressive dilatation and dysfunction. The recent overview by the ACE Inhibitor Myocardial Infarction Collaborative Group, which included observations in almost 100 000 patients with acute MI treated within 36 hours of the onset of chest pain, found a 7% reduction in 30-day mortality when ACE inhibitors were given to all patients with acute MI, with most of the benefit observed in the first week. The absolute benefit was particularly large in some high-risk groups, such as those in Killip class II or and those with an anterior MI. ACE inhibitor therapy also reduced the incidence of nonfatal MI but was associated with an excess of persistent hypotension and renal dysfunction. In the overview, more than 85% of the lives saved attributed to ACE inhibitor therapy occurred in the anterior MI subgroup, which represented 37% of the overall population.

As opposed to aspirin and reperfusion strategies, it is not critical to introduce the ACE inhibitor in the hyperacute phase of acute MI. There is benefit from ACE inhibitor therapy when administered at any time following MI, although benefit is lessened if therapy is delayed by days or weeks; therefore, a reasonable time to administer these agents is in the first 6 to 12 hours, once the patient has stabilized in the CCU. The benefits of ACE inhibitors appear to be class-specific, with little difference between agents. Specific agents and dosing recommendations are reviewed in Chapters 22 23.

Of note, ACE inhibitors also may protect against progression of atherosclerosis and the development of MI by their antiproliferative and antimigratory effects on smooth muscle cells, neutrophils, and mononuclear cells by enhancing endogenous fibrinolysis and by improving endothelial dysfunction. Studies suggest that patients treated with ACE inhibitors experience fewer MIs and episodes of unstable angina not related to hemodynamic effects and ventricular remodeling, and further studies are in progress to determine the role of such therapy in routine secondary prevention.

Catheterization and revascularization following thrombolytic therapy In patients with ST-segment elevation MI treated with thrombolytic therapy, numerous studies have failed to show a benefit for routine angiography and revascularization, whether performed early or late after MI. One randomized trial has shown a reduction in cardiac events in patients randomized to an invasive strategy after a positive predischarge exercise tolerance test. Therefore, routine angiography in all patients cannot be recommended, and catheterization should be reserved for high-risk patients with evidence of spontaneous or inducible ischemia after MI and perhaps also patients with clinical CHF or significant LV dysfunction. The indications for revascularization are identical to those described earlier for unstable angina and NQMI.

Emergency treatment of acute myocardial infarction

In addition to the standardized use of nitrates, ace-inhibitors and aspirin — as described in this and other chapters — immediate therapy for acute myocardial infarction has the objective of achieving pain relief, which is achieving with: (1) oxygen administration; (2) analgesic therapy.

Suggested readings

ACE INHIBITOR MYOCARDIAL INFARCTION COLLABORATIVE GROUP. Indications for ACE inhibitors in the early treatment of acute myocardial infarction: systematic overview of individual data from 100000 patients in randomized trials. Circulation 1998;97:2202-12.

ANTIPLATELET TRIALIST'S COLLABORATION. Collaborative overview of randomized trials of antiplatelet therapy: I. Prevention of death, myocardial infarction, and stroke by prolonged antiplatelet therapy in various categories of patients. Br Med J 1994;308:235-46.

BODEN WE, O'ROURKE RA, CRAWFORD MH, et al. Outcomes in patients with acute non-Q-wave myocardial infarction randomly assigned to an invasive as compared with a conservative strategy. N Engl J Med 1998;338:1785-92.

BRAUNWALD E ed. Heart disease: a textbook of cardiovascular medicine, 5th ed. Philadelphia: W B Saunders, 1997.

FIBRINOLYTIC THERAPY TRIALISTS' (FTT) COLLABORATIVE GROUP. Indications for fibrinolytic therapy in suspected acute myocardial infarction: collaborative overview of early mortality and major morbidity results from all randomised trials of more than 1000 patients. Lancet 1994;343:311-22.

THE GUSTO INVESTIGATORS. An international randomized trial comparing four thrombolytic strategies for acute myocardial infarction. N Engl J Med 1993;329:673-82.

HILLIS LD. Coronary artery bypass surgery: risks and benefits, realistic and unrealistic expectations. J Invest Med 1995; 43:17-27.

KULBERTUS H, PIERARD L, Myocardial infarction. In: Dalla Volta S, Bayés de Luna A, Brochier M. Dienstl F, et al. The McGraw-Hill Clinical Medicine Series: Cardiology. London: McGraw-Hill International UK, 1999, pp. 377-406.

LIBBY P. Molecular bases of the acute coronary syndromes. Circulation 1995;91:2844-50.

OLER A, WHOOLEY MA, OLER J, GRADY D. Adding heparin to aspirin reduces the incidence of myocardial infarction and death in patients with unstable angina: a meta-analysis. JAMA 1996;276:811-5.

REEDER GS, GERSH BJ. Modern management of acute myocardial infarction. Current Prob Cardiol 1996;21:585-667.

THE TIMI IIIB INVESTIGATORS. Effects of tissue plasminogen activator and a comparison of early invasive and conservative strategies in unstable angina and non-Q-wave myocardial infarction: Results of the TIMI IIIB Trial. Circulation 1994; 89:1545-56.

TOPOL EJ, SERRUYS PW. Frontiers in interventional cardiology. Circulation 1998;98:1802-20.

WEITZ JI. Low-molecular weight heparins. N Engl J Med 1997; 337:688-38.

Clinical management of heart failure

Willem J. Remme

During recent decades, heart failure has developed into what is probably the most important syndrome of cardiovascular medicine in terms of morbidity, hospitalization rate, and health care costs and mortality. Incidence and prevalence of heart failure are increasing rapidly and currently range from 1 to 2% in middle-aged patients to more than 10% in octogenarians. Hospitalization frequency and duration are extensive, with a hospitalization rate of 3 to 5 times per year in severe heart failure not being exceptional. In addition, heart failure is an expensive disease, consuming an average 1 to 2% of any national health care budget. Heart failure is also a malignant disease. Whereas in mild to moderate stages of heart failure the yearly mortality averages 10 to 20%, this figure approximates 50 to 60% in severe heart failure. As such, heart failure leads to more deaths than most cancers.

Although the etiology of heart failure varies throughout the world, the underlying etiology in most patients is ischemic heart disease, followed by heart failure due to hypertension and cardiac hypertrophy, idiopathic dilated cardiomyopathy, and heart failure related to chronic valvular disease and congenital disease. The most important risk factors are age, diabetes mellitus, hypertension, body weight, and smoking. Coronary artery disease confers a fourfold increased risk. Moreover, hypertensive cardiovascular disease with electrocardiographic (ECG) evidence of left ventricular hypertrophy increases the risk markedly.

Heart failure is typically a chronic process that results either from an initiating, acute insult to the myocardium, i.e., a myocardial infarction (MI) or inflammation, or from long-term pressure or volume overload. Less commonly, various forms of cardiomyopathy may lead to sys-

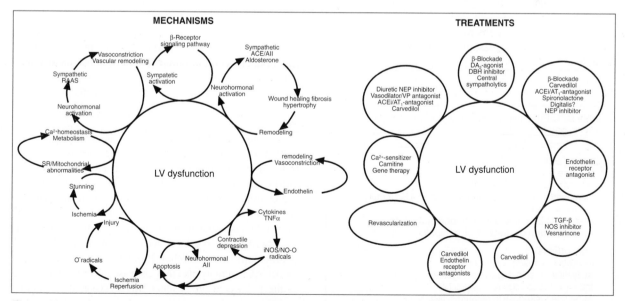

Figure 26.1 Schematic representation of the most pertinent mechanisms leading to progressive left ventricular (LV) dysfunction and heart failure and the pharmacologic interventions that may interfere with each separate mechanism (AII = angiotensin II; ACEi = ACE inhibitor; AT = angiotensin; DA$_2$ = dopamine; DBH = dopamine β-hyroxylase; iNOS = inducible nitric oxide synthase; NEP = neutral endopeptidase; NOS = nitric oxide synthase; RAAS = renin-angiotensin-aldosterone system; SR = sarcoplasmic reticulum; TNF = tumor necrosis factor).

tolic or diastolic dysfunction and subsequently to heart failure. Idiopathic dilated cardiomyopathy probably underlies 10 to 20% of heart failure cases, although its precise incidence is unknown. Less common are hypertrophic and restrictive cardiomyopathy.

Determination of (worsening) heart failure

Various mechanisms underlie the occurrence and subsequent worsening of heart failure. Of these, the most important are neurohormonal activation, cardiac remodeling, and myocardial ischemia. Contributive factors include oxidative stress and free radical production, cytokine activation and apoptosis, downregulation and/or uncoupling of various cardiac receptors, abnormalities in subcellular signaling pathways, disturbed calcium homeostasis, abnormal contractile protein expression, a disturbed energy metabolism, and an inappropriately increased heart rate. Pertinent peripheral abnormalities include abnormal endothelial function, peripheral vasoconstriction, skeletal muscle abnormalities with reduced anaerobic enzyme activity and a shift from type I slow twitch fibers to type IIB fast twitch fibers, functional renal impairment, and electrolyte disturbances.

These cardiac and peripheral alterations that underlie the occurrence and subsequent worsening of heart failure are potential targets for pharmacologic modulation of the disease (Fig. 26.1). The most pertinent changes will be discussed briefly.

Neurohormonal activation

Neurohormonal activation is one of the pivotal expressions of the heart failure syndrome. Various neurohormonal systems become activated during the process, e.g., the sympathetic system, the renin-angiotensin-aldosterone system, arginine vasopressin, natriuretic peptides, and endothelin.

Table 26.1 Potential adverse effect of sympathetic activation in heart failure

Cardiac effects
Myocyte hypertrophy
Myocyte necrosis and fibrosis
Increased myocardial oxygen demand and ischemia
Ventricular arrhythmias
Decreased β-adrenergic receptor responsiveness
  (non-uniform destruction of sympathetic innervation)

Renal effects
Increased reabsorption of sodium
Activation of renin-angiotensin system
Increased renal vascular resistance
Attenuated response to natriuretic factors

Vascular effects
Neurogenic vasoconstriction
Vascular hypertrophy

Sympathetic activation

Baroreceptor reflex dysfunction is a common observation in heart failure and leads to a loss of balance between sympathetic and parasympathetic activity. In addition, cardiopulmonary reflexes become impaired. A reduction in barocardiopulmonary receptor sensitivity in heart failure diminishes normal central inhibitory control of sympathetic outflow, vasopressin release, and renin secretion. Consequently, plasma norepinephrine levels increase and, eventually, may become a significant marker of the severity of heart failure and of prognosis. Although plasma norepinephrine levels correlate with sympathetic nerve fiber activity in patients with heart failure, circulating norepinephrine is not a very sensitive marker of overall sympathetic tone. Moreover, cardiac sympathetic activation increases significantly more than that of other organs and contributes largely to overall sympathetic tone. Measurement of circulating norepinephrine therefore may not reflect what happens in the heart. Indeed, heart rate variability determination may indicate early withdrawal of parasympathetic tone and increase in sympathetic activation not indicated by the less sensitive circulating norepinephrine level. At a relatively early stage in the heart failure process, cardiac sympathetic tone is activated, preceding generalized sympathetic activation, and contributes to various pathophysiologic processes, such as cardiac remodeling, β-receptor downregulation, abnormally increased heart rate, and myocardial ischemia. The potential adverse effects of sympathetic activation in heart failure are indicated in Table 26.1.

The renin-angiotensin system

Enhanced sympathetic outflow to the kidney as a result of diminished cardiac output should increase renin release. However, circulating renin levels are not necessarily elevated in patients with stable heart failure. In contrast, renin-aldosterone activation is observed during acute episodes or exacerbations of more severe heart failure. A secondary fall in renal output may augment blood volume and improve cardiac pump function, subsequently normalizing plasma renin-aldosterone levels. In advanced heart failure, these compensating mechanisms fail, and renin, angiotensin II, and aldosterone levels finally may increase.

The preceding concerns the circulating renin-angiotensin system. However, many organs produce components of a tissue renin-angiotensin system that may function in an autocrine or paracrine fashion. These tissue renin-angiotensin systems may behave quite differently from the circulating system. Thus, early after myocardial infarction, cardiac tissue angiotensin-converting enzyme (ACE) levels increase, leading to a local activation of the cardiac renin-angiotensin system. When heart failure ensues in this model, ACE activity also may increase in other organs, such as the kidney, in the absence of an activated circulating renin-angiotensin system.

Angiotensin II, the end product, is a strong vasoconstrictor and growth-promoting peptide, possibly involved in the process of cardiac remodeling, among other factors, such as sympathetic activation. Thus, after MI, the concentration of angiotensin II increases several-fold at the infarct site compared with noninfarcted tissue and relates to the increased expression of ACE and other components necessary for angiotensin II generation at this site. In vitro studies indicate that angiotensin II may cause a rapid induction of immediate early gene expression involved in cardiac fiber growth and the induction of fibrosis in the scar tissue or in interstitial fibrosis distinct from the infarct site. Of importance, angiotensin II receptor binding density increases during the first week after MI, as well as remote from the infarct site, at sites where fibrosis takes place. Of interest, this increase in angiotensin II receptors parallels increased high-density ACE binding. Moreover, in models of pressure overload or in genetic hypertensive animal models, there are strong suggestions that angiotensin II mediates cardiac hypertrophy. The growth- and fibrosis-promoting effects of angiotensin II are induced through angiotensin I receptor stimulation and can be blocked by angiotensin II type 1 (AT_1) receptor antagonists. In contrast, AT_2 receptor activation leads to antitrophic-antiproliferative effects and may enhance apoptosis. Both ACE inhibitors and AT_1 receptor antagonists have been shown to modulate cardiac growth and fibrosis in different models. The role of the AT_2 receptor and its modulation in this regard is less well defined. Of further importance in heart failure, angiotensin II increases central sympathetic tone, augments norepinephrine release from nerve endings, and promotes postsynaptic sympathetic tone.

Aldosterone

Aldosterone was initially believed to be important in the pathophysiology of heart failure for its ability to promote sodium retention and potassium loss. It has now become clear that aldosterone may affect the occurrence and worsening of heart failure in other ways. Aldosterone causes myocardial and vascular fibrosis, may lead to direct vascular damage, is involved in baroreceptor dysfunction, and may promote sympathetic activation and parasympathetic inhibition. It has been shown that aldosterone prevents myocardial norepinephrine uptake.

Endothelin

Like angiotensin II, endothelin is a strong vasoconstrictor and growth-promoting peptide. Endothelin-1 induces vasoconstriction by binding to ETA and ETB receptors in vascular smooth muscle cells. In contrast, it induces vasodilatation through ETB receptors present in endothelial cells. The overall effect on vascular tone therefore depends on the selective or nonselective receptor binding of endothelin. In analogy with the the effect of angiotensin II, endothelin affects calcium signaling pathways and the hydrolysis of phospholipids, tyrosine, and mitogen-activated protein kinases. As such, it has positive inotropic effects and growth-promoting properties. Endothelin-1 induces hypertrophy of cultured cardiac myocytes and is involved in left ventricular hypertrophy during pressure overload, most likely involving a local car-

diac endothelin system. In pressure overload cardiac hypertrophy, endothelin-1 production and its binding sites in the heart are upregulated. Myocardial endothelin and endothelin receptors are also expressed in models of heart failure. The cell types involved may be several, including endothelial cells, endocardium, and myocytes. Since pressure overload or stretch induces myocardial ET expression, this may suggest that myocardial ET production is an early component of cardiac remodeling. Of interest, angiotensin II induces the expression of the ETB receptor in cultured myocytes, whereas ET receptor antagonists affect the growth-promoting effects of angiotensin II in cardiac myocytes, indicating an interaction of the systems at a cellular level.

Recently, it has been indicated that chronic endothelin receptor blockade may attenuate progressive left ventricular dilatation after myocardial infarction, suggesting the potentially important role of this peptide in cardiac remodeling.

Vasopressin

Circulating vasopressin levels are increased in heart failure. Vasopressin is a potent vasoconstrictor substance and antidiuretic neurohormone. It may induce vasodilatation through vasopressin V_2 receptor stimulation. Vasopressin is secreted in direct response to changes in osmolality, as sensed by hypothalamic receptors. In heart failure, baroreceptor dysfunction plays an important role in reducing responsiveness for vasopressin production following stimuli that normally would increase plasma vasopressin. Vasopressin is likely to contribute to systemic vasoconstriction in heart failure, since several studies with a vasopressin V_1 antagonist indicate significant vasodilating effects and an improvement in cardiac pump function in patients with heart failure.

Natriuretic peptides

Basically, the natriuretic peptides can be viewed as opposing the effects of the sympathetic system, angiotensin II, and endothelin. They have vasodilating properties and inhibit vascular and, possibly, cardiac growth. In addition, they oppose the effects of the renin-angiotensin system and may enhance baroreceptor sensitivity, thereby reducing increased norepinephrine release in heart failure. Natriuretic pepides, in particular ANP, promote diuresis and natriuresis. ANP is predominantly formed in the atria (right more than left), whereas BNP is predominantly formed in the ventricles and CNP in endothelial cells. ANP and BNP production increase markedly after a cardiac insult such as after MI, and early during the transition from left ventricular dysfunction to heart failure, the local production of BNP in the left ventricle surpasses the increase in ANP at that site. In addition, natriuretic peptides are an early marker of left ventricular dysfunction, both cardiac and systemic ANP levels preceding those of other neurohormones, including norepinephrine, epinephrine, and angiotensin II. As such, natriuretic peptides such as ANP and BNP are early markers of left ventricular dysfunction and heart failure. In addition, the level of natriuretic peptide increase confers prognostic significance following MI or in patients with heart failure. It has been suggested that activation of ANP may modulate activation of other neurohormonal systems, at least during the early phase of the heart failure process. Changes in wall stress and dilatation of the heart induce cardiac natriuretic peptide secretion, although this effect may disappear over time. Thus, during a first episode of acute heart failure, a small rise in right atrial pressure results in significant ANP production, which does not further increase on a much larger increase in atrial pressure when chronic heart failure is present. Nevertheless, a correlation remains between plasma and/or cardiac venous atrial natriuretic peptide levels and cardiac function.

Cardiac remodeling

Cardiac remodeling can be defined as molecular changes and changes in myocardial gene expression that are manifested clinically as changes in size, shape, and function of the heart following cardiac injury and/or hemodynamic stress. This is a progressive process that continues even after the initial injury resolves and results in progressive systolic and diastolic dysfunction. The key components at the microscopic level include myocyte hypertrophy, interstitial fibrosis, and cell loss due to necrosis and/or apoptosis. At the macroscopic level this will lead to increased left ventricular volume and mass, a change in the shape of the left ventricle (becoming more spherical than elliptical), and as a result, systolic and diastolic dysfunction with mitral and/or tricuspid regurgitation. Other contributors to left ventricular remodeling include systolic and diastolic overload (wall stress), sympathetic activation (norepinephrine), endothelin, aldosterone, cytokines, apoptosis, decreased nitric oxide production, and oxidative stress (Tab. 26.2).

Remodeling of the heart is an early phenomenon, often linked to cardiac necrosis resulting from MI. In the acute phase, at the site of necrosis the damaged cells lengthen,

---

Table 26.2 Determinants of cardiac remodeling

Myocardial infarction
Systolic pressure overload, e.g.; hypertension, aortic valve stenosis
Diastolic pressure overload, e.g.; mitral and tricuspid insufficiency
Sympathetic activation
Local tissue renin-angiotensin activation
Cardiac endothelin
Aldosterone
Cytokine activation
iNOS/NO-O
Oxidative stress
Apoptosis

(iNOS = inducibile nitric oxide synthase.)

---

the ventricular wall thins, and infarct zone expansion occurs. This is followed at the site of necrosis by inflammation and reabsorption of dead tissue, scar formation, and continuing expansion of the site of necrosis. Thereafter, a chronic phase in the remodeling process can be observed, where at a remote site from the initial injury dilatation and reshaping of the left ventricle occur as well as hypertrophy. As a consequence, left ventricular mass increases, left ventricular volumes increase; the left ventricle becomes spherical, and the ejection fraction progressively declines. The result of this left ventricular remodeling process is that systolic wall tension and stress increase, as do diastolic wall tension and stress. Thus, myocardial oxygen consumption increases at a time when subendocardial coronary perfusion diminishes. The hemodynamic consequences are reduced fractional shortening and left ventricular ejection fraction, mitral regurgitation, and abnormalities in depolarization, leading to arrhythmias. Several clinical studies have indicated a relationship between adverse events and the increase in ventricular size following myocardial injury. In addition, a relation between mortality and the decline in systolic function exists. Thus, mortality is higher in patients with the greatest decrease in ejection fraction. Although there may not be a direct temporal relationship between the remodeling process and worsening of heart failure, in general, all patients with major adverse remodeling eventually experience progressive worsening of cardiac function. However, disease progression may occur in the absence of cardiac remodeling, because mechanisms other than the remodeling process per se have an impact on the course of disease. Nevertheless, the process of cardiac remodeling may underlie a sizable proportion of cardiovascular morbidity and mortality. Indeed, therapies that modulate the remodeling process, such as ACE inhibition, β-blockade, and carvedilol, have all shown a beneficial effect on morbidity and mortality in heart failure.

Cytokines

Activation of the immune system has been implicated in cardiac contractile dysfunction observed in conditions of septic shock, myocarditis, and cardiac allograft rejection. Several cytokines, including tumor necrosis factor α(TNFα), interleukin 2 (IL-2), and IL-6, may induce contractile dysfunction. The underlying mechanisms are not fully understood but may include increased cardiac myocyte inducible nitric oxide synthase (iNOS) activity and subsequent nitric oxide (NO) production in the heart.

In heart failure, circulating levels of TNFα increase with progressive heart failure as well as soluble TNF receptors. Although this increase may merely reflect the severity of the disease, overexpression of the cytokine may lead to cardiac dysfunction and cardiomyopathy and may be related to the occurrence of cachexia in severe heart failure.

In healthy animals, pathophysiologically relevant concentrations of TNFα lead to a time-dependent reduction in cardiac contractile behavior and to left ventricular enlargement, indicating a potential role in cardiac remodeling. In addition, transgenic mice with myocardial TNFα expression develop cardiac failure. The administration of a soluble TNFα antagonist partially restores the negative effect of the cytokine on cardiac function and size. Moreover, in vitro and in vivo studies indicate that agents such as amiodarone and amlodipine may reduce cytokine production and lower circulating cytokine levels.

Preliminary data with a TNFα receptor antagonist in patients with heart failure indicate significant improvements in left ventricular ejection fraction and in heart failure symptoms.

Apoptosis

Part of the remodeling process in heart failure, at least that which results from ischemic heart disease, is due to cardiac cell loss, either through necrosis or by apoptosis, or programmed cell death. Apoptosis is activated by various factors, including ischemia and oxidative stress, mechanical stress, cytokines, and certain neuropeptides such as angiotensin II. The precise contribution of apoptosis to heart failure is difficult to assess, partly because reported incidences show marked variability depending on the techniques used to identify the process.

Oxidative stress and heart failure

Oxygen-derived free radical production is a process common to ischemia-reperfusion and stunning. In contrast, its occurrence in heart failure has less extensively been studied. Nevertheless, since myocardial ischemia is the key etiologic process for heart failure, it has been suggested that oxidative stress induced by repetitive episodes of acute ischemia could be involved in the progression of the disease into heart failure. Potential sources of free radicals in the myocardium include a reduced state of mitochondrial carriers following partial degradation of the adenine nucleotide pool, leading to an increase in electron leakage from the respiratory chain, superoxide production by xanthine oxidase following increased hypoxanthine levels during ischemia, autoxidation of catecholamines, and superoxide production by activated neutrophils. Whether oxidative stress occurs following production of oxygen free radicals depends on the efficacy of the natural antioxidant network in the heart, which includes enzymes such as superoxide dismutase (SOD), catalase, and glutathione peroxidase and endogenous antioxidants such as ascorbic acid, cysteine, and vitamin E. During prolonged ischemia and following reperfusion, several of these antioxidant systems are under stress, including SOD and the glutathione system. Oxidative stress may occur and lead to various degrees of cell damage. Through oxidation of GSH groups in proteins and enzymes, irreversible damage leading to stunning may occur. Extensive oxidative stress may lead to irreversible damage and necrosis, and of interest, excessive oxygen free radicals may induce apoptosis. Several lines of evidence indicate that oxygen free radical production is linked to apoptosis. For instance, oxygen free radical–mediated DNA damage may lead to accumulation of p53, which is associated with apoptosis.

In addition, oxygenated derivatives of arachidonic acid, i.e., hydroperoxyeicosatetraenoic acids (HPETEs), are potent inducers of apoptosis. HPETEs are possibly involved in TNF-mediated programmed cell death. Since the cytokine TNF is increased in heart failure, this may be one of the links between oxidative stress, apoptosis, and heart failure. In addition, TNF causes expression of inducible nitric oxide synthase (iNOS), leading to production of NO, a free radical in itself, but also readily binding with molecular O_2 to form O·. Thus, links can be made between activation of TNFα and its receptors during heart failure, induction of oxygen-derived free radicals (including NO and O·), oxidative stress, and apoptosis. Oxidative stress may have deleterious effects on the heart, leading to contractile dysfunction, cell loss, and cardiac remodeling, but also in the vascular wall, particularly the endothelium, where endothelial dysfunction and apoptosis occur. Pharmacologic developments aimed at one or all three of these factors would be important in preventing worsening heart failure. In this regard, several experiments indicate that carvedilol may be a strong antioxidant, able to inhibit apoptosis in the myocardium, a process that may underlie its beneficial clinical effects in this syndrome.

Treatment

Drug therapy

Treatment options and drugs under development or evaluation are given in Table 26.3.

ACE inhibitors

ACE inhibitors have clearly become the cornerstone of heart failure therapy. Controlled trials indicate beneficial effects on morbidity, improved survival, and retardation of left ventricular remodeling (i.e., left ventricular volume

---

Table 26.3 Pharmacological treatment of heart failure

Currently accepted pharmacologic heart failure therapy
1. Angiotensin converting enzyme inhibitors (ACE inhibitors)
2. Beta-adrenoceptor antagonists
3. Diuretics
4. Cardiac glycosides
5. Vasodilator agents
6. Aldosterone receptor antagonists
7. Positive inotropic agents

Drugs under development/evaluation
1. Angiotensin II receptor antagonists
2. Renin inhibitors
3. Arginine vasopressin (AVP) antagonists
4. Endothelin receptor antagonists
5. Neutral endopeptidase inhibitors
6. h-BNP
7. Metabolic therapy

Table 26.4 Target and maintenance ACE inhibitor doses in large, controlled mortality trials with a positive outcome

	Drug	Target dose	Mean daily dose
Heart failure studies			
Consensus I, 1987	Enalapril	20 mg bid	18.4 mg
V-HeFT II, 1991	Enalapril	10 mg bid	15.0 mg
SOLVD, 1991	Enalapril	10 mg bid	16.6 mg
Post-MI studies with ALVD/CHF			
Save, 1992	Captopril	50 mg tid	NA
AIRE, 1992	Ramipril	5 mg bid	NA
TRACE, 1992	Trandolapril	4 mg qd	NA

(ALVD= asymptomatic left ventricular dysfunction; NA = not available.)

enlargement). Improved survival has been noted in mild, moderate, and severe heart failure, whereas a reduction in hospitalization for heart failure occurs in each phase. In patients with asymptomatic left ventricular dysfunction, ACE inhibitors prevent or retard the occurrence of symptomatic heart failure, as indicated by hospitalizations for this syndrome. In this subset there is no effect on mortality, though. Moreover, in patients with left ventricular dysfunction with an MI, ACE inhibitors reduce subsequent occurrence of heart failure and, in those with symptomatic heart failure post-MI, significantly improve survival. ACE inhibition significantly improves symptoms in patients with heart failure and may increase exercise capacity, although the latter is not observed consistently.

This discrepancy in the effect on symptoms versus on the progression of worsening heart failure reflects the mode of action of ACE inhibition. Either through modulation of local or circulating angiotensin II formation or by increasing bradykinin, ACE inhibitors modulate the cardiac remodeling process. In addition, ACE inhibition leads to reduced sympathetic activity and suppression of endothelin activation.

A major component of the beneficial effects of ACE inhibition may link to its anti-ischemic effects, which are identified following long-term treatment with these agents. In studies such as SOLVD and SAVE, after treatment over 6 or 12 months, a significant reduction in

recurring MI and/or unstable angina has been noted. Concomitant with the effect on heart failure, the anti-ischemic properties of ACE inhibition relate to an improvement in abnormal endothelial function, reduced neointima proliferation, and antiatherosclerotic effects. It is likely that these long-term structural anti-ischemic properties are due primarily to the increase in bradykinin or activation of bradykinin B2 reception by ACE inhibitors. Furthermore, ACE inhibition may lead to normalization of an abnormal balance between PAI-1 and t-PA, leading to fewer thrombotic episodes in concert with antiplatelet aggregating effects through a further increase in bradykinin and nitric oxide. Besides these long-term structural effects on the vascular wall, ACE inhibition, by reducing cardiac volumes, may improve myocardial oxygen demand, thereby lessening the potential for ischemia. Furthermore, it has been shown that ischemia-induced neurohormonal activation may be modulated by ACE inhibition, thereby leading to less systemic and coronary

Table 26.6 Recommended procedure for initiating ACE inhibitor therapy

1. Start with a low dose and increase dose to maintenance lavels shown to be effective in large trials (see Tab. 26.5)
2. Avoid excessive diuretic treatment before initiation of ACE inhibition, stop diuretics for 24 hours before start of treatment
3. Monitor renal function and electrolytes during the titration phase every 3-5 days until stable, thereafter every 3-6 months. Renal function deterioration may occur, but only requires interruption of treatment when substantial and/or rapidly fast occurring
4. During initiation blood pressure control is advisable when given in the morning, thereafter check blood pressure 1-2 weeks after dose increments
5. Avoid potassium-sparing diuretics. Potassium-sparing diuretics should only be considered with persisting hypokalemia. Irrespective of potassium levels spironolactone should be considered in NYHA III-IV after stabilisation of ACE inhibitor therapy
6. Avoid non steroidal anti-inflammatory drugs (NSAIDs)

Table 26.5 ACE inhibitor starting and maintenance dose ranges

Drug	Target dose	Mean daily dose
Benazepril	2.5 mg	5-10 mg bid
Captopril	6.25 mg tid	25-50 mg tid
Enalapril	2.5 mg	10 mg bid
Lisinopril	2.5 mg	5-20 mg qd
Perindopril	2 mg	5-10 mg bid
Quinapril	2.5-5 mg	4 mg
Ramipril	1.25-2.5 mg	2.5-5 mg bid

Table 26.7 Comparative pharmacology and effect on underlying mechanisms of progressive ventricular dysfunction of β_1-blockade, carvedilol and ACE inhibition, the three main classes of drugs proven to reduce mortality in heart failure

Modulation of neurohormones	β_1-blockade sympathetic > RAS	ACE inhibition RAS > sympathetic	Carvedilol RAS > sympathetic
Cardiac antiadrenergic	+	±	+
Alpha$_1$-blockade	–	–	+
Bradykinin/NO production	–	++	–
Antioxidant	–	+?	++
Inhibition of neutrophil recruitment	–	–	+
Anti-ischemic	++	+	++
Inhibition of apoptosis	–	±?	+
Modulation of cardiac remodeling	+	++	++

(RAS = renin angiotensin system; NO = nitric oxide.)

vasoconstriction during ischemia. These different mechanisms in concert are likely to significantly decrease the occurrence of myocardial ischemic events. Adverse events induced by ACE inhibition are renal insufficiency, hyperkalemia, hypertension, and edema. Except for the latter and bilateral arterial stenosis, there are, however, no absolute contraindications to initiation of ACE inhibitor treatment in heart failure. Often, hypertension, renal insufficiency, and hyperkalemia can be counteracted by slower drug titration and/or a reduction in dosage. However, the risk of hypertension and renal dysfunction increases in patients with severe heart failure, elderly patients, patients with renal dysfunction or hypernatremia, and patients receiving high dosages of diuretics. A common side effect related to bradykinin is dry cough. This may lead to withdrawal of the ACE inhibitor in approximately 15% of patients. However, in heart failure this condition is often difficult to distinguish from cough resulting from pulmonary congestion.

The optimal dose levels of ACE inhibition in heart failure are not really known. Thus far, recommendations are based on dosages that have been shown effective in the large, controlled trials (Tab. 26.4). As a consequence, the Guidelines for Treatment of Heart Failure, as published by the Task Force of the Working Group on Heart Failure of the European Society of Cardiology, suggest that ACE inhibition dosages should be increased to the target

dosages in the large, controlled trials (Tabs. 26.4 and 26.5). Preliminary data from the ATLAS trial, which compares low- (5 mg) versus high-dose (30 mg) lisinopril in heart failure, would suggest that a high dose of ACE inhibition would be better than a low dose. Although in this study the primary endpoint, a reduction in mortality, was not reached, there was a trend toward a better effect with the higher dosage and, in addition, a significantly lower hospitalization rate with the higher dosage. The side-effect profile was comparable between the low- and high-dose groups. The recommended procedure for starting an ACE inhibitor as indicated by the European Guidelines for Treatment of Heart Failure, is given in Table 26.6.

β-Blockers

Recent large, controlled studies have now without any doubt proven that long-term β-blockade has significant beneficial effects in most heart failure patients, irrespective of the underlying etiology. The US carvedilol program, CIBIS II, and provisionally, MERIT indicate that either β_1-adrenergic blockade (e.g., metoprolol, bisoprolol) or the nonselective β-adrenergic blocker and antioxidant drug carvedilol improve mortality in patients with mild, moderate, and possibly severe heart failure. Furthermore, they significantly reduce all-cause and cardiovascular hospitalizations and markedly improve car-

Table 26.8 Initiating dose, target dose and titration scheme of β-blocking agents in placebo-controlled large trials

β-Blockers	First dose (mg)	Titration scheme Total daily dose (mg)									Target dose Total daily dose (mg)
Metoprolol (MCD trial)	5	wk 1 10	wk 2 15	wk 3 30	wk 4 50	wk 5 75	wk 6 100	wk 7 150			100-150
Bisoprolol (CIBIS II)	1.25	wk 1 1.25	wk 2 2.5	wk 3 3.75	wk 4-7 5				wk 8-11 7.5	wk 12-15 10	10
Carvedilol (US trials)	3.125	wk 1 6.26	wk 2	wk 3 12.5	wk 4	wk 5 25	wk 6	wk 7 50			50

diac function, as indicated by a significant improvement in left ventricular ejection fraction. In addition, carvedilol reduces left ventricular volumes when administered in addition to ACE inhibition. In contrast, ACE inhibition alone in the latter studies had no such effect. Several smaller, controlled studies also indicate a significant improvement in left ventricular function, and overall, patients appeared to feel better. However, exercise capacity did not change in most studies, although there was a tendency toward improvement in submaximal exercise capacity. A significant correlation appears present between the negative chronotropic activity of β-blockade and its effect on maximal exercise performance. Thus, β_1-selective agents such as metoprolol, which also induces β_1-receptor upregulation during long-term treatment in heart failure, in contrast to nonselective agents such as carvedilol, allow a relative preservation of the chronotropic response to exercise. Since left ventricular function also improves, this contributes to improvements in peak exercise capacity observed with this agent. A large trial studied the effect of metoprolol on exercise capacity. The MDC trial observed an improvement in exercise capacity after long-term treatment (12 months) but not after 6 months of treatment.

The underlying mechanisms for the beneficial effects of long-term β-blockade in heart failure are several and include anti-ischemic effects, direct antiarrhythmic effects, modulation of sympathetic overactivation, protection against direct catecholamine-induced myocardial necrosis, decreased renin-angiotensin activity, and lowering of heart rate. The latter may be important, since in vitro studies indicate that, in contrast with normal tissue, increases in the stimulation frequency do not improve contractility or relaxation in myopathic tissue. In fact, with high frequencies, contractility and relaxation decline, and an optimum may be present at lower frequencies of 40 to 60 beats per minute. This would suggest that a reduction in heart rate per se induced by β-blockade may be beneficial in heart failure.

Agents that induce β_1-blocking properties in addition upregulate the β_1-receptor, which is downregulated in heart failure. Although this may improve chronotropic responsiveness and exercise capacity, increased β_1-receptor density and, possibly, responsiveness also may increase the risk of further negative effects of sympathetic overactivation on the heart. In studies that compared the effects of chronic β_1-selective blockade with metoprolol versus nonselective blockade with carvedilol, cardiac norepinephrine release indicated a reduction with the latter but unchanged norepinephrine release from the heart during long-term metoprolol administration. Nonselective β-blockade therefore may be a better choice in the treatment of heart failure. In addition, other properties may add to this pharmacologic profile. In the case of carvedilol, this would include β-blockade, which leads to vasodilatation, left ventricular unloading, and antiremodeling effects and strong antioxidant and anti-inflammatory actions, which include less oxidative stress, iNOS production, recruit-

ment of adhesion molecules, and possibly apoptosis. This complex profile theoretically would favor carvedilol in the treatment of heart failure over β_1-selective blockade. This hypothesis is currently being tested in the large COMET study, which compares the effects of carvedilol versus metoprolol in addition to standard heart failure treatment, including ACE inhibition and diuretics, on overall mortality rate as primary endpoint. The profile of carvedilol leads to another interesting hypothesis, i.e., that carvedilol may be as good as or possibly better than ACE inhibition where heart failure is concerned. In terms of mechanisms leading to cardiac remodeling, the pharmacologic profile of carvedilol may indeed compare favorably with that of an ACE inhibitor (Tab. 26.7). This hypothesis is tested in the CARMEN trial, which compares the effect of carvedilol alone versus ACE inhibition (enalapril) alone versus the combination on cardiac remodeling (left ventricular volumes and ejection fraction) and morbidity in patients with mild to moderate heart failure.

The objective of β-blockade in heart failure is to prevent or revert cardiac remodeling and worsening of heart failure, including mortality. It does not aim at an immediate effect on symptoms. Thus, β-blockade is initiated at very low dosages and titrated only to dosages that have been shown to be effective in the various trials (Tab. 26.8). Initiation should always be carried out under stable conditions. If so, titration is well tolerated in most patients, although a slight but significant increase in worsening heart failure or vasodilating hypertension or dizziness with the vasodilation has been observed. Often these can be counteracted by manipulating other heart failure drugs or by temporarily reducing the β-blocking dose. In the US carvedilol studies, the initial increase in hospitalizations for heart failure during the uptitration phase was significantly offset thereafter by a much greater reduction in hospitalizations during chronic carvedilol treatment. As with ACE inhibition, the optimal dosage of β-blockade in heart failure is as yet not defined. However, the MOCHA trial indicates that carvedilol leads to a dose-related increase in ejection fraction and a dose-related decrease in mortality, supporting the aims of the large, controlled trials to administer β-blockade in relatively high dosages.

Diuretics

In contrast to ACE inhibition and β-blockade, diuretics are only indicated for symptomatic treatment. They have no proven benefit where the prevention of (worsening) heart failure is concerned. In fact, since diuretic treatment may lead to neurohormonal activation, the argument could be that they may activate the remodeling process and thereby worsen heart failure. Alternatively, by reducing cardiac volumes and wall stress, they should lead to less remodeling. Diuretics probably should be viewed as supportive treatment in heart failure, necessary when fluid retention is present, manifest as lung congestion and peripheral edema. In the absence of these, it is questionable whether diuretics should be administered at all. Indeed, the Guidelines for Treatment of Heart Failure strongly advocate that administration of diuretics should be related to the presence or absence of fluid retention.

Thus diuretics should not be first-line treatment but should follow the administration of ACE inhibitors. The choice between a thiazide or a loop diuretic in mild heart failure is not a crucial one. However, when heart failure progresses, a loop diuretic is usually necessary. In addition, thiazide diuretics are less effective with declining renal function if the glomerular filtration rate falls below 30 ml/min and are therefore less useful in the elderly patients, in whom renal function usually is diminished. With persistent fluid retention and insufficient response of the diuretic, the dose should first be increased, and subsequently, with persistent fluid retention, loop diuretics should be administered twice daily. If fluid retention still persists, loop diuretics and thiazides can be combined, and in more severe heart failure, metolazone or spironolactone can be added.

Potassium-sparing diuretics such as triamterene and amiloride should not be prescribed in the presence of an ACE inhibitor unless there is persistent hypokalemia. In the latter situation, oral potassium supplements are less effective than potassium-sparing diuretics.

Digitalis glycosides

Digitalis glycosides are potent and highly specific inhibitors of membrane Na^+,K^+-ATPase. Subsequent enhanced Na^+ influx in the cell leads to exchange for Ca^{2+} by the Na^+/Ca^{2+} exchanger, resulting in increased intracellular calcium in the cardiocyte leading to increased inotropic force and in the vascular muscle cell leading to vasoconstriction. In addition, nanomolar concentrations of cardiac glycosides may alter the ion selectivity of sarcolemmal Na^+ channels, leading to immediate Ca^{2+} influx through a mechanism termed *slip-mode conductance*. At therapeutic levels digitalis decreases automaticity and increases the diastolic potential, whereas at higher dosages it increases automaticity and decreases the maximum diastolic potential. The latter and the increase in intracellular calcium, which leads to overloading of the calcium stores and spontaneous oscillatory release, underlie the arrhythmogenic potential of digitalis glycosides. Of interest, in heart failure, therapeutic dosages of digitalis modify the enhanced sympathetic tone. Acute digitalization with lanatoside significantly reduces sympathetic nerve activity and leads to vasodilatation instead of the vasoconstriction observed in healthy persons.

For many centuries digitalis has been the heart failure drug of choice. However, this role has now passed on to ACE inhibitors and β-blockers. Indeed, guidelines are careful to mention that there is always a role for digitalis in patients with symptomatic heart failure and atrial fibrillation, but not necessarily for patients in sinus rhythm. The reason is the narrow window between possible effects and certain adverse events. Patients with increased digitalis levels, reached because of reduced renal clearance (digoxin), hepatic insufficiency (digitoxin), or comedication with antiarrhythmics (amiodarone), frequently have adverse events, in particular serious arrhythmias. Since the therapeutic efficacy in terms of increased inotropy is questionable, this is important. Nevertheless, several medium-sized studies, such as PROVED and RADIANCE, examining the effect of withdrawal of digoxin in stable NYHA II and III heart failure patients in sinus rhythm, suggested significant worsening of symptoms compared with patients who continued. This potential beneficial effect may be due to the reduction in sympathetic overactivation caused by the drug rather than to its positive inotropic effect. Digoxin does not negatively affect mortality, nor does it improve it. In the large DIG study in approximately 6800 patients, half on active treatment, digitalis had no effect on survival. There was a trend to fewer deaths due to worsening heart failure, offset by more patients dying from other cardiac causes, including tachyarrhythmias and bradyarrhythmias. Significantly fewer patients were hospitalized for worsening chronic heart failure (CHF), the relative risk greater in patients with more severe CHF and lower ejection fractions.

The current perception of the use of digoxin in sinus rhythm would include patients with more severe heart failure not sufficiently responding to ACE inhbition, diuretics, and β-blockade. Judicious use of digoxin, recognizing the potential of increased serum levels under certain conditions, remains important (Tab. 26.9).

Vasodilators

Following the concept of increased vasal tone being a hallmark of (advanced) heart failure, many attempts have been made to develop efficient vasodilators, without much success. Taking for granted that ACE inhibitors, or for that matter other relevant neurohormonal antagonists such as angiotensin II antagonists or endothelin antago-

---

Table 26.9 Digitalis glycosides in stable CHF due to systolic dysfunction-recommendations

Digoxin
Initiating dose: 0.25 mg bid for 2 days, thereafter 0.25-0.375 mg daily (normal renal function)
Elderly: 0.0625-0.125 mg maintenance dose (occasionally 0.25 mg) depending on (low) digoxin levels. Starting dose: 0.625 mg
Renal dysfuction: digoxin clearance approximates creatinine clearance (Cockroft and Gault formula: creatinine clearance=(140–age) x weight (kg) / 72 x serum creatinine (mg, 100 ml^{-1}) (see Chap. 21)

Digitoxin
Oral loading dose 0.3 mg/day for 3 days, maintenance daily dose 0.07-0.1 mg

Monitoring digoxin levels
Elderly
Renal insufficiency
Co-medication: amiodarone, quinidine, verapamil
Insufficient drug effect
Suspected overdose

Monitoring digitoxin levels
Significant hepatic dysfunction

nists, should not be classified as vasodilators, very few compounds have really stood up to the test.

A major problem of any vasodilator without adequate antivasoconstricting hormonal properties is tachyphylaxis and tolerance. Thus early studies with α-adrenergic antagonists, notably prazosin, indicated early loss of their initial vasodilating properties. In the V-HeFT I study, this compound was subsequently shown to be without any effect on survival, whereas in contrast, the combination of hydralazine and nitrates significantly improved it. In a subsequent trial by the same investigators, this combination, however, proved inferior to the ACE inhibitor enalapril, given the same endpoint. Since the effects of nitrates and hydralazine were fully comparable in both studies of the same design and patient profile, a prudent comparison can be made, indicating no effect with prazosin and placebo, a better effect with the combination of nitrates and hydralazine, and a superior effect with ACE inhibition.

The problem with the combination is that high dosages of each compound are probably necessary, for hydralazine up to 300 mg and for nitrates up to 160 mg, introducing the problem of side effects and tolerability. Nevertheless, in situations where ACE inhibitors cannot be given, this combination may be an alternative. There are no data on the efficacy of hydralazine and nitrates in addition to ACE inhibition. To coadminister these together with ACE inhibitors theoretically may improve the patient, since the effect of the combination on cardiac function as well as on exercise capacity was shown to be better in the V-HeFT II study than with enalapril. However, no data are known on the overall effect on mortality and morbidity. Besides, in more advanced heart failure, low blood pressures may make coadministration of ACE inhibition and nitrates and hydralazine in sufficiently high dosages difficult.

Nitrates alone are often administered to patients with CHF, but the data to support this are not there. This is similarly true for hydralazine. Nevertheless, nitrates and hydralazine on their own may be prescribed for coexisting angina or hypertension, respectively.

Tachyphylaxis is a problem with nitrates in heart failure, as it is in ischemic heart disease, depending on the frequency of administration. A dosing interval of 8 to 12 hours should be introduced. Hydralazine appears to diminish the hemodynamic tolerance observed with nitrates alone, a possible mechanism in the beneficial effect of the combination.

Thus far *calcium antagonists* have not proven successful in the treatment of heart failure. Nondihydropyridine derivatives and the first-generation, immediate-acting dihydropyridines generally led to deterioration of hemodynamic and neurohormonal status of CHF. In contrast, the later-generation, slow-acting dihydropyridines have either no effect or a positive effect in selected patient populations. In V-HeFT III study, felodipine did not affect mortality or morbidity outcomes. In PRAISE I, amlodipine improved patients with idiopathic dilated cardiomyopathy. Of interest, there are suggestions that the latter drug may reduce cytokine activity in animal models

of myocarditis. A large prospective study with amlodipine, PRAISE II, is currently investigating the potential of this drug in CHF. Since in both PRAISE I and V-HeFT III calcium antagonists proved to be safe, their use can be recommended in patients with concomitant hypertension.

Aldosterone receptor antagonists

Old drugs, if they stay around long enough, may lead to new concepts in disease management. This is certainly true for spironolactone, long viewed as a potassium-sparing diuretic, but recently setting the stage for the development of a novel class in cardiovascular therapy, the selective aldosterone receptor antagonists (SARAs).

Aldosterone in the past was viewed as part of the renin-angiotensin-aldosterone system and as such received little attention on its own. It was believed to be sufficiently modulated by ACE inhibition. Now it has attracted growing interest and recognition as an important pathophysiologic mechanism in left ventricular hypertrophy and heart failure. In addition to H_2O/Na^+ retention and Mg^{2+} and K^+ loss, aldosterone is pivotal in the development of cardiac fibrosis; it reduces cardiac catecholamine uptake, reduces high-density lipoprotein (HDL) cholesterol, is involved in endothelial dysfunction, and may mediate intimal hyperplasia following angioplasty. Together these actions may significantly contribute to the development of ventricular dysfunction and heart failure and the occurrence of arrhythmias and myocardial ischemia in this setting. Spironolactone modulates these actions, as observed in various experimental settings. Since several studies have indicated that chronic ACE inhibition does not sufficiently suppress circulating aldosterone levels in hypertension and heart failure and preliminary data indicate that this is also true with angiotensin II antagonist treatment in CHF, aldosterone receptor blockade appears appropriate under these conditions. Indeed, already in the RALES dose-finding study, low-dose (25-50 mg) spironolactone therapy was found to reduce circulating ANP levels, a marker of efficacy in CHF, besides being well tolerated and not leading to hyperkalemia or renal insufficiency when administered together with ACE inhibitors.

The subsequent RALES mortality trial, which included approximately 1500 patients with advanced CHF on ACE inhibition and full diuretic therapy, was discontinued prematurely because of a very significant positive effect of spironolactone on survival as well as cardiovascular hospitalizations and worsening heart failure. This trial signifies the role of aldosterone receptor antagonism in addition to ACE inhibition and has set the stage for the evaluation of more selective antagonists, e.g., eplerenone, which lacks the hormonal side effects of spironolactone. Preliminary data indicate that the latter is efficacious in hypertension, while studies in heart failure are in progress.

Positive inotropes

Positive inotropes other than digitalis glycosides have been developed and tested extensively in the context of heart failure during the last two decades, the conviction being that where a diminished contractile function of the heart was at the basis of the disease, any intervention that could improve inotropy should have merits. Unfortunately, this has by and large not proven to be the case, not until recently, that is.

Basically, pharmacologic interventions to increase contractile force and/or contractility can be viewed as either cAMP-dependent or cAMP-independent.

cAMP-dependent drugs, the oldest to be developed, increase cAMP through increased β-adrenergic receptor stimulation or by decreasing its breakdown by cAMP-specific type III phosphodiesterases (PDEs). cAMP formation depends on the activity of adenyl cyclase, which is governed by the stimulatory β-adrenergic versus inhibitory muscarinic or adenosine receptors and the stimulatory versus inhibitory G-protein systems. Increased cAMP leads to increased cellular calcium influx through voltage-dependent calcium channels, subsequently inducing significant calcium release from ryanodine-sensitive calcium release channels in the sarcoplasmatic reticulum (SR). This enhances calcium availability to the contractile proteins and force development. cAMP increases myosin ATPase activity and contractility. Finally, it stimulates calcium uptake by the SR by protein kinase–induced activation of troponin I (reduction in calcium sensitivity) and phospholamban (calcium reuptake by SR), respectively.

Thus, both contractility and relaxation are under the direct positive influence of the second messenger cAMP, at least in the normal heart. In heart failure, several intrinsic changes diminish this potential significantly and underlie the lack of significant effect observed with cAMP-dependent inotropes. Heart failure is characterized by reduced β-receptor responsiveness due to diminished β_1-receptor density, increased β-AR kinase activity and β-receptor uncoupling, and enhanced expression of the inhibitory G-protein (G1α protein).

Thus, agents such as sympathomimetic drugs are less efficient. In addition, forskolin stimulation of adenylate cyclase activity may be reduced.

As regards PDE activity, both soluble and particulate cGMP-inhibited, cAMP-specific PDE isoforms are reduced by 30 to 50% in CHF, explaining the diminished efficacy of PDE inhibitors such as milrinone and enoximone. Consequently, hemodynamics do not consistently improve with orally active cAMP-dependent inotropes. Although this was suggested by initial, uncontrolled, short-term studies, it could not be confirmed in later, controlled, longer-term trials. Hemodynamic tolerance may occur, at least with the PDE inhibitors, after only a few weeks of treatment, most likely the result of diminishing vasodilating capacity (the result of vascular PDE inhibition) over time. Moreover, as with other CHF treatment modalities, hemodynamic efficacy does not necessarily imply improved exercise capacity, morbidity, or survival. Most studies with long-term cAMP-dependent inotropic therapy lack significant improvement in exercise capacity and, worse, all lead to significantly increased mortality. Consequently, these agents have not been further developed in heart failure, with the exception of short-term parenteral treatment in severe end-stage CHF, with a view on bridging the patient to cardiac transplantation.

cAMP-independent agents increase contractile force either by increasing cardiac cellular calcium influx or by improving calcium sensitivity toward the contractile apparatus. Increased calcium influx can be achieved by stimulating sarcolemmal sodium channels, stimulating Na+,K+-ATPase (digitalis glycosides), prolonging the action potential by blocking the delayed rectifier outward potassium channel, or administering dihydropyridine-type calcium channel enhancers and α-adrenergic agents. Of these, the sodium channel enhancers have generated the most interest in humans (besides digitalis). Vesnarinone, a complex molecule combining sodium channel stimulatory and potassium channel-blocking properties with selective PDE inhibition, has been studied extensively. Whereas initial, smaller, controlled studies indicated a beneficial effect, a subsequent larger, controlled study found a sig-

Table 26.10 Agents with calcium-sensitizing properties

	Ca²⁺-sensitizing	PDE-inhibiting	Na⁺ channel	Other
Drug evaluated in humans				
Sulmazole	+	+		
Isomazole	+	+		
UK-61.260	+?	+		
MCI-154	+	+		
Org 30029	+	+		
DPI 201-106	+		+	
Levosimendan	+			K-channel agonist
Drugs not evaluated in humans				
EMD 57033	+	-		
SCH 00013	+	+?		

(PDE = phosphodiesterase.)

nificant increase in mortality, even in the smaller dose range. Nevertheless, the compound has been shown to modulate cytokine activation, and studies with quinoline derivatives continue.

The reason for the negative effect of vesnarinone is unclear but could be related to its PDE-inhibiting properties, making it a partial cAMP-dependent agent. Also, the increase in cellular calcium may be detrimental, in a similar fashion as with digitalis glycosides, resulting from overloaded SR and arrhythmias.

This problem does not occur with calcium-sensitizing agents. Here, an increase in sensitivity for calcium, usually of troponin C, results in enhanced and, with most agents, prolonged binding, increasing contractile force but at the same time also reducing relaxation. The advantage of calcium-sensitizing agents is that they do not require more calcium to increase contractile force but are effective at normal or even reduced cytosolic calcium levels.

Calcium sensitivity increases on stretching of the cardiocyte, cellular alkalosis, and α-adrenergic stimulation. It decreases with acidosis, elevated inorganic phosphate levels, and following β-adrenergic stimulation. Since the latter are prominent features in heart failure and ischemia, the effect of calcium-sensitizing agents is more pronounced here than under normal conditions. Lowering pH in vitro improves the contractile force of drugs such as pimobendan and MCI-154. In contrast, the contractile force of cAMP-dependent agents (e.g., milrinone) diminishes under these conditions. In addition, calcium-sensitizing agents remain effective or display better effects in advanced CHF, whereas cAMP-dependent agents become more and more ineffective. Finally, increasing inotropy through calcium sensitization is more economic and less energy consuming than through cAMP-dependent actions.

In the clinical arena, calcium sensitizers by and large have shown improvements in hemodynamics as well as in exercise capacity. Unfortunately, since nearly all investigated drugs in this class are hybrids, with PDE-inhibiting effects as well (Tab. 26.10), survival does not improve, but as shown in the largest available study, the PICO trial with pimobendan, there is a tendency toward a similar negative outcome as with the cAMP- dependent drugs.

In addition, there is the negative effect on relaxation to take into account. This may be of less concern with levosimendan, a compound that increases calcium sensitivity as a function of the level of cytosolic calcium, only during the early phase of systole when calcium levels rise, hence not affecting relaxation. Moreover, levosimendan modulates ATP-sensitive potassium channels, reduces endothelin levels, and at the therapeutic dose level, has only minor PDE-inhibiting effects. Currently, clinical outcome studies are under way in severe CHF and in post-MI left ventricular dysfunction that will further define the potential role of this class of positive inotropic drugs in heart failure.

New areas of drug development

Several new pharmacologic developments are sufficiently advanced to consider them potential novel targets of heart failure therapy. However, since final proof from large controlled trials is still lacking, they have as yet not been approved or accepted in current treatment guidelines. The most important in terms of development in this category are angiotensin II receptor antagonists, endothelin receptor antagonists, neutral endopeptidase inhibitors, human b-type natriuretic peptide, and metabolic therapy, including L-propionylcarnitine, coenzyme Q10, and growth hormone.

Angiotensin receptor antagonists (see also Chaps. 22 and 23)

ACE inhibition, although an important step forward in the treatment of heart failure, still is insufficiently effective, with significant numbers of patients dying or being hospitalized for heart failure. In addition, side effects that to some extent may be bradykinin-related, such as cough, prohibit a sizable number of patients from receiving optimal or any ACE inhibitor therapy. Moreover, since ACE inhibition is often prescribed in low dosages, insufficient ACE inhibition and angiotenin II suppression occur. Moreover, angiotensin II formation may occur through other pathways bypassing ACE, thus leading to an escape of angiotensin II production despite appropriate ACE inhibition. The concept that angiotensin II receptor (AT_2 receptor) antagonism could afford an alternative approach to modulate the negative effects of angiotensin II in CHF, mainly mediated by the AT_1 receptor, therefore would seem appropriate. Hemodynamic studies with AT_1 antagonists indicate a dose-dependent persistent reduction in left ventricular filling pressure but no consistent effects on cardiac index. In addition, no consistent long-term effects on neurohormones have been observed, with some studies quoting a reduction in aldosterone and an increase in renin and others not. In medium-term studies comparing ACE inhibitors and AT_1 antagonists in CHF, no difference was observed in the effect on ejection fraction, exercise capacity, and neurohormones. Only the ELITE study, designed to compare primarily the renal effects of losartan and captopril, claimed a significant difference in survival in favor of losartan, a secondary endpoint in the study. The primary endpoint, a difference in renal function in favor of AT antagonist, was not met. This study, underpowered to detect a priori an effect on survival as the primary endpoint, has gained much interest and has led to many CHF patients receiving AT antagonists instead of ACE inhibition, largely because the tolerance to the first is perceived better than to the latter. Whether AT antagonists should be prescribed in heart failure is as yet unclear and needs to be evaluated in large controlled trials, such as ELITE 2 and Val-HeFT, that study different AT receptor antagonists as an alternative or in addition to ACE inhibition. As regards the potential efficacy of AT antagonists, there are a number of concerns. The first concern is the lack of effect on bradykinin, possibly a factor of major therapeutic importance with ACE inhibition. Second is that the alternative pathways for angiotensin II formation, including chymases, may not be relevant in the human heart. Third, the AT$_1$ receptor is downregulated in heart failure, and therefore, effective antagonism is minimized. Fourth, with AT$_1$ receptor antagonism, angiotensin II may preferentially affect the AT$_2$ receptor, which may stimulate apoptosis.

Whether the preceding concerns are real or not needs to be further studied before decisions as to individualized heart failure treatment can be made, granted that the large studies indeed do show a beneficial profile of these agents.

Endothelin antagonists

Several different endothelin (ET) receptor antagonists have been developed and studied in animal models of heart failure and in CHF patients. Both selective ETA antagonists and combined ETA and ETB blockade improve cardiac function in rodent and canine models of heart failure. Long-term treatment (9 months) with bosentan, an ETA and ETB antagonist in rats with heart failure, reduced cardiac dimensions and left ventricular collagen density and improved hemodynamics, in addition to lowering plasma catecholamines and improving survival. A similar but shorter study (8 weeks), observing comparable hemodynamic effects, indicated that bosentan also lowered left ventricular tissue ET-1 levels and ET receptor density. Selective blockade of ETA receptors in a rat CHF model also improved survival. Comparison of selective endothelin ETA and ETB antagonists in a canine heart failure model indicated a potential beneficial effect of the selective ETA antagonist in terms of hemodynamics (improved cardiac output) and increased diuresis and natriuresis, whereas in contrast, the ETB antagonist decreased cardiac output and increased systemic vascular resistance and cardiac filling pressures. In CHF patients, bosentan acutely reduces left ventricular filling pressure and systemic and pulmonary artery pressures without affecting heart rate and increases cardiac output, effects that are sustained for at least 14 days. Long-term effects on mortality and morbidity are not yet available.

Neutral endopeptidase (NEP) inhibitors

Inhibition of NEP, responsible for the rapid breakdown of natriuretic peptides and thereby increasing ANP levels, is a potential useful approach, since the peptide may lead to vasodilation and increased diuresis as well as natriuresis. In patients with mild heart failure, chronic oral administration of the NEP inhibitor candoxatril leads to a sustained increase in ANP levels, hemodynamic improvement, and enhanced diuresis and natriuresis. A recent study in CHF patients on ACE inhibitor therapy indicated that candoxatril also improved exercise capacity, although it did not affect quality-of-life measures.

Long-term NEP and ACE inhibition appears an attractive combination and has led to the development of molecules that combine both actions.

Human b-type natriuretic peptide

Nesiritide is the generic name of a new human b-type natriuretic peptide that causes cGMP-mediated natriuresis, diuresis, and neurohormonal suppression. Preliminary data indicate that nesiritide produces a rapid improvement in symptoms and dose-related increases in cardiac output and reductions in left ventricular filling pressures, comparing well with dobutamine in patients with acute exacerbations of heart failure. The drug is well tolerated, and although parenteral administration is necessary, it offers the possibility of acute CHF therapy without the need of invasive monitoring.

Metabolic therapy

l-Propionyl carnitine Carnitine is pivotal in mediating cellular fatty acid uptake and metabolism. It is located predominantly in cardiac and skeletal muscle. In heart failure, cardiac carnitine levels are decreased, and suppletion has been shown to improve cardiac function in animal models of cardiomyopathy. L-Propionylcarnitine has several advantages over carnitine in that it is more lipophilic and is better taken up by the heart, and it specifically stimulates the Krebs' cycle by an anaploretic action. In patients with asymptomatic left ventricular dysfunction, it acutely improves cardiac function. In several small, controlled studies, long-term oral administration leads to increased exercise capacity, improved left ventricular ejection fraction, and a reduction in left ventricular dimensions. However, a large, long-term, placebo-controlled trial could not confirm these observations. Only in patients with mild impairment of cardiac function was a small improvement in exercise duration noted, but not in those with more severely impaired left ventricular function.

Coenzyme Q10 Coenzyme Q10 is an important constituent of the respiratory chain reaction. In cardiac biopsies of patients with heart failure, coenzyme Q10 levels are significantly reduced, and several animal studies indicate improvement in cardiac function following coenzyme Q10 administration. In addition, hemodynamic improvement has been reported in an open, uncontrolled human study. This could not be confirmed in a long-term controlled study, suggesting that coenzyme Q10 is useful in heart failure dubious.

Growth hormone Growth hormone affects cardiac performance and wall stress by an effect on cardiac growth. Growth hormone deficiency is characterized by a reduction in ventricular wall thickness leading to increased wall stress, whereas cardiac output is decreased. Substitution therapy leads to normalization of wall thickness and improved cardiac function. Enhanced cardiac function may occur through increased calcium influx in the cardiocyte and/or enhanced responsiveness of the myofilaments to calcium.

Several open, uncontrolled studies in heart failure patients indicated acute hemodynamic improvement. Unfortunately, this could not be confirmed in a recent placebo-controlled 3-month study. Although in that study it was found that growth hormone treatment was safe and without significant side effects, no effect on cardiac function or structure was observed.

Suggested readings

CIBIS-II INVESTIGATORS AND COMMITTEES. The Cardiac Insufficiency Bisoprolol Study II (CIBIS-II): a randomised trial. Lancet 1999;353:9-13.

COHN JN, JOHNSON G, ZIESCHE S, et al. A comparison of enalapril with hydralazine-isosorbide dinitrate in the treatment of chronic congestive heart failure. N Engl J Med 1991;325:303-10.

CONSENSUS TRIAL STUDY GROUP. Effects of enalapril on mortality in severe congestive heart failure: results of the north Scandinavian enalapril survival study. N Engl J Med 1987;316:1429-35.

DUPREZ DA, DE BUYZERE ML, RIETZSCHEL ER, et al. Inverse relationship between aldosterone and large artery compliance in chronically treated heart failure patients. Eur Heart J 1998; 19:1371-6.

ISGAARD J, BERGH C-H, CAIDAHL K, et al. A placebo-controlled study of growth hormone in patients with congestive heart failure. Eur Heart J 1998;19:1704-11.

PACKER M, BRISTOW MR, COHN JN, et al, for the Carvedilol Heart Failure Study Group. The effect of carvedilol on morbidity and mortality in patients with chronic heart failure. N Engl J Med 1996;334:1349-55.

PACKER M, O'CONNOR CM, GHALI JK, et al. Effect of amlodipine on morbidity and mortality in severe chronic heart failure: prospective randomized amlodipine survival evaluation (PRAISE) study. N Engl J Med 1996;335:1107-14.

PFEFFER MA, BRAUNWALD E, MOYE LA, et al, for the SAVE Investigators. Effect of captopril on mortality and morbidity in patients with left ventricular dysfunction and myocardial infarction: results of the survival and ventricular enlargement trial. N Engl J Med 1992;327:669-77.

PITT B, SEGAL R, MARTINEZ FA, et al. Randomised trial of losartan versus captopril in patients over 65 with heart failure (evaluation of losartan in the elderly study, ELITE). Lancet 1997;349:747-52.

REMME WJ. Therapeutic strategies and neurohormonal control in heart failure. Eur Heart J 1994;15:129-38.

SWEDBERG K, ENEROTH P, KJEKSHUS J, WILHELMSEM L, for the CONSENSUS Trial Study Group. Hormones regulating cardiovascular function in patients with severe congestive heart failure and their relation to mortality. Circulation 1990;82:1730-6.

THE DIGITALIS INVESTIGATION GROUP. The effect of digoxin on mortality and morbidity in patients with heart failure. N Engl J Med 1997;336:525-35.

THE RALES INVESTIGATORS. Effectiveness of spironolactone added to an angiotensin-converting enzyme inhibitor and a loop diuretic for severe chronic congestive heart failure [randomized aldactone evaluation study (RALES)]. Am J Cardiol 1996;78:902-7.

THE SOLVD INVESTIGATORS. Effects of enalapril on survival in patients with reduced left ventricular ejection fractions and congestive heart failure. N Engl J Med 1991;325:293-302.

URETSKY B, YOUNG JB, SHAHIDI FE, et al. Randomized study assessing the effect of digoxin withdrawal in patients with mild to moderate chronic congestive heart failure: results of the PROVED trial. J Am Coll Cardiol 1993;22:955-62.

CHAPTER 27

New areas of drug development

Sebastian Harder

Cardiovascular diseases remain the leading cause of mortality and morbidity in industrial nations of the first and second world and are gaining evolving significance in third world nations. Development of new targets in treating cardiovascular diseases and improving established therapies are therefore advantageous and prestigious objectives in drug research. Clearly, the cardiovascular field covers an abundance of disease conditions as well as pharmacologic targets that cannot be referred to in detail. However, four promising drug classes that may face clinical application in the nearer future may be chosen from a large list of currently investigated drugs acting at various targets.

Endothelin antagonists may play a role as antihypertensive as well as vasodilating agents in chronic heart failure (CHF). Azimilide and related compounds may form a new class of antiarrhythmic drugs for rhythm control in atrial fibrillation. Inhibitors of neutral endopeptidases prevent breakdown of atrial natriuretic peptide (ANP), and the most promising compounds act as dual inhibitors of neutral endopeptidase (NEP) and angiotensin-converting enzyme (ACE), so-called vasopeptidase inhibitors. These agents may be useful in hypertension as well as in CHF. Proangiogenic agents may increase formation of collateral vessels in ischemic heart disease.

Before reviewing these drugs in detail, the most recent results on already known drug classes should be mentioned. Low-molecular-weight heparins have been shown effective in the treatment of unstable angina (see Chap. 25), β-blockers are finally established as core therapy of congestive heart failure (see Chap. 26), and angiotensin-receptor antagonists (AT₁) are established as useful alternatives or even adjunctive therapy to ACE inhibitors in CHF and hypertension (see Chap. 23).

There is accumulating evidence that low-molecular-weight heparins (LMWHs) are safe and effective alternatives to standard heparin in unstable coronary artery disease and that they offer practical and therapeutic advantages. The low-molecular-weight heparin Fragmin during the Instability in Coronary Artery Disease (FRISC) trial showed that dalteparin resulted in a 63% reduction in the risk of death or acute myocardial infarction (MI) compared with aspirin alone. The Fragmin in Unstable Coronary Artery Disease (FRISC) trial showed that dal-

teparin was as effective as intravenous heparin. Enoxaparin resulted in a statistically significant 16% reduction in the combined outcome of death, MI, and recurrence of angina in comparison with standard heparin in the Efficacy and Safety of Subcutaneous Enoxaparin in Non-Q-Wave Coronary Events (ESSENCE) trial.

The first pivotal results on the benefit of β-blockers in CHF were obtained with carvedilol, and the vasodilating properties of this dual α- and β-blocker have been claimed to contribute to the clinical benefit, making carvedilol an outstanding compound in comparison with other β-blockers. However, the MERIT-HF study with controlled-release metoprolol showed a 34% risk reduction for cardiovascular mortality in patients with CHF New York Heart Association class II and III (NYHA II-III), and similar results were seen with bisoprolol (CIBIS-2), making a class effect of β-blockers in CHF more propable.

The AT₁ antagonist losartan has been shown effective in CHF, although the 4.5% reduction in mortality, compared with captopril, was not confirmatory statistically and deserves larger studies. These studies are already launched with several other AT₁ antagonists (e.g., losartan: ELITE II; valsartan: ValHeft; candesartan: RESOLVD), currently available results from trials comparing AT₁ antagonists versus ACE inhibitors as well as AT₁ antagonist on top of an ACE inhibitor, do not confirm a protective activity of AT₁ antagonists.

Annual mortality rate in severe CHF remains 15%, 30-day mortality in acute coronary syndromes varies between 3 and 10%, and hypertension (as a meaningful predictor for CHF and coronary artery disease) remains uncontrolled in 30 to 50% of the hypertensive population. In other fields, e.g., revascularization in acute coronary syndromes or prevention or treatment of arrhythmias, invasive procedures (e.g., angioplasty, catheter ablation) or devices (e.g., pacemakers, implantable cardiac defibrillators) may increasingly take the place of conventional drug therapy. On the other hand, invasive approaches in revacularization generate new targets for adjuvantive antithrombotic or antiplatelet therapies, e.g., by antagonists of the fibrinogen receptor on platelets (GPIIb/IIIa inhibitors) (see Chap. 26).

Endothelin-receptor antagonists

Endothelin is a potent endothelium-derived vasoconstrictor peptide with proliferative properties. It is generated by proteolytic processing from preproendothelin to at least three mature isoforms: ET-1, ET-2, and ET-3. There are two important receptor subclasses: ETA receptors have been found predominantly in the heart and vascular smooth muscle, whereas ETB receptors are more widely distributed in the kidney, uterus, central nervous system (CNS), and endothelial cells. The binding of endothelin to its receptor leads to multiple effects predominantly on vascular and airway smooth muscle and eliciting contraction or pressor effects. Endothelin is a potent vasoconstrictor and has a long duration of physiologic action because of tight receptor binding. Elevated levels of the peptide occur in hypertension, CHF, and coronary artery disease. There are several nonspecific (ETA/ETB) or specific endothelin receptor antagonists in development. The most advanced compound that is currently in phase III trials is the nonspecific antagonist bosentan. In CHF, short-term oral bosentan therapy improved systemic and pulmonary hemodynamics in patients who were symptomatic with standard triple-drug therapy. In a study on 63 patients with symptomatic heart failure despite treatment with diuretics, digoxin, and ACE inhibitors, patients received oral bosentan (1 g bid) or placebo in a double-blind and randomized fashion over 2 weeks. Compared with placebo, bosentan on day 1 significantly decreased mean arterial pressure by 14% and capillary wedge pressure by 14.5%. Cardiac output increased by 15%, and heart rate was unchanged. After 2 weeks, cardiac output had further increased by 15%, and pulmonary wedge pressure further decreased compared with day 1. Heart rate remained unchanged.

It has been shown that endogenous endothelin exerts a vasoconstrictor tone in epicardial coronary arteries of patients with coronary artery disease. In such patients, bosentan elicited coronary vasodilation under acute conditions. Bosentan (200 mg iv) increased coronary diameter, particularly in vessels with no or mild angiographic changes, wheras coronary flow velocity did not change (see also Chap. 26).

The contribution of endothelin to blood pressure regulation in patients with essential hypertension has been studied in 293 patients with mild to moderate essential hypertension. After a placebo run-in period of 4 to 6 weeks, patients were randomly assigned to receive one of four oral doses of bosentan (100, 500, or 1000 mg once daily or 1000 mg bid), placebo, or the ACE inhibitor enalapril (20 mg qd) for 4 weeks. Compared with placebo, bosentan resulted in a significant reduction in diastolic pressure with a daily dose of 500 or 2000 mg (an absolute reduction of 5.7 mm Hg at each dose), which was similar to the reduction with enalapril (5.8 mm Hg). The effect of treatment with bosentan on blood pressure occurred without reflex neurohormonal activation.

New antiarrhythmic agents

Atrial fibrillation (AF) is the most common form of cardiac arrhythmia with a high prevalence in the aged population. An important therapeutic goal is restoration and maintenance of sinus rhythm whenever possible. Success with complex class III agents such as sotalol or amiodarone in the treatment of AF has led to the synthesis and characterization of compounds with simpler ion channel-blocking properties. Newer antiarrhythmic drugs either block a specific ionic current (e.g., dofetilide) or block multiple ionic channels (e.g., ibutilide and azimilide) in order to prolong atrial and ventricular action potentials without other specific pharmacologic effects. Of these second-generation class III drugs, ibutilide and dofetilide have demonstrated clinical efficacy in the setting of AF. However, their favorable antiarrhythmic effect seems to be counterbalanced by the incidence of proarrhythmias. A recent trial showed that the efficacy of transthoracic cardioversion for converting AF to sinus rhythm was enhanced by pretreatment with ibutilide, but sustained polymorphic ventricular tachycardia occurred in patients who had a low ejection fraction.

One very recent example of such agents is azimilide, which recently has faced clinical investigation. Like other class III agents, azimilide prolongs the resting period of the heart by blocking cardiac potassium channels. In these respects, its properties, at least in terms of its use in AF, resemble those of amiodarone. However, unlike other class III agents, the drug blocks both slow and rapid potassium channels and has little or no effect on atrioventricular (AV) conduction, which precludes the modulation of ventricular response in patients relapsing to AF. Azimilide does not affect PR or QRS interval and minimally affects hemodynamic properties such as blood pressure and heart rate. Its in vivo effects appear to be rate-independent and are maintained under ischemic or hypoxic conditions, properties of potential clinical significance. The drug is completely absorbed, and the extent of absorption is not affected by food. It can be administered once daily. Clinical data suggest that dose adjustments of azimilide are not required for age, gender, hepatic or renal function, or concomitant use of digoxin or warfarin. Unlike amiodarone, azimilide has shown no evidence of pulmonary or ocular toxicity. It has been suggested that the electrophysiologic profile of azimilide will result in a lower incidence of proarrhythmic effects, which may occur in 1 to 3% of patients treated with other class III agents. In a recently reported phase III trial, 384 patients received either azimilide 50, 100, or 125 mg orally daily or placebo. Time to symptomatic recurrence of AF was 17 days in the placebo group, 22 days in those receiving 50 mg, 41 days in those receiving 100 mg, and 130 days in those receiving 125 mg azimilide, respectively. One patient developed torsades de pointes arrhythmia while taking 100 mg azimilide. Data from open studies indicate an incidence for torsades de pointes arrhythmias of about 1%. The ongoing AzimiLide post-Infarct surVival Evaluation (ALIVE) trial examines the potential of azimilide for improving survival in post-MI patients at high risk of sudden cardiac death. The trial consists of three groups – patients receiving 75 mg azimilide orally each day, patients receiving 100 mg azimilide orally each day, and patients receiving placebo. Treatment is scheduled to be administered for a 1-year follow-up period, and all-cause mortality rate will be the primary endpoint. Pending the results of this and other pivotal trials, azimilide is expected to be the next new antiarrhythmic agent available on the market for the prevention of supraventricular arrhythmias and sudden cardiac death.

Dual neutropeptidase-ACE inhibitors

Vasopeptidase inhibition is a new concept in cardiovascular therapy. It involves simultaneous inhibition with a single molecule of two key enzymes involved in the regulation of cardiovascular function, neutral endopeptidase (NEP) and angiotensin-converting enzyme (ACE). Simultaneous inhibition of NEP and ACE increases natriuretic and vasodilatory peptides in a manner similar to atrial natri-uretic peptide and bradykinin. By simultaneously inhibiting the renin-angiotensin-aldosterone system and potentiating the natriuretic peptide system, vasopeptidase inhibitors (VPIs) reduce vasoconstriction and enhance vasodilation, thereby decreasing vascular tone and lowering blood pressure.

Omapatrilat, a heterocyclic dipeptide mimetic, is a novel VPI that demonstrates antihypertensive efficacy in animal models. In animal models of heart failure, omapatrilat is more effective than ACE inhibition in improving cardiac performance and ventricular remodeling and prolonging survival. Omapatrilat is the first VPI that entered clinical trials in hypertension and will soon do so in CHF. In mild to moderate hypertensives, omapatrilat 40 mg orally per day lowered diastolic blood pressure by 11 mm Hg compared with 10 mm Hg with 20 mg lisinopril. It has been further reported that omapatrilat also effectively reduces blood pressure in African-American patients, who are known to be more resistant to ACE inhibitors. Side effects of VPIs are expected to be similar to those of ACE inhibitors (e.g., cough). Unfortunately, clinical development of omopatrilat has been stopped due to an apparent high incidence of angioneurotic edema.

Vascular growth factors and angiogenesis blockers

Once the myocardium is under hypoxia due to narrowing of coronary arteries, it produces angiogenic peptides (e.g., fibroblast growth factor) to develop collaterals to restore the blood supply to its ischemic region. Thus, if angiogenic growth factors are supplied exogenously, the development of collaterals should be facilitated and may save the myocardium from hypoxia, thereby enhancing heart function. In addition to the experiments using recombinant protein of angiogenic factors, recent reports have shown that gene transfer of such angiogenic factors indeed restored blood supply into ischemic myocardium and enhanced its function, suggesting that such an approach may be an effective new strategy in the treatment of ischemic vascular diseases. Vascular endothelial growth factor (VEGF) promotes growth of small vessels. Inhibition of VEGF may be a meaningful target in cancer therapy, disabling vascularization of tumors and therefore inhibiting tumor growth (see Chap. 64) but it may also reduce plaque growth. On the other hand, promotion of vessel growth by VEGF may bypass stenotic coronary arteries. This therapy option may be advantageous in symptomatic patients with microvessel atherosclerosis or in those who are not eligible for angioplasty or coronary artery bypass grafting (CABG). VEGF may be released at the target by direct intramyocardial injection of the naked VEGF encoding gene, injection of an adenovirus vector encoding the VEGF gene, or intracoronary or systemic infusion of recombinant VEGF.

Gene therapy with VEGF has shown promising results in small series of patients with coronary artery disease (CAD) or peripheral arterial occlusion. In one pilot study, the safety and activity of direct myocardial gene transfer of VEGF as sole therapy for patients with symptomatic myocardial ischemia was investigated in five patients who had failed conventional therapy. Naked plasmid DNA encoding VEGF (phVEGF165) was injected directly into the ischemic myocardium via a mini-left anterior thoracotomy. Injections caused no hemodynamic changes. Postoperative cardiac output fell transiently but increased within 24 hours. All patients had significant reduction in angina (reduction in nitroglycerin use), and left ventricular ejection fraction was either unchanged ($n = 3$) or improved ($n = 2$). This initial experience with gene transfer for myocardial ischemia suggests that this approach is safe and may lead to reduced symptoms and improved myocardial perfusion in selected patients with chronic myocardial ischemia. VEGF gene therapy also has been investigated in arterial occlusion (arteritis obliterans), a distinct form of vascular occlusive disease that afflicts the peripheral arteries of young smokers and leads to persistent ulceration and pain. In a group of six patients, the above-mentioned naked plasmid DNA encoding phVEGF165 was injected intramuscularily. The ulcers that were nonhealing for more than 1 month healed completely in three patients, and nocturnal rest pain was relieved in the remaining two patients.

Results with recombinant VEGF, given intravascularly, are less convincing. A first placebo-controlled clinical trial in 178 CAD patients was carried out with purified VEGF, released in the coronary vessels by a 20-minute infusion, followed by a series of systemic infusions. After a follow-up of 2 months, no statistically significant improvements over placebo were observed for excercise time and angina. It has been speculated that the local release over a prolonged time period, as it is effected only by the gene therapy, may be critical for vessel formation. A further objection against VEGF therapy is the risk of promoting tumor growth and retinopathy in diabetic subjects. Other researchers believe that angiogenesis may be involved in the progression of atherosclerosis, and they are testing angiogenesis inhibitors similar to those used in cancer therapy (see Chap. 64) as a possible treatment for atherosclerosis.

New drug classes always hold promises that were stated somewhat enthusiastically by inspired researchers and companies. However, the clinical benefit of a new drug must be established by rigorous approaches of controlled trials and appropriate comparators. Trial designs must rely on hard endpoints that are meaningful to patient prognosis and the burden of a disease, and surrogate markers in the cardiovascular field (e.g., hemodynamic improvements) are not necessarily predictive of clinical outcome. Furthermore, the cost-effectiveness of a new therapy must be convincingly proven by appropriate measures. This constellation and the high costs for filing for approval of a new drug constitute a high hurdle for companies. Often enthusiasm declined sharply when first clinical trials were disappointing, and promising drugs vanished in drawers, sometimes merely due to pitfalls in trial design. Therefore, not all the compounds presented here may finally face clinical application.

Suggested readings

BURNETT JC JR. Vasopeptidase inhibition: a new concept in blood pressure management. J Hypertens 1999;17:S37-43.

CAPUCCI A, VILLANI GQ, ASCHIERI D, PIEPOLI M. Effects of class III drugs on atrial fibrillation. J Cardiovasc Electrophysiol 1998; 9:S109-20.

COREY A, AL-KHALIDI H, BREZOVIC C, et al. Azimilide pharmacokinetics and pharmacodynamics upon multiple oral dosing. Biopharm Drug Dispos 1999;20:59-68.

ISNER JM, BAUMGARTNER I, RAUH G, et al. Treatment of thromboangiitis obliterans (Buerger's disease) by intramuscular gene transfer of vascular endothelial growth factor: Preliminary clinical results. J Vasc Surg 1998;28:964-73.

KRUM H, VISKOPER RJ, LACOURCIERE Y, et al. The effect of an endothelin-receptor antagonist, bosentan, on blood pressure in patients with essential hypertension. Bosentan Hypertension Investigators. N Engl J Med 1998;338:784-90.

LOSORDO DW, VALE PR, SYMES JF, et al. Gene therapy for myocardial angiogenesis: Initial clinical results with direct myocardial injection of phVEGF165 as sole therapy for myocardial ischemia. Circulation 1998;98:2800-4.

MOULTON KS, HELLER E, KONERDING MA, et al. Angiogenesis inhibitors endostatin or TNP-470 reduce intimal neovascularization and plaque growth in apolipoprotein E-deficient mice. Circulation 1999;99:1726-32.

ORAL H, SOUZA JJ, MICHAUD GF, et al. Facilitating transthoracic cardioversion of atrial fibrillation with ibutilide pretreatment. N Engl J Med 1999;340:1849-54.

SINGH BN. Current antiarrhythmic drugs: an overview of mechanisms of action and potential clinical utility. J Cardiovasc Electrophysiol 1999;10:283-301.

SUTSCH G, KIOWSKI W, YAN XW, et al. Short-term oral endothelin-receptor antagonist therapy in conventionally treated patients with symptomatic severe chronic heart failure. Circulation 1998;98:2262-8.

TOSS H, LUNDAHL B, SIEGBAHN A, WALLENTIN L. Prognostic influence of increased fibrinogen and C-reactive protein levels in unstable coronary artery disease. FRISC Study Group. Circulation 1997;96:4204-10.

TURPIE AG. Low-molecular-weight heparins and unstable angina: Current perspectives. Haemostasis 1997;27:19-24.

Pulmonary diseases

CHAPTER 28

Asthma

Ivan Bakran

"Asthma is a chronic inflammatory disorder of the airways in which many cells play a role, in particular mast cells, eosinophils and T lymphocytes. In susceptible individuals this inflammation causes recurrent episodes of wheezing, breathlessness, chest tightness and cough particularly at night and/or in the early morning. These symptoms are usually associated with widespread but variable airflow limitation that is at least partly reversible either spontaneously or with treatment. The inflammation also causes an associated increase in airway responsiveness to a variety of stimuli" (*Global Initiative for Asthma*).

This new asthma definition published by the NHLBI/WHO recognizes chronic inflammation as the most important pathophysiologic element in asthma, which should be addressed accordingly by anti-inflammatory drugs.

Asthma is one of the most common chronic diseases worldwide, affecting roughly 150 million persons. The prevalence of active disease is roughly 1 to 10% in different parts of the world and is even more common in children. The prevalence of bronchial hyperresponsiveness to unspecific spasmogenes, such as metacholine, is even higher, reaching 20% of the population without clinical signs of asthma. The increase in prevalence of asthma is the consequence of increased exposure to allergens and pollutants, mainly in more affluent societies.

Disease presentation

A classification of asthma based on severity is of importance for the rational and timely prescription of drugs. Both symptoms (e.g., dyspnea, wheezing, chest tightness, and cough) and airflow limitation and its variability, measured by PEF (peak expiratory flow) or FEV_1 (forced expiratory volume in 1 second), enable asthma to be subdivided into intermittent, mild persistent, moderate persistent, and severe persistent disease. The variability of PEF may be calculated by the equation

$$\text{Daily variability} = (\text{PEF evening} - \text{PEF morning})/$$
$$(\text{PEF evening} + \text{PEF morning}) \times 100$$

Characteristics of various forms of asthma are presented in Table 28.1. The presence of one of the features of severity is sufficient to place a patient in that category.

The clinical manifestations of asthma occur as a result of airway obstruction. Airway narrowing may worsen gradually and persist despite therapy, or it can develop abruptly, leading to acute respiratory insufficiency.

Inflammatory changes in the airways are believed to initiate airway obstruction in asthma. Airway inflammation is also a primary mechanism responsible for airway hyperresponsiveness, a condition manifested by an exaggerated bronchoconstrictor response to various physical

---

Table 28.1 Classification of the asthma severity*

Intermittent asthma
Intermittent symptoms < 1 time a week
Brief exacerbations (from a few hours to a few days)
Nighttime asthma symptoms < 2 times a month
Asymptomatic and normal lung function between
  exacerbations
PEF or FEV_1 > 80% predicted, variability < 20%

Mild persistent asthma
Symptoms > 1 time a week but < 1 time per day
Exacerbations may affect activity and sleep
Nighttime asthma symptoms > 2 times a month
FEF or FEV_1 > 80% predicted, variability 20-30%

Moderate persistent asthma
Symptoms daily
Exacerbations affect activity and sleep
Nighttime asthma symptoms > 1 time a week
Daily use of inhaled short-acting β_2-agonist
PEF or FEV_1 > 60% to < 80% predicted, variability > 30%

Severe persistent asthma
Continuous symptoms
Frequent exacerbations
Frequent nighttime asthma symptoms
Physical activities limited by asthma symptoms
PEF or FEV_1 > 60% predicted, variability > 30%

---

*The presence of one of the features of severity is sufficient to place a patient in that category.
(PEF = peak expiratory flow; FEV_1 = forced expiratory value in 1 second; FEF = forced expiratory flow.)

and chemical agents. For example, wheezing and dyspnea can be provoked by environmental irritants, cold air, exercise, viral infection, exposure to allergens, or inhalation of metacholine. The level of hyperresponsiveness usually correlates with the clinical severity of the asthma and medication requirements.

According to the *Global Initiative for Asthma,* the goal of management is to achieve control of asthma, which is defined as:
- minimal (ideally no) chronic symptoms, including nocturnal symptoms;
- minimal (infrequent) exacerbations;
- no emergency visits;

Table 28.2 The long-term management of asthma: treatment in the stepwise approach (adults and children over 5 years of age)

TREATMENT
Avoid or control triggers
Step 1: Intermittent

Controller	Reliever
None needed	Short-acting bronchodilator: **inhaled β_2-agonist** as needed for symptoms, but less than once a week Intensity of treatment will depend on severity of exacerbation Inhaled β_2-agonist or cromolyn or nedocromil before exercise or exposure to allergen

Avoid or control triggers
Step 2: Mild persistent

Controller	Reliever

Daily medication
  Either **inhaled corticosteroid**, 200-500 µg, or **cromoglycate**, or **nedocromil**, or sustained-release theophylline
  Antileukotrienes may be considered
	Short-acting bronchodilator: **inhaled β_2-agonist** as needed for symptoms, not to exceed 3-4 times in one day

Avoid or control triggers
Step 3: Moderate persistent

Controller	Reliever

Daily medications
  Inhaled corticosteroid, >500 µg, and, if needed
  Long-acting bronchodilator, especially for nighttime symptoms: either long-acting inhaled β_2-agonist, or sustained-release theophylline, or long-acting oral β_2-agonist. (Long-acting inhaled β_2-agonist may provide more effective symptom control when added to low-medium-dose corticosteroid compared with increasing the steroid dose.) Consider adding antileukotriene, especially for aspirin-sensitive patients and for prevention of exercise-induced bronchospasm
	Short-acting bronchodilator: **inhaled β_2-agonist** as needed for symptoms, not to exceed 3-4 times in one day

Avoid or control triggers
Step 4: Severe persistent

Controller	Reliever

Daily medications
  Inhaled corticosteroid, 800-2000 µg or more, and
  Long-acting bronchodilator: either long-acting β_2-agonist, and/or sustained-release theophylline, and/or long-acting β_2-agonist, and
Oral corticosteroid long term
	Short-acting bronchodilator: **inhaled β_2-agonist** as needed for symptoms

Step down: Review treatment every 3 to 6 months. If control is sustained for at least 3 months, a gradual stepwise reduction in treatment may be possible

Step up: If control is not achieved, consider stepup. But first: review patient medication technique, compliance, and environment control (avoidance of allergens or other trigger factors)

(Preferred treatments are in bold print. Patients should start treatment at the step most appropriate to the initial severity of their condition. A rescue course of prednisolone may be needed at any time and at any step.)

Table 28.3 Relative potencies of topical corticosteroids

Corticosteroid	Receptor affinity	Skin blanching potency
Dexamethasone	1.0	1
Beclomethasone dipropionate	0.4	600
Flunisolide	1.8	330
Triamcinolone acetonide	3.6	330
Budesonide	9.4	980
Fluticasone propionate	18.0	1200

- minimal (ideally no) need for prn (as needed) β_2-agonist;
- no limitations on activities, including exercise;
- peak expiratory flow (PEF) circadian variation of less than 20%;
- (near) normal PEF;
- minimal (or no) adverse effects from medications.

All these goals can be achieved by patient education and developing a partnership in asthma management that assesses and monitors asthma severity with measurement of symptoms and lung function. It is of the utmost importance to establish an individual medication plan for long-term management and management of exacerbations, which also includes avoidance and control of asthma triggers.

A stepwise approach to long-term asthma pharmacologic therapy, according to its severity in adults, is presented in Table 28.2. The drugs are divided into *controllers,* taken daily on a long-term basis, and *relievers,* or rescue medication, that are used on a prn basis. Controllers include inhaled and oral corticosteroids, long-acting bronchodilators, sodium cromoglycate, nedocromil sodium, and possibly ketotifen. The mainstay of this therapy is inhaled corticosteroids (e.g., beclomethasone, budesonide, or fluticasone). The reliever of first choice is a short-acting β_2-agonist.

Drug classes

Inhaled corticosteroids are currently the most effective anti-inflammatory drugs. Beclomethasone dipropionate, fluticasone propionate, budesonide, flunisolide, and triamcinolone acetonide belong to this group of drugs.

Among many proposed mechanisms of action, the most important are interference with arachidonic acid metabolism and consequently synthesis of leukotrienes and prostaglandins, prevention of activation and migration of inflammatory cells, inhibition of cytokine production, and reduction of adhesion molecules and microvascular leakage. Relative potencies of topical corticosteroids, expressed as relative to dexamethasone, are presented in Table 28.3. Pharmacokinetic parameters of inhaled corticosteroids are presented in Table 28.4.

Inhaled corticosteroids reduce asthma symptoms, frequency, and severity of exacerbations. Patients experience a rapid improvement in lung function and quality of life. Inhaled corticosteroids reduce the need for long-term use of oral corticosteroids.

One of the main advantages of inhaled corticosteroids, though, is the significantly fewer systemic adverse effects seen in comparison with oral corticosteroids. The systemic effects depend on potency, bioavailability, first-pass metabolism in the liver, and corresponding half-life. Doses above 1 mg/d of beclomethasone dipropionate or budenoside may provoke adrenal suppression, osteoporosis, and skin thinning. It appears that glucocorticoid activity of 400 µg of beclomethasone per inhalation is equivalent to 7.5 mg of prednisolone taken orally. Fluticasone is not absorbed from the gut, and although it has twice the glucocorticoid activity of beclomethasone, doses even higher than 1 mg/d do not have systemic effects.

Dysphonia, coughing, and oropharyngeal candidiasis are the local adverse effects of inhaled corticosteroids. Mouth washing after inhalation or use of spacer devices for inhalation may prevent these local side effects.

In asthma exacerbations, a short burst of oral corticosteroids lasting for 5 to 7 days can be prescribed. The drug of first choice is methylprednisolone because of its relative short biologic half-life (up to 32 h), minimal mineralocortocoid activity, and limited effects on striated muscle. The same drug should be used for oral therapy, if indicated, on a long-term basis in persistent severe asthma. The whole daily dose (mainly 0.5 mg/kg of body weight) should be given early in the morning (at 7 A.M.). In order to minimize systemic side effects, an alternate-day schedule should be tried; i.e., the whole 48-h dose

Table 28.4 Pharmacokinetic parameters of inhaled corticosteroids

Drug	CL (liters/h)	$V_{d,ss}$ (liters)	V_d (liters)	$t_{1/2}$ (h)	F_{inh} (%)	F_{oral} (%)
Beclomethasone dipropionate	13	-	167	0.1-0.2	-	-
Flunisolide	20	96	134	1.6	39	20
Triamcinolone acetonide	29	103	107	2.0	22	23
Budesonide	12	183	339	2.8	28	11
Fluticasone propionate	10	318	776	7.8	16	<1

(CL= total body clearance; $V_{d,ss}$= apparent volume of distribution at steady state; V_d= volume of distribution during the elimination phase; $t_{1/2}$= plasma elimination half-life; F_{oral}= oral bioavailability; F_{inh}= inhalation bioavailability.)

should be given once in the morning every other day. The systemic side effects of long-term use of oral corticosteroids include steroid diabetes, osteoporosis, adrenal suppression, obesity, cataracts, arterial hypertension, skin thinning, and muscle weakness.

Sodium cromoglycate also belongs to the group of control medications for bronchial asthma. However, in comparison with inhaled corticosteroids, sodium cromoglycate is a drug of second choice, except possibly in childhood asthma. This drug inhibits in a dose-dependent fashion the IgE-mediated release of bronchoconstricting and proinflammatory mediators (e.g., leukotrienes, histamine, etc.) from human sensitized mast cells. It also has a suppressive effect on macrophages, eosinophils, and monocytes.

Inhaled prophylactically, sodium cromoglycate inhibits early- and late-phase allergen-induced bronchoconstriction or acute airflow limitation due to physical exercise (so-called exercise-induced asthma). Long-term inhalation (daily dose 20-160 mg per day) can diminish airway hyperresponsiveness. The full extent of efficacy can be judged only after a 4- to 6-week trial. Sodium cromoglycate causes only minimal side effects, namely, throat irritation and coughing after inhalation of the powder formulation.

Nedocromil sodium (daily dose: 4-16 mg/day) administered by inhalation inhibits activation and mediator release from several types of inflammatory cells, including mast cells and eosinophils. It is 4 to 10 times more potent that sodium cromoglycate in preventing induced bronchoconstriction. Nedocromil sodium can be used as maintenance therapy from the very beginning of persistent mild asthma. Nedocromil sodium is not associated with any significant adverse effects.

Ketotifen taken orally (1 mg bid) also inhibits mast cell activation and release of proinflammatory mediators. It is also a strong H_1-antagonist. No long-term effects on the chronic inflammatory changes in asthma have been demonstrated. Better results are obtained in children and young atopic adults. The therapeutic effect is not immediate, so clinical utility should be assessed after more than 2 months of treatment.

Long-acting inhaled β_2-agonists include salmeterol and formoterol. They selectively stimulate β_2-receptors, causing relaxation of airway smooth muscles. At the same time they enhance mucociliary clearance, diminish vascular permeability, and prevent mediator release from mast cells and basophils. However, it seems, on the basis of biopsy studies, that bronchial inflammation is not affected. Salmeterol and formoterol have a bronchodilating action that lasts at least 12 h, and thus they can efficiently prevent early-morning bronchoconstriction, a characteristic of asthmatic patients. Several studies report that patients do not appear to develop a tolerance to salmeterol even after months of regular treatment (for pharmacokinetics and tissue distribution, see Chap. 29).

Long-acting inhaled β_2-agonists are not rescue drugs. They are indicated primarily for chronic regular treatment as an addition to therapy when conventional doses of inhaled corticosteroids (up to 800 µg per day) fail to achieve control of the disease. The daily dose of salmeterol is 50 to 100 µg tid, and that of formoterol is 12 to 24 µg tid. Inhaled long-acting β_2-agonists cause fewer side effects than oral therapy. The side effects are caused by slight β_1 activity, such as skeletal muscle tremor, tachycardia, and hypokalemia when higher doses are used.

Oral sustained-release theophylline is an alternative drug to long-acting β_2-agonists. The precise mechanism of action of theophylline is not clear (see Chap. 29). Bronchodilation could be explained by theophylline's ability to block phosphodiesterase and therefore diminish cyclic AMP breakdown. However, theophylline inhibits both the early and late bronchoconstriction provoked by allergen inhalation. Some studies have shown that theophylline diminishes chronic asthma inflammation. The beneficial effect on airway hyperresponsiveness is very slight. The oral dose in adult asthmatics is 10 to 13 mg/kg per day in two divided doses, in the morning and evening. In smokers, because of the induced hepatic microsomes, the dose should be increased to 18 mg/kg per day. A steady-state serum concentration between 5 and 15 µg/ml (28-85 µ*M*) should be maintained during long-term theophylline treatment. A single intravenous dose of aminophylline (theophylline ethylendiamine) of 5 to 6 mg/kg can be used to effect, and thereafter, a continuous infusion can be given at a dose of 0.5 mg/kg/h.

Because of significant intra- and interindividual pharmacokinetic variations and the potential for interactions and significant adverse effects (e.g., nausea, vomiting, tachycardia, arrhythmias, hypertension, central nervous system stimulation, and seizures), it is advisable to monitor serum concentrations at the beginning of therapy and thereafter yearly if there is a good therapeutic response without adverse reactions. Monitoring is also useful when expected therapeutic aims are not achieved, when adverse reactions occur, and when interactions are feasible. Theophylline clearance is diminished by erythromycin, ciprofloxacin, allopurinol, propranolol, and cimetidine and enhanced by a high-protein diet, rifampin, phenobarbitone, and phenytoin.

The main rescue drug, or reliever, is an *inhaled short-acting β_2-agonist.* Throughout the world, the drug of first choice is salbutamol (albuterol) used with the metered-dose inhaler (MDI) on a prn basis. A single dose is 100 to 200 µg (1-2 puffs). The bronchodilatation occurs promptly, roughly 15 min after correct inhalation, and lasts for 4 to 6 h. It is the treatment of choice for acute asthmatic attacks and for the pretreatment of exercise-induced asthma. An increased daily use of salbutamol correlates with deterioration of asthma and strongly suggests the institution or intensification of regular anti-inflammatory drugs. Side effects include fine tremor (usually hands), headache, palpitations, tachycardia. nervous tension, and rarely, muscle cramps and hypokalemia with high doses.

It is very important to start home treatment of an asthma attack at the earliest possible sign of the deterioration. For mild to moderate exacerbations, 2 to 4 puffs of the short-acting β_2-agonist (salbutamol) every 20 min for the first hour is the treatment of first choice. Short-acting intravenous theophylline (e.g., aminophylline 5-6 mg/kg) may be considered an alternative to an inhaled short-acting β₂-agonist. The dose of aminophylline should be halved if the patient is already on oral slow-release theophylline. To speed the resolution of exacerbation, a parenteral corticosteroid (e.g., methylprednisolone 1 mg/kg iv) can be given.

Anticholinergics According to American and British and European guidelines, anticholinergics are the cornerstone of treatment of stable chronic obstructive pulmonary disease (COPD) and its relapses. They can be prescribed for inhalation alone in mild to moderate COPD or in combination with short-acting β₂-agonists in moderate and severe COPD. Two drugs are on the market – ipratropium bromide and oxitropium bromide – and both are nonselective M_1-, M_2-, and M_3-receptor antagonists (see Chap. 29).

These anticholinergic drugs have a slower onset of bronchodilatation than β₂-agonists. The peak effect is reached 30 to 90 min after inhalation, but bronchodilation lasts longer, up to 6 to 10 h. Oxitropium bromide may act slightly longer than ipratroprium bromide. Trials are in progress with tiotropium bromide, a selective M_1- and M_3-receptor antagonist with prolonged bronchodilating effect.

Specific immunotherapy, i.e., sc injections of specific allergen solutions, is indicated in the treatment of chronic allergic asthma when avoiding allergens is not achievable and appropriate medication fails to control symptoms. This treatment thus could be effective in asthma caused by grass pollen, domestic mites (*Dermatophagoides pteronyssinus*), animal dender, or *Alternaria* allergy. Specific immunotherapy with undefined allergens, such as house dust or bacteria, should no longer be practiced. Local adverse reactions include edema and inflammation, and the most serious systemic reaction is anaphylactic shock.

New areas of drug development

Inhaled corticosteroids are the current standard anti-inflammatory therapy for asthma. Treatment with inhaled corticosteroids is more cost-effective than other therapies. However, the tolerability of long-term use of high doses of inhaled corticosteroids (>1000 μg per day) is still a matter of concern, especially in young children. On the other hand, some patients abandon these drugs because of lack of immediate relief of symptoms.

Therefore, a number of ongoing studies are continuing to address certain issues relating to asthma treatment. A major step forward has been the introduction of a new class of anti-inflammatory drugs, namely, the *leukotriene antagonists or inhibitors*. Zafirlukast and montelukast act as leukotriene (LTD_4) receptor antagonists, and zileuton is a 5-lipoxygenase inhibitor. Leukotrienes occur naturally in the body and play a significant role in the inflammatory process that causes bronchoconstriction. The Food and Drug Administration (FDA) and major European authorities approved both drugs for the treatment of chronic asthma to prevent inflammation and asthma attacks. They are not suitable for treating acute asthma attacks, and with the exception of montelukast, they are not approved for use in children under 12 years of age. These drugs are taken by mouth (zafirlukast one 20-mg tablet bid, montelukast 10 mg at night for adults, and zileuton qid). Their exact place in chronic asthma therapy is still unknown, but it seems that they are already useful in mild to persistent asthma.

Zileuton has caused drug-induced hepatitis in 2 to 5% of patients. It also can interact with a number of other drugs. For example, erythromycin, terfenadine, and theophylline significantly decrease zafirlukast blood levels, and aspirin increases zafirlukast blood levels by 45%. When taken with warfarin, the effect of the anticoagulant is significantly increased and could cause bleeding. Montelukast is metabolized by the cytochrome P450 enzyme system, so caution should be exercised during coadministration of inducers (e.g., rifampin, phenobarbitone, etc.). Zileuton is instead an inhibitor of drug metabolism and with theophylline leads to a significant increase in blood levels.

Currently, there are no asthma treatments that can reverse the underlying cause of the disease. A promising approach is the use of recombinant human interleukin 4 (rhIL-4), which can prevent the production of immunoglobulin E. A lot of research has been devoted to selective inhibitors of phosphodiesterase izoenzymes (PDE III and IV inhibitors), which could have a potent anti-inflammatory effect. A promising field of research involves potassium channel openers, selective M1 and M3 antagonists, and inhibitors of inflammation caused by tachykinins.

Implementation of the new guidelines for chronic asthma treatment (*Global Initiative for Asthma,* NHLBI/WHO Report) will improve the outcome of this disease and the quality of life of asthmatic patients. Of some importance is patient education, which should begin at the time of diagnosis and be integrated into every step of medical care. The clinician and other members of the health care team should build a partnership with the patient and family, encouraging self-management skills to monitor the disease objectively, which also has a beneficial effect on patient compliance.

Suggested readings

BARNES PJ. Is immunotherapy for asthma worthwhile? N Engl J Med 1996;334:531-2.

BARNES PJ, PEDERSEN S. Efficacy and safety of inhaled corticosteroids in asthma. Am Rev Respir Dis 1993;148:S1-S26.

BRITTON MG, EARNSHAW JS, PALMER JBD. A twelve-month comparison of salmeterol with salbutamol in asthmatic patients. Eur Respir J 1992;5:1062-7.

BUSSE WW, MCGILL KA, HORWITZ RJ. Leukotriene pathway inhibitors in asthma and chronic obstructive pulmonary disease. Clin Exp Allergy 1999;29 (suppl 2):110-5.

CLARK B. General pharmacology, pharmacokinetics and toxicology of nedocromil sodium. J Allergy Clin Immunol 1993;92:200-2.

DOLLERY C. Albuterol. In: Therapeutic drugs. Edinburgh: Churchill-Livingstone, 1999, A59-A42.

EVANS D. To help patients control asthma the clinician must be a good listener and teacher. Thorax 1993;48:685-7.

GLOBAL INITIATIVE FOR ASTHMA. Global strategy for asthma management and prevention. NHLBI/WHO Report. NIH Publication No. 95-3659. Washington, USNIH, January 1995 (revised 1998).

GREENING AP, WIND P, NORTHFIELD M, SHAW G. Added salmeterol versus higher-dose corticosteroid in asthma patients with symptoms on existing inhaled corticosteroid. Lancet 1994;344:219-24.

ISRAEL E, COHN J, DUB L, DRAZEN JM. Effect of treatment with zileuton, a 5-lipoxygenase inhibitor, in patients with asthma. JAMA 1996;275:931-6.

SERAFIN WE. Drugs used in the treatment of asthma. In: Hardman JG, Limbird LE, Molinoff PB, Rudolf RW (eds). Goodman and Gilman's The Pharmacological Basis of Therapeutics, 9th ed. New York: McGraw Hill, 1996;659-82.

SPECTOR SL. Management of asthma with zafirlukast: Clinical experience and tolerability profile. Drugs 1996; 52(suppl 6):36-46.

WEINBERGER M, HENDELES L. Slow-release theophylline rationale and basis for product selection. N Engl J Med 1983;308:760-4.

Montelukast and zafirlukast in asthma. Drug Ther Bull 1998;36:65-8.

29

Acute and chronic obstructive lung diseases

Jurij Šorli

Diseases of the lower respiratory tract are among the most common in both children and adults. Although acute bronchitis is a relatively frequent disease, it does not present important health problem in contrast with chronic disorders. Chronic pulmonary disorders, best characterized by expiratory flow limitation, represent a significant proportion of patients in daily practice in most developed countries. In children, asthma is the most frequent manifestation, and in older patients, chronic obstructive pulmonary disease (COPD) takes priority. Both diseases present a difficult task in differential diagnosis if encountered later in life. Therapy and prognosis are different, and great care must be taken to establish proper diagnosis and to reevaluate it in time. Bronchiectasis, a focal bronchial dilatation, usually is accompanied by infection. This represents a therapeutic challenge. The infection is acquired most often, but it may be associated with congenital and/or hereditary conditions.

Seen less frequently but very important from a therapeutic point of view is the group of patients with cystic fibrosis, a monogenic disorder in the long arm of chromosome 7 resulting in decreased permeability of chloride ion transport across the lung epithelium. The disorder is more common in Caucasians, and the range of reported incidence goes from 1 in 569 newborns in the Amish population (Ohio) to 1 in 90,000 in the Asian population in Hawaii.

ACUTE BRONCHITIS

Acute bronchitis is an acute inflammation of the tracheobronchial tree that is generally self-limited with eventual complete healing and return of function. It is a common disease, usually occurring at the time or shortly after upper respiratory tract infections. It is accompanied by cough, sputum production, occasional wheeze, and slight fever. It may be serious in debilitated patients and in those with chronic lung or heart disease. Pneumonia is a critical complication.

Viral infection (influenza and adenoviruses in adults and respiratory syncytial and parainfluenza viruses in children) are believed to be the main etiologic factors. Field studies, however, have identified pathogens similar to those in community-acquired pneumonia and chronic bronchitis (*Streptococcus pneumoniae* and *Hemophilus influenzae* in up to 30% each, *Moraxella catarrhalis* in up to 10%, viruses in up to 8%, and mixed infection in up to 10%).

Rhinitis, malaise, slight fever, sore throat, and muscle pain often precede acute bronchitis. Initially the cough is dry and nonproductive; later it is abundant, mucoid, or mucopurulent. If superimposed bacterial infection takes place, the sputum may become frankly purulent.

Pulmonary signs are few in the absence of complications. Wheezing may be noted. Chest radiograph, arterial blood gases, Gram stain, and sputum culture should be done if complications are suspected or an underlying chronic respiratory disorder exists.

Treatment

Acute bronchitis needs treatment only exceptionally. Rest is indicated until the fever subsides. Oral fluids should be given during fever. An antipyretic analgesic (for children, paracetamol 10-15 mg/kg q6h; for adults, paracetamol 500 mg or aspirin 500 mg q6h) should be given only if fever is high enough to interfere with respiratory and/or cardiovascular function. The decision to use an antibiotic depends on the duration of symptoms, the purulence of sputum, and preexisting medical conditions (e.g., chronic obstructive lung disease). For complications, antibiotic therapy is identical to the treatment of community-acquired pneumonia or chronic bronchitis; in the case of protracted bronchial hyperactivity, symptomatic treatment with short-acting β_2 agonists may help (for the treatment of cough, see Chap. 30).

CHRONIC OBSTRUCTIVE PULMONARY DISEASE (COPD)

Chronic obstructive pulmonary disease (also known as *chronic obstructive lung disease,* COLD, and *chronic obstructive airways disease,* COAD) is a common term for the clinical condition characterized by persistent, partially or nonreversible airflow limitation, dyspnea, cough, and expectoration. It is not a uniform illness.

Unlike asthma, chronic obstructive pulmonary disease has shown some decrease in incidence and also in mortality in recent years in most western countries in younger cohorts. However, it is still a very important disease in older cohorts, especially in patients over 70 years of age. Up to 15 million people suffer from chronic obstructive pulmonary disease, and the disease is the fifth leading cause of death in the United States. In England, up to 7% of all deaths are attributed to chronic obstructive pulmonary disease. Chronic obstructive pulmonary disease is also a frequent reason for hospitalization (up to 15% of all admissions) and an important contributor to the health services workload (twice as high as asthma).

The etiology of chronic obstructive pulmonary disease is not fully understood. Cigarette smoking was found to be the single most important risk factor, with environmental pollution a probable additional factor. However, it is not clear why clinically significant airway obstruction develops in only 10 to 15% of smokers. Other more or less probable risk factors are bronchial hyperresponsiveness, specific occupations, adenovirus infections, low birth weight, low socioeconomic status, and excessive alcohol consumption. α_1-Antitrypsin deficiency has an important role in the development of emphysema in at least 80% of patients with homozygous α_1-antitrypsin deficiency.

In chronic airways obstructive disorders, three pathologic entities can be differentiated: (1) chronic bronchitis is a condition associated with prolonged exposure to nonspecific bronchial irritants and accompanied by mucus hypersecretion and certain structural changes in the bronchial wall; (2) chronic obstructive bronchitis is a disease of the small airways of a degree that leads to clinically significant airways obstruction, and (3) emphysema is marked by enlargement of the airspaces distal to the terminal nonrespiratory bronchioles and accompanied by destructive changes in the alveolar walls. In chronic obstructive emphysema, there is such a loss of lung recoil that airways markedly collapse on expiration.

Differentiation of severe forms of chronic obstructive pulmonary disease from chronic severe asthma is difficult, if not impossible. The disease usually starts with few or even no symptoms after 40 years of life. Later, the main characteristics of the clinical picture develop slowly: progressing symptoms of morning cough and sputum production on most days during cold periods of the year and shortness of breath on exertion due to progression of the obstructive changes. The course of the disease is also marked by relapses, usually in the form of recurrent respiratory infections. Hypoxemia, hypercapnia, pulmonary hypertension, and cor pulmonale that mark the end stage of the disease finally characterize respiratory failure.

Prognosis is related inversely to the age of patient and directly to the postbronchodilator value of the forced expired volume in 1 second (FEV_1). Three-year survival of patients over 60 years of age with an FEV_1 in the range of 40 to 49% of predicted is about 75%. In patients with an FEV_1 of less than 0.75 liter, mortality at 1 year is 30% and at 10 years is 95%. The usual yearly decline in FEV_1 in smokers is over 50 ml (normal subjects < 30 ml), but this returns to normal if the patient stops smoking.

Physical examination varies according to the severity of the disease. With more advanced disease, tachypnea and a prolonged expiratory phase of the respiratory cycle are present. Hyperresonant percussion and a low position of the diaphragm are due to emphysematous hyperinflation of the lungs. Breath sounds are reduced. Wheezes and rales are heard despite the absence of heart failure. Diagnosis is based on pulmonary function tests that give a characteristic pattern of volume-dependent airway obstruction. Forced vital capacity (FVC) is reduced, as well as the FEV_1/FVC ratio and the $FEF_{25-75\%}$.

Worsening of obstruction causes a decline in vital capacity (VC). Chest radiograph abnormalities may be minimal, but hyperlucency, hyperinflation, and a narrow, vertically oriented cardiac silhouette may be found. Flattening of the diaphragm is typical. Abnormalities of the gas exchange are common. Carbon dioxide retention (PCO_2 > 45 mmHg) is typical for so-called blue bloaters (type B patients with COPD, marked by hypoxemia, cyanosis, and right-sided heart failure). Type A patients, so-called pink puffers, have abnormal levels of ventilation for a given workload, and VO_2 is increased.

Treatment

No drug treatment has been shown to affect the natural history of chronic obstructive pulmonary disease. Therapeutic considerations must be directed toward the control of symptoms, maintenance of adequate lung function, prevention of complications, and improvement in quality of life.

Nonpharmacologic treatment

Since smoking is the most important etiologic factor in COPD, to prevent further deterioration of lung function, the patient should stop smoking. Psychologic counseling and eventual additional treatment with nicotine supplements (e.g., chewing gum or the transdermal nicotine patch) have a maximal success rate of 10 to 30% after the first year. Outdoor and indoor pollution may exacerbate symptoms and impair lung function; therefore, strict adherence to air quality regulations and guidelines must be maintained.

Both weight reduction in obese COPD patients to improve exercise capability by reducing energy requirement and prevention of malnutrition in others are advised.

Exercise is encouraged even in dyspneic patients to prevent deconditioning, but respiratory muscle training alone has not proven to bring clinically important benefit for COPD patients. Walking is preferred, but treadmill, cycling, and stair climbing also can be advised. Benefits disappear rapidly if exercise is discontinued.

Influenza vaccination generally has been associated with a reduction in mortality in the elderly but not specifically in COPD patients. The same is valid for pneumococcal vaccine. Killed influenza vaccines are recommended and should be given parenterally each fall. Pneumococcal vaccination should be repeated every 5 to 10 years.

Drug therapy

Since obstruction to airflow is the most typical characteristic of chronic obstructive pulmonary disease and causes dyspnea and diminished exercise ability, bronchodilators are the drugs of first choice. In mild forms of chronic obstructive pulmonary disease, a selective short-acting β_2 agonist followed by ipratropium bromide (often more effective) is used. These drugs should be prescribed on an "as required" basis or before exercise to enhance tolerance (see also Chap. 28).

In more advanced disease ($FEV_1 < 70\%$ predicted, $FEV_1/FVC < 88\%$ of predicted in men or <89% of predicted in women), short-acting β_2 agonists or ipratropium bromide are prescribed in regular intervals (three to four times daily) alone or in combination.

Theophyllines Theophyllines are modest bronchodilators that are the second-choice drugs in COPD. They should be used only in the case of failure of β_2 agonists and anticholinergics or as third-line drugs in severe COPD. The reason is their potentially beneficial nonbronchodilating effects in improving the strength and effectiveness of the respiratory muscles, augmenting respiratory drive, providing anti-inflamatory action, and improving right ventricular performance.

In acute, mild relapses of chronic obstructive pulmonary disease, antibiotics and systemic corticosteroids are also justified for short periods (see below).

Antibiotics Antibiotics are prescribed on empiric grounds for 7 to 14 days when the sputum becomes purulent or other signs of acute infection became apparent. The most common pathogens in COPD are *S. pneumoniae, H. influenzae, M. catarrhalis,* and viruses. Inexpensive antibiotics, e.g., amoxicillin (more expensive with clavulanic acid), and tetracyclines are the drugs of choice. Cephalosporins, macrolides, and quinolones can replace these drugs. Selection of an adequate antibiotic should be guided by local resistance patterns. Antibiotics should be started early in relapses, but prophylactic use is not justified (see below).

Corticosteroids The role of corticosteroids in chronic obstructive pulmonary disease is still under debate. Short-term trials in relapse-free periods of oral prednisolone or equivalent at 0.4 to 0.6 mg/kg per day (for 2-4 weeks) or aerosol fluticasone, beclomethasone dipropionate, flu-

nisolide, budesonide, or equivalent at greater than 2000 µg per day (for 6-8 weeks) may improve lung function in a small group of patients. Long-term use of low-dose corticosteroid aerosols did not prove beneficial in the preservation of lung function. In severe relapses, prednisone or equivalent is used for short periods in dosages of up to 0.8 mg/kg per day. Such patients must be treated in hospital or in an intensive care unit. Therapy consists of low-inspired oxygen by Venturi mask, a combination of β_2 agonists and an anticholinergic given by air-driven nebulizer, iv aminophylline, iv or oral corticosteroids, and antibiotics. Ventilatory support or mechanical ventilation is necessary in life-threatening relapses or in patients in whom maximal therapy fails to restore pulmonary function.

Oxygen Supplemental oxygen in form of long-term oxygen therapy (LTOT) for more than 15 hours per day is justified if stable patients with COPD have a PaO_2 of less than 7.3 kPa, with or without hypercapnia, and an FEV_1 of less than 1.5 liters (see Chap. 31). In the presence of pulmonary hypertension, cor pulmonale, polycythemia, or severe nocturnal hypoxemia, long-term application of oxygen is prescribed even in the presence of a stable PaO_2 of less than 7.9 kPa. The mode of application is usually through a nasal cannula, and a flow of 1.5 to 2.5 liters/min is usually adequate to achieve a PaO_2 of over 8.0 kPa. Venturi masks deliver concentrations that are more accurate, but they are less convenient to use.

Oxygen concentrations are the preferable source of oxygen in home settings because of simplicity and expense. Liquid oxygen is more expensive but offers the advantage of a portable system for travel or exercise and better mobility for the patient. In such cases, oxygen conservation delivery systems should be contemplated. Oxygen cylinders are too cumbersome and expensive and are prohibited by technical regulations in some countries. In relapses, supplemental oxygen must be prescribed according to the level of hypoxemia, and the need for ventilatory support must be considered in the case of failure.

Mucolytics and antitussives Mucolytics and antitussives are not indicated in COPD because there is no evidence that currently available mucolytics are of any benefit in clearing mucus. Antitussives are contraindicated because they suppress coughing, which is useful in clearing the respiratory tract, and some of them (opiates) may even impair ventilatory drive.

Respiratory stimulants Respiratory stimulants have no proven value in the treatment of chronic obstructive pulmonary disease. Doxapram is inferior to noninvasive supportive ventilation, and oral almitrine bismesylate can improve oxygen tension to a similar degree as a small increase in inspired oxygen. In contrast to LTOT, there are no proven long-term effects of almitrine. Use of almitrine at the recommended dose has resulted in important peripheral neuropathy.

BRONCHIECTASIS

Bronchiectasis is irreversible focal bronchial dilatation, usually accompanied by infection. It is most often acquired and associated with various conditions, either congenital or hereditary. Congenital bronchiectasis is rare. The underdeveloped lung periphery results in cystic dilatation of developed bronchi. The acquired form is the consequence of bronchial wall destruction by infection, inhalation of noxious gases, immunologic processes or inadequate nutrition of the bronchial wall, mechanical alterations secondary to atelectasis, or loss of parenchymal volume.

Increased susceptibility to recurrent or persistent lung infection is the main characteristic. Excess mucus is secreted and pooled in dilated bronchi. Cough becomes less effective. Physical findings reveal inspiratory rales over the involved region, accompanied by variable low-pitched wheezes. Chest radiograph confirms local findings. Computed tomographic (CT) scanning is useful for accurate diagnosis of bronchiectatic airways.

Treatment

Nonpharmacologic treatment

Postural drainage is regarded as the cornerstone of therapy, together with chest physiotherapy – percussion and vibration.

Drug therapy

Antimicrobial agents are also of clinical value in this chronic suppurative disease, but their role has never been properly evaluated. Sputum should be cultured periodically and the sensitivity of the causative agent(s) tested. Potential emergence of resistant *Pseudomonas* makes treatment difficult. Treatment with the antibiotics is tailored to individual requirements and can be given intermittently or continuously. Cotrimoxazole and quinolones (ciprofloxacin) are given orally because of superior penetration in usual doses. Combined therapy, if necessary parenterally, is given in resistant cases. In vitro and in vivo effects often are not identical. Bronchodilator therapy can help the clearance of airway secretions and may improve pulmonary function. Corticosteroids are indicated in the treatment of allergic bronchopulmnonary aspergillosis resulting in bronchiectasis.

CYSTIC FIBROSIS

Cystic fibrosis (CF) is an inherited multiorgan disease of the exocrine glands that usually, but not always, manifests in childhood. Cystic fibrosis affects in the first place the gastrointestinal (GI) and respiratory systems. Obstructive pulmonary disease, exocrine pancreatic insufficiency, and high sweat electrolytes characterize the process.

The gene responsible for cystic fibrosis encodes a membrane-associated protein called the *transmembrane conductance regulator* (CFTR) that is involved with chloride transport across epithelial membranes. Nearly all exocrine glands are affected. Three types of glands can be differentiated: (1) those obstructed by viscid or solid eosinophilic material in the lumen (e.g., pancreas, intestine, bile ducts, gallblader, and submaxillary glands); (2) those which produce an excess of secretions (e.g., tracheobronchial and duodenal glands), and (3) those which secrete excessive sodium and chloride (e.g., sweat, parotid, and small salivary glands). A number of other abnormalities occur, such as aspermia, infertility, and an increased incidence of abortion. The lungs are normal at birth, but soon, abnormally thick mucus secretions begin to cause obstruction, bronchiolitis, and mucopurulent plugging of the airways. *Staphylococcus* and later a mucoid variant of *Pseudomonas aeruginosa* are the most frequently isolated pathogens.

Prognosis depends on factors such as sex and race. Males and blacks with affected sites other than the respiratory tract have a better prognosis than females, whites, and those with respiratory tract involvement. Organization of care (patients treated in established care centers have a better prognosis than those treated in nonspecialized settings) is important as well. Today, about 50% of patients with CF are expected to survive up to 30 years.

Meconium ileus is the first sign, present at birth in 7 to 10% of affected infants, followed by other signs of cystic fibrosis. Pulmonary symptoms present as chronic cough, wheezing, and recurrent pulmonary infections. Cough is accompanied by vomiting, gagging, and sleep disturbances. A number of complications occur, such as retarded growth, pneumothorax, hemoptysis, and pulmonary hypertension with right-sided heart failure. Diagnosis is made by meconium examination (large amounts of serum protein and low levels of pancreatic enzymes and HCO_3), an abnormal secretin stimulation test, an elevated sodium and/or chloride concentration in sweat (>60 mEq/liter), and the most reliable, the quantitative pilocarpine iontophoresis sweat test.

Treatment

Treatment of patients with cystic fibrosis is complex. The aims are maintenance of adequate nutrition, prevention and therapy of pulmonary complications, physical activity, and psychosocial support. Enemas are given to relieve meconium ileus, pancreatic enzymes are given with each meal to address pancreatic insufficiency, and an adequate diet is provided (e.g., protein, calories, and vitamins) to maintain good nutritional status.

Nonpharmacologic treatment

In early stages of the disease, postural drainage with chest percussion should be introduced. Although evidence of direct improvement is lacking, long-term studies have shown that patients on regular chest physiotherapy improve their lung function. Psychosocial support that promotes self-confidence and the patient's ability to take control of his/her medical management is of great value. Nutrition is also an important factor in slowing progress of the disease. Supplemental pancreatic enzymes in granular or capsular form (4000-24000 units of lipase capsules daily, based on weight gain, presence or absence of abdominal cramping, and the character of stools) are given at mealtimes. Vitamins A, D, and E are supplemented on a daily basis, whereas vitamin K is given sporadically to treat bleeding complications. Caloric needs are higher than usual due to increased work of breathing, and a balanced diet is encouraged.

Drug therapy

Since lung infection is the controlling factor in terms of morbidity and mortality in cystic fibrosis, antibiotic therapy is the mainstay of treatment. Antibiotic intervention depends on clinical symptoms and should be guided by the identification of pathogens from the lower respiratory tract. In children, initial colonization usually takes place with *S. aureus* and *H. influenzae,* which is also found in adults. By early adolescence, most CF patients are infected with *P. aeruginosa* and lately also with *Burkholderia cepacia.* It is not uncommon that CF patients acquire viral infections and infections by atypical microorganisms in equal proportions as the normal population. Mycobacterial and fungal infections are rare.

Antibiotics should be prescribed early, in higher doses than for non-CF indications, and for longer periods. Higher doses are needed because sputum levels are less than half the serum concentration. Besides oral and intravenous use, aerosol and intravenous preparations often are successful. If *S. aureus* is present, the choice may include a semisynthetic penicillin, combination ampicillin and clavulanic acid, cephalosporin, clindamycin, or cloramphenicol.

Infections with *H. influenzae* should be treated with ampicillin and clavulanic acid and chloramphenicol. After colonization with *P. aeruginosa,* therapy with intravenous or aerosolized antibiotics at regular intervals (usually every 3 months) is indicated. Initially, a combination of an aminoglycoside with either antipseudomonal penicillin or a third-generation cephalosporin is used. With development of resistance or allergic reactions to penicillins or cephalosporins, carbapenems (e.g., imipenem or meropenem) may be used. Quinolones are the only effective oral antibiotics for *P. aeruginosa,* but resistance and declining clinical response follow repeated use. In aerosol application, gentamicin, tobramycin, and carbenicillin were used with success. Selection, dosage, and mode of application of some antibiotics in adults with cystic fibrosis are given in Table 29.1.

β_2 agonists and anticholinergics are frequently indicated because of wheezing and decreased lung function. Theophylline is less advisable because of gastrointestinal side effects. Corticosteroids have no measurable effect on lung function, and their use cannot be advocated in cystic fibrosis.

Mucolytics, expectorants, and cough supressants were used to alleviate chest problems with little or no success. In fact, long-term use of iodides resulted in hypothyroidism. Mucolytics such as N-acetycysteine can damage the bronchial mucosa and promote bronchitis. At present, several experimental drugs are under consideration, such as amiloride and triphosphate nucleotides. Both act by increasing salt and water availability on the epithelial surface and may improve mucus clearance. Routine vaccination against influenza, pertussis, and measles has an

Table 29.1 Antibiotics used to treat cystic fibrosis lung infections in adults

Organism	Drug	Dose (g)	Doses/day	Route
S. aureus	Cloxacillin	0.5-1.0	4	po
	Clindamycin	0.125-0.3	4	po
	Erythromycin	0.5	4	po
	Amoxicillin/ clavulanic acid	0.5	3	po
	Oxacillin	0.4	4	iv
H. influenzae	Amoxicillin	0.5	3	po
	Chloramphenicol	0.5	3-4	po
P. aeruginosa	Ciprofloxacin	0.75	2	po
	Gentamicin or tobramycin	0.08-0.12	3	iv
	Ceftazidime	3.0	4	iv
	Aztreonam	2-3.0	4	iv
	Imipenem	0.5	4	iv
	Meropenem	2.0	4	iv
	Azlocillin	5.0	4	iv
	Gentamicin	0.08-0.16	2-4	iv
	Tobramycin	0.08-0.16	2-4	iv
	Carbenicillin	2-4.0	2-4	Aerosol

important role in the prophylaxis of respiratory infections. Since the susceptibility to pneumococcus does not seem to be increased in patients with cystic fibrosis, routine vaccination against this pathogen is not justified.

Drug classes

β₂-AGONISTS

All β-agonists are administered preferentially by inhalation because of delivery close to the target and the low dose needed, thus preventing possible side effects. Inhalatory preparations include a pressurized metered-dose inhaler (PMDI), dry-powder inhalers, and solution for use in nebulizers.

The usual dosage in mild, stable chronic obstructive pulmonary disease is 1 to 2 puffs on "as required" basis and before exercise from a PMDI or dry-powder inhaler. In more advanced disease and in older patients, the dose should be elevated and given regularly, 1 to 2 puffs three to four times daily. If a β₂ agonist is inhaled from a nebulizer, the recommended dose is 1 to 2 ml of solution three to four times daily.

In relapses, inhalation from a nebulizer is recommended preferentially over inhalation from a PMDI or dry-powder inhaler. The dose should be raised to 4 to 6 inhalations (or more if required) daily of 2 ml of solution or 2 puffs from a PMDI every 4 to 6 hours (suggested doses refer to salbutamol and should be altered accordingly if another β₂ agonist is used). Combination with an anticholinergic (e.g., ipratropium bromide) always should be considered, and in the case of a poor response, intravenous methyxantines are the next choice.

There are differences in dose per puff in different preparations as a result of different drug potencies. In vitro comparisons of equivalent bronchodilating doses of different β₂ agonists showed that salbutamol and fenoterol are equally potent, terbutaline is 2.5 times less potent, and formoterol and salmeterol are 5 to 10 times more potent than albuterol or fenoterol.

Pharmaceutical forms of short-acting β₂ agonists are as follows: in PMDIs, 100 μg/puff, salbutamol and isoprenaline; 200 μg/puff, fenoterol, pirbuterol, and rimiterol; 250 μg/puff, terbutaline; 400 μg/puff, isoprenaline; 500 μg/puff, reproterol; in powder inhalers, 200 and 400 μg/puff, salbutamol; 500 μg/puff, terbutaline. Forms of long-acting β₂ agonists are as follows: in PMDIs, 25 μg/puff, salmeterol; and in powder inhalers, 50 μg/puff, salmeterol. Nebulizer solutions include 2.5 mg/2.5ml and 5 mg/ml, salbutamol; 5 mg/ml, fenoterol; 10 mg/ml, reproterol; 2.5 and 10 mg/ml, terbutaline; and 12.5 mg/capsule, rimiterol). Tablets or sustained-release tablets for oral administration are used less frequently because side effects for doses equivalent to inhaled drugs are significantly more frequent. In addition, onset of action is much delayed (15-20 min versus 2-3 min), with peak effect at between 1 and 2 hours compared to

15 minutes to 1 hour after inhalation. The recommended dosage schedule in adults is 1 to 2 tablets (salbutamol, 2 and 4 mg; terbutaline, 5 mg; reproterol, 20 mg; pirbuterol, 10 and 15 mg) bid or qid.

Compared with anticholinergic drugs, β₂ agonists are twice as potent and have a far more rapid onset of action. Use of long-acting β₂ agonists in chronic obstructive pulmonary disease has so far not been tested clinically to the extent that clear indications are proven, but their effect should be checked on an individual basis.

Pharmacokinetics and tissue distribution

Lipophilic drugs (e.g., clenbuterol) pass the airway epithelium rapidly and are retained in the tissue. Hydrophilic compounds (e.g., terbutaline, isoproterenol, fenoterol, albuterol, and salbutamol) reach lung receptors more easily from systemic administration. Deposition of the drug is a function of the inhalation technique. Even optimal inhalation technique delivers only up to 20% to the lungs, up to 70 to 80% is swallowed, and the rest is retained in the inhalation device. From this perspective, there is little difference between a PMDI and a nebulizer. The delivery of dry-powder inhalators is similar to that of PMDIs in some inhalation devices (Rotahaler) and about half in others (Diskhaler). Absorption is higher (2-3-fold increase) in smokers, after exercise, and in patients with a damaged epithelium. The mean duration of action of inhaled β₂ agonists is in the range of 4 to 6 hours. Prolonged bronchodilation over 12 hours has been demonstrated with formoterol and salmeterol. Since β₂ agonists are potent drugs, with daily doses of a few milligrams at most, one can expect that saturation of carrier mechanisms or enzyme systems would not occur at therapeutic dosages. Studies in adults and children established a linear correlation between the infusion rate of terbutaline or the dose of sustained-release tablets and corresponding plasma concentrations. There is no clear correlation between plasma concentration and bronchodilating effect; therefore, therapy with β₂ agonists should be monitored on the basis of therapeutic response and the occurrence and severity of side effects. Plasma protein binding of salbutamol and terbutaline is low (<20%) in contrast to salmeterol and clenbuterol (>90%). Salbutamol, terbutaline, and fenoterol traverse the placenta to the fetus. Equilibration is rather slow (<3 hours), but an equilibrium concentration of over 90% of that in maternal venous blood is reached. In breast milk, concentrations are negligible due to the rather high (>100 liters) volumes of distribution of β₂ agonists. In humans, sulfate conjugation is the most common metabolic pathway. Most β₂ agonists are filtered in the glomeruli, and some are also secreted by the tubular epithelium.

Pharmacokinetics is identical in normal and COPD patients and in adults and in children. The combination of a β₂ agonist and an anticholinergic in this order increases bronchodilation only slightly. If the drugs are given in reverse order, i.e., the β₂ agonist after the anticholinergic, bronchodilating effect is significantly enhanced. Combination of theophylline and a β₂ agonist has an additive effect only. The question of whether theophylline adds any measurable benefit to optimal β_2 agonist therapy is still not resolved.

Side effects

Side effects are relatively rare and dose related and are due to stimulation of extrapulmonary β receptors. Side effects are far more common with oral and iv administration than with inhalation therapy. The main side effects are muscular, cardiovascular, and metabolic, including especially unwanted changes in lung function. Muscular tremor is due to stimulation of β_2 receptors in skeletal muscle and is more pronounced in elderly patients. Tachycardia and palpitations are due to peripheral vasodilatation and secondary reflex cardiac stimulation, direct stimulation of atrial β_2 receptors, and with high doses of β_2 agonists, myocardial β_1 receptors as well. After prolonged use of a β_2 agonist, these side effects tend to diminish (tolerance).

The most pronounced and potentially serious metabolic side effect is hypokalemia, especially with hypoxia or use of diuretics. Hypokalemia is the result of combined β_2-receptor stimulation of potassium entry into the skeletal muscle cell and increased insulinemia. Increases of insulin secretion, free fatty acids, glucose, pyruvate, and lactate are seen normally only after high doses of β_2 agonists.

In severe chronic airway obstruction, hypoxemia can be enhanced by mismatch of ventilation and perfusion as a result of pulmonary vasodilation induced by β agonists. Therefore, additional oxygen in inspired air is beneficial during acute relapses of chronic obstructive pulmonary disease.

Possible relationships between high doses of β agonists and death from asthma have been suspected in the United Kingdom, New Zealand, and Canada. No similar relationship was found after high-dose prescriptions in chronic obstructive pulmonary disease.

ANTICHOLINERGICS

Anticholinergic drugs have been in use for respiratory problems for centuries. Burning leaves or roots of *Datura stramonium* in pipes or cigars were used for their bronchodilating effect in asthma. Later, the alkaloid extract atropine was popular until β agonists and methylxanthines came into use during the last 50 years. Atropine use has declined because of frequent and sometimes dangerous systemic side effects.

Better knowledge and understanding of the pathophysiology of the airways, especially in terms of cholinergic control of bronchomotor tone, opened the possibility of influencing changes induced by the disease. Synthetic atropine analogues similar to atropine but with significantly reduced side effects have been developed. They are also poorly absorbed and do not cross the blood-brain barrier. Other pharmacologic properties similar to atropine are retained, and when applied by inhalation, these agents act specifically on the respiratory tract.

Among the anticholinergics on the market, the quaternary anticholinergic drugs have a primary role. In this group, ipratropium bromide is the best studied. Another marketed compound is oxitropium bromide. Ipratropium is available as a PMDI (20 (μg/puff) and as a nebulizer solution (250 μg/ml). The dosage regimen is usually four times 2 puffs daily, but in relapses, up to 2 puffs eight times daily has been recommended.

After inhalation, the blood concentrations are too low to be measured accurately (<1% of administered dose). The half-life in the circulation is around 3 hours, and the maximal bronchodilator effect is achieved at 40 to 80 μg of inhaled ipratropium. Half the broncodilating effect occurs in the first 3 to 5 minutes and 80% in the first 30 minutes. The maximal effect occurs after 1.5 to 2 hours, and after 40 μg of inhaled ipratropium, the duration is 4 to 6 hours.

Bronchial secretion has been shown to be inhibited in rabbits after atropine aerosol at concentrations of 4×10^{-9} to 4×10^{-5} g/ml. A minimal inhibition of mucociliary transport also was noted at very high concentrations of ipratropium bromide (10^{-5} g/ml), whereas smooth muscle relaxation was achieved at doses 10^{-9} to 10^{-7} g/ml. Inhibition of salivary secretion was achieved at doses 100 times greater than the ones used to achieve maximal bronchodilatation. No tolerance (e.g., tachyphylaxis) to ipratropium has been shown, and even after prolonged use of anticholinergic agents, patients show no decline in bronchodilatation.

Clinical studies in stable COPD compared anticholinergic agents with β_2 agonists, methylxanthines, and multidrug combinations. Ipratropium typically increases FEV_1 by 15 to 25%; specific airway conductance almost doubles, and FVC decreases by 0.30 to 0.60 liter. In an early-term study in 261 patients, ipratropium was superior to a β agonist after 1, 45, and 90 days in mean peak response of FEV_1 and FVC. This response was even more evident in patients with low baseline FEV_1 values. Another study confirmed that 36 μg of ipratropium had a more durable effect than 200 μg of salbutamol. A combination of 40 μg of an anticholinergic and 200 μg of a β agonist was superior to either agent alone with respect to an increase in FEV_1 and duration of the effect. Several studies of maximal response after salbutamol proved that subsequent inhalation of 80 μg ipratropium resulted in further increase in FEV_1 and FVC. This effect was not confirmed in other studies. Comparison of continued therapy versus on-demand treatment gave conflicting results. Continuous treatment resulted in a greater FEV_1 reduction than treatment on demand (0.082 versus 0.031 liter/year). Bronchial hyperresponsiveness increased slightly but not significantly.

In acute relapses, regimens based on ipratropium, fenoterol, or a combination produced a similar bronchodilation at 45 and 90 minutes. The maximal increase in FEV_1 was 26.5%. In a crossover study, the increase in FEV_1 caused by ipratropium-orciprenaline (a nonselective β_2 agonist) was 24% when ipratropium was given first. However, there was no further increase in FEV_1 after orciprenaline. The same also was true when orciprenaline was given first.

Side effects

Side effects were best studied with ipratropium bromide. Since absorbability of the drug when delivered to the mucosal surfaces is poor, side effects are much smaller than those of atropine. In the lower respiratory tract, ipratropium has negligible effects on mucociliary clearance, ciliary activity, and mucus production, even after long-term treatment. In the upper respiratory tract, drying of the mucosa is quite frequent and can result in discomfort. The underlying mechanism is not known. In the eye, up to four times the recommended dose has no effect on intraocular pressure, pupil diameter, or accommodation. When applied directly to the eye (by mistake), ipratropium caused prolonged dilatation of the pupil, and in combination with salbutamol, this can present a serious risk in patients with glaucoma. There are no important effects on the genitourinary and cardiovascular systems even in doses up to eightfold normal.

METHYLXANTHINES

Methylxanthines such as theophylline have been used for the treatment of asthma since 1930 and are still the most widely used drugs worldwide. However, their narrow therapeutic range, relatively low efficacy as bronchodilators compared with β agonists, and high incidence of side effects with relatively low plasma levels caused a recent decline in their use. In asthma as well as in COPD, they are relegated to second- or third-line therapy.

Theophylline is a methylxanthine that is similar to caffeine. Among salts of theophylline, the most common is aminophylline (ethylenediamine), with better solubility at neutral pH. Enprofylline, the 3-propyl derivative of theophylline, is a more potent bronchodilator and may have fewer side effects. Other derivatives or salts are not in any way superior to theophylline.

The exact mechanism of action of theophylline is not certain. A number of mechanisms have been investigated and proposed: phosphodiesterase inhibition, adenosine receptor antagonism, increased epinephrine inhibition, inhibition of calcium entry/release, and inhibition of phosphoinositide hydrolysis. Phosphodiesterase inhibition has been widely held as a basis for the bronchodilating effect of theophylline, but recent investigations have shown that this effect may be more relevant in mediating the anti-inflammatory and immunomodulatory effects of theophylline. The main action of theophylline is assumed to be exerted as smooth muscle relaxation, an increase in mucociliary clearance, and prevention of microvascular leakiness. There is also some increase in contractility of the fatigued diaphragm in humans.

Pharmaceutical forms of theophylline are tablets and slow-release tablets or capsules; aminophylline is also available for iv use. Slow-release preparations are preferred because they are absorbed at a constant rate and provide steady plasma concentrations. Differences between preparations exist but are relatively minor and of no clinical significance. The usual dosing regimen for slow-release preparations is 8 mg/kg bid. In relapses, iv application is preferred. The loading dose should be 6 mg/kg over 20 to 30 minutes, followed by continuous infusion of 0.5 mg/kg per hour. If the patient was already taking theophylline, the doses should be halved. In all patients, plasma levels of theophylline should be monitored and maintained within the limit of 10 to 20 μg/ml.

Side effects

The most common side effects are anorexia, nausea, vomiting, and central toxicity, expressed as irritability or confusion. Nausea is probably due to both central effect and a local effect on gastric mucosa. It is usually present at plasma concentrations above 15 μg/ml. Acute abdominal pain, diarrhea, and gastric bleeding also have been reported. With higher plasma concentrations, arrhythmias and convulsions may be the most prominent features of theophylline toxicity. It is not uncommon that major side effects are not preceded by minor ones, and therefore, measurement of serum concentrations at regular intervals is obligatory during theophylline therapy.

ANTIBIOTICS

The importance of bacterial infections in COPD patients is generally underappreciated because of studies indicating that antibiotic treatment has little or no impact on relapses or general development of illness. This is true only as a general rule, whereas some subsets of COPD patients may benefit from antibiotic therapy. These include those with more severe illness, frequent relapses, frequent use of an antibiotic and thus danger of harboring resistant pathogens, rapid decline in FEV_1 (>100 ml/year) or high degree (<0.75 l) of FEV_1 impairment, and significant comorbidity (usually cardiovascular). In some of these patients, unsuspected bronchiectasis was established in thin-section CT scans.

The most frequent bacterial isolates in COPD relapses (in up to 50% of all patients) are *H. influenzae* (up to 60% of all bacterial isolates), *S. pneumoniae* (up to 25%), and lately, *M. catarrhalis* (up to 15%). In patients with poor health status or advanced disease, *P. aeruginosa* is also found. Many patients (about a third) also retain bacteria in their sputum between relapses, but bacterial counts are significantly lower compared with those in exacerbation. Resistance to certain antibiotics varies from country to country. In North America and most of Europe, 20 to 40% of *H. influenzae* and almost 100% of *M. catarrhalis* can be expected to be resistant to β-lactamase-mediated amoxicillin. Since antibiotic prescriptions in lower respiratory tract infections account for a large proportion of the annual health care expenditures in every country (in the United States, 4 billion dollars), misuse or inappropriate use of these agents should be avoided as much as possible. It should be stressed that antibiotics represent only a small part of the actual cost of care for COPD patients.

A wide range of antibiotics may be used in COPD relapses. These include penicillins, cephalosporins, macrolides, azalides, tetracyclines, trimethoprim-sulfamethoxazole, and quinolones. Treatment of first choice in patients with milder forms of COPD (FEV$_1$ > 50%) should be an aminopenicillin. In more advanced disease (FEV$_1$ < 50%, advanced age, >4 relapses per year, comorbidity), a penicillin plus a β-lactamase inhibitor, quinolones, a second- or third-generation cephalosporin, or a second-generation macrolide should be selected, and in chronic bronchial infection in which *P. aeruginosa* or Enterobacteriaceae are present, ciprofloxacin is the drug of first choice.

Therapy should be prescribed for 7 to 14 days in doses that ensure a ratio MIC/AUC (minimal inhibitory concentration – MIC or MIC$_{90}$ versus area under the curve – AUC 0-24 h) of more than 125 or even more than 250. Usually, dosing in penicillins and penicillin plus clavulanic acid preparations is bid to qid and in others bid. It must be noted that surveys of patient behavior established that more than 50% of patients neither took their antibiotics regularly nor completed the prescribed course of medication.

It is important to consider two pharmacokinetic issues in COPD therapy with antibiotics. The first is tissue penetration, and the second is drug metabolism and excretion. Penicillins, cephalosporins, and aminoglycosides do not penetrate bronchial mucosa and secretions (mucus) well. They rarely achieve adequate levels as compared with serum concentrations. Azalides, quinolones, and macrolides, however, are able to achieve concentrations in bronchial mucosa and secretions well in excess of serum levels. Specific ratios of mucosal tissue concentration versus MIC$_{90}$ of over 100 are achieved with certain selected drugs and respiratory pathogens (ciprofloxacin: *H. influenzae,* 162; *M. catarrhalis,* 81; *S. pneumoniae,* 4.9; clarithromycin: 85, 10, and 0.8, respectively; erythromycin: 0.9, 27, and 3.3, respectively; amoxicillin: 2.7, 45, and 2.7, respectively). The values for azithromycin are 3.89, 7.78, and 32.4, respectively, with concentrations in alveolar macrophages of 23.46 and 191.6 µg/ml.

Side effects

Typical adverse events seen with antibiotic therapy range from mild discomfort to life-threatening pseudomembranous colitis. Usual side effects include nausea, vomiting, insomnia, headaches, diarrhea, thrush, rash, photosensitivity, and Stevens-Johnson syndrome. Also of importance is interaction with other drugs used in the therapy of chronic obstructive pulmonary disease. Macrolides and quinolones (e.g., enoxacin and, to a lesser extent, ciprofloxacin) depress the cytochrome P450 pathway in the liver and reduce the elimination of, for example, theophylline.

CORTICOSTEROIDS

Use of steroids in the treatment of obstructive lung disease, notably asthma, started shortly after their discovery in the 1950s. In asthma, they remain the first-line basic therapy. Their use in COPD is more limited, and expectations that inhalation of corticosteroids would favorably influence the progressive fall in lung function were not confirmed in large-scale clinical trials.

Steroids act by interaction with specific receptors within the cytoplasm. The steroid-receptor complex is then transported to the nucleus, where it binds to specific sequences of certain target genes, resulting in increased or decreased protein synthesis. These events take some time, and, therefore, onset of action of corticosteroids is delayed for several hours after application. Prednisolone is readily absorbed after oral administration. It is metabolized in the liver. The plasma half-life is 2 to 3 hours, and the biologic half-life is approximately 32 hours. Prednisolone is up to 92% protein bound to a specific protein called *transcortin*. Only the unbound fraction is biologically active. Drugs such as rifampicin, phenobarbitone, and phenytoin lower the plasma half-life by enzyme induction.

The usual application in patients with COPD relapses is a 7- to 14-day course of prednisolone or prednisone, 30 to 40 mg daily, in a single oral morning dose. Evidence of benefit, e.g., earlier discharge from the hospital, is still lacking. A trial of corticosteroids is justified in COPD patients, however, especially if this is the first presentation of disease, if there is an evidence of a previous favorable response to steroid treatment during relapse, or in the case of failure to a maximal dose of a bronchodilator.

Inhaled glucocorticoids can have some objective effect in patients with bronchial hyperresponsiveness, but their role, contrary to the case of asthma, has not been established in chronic obstructive lung disease.

New areas of drug development

New types of anticholinergics with enhanced potency and long-lasting efficiency have been developed. Tiotropium (Ba 679 BR) has equal affinity for M1, M2, and M3 receptors and is approximately 10-fold more potent than ipratropium bromide. Clinical studies confirmed that it protects against cholinergic bronchoconstriction for over 24 hours. Tiotropium will be suitable for daily dosing, particularly in patients with COPD.

Gene transfer therapy in CF patients already has been shown to be technically feasible. The CFTR gene was transferred in vitro and in vivo using an adenoviral vector to epithelial respiratory cells, where it was expressed for days and even weeks. Systems for an efficient targeted delivery and integration have been described, and there is a significant likelihood for genetic reparation in the foreseeable future.

Suggested readings

ALBERT RA, MARTIN TR, LEWIS SW. Controlled clinical trial of methyprednisolone in patients with chronic bronchitis and acute respiratory insufficiency. Ann Intern Med 1980;92:753-8.

AMERICAN THORACIC SOCIETY. Standards for the diagnosis and care of patients with chronic obstructive pulmonary disease. Am J Respir Crit Care Med 1995;152:S77-120.

BALDWIN DR, WISE R, ANDREWS JM, et al. Azithromycin concentrations at the sites of pulmonary infection. Eur Respir J 1990;3:886-90.

BTS guidelines for the management of chronic obstructive pulmonary disease. The COPD guidelines Group of the Standards of Care Committee of the BTS. Thorax 1997;52(suppl 5):1-28.

CHAPMAN KR. The role of anticholinergic bronchodilators in adult asthma and COPD. Lung 1990;168(suppl):295-303.

CURTIS JR, DEYO RA, HUDSON LD. Health-related quality of life among patients with chronic obstructive pulmonary disease. Thorax 1994;49:162-70.

KERSTJENS HA. Stable chronic obstructive pulmonary disease. Brit Med J 1999;319:495-500.

PAUWELS R, O'BYRNE PM eds. Beta$_2$-agonists in asthma Treatment Lung biology in health and disease. New York: Marcel Dekker, 1997.

REGELMAN WE, ELLIOTT GR, WARWICK WJ, et al. Reduction of sputum *P. aeruginosa* density by antibiotics improves lung function in cystic fibrosis more than do bronchodilators and chest physiotherapy alone. Am Rev Respir Dis 1990;141:914-21.

SAINT S, BENT S, VITTINGHOFF E, GRADY D. Antibiotics in chronic obstructive pulmonary disease exacerbations: a meta-analysis. JAMA 1995;273:957-60.

SIAFAKAS NM, VERMEIRE P, PRIDE NB, et al. Optimal assessment and management of chronic obstructive pulmonary disease (COPD). Eur Respir J 1995; 8:1398-420.

VAN SHAYCK CP, CLOOSTERMAN SGM, HOFLAND ID, et al. How detrimental is chronic use of bronchodilators in asthma and chronic obstructive pulmonary disease? Am J Respir Crit Care Med 1995;151:1317-9.

Cough

William M. Corrao

Cough is one of the most frequent symptoms encountered in clinical practice by physicians. It is also the most common symptom of the most frequent human affliction, the common cold. The prevalence of cough in nonsmoking adults ranges from 14 to 23%. It is estimated that more than 1 billion dollars is spent on over-the-counter (OTC) medicines in the United States alone for the treatment of coughs and colds. This amount does not include the cost of specific therapies directed at the principal cause of a chronic cough.

To most patients, cough is an annoying symptom requiring evaluation because it causes insomnia, chest pain, headache, dizziness, syncope, fatigue, and loss of time from work and school. Physicians must recognize that cough serves two major purposes: (1) it protects the lower respiratory tract from aspirating foreign materials, and (2) it aids the lower respiratory tract in expectorating excess mucus when normal mucociliary clearance mechanisms are overwhelmed. When evaluating the patient with a chronic cough (defined as a cough of greater than 3 weeks' duration), the physician must keep these two functions in mind and not routinely prescribe "cough medicines" simply to relieve the symptom. Understanding these functions necessitates a brief review of the cough reflex.

The cough reflex is made up of five components: (1) cough receptors, (2) afferent nerves (e.g., vagal, trigeminal, glossopharyngeal, and phrenic), (3) a cough center located in the medulla, (4) efferent nerves (e.g., vagal, phrenic, intercostal, lumbar, trigeminal, facial, and hypoglossal), and (5) effector organs (e.g., diaphragm, intercostal and abdominal muscles, and muscles of the larynx, trachea, and bronchi, as well as upper airway and accessory respiratory muscles) (Tab. 30.1).

Knowledge of the human cough receptor, while studied extensively, is still far from complete and remains controversial. Receptors are found in abundance in the larynx, trachea, and larger bronchi. They are more prevalent in larger airways and are increased at the carini, where they are most likely to be stimulated by irritants. While no histologic "receptors" have been seen in the sinuses, pharynx, diaphragm, pericardium, or pleura, their existence is inferred by the high prevalence of cough in patients with diseases affecting these organs. The larynx is felt to be an important site for the initiation of both cough and bronchoconstrictive reflexes. C-fiber receptors (bronchial and pulmonary) are also felt to be important.

Table 30.1 Cough reflex

Receptor	Afferent nerves	Cough center	Efferent nerves	Effector organs
Larynx, trachea, bronchi, ear canal, pleura, stomach	Vagus	Diffusely located in medulla near the respiratory center; under control of higher center	Vagus, phrenic, intercostal, lumbar	Muscles of larynx and bronchi; diaphragm; intercostal and abdominal muscles
Nose, paranasal sinuses	Trigeminal			
Pharynx	Glossopharyngeal		Trigeminal, facial hypoglossal, and accessory respiratory muscles	Upper airways respirator
Pericardium, diaphragm	Phrenic			

Disease presentation

The diagnosis of cough involves an anatomic evaluation of the afferent limb of the cough reflex, i.e., an examination of the sites where cough receptors are prevalent. Results of this approach suggest that three conditions-postnasal drip syndromes (PNDS), bronchial asthma, and gastroesophageal reflux disease (GERD)-account for the greatest number of etiologies. Five studies prospectively examined 335 patients: 110 (33%, range 19-60%) had PNDS, 86 (26%, range 7-31%) had bronchial asthma, and 36 (11%, range 4-21%) had GERD. In some series, more than 50% of patients had two or more causes to explain the chronic cough.

POSTNASAL DRIP SYNDROMES

The most common cause of acute cough is the common cold. Excessive secretions in the nose and/or sinuses stimulate cough receptors by "dripping" into the hypopharynx resulting in mechanical stimulation of the cough receptors. The common cold can be considered part of the postnasal drip syndromes. The common cold is usually self-limited, lasting less than 14 days.

Patients typically complain of a sensation of something dripping into the throat, a "lump" in the throat, a need to clear the throat frequently, a "tickle" behind the larynx, nasal congestion, and/or rhinorrhea. Hoarseness is also encountered commonly. Cough increases while talking, when lying down, with change in temperature, and with exposures to respiratory irritants, e.g., cigarette smoke. Physical findings include nasal mucosal edema and inflammation, a granular or cobblestone appearance to the posterior nasopharynx, and mucus adherent to the posterior nasopharyngeal wall. Radiographic abnormalities of sinus radiographs include mucosal thickening, air-fluid levels, and opacification of the sinuses. Some patients may have none of these findings but respond to specific postnasal drip syndromes therapy, namely, antihistamine-decongestant preparations. Some authors have strongly suggested that a successful trial of an antihistamine-decongestant is diagnostic even in the absence of the preceding findings. Allergy testing as part of the routine evaluation for postnasal drip syndromes is not recommended unless a history of allergic symptoms is forthcoming. A history of specific exposures, e.g., animal dander, with a confirmatory skin test is certainly more useful than a positive skin test alone. A history of a recent upper respiratory tract infection is required to diagnose postviral postnasal drip syndromes, and excessive use of medications (e.g., oxymetazoline hydrochloride or cocaine) is necessary to make the diagnosis of postnasal drip syndromes secondary to medication abuse.

Treatments of general use in the disease

The best therapy for postnasal drip syndromes due to perennial rhinitis or postviral rhinitis appears to be the older-generation antihistamine-decongestant combinations. In four prospective, descriptive studies, cough was treated successfully using these combination antihistamine-decongestants. There were no placebo controls in any of these studies. In one randomized, placebo-controlled study of acute cough, the older-generation antihistamine-decongestants were effective in controlling cough. Antihistamines (see Chap. 78) act as competitive antagonists of histamine at H_1 receptors. Commonly used antihistamines include chlorpheniramine 2 to 4 mg qid, diphenhydramine 25 to 50 mg tid, tripelennamine 25 to 100 mg tid, brompheniramine 4 to 8 mg tid or qid, dexbrompheniramine 2 to 4 mg qid, triprolidine 2.5 mg tid, and azatadine 1 to 2 mg bid. These drugs are absorbed readily from the gastrointestinal tract and are metabolized in the liver by the microsomal oxidation system. Their major effect is blocking the inflammatory cascade stimulated by histamine. They also have a mild anticholinergic drying effect. Major side effects include sedation, mild confusion, impaired judgment, and urinary hesitancy and retention. These drugs are contraindicated in patients taking monoamine oxidase (MAO) inhibitors because the MAO inhibitors potentiate the antimuscarinic action of antihistamines.

Decongestants are sympathomimetic agents that cause vasoconstriction in small blood vessels and decrease secretions by means of α-adrenoceptor stimulation and parasympathetic suppression. Their primary effect is via a stimulation that causes mucosal vasoconstriction, thereby decreasing congestion and secretions. Pseudoephedrine 60 to 120 mg bid to qid and phenylpropanolamine 25 to 100 mg tid to qid are two agents commonly used in combination with antihistamines. Oxymetazoline 1 to 2 drops every 6 to 8 hours and phenylephrine 1 to 2 drops every 4 hours can be used topically in the nose. They should not be given for more than 96 hours.

Major side effects include tachycardia, hypertension, central nervous system (CNS) stimulation, and insomnia. These agents cannot be used in patients taking MAO inhibitors or tricyclic antidepressants. Rebound congestion occurs with topical drops if used for more than 4 days. Data looking at the effect of newer nonsedating antihistamine-decongestant preparations in the treatment of cough secondary to the common cold suggest that they are not as effective as the older sedating antihistamine-decongestant combinations. The newer, nonsedating antihistamines include loratadine 10 mg qd, astemizole 10 mg qd, fexofenadine 60 mg bid, and cetirizine 10 mg qd. Their mechanisms of action are similar to those of the older-type antihistamines without the CNS side effects. Fexofenadine and loratadine are available with pseudoephredrine 120 mg. Treatment for allergic rhinitis includes nasal steroids and/or cromolyn nasal sprays and all antihistamines (older and newer generations). Decongestants can be added when these combinations do not work. There are no randomized, double-blind, placebo-controlled studies looking at these therapies for cough in acute sinusitis. Clinical experience suggests that they work effectively. The treatment of chronic sinusitis is more controversial. Long-term antibiotics effective against *Streptococcus pneumoniae, Hemophilus influenzae,* anaerobes, and *Staphylococcus aureus* often need to be used for up to 4 to 6 weeks. Nasal corticosteroids (e.g., beclomethasone, fluticasone, triamcinolone, and budesonide) and decongestants are advocated. Sinus surgery using endoscopic technology is helpful when medical therapy fails. Patients must be advised that recurrence of symptoms after surgery is possible.

BRONCHIAL ASTHMA

Asthma has been known for many years to be a common cause of cough in patients of all ages (see Chap. 28). While the exact pathogenesis of asthma is unknown, it is felt to be a disease characterized by chronic inflammation of the airways, variable airflow obstruction, hyperreactive airways, and symptoms that respond to specific bronchodilator therapy. Typically, patients with asthma present with symptoms of wheezing, cough, chest pain, and dyspnea. They have reversible obstructive airways disease by spirometry and respond to bronchodilators and anti-inflammatory therapy. Patients with no previous history of bronchial asthma may present with a chronic cough of unknown etiology. When challenged with methacholine, they are found to have hyperreactive airways and may respond favorably to bronchodilator therapy. Up to 39% of children and 43% of adults present with cough as the only symptom of bronchial asthma. Cough is triggered by exercise in 78%, cold air in 44%, and upper respiratory tract infections in 100% and occurs during sleep in 72%. Most patients present with a normal spirogram. Bronchial hyperreactivity is demonstrated in nearly all patients in whom it is evaluated. Some investigators feel that a negative inhalation challenge makes the diagnosis of cough-variant asthma very unlikely. Follow-up studies in children suggest that between 9 and 75% will subsequently develop typical asthma symptoms, whereas only 50% of adults develop the more characteristic symptoms of wheezing, coughing, shortness of breath, and need for chronic asthma therapy.

Treatments of general use in the disease

The therapeutic approach to cough-variant asthma is similar to the therapy used in patients with more typical symptoms of wheezing, shortness of breath, chest pain, and cough.

Beta-agonists have been shown in prospective, descriptive studies to be beneficial. However, there are no double-blind, placebo-controlled studies looking at β–agonists alone and their effect on cough. β–Agonists can be inhaled by means of a pressurized metered-dose inhaler (PMDI) with a spacer or a dry-powder inhaler, or they can be taken orally (see Chap. 29). Commonly used β-agonists include salbutamol, metaproterenol, bitolterol, isoetharine, pirbuterol, and terbutaline 2 puffs qid. Salbutamol extentabs 4 mg bid and terbutaline 2.5 to 5 mg qid are also available for oral administration. They all work by stimulating the β-receptor, which, in turn, stimulates adenyl cyclase to generate cyclic adenosine monophosphate (cAMP) intracellularly. This increase in cAMP promotes smooth muscle relaxation. These drugs are metabolized by catechol-*o*-methyl-

transferase and monoamine oxidase. Major side effects include tremor, restlessness, tachycardia, arrhythmia, hypertension, and hypokalemia. Certain individuals with highly reactive airways cannot tolerate PMDIs because the inhaled particles trigger more coughing. In these individuals, oral β-agonists should be given.

Corticosteroids via PMDI with spacer or dry-powder inhaler can be used alone or in combination with β-agonist therapy. Inhaled corticosteroids include beclomethasone 2 to 4 puffs qid, flunisolide 2 puffs bid, triamcinolone 2 to 4 puffs qid, fluticasone 2 to 4 puffs qid, and budesonide 1 to 2 puffs qid. Major side effects include throat irritation, cough, oral candidiasis, and hoarseness. Oral corticosteroids (40-60 mg of prednisone per day) can be used as initial therapy in patients with severe symptoms; however, a positive outcome should not be used as a diagnostic test for asthma in the absence of the other diagnostic criteria because there are other nonasthmatic conditions that respond favorably to corticosteroids (e.g., chronic airway inflammation in nonasthmatics and eosinophilic bronchitis). Chromolyn sodium has been shown in one randomized, double-blind, placebo-controlled study to be effective against cough.

COUGH ASSOCIATED WITH GASTROESOPHAGEAL REFLUX DISEASE

Gastroesophageal reflux is associated with the movement of stomach "juice" to the esophagus. In many normal individuals this occurs as an asymptomatic phenomenon. Reflux becomes a disease when it leads to symptoms. Typical gastrointestinal symptoms include substernal burning, indigestion, regurgitation of digested food, dysphagia, hoarseness, choking, and chest discomfort. The respiratory symptoms include aspiration, hemoptysis, bronchiectasis, adult respiratory distress syndrome, pulmonary fibrosis, atelectasis, bronchitis, asthma, and chronic cough. Lower esophageal sphincter (LES) dysfunction is felt to be the major cause of reflux. Chronic cough has been shown to be the result of gastroesophageal reflux disease in up to 21% of patients presenting with chronic cough of unknown etiology. There is no doubt that gastroesophageal reflux disease can be a complication of chronic cough related to another etiology. This, in turn, can self-perpetuate a cough-reflux cycle. In other words, chronic cough of any etiology may cause gastroesophageal reflux disease (GERD) with cough, and gastroesophageal reflux disease all by itself may lead to cough (see Chap. 33). The diagnosis can be made on the basis of a history plus abnormalities demonstrated by barium swallow, endoscopy, and esophageal motility or esophageal pH probe monitoring. The diagnosis is confirmed with the disappearance of cough when appropriate antireflux therapy has been initiated. Children are not immune to this etiology of chronic cough. The pathogenesis of chronic cough associated with gastroesophageal reflux disease is felt to be a vagally mediated distal esophageal-tracheobronchial reflex. Many patients will not exhibit typical reflux symptoms of heartburn or acid indigestion. In anyone with cough of unknown etiology in whom no other cause can be found, examination for GERD should be carried out even in the absence of reflux symptoms.

Treatments of general use in the disease

Therapy in gastroesophageal reflux disease is to decrease the frequency and duration of reflux events and "neutralize" gastric secretions (see Chap. 33). Conservative measures include cessation of cigarette smoking and avoidance of caffeine; a high-protein, low-fat diet; weight reduction; and raising the head of the bed 4 to 6 inches. H_2 antagonists have been used successfully with these conservative measures in patients with chronic cough, with successful outcomes 80% of the time. Commonly used H_2 antagonists include cimetidine 300 to 600 mg po every 6 hours, famotidine 20 to 40 mg po qd, nizatidine 150 mg po bid, and ranitidine 150 mg po bid. They are partially metabolized in the liver and excreted in large part unmetabolized in the urine. Therefore, patients with renal impairment must have the dose reduced. Ranitidine has a prolonged half-life in patients with hepatic dysfunction. Side effects, while rare, include headaches, dizziness, nausea, myalgias, increased somnolence, and confusion in elderly patients, primarily with cimetidine.

Cimetidine inhibits the cytochrome P450 system and increases the half-life of phenytoin, theophylline, phenobarbital, cyclosporine, carbamazepine, propranolol, calcium channel blockers, quinidine, mexiletine, sulfonylureas, warfarin, and tricyclic antidepressants. The other H_2 blockers interact weakly with the P450 system, and thus they do not lead to specific drug interactions The beneficial effect on cough remains for some time after therapy is discontinued, most likely because it interrupts the perpetuating cycle of cough-induced reflux. Proton pump inhibitors (omeprazole 20-40 mg po qd and lansoprazole 15-30 mg po qd) can be tried if H_2 antagonists are not successful. The proton pump inhibitors work by blocking the H^+,K^+-ATPase pump, the ultimate mediator of gastric acid secretion. Omeprazole inhibits CYP2C19 and increases the half-life of phenytoin, diazepam, and the D-isomer of warfarin. There have been no clinically significant drug-drug interactions with lansoprazole. Major side effects include nausea, diarrhea, and abdominal pain; minor side effects include headaches, dizziness, and somnolence.

Prokinetic agents (cisapride 10-20 mg po, metoclopramide 10-15 mg po) (see Chap. 33) have been used successfully in children. Metoclopramide enhances motility of smooth muscle from the esophagus through to the proximal small intestine, thereby enhancing gastric emptying. It is a dopaminergic agonist metabolized in part by the liver, but its cellular mechanism of action is not well understood. Dosage should be decreased in patients with renal impairment. Cisapride works like metoclopramide but also stimulates the colon and may cause diarrhea. It is metabolized in the liver by hepatic N-dealkylation and hydroxylation. Side effects include extrapyramidal symptoms, anxiety, depression, and cardiovascular disorders, e.g., torsade de pointes, at times dangerous, and possibly related to CYP3A4 antagonism. It may take up to 6 months for a combination of H_2 antagonists or proton pump inhibitors and prokinetic agents to effectively eliminate cough. For patients who have failed medical therapy, laparoscopic funduplication is indicated.

POSTINFECTION COUGH

This entity may be the most difficult to diagnose specifically despite a trend to view infection as the cause of chronic cough in most patients. Since viral syndromes cause acute cough most frequently, and because many patients with PNDSs and bronchial asthma report a "cold" as triggering the initial episode of cough, postinfectious etiologies are commonly considered. In children, diagnosis becomes even more difficult because of the number of respiratory viruses and atypical organisms that can cause cough. Recently, *Chlamydia trachomatis* and *Bordetella pertussis* have been associated with the development of a chronic but self-limited cough. The pathogenesis is felt to be related to airway inflammation with or without bronchial hyperreactivity (in some series these patients have been called asthmatics because of the demonstration of bronchial hyperreactivity). Because of the uncertainties in making the diagnosis, specific therapy is lacking unless there is proof of a specific infecting agent.

Treatments of general use in the disease

Oral prednisone given for a short period of time has been successful. Inhaled corticosteroids (e.g., beclomethasone, flunisolide, fluticasone, triamcinoline, and budesonide) certainly should be considered, especially after initial success with oral corticosteroids. Macrolide antibiotics (e.g., erythromycin, azithromycin, and clarithromycin) may help if an infectious etiology is detected early in the course of the illness.

CHRONIC BRONCHITIS

The term *chronic bronchitis* defines a disorder seen primarily in patients who smoke cigarettes and/or have significant long-term exposures to dusts and other respiratory irritants. The American Thoracic Society states that patients must cough and produce mucus for most days of at least 3 months for 2 consecutive years. The cough is worse in the morning but can occur anytime day or night. The typical long-term cigarette smoker becomes so used to expectorating each day that unless questioned specifically, he/she may not even consider it abnormal. The cough is caused primarily by hypersecretion of mucus, impaired mucociliary clearance, and airway inflammation. Most patients seek medical attention when they experience an increased cough frequency, an increase in the amount of secretions, a change in the color of secretions, or increasing shortness of breath associated with cough.

Treatments of general use in the disease

Smoking cessation is an absolute necessity when trying to control this cough. When successful, cough will either disappear or decrease significantly in more than 90% of patients between 1 and 3 months after smoking cessation.

While bronchodilators, β-agonists, ipratropium bromide and theophylline are used to treat symptoms in patients with chronic bronchitis, their specific effect on cough has not been studied. Ipratropium bromide via PMDI at 2 puffs four times daily did decrease sputum production in one placebo-controlled study. Corticosteroids given orally for 7 to 10 days are used commonly to decrease airway inflammation and appear to improve symptoms, but their specific effect on cough has not been evaluated. Organic iodide has been shown to be effective, but it is not used because of a plethora of side effects. Antibiotics directed primarily towards *S. pneumoniae* and *H. influenzae* are nearly always used for exacerbations of chronic bronchitis because these organisms are grown most commonly from the sputum of these patients. Viruses and atypical organisms (*Mycoplasma, Chlamydia*) also may have a role. The most common "cocktail" used to treat these patients includes a bronchodilator, ipratropium bromide, antibiotics, and when these fail, a course of oral corticosteroids.

ANGIOTENSIN-CONVERTING ENZYME (ACE) INHIBITOR-INDUCED COUGH

With the prolific use of ACE inhibitors in the treatment of hypertension and left ventricular dysfunction, this common side effect of these agents (cough) soon became evident (see Chap. 23). It occurs frequently, more than 10% in most studies. It is a class effect of all drugs in this category; i.e., coughing with one ACE inhibitor usually means coughing with another. Therefore, switching from one ACE inhibitor to another usually does not alleviate the problem. It is not dose-related; it may appear soon after starting the drug or up to months later. Once the ACE inhibitor is discontinued, cough usually disappears within 1 week, but it may take up to 1 month before the cough disappears completely. The pathogenesis appears to be related to excess amounts of substance P and bradykinin in the tracheobronchial tree. Prostaglandins also may be involved because sulindac, nifedipine, and indomethacin decrease ACE inhibitor-induced cough. Picotamide (600 mg po bid), a thromboxane antagonist, has been shown recently to block ACE inhibitor-induced cough in a double-blind crossover study. This suggests that an imbalance between thromboxane and prostacyclin may be responsible for ACE inhibitor-induced cough. Discontinuation or substitution of the drug whit eventually an AT₁ antagonist remains the best therapy.

BRONCHIECTASIS

This once very common affliction is now encountered in very few patients. The disease entity is related to an abnormal pathology of the airways, namely, dilatation of airways, hypertrophied mucus glands, and hypersecretion of mucus. Cough with excessive production of mucopurulent secretions and a high incidence of hemoptysis is the most common symptom. The patient occasionally will wheeze, and in some children, wheezing may be the first sign of cystic fibrosis. Sputum cultures reveal a number of different organisms but most commonly *S. pneumoniae, H. influenzae, S. aureus, Pseudomonas aeruginosa* (primarily in patients with cystic fibrosis), anaerobes, and mycobacteria. The diagnosis is easily confirmed by the typical clinical history as well as an abnormal chest radiograph that usually demonstrates increased markings and/or areas of cystic formation.

Treatments of general use in the disease

It is important for the patient with bronchiectasis, as well as the physician, to realize that coughing is a beneficial symptom. It helps clear lower respiratory tract secretions. Cough has to be treated when it overwhelms the patient during an exacerbation, but it cannot be completely eliminated. Therapy consists of chest physiotherapy including percussion, postural drainage, forced expiratory techniques to strengthen cough, antibiotics, β-agonists, and theophyllines. Dornase-α, a recombinant human deoxyribonuclease given by inhalation via nebulizer 2.5 mg qd or bid, decreases the viscosity of purulent sputum by selective cleavage of DNA in purulent mucus. The antibiotics should have activity against *S. pneumoniae, H. influenzae, P. aeruginosa,* and *S. aureus* and should be given for at least 2 to 3 weeks; on occasion, months of continuous therapy are required.

PSYCHOGENIC COUGH

Psychogenic cough, or habit cough, while infrequent, is a difficult diagnosis to confirm. It is also a diagnosis of exclusion. It is seen more commonly in children but can be seen in adults. It is the rarest of all causes of chronic cough. The typical characteristics include a loud "barking seal," paroxysmal, dry cough not occurring at night. While the characteristics of the cough are typical, they are certainly not diagnostic. A conscientious effort to diagnose a specific cause must be made before telling a patient that his cough is a habit or of psychogenic etiology. Therapy includes counseling, psychiatric intervention, and behavioral modification.

Cough modifiers

After extensive evaluation, the etiology in most patients who have a chronic cough can be identified and treated specifically (Tab. 30.1). However, there are a few patients in whom cough modifiers may be necessary. Cough modifiers can be divided into antitussives and protussive agents.

The literature evaluating drugs useful in the treatment of cough using only randomized, double-blind, placebo-controlled studies in human subjects found that ipratropium bromide in chronic bronchitis, iodopropylidine glycerol in chronic bronchitis and asthma, guaimesal in acute and chronic bronchitis, and dexbrompheniramine maleate plus pseudoephedrine sulfate in the common cold have been shown to be effective antitussive drugs. Dropropizine and its L-isomer levodropropizine are two antitussives available in Europe. The mechanism of action includes affinity for H_1 and α-adrenergic receptors. Levodropropizine has weaker CNS sedative effects. Narcotic and nonnarcotic antitussives also can decrease cough by a direct effect on the cough center in the medulla.

All members of the phenanthrene alkaloid group (e.g., morphine, meperidine, codeine, and hydrocodeine) are effective antitussive medications. These drugs act as adjuncts on the opiate receptors in the cough center. They all have the common side effects of sedation, constipation, lethargy, urinary retention, and respiratory depression. Psychic dependence, physical dependence, and tolerance may develop with continuous use. Dextromethorphan 10 to 30 mg qid, diphenhydramine 25 to 50 mg every 4 hours, caramiphen 20 mg po tid, and noscapine 15 to 30 mg tid or qid belong to a group of nonnarcotic antitussive agents that have been shown to decrease cough. These agents act directly on the cough center but are not addictive. They have no CNS side effects when given in therapeutic doses.

Dextromethorphan, the D-isomer of the codeine analogue levorphanol, does not act through opioid receptors. It acts centrally by increasing the threshold to stimulate cough. It is rarely addictive. Dextromethorphan is metabolized in the liver by the cytochrome P450 system. Some individuals with genetic polymorphism of CYP2D6 metabolize dextromethorphan at a slower rate than normal. They are "poor metabolizers" (PMs) versus normal "extensive metabolizers" (EMs). This genetic polymorphism may influence the antitussive effect of dextromethorphan but does not clearly appear to affect dependence.

Protussive therapy increases cough effectiveness, i.e., airway clearance. Hypertonic saline aerosol in patients with bronchitis, amiloride aerosol in patients with cystic fibrosis, and aerosolized terbutaline in patients with bronchiectasis have been shown to be effective protussive mediators.

Table 30.2 Therapy of chronic cough

Diagnoses	Therapy
Postnasal drip syndromes	
Perennial rhinitis Post-infectious rhinitis	• First-generation antihistamine: e.g. brompheniramine, phenylpropanolamine, azatadine-pseudoephedrine • Second-generation antihistamine-decongestants (nonsedating): e.g., loratadine, pseudoephedrine
Allergic rhinitis	• Avoidance of allergens • First-generation antihistamines: e.g diphenhydramine, chlortrimeton • Nonsedating antihistamines: loratadine, cetirizine, fexofenadine astemizole • Cromolyn (nasal) • Nasal corticosteroids: beclomethasone, fluticasone budesonide • Ipratropium bromide (nasal) • Desensitization (long-term benefit)
Sinusitis	• Antibiotics (to cover S. pneumoniae, H. influenzae, anaerobes, S. aureus) • Nasal corticosteroids • Decongestants • Surgery
Cough variant asthma	• β agonists: salbutamol, metaproterenol, pirbuterol via PMDI, dry powder, oral • Inhaled corticosteroids: beclomethasone, triamcinolone, via PMDI, dry powder • Oral prednisone • Nedocromil sodium
Gastroresophageal reflux disease	• Conservative measures: raise head of bed 4-6", high protein, low fat diet, no cigarettes, no caffeine • Pharmacologic agents: H_2 blockers ranitidine, cimetidine; proton pump inhibitors-omeprazole, lansoprazole; pantoprazole; prokinetic agents: metoclopramide, cisapride • Surgery funduplication

Chronic bronchitis	• Avoid cigarette smoke and other respiratory irritants
	• Bronchodilators-β agonists, theophylline
	• Ipratropium bromide
	• Corticosteroids (oral)
	• Antibiotics
	  Simple bronchitis: amoxicillin, quinolone, second generation cephalosporin.
	  Complicated bronchitis: quinolone, second generation macrolide, amoxicillin clavulanate

BERKOWITZ RB, CONNELL JT, DIETZ AJ, et al. The effectiveness of the nonsedating antihistamine loratadine plus pseudoephedrine in the symptomatic management of the common cold. Ann Allergy 1989;63:336-9.

BRODY TM, JOSEPH L, MINNEMAN KP. Human pharmacology: molecular to clinical. St. Louis: Mosby-Year Book, 1998.

BRONSKY EA, DRUCE H, FINDLAY SR, et al. A clinical trial of ipratropium bromide nasal spray in patients with perennial nonallergic rhinitis. J Allergy Clin Immunol 1995; 95:1117-22.

CORRAO WM, BRAMAN SS, IRWIN RS. Chronic cough as the sole presenting manifestation of bronchial asthma. N Engl J Med 1979;300:633-7.

CURLEY FJ, IRWIN, RS, PRATTER, MR, et al. Cough and the common cold. Am Rev Respir Dis 1988;138:305-11.

DiPEDE C, VIEGI G, QUACKENBOSS JJ, et al. Respiratory symptoms and risk factors in an Arizona population sample of Anglo and Mexican-American whites. Chest 1991;99:916-22.

ING AJ, NGU MC, BRESLIN ABX. Pathogenesis of chronic persistent cough associated with gastroesophageal reflux. Am J Respir Crit Care Med 1994;149:160-7.

IRWIN RS, CURLEY FJ. The treatment of cough: a comprehensive review. Chest 1991;99:1477-84.

IRWIN RS, CORRAO WM, PRATTER MR. Chronic persistent cough in the adult: the spectrum and frequency of causes and successful outcome of specific therapy. Am Rev Respir Dis 1981;123:413-7.

IRWIN RS, CURLEY FJ, FRENCH CJ. Chronic cough. The spectrum and frequency of causes, key components of the diagnostic evaluation, and outcome of specific therapy. Am Rev Respir Dis 1990;141:640-7.

ISRAILI ZH, HALL WD. Cough and angioneurotic edema associated with angiontensin-converting enzyme inhibitor therapy: a review of the literature and pathophysiology. Ann Intern Med 1992;117:234-42.

JOHNSON D, OSBORN LM. Cough variant asthma: a review of the clinical literature. J Asthma 1991;28:85-90.

MALINI PL, STROCCHI E, ZANAROLI M, et al. Tromboxane antagonism and cough induced by angiotensin-converting-enzyme inhibitor. Lancet 1997;350:15-8.

POE RH, HARDEEN RV, ISRAEL RH, KALLAY MC. Chronic persistent cough. Chest 1989;95:723-8.

WITEK TJ, SCHACHTER EN. Pharmacology and therapeutics in respiratory care. Philadelphia: WB Saunders, 1994.

31

Oxygen and other ancillary therapies

Neven Tudorić

OXIGEN THERAPY

Oxygen is needed for the generation of mitochondrial adenosine triphosphate (ATP), the main source of energy necessary for vital cell functions. In the milieu of aerobic metabolism, 30 molecules of ATP from each molecule of glucose, metabolized in the presence of oxygen, will be produced. Anaerobic glycolysis produces instead only 3 molecules of ATP for each glucose molecule, with lactic acid formed as the end product. Oxygen delivery to tissues depends on alveolar ventilation, distribution of ventilation-perfusion ratio within the lungs, hemoglobin concentration and its affinity for oxygen, concentration of other ligands of hemoglobin, cardiac output, and distribution of capillary blood flow within the tissues.

Oxygen therapy can raise the partial pressure of oxygen in inhaled gas (PiO_2), which depends on the fractional percentage of inspired oxygen (FiO_2) and barometric pressure. For room air at sea level, $PiO_2 = 0.21 \times 760$ mm Hg = 160 mm Hg. After saturation with water vapor in the upper airways, the PiO_2 is slightly diluted and reaches 149 mmHg. For practical purposes, the PO_2 of inhaled gas as it enters the alveoli can be approximated by multiplying the FiO_2 by 7 (i.e., for room air, $21 \times 7 = 147$ mm Hg; for 40% O_2, $40 \times 7 = 280$ mm Hg).

Since the oxygen-carbon dioxide exchange is continuous in alveolar gas, the alveolar PO_2 (PaO_2) is considerably lower than that of inspired gas. Since total gas tension in the alveoli must remain constant, the greater the amount of carbon dioxide entering the alveoli, the lower the PaO_2. The respiratory quotient is not 1.0 but is about 0.8, so every millimeter of mercury of alveolar PCO_2 ($PaCO_2$) displaces 1.25 mm Hg of PaO_2. For clinical purposes, the $PaCO_2$ can be assumed to be equal to the arterial PCO_2 ($PaCO_2$). It follows that the PaO_2 may be calculated by the equation $PaO_2 = PiO_2 - 1.25 PaCO_2$. For room air, with $PaCO_2$ of 40 mm Hg, the $PaO_2 = 147 - 50 = 97$ mm Hg. If ventilation (V) and perfusion (Q) were perfectly matched (V/Q= 1), PaO_2 and PaO_2 would be equal. The overall V/Q ratio of the normal lung, however, is approximately 0.8. This results in a PaO_2 that is 5 to 15 mm Hg lower than the PaO_2. The difference in PO_2 between alveolus and artery ($A - aDO_2$) is a direct reflection of the degree of mismatching between V and Q, i.e., the severity of intrinsic lung disease. $A - aDO_2$ increases progressively with age.

By increasing PiO_2, oxygen therapy raises PaO_2 and the oxygen saturation of hemoglobin (SaO_2). Therefore, an oxygen lack (hypoxemia) is the main indication for oxygen therapy. For effective oxygen therapy, it is necessary to understand the causes and mechanisms of hypoxemia. Hypoxemia may be caused by four different physiologic mechanisms:

1. *Decreased PiO_2 due to living at high altitude or being in high-altitude aircraft.* The fall in barometric pressure at high altitude lowers the PiO_2, causing arterial hypoxemia despite compensatory hyperventilation. In other words, the barometric pressure at 2400 m is 560 mmHg, and PiO_2 is 117 mmHg (0.21×560). This is equivalent to breathing only 17% oxygen at sea level. The same conditions occur in the passenger cabins of commercial aircraft, which are pressurized to the equivalent of 1500 to 2400 m.

2. *Hypoventilation due to sleep apnea, neuromuscular disorders (e.g., myasthenia gravis, peripheral neuropathy, or bilateral diaphragmatic palsy), drug overdose, or head injury.* Hypercapnia is synonymous with hypoventilation. It is evident from the alveolar gas equation (see above) that hypoventilation alone can lead to hypoxemia. If the $PaCO_2$ increases from 40 to 80 mm Hg, the PaO_2 must drop by 50 mmHg (40×1.25), from 90 to 40 mm Hg. If hypoxemia is induced by alveolar hypoventilation alone (very uncommon because hypoventilation nearly always causes some atelectasis and other secondary effects), then the $A - aDo_2$ remains normal. In these cases, hypoxemia can be corrected by increasing ventilation without any increase in FiO_2.

3. *Ventilation-perfusion imbalance due to chronic obstructive pulmonary disease, asthma, most interstitial lung diseases, pulmonary edema, adult respiratory distress syndrome, athelectasis, or pneumonia.* Important reflex mechanisms exist to increase blood flow to well-ventilated alveoli and, conversely, to

reduce blood flow to poorly ventilated alveoli, thus preserving the average alveolar V ratio at around 0.8. Areas with low V/Q ratios result in hypoxemia, whereas areas with high ratios lead to wasted ventilation (dead space), which contributes to hypercapnia by causing increased work of breathing. As long as airways are not totally occluded, hypoxemia is readily corrected with small increments in FiO_2. Areas that are not at all ventilated but are still being perfused result in right-to-left shunting of blood. This is more refractory to oxygen therapy because oxygen cannot reach the diffusing surface. Such patients often must be treated with mechanical ventilation and positive end-expiratory pressure (PEEP).

4. *Impaired diffusion due to interstitial diseases.* Thickening of the alveolar capillary membrane was for many years thought to cause hypoxemia by decreasing oxygen diffusion through the thickened membrane. However, it is now realized that this is generally not the case and that the most common cause of hypoxemia in these conditions is ventilation-perfusion mismatch.

INDICATIONS FOR OXYGEN THERAPY

In most instances, oxygen is administered as a treatment for respiratory failure – either hypoxemia, tissue hypoxia, or both. Therefore, the goal of oxygen therapy is to alleviate the hypoxemia and/or the deleterious effects of end-organ dysfunction secondary to tissue hypoxia. Respiratory failure is defined as present in a patient with lung disease in whom the PaO_2 is below 60 mm Hg (8.0 kPa) when breathing air at rest at sea level. Hypoxemia can be hypercapnic (associated with carbon dioxide retention) and normocapnic (low or normal $PaCO_2$).

Hypercapnic hypoxemia can be detected predominantly in patients with chronic obstructive airway disease and is the hallmark of the "blue and bloated" patient, in whom arterial hypoxemia is associated with carbon dioxide retention, secondary polycythemia, pulmonary hypertension, and chronic cor pulmonale. In these patients, the usual strategy is to administer oxygen at a low flow rate, precisely controlled, that suffices to increase the PaO_2 to a tolerable level without abolishing the patient's hypoxic ventilatory drive. Excessive oxygen administration in the management of carbon dioxide retention is a common cause of respiratory depression as a result of antagonism to the hypoxic ventilatory drive that in these patients replaces the normal sensitivity of the respiratory center to changes in PCO_2. The goal is to achieve a PaO_2 of 50 to 60 mm Hg. This can be achieved by a slight increase in PaO_2 (10-20 mmHg) by administering approximately 24 to 28% oxygen. Changes in PaO_2 of this magnitude rarely depress alveolar ventilation, but because the initial PaO_2 is on the steep part of the oxyhemoglobin dissociation curve, oxygen saturation increases sufficiently. Serial determinations of arterial blood gases are necessary to monitor the course of arterial

hypoxemia and hypercapnia as the inspired oxygen concentration is increased to the desired level. Because of the need for precise control of the inspired oxygen concentration in managing hypercapnic hypoxemia, many physicians use Venturi masks (designed to deliver specific concentrations) in this situation. However, equally successful results can be obtained by the careful use of nasal cannulas. The FiO_2 delivered to the patient can only be estimated with nasal cannulas. Such estimates require knowledge of the total minute ventilation and the duration of inspiration and expiration.

Most patients with hypercapnic hypoxemia respond to controlled oxygen delivery with relief of arterial hypoxemia and, in conjunction with other supportive measures, improvement in clinical status. However, some patients experience progressive hypercapnia and acidosis that require an artificial airway and mechanical ventilation. After this, effective oxygenation nearly always can be achieved using an inspired oxygen concentration of less than 50% without the addition of continuous positive airway pressure (CPAP) or PEEP.

Normocapnic hypoxemia can be detected predominantly in patients with pneumonia, pulmonary edema, an acute attack of bronchial asthma, pulmonary thromboembolism, atelectasis, a large pleural effusion of rapid onset, acute lung injury, or adult respiratory distress syndrome. In these patients, high concentrations of oxygen can be administered without fear of developing carbon dioxide retention. An initial FiO_2 of approximately 40% is used and subsequently adjusted according to the results of arterial blood-gas analyses. The controlled, low-dose oxygen titration approach used for hypercapnic hypoxemic patients is not appropriate for hypoxemic patients without hypercapnia, who may remain dangerously hypoxemic if the FiO_2 is increased only gradually. In patients with hypercapnic hypoxemia, a PaO_2 of 50 to 65 mm Hg is considered optimal; in nonhypercapnic patients, the corresponding range is from 60 to 80 mm Hg. In addition to oxygen therapy, attempts should be made to reverse the underlying lung pathology. Maintaining cardiac output by the appropriate use of fluids and inotropic agents is crucial.

In contrast to patients with hypercapnic hypoxemia, in whom alveolar hypoventilation is the major indicator for ventilatory support, the primary reason for the use of mechanical ventilation in patients with normocapnic hypoxemia is a failure to oxygenate the patient at an acceptable FiO_2. The use of positive pressure helps to recruit alveoli and advantageously redistribute lung fluids. However, a decision must be made regarding the mode of ventilation because application of PEEP and CPAP may improve or worsen the degree of hypoxemia. Careful and repeated monitoring of clinical and laboratory indices of tissue oxygenation and end-organ function is required.

OXYGEN DELIVERY SYSTEMS

A number of delivery systems are available for the short-term administration of oxygen. In general, they can be divided into two major groups: low-flow and high-flow systems. The low-flow systems are not intended to provide the total inspiratory requirements of the patient. With low-flow systems, the FiO_2 entering the airways can vary greatly because it depends on the flow rate of oxygen, the tidal volume, and the respiratory rate. High-flow systems provide flow rates that are high enough to completely satisfy the patient's inspiratory demand, either by controlled entrainment of ambient air or by a high flow of oxygen.

The low-flow systems include nasal catheters and cannulas, simple oxygen masks, and masks with reservoir bags. The former two systems deliver, at a flow rate between 1 and 4 liters/min, an FiO_2 of 20 to 35%. At a flow rate of 4 to 6 liters/min of 100% oxygen, they can deliver an FiO_2 of up to 50%. Masks with reservoir bags can deliver an FiO_2 of greater then 50% to a patient who does not have an artificial airway.

The high-flow systems include jet-mixing Venturi masks, able to deliver an FiO_2 of between 24 and 40%, being relatively independent of the oxygen flow rate. They are particularly useful in treating patients with hypercapnic hypoxemia, in whom there is a danger of respiratory depression from excessive inspired oxygen concentration. T-tubes and tracheostomy collars are reserved for patients with artificial airways.

OXYGEN THERAPY IN SPECIAL CLINICAL CIRCUMSTANCES

Acute exacerbation of chronic bronchitis and emphysema

Guidelines for controlling oxygen therapy have evolved on the basis of clinical experience. They have led to the proposal that PaO_2 should be maintained at over 50 mm Hg (6.6 kPa) at minimum if arterial pH does not fall below 7.26. In patients with chronic bronchitis and emphysema, all clinical signs are unreliable. Arterial blood-gas analysis is the only certain method of diagnosing this type of respiratory failure. After the initial blood-gas analysis has indicated the severity of the condition, oxygen is given by nasal prongs at 2 liters/min, and arterial blood-gas analysis is repeated 30 to 60 minutes later. If the PaO_2 is over 50 mm Hg and the arterial pH is not lower than 7.26, controlled oxygen therapy should continue. If these limits are not achieved, then the inspired oxygen flow rate should be lowered to l liter/min by nasal prongs and the blood-gas analysis repeated in 1 hour. If a PaO_2 over 50 mm Hg cannot be achieved without the pH falling below 7.26, then a respiratory stimulant should be administered. Doxapram may be given by continuous intravenous infusion (0.5-4 mg/min of the doxapram infusion in a concentration of 2 mg/ml in 5% glucose). The aim is to increase or maintain ventilation for a short time, usually 24 to 48 hours, allowing oxygen therapy to be given at a concentration that otherwise would cause excessive hypercapnia and acidosis. Used in this way, doxapram may "buy time" while another treatment is given in an attempt to avoid the need for assisted ventilation, which should be considered if recommended limits cannot be achieved.

It should be stressed that the pH disturbance is a much better guide to the acuteness and severity of the condition than is the $PaCO_2$ level alone.

Adult respiratory distress syndrome (ARDS)

It is essential to treat this life-threatening hypoxemia with a high FiO_2, followed by repeated blood-gas analyses to be certain that the treatment is adequate. Frequently, it is possible to achieve a satisfactory PaO_2 only with an FiO_2 of 60% or more, which by itself damages the pulmonary capillary membrane if it is maintained for a long period of time. Prompt endotracheal intubation may be needed to deliver oxygen and PEEP because hypoxemia is due to the nature of the lung injury, frequently refractory to oxygen inhalation by face mask.

Acute attack of bronchial asthma

Oxygen therapy is always indicated in this situation because severe asthmatics are invariably hypoxemic. The FiO_2 is guided by the blood-gas analysis; the PaO_2 should be maintained higher than 60 mm Hg, in the 70 to 90 mm Hg range if possible. Oxygen may be given effectively by nasal prongs or, if tolerated, by Venturi mask. Since oxygen may dry the mucosa, it always should be humidified.

LONG-TERM OXYGEN THERAPY

In long-term oxygen therapy, treatment is given for most of the 24-hour day for many weeks or years – potentially for the rest of a patient's life. A number of studies have shown that long-term oxygen therapy, taken for a minimum of 15 hours per day, improves survival in patients with chronic bronchitis and emphysema complicated by chronic hypoxemia and cor pulmonale. Selection criteria for this treatment include: (1) a PaO_2 under 55 mm Hg (7.3 kPa) when awake and breathing air, (2) a forced expiratory volume in 1 second (FEV_1) of 1.5 liters or less, (3) a clinical diagnosis of chronic bronchitis and emphysema, and (4) usual episodes of ankle edema due to cor pulmonale. These findings should be constant for at least two measurements 4 weeks apart. This ensures that the patient is in a steady clinical state and that hypoxemia is not transitory due to an acute exacerbation. Before making a final decision about administration of long-term oxygen therapy, it is necessary to test the effects of oxygen by measuring the PaO_2 and $PaCO_2$ during 1-hour periods at flows of 1 to 3 liters/min. This helps in choosing the proper flow and allows determination of the level of carbon dioxide retention.

The favored method of supply is now the oxygen concentrator, a device that uses a molecular sieve and compressor to remove nitrogen from air. Concentrators yield oxygen concentrations of over 93% at flow rates of 2 liters/min when in continuous use; oxygen concentration falls to 85 to 90% at higher flow rates. The oxygen is delivered to the patient by nasal prongs.

OXYGEN TOXICITY

Continued inhalation of over 40% oxygen for more than 48 hours can reduce vital capacity with substernal distress, breathlessness, and cough even in healthy, normal volunteers. If exposure continues, adult respiratory distress syndrome develops with damage to alveolar capillary membranes and high-protein alveolar edema. This is recognized clinically by severe breathlessness, cyanosis refractory to further oxygen administration, and diffuse infiltrates on the chest radiograph. Pulmonary oxygen toxicity may be avoided if concentrations of over 40% are not given continuously for more than 24 hours.

Since patients with acute lung injury should be treated with high oxygen concentrations, owing to their severe hypoxemia, it is difficult to isolate the symptoms of the specific disease from those caused by oxygen toxicity. This means that oxygen toxicity in patients receiving high concentrations of oxygen can only be suspected. Because a protective drug treatment does not exist, it is necessary to follow the general rule of administering the lowest concentration of oxygen required for maintaining sufficient tissue oxygenation.

ANCILLARY THERAPIES IN PULMONARY MEDICINE

RESPIRATORY PHYSICAL THERAPY

Pulmonary rehabilitation programs focus on reversing a patient's disability from the chronic pulmonary disease rather than solely on reversing a chronic, progressive disease process. They attempt to return the patient to the highest possible functional capacity allowed by his/her pulmonary handicap and overall life situation. After the medical evaluation, psychosocial assessment, and goal setting, the program should be tailored to the individual and include education, chest physiotherapy instruction, exercise training, and psychosocial support. Physical therapy takes a three-pronged approach that includes relaxation exercises, sputum clearance (postural drainage), and breathing exercises.

Relaxation exercises   Chronic pulmonary patients are particularly tense and anxious individuals because of dyspnea and fear of suffocation. To relieve the constant anxiety, decrease the compensatory muscular contraction, and significantly improve the results of postural drainage and breathing, relaxation exercises are the essential first step in rehabilitation.

Sputum clearance   Sputum clearance methods can be used in patients who produce 30 ml or more of sputum daily. Methods include postural drainage, compression and percussion, thoracic expansion exercises, and the forced-expiration technique. Postural drainage (usually with vibropercussion) is indicated in patients with an inability to raise bronchial secretions as a result of structural abnormalities (e.g., bronchiectasis, cystic fibrosis, or lung abscess), in patients with acute infection and limited forced expiratory volumes (e.g., chronic obstructive pulmonary disease or pulmonary fibrosis), and in patients with poor tussive forces (e.g., old age or cachexia, neuromuscular disease, or postoperative or traumatic pain).

A specific position may facilitate optimal gravity-augmented drainage of secretions from each lobe or a segment of both lungs. Specific positioning helps the patient evacuate pooled secretions, especially when used with terminal expiratory and deep-breath coughs. Vibropercussion, using either chest clapping with a flexible wrist and cupped hands or a mechanical vibrator, helps loosen and mobilize other secretions that can be expectorated. The process is tiring, and patient rarely can tolerate more than two to three treatments per day, preferably before meals, with each treatment lasting 30 to 45 minutes.

Breathing exercises   Breathing exercises are indicated in patients with advanced chronic bronchitis and emphysema who hyperinflate during attacks of bronchospasm, exercise, or panic. The first step in the basic breathing exercises is to master abdominal breathing, including pursed-lip exhalation. Abdominal breathing is practiced while lying on the back with the legs thrown up, one hand on the chest, and the other on the abdomen. The patient breaths in deeply through the nose, letting the abdomen protrude fully as felt by the hand, and exhales slowly through pursed lips, drawing the abdomen inward. A metronome can be used, with 1s to breath in and 3 s to breath out. The chest remains stationary. Abdominal breathing can be performed against a weight on abdomen (e.g., a sandbag, hot water bottle, or book). The patient pushes the abdomen against the weight when he exhales.

Patients must be taught pursed-lip breathing by practicing exhalation against partially closed (pursed) lips, as if ready to whistle. It also can be practiced by candle blowing – the patient blows gently through pursed lips, using abdominal breathing, not extinguishing flame of candle but bending it away. Pursed-lip breathing creates a pressure within the airways that prevents bronchiolar collapse from high intrathoracic pressures. This technique, accompanied by small inhaled breaths, allows deflation of hyperinflated lungs with return to a lower work of breathing.

PRINCIPLES OF INHALED THERAPY

Inhaled therapy has several distinct advantages over other routes when treating lung disease. First of all, aerosol particles have a favorable surface-to-volume ratio. Second, there is wide dispersion and surface contact for drug diffusion. In addition, the dose is small, and the systemic absorption remains slight, thus minimizing side effects.

The onset of drug action is often rapid and the duration satisfactory.

The drug is delivered as an aerosol, which is a suspension of fine liquid or solid particles in air; the particles range in size from 0.01 to 100 µm. Most particles larger than 8 µm and all particles larger than 15 µm are deposited in the oropharynx by inertial impaction. Particles in the range of 5 to 10 µm deposit on the intrapulmonary airways down to those of about 2 µm in diameter. Smaller particles (<5 µm in diameter) reach the alveoli and are thus in the respirable range.

Therapeutic aerosols can be produced as liquid mists by metered-dose inhalers or nebulizers and as dusts by dry-powder inhalers. Metered-dose inhalers (MDI) have become the most popular type of device. The drug is dissolved or suspended in a liquid propellant, such as chlorofluorocarbon (CFC), in a sealed canister. Although medical aerosols do not contribute significantly to the CFC-induced destruction of the stratospheric ozone layer, new CFC-free propellants have been tested. It is important to demonstrate to the patient how to use the MDI as well as all other inhalers. The canister should be shaken, the mouthpiece placed in the mouth, and at the start of a slow and deep inspiration, the MDI should be activated by pressing the canister down. The breath should be held for about 10 s. Some patients may have coordination difficulties, and these can be avoided by using one of the more sophisticated breath-regulated MDIs that automatically deliver an aerosol dose to the patient at the beginning of the inspiratory cycle.

For the patient with poor technique in using MDIs, especially young children, spacers with holding chambers are helpful. In this case, the inhaler is inserted into the spacer device while its mouthpiece is placed in the mouth. The spacer device allows discharge of the drug into a chamber, where particles of the medication are held in suspension for 3 to 5 s. During this time, the patient can inhale the drug. Spacers will maximize the tracheobronchial deposition of the aerosol (approximately 15% of dose). Further, they reduce deposition in the mouth and oropharynx, decreasing cough as well as the possibility of oral candidiasis when used to deliver corticosteroids. The use of spacers for the delivery of inhaled corticosteroids has been shown to decrease the systemic bioavailability of corticosteroids and the risk of systemic side effects. In patients with good technique for MDI use, spacers will offer no additional advantages.

Dry-powder inhalers are CFC-free and breath-regulated, thus greatly reducing coordination difficulties. However, in patients with severe airway obstruction due to a low inspiratory flow rate, the effect of the therapy may be insufficient, especially during relapse. Rotahaler and Spinhaler are single-dose powder inhalers in which screwing or twisting the inhaler pierces or splits the capsule containing the medicine (see Chap. 5). A quick and deep inhalation delivers the powder to the lungs. Multidose powder inhalers such as Diskhaler and Turbohaler generally are easier to use than MDIs, and little coordination is required.

Nebulizers are devices that apply energy to a liquid to create a "wet" aerosol. They are easier to use than MDIs or dry-powder inhalers and therefore are particularly valuable for children under 5 years of age and in the treatment of acute severe asthma. The two systems in general use are the jet and ultrasonic nebulizers. The former uses a stream of compressed air or oxygen to produce aerosol by drawing up the liquid through a capillary membrane. In ultrasonic nebulizers, high-frequency sound waves focused on the surface of the drug solution produce an aerosol. This nebulizer has a higher output than a jet nebulizer but produces larger particles. In general, about 10% of the aerosol reaches the lung.

The inhaled route is used most often to administer drugs for the prevention and reversal of airway obstruction in asthma and chronic bronchitis, such as inhaled corticosteroids (e.g., beclomethasone, budesonide, flunisolide, fluticasone, and triamcinolone), cromones (e.g., sodium cromoglycate and cromolyn sodium), inhaled short-acting β_2 agonists (e.g., salbutamol, fenoterol, metaproterenol, pirbuterol, and terbutalin), inhaled long-acting β_2 agonists (e.g., salmeterol and formoterol), and anticholinergics (e.g., ipratropium bromide and oxitropium bromide). Antibiotic and mucolytic aerosols are used much less frequently.

Suggested readings

CELLI BR. Current thoughts regarding treatment of chronic obstructive pulmonary disease. Med Clin North Am 1996;80:589-609.

CHAPMAN KR. Therapeutic approaches to chronic obstructive pulmonary disease: An emerging consensus. Am J Med 1996;100:S5-S10.

FULMER JD, SNIDER GL. ACCP-NHLBI National Conference on Oxygen Therapy. Chest 1984;86:234-47.

NHLBI/WHO WORKSHOP REPORT. Global strategy for asthma management and prevention. NIH Publication 96-3659A. Washington: NIH, 1995.

RIES AL, KAPLAN RM, LIMBERG TM, PREWITT LM. Effects of pulmonary rehabilitation on physiologic and psychosocial outcomes in patients with chronic obstructive pulmonary disease. Ann Intern Med 1995;122:823-32.

TARPY SP, CELLI BR. Long-term oxygen therapy. N Engl J Med 1995;333:710-4.

Gastrointestinal diseases

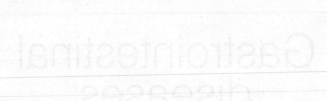

CHAPTER

32

Functional disorders of the gastrointestinal tract

Thomas R. Weihrauch

NAUSEA AND VOMITING

Nausea is a subjective sensation that is restricted to the gastrointestinal tract and is combined with the urgency to vomit. Emesis is a complex reflex of the autonomic and somatic nerve systems and the endocrine system with the goal to empty the stomach.

There are numerous causes for the symptoms of nausea and vomiting: (1) vomiting caused by various types of disorders throughout the entire digestive tract – from the pharynx to the rectum, including liver, pancreas, and bile ducts – such as inflammation, mechanical obstruction, and toxic irritation; (2) cerebral vomiting, caused by stimulation of the chemoreceptor trigger zone in the area postrema of the fourth ventricle, either mechanic (e.g., concussion, raised intracranial pressure), toxic (e.g., emetics such as morphine or apomorphine, digitalis intoxication, cytostatics, endogenous-toxic), or as a result of cerebral hypoxia (e.g., cerebral anemia or hemorrhage); (3) vomiting caused by vestibular stimulation (e.g., motion sickness, Menière's syndrome); and (4) vomiting of pregnancy, the cause of which is largely unexplained.

Treatment

In acute conditions, i.e., short-term vomiting such as occurs after inappropriate diet and excess alcohol intake or in morning sickness with occasional vomiting in early pregnancy, treatment is not necessary or may consist solely of prescribing easily digestible foods. When nausea or vomiting is marked and persistent, however, general well-being is impaired, and the condition leads to disorders of electrolyte and water balance, then treatment is necessary.

Causal therapy consists of medical, surgical, or neurosurgical treatment of the underlying disease. Symptomatic treatment is used to support specific treatment and is employed only where causal therapy is impossible.

Nonpharmacologic treatment

The diet must ensure an adequate intake of fluids and electrolytes. Where this is not possible orally, iv infu-

sions may be necessary in certain circumstances. Generally, it is advisable with an acute onset of vomiting (especially from the intestinal tract) to withdraw all food intake initially for a few hours and then subsequently to encourage the patients to drink tea and eat dry, easily digested foodstuffs (e.g., rusks and salted biscuits, if these are tolerated) as frequent small meals.

Drug therapy

Antihistamines

Antihistamines (H_1-receptor antagonists) (see Chap. 78) with a marked central nervous system inhibitory action are used as antiemetics. For motion sickness, prophylaxis about 1 hour before starting the journey is recommended. Antihistamines have varying degrees of sedative action.

Meclozine is especially suitable for the treatment of motion sickness. *Dosage:* 1 (or 2) tablets (25 mg) orally 1 hour before starting the journey and every 4 hours thereafter; where vomiting is already established, 1 suppository (50 mg) rectally.

Dimenhydrate is also used in the treatment of motion sickness, but it is also used for other forms of vomiting. *Dosage:* 1 sustained-release tablet at intervals of 8 to 10 hours, 1 suppository tid or qid, or 1 to 2 ampoules iv or im daily (sustained-release coated tablets 0.2 g, 1 suppository 0.15 g, 1 ampoule iv 0.065 g in 10 ml, 1 ampoule im 0.1 g in 2 ml).

Side effects

Side effects include drowsiness, dry mouth, and rarely, blurred vision.

Contraindications

Contraindications are urinary bladder dysfunction and glaucoma. In the first 3 months of pregnancy, antihistamines should be used only for strictly indicated conditions.

Interactions

Sedatives, tranquilizers, and alcohol may increase drowsiness; monoamine oxidase (MAO) inhibitors may increase and prolong anticholinergic effects. Cytochrome P450 interactions (see Chap. 6) are of minor significance for the above listed compounds.

Phenothiazines

Phenothiazines are neuroleptic drugs with a central sedative action (see Chap. 12). Their antiemetic activity is based primarily on their ability to block the dopamine receptors in the area postrema. They are effective against vomiting due to various causes, apart from motion sickness. Only piperazine-substituted chlorpromazine derivatives are also effective in motion sickness.

Perphenazine is also suitable as an antiemetic for the treatment of motion sickness. *Dosage:* 4 to 8 (up to 12) mg per day orally. A daily dose of 12 mg should not be exceeded in ambulatory patients.

Triflupromazine is also useful in motion sickness. *Dosage:* 10 (or 20) mg orally tid and, if necessary, 10 (or 20) mg im. Fluphenazine also may be used. *Dosage:* 1 to 2 mg per day (1 tablet = 1 mg, 1 ampoule = up to 1 mg). Daily doses of 2 mg should not be exceeded in ambulatory patients.

Side effects

Side effects include sedation, disorders of the autonomic nervous system and extrapyramidal system, allergic skin reactions, and agranulocytosis. Phenothiazines may be used in the first 3 months of pregnancy only to a limited extent on strict definition of the indications.

Contraindications

Acute intoxications may be seen with sedatives and ethanol.

Interactions

Interactions are seen with sedatives/tranquilizers, ethanol, anticholinergics, and dopamine antagonists.

Scopolamine

Anticholinergics such as scopolamine (M-cholinergic-receptor antagonists) are particularly effective in the prophylaxis of nausea and vomiting of vestibular origin (i.e., motion or sea sickness). *Dosage:* 1 plaster about 4 to 6 hours or the evening before starting the journey. The action lasts for up to 3 days. Side effects are those known for this class of substances, and the activity is potentiated by interaction with alcohol.

Dopamine antagonists

Dopamine antagonists are antiemetics that centrally block dopamine (D_2) receptors; they have an additional peripheral antiemetic action that results from their ability to increase gastrointestinal motility in hypotonic functional disorders of the gut. A dyskinetic syndrome may occur as a side effect.

Metoclopramide, a D_2-receptor antagonist, also acts at higher doses on 5-HT$_3$ receptors (see below). *Dosage:* 10 mg rectally bid or tid or 5 to 10 mg orally tid. If necessary, 10 mg im or iv qd to tid.

Alizapride also may be used. *Dosage:* 50 mg bid or tid; oral dose: 50 mg tid up to six times per day as concomitant therapy with cytostatics.

Domperidone is a D_2 antagonist that acts almost exclusively peripherally and therefore has limited central nervous side effects. *Dosage:* 10 to 20 mg tid.

Cisapride and clebopride are used mainly for their activity on gastric motility (see below).

Pharmacokinetics

See Table 32.1.

Side effects

Side effects include anxiety (mild), depression (rare), neuroleptic syndrome, ataxia (high doses), and hypotension.

Contraindications

Contraindications include pheochromocytoma, mechanical intestinal obstruction, intestinal perforation, prolactin-dependent tumors, epilepsy, extrapyramidal disorders, and comedication with MAO inhibitors.

Table 32.1 Dopamine antagonists: pharmacokinetic parameters

Drug	Oral bioavailability (%)	T_{max} (h)	Volume of distribution (l/kg)	Plasma half-life (h)	Plasma protein binding (%)
Alizapride	75-95	0.75-1.0	3.5	2-5	75
Domperidone	15-30	0.5	5.7	—	92
Metoclopramide	30-80	0.5-2.0	2.2-3.4	5.7 (normal dosage) 7.8 (high dosage)	40

Table 32.2 5-Hydroxytryptamine 3 (5-HT$_3$ antagonists): pharmacokinetic parameters

Drug	Oral bioavailability (%)	T$_{max}$ (h)	Volume of distribution (l/kg)	Plasma half-life (h)	Plasma protein binding (%)
Dolasetron	75	1.5	4.7	7-9	69-77
Granisetron	69	1.5	3	~10	~65
Ondansetron	~60	1-1.5	1.9	3-4.5	70-76
Tropisetron	50-70	1.3	4.5	7.3-8.6 (in slow metabolizers up to 30-42 h)	50-71

Interactions

Interactions may be seen with sympathomimetics. There may be decreased absorption of digoxin and cimetidine and increased absorption of levodopa, paracetamol, several antibiotics, and lithium.

Serotonin (5-HT$_3$) antagonists

These selectively block the 5-HT$_3$ receptors in the area postrema but also probably have a serotonin antagonist action on the receptors in the GI tract without the side effects of the dopamine antagonists (no dyskinesias, occasional flushing or headaches). These agents have high antiemetic potency and are used mainly for radiation and cytostatic therapy.

Ondansetron Dosage: 2 to 4 mg orally; in severe emesis, 8 to 16 mg iv every 12 hours. Oral bioavailability is about 60%, with effective blood levels detected 30 to 60 minutes after administration. Ondansetron is metabolized extensively in the liver, with a plasma half-life of 3 to 4 hours.

Granisetron This is given iv in a 3 mg dose. (10 µg/kg in cisplatin therapy, 40 µg/kg in repeat-cycle chemotherapy). Oral: 1 mg bid prevents nausea and vomiting associated with emetogenic cancer therapy. Granisetron is metabolized in the liver; about 11% appears unchanged in the urine, 48% is eliminated as metabolites in the urine, and 34% is eliminated in the feces. Plasma protein binding is about 65%.

Tropisetron This is a new derivative, given mainly in 5-mg ampoules; oral tablets are also available. This product undergoes CYP2D6-mediated polymorphic metabolism (see Chap. 6); poor metabolizers (PM) are at risk of side effects.

Dolasetron This is another new derivative, also mainly used iv, although oral doses (8 mg tid) are also available. Clinical experience is limited.

A number of randomized trials have clearly proven the value of combining 5-HT$_3$ antagonists with dexamethasone (8-20 mg daily) for potentiation of their action.

Pharmacokinetics

For details, see Table 32.2

Side effects

Side effects include headache, dizziness, musculoskeletal pain, drowsiness, sedation, anxiety, and hypotension.

Contraindications

These agents are contraindicated in children under 4 years of age and in those with a known hypersensitivity to any of them.

Interactions

No interactions have yet been identified as for other centrally active drugs, e.g., diazepam, morphine, or for other antiemetic drugs. Moreover, for concomitant drugs that induce or inhibit the cytochrome P-450 drug-metabolizing system of the liver, no dose adjustment is recommended on the basis of available data except for tropisetron and CYP2D6 substrates.

DIARRHEA

For persons eating a European diet, diarrhea generally can be defined as more than three passages of loose stools and a total stool weight of less than 250 g per day. Of approximately 9 liters of water that normally flows through the upper intestinal tract, only about 1.5 liters pass the ileocecal valve into the cecum, and only 0.15 liter is discharged via the anus daily. In the small intestine, water resorption is coupled with sodium and glucose absorption, which must be borne in mind with respect to therapy.

ACUTE DIARRHEA (DURATION <2 WEEKS)

The most frequent cause of acute diarrhea is acute gastroenteritis due to bacteria in the intestines (i.e., bacterial food poisoning). The common pathogens are *Salmonella, Shigella, Escherichia coli* (enterotoxin-producing *E. coli* are the most frequent cause of traveler's diarrhea), *Proteus, Pseudomonas aeruginosa, Yersinia enterocolitica, Campylobacter jejuni,* and *Chlamydia.* The incubation period may range from several hours to several days. Alternatively, diarrhea may arise from the toxins that have been ingested on eating contaminated food (e.g., toxins from *Staphylococcus* and *Clostridium* spp.). In this case, the incubation period is only a few hours. In addition, there are also numerous other causes, e.g., bacterial (typhoid, paratyphoid, cholera), viral (rotaviruses), antibiotic-induced (*Clostridium difficile*), parasitic (amebic, lambliasis, ascariasis), allergic (food allergies), and drug-induced (laxatives, cytostatics, antibiotics, and digitalis overdose).

Symptoms are determined by the type and severity of the noxious agents. The most frequent are mild forms of short duration (2-3 days) with acute gastroenteritis accompanied by nausea and vomiting, temperature of less than 38.5 °C, and pulpy to liquid stools. Where there is more serious impairment of general well-being, a temperature higher than 38.5 °C, and/or blood in the stools or signs of dehydration with a tendency to collapse, an immediate differential diagnosis should be carried out as the basis for causal therapy.

In acute diarrhea, diagnostic procedures do not provide any clear evidence of cause in more than 80% of patients and therefore can be omitted in uncomplicated cases. For outpatients without extensive diagnosis, if the temperature is less than 38.5 °C and there are no signs of dehydration and no blood in the stools, regression of the symptoms should occur within a week of starting symptomatic treatment. If regression does not occur, the patient should be referred for specialist examination and possibly admitted to hospital. Hospitalizations also should be considered (1) on occurrence of diarrhea within 48 hours of returning from subtropical, tropical, or endemic areas (to exclude cholera) or (2) where the temperature is higher than 38.5°C and there are signs of dehydration and/or blood in the stools.

Treatment

Treatments of general use in the disease

Rehydration

WHO formula = 2 teaspoons of NaCl, 3 teaspoons of KCl, 3 teaspoons of $NaHCO_3$, and 2 teaspoons of glucose in 1 liter of water or ready-to-use electrolyte pack, 1 sachet in 200 ml of water, or 1 teaspoon of NaCl and 4 teaspoons of sugar in 1 liter of water or potassium-containing fruit juice, Coca-Cola or lemonade (sugar and liquid) and salted pretzel sticks (carbohydrates and salt).

Diet

The diet has few restrictions and should provide adequate fluid intake.
Supportive measures include adsorbents and spasmolytics.

Antibiotics

These should be used only after appropriate evaluation.

Drug therapy

Opioid antidiarrheals agents

Loperamide This piperidine opioid triggers two opioid-receptor-mediated mechanisms: inhibition of (1) intestinal transit and (2) intestinal secretion. Loperamide has been studied extensively in acute infectious diarrhea (traveler's diarrhea) as well as in chronic diarrhea, such as Crohn's disease and chronic ulcerative colitis. In all these trials, loperamide was efficacious and superior to placebo and equal to or more potent than diphenoxylate or codeine. Loperamide acts quickly following oral administration and has a plasm half-life of 11 hours; plasma protein binding is 96.5%.

Starting dose is 4 mg for loperamide, followed by additional doses after each liquid stool, up to tid.

Diphenoxylate Diphenoxylate is also a piperidine opioid. Preparations contain 25 µg of atropine to discourage abuse. This results in unpleasant side effects such as dry mouth, blurred vision, etc. Starting dose is 2.5 mg, up to bid or tid.

Side effects

These opioid derivatives show the side effects expected with opioids; overdose may lead to constipation or even toxic megacolon. Diphenoxylate may cause CNS effects and anticholinergic side effects. Rarely, exanthemas, headache, and drowsiness are seen. Addiction is unlikely.

Contraindications

Contraindications include ileus, children younger than 2 years of age, pregnancy and breast feeding, and diarrhea accompanied by high fever and bloody stools.

Interactions

No drug interactions between loperamide and other drug have been described.

UNCOMPLICATED ACUTE DIARRHEA

Treatment

Treatment is aimed at mantaining normal electrolyte and water balance and improving the diarrhea. In severe diarrhea, modern opioids (e.g., loperamide) that do not have any central action (see above) can be used because of their advantage of rapid onset of action.

Oral rehydration

To achieve optimal oral rehydration, carbohydrates, which promote the absorption of sodium and water and thus reduce electrolyte and fluid losses, are preferred. When there is acute vomiting and diarrhea with dehydration, then parenteral feeding is needed.

Diet

Since absorption in the small intestine generally is intact in infectious diarrhea, dietary intake should be adjusted to the state of the disease; only minor restrictions are necessary for nausea, vomiting, abdominal cramps, and loss of appetite, and no restrictions are necessary for a normal appetite. In all patients, however, adequate fluid intake must be ensured.

Supportive measures

These include adsorbents (charcoal tablets) tid to qid, kaolin pectate 4 to 8 teaspoons per day, and siliciumdioxide 4 to 8 teaspoons per day. Spasmolytics may be used for severe abdominal symptoms, such as butyl-scopolamine 10 to 20 mg orally or as suppository tid. Intestinal antiseptics and bacterial substitution are not indicated because of their as yet unclear therapeutic effect. The same applies to antibiotics for mild forms of diarrhea because they prolong the excretion of pathogenic organisms, e.g., of *Salmonella* (for differential therapy of enteritis, see also Tab. 32.3).

TRAVELER'S DIARRHEA

The most frequent pathogen is enteropathogenic *E.coli* (more than 50%) transmitted by contaminated food, tap water, or ice cubes.

Treatment

Ciprofloxacin and cotrimoxazole are the drugs of choice (Tab. 32.3), combined with general measures plus loperamide (see above) as needed. Prophylaxis should be based on the advice to consume only well-cooked food, bottled drinks ("Cook it, peel it, or leave it"). Drug prophylaxis for short-term visits has been carried out successfully with fluoroquinolones (the most predictably effective antimicrobial drugs when susceptibilities are not known, e.g., ciprofloxacin), cotrimoxazole (resistance is common in tropical areas, effective in inland Mexico during summer), and doxycycline (resistance is found in many areas of the world, limiting its value).

SEVERE ACUTE DIARRHEA

Children, elderly persons, and those with impaired resistance are at particular risk for infectious diarrhea. In severe cases of diarrhea that are accompanied by temperatures above 38.5 °C, dehydration, and blood in the feces, a diagnosis of the cause and the pathogen must be attempted so that corresponding antibiotic therapy may be started. Substitution of electrolytes and water should take place, if necessary, parenterally, and the patient should be sent to hospital.

Table 32.3 Specific therapy of enteritis

Bacteria	Compound	Dosage	Application (days)
Salmonella typhi/ Paratyphi	1. Ciprofloxacin	4 x 250 mg po	14
		4 x 200 mg iv	14
	2. Ceftriaxone	1 x 2 g iv	14
Salmonella enterica	1. Ciprofloxacin	2 x 500 mg po	7
	2. Cotrimoxazole	2 x 0.96 g po	7
Shigella	1. Ciprofloxacin	2 x 500 mg po	5
	2. Cotrimoxazole	2 x 0.96 g po	5
	3. Ampicillin	4 x 500 mg po	5
Yersinia	1. Ciprofloxacin	2 x 500 mg po	7
	2. Cotrimoxazole	2 x 0.96 g po	7
Campylobacter	1. Clarithromycin	2 x 0.25 g po	7
	2. Ciprofloxacin	2 x 500 mg po	7
	3. Tetracycline	4 x 500 mg po	7
E. coli (invasive Enterocytotoxic)	1. Ciprofloxacin	2 x 500 mg po	5
	2. Cotrimoxazole	2 x 0.96 g po	5
	3. Doxycycline	2 x 100 mg po	5
Clostridium difficile	1. Vancomycin	4 x 125 mg po	10
	2. Metronidazole	4 x 500 mg po, iv	10
Vibrio cholerae	1. Tetracycline	4 x 500 mg po	2
	2. Cotrimoxazole	2 x 0.96 g po	5

Treatment

Parenteral substitution

A suitable solution is Ringer's lactate solution to which 10 to 20 mmol/liter of potassium has been added. This solution should be infused in accordance with the estimated loss, with monitoring of the hematocrit, serum electrolyte levels, and acid-base balance. The quantity infused is adjusted according to enteral losses and orally administered fluids.

Antibiotic therapy

Antibiotic therapy is now generally based on the new gyrase inhibitors, e.g., ciprofloxacin, ofloxacin, or cotrimoxazole. These generally are effective in most infectious diarrheas (for differential therapy of enteritis, see also Tab. 32.1; for kinetic data, see Chap. 38).

PSEUDOMEMBRANOUS COLITIS

The pathogenesis of pseudomembranous colitis is secondary to alterations of the intestinal flora due to the use of most antibiotics, particularly lincomycin and clindamycin but also ampicillin and tetracycline. *Clostridium difficile* can proliferate and damage the mucous membranes with its toxin. White pseudomembranes of necrotic mucosa and fibrin that cover the ulcers with granulocyte infiltration are typical. Patients in poor general conditions, and those undergoing simultaneous administration of cytostatics or immunosuppressant therapy are predisposed.

Liquid, occasionally blood-stained diarrhea, abdominal cramps, tenesmus, and fever are the leading symptoms. Dehydration, electrolyte loss, leukocytosis, an increased erythrocyte sedimentation rate (ESR), and intestinal loss of protein also occur. These symptoms occur generally 2 to 28 days after starting antibiotic therapy and up to 3 weeks after withdrawal. In the case of toxic megacolon, perforation and abscess, mortality may be high. Rectoscopy and coloscopy show whitish-yellow plaques, and toxins and organisms may be detected, particularly *C. difficile* (positive *C. difficile* toxin A test in the stools).

Treatment

Treatment in an intensive care unit is recommended because of the severity of the clinical picture: (1) infusional or transfusional treatment and, when necessary, substitution of blood or plasma (blood-stained diarrhea, exudative enteropathy) together with (2) withdrawal of the previously administered antibiotic if the underlying disease permits this.

Drug therapy

Vancomycin This is the antibiotic of choice, with response rates of 95 to 100%. Poorly absorbed after oral administration, it reaches effective therapeutic stool levels (350-500 µg with 125-mg dose). Serum levels are negligible, and there is essentially no systemic toxicity. *Dosage*: 125 mg orally qid at regular intervals. Metronidazole (dosage 500 mg qid) is also effective but occasionally may fail because of *C. difficile* resistance.

Teicoplanin Experience with teicoplanin, an alternative peptide antibiotic, is limited.

Other antibiotics are essentially ineffective.

Treatment must be continued until the stools are free of pathogens (generally after 1-2 weeks) or, if no method of detection is available, until there is clinical improvement. Relapses may occur in 10 to 20% of patients, and these must again be treated with the schedule given, which is then slowly reduced (for 1 week each, vancomycin 250 mg qid, 125 mg qid, 125 mg bid, 125 mg qd, and then 125 mg orally every second day).

Contraindications

Contraindications include impairments of the vestibular and cochlear nerves; carefully monitor hearing (including drug monitoring) and renal function, especially when given concomitantly with other neuro- or nephrotoxic drugs.

CHRONIC DIARRHEA (DURATION >2 WEEKS)

Chronic diarrhea is not a disease but a symptom, and it may be the result of a wide range of disorders or diseases. Symptoms depend on the type, severity, and course of the underlying disease. Recognition of the underlying disease is important for specific therapy.

Treatment

Symptomatic therapy cosists of general measures (e.g., diet, fluid and electrolyte administration, and adsorbents), administration of antidiarrheal agents (e.g., loperamide 2-4 mg = 1-2 capsules tid, kaolin pectate 4-8 teaspoons per day), and administration of parasympatholytics (butylscopolamine 10-20 mg tid). Causal therapy depends on the underlying cause of the diarrhea.

CONSTIPATION

Chronic constipation is diagnosed if stools are passed only every third day or less frequently and only with severe straining ("too infrequently, too difficult, too hard, too little"). A precise history therefore is necessary. However, subjective components and the subjective suffering of the person who believes himself or herself to be constipated play a major role (pseudoconstipation). Constipation generally has functional and rarely organic causes. It is frequently a component of the irritable bowel syndrome (see Chap. 35). With increasing age, women tend to suffer from constipation two to three times more frequently than men.

The etiology and pathogenesis provide starting points for causal treatment of organic causes and, to some extent, functional forms as well.

Treatment

In uncomplicated chronic constipation, the treatment regimen given in Table 32.4 has proven valuable without, however, all the measures being scientifically supported. It should be explained to the patient, and he/she should follow it strictly for at least 2 weeks. Consultation should then take place again. The vicious circle that is initiated by laxatives (i.e., laxatives-defecation-constipation-laxatives) must be interrupted.

Drug therapy

Cisapride

Cisapride is a benzamide with prokinetic properties that works on the gastrointestinal tract by facilitating acetylcholine release from postganglionic nerve endings in the myenteric gut plexus. Unlike dopamine antagonists, it also increases colonic motility. Since cisapride is devoid of dopamine antagonist activity, it does not influence prolactin nor does it cause extrapyramidal symptoms.

The bioavailability of oral cisapride is 30 to 40%. Pleak blood levels occur 2 hours after dosing, longer if cisapride is taken with food; therefore, the drug should be taken on an empty stomach. Metabolization is in the liver, i.e., by cytochrome P450 enzymes (see below); lower doses thus are necessary in hepatic insufficiency.

Table 32.4 Basic treatment of uncomplicated chronic constipation

1. In the morning, before getting up, abdominal massage along the large intestine
2. A glass of fruit juice on an empty stomach
3. For breakfast, whole-meal bread, coffee, and 2 teaspoons of linseed (whole or milled) or wheat bran (previously soaked)
4. Attempt to defecate, even in the absence of an urge, for at least 5 min daily but without straining after breakfast (conditioning in stool propulsion by gastrocolic reflex)
5. Physical exercise, particularly in patients with sedentary jobs (morning gymnastics, walking part or all of the way to work)
6. Major meals should be rich in fiber (e.g.,vegetables, fruit, salads, whole-meal bread) plus yogurt and low-fat soft cheese. Sufficient fluid intake (2 liters/d)
7. Depending on success at breakfast, give possibly an additional 2 teaspoons of linseed or wheat bran with copious fluids at the evening meal

If defecation is still unsatisfactory after a further 2 days:

8. Local evacuation aid with a small enema and further systematic adherence to 1-7 above
9. Further encouragement from the doctor and supervision of the patient
10. If laxatives cannot be avoided despite these measures, they should be administered only every second or third day

---

Dosage

10 mg orally four times daily, at least 15 minutes before meals and at bedtime. A dose increase to 20 mg four times daily may be necessary to obtain a satisfactory result. *Clebopride*, an analogue with a similar activity profile, is available in most countries. Doses vary from 0.5 mg orally to 1 mg iv in repeated doses. The product has been associated with frequent drowsiness and occasional reports of dyskinesia.

Side effects

Side effects include abdominal cramps, diarrhea, headache, dizziness, skin reactions, and exanthema.

Interactions

Through increased gastrointestinal motility, an increased absorption of drugs from the small intestine may occur, e.g., benzodiazepines, paracetamol, and oral anticoagulants. H_2 blockers and ketoconazole inhibit cisapride metabolism by way of CYP3A4 isoenzyme, resulting in high cisapride plasma concentrations with the possibility of QT-interval prolongation. A similar risk may found with macrolide antibiotics and grapefruit juice. Serious cardiac arrhythmias including ventricular tachycardia and torsades de pointes have been observed after concomitant use of these agents.

Laxative therapy

Chronic laxative abuse can lead to intestinal loss of Na, K, Ca, and H_2O, occasionally resulting in osteoporosis, hyperkalemia, and exsiccosis.

Contraindications

The major contraindications are uncomplicated chronic constipation, mechanical ileus, suspected perforation or abscess in the abdomen, and ulcerative colitis with simultaneous constipation and severe abdominal symptoms of unknown origin.

Major laxative preparations

High-fiber and swelling materials are often sufficient for the preceding indications. Linseed or wheat bran 1 to 2 teaspoons bid or tid or other high-fiber products 1 teaspoon, previously soaked, bid simultaneously with plenty of fluids (2 liters/d) are sufficient. Otherwise, there is the danger of developing ileus. Lactulose 30 to 60 ml per day or lactitol 1 sachet (10 g) in the morning and evening are adequate. Bisacodyl coated tablets or suppositories are given once daily. Herbal laxatives such as aloes, senna, and frangula are available in various preparations. Sodium picosulfate 10 to 15 drops or 1 tablet per day can be given. It is important *not* to use liquid paraffin, castor oil, or phenolphthalein-containing drugs.

Suggested readings

DOLLERY C, ed. Therapeutic drugs. Edinburgh: Churchill-Livingstone, 1991.

FELDMAN M, SCHARSCHMIDT BF, SLEISENGER MH, eds. Sleisenger and Fordtran's Gastrointestinal and liver disease, 6th ed. Philadelphia: WB Saunders, 1998.

GRUNBERG SM, HEASKETH PJ. Control of chemotherapy-induced emesis. N Engl J Med 1993;329:1790-6.

RAKEL RE, ed. Conn's Current Therapy, 1998 Philadelphia: W.B. Saunders, 1998.

RUOFF H-J, FLADUNG B, DEMOL P, WEIHRAUCH TR. Gastrointestinal receptors and drugs in motility disorders. Digestion 1991;48:1-17.

THE ITALIAN GROUP FOR ANTIEMETIC RESEARCH. Dexamethasone, granisetron, or both for the prevention of nausea and vomiting during chemotherapy for cancer. N Engl J Med 1995;332:1-5.

33

Esophagus, stomach, and duodenum

Cornelis B. H. W. Lamers

ESOPHAGUS

GASTROESOPHAGEAL REFLUX DISEASE

Gastroesophageal reflux disease (GERD) is any symptomatic clinical condition or histopathologic alteration due to reflux of gastric contents into the esophagus. At endoscopy, patients with gastroesophageal reflux disease may have various endoscopic abnormalities resulting from this reflux. In addition, some patients without reflux esophagitis at endoscopy may have histopathologic changes of the esophageal epithelium resulting from the refluxed gastric contents. Other patients with complaints of gastroesophageal reflux disease may not have any endoscopic or histopathologic abnormalities, but the alleviation of symptoms during acid-inhibitory therapy supports the diagnosis of gastroesophageal reflux disease. The damage to the esophagus is due mainly to the irritative and erosive effects of acid and pepsin, and in a minority of patients bile and pancreatic enzymes have been suggested as contributory factors.

The diagnosis of GERD is made in the presence of more or less characteristic symptoms, often accompanied by either reflux esophagitis documented by endoscopy or histopathology or increased exposure of the esophagus to acid demonstrated by intraesophageal pH monitoring. Symptom analysis, grading of endoscopic and histopathologic abnormalities, and quantitative analysis of intraesophageal pH data are used to further characterize the disease.

If heartburn is taken as a characteristic symptom of GERD, the disorder occurs very frequently. In the United States, heartburn is experienced daily in 7%, weekly in 14%, and monthly in 15% of the individuals, and the frequency is even higher in pregnant women. About 50 to 80% of patients with regular symptoms show histopathologic features of reflux esophagitis. The prevalence of reflux esophagitis in the general population is about 4%, with a slight increase seen in the older individuals. The prevalence of GERD is roughly equal in males and females, while reflux esophagitis is reported to be slightly more frequent in males than in females.

Table 33.1 Pathophysiology of gastroesophageal reflux disease

Increased gastroesophageal reflux
Transient lower esophageal sphincter relaxations
Hypotensive lower esophageal sphincter
Motility disorders
Hiatal hernia
Severe acid hypersecretion
Normal gastroesophageal reflux
Hypersensitive esophagus

Pathophysiology

Gastroesophageal reflux disease is characterized by symptoms of excess acid with or without endoscopic or histopathologic abnormalities due to gastroesophageal reflux. Table 33.1 lists the main pathophysiologic mechanisms for increased gastroesophageal reflux. In addition, some patients with characteristic symptoms that respond to pharmacologic acid inhibition show 24-hour pH-monitoring results within the normal range, suggesting a hypersensitive esophagus.

The antireflux barrier is formed by a complex mechanism in which the intrinsic pressure of the lower esophageal sphincter, the extrinsic compression produced by the crural diaphragm, and the integrity of such anatomic structures as the intraabdominal location of the sphincter and the acute angle of His are involved. In some patients with gastroesophageal reflux disease, there are no obvious anatomic abnormalities, but the reflux appears to be due to an increase in the number and length of transient lower esophageal sphincter relaxations (TLESRs). Transient lower esophageal sphincter relaxations are sphincter relaxations that are not induced by swallowing, but they may lead to low intraesophageal pH values accompanied by reflux symptoms. These transient lower esophageal sphincter relaxations are provoked by distension of the stomach and are the main pathogenetic mechanism in the majority of patients with mild to moderate gastroesophageal reflux disease.

Motility disorders of the esophageal body may result in

decreased esophageal acid clearance and, as a consequence, may increase the exposure time of the esophageal mucosa to acid. Reduced salivation also may contribute to an increased acid exposure of the esophagus. Massive hypersecretion of gastric acid, as in patients with gastrinoma (Zollinger-Ellison syndrome), is also accompanied by increased reflux symptoms. The heterogeneity and complexity of the pathogenesis of gastroesophageal reflux disease affect the therapeutic possibilities to achieve permanent cure of the disease in most of the patients.

The main symptoms related to abnormal esophageal acid exposure include heartburn, retrosternal burning or pain, and acid regurgitation. However, these symptoms also are observed frequently in subjects with normal esophageal acid exposure, suggesting that they also may be due to a hypersensitive esophagus. It has been suggested that such laryngopharyngeal symptoms as posterior laryngitis, pharyngeal pain, dental erosions, sinus problems, otalgia, and especially asthma (so-called reflux-induced or gastric asthma) may be secondary to reflux and regurgitation of acid.

Long-standing severe reflux may be complicated by the development of Barrett's esophagus and peptic strictures, which often occur in combination in a single patient. Peptic strictures may affect food transport in the esophagus and lead to dysphagia, weight loss, and food aspiration. In Barrett's esophagus, the squamous epithelium of the distal esophagus is replaced by metaplastic columnar epithelium, usually of the intestinal type. Patients with intestinal-type metaplasia of the esophagus have an increased risk for the development of adenocarcinoma (see Chap. 57). Because of the poor prognosis of esophageal adenocarcinoma, surveillance of Barrett's esophagus is recommended.

Diagnosis

The diagnosis of GERD is based on the presence of characteristic symptoms sometimes documented by endoscopy and 24-hour ambulatory pH monitoring. In addition, relief of symptoms during acid-inhibition therapy strongly supports the diagnosis, and a short course of a powerful acid-inhibitory drug often is used as a patient-friendly diagnostic tool.

At endoscopy, esophagitis usually is graded with increasing severity:
- grade 0: no abnormalities;
- grade 1: no macroscopic lesions, but erythema, hyperemia, or mucosal friability;
- grade 2: superficial erosions involving less than 10% of the mucosa of the distal 5 cm of the esophageal squamous mucosa:
- grade 3: superficial erosions or ulceration involving 10 to 50% of the distal esophagus;
- grade 4: deep ulcerations or confluent erosions of more than 50% of the distal 5 cm of the esophagus.

Although patients with more severe esophagitis often require more powerful therapy, this grading is of very limited value for the individual patient. However, for clinical trials comparing groups of patients, endoscopic grading is of great value. Esophageal pH monitoring is of limited clinical value. This measurement is clinically helpful only in patients with atypical symptoms and in those who experience insufficient symptom relief despite adequate antireflux therapy.

Treatment

The aim of treatment of gastroesophageal reflux disease is to lower the acid exposure of the esophageal epithelium and by doing that to alleviate the patient's discomfort. The esophageal acid exposure can be reduced by therapies that diminish gastroesophageal reflux, lower the acid content of the refluxate, and prevent the contact between the intraesophageal contents and the esophageal lining.

As shown in Table 33.2, the basic principles of therapy of gastroesophageal reflux disease comprise:
1. nondrug therapy: lifestyle modifications;
2. drug therapy;
3. antireflux surgery.

Treatment of the patient with gastroesophageal reflux disease should be individualized, but in general, a stepwise treatment approach can be advocated as the strategy of choice.

Step 1: lifestyle modifications The lifestyle modifications comprise elevation of the head of the bed, prevention of bending down, body weight optimization, prevention of high intraabdominal pressure, avoidance of food items known to lower the lower esophageal sphincter pressure, avoidance of heavy or fat meals before bedtime, and refraining from smoking, as well as possibly stimulating salivation by chewing gum. If these individualized recommendations for modification of lifestyle provide insufficient relief of symptoms, drug therapy as second treatment step should be added.

Table 33.2 Therapy of gastroesophageal reflux disease

Nondrug
  Lifestyle modifications

Drugs
  Drugs lowering acidity
    Antacids
    H_2-receptor antagonists
    Proton pump inhibitors
  Prokinetic agents
    Cisapride
    Clebopride
  Mucosa-protecting agents
    Sucralfate

Antireflux surgery
  Endoscopic fundoplication
  Open surgery

Step 2: drug therapy When coming to drug therapy, it has to be decided on what class of drugs to start with. Although the prokinetic agent cisapride and the mucosa-protective agent sucralfate have been shown to be superior to placebo in patients with mild gastroesophageal reflux disease, the efficacy, however, is modest in comparison with powerful gastric acid inhibitors. For this reason, most clinicians start therapy with acid-suppressive therapies, which are very effective and have an excellent safety profile. Two different strategies for acid-suppressive dug therapy can be applied. First, the so-called bottom-up or step-up approach is used, i.e., starting with low to moderate acid inhibition and, if required, moving to stronger acid suppression by either an increase in dose or a switch to a more powerful compound. Second, the top-down or step-down approach is used, i.e., starting with powerful acid-inhibitory therapy, followed by lowering the dose or switching to a less powerful compound in order to obtain the optimal (i.e., cost-effective) therapy for an individual patient. When acid-inhibitory potency is considered, proton pump inhibitors are more powerful than H_2-receptor antagonists, and the latter drugs have a stronger acid-lowering effect than the antacids.

Step 3: antireflux surgery Only a minority of patients are candidates for antireflux surgery. Possible candidates include patients who respond insufficiently to optimal medical therapy and young patients who prefer surgery to the long-term use of drugs. The best candidates are patients with troublesome regurgitation, because effect of acid-inhibitory therapies is limited in such patients, and antireflux surgery may create an efficient barrier to gastroesophageal reflux. Antireflux surgery presently is done as a laparoscopic procedure, whereas open surgery is restricted to selected patients in whom the laparoscopic approach is not feasible. However, antireflux surgery is not without side effects. Several patients suffer from dysphagia, while others have a continued need for acid-inhibitory drugs.

Drug therapy

Acid-lowering drugs

Antacids **Action and pharmacokinetics** Antacids alleviate heartburn in subjects with occasional complaints of short duration. Antacids bind the protons present in acidic gastric contents, leading to partial or complete neutralization of the gastroesophageal refluxate.

Several types of antacids are on the market. The majority contain either an aluminum or magnesium compound or a carbonate. The neutralizing capacity, possible side effects, patient preference, and cost are factors involved in the choice of the type of antacid. The main disadvantage of antacids is their short duration of action of about 1 hour. The absorption of antacids is very low. However, when used in high doses for long periods of time, various components of the antacids may be absorbed, leading to electrolyte imbalance and alkalosis. High doses of antacids therefore are contraindicated in patients with renal failure.

Antacids usually are taken only for occasional

episodes of mild heartburn. In patients with frequent or more severe complaints, the frequent dosing and possible side effects limit the use of antacids. The efficacy predominantly depends on the neutralizing capacity of the antacid. However, the effect usually lasts only 1 to 2 hours, making antacids unsuitable for the treatment of long-lasting or chronic heartburn.

Antacids may interfere with the resorption of various types of drugs by several mechanisms, including a change in gastric acidity (e.g., ketoconazole), adsorption or complex formation (e.g., tetracyclines), or influence on gastrointestinal motility (e.g., diarrhea due to magnesium-containing compounds). The combination of magnesium- and aluminum-containing compounds is advantageous because the stimulation of gastrointestinal transit by magnesium compounds is balanced by the retarding effect of aluminum compounds.

Frequent administration of high doses of antacids may lead to electrolyte imbalance, alkalosis, abnormal mineralization of bone, and renal damage. Antacids therefore should be restricted to the symptomatic therapy of occasional complaints of heartburn.

The place of antacids in the treatment of gastroesophageal reflux disease is very limited. Occasional complaints of heartburn are the only potential indication for therapy with antacids. Long-term and frequent use of high doses of antacids should be avoided due to the possibility of side effects.

Histamine H_2-receptor antagonists **Action and pharmacokinetics** Histamine H_2-receptor antagonists inhibit the binding of histamine to its receptor on the parietal cell in the body and fundus of the stomach, resulting in decreased gastric acid secretion. Histamine is produced by enterochromaffine-like (ECL) cells in the fundic mucosa, especially after stimulation with gastrin. Furthermore, there is a close interaction among the H_2 receptor, the gastrin receptor, and the muscarine M_3 receptor on the parietal cell in such a way that stimulation of one of the receptors increases the sensitivity of the other two receptors or, on the other hand, inhibition of one of the receptors reduces the sensitivity of the other two receptors for stimulation. Thus H_2-receptor antagonists inhibit the acid stimulatory action not only of histamine but also of gastrin and acetylcholine. H_2-receptor antagonists have been shown to be superior to placebo in the treatment and prevention of reflux esophagitis. For maintenance therapy, usually half of healing dose is used. Even lower doses are effective in patients with episodic heartburn. It has been shown that a dose of ranitidine as low as 75 mg relieves occasional heartburn, whereas 25 mg does not offer any clinical effect.

A number of H_2-receptor antagonists are on the market in various countries. The main pharmacologic characteristics are given in Table 33.3. H_2-receptor antagonists are well absorbed. The absorption is somewhat inhibited by the concomitant use of food or antacids. The drugs are metabolized in the liver and excreted mainly by the kidneys. Therefore, in patients with renal failure (creatinine clearance < 15 ml/min), the dose has to be reduced to about 30 to 70% of the standard dose. This dose reduction in renal failure has to be more pronounced for roxatidine and famotidine than for cimetidine.

Bioavailability is reduced by 30 to 60% by "first pass" hepatic metabolism, although this reduction is somewhat smaller for roxatidine and nizatidine. With iv dosing, complete bioavailability allows administration of lower doses of the compounds.

Dosage The dosages of oral preparations of the antagonists are given in Table 33.3. Apart from the tablets, effervescent preparations are available for cimetidine and ranitidine, and most of the H_2-receptor antagonists also have preparations for parenteral administration. For iv use, two regimens are employed, either repeated-bolus injection (e.g., 50 mg ranitidine every 6 h) or a bolus injection followed by a continuous infusion (e.g., 50 mg ranitidine followed by an infusion of 0.125 mg/kg ranitidine per hour). The total daily dose to be administered iv is usually similar to or slightly lower than the oral daily dose. Parenteral administration is used mainly for the prevention of stress ulcers in patients in the intensive care unit and in patients with bleeding ulcers, but only rarely in patients with gastroesophageal reflux desease. Some patients with gastroesophageal reflux desease need higher doses of H_2-receptor antagonists than those listed in Table 33.3. However, when high doses of H_2-receptor antagonists are needed, a low dose of a proton pump inhibitor is often more cost-effective. The effervescent forms of H_2-receptor antagonists have the advantage of a rapid onset of action, which is especially helpful in patients with heartburn who are treated on demand by H_2-receptor

antagonists. The potency of cimetidine in inhibiting acid secretion by weight is given in Table 33.3. H_2-receptor antagonists in standard doses are efficacious in patients with mild to moderate complaints of gastroesophageal reflux desease. However, patients with more severe GERD require more profound acid inhibition.

Interestingly, when H_2-receptor antagonists are studied in constant daily doses for longer time periods, there is a slight reduction in the acid-inhibitory potency. In studies using iv administration, this decrease in efficacy is demonstrable from the third or fourth day of treatment.

Cimetidine is metabolized by the cytochrome P450 enzyme system and acts as an enzyme antagonist, thus leading to increased levels of concomitantly taken drugs that are also metabolized through this enzyme system, such as warfarin, theophylline, phenytoin, diazepam, acenocoumarol, nifedipine, and propranolol (see Chap. 6). This interaction is much less for the other H_2-receptor antagonists.

H_2-receptor antagonists are remarkably safe drugs. Despite their wide use, severe side effects are extremely rare. When cimetidine is used, care should be taken to prevent possible drug interactions. However, clinically relevant drug interactions using cimetidine appear to be rare.

Proton pump inhibitors **Action and pharmacokinetics** Proton pump inhibitors (PPIs) inhibit gastric acid secretion by binding to and inhibiting the enzyme H^+,K^+-ATPase in the parietal cell. This enzyme is involved in the final step of acid secretion. Therefore, proton pump inhibitor/s inhibit acid secretion irrespective of the type of stimulus and metabolic pathway. By binding to the H^+,K^+-ATPase, proton pump inhibitor/s induce a strong and long-lasting reduction of gastric acid secretion. The maximum antisecretory action of PPIs is reached on the third to fifth day, and the effect continues for about 3 days after stopping the administration.

Table 33.3 Pharmacokinetics of H_2-receptor antagonists

Drug	T_{max} (h)	Plasma half-life (h)	Relative potency	Standard daily dose (mg)	Maintenance dose (mg)
Cimetidine	1-2.5	2.0-3.0	1	800	400
Ranitidine	2-3	2.0-3.0	4-10	300	150
Famotidine	1-3	2.5-4.0	20-50	40	20
Nizatidine	1.5	1.1-2.8	4-10	300	150
Roxatidine	3	6.0-7.0	8-20	150	75

Table 33.4 Pharmacokinetics of proton pump inhibitors

Drug	T_{max} (h)	Plasma half-life (h)	Relative potency	Standard daily dose (mg)	Maintenance dose (mg)
Omeprazole	2-4	1	1	20-40	10-20
Lansoprazole	1-3	1.5	1	30	15
Pantoprazole	2-3	1	1	40	20
Rabeprazole	3	1	1	20	10-20

The pharmacokinetics of the PPIs are remarkably similar (Tab. 33.4). Resorption is rapid, metabolization takes place in the liver, and excretion occurs mainly via the kidneys, although lansoprazole is also exerted in the feces. Recently, studies have been performed with the stable S-enantiomer of omeprazole. This esomeprazole is less dependent on the metabolism by the CYP2C19 isoenzyme than the racemic mixture of omeprazole, thus resulting in higher blood levels and a slightly stronger and less variable effect of omeprazole. The plasma half-life is increased in patients with severe renal or liver insufficiency.

The standard daily doses for patients with gastroesophageal reflux disease are give in Table 33.4. Some patients with severe gastroesophageal reflux disease require higher than standard doses. In individual patients, the dose should be tailored to relieve the symptoms, whereas in some patients split doses or night time dosing leads to better results. The lower doses of omeprazole (10 mg), lansoprazole (15 mg), and pantoprazole (20 mg) may be indicated in the maintenance treatment of patients with moderately severe gastroesophageal reflux disease. Preparations for iv administration are available for omeprazole and pantoprazole and may be used in patients with severe peptic stricture of the esophagus as a complication of gastroesophageal reflux disease. The efficacy of the various proton pump inhibitors is dose-dependent and roughly similar for the standard daily doses. Standard doses of PPIs are more effective than standard doses of H_2-receptor antagonists and are to be preferred in patients with severe gastroesophageal reflux disease.

Proton pump inhibitors undergo extensive biotransformation through the cytochrome P450 enzyme system (see Chap. 6). The major isozyme involved in the metabolism of proton pump inhibitors are CYP2C19 and CYP3A4. Due to mutations of the CYP2C19 isozyme, about 20% of Japanese, 10-15% of Chinese and Koreans but less than 5% of Caucasians and Africans are poor metabolizers of CYP2C19 substrate, thus resulting in higher plasma concentrations. Omeprazole, lansoprazole and pantoprazole undergo pronounced metabolism by CYP2C19, whereas rabeprazole and esomeprazole (see above) are less affected by mutations. CYP2C19 dependent metabolism results in higher variability in plasma concentrations and antisecretory effects and in a greater susceptibility for drug interactions when compared with the other proton pump inhibitors. As a consequence, increased levels of drugs metabolized through the CYP2C19 enzyme system have been found in studies particularly with omeprazole and lansoprazole. Therefore, drugs such as phenytoin, theophylline, diazepam, etc. should be avoided or administered with care in patients on lansoprazole or omeprazole. A possible antagonism also may be seen with macrolide antibiotics (e.g., clarithromycin).

Because of their potent acid-inhibiting properties, PPIs may affect the absorption of drugs that are better absorbed from an acidic environment, such as ketoconazole.

Proton pump inhibitors have proved to be well tolerated and safe drugs. ECL-omas reported in rats on extremely high doses of PPIs have not been reported in humans treated with proton pump inhibitor/s. However, high plasma gastrin levels are found during acid inhibition, and measurement of

plasma gastrin levels may aid in dosing of PPIs in patients with insufficient clinical response.

Because of their ability to induce profound dose-dependent and long-lasting inhibition of gastric acid secretion, the proton pump inhibitors are superior to the H_2-receptor antagonists and other drugs in the treatment of gastroesophageal reflux disease. The proton pump inhibitor/s are well tolerated and offer great benefit to patients with severe gastroesophageal reflux disease. Cost-effectiveness analyses favor proton pump inhibitor/s for severe and H_2-receptor antagonists for mild gastroesophageal reflux disease.

Prokinetics: cisapride

Action and pharmacokinetics Cisapride acts mainly by the release of acetylcholine at the myenteric plexus. The drug stimulates peristalsis, increases lower esophageal pressure, and enhances gastric emptying. After oral administration, cisapride is rapidly and well absorbed. Its bioavailability is about 40 to 50%. The maximum plasma concentration is reached after 1 to 2 hours. Almost all the drug is protein bound. The plasma half-life of the drug is about 10 hours. The drug is metabolized in the liver by N-dealkylation and hydroxylation, and the metabolites are excreted in equal amounts in feces and urine.

Dosage The dose for treatment of symptomatic gastroesophageal reflux disease is 10 mg qd or 20 mg bid daily, whereas for maintenance therapy of gastroesophageal reflux disease, 10 mg bid or 20 mg at night is advocated. The drug is to be taken about 15 minutes before meals and at bed time. Cisapride is also available as a 10-mg effervescent tablet, a 30-mg suppository, and a 1 mg/ml suspension. No iv form is available because of potential cardiac toxicity. Half dose is recommended for patients with liver or renal disease. Cisapride is about equally effective as low-dose H_2-receptor antagonists. Use of this drug therefore should be restricted to mild and moderate gastroesophageal reflux disease.

Drug interactions Due to inhibition of biotransformation, increased plasma levels of cisapride can be found during simultaneous treatment with antimycotic chemotherapeutic agents such as ketoconazole, itraconazole, miconazole, and fluconazole; the macrolides erythromycin and clarithromycin; the lipid lowering statin; the HIV protease inhibitors; all CYP3A4 antagonists (see Chap. 6). The resulting increased plasma cisapride levels can lead to prolongation of the QT interval and severe cardiac arrhythmias. The combined used of cisapride with the above-mentioned drugs should be avoided. There is evidence that some individuals may be particularly sensitive to the cardiac side effects even during therapy with cisapride alone. Furthermore, because of its effect on gastrointestinal motility, cisapride may affect intestinal absorption of various agents, including H_2-receptor antagonists, acetaminophen, and anticoagulants.

Because of cisapride's potential cardiac toxicity (prolongation of the QT interval and arrhythmias), the drug may undergo severe restriction of clinical indications.

Such may not be the case for clebopride available in most European nations.

Mucosa-protecting agents: sucralfate

Action and pharmacokinetics Sucralfate is a basic aluminum-sucrose-sulfate compound that binds to the protein of erosive and ulcerative lesions, complexing to form a protective film against aggressive factors in the esophageal luminal contents. The drug acts locally with minimal resorption and excretion via the fecal route.

In patients with gastroesophageal reflux disease, a suspension, tablets, or granules dissolved in water are preferred over undissolved tablets. The daily dose of sucralfate is 1 g, to be taken after meals and at bed time. Sucralfate can be used in patients with mild gastroesophageal reflux disease. However, the compound possesses low efficacy when compared with antisecretory agents. Sucralfate may protect the esophageal mucosa against biliary duodenogastroesophageal reflux, but the effect is often rather disappointing.

Sucralfate is reported to inhibit the resorption of some antimicrobial agents such as ciprofloxacin and tetracycline. In patients with renal failure, the small amounts of aluminum absorbed may accumulate and lead to increased plasma levels and aluminum intoxication.

The place of sucralfate in the treatment of gastroesophageal reflux disease is very modest. The efficacy is limited, and the drug may only be considered for patients in whom biliary duodenogastroesophageal reflux is involved in the pathophysiology of gastroesophageal reflux disease, e.g., in gastroesophageal reflux disease in patients with previous gastrectomy.

Treatment of complications

Barrett's esophagus Barrett's esophagus is characterized by replacement of the native squamous epithelium by metaplastic columnar epithelium. Since Barrett's esophagus, especially when intestinal metaplasia is present, is a premalignant condition, regular endoscopic screening with multiple biopsies has been recommended (see Chap. 57).

No drug therapy has been demonstrated to unequivocally replace the metaplastic columnar epithelium with normal squamous epithelium. However, since Barrett's esophagus is the result of severe gastroesophageal reflux, endoscopic esophagitis and complaints of heartburn or regurgitation usually are present. Treatment with PPIs heals the esophagitis, alleviates the heartburn symptoms, and possibly prevents extension or aggravation of the intestinal metaplasia. However, there is no evidence that treatment with PPIs inhibits the sequence from metaplasia to dysplasia to adenocarcinomas. In Barrett's patients with severe regurgitation and/or a large hiatal hernia, antireflux surgery may be considered.

Peptic strictures Reflux esophagitis of long duration may be complicated by peptic strictures leading to dysphagia. Treatment consists of endoscopic dilatation of the stricture in combination with proton pump inhibitors. It has been shown that long-term profound acid inhibition prevents recurrences of strictures once the esophagus is effectively dilated.

Extraesophageal complications of gastroesophageal reflux disease Gastroesophageal reflux and acid regurgitation may induce a number of extraesophageal complications, especially posterior laryngitis, throat pain, sinus problems, and so-called gastric or reflux-induced asthma. Therefore, in patients with these extraesophageal manifestations, the diagnosis of gastroesophageal reflux disease should be considered. If symptoms, endoscopy, or esophageal pH measurements point to the presence of gastroesophageal reflux disease, therapy with PPIs should be started, and the effect on the laryngopharyngeal and asthma symptoms should be evaluated. A positive response to PPIs preferably should be corroborated by objective measurements of pulmonary function and laryngoscopic examination.

STOMACH AND DUODENUM

PEPTIC ULCER

Peptic ulcers are defects in the mucosa of the stomach or duodenum extending through the muscularis mucosae that persist as a function of the acid-peptic activity in gastric juice. Superficial lesions that do not extend through the muscularis mucosae are called *erosions*.

An imbalance between acid-peptic activity in gastric juice and protective mechanisms of the gastroduodenal mucosa forms the basis for the development of ulcers. In other words, in patients with peptic ulcers, either the acid-peptic activity is increased or the protective mechanisms of the gastroduodenal mucosa are diminished or a combination of these factors exist. Drug therapy is aimed at interfering with these mechanisms and restoring the normal balance. This normalized balance will give the gastroduodenal mucosa the background for spontaneous healing.

In the Western world and several other parts of the world, the incidence of peptic ulcer is decreasing. This decrease is due mainly to a lower incidence of *Helicobacter pylori*–associated ulcers, especially resulting from better hygienic conditions. On the other hand, the number of elderly individuals who are regular consumers of nonsteroidal anti-inflammatory drugs (NSAIDs) for their rheumatic and musculoskeletal disorders is rapidly increasing, leading to an increase in the occurrence of NSAID-related ulcers.

Complications of peptic ulcer include bleeding, perforation or penetration, and stricture formation. Ulcer bleeding and perforation are life-threatening complications, whereas stricturing of the antropyloric area may lead to gastric outlet obstruction.

Understanding of the pathophysiology of peptic ulcers has been revolutionized by the detection and appreciation of the important role of *H. pylori* infection in the pathophysiology of ulcers. Most ulcers develop on a background of *H. pylori*-associated gastritis. Eradication of the *H. pylori* by antibiotics will normalize the gastric mucosa and create an environment favoring of ulcer healing. In addition, *H. pylori* eradication prevents recurrence of both duodenal and gastric ulcers.

For practical reasons, it is important to distinguish separate pathogenetic entities of peptic ulcer:
• peptic ulcers associated with *H. pylori* infection;
• peptic ulcers associated with the intake of NSAIDs;
• peptic ulcers due to a specific uncommon pathology, e.g., gastrinoma (Zollinger-Ellison syndrome);
• erosions and ulcers in severely ill patients in intensive care units (so-called stress ulcers).

This division of peptic ulcers on the basis of pathophysiology is of great help to clinicians in dealing with patients with ulcers in their practice.

Clinical findings

The predominant symptom of both duodenal and gastric ulcers is epigastric pain, which occurs in about 60 to 75% of patients. However, pain is equally prominent in patients with gastric complaints without an ulcer, e.g., patients with so-called nonulcer or essential dyspepsia. Other complaints, such as nausea, vomiting, heartburn, pain relief by alkali, and anorexia, are also nonspecific, and it is therefore not possible to differentiate between duodenal ulcer, gastric ulcer, and nonulcer dyspepsia on the basis of complaints only. Thus the diagnosis of peptic ulcer only can be made by imaging methods, such as a barium meal or preferably a gastroduodenoscopy.

Diagnosis

The diagnosis of peptic ulcer is made by inspection of the stomach and duodenum at endoscopy. Because of the potential for malignancy, gastric ulcers always should be biopsied extensively. Endoscopy also allows biopsies to be taken from the gastric mucosa. Histopathologic examination of such gastric biopsies is important for the diagnosis of gastritis, the demonstration of *H. pylori* infection, and to exclude other rare causes of ulcers. In addition, culturing of gastric biopsies may help to identify the *H. pylori* bacterium and to determine the sensitivity of the microorganism to the antibiotics to be used. It is important to take the biopsies both from the antrum and the duodenum, especially in patients who are treated with PPIs. It is also possible to determine the *H. pylori* status by noninvasive methods. The [^{13}C]urea breath test and measurement of specific anti-*H. pylori* antibodies in serum may help to identify *H. pylori*–positive patients. Recurrent gastric complaints in an *H. pylori*–positive patient with a history of a documented duodenal ulcer

can be managed by *H. pylori* eradication therapy without a repeated endoscopy. However, in a symptomatic *H. pylori*–positive patient with a history of gastric ulcer, endoscopy always should be performed to exclude gastric malignancy. If in a duodenal ulcer patient an infection with *H. pylori* and the use of NSAIDs are excluded, serum gastrin as a marker for gastrinoma should be measured, and biopsies should be studied carefully by histopathology to exclude rare conditions such as Crohn's disease, etc.

Treatment

The aims of therapy of peptic ulcer are as follows:
1. to alleviate symptoms;
2. to heal the ulcer and by so doing reduce the risk for ulcer complications;
3. to prevent recurrence of the ulcer.

In practice, alleviation of symptoms and healing of the ulcer can be obtained in practically any patient with peptic ulcer, provided that powerful antisecretory agents are given and the patient is compliant with the therapy. However, for prevention of ulcer recurrences, it is important to identify the cause of the peptic ulcer, such as *H. pylori* infection, NSAID use, gastrinoma, etc. If it is impossible to eliminate the cause, long-term antisecretory therapy should be started, since this therapy is also capable of preventing ulcer relapses. Gastric surgery for peptic ulcer is only indicated when ulcer complications cannot be controlled adequately by conservative means. However, debilitating gastric resections should be avoided, since simple closure of a perforation or undersewing of a bleeding ulcer is effective. These surgical procedures should be combined with long-term therapy with powerful antisecretory drugs, unless causative therapy preventing recurrent peptic ulceration can be applied effectively.

H. pylori-positive peptic ulcer

As soon as a diagnosis of peptic ulcer is made and, in cases of gastric ulcer, malignancy is excluded, antisecretory therapy is started, and *H. pylori* testing is performed. If the *H. pylori* status proves to be positive, triple eradication therapy is given for 1 week. Triple eradication therapy consists of an antisecretory antiulcer agent and two antibiotics (Tab. 33.5). As antiulcer therapy, proton pump inhibitors, bismuth subcitrate, or ranitidine bismuth citrate are used, whereas clarithromycin, amoxicillin, metronidazole, or tetracyclines are given as antibiotics. If the patient has been treated with clarithromycin or metronidazole previously, the sensitivity of the bacterium should be tested. When the bacterium is sensitive to the antibiotics and there is optimal compliance with treatment, the eradication rate is at least 90%. However, side effects of the antibiotics may interfere with compliance with this triple eradication therapy.

Table 33.5 Eradication therapy for *Helicobacter pylori*		

Triple therapy

PPI[1]	+ amoxicillin[4]	+ clarithromycin[5]
PPI[1]	+ amoxicillin[4]	+ metronidazole[6]
PPI[1]	+ clarithromycin[5]	+ metronidazole[6]
Bismuth[2]	+ metronidazole[6]	+ tetracycline[7]
RBC[3]	+ clarithromycin[6]	+ metronidazole[6]

Quadruple therapy

PPI[1]	+ bismuth[2]	+ metronidazole[6]	+ tetracycline[7]

[1]PPI, proton pump inhibitor: omeprazole 40 mg or 20 mg bid, lansoprazole 30 mg, pantoprazole 40 mg, rabeprazole 20 mg qd.
[2]Bismuth subcitrate 120 mg qd.
[3]Ranitidine bismuth citrate 400 mg bid.
[4]Amoxicillin 1000 mg bid or 500 mg tid.
[5]Clarithromycin 500 mg bid.
[6]Metronidazole 500 mg bid.
[7]Tetracycline 500 mg qd.

Table 33.5 reports frequently used triple eradication therapies for *H. pylori*, but several other combinations of an antiulcer drug and suitable antibiotics may be equally effective.

Quadruple therapy consisting of a PPIs, bismuth subcitrate, metronidazole, and tetracycline is an alternative that is useful in patients experiencing severe side effects of clarithromycin or amoxicillin.

H. pylori-negative peptic ulcer

NSAID-induced ulcer If the *H. pylori* status of the peptic ulcer patient is negative, the possibility of NSAID-induced ulcer should be taken seriously into consideration. NSAIDs inhibit prostaglandin synthesis by inhibiting prostaglandin synthase. Since prostaglandins play an important physiologic role in the integrity of the gastroduodenal mucosa and its overlying mucus layer, these drugs may affect the mucosal defense mechanism, leading to gastroduodenal ulceration.

Therefore, in a patient with a peptic ulcer, NSAID therapy should be discontinued immediately. If stopping the NSAID is not feasible due to severe rheumatoid arthritis or other musculoskeletal disease, PPIs therapy should be given. This therapy should be continued for a long time unless the patient is able to stop the NSAIDs later on. Misoprostol, a synthetic prostaglandin E_1 analogue, is an alternative for antisecretory therapy, but this therapy often is accompanied by gastrointestinal side effects, especially diarrhea. Recently, COX-2-specific NSAIDs (celecoxib, rofecoxib) have been developed that alleviate arthritic and musculoskeletal symptoms but leave the mucosal defense mechanism intact.

Gastrinoma If in an *H. pylori*-negative patient evidence of NSAID use is lacking, the possibility of a gastrinoma

should be considered. A gastrinoma is a malignant endocrine tumor of the pancreas or duodenum metastasizing to the regional lymph nodes and the liver. The tumor secretes large amounts of gastrin into the circulation, inducing marked gastric acid hypersecretion. The extremely high acid secretion may lead to often complicated peptic ulcers, diarrhea, and gastroesophageal reflux disease. The diagnosis is made by the demonstration of an elevated plasma gastrin level that further increases after administration of secretin (positive secretin stimulation test). Therapy consists of PPIs, often in high doses, while a workup is done to determine the resectability of the tumor. If resection is impossible, or if the plasma gastrin level continues to be elevated after tumor resection, lifelong proton pump inhibitor/s therapy is the treatment of choice.

In *H. pylori*-negative patients in whom there is no evidence of NSAID use or gastrinoma, further diagnostic analysis should be done, especially to exclude malignancy, Crohn's disease, and several other conditions.

Gastroduodenal pathology associated with *H. pylori* infection

Apart from peptic ulcers, *H. pylori* also may play a role in the pathophysiology of other gastric pathologies, including gastric lymphoma (maltoma), gastric adenocarcinoma, and possibly nonulcer dyspepsia. However, a considerable proportion of *H. pylori*-positive individuals have no complaints or pathophysiology other than the *H. pylori*-induced gastritis. It is presently not clear why some individuals develop complaints and/or pathology, whereas others do not. Interestingly, successful eradication of *H. pylori* by triple therapy has been reported to cure early maltoma (see Chap. 63). However, careful follow-up is mandatory.

Patients with gastric carcinoma should be treated by surgery. In patients with nonulcer or essential dyspepsia, the effect of *H. pylori* eradication therapy on symptoms is conflicting, but most studies do not point to a causative role for *H. pylori* in nonulcer or essential dyspepsia.

Drug therapy

The various drugs and their recommended dosages in the treatment of peptic ulcer are given in Table 33.6. The duration of therapy is 4 weeks for duodenal ulcer and 6 weeks for gastric ulcer. Therapy for gastric ulcer always should be followed by endoscopy. If the ulcer persists or residual lesions are present in the stomach after therapy, another set of multiple biopsies should be taken to exclude malignancy. Antisecretory agents are the preferred therapy of peptic ulcer.

Antisecretory agents

H₂-receptor antagonists and proton pump inhibitors *Pirenzepine* is a muscarine M_1 antagonist with low antisecretory action through inhibition of the muscarine M_1 receptor on the parietal cell. Owing to anticholinergic side effects, such as tachycardia, dry mouth, and visual disturbances at clinically effective antisecretory doses, the drug is not of great use in the treatment of peptic ulcer.

Mucosa-protecting agents

Mucosa-protecting agents are superior to placebo, but these agents are inferior to the antisecretory agents. *Sucralfate* is rarely used in the treatment of peptic ulcer, but this basic aluminum-sucrose-sulfate compound has some effect in the prevention of stress ulcers in the intensive care setting.

Bismuth subcitrate does not only bind to erosions and ulcers, protecting them from the acid-peptic gastric juice, but it also stimulates endogenous prostaglandin synthesis by the stomach and exerts an antimicrobial action against *H. pylori*. Because of the anti-*H. pylori* property, the drug is used in eradication regimens for *H. pylori*. Bismuth subcitrate is absorbed to a very low extent (<0.2%) and therefore is excreted mainly in the feces, giving the stools a dark color. Side effects are related mainly to the gastrointestinal tract and include nausea, diarrhea, and constipation. Therapy with bismuth compounds should last no longer than 4 weeks because long-term therapy may induce systemic toxicity. Bismuth subcitrate inhibits the absorption of tetracyclines.

Ranitidine bismuth citrate contains ranitidine and a complex of bismuth and citrate. In the gastrointestinal tract, the drug is split into ranitidine and the bismuth compound. The bismuth compound exerts mucosa-protecting and anti-*H. pylori* effects in the stomach, whereas the ranitidine inhibits gastric acid secretion. In a dose of 400 mg twice daily, ranitidine bismuth citrate is part of some eradication regimens for *H. pylori*. In combination with clarithromycin 500 mg bid and metronidazol 500 mg bid or tid, successful eradication of *H. pylori* is achieved in about 90% of infected individuals (see Tab. 33.5).

Misoprostol is a synthetic prostaglandin E_1 analogue with weak antisecretory properties. Like natural prostaglandin E_1, the drug exerts a mucosa-protecting effect by stimulating mucosal bicarbonate secretion and enhancing the integrity of the mucous layer.

The drug is rapidly absorbed and metabolized to active compounds. The T_{max} occurs at 30 minutes, metabolization takes place in the liver, and elimination is mainly by the kidney and to a smaller extent in the feces, whereas the plasma half-life is about 20 to 40 minutes. Misoprostol induces contractions of smooth muscle, including the gastrointestinal tract (abdominal cramps and diarrhea) and the uterus (risk of abortion). Although the drug is superior to placebo in the treatment of peptic ulcer, because of its rather low antiulcer efficacy and frequent side effects, it is not recommended for the treatment of ulcers. However, misoprostol therapy compensates for the prostaglandin inhibition by NSAIDs and has been shown to prevent NSAID-induced ulcers and NSAID-induced ulcer bleedings. The dose for the prevention of NSAID-induced ulcers is 200 µg bid or tid.

Treatment of complications

Peptic ulcer bleeding   Bleeding from gastroduodenal ulcer is a serious complication, with mortality rising to about 10% in the elderly. Therapy consists of endoscopic hemostatic therapy combined with potent antisecretory drugs to prevent recurrent bleeding and to heal the ulcer. Since recurrent bleeding is an important cause of mortality, surgery should be taken into consideration as a valuable alternative therapy. Remarkably, peptic ulcer bleeding stops spontaneously in 50 to 80% of patients with no early recurrences. Inhibition of gastric acid reduces the risk of clot lysis. However, the optimal antisecretory therapy is not well established. H_2-receptor antagonists have little effect on the natural history of peptic ulcer bleeding. However, it has been reported that proton pump inhibitor/s reduce the rebleeding rate and the need for surgery. The optimal dose and route of administration (intravenous, oral, intravenous followed by oral) has still to be determined.

Stress ulcer bleeding Severely ill patients in the intensive care setting may bleed from so-called stress ulcers without previous gastric complaints. Stress ulcer bleeding is a life-threatening condition that preferably should be prevented. Endoscopic therapy, acid inhibition, and surgery are therapies to be considered for bleeding stress ulcers. Prevention should be applied to patients with a high risk of stress ulcer bleeding, i.e., patients on mechanical ventilation for more than 48 hours and those with coagulopathy. Large doses of antacids have been shown to be effective, whereas the effect of sucralfate is limited. Intravenous acid inhibition seems to be the prophylactic therapy of choice for high-risk patients. Although ranitidine in a dose of 50 mg tid or qid proved to be effective,

---

Table 33.6 Drugs used in the treatment of peptic ulcer

Antisecretory agents

H₂-receptor antagonists

Cimetidine	400 mg bid or 800 mg at night
Ranitidine	150 mg bid or 300 mg at night
Famotidine	20 mg bid or 40 mg at night
Nizatidine	150 mg bid or 300 mg at night
Roxatidine	75 mg bd or 150 mg at night

Proton pump inhibitors

Omeprazole	20 mg
Lansoprazole	30 mg
Pantoprazole	40 mg
Rabeprazole	20 mg

Anticholinergics

Pirenzepine	50 mg tid

Mucosa-protecting agents

Sucralfate	1 g qd
Bismuth subcitrate	120 mg qd

Prostaglandin analogues

Misoprostol	200 µg bid or qd

the efficacy of omeprazole is reported to be superior. Further studies are needed to determine the optimal dose and regimen of antisecretory therapy in the prevention of stress ulcer bleeding.

Ulcer perforation   Ulcer perforation should be treated by surgery. However, in order to prevent relapses, the *H.* *pylori* status, the NSAID intake, and/or plasma gastrin levels have to be determined, and if possible, causative therapy should be started. If such therapy is not possible, long-term antisecretory therapy (PPIs or H$_2$-receptor antagonists) should be given.

Gastric outlet obstruction   Surgical or endoscopic dilatation should be followed by a diagnostic workup (*H. pylori* status, plasma gastrin level), followed by causative therapy or long-term acid inhibition.

Suggested readings

Bungard TJ, Kale-Pradhan PB. Prokinetic agents for the treatment of postoperative ileus in adults: a review of the literature. Pharmacotherapy 1999;19:416-23.

DeVault KR. Overview of medical therapy for gastroesophageal reflux disease. Gastroenterology Clin N Am 1999;28: 831-45.

Hawkey CJ, Tulassay Z, Szczepanski L, et al. Randomised controlled trial of *Helicobacter pylori* eradication in patients on non-steroidal anti-inflammatory drugs: HELP NSAIDs study. Helicobacter Eradication for Lesion Prevention. Lancet 1998;352:1016-21.

Houben MH, Van Der Beek D, Hensen EF, et al. A systematic review of *Helicobacter pylori* eradication therapy: the impact of antimicrobial resistance on eradication rates. Aliment Pharmacol Ther 1999;13:1047-55.

Hunt RH. Importance of pH control in the management of GERD. Arch Int Med 1999-159:649-57.

Katz PO, Castell DO. Medical therapy of supraesophageal gastroesophageal reflux disease. Am J Med 2000;S170-S177.

Kiyota K, Habu Y, Sugano Y, et al. Comparison of 1-week and 2-week triple therapy with omeprazole, amoxicillin, and clarithromycin in peptic ulcer patients with *Helicobacter pylori* infection: results of a randomized controlled trial. J Gastroenterol 1999;34:76-79.

Lee J, O'Morain C. Who should be treated for *Helicobacter pylori* infection? A review of consensus conferences and guidelines. Gastroenterology 1997;113:S99-S106.

Lieber CS. Gastritis and *Helicobacter pylori*: forty years of antibiotic therapy. Digestion 1997;58:203-10.

Penston JG. McColl KE. Eradication of *Helicobacter pylori*: an objective assessment of current therapies. Br J Clin Pharmacol 1997;43:223-43.

Peterson WL, Cook DJ. Antisecretory therapy for bleeding peptic ulcer. JAMA 1998;280:877-8.

Scheiman J, Isenberg J. Agents used in the prevention and treatment of nonsteroidal anti-inflammatory drug-associated symptoms and ulcers. Am J Med 1998;105: S32-S38.

Tanigawara Y, Aoyama N, Kita T, et al. CYP2C19 genotype-related efficacy of omeprazole for the treatment of infection caused by *Helicobacter pylori*. Clin Pharmacol Ther 1999;66;528-34,

Thompson JS, Quigley EM. Prokinetic agents in the surgical patient. J Surg 1999;177:508-14.

van Doorn LJ, Schneeberger PM, Nouhan N, et al. Importance of *Helicobacter pylori* cagA and vacA status for the efficacy of antibiotic treatment. Gut 2000:46;321-6.

34

Small bowel diseases

Gino Roberto Corazza, Rachele Ciccocioppo

The most important and obvious consequence of small bowel diseases is nutrient malabsorption. Treatment should be aimed at curing the underlying disease as well as at restoring nutritional deficiencies. The practical management of patients with celiac disease, Whipple's disease, small intestine bacterial overgrowth, giardiasis, tropical sprue, short bowel syndrome, intestinal lymphangiectasia, and lactase deficiency will be reported herein.

CELIAC DISEASE

Celiac disease (nontropical sprue, gluten-sensitive enteropathy) can be defined as a chronic disease characterized by villous atrophy, crypt hypertrophy, and T-lymphocyte infiltration of the small bowel mucosa. These lesions are triggered in genetically susceptible individuals by the ingestion of wheat gliadin and barley and rye prolamins. Mucosal abnormalities and clinical symptoms critically improve after withdrawal of these offending agents from the diet. Gliadin and prolamin ingestion induce HLA-DQ2-positive subjects to mount an abnormal immune reaction against an autoantigen recently identified in the tissue enzyme transglutaminase. In the general population, it has been shown that the real prevalence of this condition is much higher than previously thought and is close to 1 in 200.

Celiac disease can start at any age, but the clinical features of the adult form are more protean than those of the childhood counterpart. Patients with minor, transient, or apparently unrelated symptoms have been diagnosed more frequently than patients with classic malabsorption symptoms, such as diarrhea, steatorrhea, and weight loss. Celiac disease should be suspected in the presence of conditions such as anemia or anisocytosis, aphthous stomatitis, short stature, dental enamel hypoplasia, infertility, recurrent abortion, pathologic bone fractures, and unexplained hypertransaminasemia or in association with one of the diseases listed in Table 34.1. Since celiac disease may occur in 6 to 7% of first-degree relatives of known celiac patients, serologic screening within celiac disease families is strongly advisable and represents the most common method to diagnose completely silent patients.

Since the definition of celiac disease is universally given in morphologic terms, a duodenal endoscopic biopsy is essential for the diagnosis. A second biopsy is necessary to show an improvement towards normality of the previously described lesions after the withdrawal of gliadin and related prolamins. The diagnostic rate of celiac disease recently has been increased by the search for antigliadin and antiendomysium antibodies. Radiology has essentially no role in the diagnosis of celiac disease unless one of its major complications is suspected.

Treatment

Withdrawal of wheat, rye, and barley from the diet (the so-called gluten-free diet) has greatly changed the prognosis and natural history of celiac disease. Recent studies have suggested that oat cereal is neither toxic nor immunogenic for celiac patients. This has important implications because the inclusion of oats would substantially improve the fiber and nutrient content of gluten-free diets. Corn, rice, buckwheat, legumes, potatoes, and tapioca are also well tolerated and may represent an alternative source of vegetable proteins for celiac disease patients.

A gluten-free diet is followed, in most patients, by healing of small bowel lesions and resolution of symptoms. This diet must constitute a lifetime commitment, should not be undertaken as a therapeutic trial prior to biopsy, and must be as strict as possible. A gluten-free diet is easy to prescribe but difficult to follow, since wheat flour is contained in many pharmaceutical products and in numerous canned, frozen, and convenience-type processed foods that are commonly part of the western diet. Unsuspected sources of gliadin or prolamins include ice cream, salad dressings, candy bars, soups, sauces, instant coffee, catsup, and mustard. The ingestion of beer and malt foods that contain barley should be avoided.

Supplementary therapy in celiac disease is generally needed only in the initial stage, i.e., when damaged mucosa does not yet permit adequate nutrient absorption. These prescriptions must be limited as far as possible and aimed not so much at correcting specific laboratory parameters as at controlling the symptoms linked to such deficits. If necessary, however, fluids must be administered for dehydratation, albumin for edema, and vitamins,

Table 34.1 Celiac disease and frequently related disorders

Insulin-dependent diabetes mellitus
Thyroid disease
IgA deficiency
Down syndrome
IgA mesangial nephropathy
Epilepsy with cerebral calcification
Alopecia
Atopy
Inflammatory bowel disease
Primary biliary cirrhosis
Primary sclerosing cholangitis
Rheumatoid arthritis
Sarcoidosis
Bird-fancier's lung
Recurrent pericarditis
Lung cavities
Sjögren syndrome
Systemic and cutaneous vasculitis
Systemic lupus erythematosus
Polymiositis
Myasthenia gravis
Iridocyclitis or choroiditis
Macroamylasemia
Addison's disease
Autoimmune thrombocytopenic purpura
Autoimmune hemolytic anemia

iron, folic acid, and calcium for tetany and potassium and magnesium for muscle cramps.

A few patients fail to improve after a gluten-free diet. Failure to improve in terms of symptoms may be due to the superimposition of other conditions such as lactase deficiency, bacterial overgrowth, and pancreatic insufficiency that should be recognized and treated adequately. Refractory celiac disease is characterized by the lack of histologic response to a gluten-free diet not due to the presence of the classic complications of celiac disease. Refractoriness may occur from the onset or after many years of treatment. Recently, a few adult patients with antienterocyte autoantibodies and villous atrophy unresponsive to a gluten-free diet but sensitive to steroid therapy and, therefore, affected by autoimmune enteropathy have been described

When a true refractory celiac disease is considered, immunosuppressants (methylprednisolone 40-60 mg qd, azathioprine 1.5 mg/kg qd, or cyclosporine A 5 mg/kg qd) should be added to the gluten-free diet.

WHIPPLE'S DISEASE

Whipple's disease is a chronic infection with intestinal and extraintestinal manifestations caused by *Tropheryma whippelii* that has been characterized recently by polymerase chain reaction (PCR) and by sequencing of the amplification products of the 16S ribosomal RNA gene from duodenal biopsy material and classified in the Actinobacteria family. More than 90% of patients are

middle-aged Caucasian men. Host defense abnormalities such as lymphopenia, decreased monocytic phagocytosis, reduced numbers of cells expressing complement receptor type 3, and more recently, lower monocyte interleukin 12 (IL-12) production and interferon gamma (IFN-γ) secretion by mononuclear cells have been described and may represent the genetic basis of Whipple's disease.

The clinical presentation of Whipple's disease is very insidious. Malabsorption symptoms often are preceded by a chronic, migratory, and seronegative arthropathy involving predominantly the peripheral joints, but the symptoms of episodic diarrhea, steatorrhea, anorexia, and weight loss usually lead to the diagnosis. No major organ is excluded from infection by *T. whippelii*, and the systemic symptoms that occur most frequently are fever, lymphoadenopathy, hyperpigmentation, night sweats, and chronic nonproductive cough. A crucial area of involvement is the central nervous system (CNS), with such manifestations as memory disorders, ophthalmoplegia, nystagmus, myoclonia, ataxia, seizures, dementia, and personality changes.

The positive diagnosis of Whipple's disease still rests on histopathologic grounds. The jejunal biopsy classically shows a massive infiltration of the lamina propria by foamy macrophages containing highly periodic acid-Schiff (PAS)-positive granulations. Although Whipple's disease can occur in the absence of intestinal involvement, the same lesions also may be found in other involved organs. PCR analysis to detect *T. whippelii* may be useful to diagnose the infection in tissues apparently unaffected by histology.

Treatment

Prior to the use of antibiotics, Whipple's disease had a poor prognosis. Almost all antibiotics have been employed in the treatment of this disease, and although tetracyclines have been used for a long time, greater awareness of the risk of CNS relapses has led to a preference for drugs that can pass the blood-brain barrier. In most patients, antibiotic therapy leads to a dramatic improvement in the clinical state and to a lasting remission. One of the recommended treatments is daily parenteral administration of benzylpenicillin (1.2 million IU) plus streptomycin (1 g) for 15 days, followed by oral cotrimoxazole (TMP-SMX, 160 mg/800 mg) bid for 1 year. Although cotrimoxazole is significantly more efficacious than tetracycline in the treatment of cerebral Whipple's disease, this drug does not prevent cerebral relapses in all patients. For this reason, third-generation cephalosporins have been recommended, starting with parenteral administration of ceftriaxone (2 g bid), followed by oral cefixime (400 mg qd) for 1 year. Theoretically, the endpoint of treatment should be the disappearance of symptoms, as well as eradication of intra- and extracellular bacteria, even if persistence of a few PAS-positive cells in the small bowel mucosa is not an indication to continue therapy.

SMALL INTESTINE BACTERIAL OVERGROWTH

Small intestine bacterial overgrowth (SIBO) is characterized by nutrient malabsorption associated with excessive numbers of bacteria (counts > 10^6 organisms/ml of jejunal aspirate) or with the presence of colonic species such as gram-negative rods, *Bacteroides,* and *Clostridium* in the lumen of the small intestine. The two general mechanisms proposed to explain small intestinal bacterial overgrowth (SIBO) are (1) failure of clearance from the upper gastrointestinal (GI) tract of bacteria arriving by the oral route and (2) seeding of the upper gastrointestinal tract with colon contents, which can occur through an enterocolonic fistula or after resection of the ileocecal valve. In the past, when more aggressive gastrointestinal surgery was performed, anatomic abnormalities (Billroth II gastric operation, extensive resection for Crohn's disease) were the most common causes of SIBO. At present, iatrogenic hypochlorhydria, aging, and abnormalities in intestinal motility (e.g., scleroderma, intestinal pseudo-obstruction, diabetic autonomic neuropathy) predominate.

The clinical presentation depends largely on the nature of the predisposing condition, and in some cases it is difficult to establish whether symptoms are related to the underlying disease or to a secondary small intestinal bacterial overgrowth. All symptoms of malabsorption (i.e., diarrhea, steatorrhea, anorexia, abdominal discomfort, anemia, and osteoporosis) may be present. However, macrocytic anemia, due to avid bacterial binding to vitamin B_{12}, and gallstones, due to bacterial deconjugation and dehydroxylation of primary bile salts, occur more frequently in SIBO than in other malabsorption syndromes.

Diagnosis of SIBO is based on a properly collected and appropriately cultured aspirate from the lumen of the proximal small intestine. However, in clinical practice, the use of bacteriologic analysis is hampered by the need for intubation and by the numerous difficulties and high costs. Over recent years, the use of indirect methods has been considered. Intestinal juice may be examined by gas-liquid chromatography for volatile fatty acids, which are a hallmark of nonsporulating anaerobic bacteria. Other noninvasive methods, such as the [^{14}C]xylose breath test and the hydrogen breath test after glucose ingestion are still waiting for better standardization.

Treatment

Appropriate therapy of patients with SIBO must include consideration of surgery, antimicrobial chemotherapy, and nutritional supplementation. Surgically remediable localized lesions such as strictures, fistulas, postoperative blind loops, and diverticula always should be sought and, if possible, removed. In the majority of patients, however, medical treatment of SIBO is a lifelong process.

Antibiotic therapy remains largely empiric because of a lack of controlled trials. Since the overgrowth flora typically contain many different species, broad-spectrum antibiotics usually are recommended. Tetracycline (250 mg qid po) represents the first-choice drug. Although this drug has little direct influence on anaerobes, it may suppress aerobes acting as oxygen scavengers and thereby indirectly inhibit anaerobes. Symptoms usually improve within a week, and although bacterial flora can return to the pretreatment status rapidly, the clinical response can be prolonged. At any rate, repeat courses of tetracycline every 4 to 6 weeks may be instituted as symptoms recur. If treatment with tetracycline does not produce salutary effects, metronidazole (250 mg tid) represents a useful alternative because of its direct effect on anaerobes. Rifaximin, a new nonabsorbable derivative of rifamycin and, therefore, with reduced side effects, has been shown to have a satisfactory therapeutic efficacy at the dose of 800 mg per day. Drugs such as chloramphenicol and lincomycin are no longer used because of the risk of potentially dangerous side effects. Penicillin, ampicillin, aminoglycosides, kanamycin, and neomycin are usually ineffective.

Nutritional support is an important part of the therapy program. An increased dietary intake can be achieved by providing more calories (>2500 kcal per day), whereas patients with cobalamin deficiency should receive monthly injections of vitamin B_{12} (100 μg).

GIARDIASIS

Giardia lamblia is the most common intestinal protozoan parasite that affects humans and may be considered a true zoonosis (see Chap. 42). The mechanisms by which *G. lamblia* produces malabsorption are poorly understood, but possible explanations include direct mucosal injury, reduced disaccharidase activity, increased bile salt deconjugation, release of parasite products, and mucosal inflammation associated with T-cell activation and cytokine release. Secretory immunoglobulin A (IgA) is important to host protection, as confirmed by the striking association between giardiasis and IgA deficiency.

Giardiasis can present as an asymptomatic infection (and this represents the most common clinical form) or with an acute, generally short-lived and self-limiting diarrhea or, finally, with a chronic diarrhea that leads to a malabsorption syndrome. Diagnosis relies largely on the microscopic detection of trophozoites or cysts in feces after examination of three separate specimens passed on different days. However, this method is labor-intensive and time-consuming. The coproantigen-ELISA test is especially advantageous in situations where only a single-stool sample can be examined.

Treatment

Metronidazole (2 g as a single daily dose for 3 consecutive days for adults, 15 mg/kg per day in three divided doses for 10 days for children) and tinidazole (2 g as a single dose for adults, 50-75 mg/kg as a single dose for children) represent the drugs of choice because the treatment period is short and compliance is generally good. Treatment failures can occur in around 10% of patients. Paromomycin, because it is poorly absorbed, has been proposed for use in pregnancy instead of metronidazole.

TROPICAL SPRUE

Tropical sprue is characteristic of tropical areas, where it exists either as isolated cases or in an endemic form. It is an infectious disease caused by persistent, chronic intestinal contamination with one or more enteric pathogens (*Klebsiella pneumoniae, E. coli,* or *Enterobacter cloacae*) that produce toxins responsible for intestinal abnormalities. It can affect a traveler on a brief visit, but it is more likely to occur among those living in an endemic area.

The syndrome is characterized by an acute episode of diarrhea, mild abdominal cramps, and sometimes fever and malaise. After a week, a mild chronic diarrhea and secondary lactase deficiency usually remain. After a few months, severe folate depletion and a malabsorption syndrome with anorexia and weight loss develop. Sometimes a protein-losing enteropathy may occur. If untreated, tropical sprue progresses to profound emaciation and weakness. Less commonly, symptoms develop after returning to a temperate zone.

Most instances occur in young adults after tropical exposure. Intestinal biopsy in the advanced stage shows nonspecific abnormalities such as partial villous atrophy, the severity of which does not correlate with that of diarrhea or the degree of malabsorption.

Treatment

Combined therapy with folic acid (5 mg per day po) and tetracycline (250 mg po qid) results in both clinical improvement and healing of the intestinal lesion, although relapses may occur occasionally. Patients with chronic disease should be treated for as long as 6 months.

SHORT BOWEL SYNDROME

Short bowel syndrome (SBS) can be defined as a malabsorption syndrome that results from extensive intestinal resection. In fact, resection of a short segment of the small intestine has chronic consequences only if the ileum, which is the site of active transport of bile salts and vitamin B_{12}, is removed. Serious and life-threatening nutritional deficiencies occur if more than 50% of the small bowel is resected.

If the resection has been extensive, diarrhea, dehydration, and electrolyte deficiencies may be prominent in the early postresection period. Diarrhea may be worse after removal of the distal ileum owing to the secretory effect of bile salts on the colonic mucosa. In the so-called intermediate phase, malabsorption symptoms (weight loss and nutritional deficiencies) dominate. The late phase depends on the capacity of the residual intestine to adapt and to increase the absorptive surface area.

The clinical symptoms are those of a severe malabsorption syndrome. In patients with ileal resection, there is an increased incidence of cholesterol gallstones and a propensity for oxalate renal stones to develop (owing to colonic hyperabsorption of oxalate in the presence of steatorrhea). If protein-calorie malnutrition is severe enough, hepatic changes of kwashiorkor develop. Bone loss is particularly severe as a result of calcium loss and vitamin D malabsorption. Lactic acidosis is a rare but serious complication due to fermentation within the residual lumen brought about by bacterial overgrowth.

Treatment

In the acute phase, the main therapeutic problem is to prevent the massive diarrhea that leads to fluid and electrolyte imbalances. Treatment, therefore, consists of replacement with Ringer's lactate and glucose solution at a volume that correlates with the amount of fluid lost. On the third postoperative day, total parenteral nutrition can be started. Depending on the patient's condition, in a period of time ranging from 5 days to 2 weeks, the adaptation phase may begin with oral nutrition.

There is a significant correlation between the length of the remaining bowel and the duration of the need for nutritional support. The minimum length to maintain nutritional integrity for enteral feeding seems to be 110 to 150 cm when associated with colectomy and 50 to 70 cm if the colon is left intact. Metabolic and nutritional markers should be measured frequently. In the maintenance phase, the diet must contain at least 45 to 60 kcal/kg per day, divided into many small meals and without separating liquids from solids. Furthermore, patients need oral supplementation of calcium, magnesium, zinc, vitamins, minerals, and trace elements.

In the management of specific patients, several drugs may be useful, such as loperamide to slow intestinal transit (4-16 mg per day) and H_2-receptor antagonists or proton pump inhibitors to reduce gastric acid output and secretory diarrhea (ranitidine 300-600 mg per day or omeprazole 20-40 mg per day) (see Chap. 33). Somatostatin and its analogue, octreotide, can reduce the fecal fat output, prolong intestinal transit time, and increase the absorption rate. Because octreotide may produce tachyphylaxis within weeks, it should be given during the adaptation phase but not during the mainteinance phase. Cholestyramine binds bile acids and is effective in bile salt diarrhea, but pancreatic enzymes may be needed. Metronidazole or rifaximin is indicated in the case of superimposed bacterial overgrowth.

INTESTINAL LYMPHANGIECTASIA

The primary form of intestinal lymphangiectasia is a rare disorder of unknown etiology that affects children and young adults, characterized by dilated lymphatic vessels within the small bowel wall. The secondary form is due to lymphatic obstruction of the bowel that occurs later in life as a consequence of constrictive pericarditis, right-sided heart failure, Crohn's disease, abdominal tubercolosis or sarcoidosis, intestinal lymphoma, retroperitoneal malignancies, and systemic lupus erythematosus. In many primary cases there are lymphatic abnormalities elsewhere in the body that may be clinically apparent or documented by lymphangiography.

Most patients present with a protein-losing enteropathy (e.g., edema, diarrhea, low levels of serum immunoglobulins, transferrin, ceruloplasmin, and lymphocytes). Gastrointestinal symptoms are uncommon and, when present, are mild. Despite the reduced levels of immunoglobulins and lymphocytes, opportunistic infections seldom occur.

The main laboratory features include low concentrations of albumin and immunoglobulins, lymphopenia, and mild steatorrhea. The diagnosis usually is based on jejunal biopsy that shows the dilated lacteals inside distorted villi. Protein loss is measured by giving ^{51}Cr-labeled proteins intravenously and evaluating the fecal isotope excretion on the subsequent days.

Treatment

Some reports have demonstrated clinical improvement with surgical treatment or with a low-fat, medium-chain triglyceride–supplemented diet. Antiplasmin therapy with *trans*-4-aminomethyl cyclohexane carboxylic acid (*trans*-AMCHA, 2-4 g/d) has been shown to have a dramatic effect both on serum protein levels and on circulating immunoglobulins and lymphocytes. This therapy must be carried out for life, but in other patients subsequently described, this regimen was ineffective despite an increment in the daily dose. In primary intestinal lymphangiectasia sustained by an inflammatory state, steroids (prednisolone 30 mg qd) have been successful. Finally, because somatostatin receptors have been found in normal gut lymphoid tissue, octreotide (100 µg bid) may be considered a useful alternative.

LACTASE DEFICIENCY

Lactase deficiency (LD) is a characteristic of the adult small intestine in many geographic areas (southern Italy, Mediterranean basin, Africa, Middle East). As a consequence, the digestion and absorption of lactose, the major sugar in milk and dairy products, are hampered. The malabsorbed lactose undergoes anaerobic bacteria fermentation in the colon, with the production of short-chain fatty acids, hydrogen, CO_2, and methane responsible for the symptoms of lactose intolerance, such as abdominal cramps and distension, bloating, excessive flatus, and occasionally, watery diarrhea. The degree of discomfort depends on the amount of lactose ingested, rather than on individual sensitivity.

The measurement of hydrogen in the expired air after lactose ingestion (the hydrogen breath test) is the usual way to detect lactose malabsorption.

Treatment

Complete withdrawal of milk is usually not required because lactase deficiency is seldom absolute. Patients with LD can lower their symptoms by ingesting milk with solid foods, which contributes to a delay in gastric emptying and thus graduates the delivery of lactose to the small bowel. Alternatively, such patients tolerate prehydrolyzed milk with exogenous lactase or yoghurt that contains a minor amount of lactose.

Suggested readings

BAC DJ, VAN HAGEN PM, POSTEMA PTE, et al. Octreotide for protein-losing enteropathy with intestinal lymphangiectasia. Lancet 1995;345:1639.

CATASSI C, RATSCH IM, FABIANI E, et al. Coeliac disease in the year 2000: exploring the iceberg. Lancet 1994;343:200-3.

CORAZZA GR, GASBARRINI G. Coeliac disease in adults. Baillières Clin Gastroenterol 1995;9:329-50.

CORAZZA GR, VALENTINI RA, FRISONI M, et al. Gliadin immune reactivity is associated with overt and latent enteropathy in relatives of celiac patients. Gastroenterology 1992;103:1517-22.

CORAZZA GR, VENTRUCCI M, STROCCHI A, et al. Treatment of small intestine bacterial overgrowth with rifaximin, a non-absorbable rifamycin. J Int Med Res 1988;16:312-6.

DIETERICH W, EHNIS T, BAUER M, et al. Identification of tissue transglutaminase as the autoantigen of coeliac disease. Nature Med 1997;3:797-801.

DURAND DV, LECOMTE C, CATHEBRAS P, et al. Whipple disease: Clinical review of 52 cases. Medicine 1997;76:170-84.

FARTHING MJG. Giardiasis. Gastroenterol Clin North Am 1996; 25:493-515.

HILL DR. Giardiasis. Issues in diagnosis and management. Infect Dis Clin North Am 1993;7:503-25.

JEEJEEBHOY KN. Therapy of the short-gut syndrome. Lancet 1983;1:1427-30.

KEINATH RD, MERRELL DE, VLIETSTRA R, DOBBINS WO III. Antibiotic treatment and relapse in Whipple's disease. Gastroenterology 1985;88:1867-73.

MINE K, MATSUBAYASHI S, NAKAI Y, NAKAGAWA T. Intestinal lymphangiectasia markedly improved with antiplasmin therapy. Gastroenterology 1989;96:1596-99.

RELMAN DA, SCHMIDT TM, MACDERMOTT RP, FALKOW S. Identification of the uncultured bacillus of Whipple's disease. N Engl J Med 1992;327:293-301.

SINGER R. Diagnosis and treatment of Whipple's disease. Drugs 1998;55:699-704.

TRIER JS. Celiac sprue. N Engl J Med 1991;325:1709-19.

35

Large bowel diseases

Sandro Ardizzone, Gabriele Bianchi Porro

Inflammatory bowel disease, irritable bowel disease, and diverticular disease of the colon are among the most common human diseases. *Irritable bowel syndrome* refers to a well-recognized symptom complex arising from interactions among the digestive tract, the psyche, and luminal factors. Alterations in function also have been reported in extraintestinal organs containing smooth muscles, such as the urinary bladder and the bronchus. Similarly, *in inflammatory bowel disease*, while ulcerative colitis is typically an inflammatory condition involving exclusively the large bowel, Crohn's disease may affect any segment of the alimentary tract, from mouth to anus, at times assuming the nature of a systemic disease.

Substantial progress has been made during the past decade in understanding the nature and treatment of these diseases. However, until the exact underlying pathogenetic mechanisms are clarified, the medical treatment of these condtions stands on an empiric basis. The physician must continue to recognize the individual circumstances of each patient and balance the benefits of prolonged therapy against side effects and costs or, as in the case of inflammatory bowel disease, benefits from surgical treatment.

INFLAMMATORY BOWEL DISEASE

Inflammatory bowel disease (IBD) is a general term for a group of chronic inflammatory disorders of unknown etiology involving the gastrointestinal tract. Chronic inflammatory bowel disease may be divided into two major groups, *ulcerative colitis* and *Crohn's disease,* characterized by recurrent inflammatory involvement of intestinal segments with several manifestations often resulting in a unpredictable course.

Inflammatory bowel diseases generate important economic issues in industrialized countries despite the relatively low number of people suffering from these conditions. The burden of disease is assessed by economists with reference to the mortality and morbidity associated with the disease. These induce costs in terms of direct medical expenses for managing the disease, expenses paid out of pocket by patients, and losses of working time and productivity. These costs were estimated in two countries:

the United States and Italy. In the United States, an overall disease burden of US$ 1.8 to 2.6 million in 1990 was estimated. In Italy, the cost was the equivalent of US$ 285 thousand for the same period. Available evidence seems to suggest a striking similarity in the cost of treating inflammatory bowel disease in the United States and Italy, although ulcerative colitis seems to be more expensive in Italy and Crohn's disease more expensive in the United States.

Ulcerative colitis and Crohn's disease are chronic inflammatory diseases usually associated with recurrent attacks alternating with complete remission of symptoms. In Western Europe and the United States, ulcerative colitis has an incidence of approximately 6 to 8 cases per 100 000 population and an estimated prevalence of approximately 70 to 150 per 100 000. Estimates of the incidence of Crohn's disease are approximately 2 cases per 100 000 population, and the prevalence is estimated at 20 to 40 cases per 100 000. While peak occurrence of both diseases is between the ages of 15 and 35 years, it has been reported in every decade of life. A familial incidence of inflammatory bowel disease has been recorded.

In *ulcerative colitis* there is an inflammatory reaction involving primarily the colonic mucosa. In general, the colon appears ulcerated, hyperemic, and usually hemorrhagic. A striking feature of the inflammation is that it is uniform and continuous with no intervening areas of normal mucosa. The rectum is usually involved, and the inflammation extends proximally in a continuous fashion but for a variable distance. In its most limited form it may involve only the rectum (proctitis), whereas the entire colon is involved in its most extended form (pancolitis).

In contrast to ulcerative colitis, *Crohn's disease* is characterized by chronic inflammation extending through all layers of the intestinal wall and involving the mesentery as well as regional lymph nodes. The bowel may appear thickened and leathery with a narrowed lumen leading to stenosis, with varying degrees of intestinal obstruction. In contrast to ulcerative colitis, the distribution of the inflammation is often discontinuous; severely involved segments of bowel are separated from each other by intervening segments of apparently normal bowel, producing "skip areas." The rectum may be spared in approximately 50% of patients with Crohn's disease of the colon. In sharp contrast, in ulcerative colitis, the involvement is contiguous, and the rectum is almost always affected. In most series reporting the distribution of Crohn's disease, approximately 30% involve the small intestine (usually the terminal ileum) without colonic disease, 30% only colonic involvement, and 40% ileocolic involvement, usually the ileum and right colon.

Although it is possible to make a correct diagnosis most of the time, a definite distinction between ulcerative colitis and Crohn's disease may not be possible in 10 to 20% of patients.

The major symptoms of ulcerative colitis are bloody diarrhea and abdominal pain, often with fever and weight loss in more severe cases. When the disease is mild, there may be one or two semiformed stools containing little blood, with no systemic manifestations. In contrast, the patient with severe disease may have frequent liquid stools containing blood and pus, complain of severe cramps, and demonstrate symptoms and signs of dehydration, anemia, fever, and weight loss.

The clinical presentation of Crohn's disease will largely reflect the anatomic location of the disease and to some degree will predict which complications of the disease may develop. The major clinical features of Crohn's disease are fever, abdominal pain, diarrhea often without blood, and generalized fatigability. There may be associated weight loss. With colonic involvement, diarrhea and pain are the most frequent symptoms. Rectal bleeding is distinctly less common than with ulcerative colitis, and this reflects the fact that the rectum is spared in many patients and indicates the transmural nature of the disease. Severe anorectal complications such as fistulas, fissures, and perirectal abscess may be seen.

Complications of both diseases may be local or systemic. Local complications consist of intestinal obstruction (more frequent in Crohn's disease than in ulcerative colitis), fistula and abscess formation (a frequent complication of Crohn's disease), and intestinal perforation. In addition, toxic dilatation of the colon and the development of carcinoma may complicate both ulcerative colitis and Crohn's disease.

Treatment

Treatments of general use in the disease

In general, the treatment of both ulcerative colitis and Crohn's disease shares certain common principles. Initial treatment of all forms of uncomplicated inflammatory bowel disease is primarily medical, and the principles of medical therapy are similar. There are certain important differences, however, between ulcerative colitis and Crohn's disease; namely, the response to drug therapy may change, complications often differ, and the prognosis after surgical therapy is not the same.

Corticosteroids, sulfasalazine, its derivative 5-aminosalicylic acid, and immunosuppressants are the mainstays of medical treatment of inflammatory bowel disease. In addition, the medical management of patients affected with inflammatory bowel disease includes a supportive therapy aiming at further lessening the symptoms of disease. This consists in using antispasmodics, antidiarrheal agents, sedatives and antidepressants, analgesics, dietary manipulation, and psychotherapeutic measures. Finally, IBD patients, especially those with Crohn's disease, may require surgical treatment.

Nonpharmacologic treatment

Supportive therapy

Considerable effort has been given to the search for a *diet* that may be beneficial in inflammatory bowel disease. However, there is no reliable evidence for a specific inflammatory bowel disease diet. There are, however, at least two rules to observe when offering dietary advice to patients with inflammatory bowel disease: (1) eat well and maintain adequate caloric intake, and (2) avoid only those foods which clearly provoke symptoms or complications.

Irritable bowel syndrome (IBS) is common in the general population and frequently complicates ulcerative colitis and Crohn's disease. It is therefore useful to identify the inflammatory and noninflammatory symptoms in individual patients with inflammatory bowel disease. Abdominal cramping, diarrhea, and constipation occur not infrequently as a consequence of irritable bowel syndrome rather than inflammatory bowel disease. In these patients, it may be useful to administer *anticholinergic preparations* (e.g., hyoscyamine, propantheline, belladonna alkaloids, etc.), especially in Crohn's disease. These agents should be used with caution and should be avoided in the presence of severe colitis, thus lessening the risk of toxic megacolon or severe obstruction.

IBD diarrhea generally is treated by controlling the underlying inflammatory process with the specific agents described in this chapter (see below). In some cases, however, additional symptomatic medication is indicated to relieve the rectal urgency and frequent bowel movements. The most useful *antidiarrheal agents* include diphenoxylate, loperamide, codeine, paregoric, and deodorized tincture of opium. Thanks to the fact that it has no effect on the central nervous system (CNS), loperamide is the preferred antidiarrheal agent used in clinical practice (see also Chap. 32). Antidiarrheal agents, however, must be used with caution in patients with severe colitis to avoid the possible induction of toxic megacolon. Antidiarrheal medications may be useful for the treatment of diarrhea in IBD patients with intestinal resection. Cholestyramine is the treatment of choice for bile salt-induced diarrhea, whereas fatty acid-induced diarrhea responds to restriction of dietary fat.

Analgesics are rarely necessary for ulcerative colitis because the inflamation usually is limited to superficial layers of the gut, whereas pain receptors are localized in the serosa and peritoneum. D-propoxyphene and paracetamol are of little help in controlling the abdominal pain of Crohn's disease. Opiates may increase bowel spasm, and after providing initial relief, more abdominal pain may follow. Moreover, they may precipitate a toxic mega-colon. The best therapy for abdominal pain in Crohn's disease is treatment of the inflammatory state. The use of aspirin and other nonsteroidal anti-inflammatory drugs (NSAIDs) is controindicated in IBD patients because of the possibility of increasing intestinal inflammation and exacerbating inflammatory bowel disease.

Considering that there is no psychologic profile that predisposes patients to the development of inflammatory bowel disease, sedative and anxiolytic drugs are not pre-scribed routinely. They should be limited to individual sit-uations and their use monitored for additive potential.

Drug therapy

Several important criteria should be used when choosing the most correct therapeutic approach to patients affected by inflammatory bowel disease: (1) aims of treatment, (2) determining the extent and localization of the disease, (3) grading activity, and (4) defining clinical pattern. Moreover, patient compliance, risks and benefits, and pharmacoeconomic considerations are also important fac-tors affecting the choice of therapy.

Aims of therapy The clinical state of a patient with active inflammatory bowel disease reflects many different fac-tors: the primary disease process of gut inflammation, confined to the mucosa in ulcerative colitis and spreading through the thickness of the wall in Crohn's disease; the metabolic consequences, such as protein-losing enteropa-thy and hypoalbuminemia, anemia, hypokalemia, hypocalcemia, and hypomagnesemia; and the structural abnormalities that arise, such as strictures, perforations, fistulas, and abscesses. Therapy of the patient involves, usually as a priority, treatment of these consequences of inflammation by transfusion and replacement of such losses as minerals, vitamins, and so on.

Extent and anatomic distribution of inflammatory bowel disease Establishing the extent and localization of ulcera-tive colitis and Crohn's disease, respectively, is an impor-tant diagnostic and clinical step in the evaluation of IBD patients because of its therapeutic implications. Colonoscopy and radiology are the primary diagnostic tools used to define the extent and anatomic distribution of inflammatory bowel disease. In ulcerative colitis, the extent of colonic involvement during the first attack has been found to be reasonably uniform in several large series of patients. Approximately 30% of ulcerative colitis patients have disease limited to the rectum, about 40% have disease that extends above the rectum but not beyond the hepatic flexure (so-called subtotal colitis), while the remaining 30% develop total colitis. However, in some population-based surveys, more than half the patients present with dis-ease extending from the rectum to the splenic flexure. Crohn's disease may affect any part of the alimentary tract from mouth to anus. About one-third of patients have involvement confined to the small bowel (regional enteri-tis), usually involving the terminal ileum (ileitis). Nearly half have involvement of both small and large bowel (ileo-colitis), usually in continuity. In about 20% of patients, dis-ease is confined to the colon alone. Perianal lesions occur in approximately one-third of patients but are only rarely the presenting or sole site of Crohn's disease.

Grading of disease activity Disease activity indices are prediction rules used to measure the activity of disease objectively so as to judge response in clinical trials. However, the use of these indices in clinical practice is limited, especially in Crohn's disease, because they are intended to make the clinical global assessment objective, a prerogative with which most clinicians do not agree. In ulcerative colitis, the activity of the disease is usually assessed primarily on the basis of clinical features. The Truelove and Witts classification of mild, moderate, or severe disease, based on certain clinical parameters and laboratory findings (e.g., number of bowel movements, fever, presence of tachycardia, anemia, and sedimention rate), is the most widely used clinical activity index in gastroenterologic practice.

In Crohn's disease, the *Crohn's disease activity index* (CDAI) was developed in the United States during the 1979 National Cooperative Crohn's Disease Study to assess objectively the response to therapy among patients studied at many participating centers. Seven-day symp-toms were recorded, as were hematocrit, an abdominal mass, use of opiates for diarrhea, extraintestinal manifes-tations, and body weight. These values were weighted by derived regression coefficients. A CDAI of less than 150 signified quiescent disease, and a CDAI of greater than 450 signified severe disease.

Clinical pattern of inflammatory bowel disease The course of ulcerative colitis follows a reliable clinical pat-tern. After the first episode, most patients (approximately two-thirds) subsequently experience recurrent attacks. A small minority, from 7 to 15%, never achieves satisfacto-ry remission and continues with symptoms to a greater or lesser degree (steroid-resistant patients), whereas others have a steroid-dependent disease.

Crohn's disease is a naturally remitting and relapsing dis-ease, and patterns of disease activity may be very different among patients. Remission may be continuous for over 20 years after one or two flare-ups in up to 20% of patients. Approximately 30% of patients who achieve remission will relapse within 1 year, and 40% will relapse within 2 years. Other patients who present with active aggressive disease never achieve remission. Aggressive disease is characterized by the short duration of disease before initial surgery and is usually associated with severely active disease and impor-tant complications such as abscess and perforation. Another population of Crohn's disease patients is characterized by a long duration of disease prior to initial surgery, with the most important complications being a fixed stenotic bowel segment or chronic active disease refractory to therapy. Surgery does not cure Crohn's disease but can be very help-ful in the management of severe or persistent complications.

Commonly, the pregnant patient with inflammatory bowel disease is advised by her obstetrician to discontinue sulfasalazine (SSZ), 5-aminosalicylic acid (5-ASA), corticosteroids, and other drugs in the interest of patient and fetus safety. Sulfasalazine and corticosteroids have been used consistently throughout pregnancy without causing harm to the fetus or newborn baby. In one large series, sulfasalazine and conventional steroids did not alter the rates of spontaneous abortion and prematurity or fetal weight. The incidence of fetal complications was lower than in the general population. Although a later report suggested that fetal complications may be higher in a medically treated group, this is more likely to be caused by disease activity and not by the effects of drug therapy alone. Few data are available concerning the safety of the several 5-ASA formulations during pregnancy. Two studies, evaluating 38 pregnancies, have shown the safety for mother and fetus of oral and topical 5-ASA. However, a recent French national survey showed one case of renal disease in a newborn baby and three newborns with congenital malformations (i.e., congenital cataract, thumb malformation, cardiac malformation).

Drug classes

CORTICOSTEROIDS (Tab. 35.1): OLD STEROIDS

Synthetic glucocorticoids such as prednisone, methylprednisolone, and hydrocortisone are the most commonly used corticosteroids in the treatment of inflammatory bowel disease.

Dosage

Prednisone is available as 5- and 25-mg tablets. Oral administration of this steroid is particularly indicated in patients with moderately active disease, generally at dosages of 20 to 25 mg per day, preferably in the morning, for an average of 4 weeks, and it must be tapered over 2 to 4 weeks depending on symptom resolution. Methylprednisolone is available in injectable form, at dosages of 20 or 40 mg. This formulation is indicated in the treatment of moderate to severe disease. Dosage and duration of therapy are variable: in patients with moderate disease, 20 to 40 mg per day, preferably in the morning, may be a starting dose, with a treatment duration of 30 days. In the case of severe or fulminant disease, this dosage must be increased to 60 mg per day for 7 to 10 days depending on the clinical response. These dosages must be tapered every 5 to 7 days until suspension. Hydrocortisone is available in injectable and rectal formulations. In its injectable form, it is available in dosages of 100 to 1000 mg. Its use is indicated in the treatment of severe or fulminant disease, at a dose of 100 mg tid for 7 to 10 days. In the rectal form, hydrocortisone may be administered as both enema (100 mg/60 ml) or foam (125 mg/50 ml) for a variable period of 3 to 6 weeks. Adrenocorticotropic hormone (ACTH), available in injectable form (0.25, 1, and 2 mg), may be useful in the treatment of severe ulcerative colitis where no steroids have been given during the previous 30 days.

Corticosteroids are in general rapidly and fairly completely absorbed from the gastrointestinal tract. When given orally, approximately 80% of prednisolone, 70% of methylprednisolone, and 50% of hydrocortisone are absorbed. Bioavailability is enhanced if lipophilic groups on the D portion of the steroid ring structure are substituted. Prednisolone is the most commonly used oral corticosteroid in the treatment of inflammatory bowel disease. After rapid absorption from the proximal gastrointestinal tract (upper jejunum), prednisone is metabolized to prednisolone with reduction by an 11-hydroxydehydrogenase.

Table 35.1 Corticosteroids commonly used in the treatment of inflammatory bowel disease

	Oral forms	Injectable forms	Others
Hydrocortisone sodium succinate	–	100-1000 mg	100 mg E 125 mg F 25 mg S
Prednisone	5 mg 25 mg	– –	–
Prednisolone sodium phosphate	–	20 mg	5 mg S 20 mg S 20 mg E
Methylprednisolone acetate	–	20-40 mg	–
Methylprednisolone sodium succinate	4 mg	8, 20, 40 mg	–
Budesonide	3 mg	–	0.5 mg S 2 mg E
Beclomethasone dipropionate	–	–	3, 5 mg E
Prednisolone (as metasulfobenzoate sodium)	–	–	20 g F
Tixocortol pivalate	–	–	250 mg E
Fluticasone	20 mg	–	–

(E = enema; S = solution; F = foam.)

Peak plasma concentrations occur in 30 minutes to 2 hours.

The most commonly used parenteral formulations are prednisolone, methylprednisolone, and hydrocortisone.

The pharmacokinetic activity of methylprednisolone is similar to that of prednisolone, as described earlier. An alternative to the synthetic steroids is ACTH, which may be administered im or iv. Adrenocorticotropic hormone is absorbed rapidly from muscle and, with a plasma half-life of 15 minutes, is cleared rapidly from the circulation.

Hydrocortisone alcohol remains the most frequently used topical steroid preparation. Although hydrocortisone enemas have been reported to have little systemic absorption and therefore to have little risk of systemic side effects, it has been demonstrated that the bioavailability of a retention enema of at least 8 hours'duration is almost similar to that of an equivalent oral dose, with 50 to 90% available to the systemic circulation. Prolonged topical administration of hydrocortisone is associated with a significant risk of adrenal suppression and exogenous hyperadrenalism.

CORTICOSTEROIDS (Tab. 35.1): NEWER TOPICAL STEROIDS

The frequent side effects associated with corticosteroid use has prompted the development of rectal and oral agents that provide certain advantages over currently available steroids by achieving equivalent or superior efficacy with a lower adverse event profile. The absence of toxicity, and in particular, the lack of suppression of the hypothalamic-pituitary-adrenal axis of these newer topical agents, relates to their low systemic bioavailability owing to extensive "first pass" metabolism in the liver, lack of rectal absorption, or both mechanisms. All these account for the low frequency of systemic effects. Moreover, these new drugs should have a high intrinsic glucocorticoid activity, high topical potency, and good metabolic stability in the bowel. Prednisolone metasulfobenzoate, tixocortol pivalate, fluticasone propionate, beclomethasone dipropionate, and budesonide are all considered to fulfill these requirements.

Pharmacokinetics

Rectal and oral prednisolone metasulfobenzoate has a low absorption compared with prednisolone-21-phosphate. The larger molecule probably gives a slower release of prednisolone. Prednisolone metasulfobenzoate has been shown to give higher rectal tissue levels than rapidly absorbed systemic steroids in patients with ulcerative colitis. Beclomethasone 17,21-dipropionate has little systemic glucocorticoid activity with oral or rectal administration despite having marked anti-inflammatory activity (500 times the anti-inflammatory potency of dexamethasone) on the skin and efficacy in enema form similar to that of prednisolone. Budesonide, a nonhalogenated glucocorticoid, also undergoes rapid liver biotransformation, affording low systemic availability (approximately 15%) with oral or rectal administration. Its anti-inflammatory

effect is optmized by a $16\alpha,17\alpha$-acetyl group asymmetric substitution, rendering it 5 times more potent than triamcinolone, which has instead a $16\alpha,17\alpha$-acetonide group. Budesonide is metabolized by the cytochrome P450 3A (CYP3A) enzymes in the human liver. Tixocortol pivalate, a cortisol derivative in which the 21-hydroxyl group has been modified with a thiol group-pivalic acid esterification, exhibits topical anti-inflammatory activity similar to cortisol but does not induce a measurable systemic glucorticoid effect when given orally or rectally.

Dosage

The newer topical steroids are available in both rectal and oral forms: prednisolone metasulfobenzoate as rectal foam, at a dosage of 20 mg per day; beclomethasone dipropionate as an enema, at a dosage of 3-5 mg per day; budesonide as oral capsules, at a dosage of 3,6, and 9 mg per day, as an enema, at a dosage of 2, mg per day, or as a suppository, at a dosage of 0.5 mg bid; tixocortol pivalate as an enema at a dosage of 250 mg per day; and fluticasone as an oral formulation, at a dosage of 20 mg per day.

Indications

Both rectal and oral formulations of these topical agents are indicated in the treatment of active distal ulcerative colitis, whereas oral administration is limited to treatment of active Crohn's disease. The duration of the treatment is variable: from 2 to 9 weeks in ulcerative colitis and from 4 to 16 weeks in active Crohn's disease.

Side effects

Although infrequent, the drug-related adverse effects include nausea, abdominal distension, fatigue, and perianal irritation.

Contraindications

Drug hypersensitivity.

SULFASALAZINE

Sulfasalazine (SSZ) was developed in the 1930s to combine the known anti-inflammatory properties of salicylates with the recently discovered antimicrobial qualities of sulfa drugs. The SSZ molecule consists of sulfapyridine attached by an azobond to 5-aminosalicylic acid (5-ASA) (Fig. 35.1). The new compound was tested in rheumatoid arthritis and in ulcerative colitis, which was then thought to be possibly of infectious origin. Early studies with sulfasalazine suggested great benefit from the drug. Since then, sulfasalazine has become a mainstay of medical therapy for inflammatory bowel disease.

Sulfasalazine is available as tablets at a dosage of 500 mg. The daily dosage is variable and ranges from 2 to 4 g

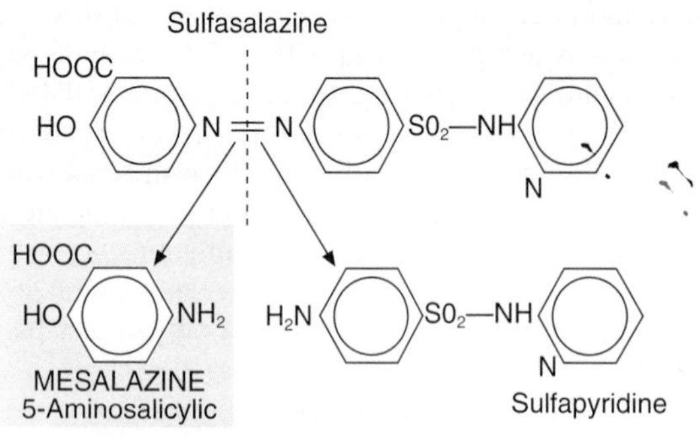

Figure 35.1 Structural formula and metabolism of sulfasalazine.

in quiescent disease to 3 to 6 g in active disease. The drug is usually given bid or tid.

After oral administration, the unchanged drug is absorbed to a limited extent. The absorption that does take place occurs mainly in the upper gastrointestinal tract. Several studies have demonstrated that not more than 30% of ingested sulfasalazine is absorbed in the small intestine and that most reaches the colon unchanged. However, up to 80% of this absorbed SSZ enters the enterohepatic circulation and is returned to the small intestine by the bile. This returned SSZ is equivalent to around 20% of the oral dose, so eventually about 90% of the original dose reaches the colon. The absorbed SSZ that does not reenter the small intestine finds its way into the systemic circulation, where blood levels can range from 2 to 10% of the original dose. After a 2-g dose of SSZ, the drug can be detected in serum within 6 hours. Following repeated daily doses, steady-state serum levels are achieved within 4 to 5 days. The initial metabolism of sulfasalazine takes place in the colon through the activity of a wide range of colonic bacteria. These bacteria have the ability to split the azo bond because they posses an intracellular azoreductase that reduces and breaks the azo bond. Sulfasalazine generally is ineffective in the treatment of isolated ileitis, presumably because this relatively germ-free area lacks bacterial azoreductase. The cleavage of the azo bond then releases the two major metabolites, 5-ASA and sulfapyridine. Approximately one-third of 5-ASA is acetylated to N-acetyl-5-amino salicylic acid in the colon. The hepatic metabolism of sulfasalazine consists of an N-acetylation and ring hydroxylation and a final conjugation with glucouronic acid. Slow acetylators may be expected to show a higher than average serum concentration of sulfapyridine for a longer period of time when compared with fast acetylators. Sulfapyridine seems to be responsible for most of the side effects associated with sulfasalazine, although adverse reactions with 5-ASA therapy are being recognized increasingly. Because only minor amounts of unchanged SSZ reach the systemic circulation, as little as 2 to 10% of the dose can be recovered unchanged from

the urine. In normal subjects, around 1% can be recovered from the feces. However, in patients with colitis, up to 7% of the dose has been recovered from the feces. Two-thirds of the 5-ASA resulting from the bacterial cleavage of SSZ is excreted unchanged in the feces. Of the sulfapyridine present in sulfasalazine, two-thirds can be recovered from the urine, as sulfapyridine and its metabolites, and the rest can be recovered from the feces. If given separately, 5-ASA and SSZ are absorbed proximally, metabolized, and excreted in the urine, never reaching the distal small intestine or colon. It is the azo bond, therefore, that allows for transport of SSZ to the distal small intestine and colon without significant absorption.

Indications

In ulcerative colitis, SSZ is indicated in the treatment of mild to moderate distal or total disease at a variable dosage of 2 to 4 g per day and in preventing relapse when the disease is quiescent at a dosage of 2 g per day. In Crohn's disease, SSZ may be used in the treatment of moderately active ileocolitis and colitis at a dosage of 4 to 6 g per day and in maintenace treatment of remission, when the disease is localized to the colon, at a dosage of 2 to 3 g per day.

Side effects

The incidence of side effects related to SSZ is high and dose-related, similar to therapeutic effects. Up to 45% of patients report side effects from SSZ. By far the greatest majority of these effects are intolerance, not allergy, and relate to the sulfapyridine moiety correlating with the acetylator phenotype. The most common but less severe adverse reactions to sulfasalazine include nausea, vomiting, dyspepsia, anorexia, and headache. More severe reactions are uncommon and include generalized allergic response, various skin eruptions, pancreatitis, pneumonia, hepatotoxicity, drug-induced connective tissue disease, and neurotoxicity. Hematologic effects, including bone marrow suppression, hemolytic anemia, and megaloblastic anemia, are uniformly related to the sulfapyridine moiety. The latter have been attribuited to sulfapyridine and inibition of folate absorption from the diet. To reduce dyspepsia, SSZ therapy should be initiated slowly and given with meals. One program begins with 500 mg on the first day, adding an additional 500 mg each day until the chosen therapeutic dose per day is reached. Minor allergic manifestations such as fever or rash can be overcome by discontinuation of the drug or by a process of gradual desensitization – readministering one-eighth of a tablet daily and then doubling the dose every 3 days until the desired therapeutic dosage is achieved.

SSZ treatment is contraindicated in all patients with hypersensitivity to salicylates and with known or probable glucose-6-phosphate dehydrogenase deficiency.

Interactions

It has been suggested that the concomitant use of antibi-

Table 35.2 Oral and topical formulations of 5-aminosalicylic acid

Azo-bond formulations, 5-ASA delivery
Olsalazine, colon
Ipsaladine, colon
Balsalazine, colon

Mesalazine formulations, coated with
pH-sensitive Eudragit L, ileum-colon
pH-sensitive Eudragit S, distal ileum-colon
semipermeable ethyl, small bowel-colon
cellulose membrane

otics may slow SSZ metabolism by inhibiting intestinal breakdown of the azo bond. Conversely, it has been shown that bacterial overgrowth in the setting of stasis, blind loop, or diverticular disease affords more rapid metabolism and absorption. Absorption of iron is inhibited if it is taken concurrently with sulfasalazine because iron is chelated by sulfasalazine. Concomitant administration of sulfasalazine and digoxin decreased digoxin bioavailability by as much as 25%.

5-AMINOSALICYLIC ACID

5-Aminosalicylic acid (ASA) has been recognized as the active moiety of sulfasalazine, acting topically on the colonic mucosa. This has led to the development of new oral 5-ASA formulations that do not contain the sulfa component (Tab. 35.2). In some of these, sulfapyridine simply has been replaced by another carrier and linked to the 5-ASA molecule by a nitrogen bridge: (1) another 5-ASA in *olsalazine* and (2) 4-aminobenzoylglycine and 4-aminobenzoyl – alanine linked, respectively, in *ipsalazine* and *balsalazine*. As in the case of sulfasalazine, however, 5-ASA is released into the colon by these formulations only after bacterial splitting of the nitrogen bond. To obviate the need for bacterial splitting, other formulations have been developed in which 5-ASA is not linked to any carrier. In these gastrointestinal formulations, 5-ASA is coated either with a semipermeable ethyl cellulose membrane that releases the drug throughout the intestine in a time- and pH-dependent manner or, as in the case of mesalazine, with a pH-sensitive acrylic resin (Eudragit S or Eudragit L) that retards release of the active molecule, especially in the colon, at a pH of greater than 6. Moreover, the fact that 5-ASA is only partially absorbed on rectal administration has promoted the development of topical formulations of 5-ASA, now available as enemas, foam, and suppositories.

Oral 5-ASA is available as tablets at dosages of 250, 400, 500, and 800 mg, whereas topical formulations include mesalazine enemas, suppositories, and foams. Enemas are buffered to an acidic pH (4.5) to minimize absorption and contain antioxidants to prevent 5-ASA oxidation; they are supplied as a 50- and 100-ml suspension containing 2 and 4 g of 5-ASA, respectively. Other 5-ASA enemas are prepared in the same way; these enemas contain 1, 2, or 4 g of 5-ASA in a 100-ml suspension

at pH 4.8. 4-ASA enemas contain 2 g of 4-ASA (a more soluble isomer of 5-ASA). A mesalazine foam also has been formulated at a dosage of 2 and 4 g. Suppositories contain 500 mg 5-ASA in a wax matrix.

Pharmacokinetics

5-Aminosalicylic is oxidized in the stomach and efficiently absorbed with little or none reaching the colon. Absorbed 5-ASA undergoes acetylation in the liver (as well as in the intestinal lumen and within epithelial cells before absorption), and both acetylated 5-ASA and the small fraction of remaining free 5-ASA are then excreted in the urine. Acetylation slows renal excretion and therefore extends the serum half-life of 5-ASA. 5-ASA is only partially absorbed on rectal administration.

Indications

Topical formulations of 5-ASA are most effective for proctitis or distal ulcerative colitis, whereas their effectivenes has not been well studied in Crohn's disease. Moreover, they are effective in maintaining remission of distal ulcerative colitis. Oral formulations of 5-ASA share an efficacy similar to that of sulfasalazine but are more expensive. Oral 5-ASA can induce remission of both ulcerative colitis and Crohn's disease and is effective in maintaining remission in both disease. Finally, oral 5-ASA formulations are effective in the prevention of postoperative recurrence in Crohn's disease.

Side effects

5-ASA acid is well tolerated by 80 to 90% of patients allergic to or intolerant of SSZ. However, 10 to 20% of patients who are SSZ intolerant have similar reactions to other 5-ASA formulations, indicating that the 5-ASA moiety is responsible for adverse events in some patients taking sulfasalazine. Caution therefore should be used in administering 5-ASA to patients who have had severe reactions to sulfasalazine. Both topical and oral forms have been associated with pneumonitis, pericarditis, myocarditis, a Kawasaki-like syndrome, pancreatitis, and paradoxical exacerbation of colitis. Serious but less well substantiated effects include possible hearing impairment and nephrotoxicity. Cross-reactivity in those allergic to aspirin also may be seen. As a potentiator of ileal chloride secretion, olsalazine has been implicated in causing often intolerable watery diarrhea, particularly in patients already suffering extensive colitis. The most common complication associated with topical preparations is anal irritation.

Contraindications

5-Aminosalicylic acid treatment is contraindicated in all patients with hypersensitivity to salicylates and glucose-6-phospate dehydrogenase deficiency.

IMMUNOMODULATORS

Immune modifier therapy in patients with inflammatory bowel disease has been the subject of great controversy. Over the last 5 years, knowledge has grown considerably, and there are now four immune-modifying agents for which adequate data from controlled clinical trials exist: azathioprine (AZA), 6-mercaptopurine (6-MP), cyclosporin A (CsA), and methotrexate (MTX).

Azathioprine (AZA) and 6-mercaptopurine (6-MP)

AZA and 6-MP are the most common immunosuppressive agents used in the treatment of inflammatory bowel disease. Several open and controlled clinical trials have demonstrated their efficacy in a particular subgroup of patients suffering from either ulcerative colitis or Crohn's disease.

AZA and 6-MP are available as tablets at a dosage of 50 mg. The usual dosage of AZA is 2 mg/kg per day and 1.5 mg/kg per day for 6-MP, starting with a dose of 25 mg per day for the first 3 days, after a complete blood count (CBC); the dose is slowly increased by 25 mg every 3 days, after a CBC count check each time. Afterwards, a CBC should be obtained weekly for 4 weeks, biweekly for 4 weeks, and then every 1 to 2 months for the duration of treatment. Liver enzymes should be monitored every 3 to 4 months for the first year and every 4 to 6 months thereafter. Once a patient has responded to AZA or 6-MP, these agents should be continued for several years.

Pharmacokinetics (see also Chap. 49)

AZA is a prodrug that is converted quickly to 6-MP via a nonenzymatic nucleophilic attack by sulphydryl-containing compounds, such as glutathione present in erythrocytes and other tissues. Three enzyme systems then compete to metabolize 6-MP: xanthine oxidase and thiopurine methyltransferase, which break down 6-MP to inactive metabolites, and hypoxanthine phosphoribosyl transferase. This is followed by several other enzymes that convert 6-MP to inactive metabolites and to the 6-thioguanine nucleotides. The half-lives of AZA and 6-MP in plasma are very short, ranging from 1 to 2 hours. In contrast, the half-life of the thioguanine nucleotides in erythrocytes is prolonged (3-13 days), and the time required to reach the steady state may help to explain the clinical observation that prolonged treatment (3-4 months) with AZA and 6-MP for inflammatory bowel disease is required before there is a therapeutic response. Both AZA and 6-MP have poor oral bioavailability: 50% and 16%, respectively. It is important to note that AZA is 55% 6-MP by molecular weight and that 88% of AZA is converted to 6-MP. Thus a conversion factor of 2.07 should be used to convert a dose of 6-MP to AZA.

Indications

In ulcerative colitis, AZA and 6-MP have a steroid-sparing effect, reduce recurrence and colectomy rates in steroid-dependent and steroid-resistant disease, may enhance steroid-induced remission, and appear to have a role in maintaining remission. In Crohn's disease, AZA and 6-MP have a similar steroid-sparing effect, may work cooperatively with steroids to induce remission, can induce and maintain prolonged remission, promote fistula healing, and as suggested recently, seem to prevent postoperative recurrence.

Side effects

Side effects resulting from treatment with AZA and 6-MP can be divided into two categories: allergic reactions that appear to be dose-independent (e.g., pancreatitis, fever, rash, arthralgias, malaise, nausea, and diarrhea) and non-allergic reactions that are probably dose- and metabolism-dependent (e.g., leukopenia, thrombocytopenia, infection, hepatitis, and malignancy). One large study reported the following frequency of side effects during treatment of inflammatory bowel disease with 6-MP: overall risk, 15%; pancreatitis, 3%; bone marrow depression, 2%; infection, 7%; hepatitis, 0.3%; and miscellaneous allergic reactions, 2%.

Contraindications

The use of AZA and 6-MP is contraindicated in patients with hypersentivity to these drugs and in patients with diffuse fungal infection, tuberculosis, and other severe septic conditions.

Interactions

Because the parent drugs and their metabolites are excreted in the urine, all dose-related toxicities may be potentiated by renal failure. Inhibitors of xanthine oxidase, such as allopurinol, may interfere with the oxidation of either AZA or 6-MP and thereby increase plasma levels and potentiate toxicity.

Cyclosporine A (CsA) (see also Chap. 75)

Cyclosporine A has revolutionized the field of transplantation and has a recognized mode of action, selectively inhibiting T-cell function. Because of the compound's toxicity and profound level of immune suppression, CsA was first tested in an uncontrolled manner in the treatment of IBD patients, providing encouraging results, especially in the treatment of chronically active Crohn's disease. However, the results of controlled studies have limited its use to only some clinical situations.

Dosage

CsA is available as a liquid solution (100 mg/ml), in injectable form (250 mg/5 ml), or gelatin capsules (25, 50, and 100 mg). Recently, a new microemulsion formulation with improved bioavailability not dependent on the presence of bile for absorption has became available. Most centers using high-dose CsA for inflammatory bowel disease have initiated therapy with continuous iv infusion at a dose of 4 mg/kg per day (equivalent to 16 mg/kg per day oral). However, it is unclear whether initial therapy with iv CsA is superior to oral therapy after accounting for differences in whole-blood CsA concentrations. If the initial therapy is to be oral, a starting CsA dose of 8 to 10 mg/kg per day is reasonable. Patients receiving iv CsA should have a whole-blood CsA concentration and serum electrolytes determined daily or, at least, every other day, whereas patients receiving oral CsA can have these parameters determined weekly. The CsA dose should be adjusted to achieve whole-blood CsA concentrations of between 251 and 350 ng/ml. The CsA dose also should be adjusted downward to maintain a serum creatinine concentration not greater than 30% above baseline, and patients with a serum cholesterol level of less than 120 mg/dl should not be treated with CsA to avoid severe nephrotoxicity and the risk of seizures. The total duration of CsA therapy should not exceed 4 to 6 months, and treatment with another remission maintenance drug should be initiated. For pharmacokinetics and side effects, see Chapter 75.

Indications

The efficacy of CsA for treatment of inflammatory bowel disease remains controversial. Nevertheless, it appears that high-dose CsA may be beneficial in severe active ulcerative colitis and possibly in severe active Crohn's disease and fistulizing Crohn's disease.

Contraindications

The use of CsA is contraindicated in patients with hypersensitivity to this drug and in patients with diffuse fungal infection, tuberculosis, and other severe septic conditions.

Interactions

There have been many descriptions of the effects of other drugs on the disposition of CsA, but only a few of these interactions appear to be clinically relevant. Accelerated clearance of CsA has been demonstrated in patients receiving phenytoin, phenobarbital, trimethoprim-sulfamthoxazole, and rifampin, presumably as a result of induction of hepatic P450 systems. Decreased clearance of CsA has been associated with concurrent administration of aminoglycoside antibiotics, erythromycin, ketoconazole, and amphotericin B; this engenders a higher risk of toxicity from CsA if its concentration in blood is not carefully monitored.

Methotrexate (MTX)

MTX has been used mainly as a chemotherapeutic agent for some cancers and in the management of severe psoriasis and advanced rheumatoid arthritis. Recently, MTX has been investigated as a treatment for inflammatory bowel disease and as a potential steroid-sparing drug.

MTX is available as tablets (5 mg) or in injectable form (25 and 500 mg). The two controlled trials of MTX in Crohn's disease used doses of 5 mg orally three times per week and 25 mg per week im. Thus, MTX doses of 15 to 25 mg per week, administered either orally or im, appear to be reasonable. The initial phase of MTX therapy for either steroid-sparing or steroid-refractory indications probably should last 12 to 16 weeks. During this initial phase of MTX therapy, patients should have serum liver enzymes and a CBC determined every 2 to 4 weeks to monitor for hepatotoxicity and bone marrow suppression. For those patients who respond to a 12- to 16-weeks course of MTX and who do not experience limiting side effects, a decision must be made regarding remission maintenance therapy. If MTX is continued for maintenance of remission purposes, then a CBC should be obtained every 4 weeks and serum liver enzymes every 4 to 6 weeks (see below) for the duration of MTX therapy.

Indications

The efficacy of MTX for the treatment of inflammatory bowel disease remains to be established. To date, the data coming from two controlled trials seem to indicate the effectiveness of MTX therapy for either steroid-sparing or steroid-refractory Crohn's disease. Further studies are necessary to better define the exact therapeutic role of MTX, if any.

Side effects

The most commonly reported toxic effects from parenteral MTX in inflammatory bowel disease include nausea, diarrhea, and stomatitis in 10% of patients. Minor leukopenia or transaminase elevation and hair loss were seen in a smaller number of patients. Serious potential toxicites are rare but include hypersensitivity pneumonia and hepatic fibrosis. The former is a rare allergic response to MTX that typically presents with cough and progressive shortness of breath. Pulmonary infiltrates or intestinal pneumonitis patterns are variable on chest radiographs, and diffusion capacity is markedly diminished. MTX therapy should be discontinued at any suggestion of pulmonary toxicity, and high-dose steroids should be administered.

Contraindications

Hypersensitivity to MTX, diffuse fungal infection, tuberculosis, and other severe septic conditions are all contraindications to MTX therapy.

Drug interactions

Since approximately 35% of MTX is bound to plasma proteins, free drug levels and consequent toxicity may be increased. The portion of each dose of MTX that is normally excreted rapidly gains access to the urine by a combination of glomerular filtration and active tubular secretion. Therefore, the concurrent use of drugs that reduce renal blood flow (e.g., NSAIDs), are weak organic acids (e.g., aspirin or piperacillin), or are nephrotoxic (e.g., cisplatin) can delay drug excretion and lead to severe myelosuppression.

ANTIBIOTICS

The role of antibiotic agents in the treatment of inflammatory bowel disease is unclear. Metronidazole is the only antibiotic of proven benefit in the treatment of Crohn's ileocolitis, colitis, perianal disease, and postoperative Crohn's disease. However, recent data coming from case reports, open studies, and very few controlled trials suggest that ciprofloxacin and antituberculosis agents also may be effective in treating IBD patients.

Metronidazole

Metronidazole is formulated as 250- and 400-mg tablets for oral administration. The drug is also available in forms for iv infusion (500 mg). In inflammatory bowel disease, many different dosage schedules have been used. In active Crohn's disease and in perianal disease, oral metronidazole was used at dosages varying from 10 to 15 mg/kg per day from 10 days to 16 weeks. In ulcerative colitis in remission, 600 mg per day for a 1-year follow-up period was effective in preventing relapse.

The drug is usually completely and promptly absorbed after oral administration, reaching concentrations in plasma of about 10 µg/ml approximately 1 hour after a single 50 mg dose. Repeated doses every 6 to 8 hours result in some accumulation of the drug. The half-life of metronidazole in plasma is about 8 hours, and its volume of distribution is approximately that of total body water. About 10% of the drug is bound to plasma proteins. Metronidazole penetrates well into body tissues and fluids, including vaginal secretions, seminal fluid, saliva, and breast milk. Therapeutic concentrations are also achieved in cerebrospinal fluid. Both unchanged metronidazole and several metabolites are excreted in various proportions in the urine after oral administration of the parent compound. The liver is the main site of metabolism, and this accounts for over 50% of the systemic clearance of metronidazole. Small quantities of reduced metabolites, including ring-cleavage products, are formed by the gut flora. The urine of some patients may be reddish-brown due to the presence of unidentified pigments derived from the drug.

In ulcerative colitis, metronidazole is not useful for active disease; it may have a role in maintaining remission, but it has not been studied extensively. In Crohn's disease, metronidazole is effective in treating ileocolitis and colitis but not isolated ileal disease; it promotes healing of perianal disease. Its role in the maintenance of remission is unclear. Finally, metronidazole is acceptable as a component of the intensive therapy for fulminant colitis or toxic megacolon.

Dose-related nausea, anorexia, and a sensation of a "furry" tongue (glossitis) may occur with metronidazole therapy. All routes of administration may result in a bothersome metallic taste. A common worsening side effect with metronidazole therapy is peripheral neuropathy, which develops most frequently at doses greater than 1 g per day. Although it is usually completely reversible with dose reduction or cessation, prolonged and severe neuropathy may develop. Metronidazole therapy is contraindicated in pregnant women and in children.

Metabolism of metronidazole may be significantly accelerated by concurrently administered medications, notably prednisone and phenobarbital. Ingestion of alcohol during treatment with metronidazole can produce a disulfiram-like effect and cause nausea and vomiting and therefore should be avoided. Moreover, metronidazole can increase the effects of oral anticoagulants.

New areas of drug development

For years, the treatment of inflammatory bowel disease has been limited to sulfasalazine and corticosteroids. Recent insight into the pathogenesis of inflammatory bowel disease has opened new options for treatment. Biopsy specimens of affected tissue in ulcerative colitis and Crohn's disease have shown lymphocytic and neutrophilic infiltration, the hallmarks of inflammation. Modalities currently under investigation include the extensively studied immunosuppressive agents and lipoxygenase inhibitors and less well-studied, emerging therapies, such as oxygen-derived free radical scavengers, immunoglobulins, lidocaine, T-cell apheresis, anti-tumor necrosis factors antibody, and CD4 antibody. Putative infectious etiologies also abound and have prompted many trials of antimycobacterial and antibacterial agents. Nutritional deficiencies also have been proposed as aggravating or causative factors in these diseases, bringing about the study of the short-chain fatty acids and glutamine as possible treatments. The hypercoagulable state of some patients with inflammatory bowel disease points toward hypercoagulability as an underlying cause. In this context, heparin has been tested as a possible approach. Some researchers proposed that local bleeding and inflammation stem from inherent clotting cascade deficiencies, a possibility that has led to factor XIII trials with mixed results.

THE IRRITABLE BOWEL SYNDROME

The irritable bowel syndrome (IBS) is a functional disorder of the gastrointestinal tract for which there is no known anatomic or biochemical cause. Irritable bowel syndrome is, without a doubt, the most common gastrointestinal disorder seen by gastroenterologists in practice.

During the last decade, epidemiologic, physiologic, and psychosocial data have emerged to improve our understanding of this disorder and its treatment. The irritable bowel syndrome is now believed to result from dysregulation of the intestinal motor, sensory, and CNS functions. Symptoms are due to both disturbances in intestinal motility and enhanced visceral sensitivity. Psychosocial factors, although not part of the irritable bowel per se, play an important role in modulating the illness experience and its clinical outcome.

IBS affects 14 to 24% of women and 5 to 19% of

men, with a decrease in reporting frequency among older people. The prevalence appears similar in whites and blacks but may be lower in Hispanics. Although up to 70% of people with irritable bowel syndrome symptoms do not seek medical attention, IBS accounts for 12% of primary care and 28% of gastroenterologic practice (41% of all functional gastrointestinal disorders).

The predominant history is chronic constipation, diarrhea, or both. Typical patients describes watery diarrhea occurring intermittently for months or years (predominant diarrhea). The diarrhea is usually worse in the morning on arising or after breakfast. After the passage of three or four loose stools with excessive mucus, the patient may feel well for the remainder of the day. The diarrhea may last for weeks or months and then disappear spontaneously for variable periods of time. Some patients describe "pencil-like," pasty stools rather then diarrhea.

Another typical presentation is that of chronic abdominal pain (predominant pain) with constipation (predominant constipation) or with alternating constipation and diarrhea. These patients describe intermittent crampy lower abdominal pain, often over the sigmoid colon, which is usually relieved by the passage of flatus or stool. Patients may describe excessive bloating that is not discernible to the physician.

The evidence is now clear that physiologic disturbances occur in at least a subset of patients, suggesting that symptoms are neither imagined nor just the product of chronic complaining. However, a plausible disease model that takes into account all the known abnormalities has yet to be derived, and none of the abnormalities is specific enough to be used as a diagnostic criterion. The mechanisms identified to date that may be linked to specific symptoms in the IBS are (1) abnormal visceral perception, (2) altered gut motor function, (3) extraintestinal motor dysfunction, (4) autonomic nervous system abnormalities, and (5) psychologic factors.

The absence of pathognomonic features has made the IBS a diagnosis of exclusion. Moreover, because no physiologic phenomenon permits the clinician to identify ISB, the disorder must be diagnosed by its symptoms. An international working party, in 1989 and again in 1992, elaborated the following criteria: at least 3 months' continuous or recurrent symptoms of abdominal pain that is relieved by defecation, or associated with a change in stool consistency, or associated with a change in stool frequency with altered stool frequency (>3 times per day or <3 times per week), altered stool form, altered stool passage (straining, urgency, incomplete evacuation), passage of mucus, or abdominal bloating.

Treatment

Treatments of general use in the disease

The variability of the presenting complaints and the lack of confirmatory diagnostic tests make the diagnosis more difficult. Following the exclusion of organic disease, the aim of therapy is amelioration of symptoms by the selective introduction of dietary, psychologic, and pharmacologic techniques designed to reduce the factors triggering symptoms and suppressing existing symptoms. The treatment strategy is based on the nature and severity of the symptoms, the degree of physiologic disturbance and functional impairment, and the presence of psychosocial difficulties affecting the course of the illness.

Nonpharmacologic treatment

It is important that physicians establish their credibility with patients on the first visit by means of a careful history, physical examination, and sigmoidoscopy. This approach not only permits a confident diagnosis but also is believed to have a therapeutic effect. The history and physical examination should result in a firm diagnosis, which is vital if the patient is to have confidence in any therapeutic plan. Many patients receive the impression that their physician considers the IBS a psychosomatic problem. There is ample evidence from both physiologic and psychologic studies that it is not. Several studies have demonstrated that people who have IBS but who have not sought medical attention for their symptoms have no more psychopathology than control subjects without irritable bowel syndrome. People with IBS who do become patients score higher than normal subjects and IBS nonpatients on tests of psychologic distress and neuroticism, but so also do patients with lactose malabsorption who seek medical attention. Furthermore, physiologic studies of IBS patients demonstrate altered visceral perception and altered motility (see above), indicating that the problem lies in the gut, not in the mind. It is important that the physician is aware of this information and imparts it to the patient.

Diet

Most physicians employ bran or other commercial bulking agents as a method of increasing dietary fiber. Bran's laxative effect has been known since early times. Although the several controlled trials available do not strongly support the use of bran, they do show that its use provides some improvement in constipation and, perhaps, relief of abdominal pain. Bran is cheap and unlikely to do harm, although some users experience increased bloating or diarrhea. The physician is best able to assess compliance if the patient starts with 1 tablespoon of bran tid with meals and subsequently adjusts the dose as necessary. Alternatively, the patient may take 15 to 20 g per day of a bulk-forming agent such as psyllium, ispagula, sterculia, mucillaginous seeds, or methylcellulose. The use of fiber involves a long commitment, and patients should judge its benefit on the basis of changes in stool consistency and frequency.

Except for trials studying the effct of dietary fiber, no controlled trials have evaluated the impact of diet on IBS symptoms. Studies indicate that some individuals with postprandial pain have a cholinergically mediated and exaggerated gastrocolic response to fat ingestion that involves increased colon contractions. Thus, a high-protein, low-fat diet may be effective. Frank lactose intolerance is unusual in Caucasians, but lactose may produce postprandial bloating and diarrhea. Occasionally, this may occur on a milk-free diet. The clinician should determine whether certain foods (particularly lactose, fructose, caffeine, fatty foods, alcohol, sorbitol gum, and gas-producing foods such as cabbage and beans) exacerbate the symptoms.

Drug therapy

Drug use is targeted toward the predominant symptoms, usually abdominal pain, diarrhea, or constipation. Prescription medication is not recommended routinely because IBS is a chronic disorder; most drugs have side effects; no drug is of proven benefit for the IBS, and the placebo response is impressive in the IBS. Consequently, placebo-controlled trials are essential for determining whether a drug is truly efficacious. Studies on several of the many drugs used in the treatment of IBS demonstrate a placebo response that ranges from 30 to 65%. This is consistent in all IBS studies. Placebos may be useful in certain instances, and the placebo response serves as a reminder of the beneficial effects of the successful physician-patient encounter.

Drug classes

DRUGS USED IN PREDOMINANT PAIN

Antispasmodic drugs are used most frequently to treat the pain symptoms in IBS. Table 35.3 shows the major kinetic parameters of the most commonly employed antispasmodic drugs in the treatment of the IBS.

Classic anticholinergics (atropine) and newer anticholinergics, such as tertiary and quaternary ammomium compounds, are the most extensively studied classes of drugs in the treatment of the ISB. The rationale lies in their ability to reduce stimulated colonic motor activity through inhibition of cholinerigic receptors. Such receptors are divided into nicotinic (N) receptors, located at the neuromuscolar junction and autonomic ganglia, and muscarinic receptors (M), subdivided into M_1 (present in the autonomic ganglia and in the CNS), M_2 (heart), and M_3 (smooth muscle and various glands) receptors. Some anticholinergics, such as the classic ones, act on both M and N receptors but act on N receptors only at a high dose.

Classic anticholinergics include atropine, scopolamine (hyoscine), and other belladonna alkaloids, available as oral, injectable, suppository, or transdermal forms. They are absorbed rapidly from the gastrointestinal tract and enter the circulation when applied locally to the mucosal surfaces. Absorption from intact skin is limited, although efficient absorption does occur in the postauricular region. Atropine has a half-life of appoximately 4 hours; hepatic

metabolism accounts for the elimination of about half of a dose, and the remainder is excreted unchanged in the urine.

Some tertiary and quaternary ammonium compounds used for pain relief in IBS include cimetropium bromide, hyoscyamine sulfate, octilonium bromide, pinaverium bromide, prifinium bromide, dicyclomine hydrochloride, methscopolamine bromide, homatropine methylbromide, methantheline bromide, propantheline bromide, anisotropine methylbromide, clidinium bromide, glycopyrrolate, isopropamide iodide, mepenzolate bromide, and trihexethyl chloride. These compounds differ from each other in that tertiary ammonium derivatives are electrically neutral, are well absorbed, and pass the blood-brain barrier, whereas quaternary compounds are hydrophilic, incompletely absorbed, and do not pass the blood-brain barrier. None of these products are significantly metabolized.

Anticholinergics are usually given orally three to four times daily, but anticholinergic effects, such as dry mouth, blurred vision, restlessness insomnia, urinary hesitancy, and constipation, can be dose-limiting. In particular, in view of the cholinergically mediated gastrocolonic response, the patient who has predictable abdominal pain after meals may benefit from administration of an antispasmodic drug before the meals (e.g., dicycloverine 10-20 mg 30 minutes before meals). This should ensure a maximum anticholinergic blockade at the time symptoms are expected and minimize exposure to side effects.

NONANTICHOLINERGIC DRUGS

Mebeverine is a nonanticholinergic (papaverine-like) antispasmodic, the mechanism of action of which is not clearly elucidated but may involve a calcium channel blockade. Overall, mebeverine is superior to placebo in terms of relieving abdominal pain, abdominal distention, and disordered bowel function at doses ranging from 100 mg four times daily to 135 mg six times daily, and it is also more effective on pain than dicyclomine. Because IBS affects the colon and small intestine, a new mebeverine microgranular formulation (mebeverine 200 mg SR) has been developed that releases mebeverine over the whole gut. The efficacy of this innovative galenic formulation has been demonstrated in different clinical trials. Peppermint oil, available in enteric-coated capsules, also may have an antispasmodic action. Few reliable data regarding the comparative effectiveness of these medications in IBS are available. In a controlled European study, trimebutine, a peripherally acting enkephalin analogue, was better than mebeverine in controlling the frequency and duration of lower abdominal pain episodes among IBS patients, but neither drug was tested against placebo.

ANTIDEPRESSANT AGENTS

This drug class may be useful in the treatment of pain in IBS patients. Relatively small doses of tricyclic antidepressants (e.g., amitriptyline, trimipramine, or

Table 35.3 Antispasmodic drugs: major kinetic parameters

	Time to maximal blood level (h)	Half-life (h)	Excretion (h)
Classic anticholinergics (atropine, etc.)	1	4	85-90% in urine
Tertiary ammonium compounds			
bromide	1.5-2	1.5	50% in urine
Pinaverium bromide	0.5-1	3.5	87% in feces
Prifinium bromide	1	2	48% in urine
Quaternary ammonium compounds (methantheline bromide, propantheline bromide, etc.)	0.5-1.5	3	>90% in urine
Nonanticholinergic drugs			
Trimebutine	1-6	2	85% in urine

desipramine) seem to be an effective treatment for some patients, especially those with intractable pain. Antidepressants may provide a remission even though the physician cannot determine with certainty whether depression is present. The benefit of these drugs may be due to their antidepressant, analgesic, sedating, or anticholinergic properties. They should be started in small doses with graded increases (e.g., amitriptyline may be given at a dose of 75 mg at bedtime). Most patients with IBS respond to lower doses, and the risk of serious side effects such as cardiovascular toxicity is minimized.

OTHER AGENTS

Anxiolytic drugs such as the benzodiazepines ought to be reserved for anxiety because there is no evidence to support them as a primary treatment of the IBS. Calcium channel blockers reduce colonic motility and myoelectric spike potentials following meals. If the physician believes that this activity is important in the genesis of IBS symptoms, then he/she might rationally test their benefit. However, the results of limited clinical trials of these drugs are not encouraging, with the exception of pinaverium bromide, a selective blocker of the calcium channel of the intestinal smooth muscle cells, without significant effect on myocardial cells. In several placebo-controlled trials, this drug was better than placebo as far as abdominal pain and constipation are concerned at a dose of 50 mg three times daily. Side effects were similar to those reported with placebo.

DRUGS USED IN PREDOMINANT CONSTIPATION

As mentioned earlier, dietary fiber is the standard long-term treatment for constipation-predominant IBS. Therefore, pharmacologic agents should only be considered for short-term relapses. The use of fiber is thought to

result in softer, bulkier stools while retaining water and decreasing transit time. An increased stool weight also may result from stimulation of colonic bacterial proliferation. The increased stool mass in turn leads to faster transit and reduced water absorption by the colonic mucosa. Weight for weight, fiber from unprocessed bran produces almost double the stool weight achieved with carrots, cabbage, and apples. Several semisynthetic bulk laxatives are available, such as those containing psyllium, hydrophilic mucilloid, ispagula, and sterculia gum. These preparations are effective, convenient, and widely used.

Generally, laxatives should be avoided in patients with IBS. Not only do they have undesirable side effects, but they may exaggerate the swings from constipation to diarrhea. Occasionally, however, constipation may be severe and unresponsive to fiber. In this case, osmotic laxatives are preferable to stimulants because the latter may damage the myenteric ganglia. Milk of magnesia 30 to 45 ml at bedtime acts overnight to produce a bowel movement in the morning. Lactulose 15 to 30 ml is a useful backup treatment, especially in the elderly. Laxatives also can be administered rectally as a suppository or enema, e.g., glycerol (glycerin), saline, or bisacodyl.

Pharmacologic agents should be considered only for short-term exacerbations. Cisapride, a prokinetic drug, at a dosage of 30 to 40 mg per day facilitates acetylcholine release from the myenteric plexus. (See Chap. 33) While used primarily for dyspeptic symptoms related to gastric stasis, studies also have reported efficacy for constipation and constipation-predominant IBS.

DRUGS USED IN PREDOMINANT DIARRHEA

For functional diarrhea, antidiarrheal agents are useful in moderate to severe cases. General adsorbents (e.g., kaolin, pectin, and aluminum hydroxide) are used widely for symptomatic control of diarrhea, but there is little evidence that they are effective. Opioid antidiarrheal drugs include morphine, codeine phosphate, diphenoxylate, and loperamide. The antidiarrheal effect of these agents is generally attributed to their action on intestinal and colonic motor activity to prolong transit time. They also have been shown to inhibit intestinal secretion and/or to increase fluid and electrolyte absorption. With the exception of loperamide, the central analgesic properties of these agents contribute to their adverse effects and preclude their use in patients with liver failure. Loperamide does not cross the blood-brain barrier; it decreases intestinal transit, enhances intestinal water and iron absorption, and strengthens rectal sphincter tone, thereby improving the diarrhea, urgency, and fecal soiling. Loperamide (2-4 mg qid) is preferred over diphenoxylate, codeine, or other narcotics for treating patients with IBS with predominant diarrhea, incontinence, or both. Further, in diarrhea-dominant IBS, small doses of cholestyramine (4 g per day) sometimes may be of help, since it is constipating even in the absence of bile salt malabsorption. Table 35.4 shows the drugs targeted at specific IBS symptoms.

DIVERTICULAR DISEASE OF THE COLON

Colonic diverticula, or diverticulosis of the colon, are by far the most common diverticula of the gastrointestinal tract and occur in about 50% of western populations over 60 years of age. Most of such diverticula are acquired pseudodiverticula resulting from herniation of mucosa and submucosa through the muscular layer of the colon, often between the mesenteric and lateral taeniae. Rarely, diverticula of the cecum and the ascending colon are congenital and are true diverticula. Far more commonly, diverticulosis is acquired and most frequently involves the sigmoid colon but, in decreasing order, may involve the descending, trasverse, and ascending colon.

Many patients with diverticulosis are unaware of diverticula or are made aware of them through barium enemas or colonoscopy done for various reasons. The exact percentage of patients who eventually experience symptoms is variously estimated from 5 to 25%. The wide variation in estimated symptom frequency is in part due to the inability to separate the symptoms of diverticulosis from those of IBS, whether they be considered etiologically related or simply coexistent. Symptoms attributed to diverticulosis include diarrhea, constipation, alternating diarrhea and constipation, intestinal distenstion, and abdominal pain; they are similar to those of the IBS.

The treatment of uncomplicated diverticulosis is undertaken to relieve symptoms and to prevent or postpone complications. The aim of the diet is to normalize bowel function and to avoid food ingredients that might tend to increase discomfort, possibly highly seasoned foods or lactose-containing foods in patients with lactose intolerance. Efforts to increase fecal bulk are linked to increased fiber intake. A possibility is to let people eat normally and supplement the diet with bulking agents, such psyllium or methylcellulose, wheat bran, or combinations (see Drugs

Table 35.4 Drugs targeted at specific IBS symptoms

Symptom	Agent	Usual daily dose
Predominant pain	*Antispamodics*	
	Dicyclomine	10-20 mg before meals
	Mebeverine	135 mg tid-qid
	Trimebutine	150 mg tid-qid
	Octilonium bromide	40 mg tid-qid
	Pinaverium bromide	50 mg tid
	Prifinium bromide	30 mg tid-qid
	Butylscopolamine bromide	10 mg tid-qid
	Cimetropium bromide	50 mg bid-tid
	Antidepressants	
	Amitriptyline	25 mg qd
	Imipramine	25 mg qd
	Fluoxetine	20 mg qd
Predominant constipation	*Bulk producers*	
	Mucillaginous seeds, gums	5-10 g
	Ispagula/sterculia	5-10 g
	Psyllium	7 g
	Unprocessed bran	1-4 g
	Methylcellulose	3-6 g
	Colonic stimulants or irritants	
	Senna	0.25-2 g
	Bisacodyl	5-15 mg
	Phenolphthalein	50-250 mg
	Osomotic agents	
	Magnesium sulfate	5-15 g
	Lactulose	15-30 ml
	Others	
	Microdose enemas (sodium citrate, surface active agents, glycerol)	5 ml
	Prokinetics	
	Cisapride	10 mg bid-qid
Predominant diarrhea	Loperamide	2-4 mg qid (max 16 mg)
	Cholestyramine	4 g tid

Used in Predominant Constipation).

The effectiveness of agents that might directly inhibit muscular contraction in the affected colon remains in doubt for lack of direct physiologic observation and controlled therapeutic trials. Musculotropic agents such as mebeverine and trimebutine, which inhibit normal sigmoid motility, have been shown to give significant symptomatic relief. Prompt relief of pain has been reported to follow iv injection of glucagon, whose role as a smooth muscle relaxant is now familiar to radiologists (see also Drugs Used in Predominant Pain).

When the direct relief of pain is required temporarily, the choice of an analgesic is critical. Morphine has been observed to directly raise intraluminal pressure in the sigmoid colon and to cause marked distention of the diverticula themselves, presumably increasing the risk of perforation. Consequently, the use of any opiate is contraindicated.

ARDIZZONE S, BIANCHI PORRO G. A practical guide to the management of distal ulcerative colitis. Drugs 1998;55:519-42.

ARDIZZONE S, MOLTENI P, BOLLANI S, BIANCHI PORRO G. Guidelines for the treatment of ulcerative colitis in remission. Eur J Gastroenterol Hepatol 1997;9:836-41.

CAMILLERI M, PRATHER CM. The irritable bowel syndrome. Mechanisms and a practical approach to management. Ann Intern Med 1992;116:1001-8.

DROSSMAN DA, THOMPSON WG. The irritable bowel syndrome. Review and a graduated multicomponent treatment approach. Ann Intern Med 1992;116:1009-16.

DROSSMAN DA, WHITEHEAD WE. Irritable bowel syndrome. A technical review for practice guideline development. Gastroenterology 1997;112:2120-37.

HANAUER S, MEYERS S. Management of Crohn's disease in adults. Am J Gastroenterol 1997;92:559-66.

HEATON KW. Diet and diverticulosis. New leads. Gut 1985;26:541-3.

KORNBLUTH A, SACHAR DB. Ulcerative colitis practice guidelines in adults. Am J Gastroenterol 1997;92:204-11.

PATTEE PL, THOMPSON WG. Drug treatment of the irritable bowel syndrome. Drugs 1992;44:200-6.

PEARSON DC, MAY GR, FICK GH, et al. Azathioprine and 6-mercaptopurine in Crohn's disease: A meta-analysis. Ann Intern Med 1995;122:132-42.

SANDBORN WJ. A review of immune modifier therapy for inflammatory bowel disease: azathioprine, 6-mercaptopurine, cyclosporine, and methotrexate. Am J Gastroenterol 1996;91:423-33.

SANDBORN WJ. A critical review of cyclosporine therapy in inflammatory bowel disease. Inflammatory Bowel Dis 1995;1:48-63.

STEPHEN AM, CUMMINGS JH. Mechanisms of action of dietary fibre in the human colon. Nature 1980;284:283-4.

SUTHERLAND LR, ROTH DE, BECK PL. Alternatives to sulfasalazine: A meta-analisys of 5-ASA in the treatment of ulcerative colitis. Inflammatory Bowel Dis 1997;3:65-78.

THIESEN A, THOMSON BR. Review article. Older systemic and newer topical glucocorticosyteroids and the gastrointestinal tract. Aliment Pharmacol Ther 1996;10:487-96.

36

Use of drugs in liver disease

Jürg Reichen, Stephan Krähenbühl

THE HEPATIC CLEARANCE OF DRUGS

The liver provides the most efficient site for drug clearance, particularly by converting lipophilic to hydrophilic substrates (see also Chap. 3). The hepatic clearance of endo- and xenobiotics is governed by the hepatic perfusion Q and by the hepatic extraction coefficient E:

$$CL_{hep} = Q \times E \qquad (36.1)$$

Extraction, in turn, is determined by so-called intrinsic clearance (CL_{int}), a measure of transport or metabolic capacity:

$$CL_{int} = V_{max}/K_m \qquad (36.2)$$

where K_m is the Michaelis-Menten constant, and V_{max} is the maximal velocity of the transport or metabolic process governing removal of the drug. Equation (36.2) also can be written as a function of the easily obtainable parameters of Eq. (36.1) as

$$CL_{int} = (Q \times E)/(1 - E) \qquad (36.3)$$

Combining Eqs. (36.1) and (36.3) yields the following equation:

$$CL_{hep} = (Q \times CL_{int})/(Q + CL_{int}) \qquad (36.4)$$

Equation (36.4) is quite important in predicting the effect of intrinsic clearance (CL_{int}) on hepatic clearance. If the intrinsic clearance is very high ($CL_{int} \gg Q$), clearance is governed by hepatic blood flow (and as a matter of fact can be used to measure Q); the clearance of such substances is said to be flow-limited. In contrast, the hepatic clearance of compounds with a low intrinsic clearance ($CL_{int} \ll Q$) is independent of hepatic perfusion and is said to be enzyme-limited. For substances with intermediate intrinsic clearance or extraction, there is a hyperbolic relation between hepatic clearance and hepatic perfusion within the physiologic range of hepatic blood flow (Fig. 36.1). These equations have to be corrected for protein binding and/or erythrocyte/plasma distribution ratios, yielding

$$CL_{hep} = (Q \times f_u \times CL_{int})/(Q + f_u CL_{int}) \qquad (36.5)$$

where f_u is the unbound fraction of the drug.

Equation (36.1) predicts that the first pass metabolism of drugs is markedly affected by perfusion and that extraction efficiency tends to fall when perfusion increases. This is not observed in the cirrhotic liver, however. Based on this observation, the *intact hepatocyte theory* was put forward to explain the impaired drug metabolism in chronic liver disease. In this model, the liver is made up of a reduced number of hepatocytes with a normal enzyme content. The hepatocytes are only partially perfused because of intrahepatic shunting. According to the intact hepatocyte theory model, the actual extraction efficiency is given by

$$E_{actual} = E_{true} \times f_m \qquad (36.6)$$

where f_m is the fraction of flow Q actually perfusing the hepatocytes. This model has now been proven to be true in different models of liver disease in the rat and recently in humans.

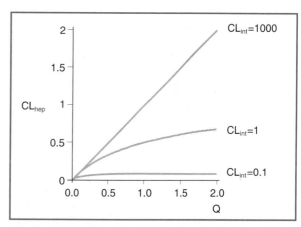

Figure 36.1 Relationship between hepatic clearance (CL_{hep}) and perfusion (Q) as a function of intrinsic clearance (CL_{int}). For a high intrinsic clearance, hepatic clearance equals flow; the clearance of these drugs is therefore called *flow-limited*. The converse is true for drugs with a low intrinsic clearance; in this case, hepatic clearance is independent of hepatic flow in the physiologic range and is called *enzyme-limited*. For further details and the governing equations, see text.

Table 36.1 Hepatic clearance is a function of intrinsic clearance and hepatic perfusion, both of which can be altered in chronic liver disease

Alterations in intrinsic clearance	Alterations in hepatic flow
Reduced liver cell number	Alterations in total flow
Alterations in enzyme content	Portosystemic shunting
Alterations in membrane lipid content	Sinusoidal capillarization
Alterations in protein binding	

ALTERATIONS OF HEPATIC PERFUSION AND OF INTRINSIC CLEARANCE IN LIVER DISEASE

The intact hepatocyte theory places much emphasis on the reduction in cell number and intra- and extrahepatic shunting to explain altered clearance of xenobiotics in liver disease. There are, however, many other factors that contribute to alterations in the hepatic clearance of drugs. These factors are listed in Table 36.1 and will be considered in more detail in the following paragraphs.

Reduced liver cell number

Morphometric analysis has shown that the hepatic clearance of the low-extraction compound aminopyrine depends on liver cell mass as determined by stereologic analysis. This also has been shown in humans by estimating the volume fraction of hepatocytes stereologically on a liver biopsy; this allows calculation of the liver cell mass by multiplying the hepatocyte fraction for liver volume as determined by computed tomographic (CT) scanning. The importance of liver cell mass is also emphasized by the finding that liver volume determines the hepatic clearance of indocyanine green in children.

Alterations in enzyme content

Although the intact hepatocyte theory postulates that liver enzyme content per hepatocyte is normal in cirrhosis, this is clearly not the case. Unfortunately, different liver diseases appear to affect phase I and II enzymes (see Chap. 3) to a different extent, making predictions about drug disposition in chronic liver disease extremely difficult. Thus, different isoenzymes are affected to different degrees in animals with cirrhosis, and these alterations depend on the model used to induce cirrhosis. The situation appears to be similar in humans. In cirrhotic human livers explanted at transplantation, total cytochrome P450 content is decreased; CYP1A2-mediated activity is decreased in all forms of cirrhosis, whereas CYP2E1 and CYP2C are decreased only in patients with cholestatic liver disease and CYP3A only in those with noncholestatic disease. Other studies also have suggested that not only CYP1A2 but also CYP2E1 are decreased in all cirrhotic livers, with apparently no difference between cholestatic and noncholestatic liver disease. Most of these changes are due to pretranslational alterations. In the case

of CYP2E1, posttranslational modifications also seem to occur.

A novel area of investigation that attempts to explain the altered drug handling in the course of liver disease has been the analysis of antibody occurrence during chronic inflammatory disease. These antibodies, generally known as *kidney, liver, microsomal type-1 (LKM-1) antibodies,* which are identified by indirect immunofluorescence, define a group of patients with type 2 autoimmune hepatitis, distinct from type 1, where antiactin and antinuclear antibodies are present in patients' sera. Sera from patients with type 2 hepatitis react with a nonglycosylated 50-kDa protein identified on CY2D6 (see also Chap. 3). Anti-CYP2D6 reactivity may be responsible for a significant impairment of metabolism of the large number of substrates of the polymorphic cytochrome, even leading to a metabolic behavior not different from the PM phenotype and independent of the degree of liver damage. LKM-1 antibodies also may be associated with hepatitis C virus infections.

Similar to phase I reactions, phase II enzymes are altered to a different extent by chronic liver disease. Based on the finding that morphine glucuronidation is maintained even in advanced liver disease, it was assumed for some time that phase II enzymes are normal in chronic liver disease. This is clearly not the case, since phenolic and acyl glucuronidation for diflunisal, for example, is reduced. By investigating different conjugation pathways in liver biopsies from patients with chronic liver disease, it could be shown that glucuronidation is maintained, whereas sulfotransferase, acetyltransferase, glutathione transferase, and thiomethyltransferase activities are all decreased to a varying degree. In addition, the activity of phase II enzymes, particularly uridine glucuronyltransferase (UGT), may be affected by the development of antibodies in the course of liver disease. Such antibodies have been identified recently with the LKM-3 antibody, specifically occurring in a large percentage of patients with hepatitis D. The impact of anti-UGT antibodies on drug handling has as yet to be defined.

Alterations in membrane lipids

Membrane lipid content and thus the function of certain membrane-bound enzymes are altered in animals with cirrhosis. These lipid changes are associated with altered membrane fluidity and correlate with functional impairment. Such changes are not restricted to the liver but are also found, for example, in the heart, where they may contribute to altered receptor function, and in the kidney, where they are associated with sodium retention. Similar changes appear to occur in human cirrhosis, as judged from the lipid composition of erythrocyte membranes.

Alterations in protein binding

Intrinsic clearance depends on the free concentration of drug, as predicted by Eq. (36.5). Protein binding of some drugs is concentration-dependent, and this has to be taken into account when predicting alterations in clearance. It is obvious that the free fraction of drugs binding to albumin will be increased in end-stage liver disease; this will apply mostly to very lipophilic and/or acidic drugs. Theoretically, hepatic clearance should increase for highly albumin-bound drugs with a low intrinsic clearance when their free fraction increases (see Eq. 36.5); these are drugs with so-called binding-sensitive clearance. However, it is difficult to predict volume of distribution and alterations in clearance on the basis of albumin concentration alone because correlation is poor and not all drugs are affected. Drugs with a pK_a in the alkaline region bind to acidic α_1-glycoprotein, an acute-phase protein whose serum concentration can be decreased or increased depending on the severity of liver disease and the presence of complicating conditions such as acute infections.

Alterations in total hepatic blood flow

Hepatic blood flow is increased early in chronic liver disease due to a hyperdynamic circulation syndrome. Late in the disease, portal perfusion is usually markedly reduced. Nevertheless, extraction of flow-limited compounds decreases, leading to an increased bioavailability of such drugs (see below). This apparent paradox is explained by the development of portosystemic shunts and sinusoidal capillarization (see below) leading to a decrease in nutritional flow as described by Eq. (36.6). Unfortunately, there is no reliable test to predict nutritional flow in cirrhosis (see above). This is due in particular to the fact that hepatic perfusion is often measured using the clearance of high-extraction compounds; this is decreased and may lead to an overestimation of hepatic perfusion when extraction is low.

Portosystemic shunting

From Eqs. (36.1) and (36.5) it is evident that portosystemic shunting -either extra- or intrahepatic – will markedly reduce extraction. The degree of portosystemic shunting can be assessed by isotopic technologies. Serum bile acids correlate well with portosystemic shunting, as determined by such techniques.

Sinusoidal capillarization

Sinusoidal capillarization, i.e., the formation of a basement membrane-like structure between the endothelial cell layer and the space of Disse, has been known for over 30 years; its functional equivalent was described later by using the multiple indicator dilution technique. In alcoholic liver disease, there is a loss of fenestrae before true capillarization occurs. Although the functional significance of this phenomenon has not been assessed yet, it stands to reason that it will have similar implications on liver function. Sinusoidal capillarization is a main determinant of liver function in animals with liver cirrhosis for both high- and low-extraction compounds.

ALTERATIONS IN PHARMACOKINETICS

From the theoretical considerations presented earlier, it is easily deduced that there can be profound alterations in

Table 36.2 Drugs with liability for adverse effects due to a high hepatic extraction (flow-limited clearance)

Compound	Extraction efficiency (%)
Bromocriptine	95
Chlormethiazole	76
Dehydroergotamine	95
Doxepin	75
Ergotamine	95
Fluorouracil	80
Imipramine	75
Isosorbide dinitrate	90
Labetalol	80
Lidocaine	70
Morphine	75
Nitroglycerin	95
Pentazocine	90
Propoxyphene	80
Propranolol	80
Verapamil	85

the pharmacokinetics of different drugs in chronic liver disease. Thus the effects of Eq (36.6) on Eq (36.1) predict a loss of the first-pass effect in chronic liver disease, flow-limited compounds being the most affected. The practical consequence of this prediction is the need for dosage adjustment of both loading and maintenance doses. There are few compounds, however, where a narrow therapeutic range makes this more than a theoretical consideration. Thus benzodiazepines with a high hepatic extraction such as midazolam or triazolam (Tab. 36.2) or oral morphine can lead to increased sedation, up to respiratory failure. Examples of drugs with flow-limited clearance are listed in Table 36.2.

Table 36.3 Cytochrome P450 isoenzymes and some typical substrates with enhanced risk for altered pharmacokinetic behavior in chronic liver disease

Isoenzyme	Substrates
1A2	Amitriptyline Imipramine Theophylline

2C	Diazepam
	NSAIDs such as
	  ibuprofen, naproxen,
	  diclofenac, oxicams

2E1	Ethanol Halogenated anesthetics Isoniazid Paracetamol
3A	Cyclosporin A Macrolide antibiotics Lidocaine Midazolam Nifedipine Tacrolimus Testosterone

Even more difficult is prediction of the disposition of drugs whose clearance is enzyme-limited, since cirrhosis affects different enzyme systems to different degrees (see above). One can predict that drugs predominantly metabolized by CYP3A will be affected in noncholestatic cirrhotic liver disease, whereas compounds metabolized by CYP2E1 will be affected in cholestatic liver disease. A few compounds with liability for such alterations are given in Table 36.3.

The decrease in drug-metabolizing enzymes can lead not only to a prolonged residence in the body but also to decreased efficacy; this is particularly true for different prodrugs that are insufficiently activated to their active congener. Thus, a reduced activation of famciclovir to penciclovir has been observed in patients with chronic liver disease (see Chap. 70). The same holds true for the ACE inhibitors enalapril and spirapril.

ALTERATIONS IN PHARMACODYNAMICS

Pharmacodynamic response to a variety of drugs is altered in cirrhosis. Clinically, the most relevant of such changes are those to vasoconstrictors, diuretics, and sedatives.

The blunted response to vasoconstrictors such as angiotensin II, α- and β-agonists, or endothelin is important in the understanding and treatment of portal hypertension but does not give rise to clinically important problems. In contrast, an altered pharmacodynamic response to diuretics may have important consequences. The response to the loop diuretics furosemide and torasemide is blunted in patients with cirrhosis, in particular when ascites is present. However, the blunted response to torasemide is overcome in part by its alterations in pharmacokinetics leading to prolonged delivery of active drug and metabolites to the distal tubule, thereby maintaining activity. This explains the clinical observation that torasemide may be more effective in the treatment of ascites than furosemide.

Sedative compounds must be used carefully in the patient with liver disease because many may be subject to pharmacokinetic and pharmacodynamic alterations; in particular, benzodiazepines can induce hepatic encephalopathy. Conversely, benzodiazepine antagonists may display potentially beneficial effects in patients with liver encephalopathy (see Chap. 15). Part of this is due to an altered brain sensitivity to benzodiazepines in particular in patients with significant portosystemic shunting and/or markedly decreased liver function. Patients with less severe liver disease have been reported not to have altered pharmacodynamic response to benzodiazepines.

PREDICTION OF ALTERED PHARMACOKINETICS OR PHARMACODYNAMICS

Conventional liver tests such as determination of transaminases or other enzymes have no value in predicting patients in whom the pharmacokinetics of a given drug will be altered. Therefore, there have been many attempts to predict drug clearance with so-called dynamic or quantitative liver function tests in particular using xenobiotics. Since the initial proposal by Brodie to use antipyrine as a model compound, in view of the multiplicity of metabolic pathways responsible for the metabolic handling of this drug, a large number of different model compounds have been proposed. These have been discussed in a number of recent reviews.

In general, the use of model compounds to predict pharmacokinetic behavior in patients with chronic liver disease has been disappointing. While there is good correlation between different aspects of hepatic function and alterations in drug disposition, the variability is too large to make them a useful tool for clinical practice. This may be due to the fact that such dynamic function tests can measure a particular aspect of liver metabolism, only contributing but not fully determining the fate of the drug. If this conclusion is accepted, then one may predict that model compounds metabolized by a particular CYP450 isoenzyme could be useful in predicting the kinetics of drugs with a narrow therapeutic index that are metabolized by the same CYP450. A good predictor example of this may be the erythromycin breath test; erythromycin is metabolized by CYP3A, and by the use of this test, an acceptable prediction of cyclosporine clearance has been obtained (see also Chap. 75). In contrast, "global" metabolic tests to predict hepatic clearance of xenobiotics have been rather disappointing. Recently, the MEGX test has gained some popularity because it is – in contrast to older tests such as the galactose elimination capacity or the aminopyrine breath test – easily performed and does not require special equipment. It measures the formation of a metabolite – monoethylglycinexylidide (MEGX) – after intravenous injection of a bolus of lidocaine. Formation of MEGX is the deethylation product catalyzed by CYP3A4. Usually, a single sample is obtained after administration of the lidocaine bolus, and MEGX is determined by an immunofluorescence polarization assay (TDx). It has been proposed as a criterion for donor selection and prioritization of transplant candidates; both indications have been severely criticized in the literature, however. Although the formation of MEGX is mediated by CYP3A4, it is clearly less reliable than the erythromycin breath test to predict the clearance of cyclosporine or tacrolimus.

Some of these "global" metabolic tests, including antipyrine clearance, the aminopyrine breath test, and the galactose elimination capacity, have been used as surrogate markers to judge the success of therapeutic interventions in chronic liver disease.

Hepatic perfusion can be assessed with the indocyanine green (ICG) clearance, provided its extraction efficiency is not too markedly reduced. ICG has never been shown to reliably predict the clearance of high-extraction compounds, however. In contrast, it may be useful for patient selection for resection in hepatocellular carcinoma. Serum bile acid levels and sorbitol clearance are proven indicators of portosystemic shunting. Again, no data are available to judge their value in dose adjustment in patients with chronic liver disease.

INCREASED SUSCEPTIBILITY
TO ADVERSE EVENTS

Altered pharmacokinetics and/or pharmacodynamics could lead to an increased susceptibility to adverse events in patients with chronic liver disease. Indeed, many manufacturers warn about the use of compounds with potential for hepatotoxicity in patients with known liver disease. With a few exceptions, this is not correct, however. Patients with preexisting liver disease are not more prone to hepatotoxicity, but if they develop hepatotoxicity, hepatic failure may occur because of their limited functional reserve.

An exception to this statement is paracetamol, which even at therapeutic doses can induce severe, even fatal liver disease in patients with preexisting disease, in particular in patients abusing alcohol. Two factors play a key role in this phenomenon. First, glutathione stores are reduced in chronic liver disease and in patients with alcohol abuse. Second, the induction of CYP2E1 by alcohol is also responsible for the formation of the toxic metabolite.

Drug accumulation in patients with chronic liver disease is thought to be responsible for an increased incidence of seizures in patients treated with pefloxacin.

Indeed, the clearance of pefloxacin is decreased, and the expected decrease can be estimated by the Child-Pugh criteria. A similar mechanism may be responsible for the β-lactam antibiotic-induced neutropenia.

Renal function is often affected in patients with liver disease. It is not surprising, therefore, that nephrotoxic drugs are often the cause of adverse events in such patients. Two classes of compounds are of particular risk, namely, nonsteroidal anti-inflammatory drugs (NSAIDs) and aminoglycosides. The kidney of the cirrhotic patient depends on prostaglandins to maintain renal perfusion; cycloxygenase inhibition induces an immediate reduction in renal perfusion and function. This is most dangerous in patients with ascites on diuretic therapy; it can happen even in patients without ascites, however. NSAIDs also can induce acute renal failure in binge drinkers without liver disease.

Aminoglycosides are more nephrotoxic in patients with obstructive jaundice. Monitoring of serum bilirubin levels may provide a good predictor for this dangerous adverse event.

Suggested readings _____

BOLDYS H, HARTLEB M, RUDZKI K, et al. Effect of propranolol on portosystemic collateral circulation estimated by per-rectal portal scintigraphy with technetium-99m pertechnetate. J Hepatol 1995;22:173-8.

BUTERS JTM, ZYSSET T, REICHEN J. Metabolism of antipyrine in vivo in two rat models of liver cirrhosis: its relationship to intrinsic clearance in vitro and microsomal membrane lipid composition. Biochem Pharmacol 1993;46:983-91.

DUCLOS-VALLÉE J-C, NISHIOKA M, HOSOMI N, et al. Interferon therapy in LKM-1 positive patients with chronic hepatitis C: follow-up by a quantitative radioligand assay for CYP2D6 antibody detection. J Hepatol 1998;28:965-70.

DURAZZO M, PHILIPP T, VAN PELT FNAM, et al. Heterogeity of liver-kidney microsomal autoantibodies in chronic hepatitis C and D virus infection. Gastroenterology 1995;108:455-62.

GEORGE J, LIDDLE C, MURRAY M, et al. Pre-translational regulation of cytochrome P450 genes is responsible for disease-specific changes of individual P450 enzymes among patients with cirrhosis. Biochem Pharmacol 1995;49:873-81.

GEORGE J, MURRAY M, BYTH K, FARRELL GC. Differential alterations of cytochrome P450 proteins in livers from patients with severe chronic liver disease. Hepatology 1995;21:120-8.

KAKIMOTO H, IMAI Y, KAWATA S, et al. Altered lipid composition and differential changes in activities of membrane-bound enzymes of erythrocytes in hepatic cirrhosis. Metabolism 1995;44:825-32.

KAWASAKI S, IMAMURA H, BANDAI Y, et al: Direct evidence for the intact hepatocyte theory in patients with liver cirrhosis. Gastroenterology 1992;102:1351-5.

MURRY DJ, CROM WR, REDDICK WE, et al. Liver volume as a determinant of drug clearance in children and adolescents. Drug Metab Dispos 1995;23:1110-6.

PACIFICI GM, VIANI A, FRANCHI M, et al. Conjugation pathways in liver disease. Br J Clin Pharmacol 1990;30:427-35.

REICHEN J: MEGX test in hepatology. The long-sought ultimate quantitative liver function test? J Hepatol 1993;19:4-7.

REICHEN J. Assessment of hepatic function with xenobiotics. Semin Liver Dis 1998;25:189-201.

ROBIN DW, LEE MH, HASAN SS, WOOD AJJ. Triazolam in cirrhosis: pharmacokinetics and pharmacodynamics. Clin Pharmacol Ther 1993;54:630-7.

RYAN J, SUDHIR K, JENNINGS G, et al. Impaired reactivity of the peripheral vasculature to pressor agents in alcoholic cirrhosis. Gastroenterology 1993;105:1167-72.

TURGEON DK, LEICHTMAN AB, LOWN KS, et al. P450 3A activity and cyclosporine dosing in kidney and heart transplant recipients. Clin Pharmacol Ther 1994;56:253-60.

New areas of drug development

Sandro Ardizzone, Gabriele Bianchi Porro

During recent years, much progress has been made in the pharmacologic treatment of gastrointestinal diseases. Increasing knowledge of pathogenetic mechanisms has produced different agents capable of controlling clinical manifestations and, at least in certain cases, modifying the natural history of the disease.

Since the introduction of cimetidine in the late 1970s, H_2-receptor antagonists (e.g., ranitidine, famotidine, roxatidine, etc.) have been used extensively for the treatment of peptic ulcer. The greater degree of inhibition of gastric acid secretion obtained by proton pump inhibitors (e.g., omeprazole, lansoprazole, pantoprazole, rabeprazole) has given higher and faster rates of gastric and duodenal ulcer healing. The discovery of the association between *Helicobacter pylori* infection, gastritis, and peptic ulcer has revolutionized the medical treatment of gastric and duodenal ulcers. Although drug treatment of *H. pylori* infection has resulted in eradication of the bacterium in over 70% of patients, the cost-effectiveness ratio needs improvement.

Because of a lack of knowledge of the exact disease mechanism, the treatment of inflammatory bowel diseases (IBD) has for years been limited to sulfasalazine, 5-aminosalicylic acid, and corticosteroids employed empirically to control the inflammatory activity. Recent insight into the pathogenesis of IBD has opened new options for treatment. Biopsy specimens of affected tissue in ulcerative colitis (UC) and Crohn's disease (CD) have shown lymphocytic and neutrophilic infiltration, the hallmarks of inflammation. Modalities currently under investigation include the extensively studied immunosuppressive agents and lipoxygenase inhibitors and less well-studied, emerging therapies such as oxygen-derived free radical scavengers, immunoglobulins, lidocaine, T-cell apheresis, antitumor necrosis factor antibody, and CD4 antibody. Putative infection etiologies also abound and have prompted many trials of agents ranging from antimycobacterials to antibacterials. The hypercoagulable state of some patients with IBD points toward hypercoagulability as an underlying cause. In this context, heparin has been tested as a possible approach.

This chapter briefly reviews the main areas of drug research, exploring more intimately the mechanisms associated with the development of upper and lower gastrointestinal diseases and providing identification of a host of potential alternative and sometimes experimental forms of drug therapy.

Esophageal motor disorders

The most important recent contribution with respect to achalasia relates to the applicability of botulinum toxin. Intrasphincteric botulinum toxin is being used increasingly for the treatment of achalasia; the presumed action is the blockade of acetylcholine release, which reduces resting lower esophageal sphincter (LES) pressure. Achalasia of the esophagus, however, is a lifelong condition that requires long-term reduction in LES pressure and improvement in esophageal emptying. It is not clear how long the effects of a single injection or repeated injections may last. The advantage of botulinum toxin therapy is that except for the minimal risk of endoscopy, there are no major side effects; such therapy thus may have a role in a select group of patients with achalasia. Whether it will replace pneumatic dilatation, which provides sustained improvement for a long time with minimal risk, remains to be seen. One study has indicated that botulinum toxin may be helpful in the short-term treatment of patients with diffuse esophageal spasm.

As far as gastroesophageal reflux disease (GERD) is concerned, improvement and sophistication of the motor function analysis through computer-assisted assay with superior sensors and sleeves have contributed to unraveling the intricate mechanisms governing the LES and the motor patterns in the esophagus. In particular, attention has been focused on the complexities of reflex inhibition of sphincter tone, responsible for transient LES and crural relaxation of a sufficient degree to allow reflux to occur. Thus the role of nitric oxide in the final pathway leading to LES relaxation and its potential for modulation generated much excitement. The spin-off of the discovery of transient LES relaxation may provide an attractive area for novel drug development.

Helicobacter pylori infection

To date, no single agent has proven effective in eradicating *H. pylori*. In 1988, the treatment consisted of colloid bismuth subcitrate for 8 weeks along with treatment with tinidazole for 10 days, and this achieved a 70% eradication rate. This was increased by the addition of a second antibiotic, creating the first triple therapy. It was then shown that the bismuth component could be replaced with a proton pump inhibitor or an H_2 antagonist and that the duration of the triple therapy could be reduced to 7 days. Such treatment achieved eradication rates of between 85 and 95%. The further addition of colloid bismuth subcitrate to produce a quadruple therapy increased the eradication rate even when given for a shorter period of time. However, one would have to conclude that the treatments for this infection are far from ideal and that a simpler, more effective treatment with fewer side effects is desired. Moreover, considering that *H. pylori* infection affects more than 50% of the world's population, the control of an infection of this high prevalence cannot be achieved with conventional antibiotics but rather by measures preventing its spread or causing immunization. A considerable amount of research has been conducted on potential vaccines against *H. pylori*, but therapeutic or prophylactic vaccines remain some way off. The cloning of the entire *H. pylori* genome in 1997 should open up new approaches to treating the infection by revealing new targets for vaccines. The description of the genome will increase our understanding of the biochemistry of the organism and may identify processes that can be targeted by new drug therapies. Understanding the molecular biology of the organism also should be useful in elucidating the mechanism of antibiotic resistance and in identifying prevention methods.

Gut infections

Although most intestinal infections are self-limiting and do not require specific treatment other than supportive therapy (i.e., fluid and electrolytes replacement), the natural history of some infections, particularly when associated with clinically severe disease, is altered by antibiotics. Antidiarrheal drugs are still used widely for the treatment of infective diarrheal disease, but their efficacy is modest, and as yet there is no antisecretory agent available in clinical practice to reduce fluid and electrolyte losses. There are a number of potential targets for antisecretory drugs in the intestine; previous preliminary studies have indicated that calcium-calmodulin inhibitors can reduce secretory diarrhea. Zaldaride maleate is such a drug, and its efficacy has now been confirmed in patients with travelers' diarrhea. This agent is currently under evaluation in other acute infective diarrheas and in patients with HIV/AIDS. A number of other agents have been shown to have antisecretory activity in animal or human models of secretory diarrhea. These include the enkephalinase inhibitor acetorphine, the $5\text{-}HT_3$ receptor antagonist granisetron, and the sigma agonist igmesine. Acetorphan's antisecretory activity is thought to reside in its ability to increase the half-life of endogenous opioids,

whereas the $5\text{-}HT_3$ receptor antagonists and igmesine may work by inhibiting local neural reflexes in the intestine, activated by secretory enterotoxins.

Irritable bowel syndrome

The presently available pharmacologic treatments for irritable bowel syndrome (IBS) are not completely satisfactory, probably reflecting the limited understanding of the underlying pathophysiologic mechanisms and also because of the lack of objective markers of diagnosis and efficacy. The high placebo response rate observed in many trials of IBS therapies is also a confounding variable in the assessment of drug efficacy. New lines of research basically lead into three directions: (1) new drugs affecting gut motility, such as $5\text{-}HT_3$ antagonists, $5\text{-}HT_4$ agonists, and CCK receptor antagonists, (2) hormonal peptides, such as octreotide and leuprolide, and (3) drugs reducing visceral sensitivity.

New drugs affecting gut motility

In the intestine, serotonin (5-hydroxytryptamine, 5-HT) is contained in enterochromaffin cells and in a subset of descending interneurons. 5-HT markedly affects intestinal motility by activating receptors located on the effector cells, nerves, or both. $5\text{-}HT_3$ and $5\text{-}HT_4$ are among the best characterized receptors are among the best; in particular, drugs able to inhibit $5\text{-}HT_3$ receptors are antiemetic and motor-inhibiting compounds (e.g., ondansetron, granisetron, and dolasetron), whereas drugs active on $5\text{-}HT_4$ receptors have stimulatory effects on peristalsis. Some compounds share both $5\text{-}HT_3$ antagonism and $5\text{-}HT_4$ agonism. $5\text{-}HT_3$ receptors are present in the gut, where they are believed to play a role in nociception by modulating the afferent side of visceral reflexes. In addition, $5\text{-}HT_3$ receptors have been described on efferent neurones in both the autonomic and enteric nervous systems. Stimulation of these receptor sites leads to the release of acetylcholine and substance P, both excitatory transmitters for gastrointestinal sensitivity. Few, rather small studies provide conflicting results on the efficacy of $5\text{-}HT_3$ antagonists in the treatment of diarrhea-predominant IBS patients. Larger clinical studies with these compounds are at present ongoing. The experience with $5\text{-}HT_4$ agonists is still at a preclinical stage, but preliminary results with this class of drugs shall soon be available.

Cholecystokinin (CCK) at physiologic and pharmacologic doses stimulates intestinal motility; specific and potent structurally unrelated CCK antagonists have been developed, some of which are highly selective for receptor subtypes A and B. The only CCK-A receptor antagonist that is under clinical evaluation is loxiglumide, a 5-oxopentanoic acid. A randomized, placebo-controlled, double-blind crossover study with this compound has shown that this drug selectively delays transit of the ascending colon in IBS patients, whereas it does not exert any effect on healthy controls, whatever the colonic site. Future studies with loxiglumide, as well as with its dextroisomer, dexloglumide, will specifically address the problem of reducing visceral hyperanalgesia in IBS patients (see Chaps. 51 and 66).

Octreotide has been shown to be of therapeutic benefit in various conditions (e.g., acromegaly, neuroendocrine tumors, etc.). It also has been shown to have a profound inhibitory effect on small bowel transit, increasing mouth-to-cecum transit time in both healthy subjects and IBS patients. Recent data suggest that octreotide acts on visceral sensory thresholds through modulation of peripheral nociceptors located either in the gut wall, in the afferent pathways to the central nervous system (CNS), or in the CNS itself. Any of these components may be involved because somatostatin receptors have been identified in human brain tissue, in peripheral nerves, as well as in the gut mucosa.

The therapeutic rationale of *leuprolide*, a molecular analogue of gonadotropin-releasing hormone (GNRH), relates to exacerbation of IBS during the postovulatory phase of the menstrual cycle. Leuprolide may suppress, through hypothalamic-pituitary feedback mechanisms, the release of ovarian hormones that affect gut motility through action on the CNS or the enteric nervous system. Leuprolide could affect neurons in the brain or spinal cord similar to the action of the thyrotropin-releasing hormone (TRH has well-documented effects on gastric motility and acid secretion). Another possibility is direct action on neural elements of the enteric nervous system; the microcircuits of the enteric nervous system use the same synaptic neurotrasmitters as the brain and spinal cord. The efficacy of leuprolide in IBS treatment has been reported especially in premenopausal women.

Modulation of visceral sensitivity

Parallel with the renewed interest in the pathophysiologic role of hyperanalgesia in IBS, there has been growing interest in the modulation of visceral sensitivity as a therapeutic target for some IBS patients. Pure modulators of gut sensitivity are not available as yet, but pharmacologic research has at least focused on this target. It is known that repeated stimulation of afferent fibers increases second-order neuronal responsiveness by producing prolonged changes in spinal cord physiology (central *neuroplasticity*) through the release of first-order stimulatory neuropeptides (e.g., substance P), neurokinin, calcitonin gene-related peptide (CGRP), and excitatory amino acids such as glutamate. These substances increase membrane excitability and activate postsynaptic receptors, leading to increased release of intracellular Ca^{2+}. Future selective receptor antagonists (e.g, NMDA, substance P, or CGRP antagonists) may prevent the development of central neuroplasticity and sensitization.

Visceral sensitization is also centrally amplified via a decrease in descending inhibitory modulation of perception through an action of CNS centers on dorsal horn second-order neurons; the neurotransmitters involved in this descending modulation include norepinephrine (acting on α_2-adrenoceptors), serotonin (interacting with 5-HT receptors), and opioid peptides (interacting with β-opioid receptors). Future research should focus on the relative role of drugs, such as the new SSRI (serotonin-reuptake inhibitor) antidepressants versus β-opioid agonists, to block or prevent visceral nociception.

Inflammatory bowel disease

While the etiology of inflammatory bowel disease (IBD) remains unknown, certain features of this disease have suggested several areas of possible importance, such as familial or genetic, infectious, immunologic, and inflammatory factors. Whether or not IBD is a response to unique or multiple noxious factors is unclear, and IBD appears as a "puzzle" whose composition is difficult until the different pieces are recognized and integrated correctly.

Without knowledge as to the exact mechanism of the disease, for years the treatment of IBD has been limited to sulfasalazine, 5-aminosalicylic acid, and corticosteroids employed empirically to control the inflammatory activity.

Recent insights into the pathogenesis underlying Crohn's disease (CD) and ulcerative colitis (UC) have opened new treatment options, providing the identification of a host of new therapeutic agents potentially interacting with or interrupting specific genetic, immunoinflammatory, infectious, vascular, and neural targets.

Genetics

There is ample evidence that CD and UC are in part the result of genetic predisposition, and as related to the pathophysiology of IBD ultimately, genes control immunologic function. Many studies have examined the association between IBD and HLA class I and II alleles. More recently, genes outside the HLA system have come under scrutiny in the search for IBD genes. Considering the central role of cytokines in modulating intestinal inflammation, it is not surprising that a number of investigators have looked for mutations or genetic polymorphisms in cytokine genes.

Several recent studies have shown that allele 2 of the *IL-1ra* gene is associated with UC. Others have shown a strong association between a specific tumor necrosis factor (TNF) microsatellite haplotype and CD. Recent genome-wide searcher reported susceptibility loci for CD on chromosome 16 and for IBD on chromosomes 3, 7, and 12. Within the susceptibility region of chromosome 16 are genes involved in cell adhesion (CD 11 integrin cluster, CD19, sialophorin), as well as the interleukin-4 (IL-4) receptor.

Regardless of whether one or several genes are involved in the pathogenesis of IBD, there is considerable optimism that these studies will lead to the definitive identification of susceptibility genes in IBD, with immediate clinical and therapeutic benefit. Cell and gene therapy could be performed by treating targeted cells with various factors or cytokines ex vivo or by inserting/deleting targeted genes in isolated cells ex vivo followed by reintroduction into the host. Alternatively, genetic manipulation may be accomplished by means of viral or plasmid vectors in vivo. Vectors also may be designed to produce antisense RNA after incorporation by targeted cells. This may effectively inhibit production of protein in a manner analogous to antisense oligonucelotides administered exogenously. Very few data are available concerning the application of this method in IBD therapy.

Interesting results have been obtained both in animals and in CD patients. Moving from the concept that T-helper 1 (Th1) responses, characterized by the production of cytokines such as IL-2, interferon-γ (IFN-γ), and tumor necrosis factor-β (TNFβ), can be dramatically downregulated by T-helper 2 (Th2) cytokines such as IL-4 and IL-10 (see below), a recent study attempted to find out whether IL-4 prevents trinitrobenzene sulfonic (TNBS) acid colitis in rats by using a recombinant human adenovirus 5 vector expressing murine IL-4 (Ad5 IL-4). The virus was given ip and it infected cells in the liver, diaphragm, and colon, also elevating IL-4 serum concentrations. Rats given the Ad5 IL-4 vector had less tissue injury, lower mucosal IFN-γ concentrations, less inducible nitric oxide synthase, and fewer neutrophils in the mucosa than rats given a control viral vector.

Aiming to possibly interfere with the activation of immune and inflammatory cells, as well as the trafficking of these cells to the site of inflammation, thereby suppressing disease expression, the efficacy and safety of ISIS 2302, an antisense inhibitor of intercellular adhesion molecule-1 (ICAM-1), implicated in leukocyte recruitment, was tested in a randomized, double-blind study in patients with steroid-dependent CD. The results showed that a significantly higher proportion of patients treated with ISIS 2302 achieved remission in comparison with the placebo group at the end of the 1-month treatment phase.

Immunoinflammatory factors

CD4[+] T cells regulate critical aspects of the specific immune response and have been classified as either T-helper 1 (Th1) or T-helper 2 (Th2) on the basis of their ability to elaborate specific cytokines. Th1 cells are responsible for cell-mediate immune responses and secrete IL-2 and INF-γ. Th2 cells, in contrast, secrete IL-4, IL-5, IL-6, IL-10, and IL-13. These subsets regulate each other reciprocally through key cytokines. IFN-γ produced by Th1 cells suppresses development of Th2, whereas IL-4, IL-10, and IL-13 secreted by Th2 cells inhibit Th1 responses. Thus, for example, inhibition of Th1 responses could represent a significant goal in the treatment of IBD, especially of CD, where the evidence of an involvement of Th1 is strongest. At least four therapeutic strategies have been developed: (1) inhibition of CD4 itself, (2) administration of immunomodulatory (primarily Th2) cytokines, (3) neutralization of cytokines that direct the response toward Th1, and (4) blocking of costimulatory signals that play a role in initiating the Th1 response.

Anti-CD4 antibodies have been used in a variety of autoimmune diseases and also have been tried in CD and UC. A CD4 depleting antibody (cM-T412) was tested in two open studies on CD and UC patients with severe steroid-refractory disease. Both CD and UC patients achieved clinical and endoscopic improvement/remission after a variable treatment period of 7 to 11 days.

In the other three open trials, CD4 nondepleting antibodies (MAX.16H5 and B-F5) were administered to a total of 16 CD and 9 UC patients with active disease. Five of the 9 UC patients achieved remission versus only 6 of the 16 CD patients. Thus, depleting antibodies to CD4 seems to be more effective therapy than nondepleting antibodies. However, concerns over long-term depression of CD4 counts and the risk of opportunistic infections could prevent widespread use of these agents.

Immunomodulatory cytokines

IL-10 is produced by Th2 cells and suppresses the production of IL-2 and IFN-γ by Th1 cells. Gene-targeted IL-10–deficient mice develop severe transmural and granulomatous inflammation of the small and large bowels, reminiscent of Crohn's disease, and inflammation can be prevented by the administration of IL-10. Lamina propria mononuclear cells obtained from patients with IBD appropriately downregulate the secretion of IL-1 and TNF when treated with IL-10. A multicenter, randomized, double-masked, placebo-controlled study of recombinant IL-10 in steroid-refractory CD has been reported. Forty-five patients were assigned to receive iv IL-10 at 0.5, 1, 5, 10, or 25 µg/kg per day or placebo daily for 7 days. Remission was achieved in 50% of patients treated with IL-10 versus 23% in the placebo group. Treatment was well tolerated, except for reports of headache and nausea. Similarly, multiple doses (1, 5, 10, and 20 µg/kg per day) of IL-10 were found effective in the treatment of mild to moderately active CD in a 28-day placebo-controlled, double-blind trial.

Trasforming growth factor-β TGF-β may be produced by T cells as well as many other varieties of cells of both hematopoietic and nonhematopoietic lineages. Enhanced expression of TGF-β message is found in the cells of the lamina propria in both UC and CD, and several studies have demonstrated a potent suppressive effect of TGF-β on Th1 effector cells. No clinical trials are available in the treatment of IBD.

Anti-IFN-γ IFN-γ is elevated in all genetic animal models of IBD and seems to be critical to the development of Th1 responses. Surprisingly, anti-IFN-γ has been administered to the IL-10 knock-out mouse without benefit. Its use in human disease has not been reported.

Anti-IL-12 IL-12 is produced by monocytes-macrophages and lymphocytes after activation by bacterial challenge or proinflammatory cytokines (see Chap. 75) and may induce CD4[+] cells to differentiate as Th1 cells. Therefore, neutralization of IL-12 may be beneficial in IBD, and studies in animals show that administration of anti-lL-12 leads to an impressive improvement in colitis even after 20 days from induction of the disease.

Proinflammatory cytokines: IL-1 and tumor necrosis factor-β

IL-1 and TNFβ share a multitude of proinflammatory properties critical to the amplification of mucosal inflammation in IBD. Enhanced expression of IL-1 and TNFβ was found in IBD, and a crucial role of TNFβ was suggested for the genesis of these diseases. TNFβ appears to stimulate granuloma formation and therefore may play a role in the pathogenesis of CD. Moreover, along with IL-6, IL-1 and TNFβ may contribute to the constitutional symptoms of IBD and lead to the generation of acute-phase proteins. It thus may be expected that inhibition of these cytokines will provide effective treatment of IBD.

In the case of IL-1, the proinflammatory effects are limited naturally by endogenous IL-1 receptor antagonists (IL-1ra), suggesting a therapeutic role for IL-1ra, especially since it ameliorates experimental colitis in rabbits. So far no results have been published concerning the potential efficacy of IL-1ra in the treatment of human IBD.

Blockade of TNF activity   Studies of neutralizing anti-TNF antibodies have shown promising efficacy in CD. A series of 10 refractory CD patients were treated with a single infusion of cA2, a chimeric monoclonal anti-TNF antibody. Onset of action was rapid (within 2 weeks), and 9 of the 10 patients had a complete response, with an average of 4 months before relapse occurred. The endoscopic appearance of the mucosa also was significantly improved at 4 weeks. This open-label experience was confirmed recently in a double-blind, parallel-arm study of patients with chronic active CD not responding to standard therapy who were randomized to receive one of the three dose levels of cA2 (5, 10, or 20 mg/kg per day) or placebo for 4 weeks. When all groups were combined, the clinical remission rate (CDAI < 150) was 33% in the cA2 groups versus 4% in the placebo group (p < 0.05). Serious adverse events were few, and overall the infusion was well tolerated by the patients.

CDP571, a humanized IgG4 anti-TNF antibody, also has been studied in 31 patients with moderately active CD. Patients were randomized to receive a single infusion of either 5 mg/kg of CDP571 or placebo in a 2:1 ratio. Two weeks after the infusion, there was a statistical improvement in the Harvey-Bradsahw score among treated patients, with a median score of 10 before treatment versus 5 after treatment (p < 0.001). The median Harvey-Bradshaw score remained unchanged among placebo-treated patients (6.5 at both time points).Two weeks after treatment, 6 patients met criteria for remission versus none in the placebo group.

Microbial etiology

Microbial agents appear to be intimately involved in the pathogenesis of IBD. Although present data do not convincingly incriminate a single, persistent pathogen as a universal cause of IBD, this hypothesis should still be considered. During the last few years, *Mycobacterium paratuberculosis,* measles virus, and *Listeria monocytogenes* have been implicated. In particular, it has been proposed that CD may be a persistent measles virus-induced granulomatous vasculitis. Moreover, paramyxovirus-like

structures were visualized in the vascular endothelium of CD patients, and measles virus antigen and mRNA were localized to granulomas and endothelial cells by immunohistochemistry and in situ hybridization. However, the interpretation of epidemiologic studies implicating the measles virus in CD has been challenged; the presence of the measles virus has not been confirmed by independent investigators, and a measles viral genomic sequence could not be detected in intestinal tissue from CD patients by nested polymerase chain reaction (PCR). Thus, despite extensive investigation of these and other organisms over the past four decades, no single specific infection has been shown convincingly to be critical to the pathogenesis of IBD.

Vascular factors

Tissue vascularization can affect the morphology and function of the bowel in different ways, including an anomalous blood supply, coagulation disorders, and vasculitis. All these mechanisms ultimately result in more or less extensive hypoxemia and subsequent damage to the mucosa and/or the deeper layers of the bowel wall. Thrombotic phenomena, formation of microthrombi, and occlusive fibrinoid lesions of arteries supplying areas of CD-affected intestine, with granulomas in the wall and lumen of the blood vessels and vascular lesions, were demonstrated in a prospective study on specimens from 15 patients prepared by heparin-saline perfusion. Thus, multifocal gastrointestinal infarction has been proposed as the pathogenetic mechanism for CD. As far as UC is concerned, evidence supports the existence of a thrombotic process including a hypercoagulable state, increased incidence of thromboembolic events, and ischemic complications such as toxic megacolon and pyoderma gangrenosum. The reported efficacy of heparin administration, at doses of 10 000 to 36 000 units per day, in the treatment of patients with refractory UC supports the vascular theory .

Neural-immune interactions

There is growing evidence that the nervous system influences the immune system and that the nervous, endocrine, and immune systems communicate with one another via neuropeptides, hormones, and cytokines. Animal studies have shown that mucosal inflammation can lead to alterations in neuroenteric function, and human studies have shown that vasoactive intestinal peptide-containing nerve fibers are reduced in both UC and CD and that substance P is elevated in IBD mucosa. Although much remains to be learned about the role of nerves in IBD, preliminary studies using topical anesthetic and autonomically active drugs such as clonidine and nicotine in UC indicate that neuromodulation may be a viable therapeutic option.

Suggested readings

American Society for Gastrointestinal Endoscopy. Technology Assessment Status Evaluation: botulinum toxin therapy in gastrointestinal endoscopy. November, 1996. Gastroint Endosc 1998;47:569-72.

ARDIZZONE S, BOLLANI S, MANZIONNA G, BIANCHI PORRO G. Inflammatory bowel disease approaching the 3rd millennium: pathogenesis and therapeutic implications. Eur J Gastroenterol Hepatol 1999;11:27-32.

FARTUHING MJG. Gut infections. Eur J Gastroenterol Hepatol 1999;11:17-20.

MCCOLL KEL. Helicobacter pylori, 1988-1998. Eur J Gastroenterol Hepatol 1999;11:13-6.

MITTAL RK, BALABAN DH. The esophagogastric junction. N Engl J Med 1997;336:924-32.

PACE F, MOLTENI P. IBS. Future development and research. In: Stockbrügger R, Pace F, eds. The irritable bowel syndrome manual. London: Mosby-Wolfe Medical Communications, 1999, pp 103.

SANDS BE. Biologic therapy for inflammatory bowel disease. Inflamm Bowel Dis 1997;3:95-99.

Infective and anti-infective agents

Basis of antibiotic therapy for major infections

Pramod M. Shah, Cesare R. Sirtori

β-LACTAMS

β-Lactam antibiotics, traditionally penicillins and, in more recent years, cephalosporins, carbapenems, and monobactams, are antagonists of cell wall biosynthesis in gram-positive and gram-negative bacteria. They bind specific cell wall proteins involved in biosynthetic processes in the cell. Since the cell wall is structurally predominant in gram-positive organisms, these are the microbial species more sensitive to the classic penicillins (penicillin G, phenoxymethylpenicillin, oxacillin) and in general to all β-lactams, with the exception of aztreonam. However, second-generation aminopenicillins, e.g., ampicillin and amoxicillin, as well as parenteral penicillins, e.g., those belonging to the ureidopenicillin group (azlocillin, mezlocillin), and finally, the third-generation cephalosporins, some of which also present a prolonged elimination half-life, have a more extended spectrum of activity because of an improved interaction with the cell wall in gram-negative organisms. These drugs may show remarkable activity against bacteria such as *Proteus, Pseudomonas, Klebsiella,* and others.

Penicillins

Mode of action and classification

Penicillins constitute one of the most important groups of antibiotics and, historically, are the forerunners of all microbially derived antibiotics. The observation of Alexander Fleming in 1928 that *Staphylococcus* could be lysed by a fungus belonging to the genus *Penicillium* opened the way to the development of all the major antibiotics available today. Penicillins act mainly by binding to penicillin-binding proteins (PBPs). PBPs have variable affinity for the different β-lactams, and while most PBPs are responsible for cell wall biosynthesis, some, e.g., PBP2, may cause delayed bacterial lysis; PBP3 may lead to the production of long, filamentous bacterial forms. Traditional penicillins (e.g., penicillin G) and the penicillinase-resistant penicillins (e.g., methicillin, oxacillin, flucloxacillin) are mainly active on

gram-positive bacteria and differ in kinetics, also allowing the use of retard formulations, the best known of which is the penicillin G-benzathine suspension, usually given in doses of 1.2 million units intermuscularly every 2 weeks for the prevention of streptococcal infections. Aminopenicillins (e.g, ampicillin, amoxicillin) and their congeners have an improved interaction with gram-negative species and are more widely used for respiratory, urinary tract, and *Salmonella* infections. Finally, the carboxy- and ureidopenicillins (e.g., carbenicillin, mezlocillin, piperacillin, and others) mainly have activity on gram-negative species.

Spectrum of activity

The spectrum of activity of the major penicillins is directed toward gram-positive cocci, particularly *Streptococcus* spp., and *Staphylococcus aureus* for β-lactamase-resistant penicillins (e.g., oxacillin, flucloxacillin). Broad-spectrum aminopenicillins show significant activity against the major gram-negative organisms, e.g., *Proteus mirabilis, Escherichia coli,* and *Hemophilus influenzae,* whereas the newer extended-spectrum penicillins (e.g., mezlocillin and others) show a useful antimicrobial activity against *Pseudomonas, Klebsiella,* and other gram-negative species as well.

Mechanism of resistance

Resistance to penicillins, as for most β-lactams, is through bacterial β-lactamases. β-Lactamases are a series of enzymes that can be either *restrictive,* i.e., active only on specific penicillins, most often aminopenicillins (e.g., ampicillin, amoxicillin), or *broad spectrum,* hydrolyzing a variety of β-lactams. In the case of gram-positive bacteria, β-lactamases are secreted extracellularly, may be transferred (e.g., by *Staphylococcus*), and frequently are induced by substrates. Gram-negative β-lactamases are instead located intracellularly on the surfaces of the inner membrane, thus allowing maximal contact with sensitive antibiotics. β-Lactamases from gram-negative bacteria may be either plasmid transferable or chromosomally encoded.

Table 38.1 Pharmacokinetics, usual daily doses, and toxicities of penicillins

Drug	Mode of application and dose	Bioavailability (%)	$t_{1/2}$	Notes: major elimination route and untoward effects
Penicillin G Benzylpenicillin	Parenteral (iv or im) 15-30 million units	–	0.5	Renally eliminated, CSF penetration at high dose. Untoward effects: GI tract, allergic reactions, seizures
Phenoxypenicillins	Oral 1.2-3 million units	60-70	0.5	Renally eliminated. Intraindividual variations in absorption. Untoward effects: GI tract, allergic reactions
Amoxicillin	Oral or iv 1.5-3.0 g	74-92% after oral dosing	1	Renally eliminated, sufficient CSF penetration at high dose. Untoward effects: GI tract, allergic reactions
Ampicillin or ampicillin-prodrugs	Oral or iv 3.0-15.0 g	50% after oral dosing >80% in case of prodrugs	1	Renally eliminated. Untoward effects: GI tract, allergic reactions
Amoxicillin + clavulanic acid	Oral or iv 1.875-3.75 g	60% after oral dosing	1	Renally eliminated. Untoward effects: GI tract, allergic and hepatic reactions. Clavulanic acid daily dose restricted to 600 mg
Oxacillin	Oral or iv 3.0-6.0 g	50% after oral dosing	0.4	Renally eliminated, poor CSF penetration even at high dose. Untoward effects: GI tract, allergic and hepatic reactions
Flucloxacillin	Oral or iv 3.0-6.0 g	50% after oral dosing	0.75	Renally eliminated, poor CSF penetration even at high dose. Untoward effects: GI tract; allergic and hepatic reactions
Mezlocillin or piperacillin or azlocillin	Parenteral 6.0-12.0 g	–	1	Renally eliminated, sufficient CSF penetration at high dose. Untoward effects: GI tract; allergic reactions

($t_{1/2}$ = elimination half-life in hours; CSF = cerebrospinal fluid levels in case of inflamed meninges; GI tract = gastrointestinal tract, mainly diarrhea, nausea, vomiting.)

More recently, bacterial resistance to β-lactams has been related to molecular alterations of the PBPs responsible for the interaction between β-lactams and bacterial cell walls. Homologous recombination events have allowed structural modifications in the PBPs, thus reducing sensitivity to major penicillins. In addition (see below for cephalosporins), there may be a significant induction of PBPs of reduced sensitivity, thus creating a "mechanical" obstacle to drug penetration into sensitive cells (Tab. 38.1).

Injectable cephalosporins

Mode of action and classification

Cephalosporins, originally isolated from a fungal species different from *Penicillium* by Brotzu in 1948, provide a more varied series of compounds because of the possibility of chemical substitutions both on the side chain of the β-lactam nucleus and on the six-member dihydrothiazine ring. Substitutions on the β-lactam nucleus are frequently (but not always) associated with changes in the spectrum, whereas substitutions on the so-called cephem nucleus frequently associate with kinetic changes (oral products generally have very small substituents, i.e., methyl or chloride groups). The explosive growth of cephalosporins makes it difficult to provide a generally acceptable classification. Injectable products have undergone a progressive evolution, i.e., from first-generation agents (e.g., cephalothin, cefazolin) with a spectrum of activity similar to that of the penicillins up to third-generation agents with markedly improved activity against major gram-negative organisms.

Spectrum of activity

Injectable cephalosporins have progressed from first-generation agents (e.g., cephalothin, cefazolin) with a spectrum of activity similar to that of penicillins to second-generation agents (e.g., cefuroxime, cefoxitine, ceftizoxime, cefmenoxime, and cefotiam) with additional activity against gram-negative species, such as *E. coli,*

Table 38.2 Pharmacokinetics, usual daily doses, and toxicities of parenteral cephalosporins

Drug	Usual dose (g)	$t_{1/2}$	Notes: major elimination route and untoward effects
Cephalothin	6.0-8.0	0.4	Renally eliminated, poor CSF penetration. Untoward effects: GI tract, allergic reactions
Cefazolin	4.0-6.0	1.5	Renally eliminated, poor CSF penetration, sufficient biliary concentrations. Untoward effects: GI tract, allergic reactions
Cefamandol	4.0-6.0	0.5	Renally eliminated, CSF penetration (?), sufficient biliary concentrations. Untoward effects: GI tract, allergic reactions, alcohol intolerance
Cefuroxime	2.25-4.5	1.2	Renally eliminated, sufficient CSF penetration, sufficient biliary concentrations. Untoward effects: GI tract, allergic reactions
Cefoxitine	4.0-6.0	0.45	Renally eliminated, CSF penetration (?), sufficient biliary concentrations. Untoward effects: GI tract, allergic reactions
Cefotaxime	4.0-6.0	1	Renally eliminated, sufficient CSF penetration, sufficient biliary concentrations. Untoward effects: GI tract, allergic reactions
Cefotiam	4.0-6.0	0.45	Renally eliminated, sufficient CSF penetration (?), sufficient biliary concentrations. Untoward effects: GI tract, allergic reactions
Ceftriaxone	2.0-4.0	12	Renal and biliary elimination, sufficient CSF penetration, high biliary concentrations. Untoward effects: GI tract, allergic reactions; biliary sludge or calculi
Ceftizoxime	4.0-6.0	1.2	Renally eliminated, sufficient CSF penetration, sufficient biliary concentrations. Untoward effects: GI tract, allergic reactions
Cefmenoxime	4.0-6.0	1.2	Renally eliminated, sufficient CSF penetration, sufficient biliary concentrations. Untoward effects: GI tract, allergic reactions
Cefodizime	2.0-4.0	2.5	Renally eliminated, sufficient CSF penetration, sufficient biliary concentrations. Untoward effects: GI tract, allergic reactions
Cefoperazone	4.0-6.0	1.2	Renal and biliary elimination, sufficient CSF penetration, high biliary concentrations. Untoward effects: GI tract, allergic reactions, alcohol intolerance.
Ceftazidime	4.0-6.0	2	Renally eliminated, sufficient CSF penetration, sufficient biliary concentrations. Untoward effects: GI tract, allergic reactions
Cefepime	4.0-6.0	2	Renally eliminated, sufficient CSF penetration, sufficient biliary concentrations. Untoward effects: GI tract, allergic reactions
Cefpirome	4.0-6.0	2	Renally eliminated, sufficient CSF penetration, sufficient biliary concentrations. Untoward effects: GI tract, allergic reactions

($t_{1/2}$ = elimination half-life in hours; CSF = cerebrospinal fluid levels in case of inflamed meninges; ? = insufficient data or data not available; GI tract = gastrointestinal tract, mainly diarrhea, nausea, vomiting.)

Klebsiella, Proteus, H. influenzae, and *M. catarrhalis.* The activity of these newer antibiotics against gram-positive organisms is generally reduced versus the first-generation products; drugs such as cefoxitine show, in addition, some activity against anaerobes, e.g., *Bacteroides fragilis.* Finally, the third-generation agents (e.g., cefotaxime, ceftriaxone, and certazidime) show still improved activity against Enterobacteriaceae, *Pseudomonas aeruginosa, Serratia,* and *Neisseria gonorrhoeae.* These antibiotics maintain an acceptable activity against major gram-positive organisms and, in the case of cefepime, may provide improved resistance against β-lactamases. However, it should be kept in mind that the classification is still under debate and that ceftizoxime, cefmenoxime, and cefotiam, for example, are considered to be third-generation cephalosporins in some countries.

Mechanism of resistance

Resistance to cephalosporins is similar to that to penicillins. However, in addition to hydrolysis by lactamases, particularly chromosomally encoded lactamases, the alterations in PBPs are more prevalent as a cause of resistance than with the penicillins. Cephalosporins of the third generation, because of an increased affinity and capacity of induction of PBPs, may lead in particular to PBP accumulation inside the bacterial cell wall, thus creating a mechanical obstacle to the passage of the cephalosporin (*filter effect*). This may, at times, require the addition of a drug with a positive interaction, e.g., an aminoglycoside.

Pharmacokinetics, usual daily doses, and toxicities

Together with the parenteral penicillins, parenteral cephalosporins are the mainstay for treating infections in hospitalized patients. They are well tolerated. The most frequent side effect is loose bowels or diarrhea. Rare untoward effects include allergy, allergic neutropenia, a positive direct Coombs' test, and bleeding disorders (e.g., prolongation of the prothrombin time). There is a low potential risk for nephrotoxicity, especially when the agent is used in combination with other nephrotoxic drugs such as an aminoglycoside (Tables 38.2 and 38.6).

Oral cephalosporins

Classification and spectrum of activity

Oral cephalosporins are characterized by low-molecular-weight substituents on the dihydrothiazine ring and may, again, be classified according to generation, although most oral cephalosporins share a spectrum of activity quite similar to that of aminopenicillins, with, however, improved resistance against β-lactamases. Cephalexin, cephradine, cefaclor, and cefadroxil, all first-generation compounds, have a maximal activity against gram-negative cocci, whereas second- and third-generation agents such as cefixime, cefdinir, and loracarbef provide improved activity against gram-negative enterobacteria, generally not including *P. aeruginosa* or *Serratia*. Cefpodoxime-proxetil and cefuroxime-axetil/pivoxil are oral formulations of two major injectable cephalosporins with a spectrum of activity similar to the parent compounds (second-generation injectables).

Mechanism of resistance

Generally, this is similar to that of either the aminopenicillins (e.g., cephalexin, cefadroxil) or of the parent injectable drug.

Pharmacokinetics, usual daily doses, and toxicities

Oral cephalosporins are variably absorbed from the gastrointestinal tract, and this may at times result in relatively low serum concentrations and a high rate of gastrointestinal untoward effects. Some of the derivatives have longer serum elimination half-lives, permitting twice-daily applications. The risk of cross-allergy with penicillins is low (Tab. 38.3).

Carbapenems and monobactams

Mode of action and classification

Carbapenems (e.g., imipenem and meropenem) are characterized by a β-lactam ring with a substituent that has a different structure from that of the penicillins or cephalosporins, whereas the only monobactam (aztreonam) has a monocyclic structure with a thiazol ring substituent.

Imipenem and meropenem are both thienamycin derivatives from *Streptomyces cattleya*. The two compounds differ because imipenem, being hydrolyzed by a dipeptidase found in the proximal renal tubules, needs concomitant administration of the dipeptidase inhibitor cilastatin, whereas meropenem may be administered alone. Imipenem potentially has the widest spectrum of activity among all antibiotics, whereas meropenem, with a similar in vitro activity against gram-negative organisms, may show less activity against gram-positive cocci. Aztreonam, finally, has selective activity against gram-negative organisms and displays no activity against gram-positive organisms.

Spectrum of activity

Imipenem has an excellent in vitro activity against aerobic and anaerobic microorganisms, including gram-positive cocci, e.g., *E. faecium*, generally resistant to other β-lactams. Most strains of *Pseudomonas* and *Actinetobacter* are inhibited, whereas *S. maltophilia* is resistant. Anaerobes generally are highly susceptible. Meropenem, as indicated, has similar in vitro activity, with somewhat lesser activity against gram-positive cocci. Finally, aztreonam has an excellent activity against Enterobacteriaceae and *P. aeruginosa* but is totally inactive against gram-positive bacteria.

Mechanism of resistance

Mechanism of resistance is essentially related to PBP mutations. All three agents are poorly sensitive to β-lactamases.

Table 38.3 Pharmacokinetics, usual daily doses, and toxicities of oral cephalosporins

Drug	Bioavailibility (%)	Daily dose (g)	$t_{1/2}$	Notes: major route of elimination and untoward effects
Cephalexin	100	3.0	1	Renal elimination. Untoward effects: GI tract, allergic reactions.
Cephradine	95	3.0	1	Renal elimination. Untoward effects: GI tract, allergic reactions
Cefadroxil	85	2.0-3.0	1.5	Renal elimination. Untoward effects: GI tract, allergic reactions
Cefaclor	90	1.5-3.0	1	Renal elimination. Untoward effects: GI tract, allergic reactions, serum sickness
Cefprozil	90	1.0-1.5	1	Renal elimination. Untoward effects: GI tract, allergic reactions
Cefixime	<50	0.2-0.4	3.8	Renal elimination. Untoward effects: GI tract, allergic reactions
Cefuroxime-axetil	>50	1.5	2	Renal elimination. Untoward effects: GI tract, allergic reactions
Cefpodoxime proxetil	>50	0.8	2.8	Renal elimination. Untoward effects: GI tract, allergic reactions
Cefetamet-pivoxil	>50	1.0	3	Renal elimination. Untoward effects: GI tract, allergic reactions
Ceftibuten	70	0.4	2.5	Renal elimination. Untoward effects: GI tract, allergic reactions
Cefdinir	<50	0.6	2	Renal elimination. Untoward effects: GI tract, allergic reactions
Loracarbef	90	0.4-0.8	1	Renal elimination. Untoward effects: GI tract, allergic reactions

($t_{1/2}$ = elimination half-life in hours; GI tract = gastrointestinal tract, mainly diarrhea, nausea, vomiting.)

Table 38.4 Pharmacokinetics, usual daily doses, and toxicities of carbapenems and monopenems

Drug	Daily dose (g)	$t_{1/2}$	Notes: major elimination route and untoward effects
Imipenem (+ cilastatin)	1.5-3.0	1	In combination with cilastatin, higher renal concentrations. Untoward effects: GI tract, CNS intolerance (e.g., seizures, dizziness, nausea)
Meropenem	3.0 g	1	Renal elimination. Untoward effects: GI tract
Aztreonam	3.0-6.0	1	Renal elimination. Untoward effects: GI tract

($t_{1/2}$ = elimination half-life in hours; GI tract = gastrointestinal tract, mainly diarrhoea, nausea, vomiting.)

Pharmacokinetics, usual daily doses, and toxicities

In many hospitals, the use of carbapenems is restricted. Major indications are severe and/or nosocomial infections and infections in immunocompromised hosts (e.g., fever of unknown origin in neutropenia). Most frequent untoward effects (UEs) are loose bowels and diarrhea. Rare UEs include allergy, allergic neutropenia, a positive direct Coombs' test, and bleeding disorders (e.g., prolongation of the prothrombin time). Imipenem is always combined with cilastatin (an inhibitor of renal dipeptidase) to inhibit its renal metabolism. There is some evidence that cilastatin might have an additional nephroprotective effect (Tab. 38.4).

Major drug interactions of β-lactam antibiotics

Beta-lactams are not metabolized and generally are poorly protein bound, thus carrying a minimal risk of interactions. However, serious bleeding reactions have been reported with several of these agents, generally given parenterally at high doses. The mechanism appears to be related to hypoprothrombinemia, thrombocytopenia, and platelet dysfunction. This risk therefore requires caution in the concomitant use of parenteral β-lactams with anticoagulants.

β-LACTAMASE INHIBITORS

β-Lactamase inhibitors possess very little activity against the major clinically relevant bacteria. These agents are combined with other penicillins because they "protect" them against inactivation by β-lactamases produced by bacteria. At present, three inhibitors (all β-lactams) are available: clavulanic acid (CL) in fixed combination with amoxicillin (in most countries) and ticarcillin (in some countries), tazobactam (TZ) in fixed combination with piperacillin, and sulbactam (SU) generally in combination with ampicillin (for parenteral application) or with sultamicillin (for oral use). In some countries, sulbactam is also available as a free compound and can be combined with other β-lactams (such as piperacillin, mezlocillin, or cephalosporins). The inhibitors maintain the activity of the

Table 38.5 Site and characteristic of β-lactamases and sensitivity to β-lactamase inhibitors

Site of resistance	β–lactamase type	Bacteria	Inhibition by CL, SU, TZ,
Plasmid	TEM-1	*S. aureus*, *E. coli*, *Hemophilus* spp., *N. gonorrhoeae*, *Salmonella* spp., *Shigella* spp.	Yes
Plasmid	TEM-2	*E. coli*	Yes
Plasmid	TEM-3 to 8	*Klebsiella* spp.	Yes
Plasmid	SHV-1	*Klebsiella* spp.	Yes
Plasmid	SHV-2 to 5	*Enterobacteriaceae*	Yes
Plasmid	OXA-1, -2, and -3	*E. coli*	Variable
Plasmid	PSE-1, -2, and -3	*Pseudomonas* spp.	Variable
Chromosomal	Type 1a	*Enterobacter* spp., *Citrobacter* spp., *Serratia* spp.	No
Chromosomal	Type 1d	*Pseudomonas* spp.	No
Chromosomal	Type IV, K1	*Klebsiella* spp., *Bacteroides* spp.	Yes

(CL= clavulanic acid; SU= sulbactam; TZ= tazobactam.)

β-lactam against most β-lactamase-producing bacteria (Tab. 38.5) and, for example, render penicillin-resistant (but oxacillin-sensitive) staphylococci sensitive to penicillin.

The pharmacokinetic properties (absorption after oral application, elimination half-life, etc.) of the inhibitors is very similar to those of the combination agent, and the dosing is influenced by this latter. Because of their broader spectrum of activity, the inhibitors are indicated in infections where resistance is frequently due to β-lactamase production, e.g., in a hospital setting or in postoperative infections. As with the penicillins, the most frequent UEs are gastrointestinal tract problems and allergy.

AMINOGLYCOSIDES

Mode of action and classification

Aminoglycosides consist of two or more amino sugars joined by a glycoside linkage to a hexose nucleus, generally in the central position. These drugs originally were derived from *Streptomyces* and, later on (e.g., amikacin) were developed by semisynthetic technologies. Aminoglycosides act by interfering with cellular protein synthesis by altering the fidelity of translation of mRNA at the ribosomal level. However, it is as yet unclear how alterations in protein synthesis may lead to such a rapidly lethal effect on cells. Since this is in large part accounted for by cellular swelling, which depends on the concentration of antibiotic, it is hypothesized that in addition to altering mRNA translation, aminoglycosides may be transported into cells by an energy-dependent mechanism in two phases. The first phase leads to contact between the aminoglycoside and polysomes, thus directly interfering with protein synthesis; aberrant proteins, being inserted into cell membranes, will then lead to altered permeability and further enhance aminoglycoside transport. In the second phase, which is energy-dependent, aminoglycoside transport is linked directly to cytoplasmic membrane disruption and ensuing cell death.

Spectrum of activity

Aminoglycosides typically display a spectrum of activity encompassing major gram-negative bacteria, including *Enterobacter* spp., *E. coli, K. pneumoniae, P. mirabilis, Providencia, Pseudomonas,* and *Serratia* spp., as well as major gram-positive cocci, including *S. aureus* and *Enterococcus faecalis.* This type of spectrum encourages wide use of aminoglycosides in the hospital setting and, unfortunately, also in outpatient treatment, with the consequence of spreading plasmid-mediated resistance. Aminoglycosides are mostly recommended in combination with parenteral penicillins or cephalosporins in severe infections because such combinations are expected to be synergistic, although in vitro data are available only for some of the compounds against limited species of pathogens. Although clinical proof of synergy is limited, most experts would recommend aminoglycosides in combination with β-lactams in severe sepsis, septic shock, and infections due to "less sensitive" organisms such as *Pseudomonas* and *Enterobacter* species. Streptomycin is presently recommended only for the treatment of tuberculosis, and spectinomycin is recommended only in gonococcal infections.

Mechanism of resistance

Aminoglycosides undergo enzymatically determined changes in their structure, carried out by phosphorylating, adenylating, or acetylating enzymes, that affect hydroxyl or amino groups in the molecules. These enzymatic processes lead to antimicrobial ineffectiveness and are acquired primarily by conjugation or DNA transfer as plasmids or resistance transfer factors. Wide diffusion of plasmids has led to widespread active resistance by major gram-negative bacteria. The development of semisynthetic aminoglycosides, such as amikacin, has somewhat improved resistance, but it is still prudent to combine the use of aminoglycosides with drugs acting via different mechanisms (e.g., β-lactams) for severe gram-negative infections.

Other mechanisms of resistance are secondary to failure of the drugs to penetrate the cytoplasmic inner membrane (permeability barrier), which occurs in particular in

Table 38.6 Pharmacokinetics, usual daily doses, and toxicities of aminoglycosides

Drug	Usual daily dose	$t_{1/2}$	Notes: major elimination route and untoward effects
Gentamicin	2-3 mg/kg	2	Renal elimination, low CSF penetration. Untoward effects: nephrotoxicity, ototoxicity
Tobramycin	2-5 mg/kg	2	Renal elimination, low CSF penetration. Untoward effects: nephrotoxicity, ototoxicity
Netilimicin	2-5 mg/kg	2	Renal elimination, low CSF penetration. Untoward effects: nephrotoxicity, ototoxicity
Amikacin	10-15 mg/kg	2.3	Renal elimination, low CSF penetration. Untoward effects: nephrotoxicity, ototoxicity
Streptomycin	15 mg/kg	2.5	Renal elimination. Untoward effects: neurotoxicity and ototoxicity
Spectinomycin	2.0-4.0 g	2.5	Renal elimination. Untoward effects: headache, nausea, vomiting
Kanamycin	2.0-4.0 g	NA	Recommended for topical use only
Neomycin	2.0-4.0 g	NA	Recommended for topical use only
Paromomycin	1.0-2.0 g	NA	Recommended for topical/enteral use only

($t_{1/2}$ = elimination half-life in hours; CSF = cerebrospinal fluid levels in case of inflamed meninges are higher; NA = not applicable.)

Table 38.7 Classification of sulfonamides according to their serum elimination half-life in hours

Group	Generic	$t_{1/2}$	Protein binding (%)
Short-acting	Sulfacarbamide	2-3	5-7
	Sulfisomidine	7	50-80
	Sulfisoxazole	6	85
Intermediate	Sulfadiazine	8-13	30-45
	Sulfaphenazole	11	99
	Sulfamethoxazole	9-11	70-80
Long-acting	Sulfadimethoxine	40	80-99
	Sulfamethoxydiazine	38	70-85
	Sulfamethoxypyridazine	36	80-95
	Sulfaperin	37	70-95
Ultra-long-acting	Sulfalene	60-80	45-80
Nonabsorbable after oral dosing	Formo-sulfathiazole	NA	NA
	Sulfaguanidine		
	Sulfaguanole		
	Sulfaloxylic acid		
Topical	Mafenide (sulfamylon)	–	–

($t_{1/2}$ = elimination half-life in hours; NA = not applicable.)

bacteria growing under anaerobic conditions, as well as resistance from alterations in ribosomal structure, resulting from single-step mutations in, for example, *E. coli*. This last mechanism is well known from the initial development of streptomycin.

Pharmacokinetics, usual daily doses, and toxicities

Aminoglycosides are parenteral antibiotics given iv o im; however, kanamycin, neomycin, and paramomycin are not recommended for parenteral application and are used as oral "topical antimicrobials" because they are not absorbed in the gastrointestinal tract. Studies have shown that despite the short half-life, the daily dose can be given just once as a short infusion. However, this form of treatment has not been investigated sufficiently in many clinical situations. Patient groups for whom such evidence is not well established include: pregnant women; patients with burns, ascites, or renal failure; and patients with meningitis, endocarditis, or osteomyelitis. Aminoglycosides are nephrotoxic and ototoxic drugs and thus should be used with special precautions. Regular monitoring of serum drug levels is recommended if high doses are used or if the drugs are used in patients with a potential for renal failure or for longer than 5 days. Very little is known about the safety of this approach in neutropenic hosts, especially those with *P. aeruginosa* infections (Tab. 38.6). Care should also be given for the frequent combination with β-lactams (see above).

Major drug interactions

Aminoglycosides are not metabolized and are excreted only by the renal route. The risk of metabolic-kinetic interactions is therefore minimal. In view of the potential nephro- and/or ototoxicity of these agents, care should be taken in their combined use with loop diuretics (e.g., ethacrynic acid and furosemide).

SULFONAMIDES AND TRIMETHOPRIM DERIVATIVES

Mode of action and classification

Sulfonamides were the first antimicrobials used successfully as systemic agents for the treatment of infections. Ever since then, a large number of derivatives have been developed, and many of them are still in use. In the early days of development, it became apparent very quickly that the antimicrobial properties, protein binding, and tolerance differed widely among the derivatives. Major UEs were and still are allergic reactions, hepatotoxicity, crystalluria, and polyneuritis. Today, sulfonamides generally are used in combination with trimethoprim derivatives because the combination has been shown to be more potent in vitro and is active also against many bacteria that are resistant to sulfonamides. Whether the combination prevents the development of resistance is a matter of controversy. Based on clinical applications, the sulfonamides can be grouped according to their serum elimination half-life (Tab. 38.7). Agents such as sulfacetamide, silver sulfadiazine, and particularly, mafenide (amino-*p*-toluene-sulfonamide) are employed only for topical use. Mafenide acetate cream is particularly effective for the local treatment of burns, preventing colonization by a wide variety of gram-positive and gram-negative bacteria.

Sulfonamides act as classic competitive analogues of *para*-aminobenzoic acid (PABA), preventing normal bacterial use of PABA for the synthesis of folic acid. They are commonly used in fixed-dose combinations with folate reductase antagonists, the major one being trimethoprim (other antagonists, e.g., tetroxoprim, are now seldom used).

Trimethoprim is available as a mono compound or mostly in combination with a sulfonamide. After oral application, it is almost completely absorbed. The serum elimination half-life is 12 hours, and it is 45% protein bound and eliminated mainly via the kidneys. The most common combination is with sulfamethoxazole (cotrimoxazole). Other sulfonamides available in combination with trimethoprim are sulfamerazine, sulfametrol and sulfadiazine.

Most combination products (e.g., sulfonamide derivative + trimethoprim) are available for both oral and parenteral application. They are the treatment of choice for infections due to *Pneumocystis carinii* (seen almost exclusively in immunocompromised or HIV-infected patients; see Chap. 42) and one of the well-accepted alternatives for the treatment of urinary tract infections and salmonellosis. Their use in lower respiratory tract infections (other than *P. carinii*) is controversial.

Spectrum of activity

Use of sulfonamides is now essentially restricted to sulfa derivatives for the treatment of inflammatory bowel disease (see Chap. 35) or sulfonamides for topical use, e.g., sulfacetamide, silver sulfadiazine, and mafedine (sulfamylon). Sulfadoxine, in view of its very long elimination half-life (7-9 days), is used in combination with pyrimethamine in the prophylaxis and treatment of malaria (see Chap. 42).

Mechanism of resistance

The mechanism of resistance to sulfonamides is by random mutation and selection or through transfer of resistance by plasmids. There are numerous possibilities, ranging from altered enzyme systems using PABA, to an increased capacity for inactivation, to development of alternative metabolic pathways for the synthesis of essential metabolites, to increased production of drug antagonists.

Major drug interactions

Sulfonamides may potentiate oral anticoagulants, sulfonylurea antidiabetics, and hydantoin anticonvulsants, primarily by inhibiting metabolism. This effect is most marked with the longer-acting agents. Trimethoprim inhibits sodium channels in the distal kidney tubule and may lead to hyperkalemia or hyponatremia when combined with thiazide diuretics. Severe hyperkalemia has been noted particularly in the elderly and in AIDS patients.

TETRACYCLINES

Mode of action and classification

Tetracyclines are bacteriostatic antibiotics that classically inhibit bacterial protein synthesis by binding to the 30S ribosomal subunit and preventing access of aminoacyl tRNA to the acceptor A site on the mRNA-ribosome complex. Antibiotics gain access to ribosomes by passive diffusion or active transport by an energy-dependent system. The additional possibility of impairment of protein synthesis in mammalian cells has been used, apparently with some advantage, for the treatment of immunologically mediated diseases, such as rheumatoid arthritis, e.g. by the use of minocycline (see Chap. 45).

There are four major tetracycline derivatives: tetracycline, oxytetracycline, doxycycline, and minocycline (Tab. 38.8). The major differences among these derivatives are of a pharmacokinetic nature, since the antibacterial spectrum is very similar, with little differences in potency against certain bacterial species. All oral derivatives should not be coadministered with antacids or milk because the absorption of tetracyclines in the gastrointestinal tract is markedly reduced.

Table 38.8 Pharmacokinetics, usual daily doses, and toxicities of major tetracyclines

Drug	Mode of application and dose	Bioavailability (%)	$t_{1/2}$	Notes: major elimination route and untoward effects
Tetracycline	Oral 0.25-0.5 g tid	30-40	8-9	Renal and biliary elimination; sufficient CSF penetration. Untoward effects: GI tract, photosensitivity, increased intracranial pressure, if given as iv bolus neuromuscular block
Oxytetracycline	Oral 0.25-0.5 g tid	30-40	8-10	Renal and biliary elimination; sufficient CSF penetration. Untoward effects: GI tract, photosensitivity, increased intracranial pressure, if given as iv bolus neuromuscular block
Doxycycline	Oral or iv 0.1 g qd or bid	75	16-18	Renal and biliary elimination; sufficient CSF penetration. Untoward effects: GI tract, photosensitivity, increased intracranial pressure, if given as iv bolus neuromuscular block
Minocycline	Oral 0.25 g qd	Almost 100	12-15	Renal and biliary elimination; sufficient CSF penetration. Untoward effects: GI tract, photosensitivity

($t_{1/2}$ = elimination half-life in hours; CSF = sufficient cerebrospinal fluid levels in case of inflamed meninges; GI tract = gastrointestinal tract, mainly diarrhea, nausea, vomiting.)

These agents also are contraindicated in pregnancy and in children younger than 12 years of age because of the danger of discoloration of the teeth.

BASIS OF ANTIBIOTIC THERAPY FOR MAJOR INFECTIONS • 401

Spectrum of activity

Tetracyclines generally are effective against major gram-positive microorganisms, less so against gram-negative species. Activity against *S. pneumoniae, N. gonorrhoeae,* and *N. meningitidis,* although still significant, is plagued by frequent resistance, and tetracyclines are not indicated for any of these infections. Such is the case also for most highly pathogenic gram-negative organisms (e.g., *Pseudomonas* and others). In contrast, tetracyclines retain significant activity against anaerobes such as *Brucella,* where they are the drugs of first choice, *H. ducreyi* (chancroid), and *Vibrio cholerae.* They inhibit the growth of major intracellular organisms including *Helicobacter pylori, Chlamydia, Mycoplasma,* and others.

Mechanism of resistance

Resistance to tetracyclines is generally plasmid-mediated and inducible. The major mechanisms are related to decreased accumulation because of reduced antibiotic influx or acquisition of an energy-dependent efflux pathway. Other apparently less significant mechanisms may be related to decreased access to the ribosome because of the presence of ribosome-protective proteins or enzymatic inactivation. Because of huge differences in resistance in terms of other frequent pathogens, local epidemiologic data should be consulted before prescribing tetracyclines.

In view of the prolonged elimination half-life and wide distribution, minocycline is frequently used for a multi-bacterial chronic disease such as acne.

Major drug interactions

Long- acting tetracyclines, e.g., minocycline, may exert a mild drug-inducing effect, thus reducing the effectiveness of concomitantly given medications. Tetracyclines are powerful heavy-metal chelators, reducing calcium absorption and, by being deposited in the skeleton, potentially leading to tooth discoloration.

QUINOLONES

Mode of action and classification

Nalidixic acid was the first quinolone to be introduced into clinical use. Because of its limited spectrum of activity to gram-negative organisms only, poor pharmacokinetic properties, rapid development of resistance, and poor tolerance, its use has dwindled nowadays. Other derivatives such as cinoxacin, rosoxacin, and pipemidic acid followed. They are used mainly for urinary tract infections, but since the development of fluorinated quinolones, markedly more active not only against gram-negative organisms but also against many clinically relevant gram-positive organisms, their use also has fallen. Newer fluorinated quinolones, such as

---

Table 38.9 Pharmacokinetics, usual daily doses, and toxicities of quinolones

Drug	Mode of application and dose	Bioavailability (oral, %)	$t_{1/2}$	Notes: major elimination route and untoward effects
Cinoxacin	Oral 1.0 g	80-90	1.5	Renal. Untoward effects: GI tract, CNS, phototoxicity, recommended for urinary tract infections only
Ciprofloxacin	Oral and iv 0.25-1.5 g	60-70	4-5	Renal. Untoward effects: GI tract, CNS, phototoxicity, interaction with theophylline
Enoxacin	Oral 0.25 g bid	79	6	Renal. Untoward effects: GI tract, CNS, phototoxicity, more pronounced interaction with theophylline
Fleroxacin	Oral and iv 0.4 g qd or bid	100	9-11	Hepatic. Untoward effects: GI tract, CNS, phototoxicity, interaction with theophylline
Levofloxacin	Oral and iv 0.5-1.0 g	100	7	Renal. Untoward effects: GI tract, CNS, phototoxicity, no relevant interaction with theophylline
Lomefloxacin	Oral 0.4 g	95	8	Renal. Untoward effects: GI tract, CNS, higher rate of phototoxicity, interaction with theophylline
Nalidixic acid	Oral 3-4 g	60-80	4-5	Renal. Untoward effects: GI tract, CNS, phototoxicity, rapid development of resistance under treatment; use is not recommended any more
Ofloxacin	Oral and iv 0.2-0.4 g	100	7	Renal. Untoward effects: GI tract, CNS, phototoxicity, no relevant interaction with theophylline
Pefloxacin	Oral and iv 0.4 g	100	10	Hepatic. Untoward effects: GI tract, CNS, higher rate of phototoxicity, interaction with theophylline
Moxifloxacin	Oral 0.4 g	91	12	Hepatic and renal. Untoward effects: GI tract, CNS, low incidence of phototoxicity, no relevant interaction with theophylline

($t_{1/2}$ = elimination half-life in hours; GI tract = gastrointestinal tract, mainly diarrhea, nausea, vomiting; CNS = central nervous system: seizures, insomnia, acute psychotic reaction.)

ciprofloxacin and ofloxacin and many others, show markedly enhanced activity against gram-positive cocci. Most are available both for parenteral and oral administration (Tab. 38.9).

Quinolones primarily affect topoisomerase II (DNA gyrase, TOP II) in gram-negative organisms and topoisomerase IV (TOP IV) in gram-positive organisms. These enzymes are responsible for the introduction of negative supercoils into DNA (TOP II) or separation of plasmids and daughter chromosomes after duplication (TOP IV). Negative supercoiling allows tight packing of the DNA and is necessary for transcription, replication, and repair of DNA. TOP II and TOP IV are highly homologous in structure, mechanism, and function. For the introduction of negative supercoils or the separation of two DNA strands, one strand (so-called gate strand) has to be separated completely from the other to pass through the break; the break is then resealed. Quinolones act on the A subunit of TOP II or TOP IV that carries out the strand-cutting function. Inhibition of TOP II and TOP IV occurs at concentrations that correlate well with those required to inhibit bacterial growth (0.1–10 µg/ml). Eukaryotic cells, because of their different organization of DNA, are poorly affected by quinolones.

Spectrum of activity

Quinolones have bactericidal activity against most common gram-negative bacteria, particularly those seen in urinary tract infections. For this reason, the earlier developed molecules, e.g., nalidixic acid or pefloxacin, are still used essentially only for this indication. The newer fluoroquinolones, e.g., ofloxacin, which are still rapidly bactericidal in vitro, are considerably more potent against gram-negative species, e.g., *E. coli,* as well as

Salmonella, Shigella, and *Enterobacter* spp.

In general, activity against gram-positive organisms is limited. However, the newer fluoroquinolones, e.g., sparfloxacin, moxifloxacin, and levofloxacin, have good activity against staphylococci, including methicillin-resistant strains, and have satisfactory activity against *Streptococcus pneumoniae*. Interestingly, several intracellular bacteria are inhibited by fluoroquinolones, including *Chlamydia, Mycoplasma, Legionella,* and *Brucella*. These products are also active against atypical mycobacteria, including *M. kansasii* and *M. fortuitum*. Some of the newer quinolones, e.g., gatifloxacin, gemifloxacin and moxifloxacin, are active in vitro against anaerobes.

Mechanism of resistance

Quinolones, because they are fully synthetic molecules and thus "not recognized" by bacteria, may be considered as active against all bacterial species. However, clinically relevant resistance has emerged rapidly among methicillin-resistant *S. aureus* and recently also *E. coli,* as well as other gram-negative organisms. Basically, two different mechanisms of resistance that affect all quinolones are known: target modification and active efflux. Point mutations at residues that are well conserved among various species in the so-called quinolone resistance-determining region of the A subunit of TOP II and TOP IV lead to a decrease in the affinity of the drug for the enzyme-substrate complex. Point mutations in the B subunit also have a role in decreased binding. Active efflux by multidrug-resistance pumps, e.g., NorA (staphylococci) and AcrAB (*E. coli*), reduce intracellular drug concentrations substantially. In many clinical isolates, both mechanisms are active. The incidence of resistant mutants is lower with the newer quinolones, e.g., ciprofloxacin, versus the older compounds, e.g., nalidixic acid. Most anaerobic microorganisms are resistant to floroquinolones, except for the case of the newer fluoroquinolones, such as moxifloxacin, and levofloxacin.

Table 38.10 Clinical classification of quinolones

Group	Mode of application and clinical indication	Derivative
I	Only orally applicable and useful only in uncomplicated urinary tract infection; use of this group is presently discouraged	Nalidixic acid, cinoxacin, pipemidic acid
II	Only orally applicable and recommended for limited indications: only urinary tract infections, gonorrhea only urinary tract infections, gonorrhea, and enteritis only pneumonia community acquired pneumonia, sinusitis, AECB, SSSI	Enoxacin, pefloxacin Norfloxacin Sparfloxacin Moxifloxacin
III	Oral and parenteral application; in highest dose may be used in severe systemic infections	Ciprofloxacin, fleroxacin, levofloxacin, ofloxacin
Under development	Classification at the present time not possible	Gatifloxacin[1], gemifloxacin, sitafloxacin, moxifloxacin

[1] Launched in the US, in Europe under development.

Quinolones are well absorbed after oral administration, and many of the untoward effects are common to all of them, but the rates are different (Tab. 38.9). Because cartilage damage has been seen in animal studies, all quinolones are contraindicated in pregnancy and in young people. These drugs also should be used with caution in patients with a history of seizures and insomnia. The daily dose depends mainly on the site of infection. In patients with altered renal excretion, lower doses are recommended for urinary tract infections, and generally higher (parenteral) doses are necessary for the treatment of systemic infections, e.g., of the lower respiratory tract. Coadministration with antacids, ferrous sulfate, and sulcralfate may result in lower absorption from the gastrointestinal tract, and an adequate time interval between quinolone administration and administration of the aforementioned drugs should be observed. Use of trovafloxacin has been associated with severe liver impairment, and the drug has been withdrawn from the world market. Based on clinical indications, the quinolones may be classified into different groups (Tab. 38.10).

Major drug interactions

Fluoroquinolone absorption can be reduced significantly by divalent or trivalent cation formulations, e.g., Al/Mg-containing antacids and, in particular, oral iron preparations. These can, at times, lead to treatment failures. Such interactions should be minimized by staggering dosing of the fluoroquinolone and the interacting agents. Some quinolones, in particular enoxacin, ciprofloxacin, and to a lesser extent, norfloxacin, inhibit the metabolism of theophylline by CYP1A2, resulting in theophylline accumulation and toxicity. The newer fluoroquinolones do so to a lesser extent. Coadministration of cimetidine may aggravate the interaction (see Chap. 6). There are case reports of pharmacodynamic interactions of fluoquinolones with cyclosporine A and tacrolimus, resulting in nephrotoxicity.

MACROLIDES, LINCOSAMIDES, FUSIDIC ACID, QUINUPRISTIN/DALFOPRISTIN

This is a group of heterogeneous antibacterial agents that are active mainly against gram-positive cocci and, in the case of macrolides, also against some of the so-called atypical pathogens, such as *Mycoplasma, Chlamydia,* and *Legionella.* All macrolides and lincosamides have a similar profile of UEs, are cross-resistant, and are cross-allergic. The newer compounds, e.g., azithromycin, clarithromycin, and roxithromycin, have better pharmacokinetic parameters after oral administration than erythromycin; however, not all are available for parenteral application. Spiramycin is used mainly for treating toxoplasmosis in pregnancy and rarely for other indications.

Macrolides are bactericidal antibiotics that inhibit protein synthesis by binding reversibly to the 50S ribosomal subunit. This site of action is shared with chloramphenicol (see below), and there may be competition between the two drug classes. Accumulation of macrolides occurs to a far larger extent (about 100 times more) in the case of gram-negative organisms. These large molecules permeate cells far better in the nonionized form, and a higher antimicrobial activity is observed at an alkaline pH.

Fusidic acid, a steroid molecule that is poorly absorbable orally, is still used in combination with other drugs in severe staphylococcal infections.

Spectrum of activity

Macrolides typically are used as alternatives to β-lactams for major gram-positive bacteria, e.g., *S. pyogenes* and *S. pneumoniae,* although resistance to macrolides appears to be increasing. Staphylococci generally are sensitive to erythromycin and major macrolides, but inhibitory concentrations are relatively high. Furthermore, there appears to be cross-resistance among major macrolides. On the other hand, the significant tissue penetration of these highly lipid-soluble molecules allows them to reach very high tissue concentrations, even in the presence of relatively low plasma drug levels.

Activity against most aerobic enteral gram-negative bacilli is essentially negative, with the exception of *N. meningitidis* and, particularly, *N. gonorrhoeae.* The elevated tissue and bacterial penetration makes them drugs of first choice against *Pasteurella multocida, Borrelia* spp., and *Bordetella pertussis,* whereas resistance is common for anaerobes such as *B. fragilis.* They are again drugs of first choice against intracellular bacteria such as *Legionella pneumophila, Chlamydia trachomatis,* and atypical mycobacteria such as *M. kansasii* and *M. intracellulare.* Finally, macrolides are now included routinely in combination therapy against *Campylobacter* spp., particularly *H. pylori.* For this indication (see Chap. 33), clarithromycin now has the widest acceptance. Newer agents such as azithromycin, although somewhat less active than erythromycin against the gram-positive organisms, display a more significant activity against *H. influenzae* and *Campylobacter* spp., as well as against *Pasteurella multocida, L. pneumophila, B. burgdorferi,* and *Fusobacterium* spp. In view of the very significant tissue penetration, the achievement of serum concentrations of 0.2 to 4 μg/ml is generally adequate for antibacterial activity. The activity of fusidic acid is limited to severe staphylococcal infections.

Mechanism of resistance

Resistance to macrolides is believed to result from three types of plasmid-mediated alterations: decreased cell permeability to the agents, production of a methylating enzyme, inducible or constitutive, that modifies the ribosomal target, and finally, hydrolysis of macrolides by specific esterases in Enterobacteriaceae. There is, furthermore, the possibility that the bacterial target is modified by mutations, and an efflux mechanism also may result in resistance.

Major drug interactions

Macrolides are CYP3A4 substrates, and their metabolism can be inhibited by drugs as cimetidine (also associated with short-term deafness when given with high-dose erythromycin) and ritonavir, used for AIDS infection (see Chap. 40). The use of macrolides, conversely, can significantly increase blood levels of drugs handled by this microsomal system, particularly nonsedating antihistamines, cisapride, and others (see Chap. 6). Dose-dependent prolongations of the QTc interval and, rarely, torsades de pointes have been seen with these drug combinations. Inhibition of CYP3A4 metabolism also has been associated with carbamazepine toxicity.

Quinupristin/dalfopristin

A special case among drugs chemically related to macrolides is that of streptogramin antibiotics. These consist of two types of molecules, belonging to groups A and B. The group B molecule quinupristin and the group A molecule dalfopristin are the first water-soluble semisynthetic streptogramins, now available in the United States and soon to enter major markets (Synercid, at 30:70 ratio of each component). Quinupristin/dalfopristin (Q/D) acts at the ribosomal level, and the two components affect different steps of ribosomal metabolism, thus theoretically leading to an extremely low risk of resistance (see Tab. 38.11). In view of the high water solubility, the combination is currently used intravenously for major infections not responding to glycopeptide antibiotics. Such is the case, particularly, for gram-positive enterococci (e.g., *E.*

Table 38.11 Pharmacokinetics, usual daily doses, and toxicities of macrolides, lincosamides, and quinupristin/dalfopristin

Drug	Mode of application and dose	Bioavailability (oral, %)	$t_{1/2}$	Notes: major elimination route and untoward effects
Azithromycin	Oral and parenteral 0.5 g	35%	>48	3-5% of the dose appears in urine in the first 24 h; extremely slow elimination rate. Untoward effects similar to those of erythromycin
Erythromycin	Oral and parenteral 0.5-1.5 g	20[1]	2	Absorption rate differs from derivative to derivative; 20-30% biliary elimination; after oral administration 2-5% appears in urine, 12-15% after iv dosing. Untoward effects: GI tract; intrahepatic cholestasis (estolate derivative); ototoxicity
Clarithromycin	Oral and parenteral 0.5 g	50	4-5	Fecal elimination, 30% appears in urine. Untoward effects similar to those of erythromycin
Dirithromycin	Oral 0.5 g	10	40	Fecal elimination, 1-2% appears in urine. Untoward effects similar to those of erythromycin
Roxithromycin	Oral 0.3 g	60	10	Fecal elimination, <10% appears in urine. Untoward effects similar to those of erythromycin
Spiramycin	Oral 1.0-1.5 g	?	2-3	Fecal elimination, 5-10% appears in urine. Untoward effects similar to those of erythromycin
Lincomycin	Oral and parenteral 7.5 mg/kg	40	4-5	Metabolism in liver, 10% appears in urine after oral administration, 38% after parenteral application. Untoward effects: GI tract, mainly diarrhea, pseudomembranous colitis (*C. difficile*), cardiotoxicity if rapidly infused
Clindamycin	Oral and parenteral 1.5-3 g	80	2-4	Metabolism in liver; 15-35% appears in urine after oral administration, 20-40% after parenteral application. Untoward effects: GI tract, mainly diarrhea, pseudomembranous colitis (*C. difficile*), cardiotoxicity if rapidly infused
Fusidic acid	Oral and parenteral 1.0-1.5 g	?	4-6	Metabolism in liver, 1% appears in urine. Untoward effects: GT tract, hyperbilirubinemia
Quinupristin /dalfopristin	Parenteral; possibly oral 7.5 mg/kg q8h or q12h	—	1	Biliary elimination (quinupristin excreted unchanged, dalfopristin metabolized). Untoward effects: venous intolerance, arthralgia/myalgia, and elevated transaminases in lesser percentages; no alterations in hematologic or other biochemical parameters

($t_{1/2}$ = elimination half-life in hours; GI tract = gastrointestinal tract, mainly diarrhea, nausea, vomiting; CNS = central nervous system: seizures, insomnia, acute psychotic reaction.)
[1]Succinate derivative.

faecium, but not *E. faecalis,* which is resistant to Q/D); the drug is currently undergoing an extensive evaluation in order to determine the validity of a more generalized approach to, for example, staphylococci. An oral form of streptogramin is being developed, apparently with satisfactory activity.

Q/D is currently used for the parenteral treatment of severe glycopeptide-resistant enterococcal infections at daily doses of 7.5 mg/kg. The elimination half-life is similar for the two components, i.e., approximately 1 hour for quinupristin and 0.4 to 0.5 hour for dalfopristin. Both compounds are eliminated primarily through the bile into the feces, quinupristin being excreted mainly unchanged and dalfopristin being metabolized extensively. Toxicity is mainly related to venous intolerance (5% of the patients), followed by arthralgia/myalgia and elevated transaminases in lesser percentages. No alterations in hematologic or other biochemical parameters have been noted. Association of Q/D with cyclosporine A has led to marked elevations (up to 3-fold) in cyclosporine blood levels.

GLYCOPEPTIDES

Only two relevant glycopeptide derivatives are available for clinical use: vancomycin and teicoplanin. They are active only against gram-positive bacteria and are drugs of choice for the treatment of infections caused by staphylococci that are resistant to methicillin (oxacillin) and of pseudomembranous enterocolitis caused by *Clostridium difficile* toxin.

Mode of action

Glycopeptides act in a similar way as penicillins by inhibiting the synthesis of the cell wall in sensitive bacteria, particularly by binding the D-alanyl-D-alanine terminus of cell wall precursor units. The drugs are thus rapidly bactericidal for dividing microorganisms. The extreme potency of these drugs and their toxicity do not indicate a wide use outside the most sensitive strains, particularly *S. aureus.*

Spectrum of activity

Vancomycin and teicoplanin are active primarily against gram-positive bacteria, particularly *S. aureus* and *S. epidermidis,* including strains resistant to methicillin. There is the possibility of a synergism between vancomycin and aminoglycosides in the case of more severe infections. The susceptibility of other gram-positive strains is generally of clinical value only for *S. viridans,* which is highly susceptible, as are most *Enterococcus* spp. In this latter case, vancomycin has not been bactericidal and needs the addition of a synergistic aminoglycoside. Plasmid-mediated resistance in gram-negative cocci, may be transferable and should be evaluated with care in the hospital setting. Of concern is the appearance of vancomycin-non-susceptible staphylococci (Tab. 38.12).

Mechanism of resistance

There are three major types of resistance. The VAN A phenotype is inducible, and VAN B is constitutive, as is VAN C, this last of lesser clinical significance. The VAN A phenotype confers resistance to both teicoplanin and vancomycin and has been identified particularly in gram-positive enterococci (e.g., *E. faecalis*). The VAN B phenotype, generally of a lower level, may be induced by vancomycin, maintaining sensitivity to teicoplanin. Finally, the VAN C phenotype again confers only resistance to vancomycin but is of minor significance.

Side effects

Vancomycin is associated with hypersensitivity reactions, e.g., chills, rash, and fever. The intravenous injection may be followed by significant flushing (red man syndrome). The more significant secondary effect of glycopeptide antibiotics is auditory impairment, not always permanent, and nephrotoxicity. These latter effects are evident to a lesser extent with teicoplanin.

Table 38.12 Pharmacokinetics, usual daily doses, and toxicities of glycopeptide antibiotics

Drug	Mode of application and dose	Bioavailability (oral, %)	$t_{1/2}$	Notes: major elimination route and untoward effects
Vancomycin	iv infusion 2 g	–	6	Renal elimination; CSF penetration 10-20% in inflamed meninges. Untoward effects: fever, uriticaria (so-called red man syndrome, if infused rapidly), oto- and nephrotoxicity
Vancomycin	po 0.5-0.1 g	<10	NA	Not absorbed after oral application; oral administration in *C. difficile* toxin mediated enterocolitis
Teicoplanin	iv or im 7.5-15 mg/kg	–	>70	Renal elimination; no CSF penetration. Untoward effects: uriticaria (no red man syndrome, as in case of vancomycin)

($t_{1/2}$ = elimination half-life in hours; CSF = cerebrospinal fluid concentration; NA = not applicable)

Major drug interactions

As in the case of aminoglycosides, glycopeptides, being nonmetabolized and only undergoing renal excretion, have a minimal risk of interactions. However, in view of the potential for oto- and nephrotoxicity, caution should be used in the concomitant administration of loop diuretics or aminoglycoside antibiotics.

CHLORAMPHENICOL

Chloramphenicol is an antibiotic originally produced by *Streptomyces venezuelae* and is now available by chemical synthesis. It is widely used, particularly in the third world, because of a broad spectrum of activity that includes anaerobic infections, rickettsial diseases, brucellosis, and typhoid fever, as well as in view of its very low cost.

Mode of action

Chloramphenicol (CAF) inhibits protein synthesis in bacteria by binding reversibly to the 50S ribosomal subunit, thus preventing the binding of the amino acid–containing end of aminoacyl tRNA. The interaction between peptidyltransferase and the amino acid substrate cannot occur, and peptide bond formation is inhibited, thus arresting bacterial growth. The site of action is near that of macrolide antibiotics, that are antagonized by concomitant CAF treatment. The possibility of a modest activity on mammalian ribosomes explains the significant risk of hematologic toxicity, namely, aplastic anemia, that has curtailed wider use of CAF.

Mechanism of resistance

Resistance of gram-positive and gram-negative microorganisms is plasmid-mediated by at least three types of acetyltransferases. Prevalence of resistance may be as high as 50% or more in some hospitals.

Spectrum of activity

CAF possesses a fairly wide spectrum of activity, including gram-negative organisms, particularly *N. gonorrhoeae* and *H. influenzae,* where the drug is primarily bacteriostatic, although it may become bactericidal at high concentrations. Most anaerobic bacteria and gram-positive cocci are inhibited at concentrations achievable with standard doses of the drug, whereas high concentrations are required for *S. pyogenes* or *S. pneumoniae*. Among major Enterobacteriaceae, resistance is relatively common, and the drug is now of lesser significance, except for *S. typhus* and *V. colerae* infections and shigellosis. In underdeveloped countries, CAF is used mainly for anaerobic infections and typhoid fever, where clinical improvement is rapid at doses of 1 g four times daily for 2 to 3 weeks, and bacterial meningitis due to *H. influenzae,* rickettsial diseases, and brucellosis as an alternative to the tetracyclines.

Pharmacokinetics, toxicity, and major drug interactions

CAF is well absorbed after oral administration, eventually after hydrolysis of the prodrug (generally palmitate ester). Peak concentrations occur after 2 to 3 hours, and the half-life is around 4 hours, unchanged in the case of renal failure, whereas it may be raised in liver insufficiency. CAF use has been associated with bone marrow toxicity, with a low incidence (approximately 1 in 30,000 or more courses of therapy). Aplastic anemia accounts for more than 70% of the cases. Mortality from this side effect is higher the longer the interval between the last dose of the drug and the appearance of symptoms. This risk should not contraindicate use in situations where the drug is necessary but should caution against use in undefined situations.

CAF is an irreversible inhibitor of all major CYP 450 enzymes and may prolong the half-life of a variety of drugs, including anticoagulants, phenytoin, sulfonylureas, etc. Severe toxicity and death may follow lack of recognition of these potential interactions. Metabolism of CAF is conversely affected by major drug inducers, including antiepileptics and rifampin, which may markedly reduce the antibacterial activity of this agent.

RIFAMYCINS

To the group of ansamycins belong two clinically important compounds: rifampin (rifampicin) and rifabutin. Whereas rifampin inhibits only bacterial RNA polymerase, rifabutin is also active against bacterial DNA synthesis. Because of this second mechanism, rifabutin is also active against some rifampin-resistant mycobacteria and as such is widely used in AIDS superinfections. Both are bactericidal on multiplying bacteria. The main indication for these drugs is mycobacterial infections; however, in some instances they are also recommended in the treatment of severe staphylococcal or *Legionella* and *Brucella* infections, albeit as in mycobacterial infections always in combination with other agents, because there is a rapid development of resistance. Mycobacteria in Europe generally are sensitive to rifamycins; however, in tropical countries and in the United States, an increasing incidence of resistance is reported. Both compounds are present in high concentrations in cells and are active against intracellular pathogens.

Spectrum of activity

Rifampin is highly active against most strains of *M. tuberculosis,* as well as on gram-positive cocci (e.g., staphylococci, streptococci, and enterococci), gonococci, meningococci, *H. influenzae, Legionella, Brucella, Bacteroides,* and *Chlamydia*. Some mycobacteria (such as *M. leprae, M. kansasii,* and *M. avium-intracellulare*) and most gram-negative bacteria are moderately sensitive. Rifabutin is more active in vitro than rifampin against *M. tuberculosis* and especially against *M. avium-intracellulare,* which makes it the agent of choice in the treatment of so-called atypical mycobacterial infections, especially in AIDS patients.

Table 38.13 Pharmacokinetics, usual daily doses, and toxiticities of rifamycins

Drug	Mode of application and dose	Bioavailability (oral, %)	$t_{1/2}$	Notes: major elimination route and untoward effects
Rifampin (rifampicin)	Oral and parenteral 0.3-0.6 g	40-60	2-5 h (progressively reduced with continued use)	Almost complete absorption after oral dosage; biliary elimination (40%); renal elimination up to 30%; $t_{1/2}$ increases to 4-7 h in hepatic insufficiency; in case of inflamed meninges sufficient cerebral concentrations; desacetyl-rifampin is the major metabolite. Rifampin is eliminated via hemodialysis. Untoward effects: the most frequent are hepatic (rise in transaminases)
Rifabutin	Oral 0.45-0.6 g	12-20	40	Biliary and renal elimination, dose reduction in patients with renal untoward insufficiency. The most frequent untoward effect is hepatic rise in transaminases; when given with inhibitors of HIV proteases, leukopenia may develop

Major drug interactions

Both rifampin and rifabutin are powerful inducers of drug-metabolizing enzymes (see Chap. 6) and as such may reduce the activity of concomitantly given drugs. Inactivation of oral contraceptives by rifampin, with obvious consequences, has become a classic example of this type of interaction. Caution should be used in concomitant treatment with anticoagulants, anticonvulsants, and hypoglycemic sulfonylureas. When given with protease inhibitors in AIDS patients, particularly with ritonavir, rifabutin metabolism is markedly reduced, and the occurrence of leukopenia has been reported (Tab. 38.13).

Suggested readings

BALL P, GEDDES AM, ROLINSON GN. Amoxicillin clavulanate: An assessment after 15 years of clinical application. J Chemother 1997;9:167-98.

BEAUCAIRE G. Clinical activity of cefepime in severe infections.Clin Microbiol Infect 1999;5:S6-14.

BERGOGNE-BEREZIN E. Current trends and new perspectives in antibiotic therapy. Chemotherapy 1989;1:285-92.

BRYSKIER A, CHANTOT J-F. Classification and structure-activity relationship of fluoroquinolones. Drugs 1995;49:16-28.

CARBON C. Quinupristin/dalfopristin: a review of its activity in experimental animal models of infection. J Antimicrob Chemother 1997;39:115-9.

CATO A, CAVANAUGH J, SHI H, et al. The effect of multiple doses of ritonavir on the pharmacokinetics of rifabutin. Clin Pharmacol Ther 1998;63:414-21.

GREGG CR. Drug interactions and anti-infective therapies. Am J Med 1999;106:227-37.

KUHLMANN J, DALHOFF A, ZEILER HJ. Quinolone antibiotics. In: Handbook experimental pharmacology, Berlin: Springer Verlag, 1998:127.

LIPSKY BA, BAKER CA. Fluoroquinolone toxicity profiles: A review focusing on newer agents. Clin Infect Dis 1999;28:352-64.

NORRBY SR. New fluoroquinolones: towards expanded indications? Curr Opin Infect Dis 1997;10:440-3.

ROLINSON GN. Forty years of β-lactam research. J Antimicrob Chemother 1998;41:589-603.

SHRYOCK TR, MORTENSEN JE, BAUMHOLTZ M. The effects of macrolides on the expression of bacterial virulence mechanisms. J Antimicrob Chemother 1998;41:505-12.

STRUELENS MJ, BYL B, VINCENT J-L. Antibiotic policy: a tool for controlling resistance of hospital pathogens. Clin Microbiol Infect 1999;5:S19-24.

ZEMBOWER TR, NOSKIN GA, POSTELNICK MJ, et al. The utility of aminoglycosides in an era of emerging drug resistance.Int J Antimicrob Agents 1998;10:95-105.

Microbial infections

Pramod M. Shah, Emilio Bouza

RESPIRATORY TRACT INFECTIONS

Respiratory tract infections (RTIs) are the most frequently diagnosed infections and a very frequent reason for antimicrobial precriptions, although the majority are viral and thus do not require antibacterial agents. Unfortunately, there is as yet no clinical or laboratory test available that discriminates between the two etiologic agents.

UPPER RESPIRATORY TRACT INFECTIONS

Acute pharyngitis and tonsillitis

Etiology

Group A beta-hemolytic streptococci are the major etiologic pathogens in acute pharyngitis and tonsillitis. However, in recent years, group C streptococci also have been reported with increasing frequency. Very rarely, *Mycoplasma pneumoniae* or *Neisseria gonorrhoeae* (special risk groups) are isolated. Recently, *Chlamydia pneumoniae* has been reported in acute cases of pharyngitis. In temperate zones, the incidence is higher in the cooler months, since the transmission of streptococci via droplets requires close contact with an infected person.

Clinical findings and diagnosis

The incubation period is usually 3 to 5 days, and most infections are mild and/or nonbacterial. Clinical findings frequently are not indicative of the causative organism. Major clinical symptoms include acute onset with fever, sore throat, and dysphagia. Rhinitis, conjunctivitis, and cough are often present but nonspecific. Regional lymph nodes may be enlarged and tender. Helpful in the diagnosis of streptococcal throat infection are a red uvula and a yellowish (pus) exudate. Most upper respiratory tract infections (URTIs) are self-limited and do not require any specific antibacterial treatment. A specific diagnosis can be established only by isolating streptococci in throat swab. However, a positive culture does not differentiate between acute infection and an asymptomatic carrier state. Serology is not helpful in acute disease, and antibodies are detectable only in the convalescent stage. An elevated white blood count (>12 000/μl) with shift to the left and an elevated C-reactive protein (CRP) level can help to establish the diagnosis.

Treatment

Antibacterial treatment is essential to prevent late sequelae of group A streptococcal infection such as rheumatic fever or poststreptococcal glomerulonephritis. Many antibiotics have proved to be effective in this infection. However, since all hemolytic streptococci are highly sensitive to penicillin G, oral penicillins are still the drugs of choice. If a high dose is used (1-2 million units), penicillin can be given twice daily in adults. In patients who are allergic to penicillin, macrolides should be prescribed. However, it should be kept in mind that in some regions, these microorganisms have shown resistance to macrolides. Until further studies are available, antibacterial treatment should be a full 10 days, except for drugs with extremely long elimination half-lives, such as azithromycin, which may be given for 3 days (Tab. 39.1). Oral cephalosporins are also active but are expensive and should be prescribed only in patients who do not tolerate penicillins or macrolides. Use of quinolones is discouraged.

Table 39.1 Treatment of streptococcal pharyngitis or tonsillitis

Drug (class)	Dosage	Duration
Oral - Penicillin	1-2 million units bid 30 min before meal or 2 h after	10 days
Erythromycin	250-500 mg tid to qid	10 days
Roxithromycin	150-300 mg qd	10 days
Clarithromycin	250 mg tid	10 days
Azithromycin	0.5 g on day 1, followed by 0.25 g	3 days

Diphtheria

Etiology

Diphtheria was almost totally eradicated in developed countries but has reemerged in the eastern hemisphere as a result of a breakdown of public health services. It is a serious disease with high mortality rate (5-10%). Most cases occur in nonimmunized persons and elderly persons with waning immunity. In recent years, a few imported cases in travelers to eastern European countries have been reported. The disease is caused by toxin of *Corynebacterium diphtheriae*.

Clinical findings and diagnosis

The incubation period is 1 to 7 days. Systemic reactions are rare in mild or uncomplicated disease. Disease can present as an upper respiratory tract infection (pharyngeal and laryngeal) or occasionally as cutaneous diphtheria (wound diphtheria). In upper respiratory diphtheria, small whitish exudates are seen at first, and they coalesce to form an extensive thin exudate that extends to cover the tonsils and palate. The membranes become thicker and are more firmly attached to the underlying tissue. The complications in diphtheria are a result of the spreading of the membranes to respiratory tract mucosa, with occlusion of the airways and resulting tachypnea, dyspnea, cyanosis, and death. The reaction to toxin leads to myocarditis (signs of decompensation and arrhythmia) and peripheral neuritis (early in disease, paralysis of the soft palate; 2-6 weeks later, cranial nerve dysfunction). Microscopy and culture of the exudate or membrane can establish the diagnosis.

Treatment

In suspected cases, treatment with antitoxin should be started promptly: 200 to 1000 units/kg of body weight is recommended. Additionally, penicillin (1 million units every 6-8 hours) or a macrolide (erythromycin 0.5 g three times daily) should be prescribed to eliminate the bacteria and the production of further toxin. Patients should be kept in isolation for the first few days.

Otitis media

Bacterial otitis media, or otitis media acuta (OMA), is an infection and inflammation with the presence of purulent discharge in the middle ear. It is probably the most frequent bacterial infection seen by pediatricians. It is mainly a disease of childhood, and almost 40% of antibiotics prescribed in children up to age 10 years are for the treatment of otitis media acuta.

Treatment

Treatment with antibacterial agents is a controversial issue. The Dutch College of General Practitioners recommends only symptomatic treatment for the first three days for patients under 2 years of age (paracetamol with or without decongestant nose drops). If symptoms (fever and/or pain) continue, patients should be reevaluated, and an antibiotic should be prescribed. In the empirical therapy of children weighing less than 20 kg, amoxicillin (40 mg/kg/day in three divided doses) or amoxicillin plus clavulanate or an oral cephalosporin with activity against *H. influenzae* is recommended. In patients allergic to beta-lactams, macrolides (e.g., erythromycin 30-40 mg/kg/day, clarithromycin, roxithromycin, or azithromycin) or cotrimoxazole are good alternatives.

Otitis externa

Otitis externa (OE) should be distinguished from otitis externa maligna (OEM), which is the more severe form, occurring mainly in elderly diabetic patients, and is associated with a high mortality rate (up to 20%). Almost all cases of otitis externa and otitis externa maligna are caused by *Pseudomonas* spp. The pathogens are often resistant to a number of antimicrobial agents, and treatment should be based on sensitivity patterns.

Clinical findings and diagnosis

Otitis externa is a superficial infection of the external auditory canal. The main symptoms are pain, itching, and fullness of the ear; on examination, moderate exudate, erythema, and edema are present. In contrast, otitis externa maligna is a severe infection. Despite the fact that more than 90% of the patients are diabetic, there is no correlation between the severity of the disease and the severity of the diabetes. If not treated, the infection spreads to the surrounding soft tissue and bone (osteomyelitis) and may progress to multiple cranial nerve palsies, thrombosis of the jugular vein, and meningitis. Microbiology of ear exudate is essential for appropriate treatment. *Pseudomonas aeruginosa* is isolated in more than 95% of the reported patients; however, in selected cases, *Staphylococcus aureus, Aspergillus fumigatus, Proteus mirabilis,* or *Klebsiella* spp. have been implicated.

Treatment

Otitis externa generally responds well to gentle cleansing or irrigation. In occasional cases, antimicrobial drops containing polymyxin or neomycin and hydrocortisone may be required. Surgical debridement may be indicated in more advanced cases. Systemic antipseudomonal antibiotics are the mainstay of therapy. Treatment should be prolonged and exceed 12 weeks in many cases. With the development of quinolones with excellent activity against *Pseudomonas* spp., initial parenteral treatment can be switched to oral. Topical application of newer antimicrobial agents has not been studied systematically but remains a controversial issue (Tab. 39.2).

Table 39.2 Antibiotic treatment of otitis externa maligna

Antibiotic	Dosage	Notes
Azlocillin or piperacillin	4-6 g tid	Combination with an appropriate aminoglycoside is often recommended
Aztreonam	2-4 g tid	Combination with an appropriate aminoglycoside is often recommended
Ceftazidime	2 g tid	Combination with an appropriate aminoglycoside is often recommended
Ciprofloxacin	400 mg tid	After 1 to 2 weeks of parenteral treatment, change to 750 mg bid orally

Sinusitis

Sinusitis – both acute and chronic – is a common problem (1.4% of 30 000 patients consulting a general practitioner in Sweden were diagnosed with sinusitis), often seen in patients with the common cold, allergies, or anatomic abnormalities of the nose. Severe complications include meningitis and brain abscess. As with other upper respiratory, tract infections, the use of antibacterial agents is a controversial issue because the etiology is viral in many instances.

Etiology

The most frequent isolates cultured in acute cases of sinusitis are *Streptococcus pneumoniae* and *Hemophilus influenzae;* anaerobes and aerobic streptococci and rarely *S. aureus* may be involved. In children, additionally, *Branhamella catarrhalis* has been cultured from maxillary sinus aspirates.

Clinical findings and diagnosis

Pain over the sinuses, fever, and persistent purulent nasal discharge, together with headache and symptoms of nasal obstruction, are the main clinical symptoms. Culture of a direct sinus aspirate is the best procedure to establish the etiologic diagnosis, but is not tolerated by many patients. A nasal swab could allow identification of the pathogen involved and should be performed if aspiration is not possible. Sonography and occasionally x-rays are performed to confirm the diagnosis.

Treatment

Appropriate antimicrobial treatment is amoxicillin, a beta-lactamase inhibitor, or a macrolide. Tetracyclines are cheap and well tolerated and can be prescribed if the resistance of the pneumococci is low.

LOWER RESPIRATORY TRACT INFECTIONS

Acute infectious bronchitis

Acute infectious bronchitis is an inflammatory condition of the tracheobronchial tree that usually is associated with a generalized respiratory infection. It is a seasonal disease with higher incidence in the winter months. Etiology and clinical presentation are discussed in Chapter 29.

Treatment

Postural drainage is indicated during acute infection, as well as the use of an aerosol bronchodilator and a humidifier. Cough-suppressant drugs are rarely indicated. The use of corticosteroid therapy is debated, but many patients improve after their use.

Antimicrobial prophylaxis may be indicated in patients with more than four relapses per year. Such agents may be prescribed daily or for 4 days per week during the winter months, or a 7-day course can be given at the first sign of a "chest cold."

Oral antibacterial therapy is usually recommended. A course of an oral agent for 7 to 10 days is usually sufficient for most acute flare-ups. Initial choices include doxycycline (100-200 mg daily), trimethoprim-sulfamethoxazole (160-800 mg twice daily), amoxicillin-clavulanate (250-125 mg three times daily), or a macrolide. Quinolones (high dose) and oral cephalosporins also have been studied. However, their use should be restricted in patients who fail on primary treatment or show evidence of resistant organisms.

Nosocomial pneumonia and pneumonia in the immunocompromised host

Nosocomial acquired pneumonia (NAP) is an infection of the lung parenchyma not present at admission and acquired during a hospital stay. Nasocomial acquired pneumonia is the cause of 10 to 20% of all nosocomial infections and occurs in 5 to 10 per 1000 hospital discharges. This incidence is 20 times higher for patients admitted to intensive care units (ICUs) and represents the first cause of death attributable to nosocomial infection. It prolongs hospital stay by a mean of 7 to 9 days per patient.

Etiology

Many factors can influence the etiology of nosocomial acquired pneumonia, but a general estimate is offered in Table 39.3. In a high percentage of patients (up to 30%), infection may be polymicrobial, especially in ventilated patients. At the same time, it must be remembered that in 30 to 50% of all cases of nosocomial acquired pneumonia, an etiologic diagnosis is not reached. Among gram-negative organisms, *P. aeruginosa* and *Acinetobacter baumanii* are frequent in ICUs. *H. influenzae* is very common as a cause of early-onset pneumonia (72 hours) in ventilated

Table 39.3 Microorganisms and empirical therapy of severe nosocomial acquired pneumonia

Microorganisms	Drugs
Enterobacteriaceae (Enterobacter, Klebsiella)	Ceftazidime or cefepime or anti-Pseudomonas penicillin or carbapenem
P. aeruginosa	+
Acinetobacter	aminoglycoside or ciprofloxacin
MRSA (methicillin resistant Staphylococcus)	or aztreonam ± vancomycin

patients. *Klebsiella, Escherichia coli,* and other *Enterobacteriaceae* are the most common gram-negative organisms in nonventilated patients.

Gram-positive organisms, particularly *S. aureus,* are an increasing cause of pneumonia in patients with cranioencephalic trauma and low levels of consciousness. In many institutions, a high proportion of *S. aureus* isolates are resistant to all β-lactam drugs. Other agents are quantitatively less important but may affect very severely a particularly compromised subgroup of hospitalized patients (viruses, fungi, *Pneumocystis carinii,* and even *Mycobacterium tuberculosis*).

Clinical findings and diagnosis

From a clinical point of view, nosocomial acquired pneumonia can be subdivided into large groups depending on

the presence or absence of severity criteria ranging from the necessity of ICU admission and mechanical ventilation up to a rapidly evolving clinical condition with shock. Diagnosis is based on chest x-ray and, for all nosocomial pneumonias, requires that an attempt at a diagnostic etiologic approach should be made.

Treatment

Treatment can be subdivided into three areas: empirical therapy in nosocomial acquired pneumonia that is not severe, empirical therapy in severe nosocomial acquired pneumonia, and etiologically guided treatment. General rules include:

1. the patient's underlying diseases and conditions clearly orient toward certain microorganisms;
2. knowledge of epidemiologic conditions in the institution and the antimicrobial susceptibility patterns of the most common microorganisms is essential;
3. knowing the type and duration of nosocomial instrumentation is essential. Particularly in ventilator-associated pneumonia (VAP), early (3-4 initial days) and late (5 or more days) pneumonias have different etiologic agents;
4. a good history of prior antimicrobial therapy should be obtained. A neutropenic patient with fever and pulmonary infiltrates despite broad antibacterial therapy probably has a fungal infection;
5. therapy should be started early in all cases of nosocomial acquired pneumonia.

Empirical therapy in nonsevere nosocomial acquired pneumonia The most frequent microorganisms isolated before the fifth day of hospital stay are *H. influenzae, S. pneumoniae,* and methicillin-sensitive *S. aureus.* In this situ-

Table 39.4 Etiologic agents of nosocomial acquired pneumonia and their specific treatment

Microorganism	First-line treatment	Alternative
Chlamydia pneumoniae	Doxycycline	Macrolides, quinolones
S. aureus Meti-S*	Cefazolin ± rifampin	Cloxacilin, cotrimoxazole
S. aureus Meti-R***	Vancomycin ± rifampin	Teicoplanin, cotrimoxazole
S. pneumoniae Peni-S*	Penicillin	Macrolides, fourth-generation quinolones
S. pneumoniae Peni-I**	Ceftriaxone	Penicillin iv, high doses, fourth-generation quinolones. Macrolides
S. pneumoniae Peni-R***	Ceftriaxone	Vancomycin, fourth-generation quinolones
Enterobacteriaceae	Second-, third-generation cephalosporins ± Aglx	Aztreonam, amox-clav, quinolones
P. aeruginosa	Anti-Pseudomonas-β-lactam + Aglx	Aztreonam + Aglx, carbapenem, cipro + Aglx
A. baumanii	Carbapenem ± Aglx	
Legionella spp.	Erythromycin ± rifampin	Cipro, doxy + rifa
H. influenzae	Ceftriaxone	Amox-clav, quinolones
Anaerobes	Amox-clav or piper-tazo	Carbapenem

(Aglx = aminoglycoside; Peni= penicillin; Meti= methicillin; S= sensitive; I= intermediate; R= resistant.)

ation, second- (e.g., cefuroxime) and third-generation cephalosporins without antipseudomonal activity (e.g., cefotaxime, ceftriaxone) and combinations of beta-lactam drugs with beta-lactamase inhibitors are adequate. In patients allergic to penicillins, fluoroquinolones and combinations of macrolides and aztreonam are adequate.

In patients with additional risk factors, other etiologic possibilities should be considered in the empirical treatment: anaerobes should be suspected in patients with massive aspiration, poor oral hygiene, or putrid secretions. These patients may require penicillins with beta-lactamase inhibitors or carbapenem. In institutions with a high rate of multiresistant organisms, glycopeptides should be included in the empirical treatment, awaiting laboratory results. High-dose cotrimoxazole may be one alternative.

Suspicion of *Legionella* infection requires the administration of macrolides plus rifampicin. In the opinion of experts, however, fluoroquinolones may be a better alternative.

Finally, the presence of *Pseudomonas* requires combined treatment with beta-lactam drugs associated with an aminoglycoside (Aglx) or ciprofloxacin.

Empirical therapy in severe nosocomial acquired pneumonia In patients with severe pneumonia, microorganisms such as *P. aeruginosa* and *Acinetobacter* spp., as well as multiresistant organisms, are more frequent. In this group, empirical therapy is frequently a combination treatment. This is justified by the frequent polymicrobial etiology of pneumonia in this group of patients and by the potential synergy of some combinations against *P. aeruginosa* (Tab. 39.3).

Etiologic therapy Once the etiology and antimicrobial susceptibility of a patient with nosocomial acquired pneumonia are known, it is time to adjust treatment to the more specific, more active, more effective, less toxic, and less expensive drug (Tab. 39.4). Parenteral treatment should be started, but some drugs, such as the fluoroquinolones, permit an oral switch as soon as the patient is stable.

The duration of treatment is a controversial issue. The most severe cases should be treated for at least 2 to 3 weeks, depending on the clinical evolution. Duration should be 3 weeks in all cases of nosocomial acquired pneumonia caused by *L. pneumophila, P. aeruginosa,* or *Acinetobacter* spp.

URINARY TRACT INFECTIONS

Urinary tract infections (UTIs) are a very frequent cause of morbidity and mortality, may involve patients of all ages, with or without underlying or predisposing conditions, and may be located at different levels of the urinary tract. Urinary tract infections acquired in the community may affect up to 3% of schoolgirls. Most women will have at least one urinary tract infection in their lifetime, particularly during the period of onset of sexual activity, and asymptomatic bacteriuria may occur in up to 40 to 50% of elderly men and women. Nosocomially acquired urinary tract infection is most frequently associated with indwelling bladder catheterization and has a prevalence of between 8 and 15% of all hospitalized patients. Lower urinary tract infection

include urethritis, cystitis, and prostatitis, and upper urinary tract infections include uretheral infection, pyelonephritis, and parenchyma and/or perinephric infections.

The term *significant bacteriuria* ($>10^5$ CFU [colony forming units] /ml of urine detected in culture) is used to describe young women with cystitis and may not apply to other circumstances. Any number of bacteria is significant in urine obtained by direct puncture techniques or during surgical procedures. At the same time, significant bacteriuria may be absent in some cases of true urinary tract infection due to the administration of prior antimicrobial agents and in patients with recently introduced indwelling bladder catheters. In cases of candiduria, figures ($\geq 10^3$ CFU/ml) may be significant. The most frequent reason for a false-positive significant bacteriuria is an inadequately obtained or transported urine culture; urine should be plated within 2 hours after voiding. Usually, contaminated urines grow a polymicrobial flora, and normally, more than two different species of bacteria in a urine culture is suggestive of contamination.

Etiology

The most frequent microorganisms in urinary tract infections are those belonging to the family Enterobacteriaceae, particularly *E. coli,* followed by nonfermenter gram-negative bacilli, particularly *P. aeruginosa.* In certain groups of patients, gram-positive cocci play an important role. *S. saprophyticus,* a novobiocin-resistant coagulase-negative staphylococcus, accounts for 10 to 15% of acute urinary tract infections in young females. In other groups of patients, the enterococcus group, *S. aureus,* and group B streptococci are important.

Candiduria is almost always significant and implies the presence of underlying diseases (diabetes mellitus), the prior administration of antibacterial agents, the presence of indwelling catheters, or a combination of these and other factors. The presence of repeatedly negative urine cultures in otherwise symptomatic patients should suggest the presence of undetected microorganisms such as *Ureaplasma urealyticum, Mycoplasma hominis, M. tuberculosis,* or adenovirus.

Clinical findings and diagnosis

Factors influencing the presence of urinary tract infection by the host include female gender, sexual activity, prostatic enlargement, lack of circumcision, pregnancy, obstruction, neurogenic bladder dysfunction, and vesicoureteral reflux. Bacterial factors that influence the incidence of urinary tract infection include bacteria belonging to certain specific serogroups and adherence ability to uroepithelial cells by fimbriae or pili that mediate attachment to the digalactoside portion of glycosphingolipids present on the uroepithelium. Clinically, there are no reliable manifestations or valid tests to clearly differentiate upper from lower urinary tract infection. Symptoms can be divided into general (fever, malaise) and local (lumbar pain, dysuria, nocturia, etc.). Clinical symptoms and signs of pyelonephritis, though usually suggestive, do not always indicate upper urinary tract infection.

Patients with dysuria, frequency, urgency, and suprapubic pain usually have cystitis. Symptoms of acute pyelonephritis generally develop rapidly and include high fever, chills, nausea, vomiting, and diarrhea and normally respond to adequate treatment in 3 to 4 days. In women with urethral syndrome and without significant bacteriuria, infection with sexually transmitted pathogens (such as *C. trachomatis, N. gonorrhoeae,* or herpes simplex virus) or low-count bacterial cystitis should be considered.

In patients with bladder catheters, the prevalence of urinary tract infection increases 3 to 5% per day of catheterization. In general, the responsible microorganisms include *Proteus, Klebsiella, Serratia, Enterobacter,* and *Pseudomonas* that display markedly greater antimicrobial resistance, and the microorganisms reach the bladder either by intraluminal route or the periurethral route.

A direct microscopic examination of a fresh voided urine and the urine sediment is an essential first step. The presence of pyuria is a highly sensitive and specific indicator of urinary tract infection. When white blood cell casts are visible, the source of the infection is in the upper urinary tract. Other than this, the presence of an abnormal urinary sediment is neither highly sensitive nor highly specific for the diagnosis of urinary tract infection when compared with the presence of significant bacteriuria.

The first microbiologic step is to stain an unspun drop of urine with the Gram technique. The presence of one or more bacteria per high-power immersion field correlates very well with growth of ($\geq 10^5$ CFU/ml in culture), and this simple technique permits a clear orientation for initial therapy. Urine cultures should be performed systematically. An unexpected negative culture may be due to prior antimicrobial administration, presence of a low number of bacteria or microorganisms not recovered by the conventional technique (e.g., *Chlamydia, N. gonorrhoeae, M. tuberculosis,* etc.).

An uncomplicated urinary tract infection affecting for the first time a sexually active young woman does not require imaging techniques, but complicated urinary tract infection, including as such a primary infection in a male younger than 50 years, requires at least confirmation of patency of the urinary tract and demonstration of normal renal function.

Treatment

In young patients with uncomplicated cystitis, a single dose or a short course (1-3 days) of treatment may be all that is required. Beta-lactam drugs, cotrimoxazole, or one of the quinolones may be the most adequate choice. However, in some areas, resistance of *E. coli* to amoxicillin is seen in close to 50% of isolates, resistance to cotrimoxazole is in the same range, and resistance to fluoroquinolones may reach 20% of isolates. Single-dose therapy is safe only for women with acute uncomplicated cystitis whose posttreatment follow-up can be ensured. A 3-day course of therapy appears to preserve the low rate of side effects of single-dose therapy while improving efficacy.

In patients with complicated urinary tract infection who require hospital admission, parenteral treatment should be initiated until the etiology of the infection, evolution of the patient, and availability of adequate oral agents are ensured. A 7- to 14-day course of cotrimoxazole, a fluoroquinolone, or a third-generation cephalosporin plus or minus an aminoglycoside is usually adequate.

In pregnancy, all urinary tract infections, including asymptomatic bacteriuria, have to be treated.

Quinolones are contraindicated in children younger than 7 years of age and in pregnancy.

CONDITIONS ASSOCIATED WITH URINARY TRACT INFECTIONS

Prostatitis

Prostatitis, an inflammatory condition of the prostate gland, can be acute or chronic and caused either by bacteria or other etiologic agents. Acute bacterial prostatitis is characterized by fever, chills, dysuria, and a painful prostate usually caused by the common urinary tract infection pathogens. A urine Gram stain is usually informative, and treatment requires administration of antimicrobial agents with good penetration into the prostatic tissue, as is the case with cotrimoxazole or fluoroquinolones, but other agents are also active in the acutely inflamed tissue. A chronic form of bacterial prostatitis should be considered in men with recurrent bacteriuria. The basic diagnostic test is the comparison of bacterial counts in urine cultures of samples obtained before, during, and after a prostatic massage. Treatment (cotrimoxazole, quinolones) administered for long periods of time (6-12 weeks) and preferentially by the oral route is required

Perinephric and renal abscesses

Renal and perinephric abscesses arise either as a consequence of hematogenous seeding of the kidneys (preferentially associated with *S. aureus*) or as a consequence of an unresolved urinary tract infection involving the renal parenchyma (most frequently caused by Enterobacteriaceae and other gram-negative rods). They commonly occur as a consequence of obstruction caused by nephrolithiasis. The organisms most frequently encountered are *E. coli, Proteus* spp., *Klebsiella* spp., and *Candida* spp.

Fever, flank pain, and abdominal pain are the most common clinical manifestations, and a perinephric abscess should be suspected particularly when such symptoms persist after 3 to 5 days of adequate therapy for acute pyelonephritis. Echography and computed tomographic (CT) scan are the procedures of choice. Treatment requires drainage (percutaneous may be adequate) of pus and antibiotic treatment in hospital.

SKIN AND SOFT TISSUE INFECTIONS

Skin and soft tissue infections (SSTIs) are some of the most frequent infections not only in the outpatient setting but also in hospitalized patients (see also Chap. 76). The normal skin offers a good defense against infection, but even a minor (nonvisible) trauma could be a portal of entry for microbes. Infections occur in all age groups. The most appropriate empirical treatment can be chosen on the basis of close inspection, which readily allows classification of infection and prediction of the most frequent pathogens (Tab. 39.5).

Infection of the skin may occur accidentally or postoperatively, depending on the type of operation (clean or contaminated), length of operation, and underlying disease of the host, may affect preexisting skin lesions (such as dermatitis, postburn injury), or may be a manifestation of a systemic infection (hematogenous dissemination in bacteremia, endocarditis, or meningitis). Many skin infections are superficial and require no antibacterial treatment.

Etiology

S. aureus is the most frequent pathogen in folliculitis, furuncles, carbuncles, paronychia, and most posttraumatic wound infections. Resistance to penicillin is high (>80%) even in the ambulatory setting, and an increasing incidence of methicillin resistance is reported from many centers worldwide.

Hemolytic streptococci (group A) are uniformly sensitive to penicillin, which is the drug of choice. Oral cephalosporin (e.g., cephalexin) or clindamycin is an alternative in patients who are allergic to penicillin. The rate of resistance to macrolides varies widely from country to country (Japan 72% in 1979, Australia 17%), so these agents should be prescribed empirically only where no or low rates are reported.

Clinical findings and diagnosis

Clinical symptoms depend widely on the extent of skin involvement and the host's systemic reaction to the infect-

ing agent. The most common agents include *S. aureus* and hemolytic streptococci (see Tab. 39.5).

Cellulitis   Both *S. aureus* and group A streptococci can cause cellulitis, which begins as a superficial skin infection. In most patients there is a history of minor skin trauma. Lesions are warm, erythematous, edematous, and painful. Within 48 to 72 hours, the infection tends to spread to the regional lymph nodes and via the bloodstream. In rare instances, other pathogens such as *Erysipelothrix rhusiopathiae* (occurring almost exclusively in butchers, fishermen, or hunters), *Corynebacteria diphtheriae,* etc. may be isolated.

Gas gangrene   This occurs generally as a result of wound contamination with a mixture of pathogenic and ubiquitously occurring *Clostridium* spp., such as *C. tetani* and *C. perfringens.* It develops in necrotic tissue after extensive damage to muscle. Once established, the infection spreads very rapidly and results in extensive damage to previously uninvolved tissue. In advanced stages, patients are septic. Bacteria are readily detected on microscopy, and the exudate should be transported to the laboratory under anaerobic conditions. In addition to prompt antimicrobial treatment, early surgical intervention is essential.

In most skin infections it should be possible to obtain adequate material for bacteriology. Culture and sensitivity determination are essential for appropriate antimicrobial treatment, since resistance patterns, especially for *S. aureus,* vary widely from country to country or even within a defined geographic region.

Treatment

Empirical treatment – depending on the type of infection – is listed in Table 39.5. Surgical consultation should be arranged for all patients with extensive pus formation, since drainage is mandatory in such instances.

Table 39.5 Infection of skin and soft tissue, most frequent pathogen and empirical treatment

Organism and infection	Empirical antimicrobial treatment	Other pathogens to be considered
Pyoderma gangrenosum	Oxacillin or flucloxacillin 1-2 g tid Clindamycin 0.3-0.6 g tid Cephalexin 1.0 g tid	–
Post traumatic wound infections	Oxacillin or flucloxacillin 1-2 g tid Clindamycin 0.3-0.6 g tid Cephalexin 1.0 g tid	*Clostridium perfringens,* coliforms, *P. aeruginosa*
Gas gangrene, myositis	Penicillin iv 5-10 million units q6-8 h	*Clostridium perfringens*

BONE AND JOINT INFECTIONS

Osteomyelitis

This inflammatory process of bone and bone marrow is caused mostly by pyogenic bacteria but may be caused by other bacteria or fungi. Classification according to pathogenesis is clinically most helpful: (1) hematogenous osteomyelitis, (2) contiguous focus osteomyelitis, (3) peripheral vascular disease-associated osteomyelitis, and (4) foreign body-associated osteomyelitis. In the past, osteomyelitis usually was hematogenous, seen most commonly in children, and *S. aureus* was the most frequent pathogen. This pathogen can survive intracellularly for a long time, thus explaining the difficulties in curing the infection and the persistence of osteomyelitis.

Etiology

Hematogenous osteomyelitis develops after bacteremia, and *S. aureus* is the most frequent microorganism. Occasionally, streptococci or gram-negative rods (elderly patients) are encountered. Contiguous focus osteomyelitis is associated with an open fracture or bone surgery.

The organisms involved depend on the contamination. Both gram-positive cocci and gram-negative rods have been cultured, and infections tend to be polymicrobial. Peripheral vascular disease-associated osteomyelitis is found in patients with diabetes or vascular insufficiency and is localized almost exclusively in the feet. The infection tends to be polymicrobial (streptococci, staphylococci and anaerobes).

In foreign body-associated osteomyelitis, the most frequent pathogens are coagulase-negative staphylococci or *Propionibacterium* spp., but other pathogens such as gram-negative rods may be encountered as well.

Other pathogens to be considered are *Salmonella, Streptococcus pneumoniae, Enterobacteriaceae*, or *P. aeruginosa* (nosocomial infection); *Pasteurella multocida* or *Eikenella corrodens* (human or animal bites); *M. tuberculosis* or *Bartonella henslae* (AIDS); and *Brucella* spp., *Coxiella burnetii*, or other organisms found in specific geographic areas.

Table 39.6 Antibacterial treatment of osteomyelitis or arthritis in adults

Bacteria	Drug of choice	Alternative
Gram-positive cocci[1]		
Penicillin sensitive	Penicillin G (5-10 million units) tid or qid	First-generation cephalosporin (e.g., 2 g cefazolin or cefuroxime 1.5 g tid) or clindamycin 0.6 g tid
Penicillin resistant	First-generation cephalosporin (e.g., 2 g cefazolin or cefuroxime 1.5 g tid) or flucloxacillin (2 g qid or tid)	Clindamycin 0.6 g tid or glycopeptide
Methicillin resistant	Vancomycin (1 g bid or tid) or teicoplanin (10-15 mg/kg q24h) in combination with rifampicin 0.45-0.6 g bid or qd	Clindamycin + rifampicin or quinupristin/dalfopristin
Enterobacteriaceae	Quinolone orally (e.g., ciprofloxacin 750 mg or levofloxacin 500 mg bid)	Third-generation cephalosporin (e.g., cefotaxime 2 g tid) or aztreonam (2 g tid)
Pseudomonas aeruginosa	Piperacillin (4 g tid) + an aminoglycoside	Ciprofloxacin (750 mg tid) or ceftazidime (2 g tid) + an aminoglycoside
Mixed aerobic and anaerobic infection	In addition to one of the above, clindamycin (0.6 g tid)	Carbapenem
Neisseria gonorrhoeae		
Penicillin sensitive	Penicillin G (5-10 million units) qid or tid	Quinolone
Penicillin resistant	Quinolone	Third-generation cephalosporin (e.g., ceftriaxone 2 g bid or qd im) or spectinomycin (2-4 g qd im)
Haemophilus influenzae (mostly infants)		
Ampicillin sensitive	Ampicillin	Cefotaxime
Ampicillin resistant	Cefotaxime	Amoxicillin + clavulanate

[1] Staphyloccoci or streptococci.

Clinical findings and diagnosis

The classic signs – i.e., acute onset with fever, rigors, and bone pain – are seen less frequently nowadays. This is probably due to early antimicrobial treatment of extraosseous bacterial infections. Local symptoms depend on the affected bone, and systemic manifestations (e.g., fever, chills, night sweats, malaise, etc.) are reported in less than 50% of patients. In any patient with low-grade fever and/or nonspecific complaints (e.g., malaise, night sweats, weight loss), an elevated erythrocyte sedimentation rate (ESR) and C-reactive protein level, osteomyelitis should be included in the differential diagnosis. Identification of the causative microorganism is essential for proper treatment, since many pathogens could be multiply resistant, especially *S. aureus*. X-ray-guided needle biopsy or surgical sampling should be performed prior to initiation of treatment.

Treatment

Optimal prolonged treatment (for at least 4 weeks) is essential in all cases of osteomyelitis (Tab. 39.6). Whether a longer treatment duration could reduce the rate of relapse remains controversial. The choice of antibiotic should be based on sensitivity patterns, and bactericidal agents are preferred. Synergistic combinations, such as a beta-lactam or clindamycin plus rifampicin (in staphylococci) or a β-lactam plus an aminoglycoside (in *Pseudomonas*), are recommended in certain instances.

In prosthetic joint surgical procedures, adequate precautions (i.e., surgery under highly sterile conditions, perioperative prophylaxis, and topical association of antimicrobials in bone cement) should be taken to prevent infection because infections associated with foreign bodies are difficult to cure.

Arthritis

Inflammation of a joint could be present in the course of an infection at a distant site (e.g., enteritis or a viral syndrome). Noninfectious processes such as gout can mimic septic arthritis. Prosthetic joint infections are very difficult to diagnose because they are insidious in onset.

In adults, infants (<3 months) and children (2-15 years) with arthritis and in patients with pyogenic arthritis, *S. aureus* and streptococci are encountered most frequently. *H. influenzae* infection occurs almost exclusively in children aged 3 to 24 months. In infections associated with foreign bodies (prosthetic joint), coagulase-negative staphylococci may be found. Gonococcal arthritis (affecting a single joint) is probably the most common cause of septic arthritis in the adolescent age group.

For therapy in addition to antibacterial treatment (Tab. 39.6), adequate drainage is mandatory, and surgical consultation should be sought very early in the disease course.

GASTROINTESTINAL AND INTRAABDOMINAL INFECTIONS

Bacterial gastroenteritis

Gastroenteritis may be due to infectious (viral, bacterial, or parasitic) or noninfectious agents. Symptoms can be limited to the upper gastrointestinal tract, with nausea, vomiting, cramping, and abdominal pain being the main symptoms (e.g., staphylococcal or *Bacillus cereus* food poisoning). Involvement of lower gastrointestinal tract is accompanied by diarrhea, which may be profuse, as in the case of cholera.

Etiology

The etiology of gastroenteritis, a food-borne disease, remains unknown in up to 50% of cases, and in many instances, the disease is of viral origin. The most frequent bacterial pathogens (in order of frequency in Europe) are *Salmonella* spp. (both in imported and endogenous cases), *Campylobacter* spp., *Yersinia* spp., and *Shigella* spp. In recent years, *Vibrio cholerae* epidemics have been reported in South America, Africa, and the Indian subcontinent (where it is endemic in many areas).

Clinical findings and diagnosis

The main symptoms are nausea accompanied by vomiting, abdominal pain, and at times systemic reactions such as fever with chills in the compromised host (e.g., elderly persons, patients with AIDS). Most pathogens can be isolated easily from stool, and identification of the causative microorganism is essential for proper treatment, since many of the pathogens can be multiply drug resistant. Serology plays a very minor role in the management of acute bacterial gastroenteritis.

Treatment

In healthy individuals, gastroenteritis is mostly a self-limited disease and requires no antimicrobial treatment (Tab. 39.7). Only fluid and electrolyte supplementation are required to prevent dehydration. Quinolones are at present the most active in vitro and clinically most effective drugs in salmonellosis and shigellosis. Resistance of these organisms to quinolones is rare. Treatment duration in salmonellosis (especially *S. typhii*) is 7 to 10 days and as short as a single administration in shigellosis. The goal of treatment is not only to cure the patient but also to eliminate the pathogen and thus interrupt transmission to other persons. The role of quinolones in treating other bacterial agents (e.g., *Campylobacter, Yersinia*) has been studied only in small number of patients.

The so-called food poisonings are due to exotoxins produced by the bacteria (*S. aureus, B. cereus, C. perfringens*), and only supportive treatment is required.

In traveler's diarrhea, antimicrobial agents are recommended only in compromised hosts or in severe disease (high fever and/or bloody stools). The use of antibacterial agents in enterohemorrhagic *E. coli* infections is a controversial issue. In some reports, the course of the disease was dilatory if antimicrobial agents were prescribed. However, since most patients present with systemic signs of severe infection (i.e., fever, rigors, and shock or preshock), clinicians tend to prescribe an antibiotic.

Prevention

Effective vaccination is available only for typhoid fever; however, almost all bacterial gastroenterites can be prevented if hygienic recommendations are followed closely.

Helicobacter pylori infection (see Chap. 33)

Antibiotic-associated diarrhea (see also Chap. 35)

Almost all antibiotics can cause diarrhea as a result of changes in the resident microbial flora. Most cases are mild, and discontinuation of the antibiotic results in prompt recovery. In a few instances (e.g., debilitated patients, patients who have undergone bowel surgery), overgrowth with toxin-producing *C. difficile* and progression to pseudomembranous colitis may occur. The infection is often acquired nosocomially and occurs in clusters. The use of gloves and proper hand washing should help prevent nosocomial transmission.

Clinical findings and diagnosis

Pseudomembranous colitis may occur in patients who are taking antimicrobials or in those who have taken them in the last 2 to 8 weeks. Persisting severe bloody diarrhea together with abdominal cramping is characteristic of *C. difficile*-associated (see also Chap. 35) pseudomembranous colitis. Since carriage state with *C. difficile* in healthy persons is known, the presence of toxins in stool has to be demonstrated to establish the diagnosis. The role of endoscopy is still being debated, but it is helpful in confirming the diagnosis in severe cases.

Treatment

Antimicrobial agents should be discontinued, and either oral metronidazole (0.4-0.5 g tid) or oral vancomycin (0.125-0.25 g q6h) is the preferred treatment. Only in rare and severe cases should metronidazole or vancomycin be given parenterally.

Biliary tract infections

Cholecystitis and cholangitis are treated primarily by surgeons, and antibiotics play a supplementary role in preventing sepsis or septic complications. In most cases (over 80%), some sort of obstruction (calculi) is present, but acute gallbladder infection may occur spontaneously. Enteric organisms (predominantly *E. coli*) and occasionally enterococci or rarely anaerobes are cultured from bile. In postoperative or postendoscopy patients or patients with tumors of the biliary tract, other organisms such as *P. aeruginosa* may be encountered. Perioperative prophylaxis in high-risk patients (e.g., geriatric patients, reoperation patients, patients with tumors) helps reduce the rate of postoperative complications.

With the introduction of ultrasonography in general practice, biliary tract obstruction can be readily ruled out. X-ray (intravenous cholangiography or endoscopic retrograde cholangiography) is only for patients with complicated disease. If possible, intraoperatively or endoscopically obtained bile should be cultured in all instances so as to collect epidemiologic data for future empirical treatment.

Treatment

The drug prescribed should achieve high and active biliary concentrations. Since bile for culturing is generally not available, presumptive treatment is directed against the most frequent cause, i.e., *E. coli*. In acute and first episodes, *E. coli* is highly susceptible to quinolones (e.g., ciprofloxacin 0.5 g or levofloxacin 0.5 g q12h), which are

Table 39.7 Antibacterial treatment of gastroenteritis in adults

Bacteria	Treatment of choice	Alternative
Salmonella or *Shigella* spp.	Quinolones	Cotrimoxazole or ampicillin or chloramphenicol
Campylobacter spp.	Erythromycin (0.5 g tid)	Quinolones
Yersinia spp.	Tetracycline (0.25 g qid)	Quinolone or cotrimoxazole
Escherichia coli enteroinvasive, toxigenic	Quinolones	Cotrimoxazole
Vibrio cholerae	Quinolones	Tetracycline or cotrimoxazole

the drugs of choice. Alternative agents include ampicillin (2 g tid) or first-generation cephalosporins (e.g., 2 g cefazolin or 1.5 g cefuroxime q8-12h). In chronic cases or after invasive procedures, *P. aeruginosa* may be involved; here, ciprofloxacin (200 mg iv q8-12h), an acyl-ureido penicillin (piperacillin 4 g tid), or ceftazidime (2 g tid) is recommended. In all instances, surgical treatment should be considered to remove the obstruction.

Peritonitis

This localized or general inflammation of the peritoneal cavity may be due to bacteria, fungi, protozoa, or chemicals. The pathogenesis is complex. It is primarily a surgical disease, associated with high mortality. Microorganisms involved are of colonic origin, and the infection is polymicrobial. Peritonitis can develop as a result of perforating abdominal trauma, perforation of a gastric or duodenal ulcer, in ulcerative colitis, or as a result of vascular insufficiency resulting in ischemic necrosis. Peritonitis during continuous ambulatory peritoneal dialysis (CAPD) generally has an insidious onset and is often monomicrobial.

A wide range of bacterial organisms are cultured in diffuse peritonitis. A mixture of coliforms, enterococci, and gram-negative anaerobes is recovered. In continuous ambulatory peritoneal dialysis peritonitis, gram-positive cocci (very frequently coagulase-negative staphylococci) are the most frequent bacterial pathogen, accounting for one-third to one-half of all cases, whereas gram-negative bacteria account for one-fifth to one-third of all cases. Tuberculous peritonitis is a rare disease. It manifests as a more subacute disease (subfebrile temperatures, night sweats, weight loss, and prostration).

Clinical findings and diagnosis _____

These will depend on the extent of involved tissue and the underlying disease. The local symptoms are localized or generalized pain, with rebound tenderness and muscle guarding or rigidity (boardlike abdomen in severe cases). The more systemic signs are fever, tachycardia, distention of the abdomen, and sepsis followed by septic shock.

In order to establish the etiology, intraoperatively obtained material or ultrasound-guided needle aspirate should be cultured aerobically and anaerobically.

Treatment _____

The cause of peritonitis should be looked for. Laparotomy is essential to drain the pus and remove necrotic tissue, which offers excellent growth conditions for bacteria. High-dose parenteral antibacterials (generally in combination that also cover anaerobes) are essential. Recommended drugs include piperacillin plus tazobactam (4.5 g tid) or carbapenem (imipenem or meropenem 1 g tid) or clindamycin (0.6 g tid) in combination with gentamicin (2-4 mg/kg of body weight once a day or in three divided doses). Quinolones (e.g., ciprofloxacin 0.2-0.4 g tid) or third-generation cephalosporins (e.g., cefotaxime 2 g tid)

that have excellent activity against coliforms need to be combined with metronidazole (0.4-0.5 g tid).

Continuous ambulatory peritoneal dialysis peritonitis can be treated with antimicrobial agents incorporated in the dialysis fluid (e.g., initially 1 g cefazolin or 2 g vancomycin, followed by 0.25 g cefazolin q6h or 0.1-0.5 g vancomycin q24h intraperitoneally) in addition to systemic treatment. Staphylococci (often methicillin-resistant) are the most frequent organisms, and empirical treatment is directed against these pathogens: vancomycin (1.5 g initially, followed by 1.0 g once a week) is recommended while awaiting the sensitivity report. Frequently, there is a need to remove and replace the infected foreign body.

SEPSIS, BACTEREMIA AND ENDOCARDITIS

Concepts and definitions regarding sepsis have evolved considerably during the present decade. At present, sepsis is a very broad (and to a certain point, imprecise) entity that requires the presence of a systemic inflammatory response syndrome (SIRS) attributable to an infection. A systemic inflammatory response syndrome implies a systemic response to an external offense and is defined by the presence of at least two of the following: fever, tachycardia, tachypnea, or an elevated white blood cell count (Tab. 39.8).

This symptomatic complex begins as a nonspecific response to an external insult, in the case of sepsis against the components or metabolic products of microorganisms, and it is caused by a complex set of different immunologic mediators. Sepsis, if unresolved or uncontrolled, may evolve successively to severe sepsis, septic shock, and multi-organ system failure. These stages can be reached progressively and have an increasingly severe prognosis. The risk of concomitant bacteremia increases from the lower to the higher stages, but it does not clearly convey a more grim prognosis in the different stages.

At present, we call *bacteremia* the presence of viable bacteria in blood. This generally includes the concept of *fungemia* (presence of viable fungi in blood) and in recent years the concept of *mycobacteremia* (presence of viable mycobacteria in blood). *Infective endocarditis* means the presence of active infection in the valvular or extravalvular endocardium.

Clinical findings and diagnosis _____

The concept of sepsis is too broad for a practical therapeutic approach. Comments should be limited to a systematic approach to patients with severe infection of unknown etiology, suspected to be bacteremic. A systematic approach should be followed taking into consideration, at least, the following factors: patients should be classified into those without underlying diseases and those with compromising diseases (either local or general). Patients with general compromise are better subdivided into those

Table 39.8 Underlying condition, clinical manifestions and etiology of sepsis

Groups of microorganisms	Some clinical characteristics
Virus	Children, or immunocompromised adults. Skin manifestations
Bacteria	
Chlamydia	Previously healthy. Genital or ocular disease, respiratory syndromes
Rickettsia	Previously healthy. Skin lesions, epidemiologic antecedents
Mycoplasma	Previously healthy. Usually young. Genital or respiratory diseases
Spirochetes	Previously healthy. Relapsing fevers, skin or genital lesions
Gram-positive	All types of patients. Classic pyogenic infections. Acute
Gram-negative	All types of patients. All syndromes. Classic pyogenic infections. Acute
Anaerobes	Postoperative, posttraumatic. Foul smelling. Necrotic
Mycobacteria and other higher bacteria	Normal or compromised patients. Respiratory chronic, slowly evolving diseases
Fungi	Normal host in endemic areas. Compromised host (e.g., neutropenic) universally
Parasites	Normal host. Travel associated HIV. Intestinal

with and without neutropenia. A thorough antecedent history of the patient (e.g., recent trips, residence, habits, drugs, sexual orientation, etc.) should be taken. After an adequate physical examination, patients should be classified in one or more syndromic groups depending on the data about focal disease that are available (e.g., fever plus cough plus an increase in sputum production = respiratory syndrome). Once a syndromic diagnosis in a certain type of patient is reached, the number of etiologic possibilities is considerably reduced. For instance, in a 25-year-old, previously healthy patient with a very severe neurologic, meningeal syndrome, *N. meningitidis* and *S. pneumoniae* are the two more important microorganisms to search for and to treat empirically. Microorganisms seen most frequently under certain conditions are listed in Table 39.8. This not only allows a systematic approach but also serves as a reminder of easily forgettable secondary problems.

Finally, diagnostic and therapeutic maneuvers must be selected, particularly tests and therapeutic decisions regarding empirical treatment.

Treatment

All patients with severe sepsis or a more evolved syndrome are entitled to receive antimicrobial drugs empiri-

cally after obtaining adequate diagnostic clinical samples. The choice of drugs should be based on the probable source of infection, Gram-stained smears of appropriate clinical specimens, and the patient's immune status according to current patterns of bacterial resistance in the hospital and in the community.

Third-generation cephalosporins (e.g., cefotaxime, ceftizoxime, cefepime, ceftriaxone, ceftazidime), imipenem, meropenem, or aztreonam can be used to treat sepsis caused by many strains of gram-negative bacilli. Ceftazidime has less activity against gram-positive cocci. Cephalosporins other than ceftazidime and cefepime have limited activity against *P. aeruginosa*. Imipenem, meropenem, and aztreonam are active against most strains of *P. aeruginosa,* and imipenem and meropenem are active against anaerobes. Aztreonam has no activity against gram-positive bacteria and anaerobes.

For initial treatment of life-threatening sepsis in adults, a third-generation cephalosporin (e.g., cefotaxime, ceftizoxime or ceftriaxone, cefepime), piperacillin/tazobactam, meropenem, or imipenem, each together with an aminoglycoside, is adequate therapy. When methicillin-resistant staphylococci (MRSA) are suspected, treatment with vancomycin or teicoplanin (e.g., aminoglycoside or rifampin) is often recommended.

For intraabdominal or other infections likely to involve anaerobes, treatment should include either ticarcillin/clavulanic acid, ampicillin/sulbactam, piperacillin/tazobactam, imipenem, meropenem, cefoxitin, or cefotetan, each with or without an aminoglycoside, or alternatively, metronidazole or clindamycin, together with an aminoglycoside. When the source of bacteremia is thought to be in the biliary tract, the possibility of *Enterococcus* spp. as an etiologic agent leads some clinicians to prefer penicillin derivatives such as piperacillin, piperacillin/tazobactam, or ampicillin/sulbactam plus metronidazole, each with or without an aminoglycoside.

In neutropenic patients, suspected sepsis and bacteremia should be treated with ceftazidime, imipenem, meropenem, or cefepime alone or, in more seriously ill patients, with an aminoglycoside. Single daily doses of amikacin and ceftriaxone or, alternatively, piperacillin/tazobactam (4.5 g tid or qid) plus amikacin may be equally effective. Addition of vancomycin from the very beginning to the other drugs in these circumstances has not improved outcome.

Bacteremia and its guided treatment

Approximately 15 to 75% of the episodes of sepsis will have demonstrable bacteremia. Bacteremic patients may have a very poor outcome unless adequate therapy is undertaken rapidly. Bacteremia occurs in between 15 and 30 of every 1000 hospitalized patients, and its incidence has been increasing, probably due to aging of the population, the increasing longevity of patients with chronic diseases, and the relatively high frequency of this condition among patients with AIDS.

Etiology

In recent years, gram-positive organisms (particularly *S.*

aureus, S. epidermidis, and *Enterococcus* spp.) represent slightly more than 50% of all bacteremic episodes. Gram-negative organisms were stabilized in number in recent years, and *E. coli* represents the single most common isolate responsible for bacteremia.

Anaerobic bacteria have been decreasing recently and now represent no more than 5% of all bacteremic episodes. The reasons may be improved diagnostic imaging techniques and better and quicker surgical procedures. Fungemia represents from 3 to 10% of all bloodstream infections that can be documented and has been increasing recently. Mycobacteremia is more than anecdotal in patients with tuberculosis and in those with nontuberculous mycobacterial diseases.

Clinical findings and diagnosis

Fever, hypothermia, hyperventilation, and abnormal CNS function (e.g., disorientation, confusion) are often early signs of sepsis. Hypotension and septic shock occur in at least 20% of all episodes. Diffuse intravascular coagulation (DIC) and skin lesions are less common, and occasionally, skin lesions may be suggestive of specific pathogens such as *N. meningitidis* (hemorrhagic lesions) or *P. aeruginosa* (ecthyma gangrenosum). Gastrointestinal manifestations and other focal signs depend on the extension of organ involvement.

Major complications include pulmonary complications (e.g., ventilation-perfusion mismatching, alveolocapillary leak, decreasing compliance, and arterial hypoxemia and the adult respiratory distress syndrome), septic shock, renal complications (e.g., oliguria, azotemia, proteinuria), coagulation abnormalities (e.g., thrombocytopenia in 10-30% and DIC), and neurologic emboli. Abnormalities include leukocytosis or leukopenia, thrombocytopenia, hyperbilirubinemia, proteinuria, respiratory alkalosis evolving to metabolic acidosis, and, frequently, hyperglycemia.

Definitive diagnosis requires blood cultures (two to three blood samples from different venipuncture sites), which should be kept incubated at least over 5 days using new techniques with continuous agitation. If fastidious microorganisms are suspected, incubation may be prolonged up to 4 weeks.

Treatment

Treatment is urgent and requires treatment of local infection, hemodynamic and respiratory support, administration of antimicrobal agents, and other measures. Removal or drainage of a focal source of infection is essential and may include withdrawal of intravenous and bladder catheters, prosthetic devices, and abscesses; adequate organ perfusion (systolic pressure > 90 mm Hg); and oxygen delivery (ventilator therapy). Urine output should be kept over 30 ml/h by continuous administration of fluids. If this can be achieved only by volume infusion, inotropic and vasopressor therapy is indicated. Antimicrobial chemotherapy should be initiated immediately after blood and other samples have been taken for culture and modified when results

of blood cultures and antimicrobial susceptibilities are known. When the condition is stabilized, the regimen often can be simplified, and a single antimicrobial agent is usually adequate. Sequential intravenous and oral therapy may be appropriate in many circumstances. Duration of therapy is at least 1 week but is influenced by factors such as the site of infection, surgical drainage, the patient's underlying disease, and the antimicrobial susceptibility of the bacterial isolates.

There is no reason to continue with glycopeptides in patients with isolates of *Staphylococcus* spp. susceptible to methicillin or corresponding β-lactam. Many enterococcal strains are now resistant to penicillins, streptomycin, gentamicin, and even vancomycin. They may require teicoplanin (not always cross-resistance with vancomycin), chloramphenicol, doxycycline, fluoroquinolones, or a combination of quinupristin/dalfopristin. Most bacteremic infections caused by *P. aeruginosa* should be treated with a combination of a β-lactam drug and an aminoglycoside.

Most cases of "simple" *Candida* fungemia (associated with intravenous catheters) can be treated with the removal of the catheter and fluconazole, especially isolates of *C. albicans* cultured from patients not previously treated with azole derivatives (see Chap. 41).

Prognosis

At the present time, drugs that neutralize bacterial endotoxin or that interfere with mediators of the inflammatory response can be considered only experimental. Mortality from bacteremic infections varies from 10 to 50% or more and is clearly related to the underlying disease of the patient and the severity of the septic episode. Mortality is much higher in patients with septic shock and multi-organic system failure. Polymicrobial bacteremia and fungemia also correlate with a poor prognosis.

Endocarditis

Infective endocarditis is an infectious disease of the endocardium (valvular or extravalvular) that is virtually always fatal if untreated. Infective endocarditis can be classified on the basis of different concepts, but three distinct clinical types deserve special mention: infective endocarditis of native valves, infective endocarditis in intravenous drug abusers (IVDA), and infective endocarditis in prosthetic valves. Clinically, infective endocarditis may be classified as acute, subacute, or chronic. Finally, the etiologic agent is an appropriate way of classifying infective endocarditis.

Etiology

Most frequent agents of infected endocarditis on native valves are streptococci, *Enterococcus* spp., and *S. aureus.* Other bacteria include the so-called HACEK group (*Hemophilus, Actinobacillus, Cardiobacterium, Eikenella*

of the list.

and *Kingella*) and more uncommonly *S. pneumoniae*, *N. gonorrhoeae*, *Brucella* spp., fungi and others. In intravenous drug abusers, *S. aureus* causes more than 50% of cases, and in these patients, microorganisms such as *P. aeruginosa* or *Candida* spp. are less uncommon.

The etiology of prosthetic valve endocarditis (PVE) varies according to the postoperative period in which it is acquired. Early-onset endocarditis (within 60 days of surgery) is usually caused by *S. epidermidis* and other microorganisms acquired during the operative procedure or during perioperative episodes of bacteremia/fungemia. Intermediate-onset endocarditis (onset between 60 days and 1 year postoperatively) may be caused by pathogens either of the early or the late period. Late-onset endocarditis (after 1 year) is mainly caused by the same pathogens as in natural valve endocarditis, with streptococci at the head

Clinical findings and diagnosis

Among predisposing conditions, rheumatic fever is becoming very uncommon in developed countries, whereas congenital heart disease, mitral valve prolapse and degenerative heart disease are rising. At the present time, between 20 and 50% of infective endocarditis has no known predisposing condition. Clinical features of infective endocarditis are the consequences of growing vegetations, persistent bacteremia, septic emboli and immune reactions. The most common clinical manifestations are fever, skin lesions, retinitis, cardiac murmurs, liver and spleen enlargement and neurologic manifestations. Renal failure and heart failure are signs of severity.

The most important steps in the diagnosis of endocarditis is confirmation of the etiologic agent with blood cul-

Table 39.9 Recommendations for treatment of infective endocarditis

Microorganisms	Antimicrobial	Dose	Length
S. aureus Methicillin S			
Native valve L side	Cloxa + Genta	2-4 g qid iv + 1 mg/kg tid iv	4-6 w/5 d
Native valve L side	Cefaz + Genta	2-4 g tid iv + 1 mg/kg tid iv	4-6 w/5 d
Native valve L side	Vancomycin	15 mg/kg bid (up to 2 g/day)	4-6 w
Native valve R side	Cloxa	2-4 g qid iv	4 w
Native valve R side	Cloxa + Genta	2-4 g qid iv + 1 mg/kg tid iv	2 w/2 w
Native valve R side	Cloxa iv (po)	2-4 g qid iv + 500 mg qid po	2 w/2 w
Native valve R side	Cefaz + Genta	2-4 g tid iv + 1mg/kg tid iv	4-6 w/1 w
Native valve R side	Vanco + Rifa	15 mg/kg bid (up to 2 g)+ 600 mg po	4 w/1w
Native valve R side + stable patient	Ciprofloxacin + Rifa	750 mg po bid + Rifa 300 mg po bid	4 w
Prosthetic valve endocarditis	Cloxa + Genta + Rifa	2-4 g qid iv + 1 mg/kg tid iv + 900 mg po	4-6 w/2 w/4-6 w
S. aureus Methicillin R			
Native valve	Vancomycin	15 mg/kg bid (up to 2 g/day)	4-6 w
Prosthetic valve endocarditis	Vanco + Genta + Rifa	15 mg/kg bid (up to 2 g) + 1 mg/kg tid iv + 900 mg po	4-6 w/2 w/4-6 w
Streptococcus (Pen MIC≤0.1 mg/ml)			
	Penicillin G	2-3 mU/q4h iv	4 w
	Cefazolin	2 g tid iv	4 w
	Pen G + Genta	2-3 mU/q4h iv+1 mg/kg tid iv	2 w
	Ceftriaxone	2 g qd/iv or im	4 w
	Ceftriaxone (ampicillin)	2 g qd/iv or im 1.0 g po qid	2 w
	Ceftriaxone + Genta	2 g qd/iv or im+1 mg/kg tid iv	2 w
	Vancomycin	15 mg/kg bid (up to 2 g)	4-6 w
Streptococcus (Pen MIC>0.1<0.5 μg/ml)	Penicillin G + Genta	3-4 mU/q4h iv+1 mg/kg tid iv	2 w
Enterococcus and **Streptococcus** (Pen MIC>0.5μg/ml)			
	Ampi + Genta	2-5 g iv qid or tid +1 mg/kg tid iv	4-6 w
	Vanco + Genta	15 mg/kg bid (up to2g)+ 1 mg/kg tid iv	4-6 w
HACEK group	Ceftriaxone	2 g iv/im	4 w
	Cefotaxime	2 g tid iv	

(S = sensitive; R = resistant; Cloxa = cloxacillin; Cefaz = cefazolin; Genta = gentamicin; Rifa = rifampin; Vanco = vancomycin; mU = million units.)

tures or other techniques and demonstration of endocardial involvement with imaging techniques. In the present decade, better cardiologic imaging methods and progress in microbiologic diagnosis have led to the acceptance of new diagnostic criteria of infective endocarditis. The most widely followed criteria, Durack's criteria, take into diagnostic consideration the type of patient (e.g., intravenous drug abuser), the number of positive blood cultures, and the nature of the isolated microorganisms, as well as echocardiographic findings. The inclusion of transesophageal echocardiography has been a very significant step ahead in the diagnosis of infective endocarditis.

Treatment

General principles of treatment include the use of microbicidal drugs in high concentrations and for long periods of time. With certain exceptions, administration of antibiotics should be intravenously and on most occasions in a hospital setting. Table 39.9 includes some of the present recommendations for treatment. In patients with unknown microorganisms, treatment should cover *Enterococcus* in patients with native valve endocarditis, *S. aureus* in intravenous drug abusers, and methicillin-resistant *S. epidermidis* in patients with prosthetic valves. Outpatient therapy has been used successfully with stable individuals who are not intravenous drug users and are highly motivated.

Indications for surgery include unavailability of microbicidal therapy (fungal endocarditis), microbiologic failure (persistence of positive blood cultures), relapse after appropriate therapy, heart failure, valve-ring abscess, large vegetations (doubtful), atrioventricular block, and major emboli.

Lyme borreliosis

Lyme borreliosis (LB) has been reported mainly from the northern hemisphere. It is widespread throughout nearly all countries of Europe, Asia, and North America, affecting all age groups. It is transmitted by ticks (*Ixodes ricinus*) from various intermediate and small mammals, including rodents. Infected ticks are spread by birds during their migratory flights. The activity of ticks is seasonal, and in Europe, most patients get infected in the period between the end of May and the end of July. In up to 50% of patients, the tick bite goes unnoticed. Removal of the tick within the first 24 to 48 hours of feeding may prevent transmission of the *Borrelia*. Antibody against *Borrelia burgdorferi* has been detected in symptom-free persons at high risk for tick bites. *B. burgdorferi sensu stricto*, *B. garinii*, and *B. afzelii* can cause Lyme borreliosis in humans

Clinical findings and diagnosis

Three clinical stages, which can overlap, are known. The first two manifestations can occur within a few weeks or months after the tick bite. The third (late) stage appears several months or years later and is characterized by chronicity. Clinical presentation depends on the stage of Lyme borreliosis (Tab. 39.10). Serology is the only diagnostic method routinely available and may pose difficulties in interpretation, especially when no tick bite is remembered by the patient. Some specialized laboratories offer service for culturing the organism from tissue biopsies or cerebrospinal fluid samples.

Treatment

If the tick is removed promptly (within 48 h), the risk of infection is minimized. Treatment depends on the stage of disease. Despite adequate treatment, the disease can

---

Table 39.10 Clinical stages of Lyme borreliosis and treatment options

Stage	Drug of choice	Alternative
Stage I (early localized form) Erythema migrans Non characteristic flulike symptoms	Doxycycline 0.1 g bid for 14-21 days	Penicillin V 1-2 million units tid or qid Amoxicillin 0.5-1.0 g tid Erythromycin 0.5 g tid Ceftriaxone 2 g iv qd
Stage II (early disseminated form) Lymphadenosis cutis benigna Neurologic manifestations (Bannwarth syndrome, meningitis, encephalitis, radiculoneuritis) Cardiac manifestations (carditis with AV block) Rheumatoid manifestations (arthralgia, arthritis, myalgia)	Penicillin G 5-10 million units iv tid for 14-21 days	Ceftriaxone 2 g iv qd for 14-21 days Cefotaxime 2 g iv tid for 14-21 days Doxycycline 0.1 g bid for 30 days
Stage III Late neurologic manifestations (peripheral neuritis, subacute encephalopathy, progressive encephalomyelitis) Acrodermatitis chronica atrophicans	Penicillin G 5-10 million units iv tid for 14-21 days	Ceftriaxone 2 g iv qd for 14-21 days

progress, and other features of the disease may develop. Thus, 1.2% of over 700 patients treated in randomized studies progressed to develop neurologic features, and 1% developed arthritis. High-dose penicillin or tetracyclines act more rapidly than erythromycin. Doxycycline is preferred in patients in stage I, penicillin G (iv) in stages II and III. Ceftriaxone is a good alternative. If patients do not tolerate doxycycline or a beta-lactam, erythromycin may be used. Treatment should be for at least 14 days; 21-day treatment is preferable. Regardless of the treatment given, many patients still complain of some late manifestations.

Preventive treatment with an antimicrobial agent (e.g., doxycycline 0.1 g bid for 3-5 days) immediately after the tick bite, before any symptoms of disease manifest themselves, is a controversial issue. In some small studies manifestations of disease were prevented.

Prevention

Vaccines have undergone clinical trials in the United States and have been shown to be safe and effective. However, they are not expected to be effective in Europe because of genetic diversity in European strains.

CENTRAL NERVOUS SYSTEM INFECTIONS
Meningitis

Until the early twentieth century, purulent bacterial meningitis was a fatal disease. With the introduction of antibiotics, meningitis became a curable infection, but morbidity and mortality and neurologic sequelae remain high.

Etiology

The most frequent bacterial pathogens are *N. meningitidis* (older children and young adults), *S. pneumoniae* (older adults, patients with head trauma in their history), and *H. influenzae* (children 1 month to 4 years until the introduction of a vaccine against *H. influenzae* type B). In immunocompromised hosts, other rare pathogens such as *Listeria* and, in patients with a nosocomially acquired infection or those with foreign bodies (e.g., cerebral shunt), gram-positive cocci (staphylococci) or gram-negative bacilli (after neurosurgery) are encountered. In developing countries, *M. tuberculosis* plays an important role.

Clinical findings and diagnosis

Bacterial meningitis is a serious and potentially life-threatening disease that starts acutely with fever, severe headache, malaise, nausea, vomiting, and altered mental state with seizures. The presence of skin lesions (petechiae) is a pointer to meningococcal meningitis. In many patients with pneumococcal meningitis there is a history of head trauma (e.g., a traffic accident with skull fracture) or otitis. *Listeria* are encountered in patients with impaired cellular immunity or liver cirrhosis. The disease progresses rapidly, and patients go into septic shock.

Blood and cerebrospinal fluid (CSF) cultures are mandatory in all patients with suspicion of meningitis. However, treatment with an antimicrobial agent should not be delayed to secure appropriate material. Besides other routine tests performed in severe cases, C-reactive protein levels should be determined. High concentrations are reported in bacterial meningitis, whereas lower concentrations (<5 mg/dl) are suggestive of a viral pathogen. The fastest results are available via microscopy of Gram-stained cerebrospinal fluid sediment and detection of antigen of the most frequent bacterial (*S. pneumoniae, H. influenzae, N. meningitidis*) pathogens.

Treatment

Treatment should be based on the clinical presentation (patient population, skin lesions, etc.) and microscopy of cerebrospinal fluid sediment, which helps predict the most frequent pathogen. The appropriate antimicrobial is listed in Table 39.11. Duration of treatment is 7 days in infections with *H. influenzae* and *N. meningitidis*, 10 to 14 days with *S. pneumoniae*, 14 to 21 days with *Listeria*, and 21 days with gram-negative bacilli (other than *H. influenzae*).

The coadministration of corticosteroids in acute purulent bacterial meningitis remains a controversial issue. Dexamethasone (1.2 mg/m^2 qid for 4 days) appears to be safe in children. In adults, however, even though sufficient data are missing, it may be reasonable to consider its use if a high number of organisms are present in cerebrospinal fluid on microscopy or in adults with poor prognostic factors such as coma or stupor.

Preventive treatment of contacts (e.g., close family members, peers in school or day-care centers) and carriers is indicated in clustering of meningococcal and *H. influenzae* meningitis. In adults, a single dose of a quinolone (ciprofloxacin 0.5 g or ofloxacin 0.4 g) is sufficient to eliminate carriage. In children, rifampicin (20 mg/kg of body weight for 3-5 days) is recommended.

Prevention

H. influenzae type B vaccination has almost totally eradicted meningitis with this pathogen in children. Available quadrivalent meningococcal vaccine containing serotypes A/C/Y/W-135 is effective; however, in most European countries, serotype B is more frequent. Meningococcal vaccine should not be used in the place of chemoprophylaxis in close contacts.

Brain abscess

Although of rare occurrence and often difficult to diagnose early in the disease, it is important to reach an early diagnosis of brain abscess because aggressive treatment can markedly reduce morbidity and mortality. Noninvasive diagnostic procedures (CT scan or MRI) have facilitated early diagnosis. Predisposing factors are (1) infection of adjacent, contiguous meningeal structures (often middle ear infection), (2) hematogenous dissemination from a distant focus (e.g., endocarditis) and (3) trauma (after neurosurgery or head injury).

Etiology

Brain abscesses tend to be polymicrobial. Both aerobes and strict anaerobes can be recovered. Among culture-positive cases (85%), 57% are predominantly anaerobes, 22% are mixed infections with aerobes and anaerobes, 35% are monoinfections with anaerobes, and 42% are monoinfections with only aerobes. The most frequent anaerobic organisms are *Bacteroides* spp., *Fusobacterium* spp., or anaerobic cocci; *Clostridium* spp. are rarely found. Enterobacteriaceae (such as *Proteus* spp., *E. coli, Enterobacter* spp.) are reported in 29%, *S. aureus* in 15%, nonhemolytic streptococci in 19%, and *Hemophilus aphrophilus* in 9%. Other bacteria such as *M. tuberculosis, Salmonella* spp., or *S. pneumoniae* are reported in less than 1% of cases.

Table 39.11 Meningitis: pathogen and intravenous treatment

Bacteria	Treatment of choice	Alternative
Neisseria meningitidis	Penicillin G 5 million units tid or qid	Third-generation cephalosporin (e.g., ceftriaxone 2 g bid or qd)
Streptococcus pneumoniae		
1. Penicillin sensitive	1. Penicillin G 5 million units tid or qid	Third-generation cephalosporin (e.g., ceftriaxone 2 g bid or qd)
2. Penicillin resistant	2. Cefotaxime (2 g tid or qid)	
	3. Cefotaxime 300 mg/kg/24 h divided q6h or vancomycin 1000 mg/12 h + IT vancomycin	
Haemophilus influenzae		
1. Ampicillin sensitive	1. Ampicillin 5 g tid or qid	Third-generation cephalosporin (e.g., ceftriaxone 2 g bid or qd)
2. Ampicillin resistant	2. Third-generation cephalosporine (e.g., ceftriaxone 2 g bid or qd)	
Listeria species	Ampicillin 5 g tid or qid	Cotrimoxazole or vancomycin + aminoglycoside
Enterobacteriaceae	Third-generation cephalosporin (e.g., ceftriaxone 2 g bid or qd) in combination with an aminoglycoside	1. Meropenem (1-2 g tid) in combination with an aminoglycoside 2. Ciprofloxacin 400 mg tid
Pseudomonas aeruginosa	Ceftazidime 2 g tid or qid in combination with an aminoglycoside	1. Meropenem (1-2 g tid) in combination with an aminoglycoside 2. Ciprofloxacin 400 mg tid
Staphylococcus aureus		
1. Penicillin sensitive	1. Penicillin G 5 million units aminoglycoside tid or qid	1. and 2. Fosfomycin (10 g tid)
2. Penicillin resistant	2. Oxacillin 2-4 g qid or cefuroxime 1.5 g tid	
3. Methicillin resistant	3. Vancomycin (1 g tid) in combination with rifampicin (0.6 g bid)	3. Imipenem (1 g tid, risk of seizures) in combination with rifampicin (0.6 g bid)

(IT = intrathecal.)

Clinical findings and diagnosis

Symptoms vary from patient to patient and are often nonsuggestive: headache, alteration in level of consciousness with focal neurologic deficit, nausea and vomiting, and fever and chills. The disease develops gradually, and the duration of symptoms can be 14 days to 2 (or more) months. In some patients, a recent history of seizures is present.

A high degree of suspicion on the part of the clinician is necessary. Lumbar puncture is not helpful and is contraindicated. CT scan is the diagnostic procedure of choice, and if possible, a stereotactic CT-guided aspiration of pus should be undertaken and the aspirate submitted for microscopy and culture.

Treatment

Optimal therapy for brain abscess is not established and depends on clinical grounds. In "less severe" cases (e.g., mild case with cerebritis or smaller lesions), antimicrobial treatment alone can be initiated under close observation. Neurosurgical consultation should be sought at an early stage of the disease. Presumptive antibiotic treatment in "primary" abscesses (i.e., not postoperative abscesses) always should cover anaerobic organisms as well. High-dose penicillin (5-10 million units iv tid or qid) plus a third-generation cephalosporin (e.g., cefotaxime 2 g iv tid or qid) in combination with metronidazole (0.5 g iv tid) should be initiated, pending culture results. In patients who do not tolerate beta-lactams, chloramphenicol can be given. Based on in vitro activity and pharmacokinetic properties (cerebrospinal fluid level), carbapenems (e.g., meropenem 1-2 g iv tid) or a quinolone (e.g., ciprofloxacin 0.4 g iv tid) in combination with metronidazole may be a good alternative; however, no clinical experience is available.

OTHER FREQUENT INFECTIONS

Tuberculosis

Tuberculosis is caused by bacteria belonging to the *Mycobacterium tuberculosis* complex. The disease affects more than 1 billion people worldwide, and there are probably 8 to 10 million new cases of tuberculosis per year. Despite modern chemotherapy, approximately 3 million deaths are attributed to tuberculosis annually. A recent increase in the incidence of tuberculosis after years of steady decrease probably was due to infection by the human immunodeficiency virus (HIV), migratory movements and social problems such as poverty and drug abuse.

Etiology

Tuberculosis is caused by bacteria belonging to *M. tuberculosis* complex, i.e., *M. tuberculosis* itself, *M. bovis,* and *M. africanum* (isolated in Africa).

Clinical findings and diagnosis

Tuberculosis is transmitted by air from patient to patient and only occasionally nowadays by raw, unpasteurized milk (containing *M. bovis*). Other routes are uncommon. Crowding, malnutrition, alcoholism and poverty are factors associated with transmission of the tubercle bacilli. After contact, most patients develop the infection but not the disease. The risk of developing the disease depends largely on bacterial load, individual susceptibility, and individual immunity. If disease follows immediately after infection, it is called *primary tuberculosis* (more common in children). Most cases of clinical tuberculosis, however, occur in the first year after infection or as a reactivation of infection acquired earlier in life (*secondary tuberculosis*).

The most important predisposing conditions to tuberculosis are HIV coinfection and silicosis; lymphoma, leukemia, other malignant neoplasms, solid organ transplantation, chronic renal failure and hemodialysis; diabetes mellitus and malnutrition.

Clinical manifestations of tuberculosis traditionally are divided into pulmonary (more than 80% of the non-HIV-infected patients) and extrapulmonary (present in up to 50% of HIV-infected patients). Pulmonary manifestations include fever, cough, night sweats, weight loss, weakness, bloody sputum, hemoptysis, and pulmonary infiltrates, usually located in the upper lobes. The extent of lung involvement varies from small infiltrates to extensive cavitary disease.

Extrapulmonary tuberculosis may cause manifestations in practically all organs. The most commonly involved sites are the lymph nodes, pleura, genitourinary tract, bones and joints, meninges and peritoneum. Less common are eye disease, otitis, nasopharyngeal involvement and cutaneous, adrenal and congenital disease.

Miliary tuberculosis is due to hematogenous spread of tubercle bacilli and causes generalized nonspecific and protean manifestations depending on the predominant site of involvement.

Diagnostic maneuvers can be divided into imaging techniques and etiologic determination. Among the imaging techniques, the chest x-ray is the first step and may show typical (upper lobe infiltrates with cavitation) or atypical presentations (particularly common in HIV-infected patients). Acid-fast bacilli (AFB) microscopy is positive in only approximately 50 to 60% of all specimens, and all samples submitted for microscopy should be systematically cultured. More sophisticated molecular techniques are a clear improvement but also are associated with false-positive and false-negative results. Definitive diagnosis depends on the isolation and identification of *M. tuberculosis* or other bacteria from the complex in culture.

Skin testing with tuberculin antigen is of limited value in the diagnosis of active tuberculosis but very useful for screening of patients with prior contact with the bacillus (exception in HIV-infected or immunosuppressed patients). Drug susceptibility testing should be performed routinely in all initial isolates, isolates of treatment failures, and isolates of all recurrences.

Treatment

Combined treatment administered under direct supervision during a long period of time is essential for the cure of tuberculosis. Available drugs are summarized in Table 39.12. The five first-line agents are isoniazid, rifampicin (and derivatives such as rifabutin and rifapentine), pyrazinamide, ethambutol, and streptomycin. Second-line drugs, owing to a lower degree of efficacy and higher intolerance and toxicity, include aminoglycosides (e.g., kanamycin, amikacin, and capreomycin), quinolones (e.g., ofloxacin, ciprofloxacin, sparfloxacin, levofloxacin), ethionamide, cycloserine, para-aminosalicylic acid (PAS), clofazimine, thiacetazone, and amoxicillin-clavulanic acid.

Regimens (Tab. 39.13) should include an initial aggressive phase against actively multiplying bacilli to be continued by a sterilizing phase required to eliminate semidormant "persisters". One drug (when available) from each group in ascending order should be given, up to 3 drugs for susceptible microorganisms and 5 or more in cases where resistant strains are suspected (at least 3 effective drugs should be prescribed when no in vitro data are available). One of regimens of choice for all forms at all ages is the combination of isoniazid (INH), rifampicin (RIF), and pyrazinamide (P) (2 months) followed by a INH + RIF (4 more months).

Treatment is most commonly given daily, although intermittent regimens produce equivalent results. For patients with sputum-negative pulmonary tuberculosis, the duration of treatment may be reduced to a total of 4 months. Supervision increases the proportion of patients completing treatment and diminishes the risk of developing resistance. Monitoring response requires monthly cultures until cultures become negative and controls for drug toxicity (Tab. 39.14).

Treatment failure should be suspected when a patient's sputum cultures remain positive after 3 months or when acid-fast bacilli smears remain positive after 5 months. The following principles should guide the treatment of resistant or multidrug resistant (MDR) tuberculosis:
1. specialized personnel and units should be employed;
2. patients should be kept in isolation;
3. psychologic support should be provided;
4. the best drugs available should all be employed without "reserve for the future";
5. the selection requires a very good clinical drug history;
6. a complete microbiologic history should be available;
7. surgery should be reserved for patients with localized disease, good residual lung function, and less than three effective drugs available for therapy;
8. not more than a single drug from each group;
9. no less than three drugs with ensured activity should be employed. Initially, until susceptibility tests are available, five or more drugs should be administered.

The regimen of choice for pregnant women is 9 months of treatment with INH and RIF supplemented by ethambutol for the first 2 months. Table 39.15 contains orientations for the use of drugs during pregnancy meningitis, renal insufficiency or failure.

Prevention

The best way to prevent tuberculosis is the rapid detection and treatment of active cases. Preventive chemotherapy or bacille Calmette-Guérin (BCG) vaccination is used. INH in a dose of 5 mg/kg per day (up to 300 mg) should be given for 6 to 12 months. A longer course is recommended for persons with HIV infection and for those with abnormal chest radiographs. Risk factors for the development of tuberculosis among purified protein derivative (PPD)-positive patients are the following: patients with gastrectomy

---

Table 39.12 Most commonly available antituberculous drugs

Drug	Formulation	Dosage/day	Tolerability
Isoniazid (INH)	50,150 mg (tabl)	Up to 300 mg	Good
Rifampicin (RIF)	300 mg (tabl)	Up to 600 mg	Good
Pyrazinamide	400, 500 mg (tabl)	1200-1600 mg	Good
Ethambutol	100, 400 mg (tabl)	800-1200 mg	Good
Streptomycin	1 g (vial)	750-1000 mg	Fair
Kanamycin	1 g (vial)	750-1000 mg	Poor
Amikacin	1 g (vial)	750-1000 mg	Poor
Capreomycin	1 g (vial)	750-1000 mg	Poor
Ethionamide	250 mg (tabl)	500-750 mg	Fair
Cycloserine	250 mg (tabl)	500-750 mg	Fair
Ciprofloxacin	250, 500, 750 (tabl)	1000-1500 mg	Good
Ofloxacin	200 mg (tabl)	600-800 mg	Good
PAS	500, 4000 (gram)	10000-12000 mg	Fair
Rifabutin	300 mg (tabl)	Up to 600 mg	Good

Table 39.13 Selection of treatment regimens (see text for explanations)

Drug	Group	mg/day	Months	Other
Isoniazid	Group 1	Up to 300	6-9	Of first choice
Rifampicin	Group 2	Up to 600	6-9	Of first choice
Pyrazinamide	Group 3	1200-1600	3-24	Of first choice
Streptomycin	Group 4	750-1000	2-3	Useless in amikacin or kanamycin-resistant strains
Kanamycin	Group 4	750-1000	2-3	Can be active against streptomycin-resistant strains
Amikacin	Group 4	750-1000	2-3	Cross-resistance with kanamycin
Capreomycin	Group 4	750-1000	2-3	No cross-resistance with other aminoglycosides
Ethambutol	Group 5	800-1200	3-24	Less active than prior group
Ethionamide	Group 6	500-750	3-24	
Cycloserine	Group 7	500-750	3	
Ciprofloxacin	Group 8	1000-1500	3-24	Cross-resistance with quinolones
Ofloxacin	Group 8	600-800	3-24	Cross-resistance with quinolones
PAS	Group 9	10000-12000	3-24	

treated with corticosteroids, patients in hemodialysis, transplant patients, and other immunocompromised patients. Contraindications to INH chemoprophylaxis include severe liver disease or prior INH hepatitis, high alcohol intake, chronic use of other potentially hepatotoxic drugs (e.g., diphenylhydantoin) and peripheral neuropathy.

The BCG vaccine is recommended for routine use at birth only in countries with a high tuberculosis prevalence.

Diseases caused by nontuberculous mycobacteria

Nontuberculous mycobacteria (NTM) are all microorganisms belonging to the genus *Mycobacterium,* with the exceptions of *Mycobacterium leprae* and mycobacteria of the tuberculosis complex. Nontuberculous mycobacteria (also referred as *atypical mycobacteria* or *mycobacte-*

ria other than tuberculosis, MOTT) are ubiquitous in nature and may be colonizers and a cause of laboratory contamination, but they also can be agents responsible for human disease.

The initial identification and classification of nontuberculous mycobacteria relies on the speed of growth, morphology, and the ability of isolates to produce pigments with or without light stimulation. Because of the slow growth of some species, precise identification can require up to several months to complete.

Since the discovery of the high incidence of disseminated infections due to *Mycobacterium avium* complex (MAC) in advanced AIDS patients, human diseases caused by nontuberculous mycobacteria are best divided into disseminated infections, usually involving AIDS or other severely immunocompromised patients, and local infec-

Table 39.14 Most frequent untoward effects and toxicity

Drug	Untoward effects	Control
Isoniazid	Hepatitis, neuropathy, drug interactions	Monthly
Rifampicin	Hepatitis, hemorrhage, flu syndrome, microsomal induction, staining of ocular lenses	Monthly
Pyrazinamide	Rash, hepatitis, hyperuricemia	Symptomatic
Ethambutol	Optic neuritis	Avoid in children
Streptomycin	Ototoxicity	Every 2 weeks
Kanamycin	Oto- and nephrotoxicity	Every 2 weeks
Amikacin	Oto- and nephrotoxicity	Every 2 weeks
Capreomycin	Oto- and nephrotoxicity	Every 2 weeks
Ethionamide	Liver toxicity, metallic taste, abdominal pain	Monthly
Cycloserine	Psychosis, seizures, rash	Monthly
Ciprofloxacin	Dizziness, hypersensitivity, CNS	Monthly
Ofloxacin	Dizziness, hypersensitivity, CNS	Monthly
PAS	Liver toxicity, abdominal pain, Na load	Monthly

tions, which may involve normal hosts or persons with local defense defects such as catheters or other prosthetic devices. In immunocompromised hosts, the majority of cases is due to *Mycobacterium* avium complex, but *M. genavense, M. kansasii, M. xenopi, M. simiae, M. scrofulaceum, M. malmoense* and *M. celatum* and others are also occasionally responsible. The origin of nontuberculous mycobacteria is the environment, and there is no evidence for nosocomial spread of nontuberculous mycobacteria from patient to patient.

Clinical findings and diagnosis

In HIV-infected patients, the CD4 lymphocyte count at the time of diagnosis is usually less than 50 CD4/l. Clinical manifestations are not distinctive and may include prolonged fever, weight loss, spleen and liver enlargement, pulmonary manifestations and diarrhea. Signs of medullary involvement, particularly anemia and leukopenia, are frequently present.

Other patients who occasionally have disseminated infections with nontuberculous mycobacteria are immunosuppressed for other reasons, including transplantation, hematologic malignancies, and treatment with corticosteroids. Blood and bone marrow cultures are frequently positive and constitute the key test for the diagnosis. Lysis centrifugation techniques and other simpler procedures are adequate.

Treatment

Since the in vitro tests are usually slow and do not always correlate with clinical results, treatment should be based on prior clinical studies and consist in the combination of two or more drugs with known clinical activity during long periods of time.

Available active drugs for *Mycobacterium avium complex* include clarithromycin, azithromycin, ethambutol, ciprofloxacin, amikacin, and rifabutin. One of the most popular, all-oral regimen includes clarithromycin (500 mg bid) or azithromycin (500 mg/day) plus ethambutol (15-25 mg/kg) with or without rifabutin (300 mg/day). Addition of amikacin in multidrug regimens does not confer additional benefits and should be reserved for patients with resistance to the former drugs.

Drugs should be administered indefinitely in patients in whom profound immunodeficiency persists, but the prospects for withdrawal of the drugs probably rely on the efficiency of antiretroviral therapy in the future. Granulocyte-macrophage colony-stimulating factor and α-interferon may act synergistically with antibiotics against *Mycobacterium* avium complex.

Prevention

This is only recommended for HIV-infected patients with CD4+ counts of less than 500/μl. Drugs with reported activity include rifabutin (300 mg/day), clarithromycin (500 mg once or twice daily), and azithromycin (1200 mg weekly).

Syphilis

Syphilis is a sexually transmitted disease caused by *Treponema pallidum*. Less common modes of transmission include nonsexual contact, intrauterine infection, and infection after blood transfusions. Syphilis steadily declined in developed countries after World War II and predominantly involves young adults of lower social classes. Congenital syphilis now includes all live or stillborn infants delivered to women with untreated or inadequately treated syphilis at delivery. An early detection of syphilis in pregnant women and in groups at particular risk for the infection, as well as in sexual partners of diagnosed patients, is essential.

Table 39.15 Precautions with antituberculous drugs during pregnancy in CNS infection and in renal failure

Drug	Pregnancy	Cerebrospinal fluid entry	Renal failure
Isoniazid	Safe	Always	Same dose
Rifampicin	Safe	Inflammation	Same dose
Pyrazinamide	Avoid	Always	Reduce
Ethambutol	Safe	Inflammation	Reduce
Streptomycin	Avoid	Inflammation	Reduce
Kanamycin	Avoid	Inflammation	Reduce
Amikacin	Avoid	Inflammation	Reduce
Capreomycin	Avoid	Inflammation	Reduce
Ethionamide	Avoid	Always	Same dose
Cycloserine	Avoid	Always	Reduce
Ciprofloxacin	Avoid	Inflammation	Reduce
Ofloxacin	Avoid	Inflammation	Reduce
PAS	Safe	Inflammation	Insufficient data

Etiology

T. pallidum are spiral-shaped microorganisms that belong to the family Spirochetaceae and the genus *Treponema*. *T. pallidum* subspecies *pallidum* is the etiologic agent of syphilis, while the subspecies *pertenue* causes yaws the subspecies *endemicum* causes bejel, and *T. carateum* causes pinta (nonvenereal treponematosis).

Clinical findings and diagnosis

Active, symptomatic periods followed by latency are characteristic of syphilis. The classic stages of syphilis are the primary lesion, the secondary bacteremic stage (characterized by disseminated mucocutaneous lesions), a latent subclinical period, which may or may not be followed by a tertiary stage (with progressive destructive mucocutaneous and systemic lesions).

The chancre, or primary lesion, appears at the site of inoculation after 7 to 30 days of incubation and usually heals after 2 to 6 weeks. If the primary lesion is untreated, secondary manifestations may appear from 6 weeks to several months after healing. This means a bacteremic stage with treponemal invasion of the skin with maculopapular skin rash, lymphadenopathy and invasion of the central nervous system (CNS) and many other structures.

After the secondary lesions subside (within 2-6 weeks), the infection enters the latent stage, detected only serologically. About two-thirds of the patients "recovered" spontaneously in the preantibiotic era, and the remaining third developed clinically apparent tertiary disease. Tertiary syphilis is an obliterative small-vessel endarteritis involving, among others, the vasa vasorum of the ascending aorta and the CNS.

T. pallidum is not demonstrable by Gram stain or culture. The diagnosis of acute lesions relies on dark-field examination, which shows characteristic motile organisms. Other morphologic techniques include direct immunofluorescence, silver staining techniques, and experimentally, polymerase chain reaction (PCR) techniques. For nonacute lesions, serology procedures are the diagnostic key. There are two types of antibodies to be detected: a group of antilipid "reaginic" nonspecific antibodies (nontreponemal screening tests) and a group of specific antitreponemal antibodies measured with treponemal tests. Both are reactive with all treponemal diseases. Nontreponemal tests include RPR, ART, VDRL, and TRUST, in which flocculation is detected macro- or microscopically. These tests are used for initial screening as well as for quantitation of antibodies. They are highly sensitive but only partially specific.

Treponemal tests include a fluorescent assay (FTA-ABS), microhemagglutination assays (MHA-TP and TPHA), and immobilization techniques (TPI). They are very specific when used for confirmation of positive nontreponemal tests but should not be used for screening.

Treatment

Treatment of syphilis is summarized in Table 39.16. Cerebrospinal fluid examination should be performed in the evaluation of latent syphilis of unknown duration, in suspected neurosyphilis, and in HIV-positive patients and patients with late complications.

Parenteral penicillin G remains the drug of choice for treating all stages of syphilis Primary, secondary, or latent syphilis known to be of less than 1 year's duration can be treated effectively with an intramuscular injection of benzathine penicillin G. Syphilis in pregnant women should be treated with penicillin in doses appropriate to the stage of the disease. When pregnant women with syphilis are allergic to penicillin, hospitalization and desensitization are recommended. A positive serologic test for syphilis in a newborn without stigmata of syphilis may be due either to passive transfer of maternal antibodies or to prenatal infection. If there is no definite history of adequate treatment of the mother with penicillin during the pregnancy, prompt treatment of seroreactive infants is recommended. Some clinicians feel that HIV-infected patients with syphilis and normal cerebrospinal fluid require higher doses or longer treatment with penicillin than usual.

The VDRL quantitative test should progressively decline in the year following adequate therapy, becoming negative by 12 months in 50% of patients.

Table 39.16 Treatment of syphilis

Stage	Drug	Dose	Duration
Prevention after a positive contact primary or secondary	Pen G benzathine Tetracycline Doxycycline	2.4 million units im 500 mg qid 100 im bid	Single dose 2 weeks 2 weeks
Latent or tertiary without	Pen G benzathine Tetracycline Doxycycline	2.4 million units im 500 mg qid 100 im bid	One dose/w, 3 consecutive 4 weeks 4 weeks
Neurosyphilis or cerebrospinal fluid abnormal	Pen G aqueous	2-3 million units iv every 4 h	2 weeks
Syphilis in pregnancy	As per stage No tetracyclines!		

AMERICAN THORACIC SOCIETY. Hospital-acquired pneumonia in adults: diagnosis, assessment of severity, initial antimicrobial therapy and preventing strategies. Am J Respir Crit.Care Med 1996;153:1711-25.

BARQUET N, DOMINGO P, CAYLÀ JA, et al. Prognostic factors in meningococcal disease-development of a bedside predictive model and scoring system. JAMA 1997;278:491-69.

BOHNEN JMA, SOLOMKIN JS, DELLINGER EP, et al. Guidelines for clinical care: anti-infective agents for intra-abdominal infection. Arch Surg 1992;127:83-9.

BOUZA E, ALBADALEJO J, CERCENADO E, et al. Evolution of the isolates of the genus mycobacterium in a general hospital. Impact of the human deficiency virus epidemic. J Clin Microbiol 1997;35:1013-15.

CHRISTOU NV, TURGEON PL, WASSEF R, et al. Management of intra-abdominal infections. Arch Surg 1996;131:1193-201.

FINCH RG. Skin and soft-tissue infections. Lancet 1988;1:164-8

FINK MP, NIEDERMAN MS, SNYDMAN DR, et al. Treatment of severe pneumonia in hospitalized patients: results of a multi-center, randomized double-blind trial comparing intravenous ciprofloxacin with imipenem-cilastatin. The Severe Pneumonia Study Group Antimicrob Agents Chemother 38:547-57.

GANSTRÖM M. Tick-borne zoonoses in Europe. Clin Microbiol Infect 1997;3:156-69.

GORDON SM, EATON ME, GEORGE R, et al. The response of symptomatic neurosyphilis to high-dose intravenous pencillin G in patients with human immunodeficiency virus infection. N. Engl J Med 1994;331:1469-73.

LEW DP, WALDVOGEL FA. Osteomyelitis. N Engl J Med 1997;336:999-1007.

KAISER AB. Surgical-wound infection. N Engl J Med 1991;324:123-4.

KAUFHOLD A. Randomized evaluation of benzathine penicillin V twice daily versus potassium penicillin V three times daily in the treatment of group A streptococcal pharyngitis. Eur J Clin Microbiol Infect Dis 1995;14:92-8.

KUNIN CM. Urinary tract infection in females. Clin Infect Dis 1994;18:1-6.

SCHAAD UB, LIPS U, GNEHM HE, et al. Dexamethasone therapy for bacterial meningitis in children. Swiss Meningitis Study Group. Lancet 1993; 342:457-61.

WOLINSKY E. Mycobacterial lymphadenitis in children: A prospective study of 105 nontuberculous cases with long-term follow-up. Clin Infect Dis 1995;20:954-61.

Viral infections

Thomas Stamminger

GENERAL PRINCIPLES OF ANTIVIRAL THERAPY

Viruses are distinguished from other microbes by their simple organization and unique mode of replication. Whereas other microbes multiply by binary fission, viruses lack the machinery for using and transforming energy and for protein synthesis. Accordingly, multiplication of viruses can take place only after infection of cells, where the machinery of the host cell is used to make the constituents of viruses. This is a major drawback for antiviral strategies because extracellular viruses are not amenable to chemotherapy. They can only be inactivated by physical treatment or treatment with virucidal agents that result in protein denaturation or disruption of lipid bilayers. This, however, affects both host tissues and virus simultaneously and therefore is useful only in discrete mucocutaneous infections such as warts.

As a result of the dependence of viruses on host metabolic functions, the intracellular targeting of viruses has to be very specific so as to distinguish infected from noninfected cells. Although still more prophylactic strategies are available (e.g., vaccination) to prevent viral infections, the molecular characterization of viral replication has revealed virus-specific events that can be inhibited by antiviral drugs. Most current antiviral agents inhibit viral nucleic acid synthesis. In addition, virus-encoded proteases recently proved to be important target molecules. Since viruses differ in their mode of replication, antiviral agents typically have a restricted spectrum of activity. Thus, a diagnosis of the infecting virus often is required before antiviral chemotherapy is initiated. This is especially important because most compounds, although inhibiting virus-specific events, also affect host cell functions and therefore are associated with a varying degree of toxicity.

Another problem with antiviral chemotherapy is the ability of certain viruses to cause persistent infections by either integration of the viral genome into the host chromosome or by establishing latency, during which replication is either absent or minimal. At present, the available antiviral drugs are not effective in eliminating these nonreplicating or latent viruses. This is of major importance because latent viruses form a reservoir for recurrent infections that results in a reappearance of viral replication as soon as the drug is removed. This often can be observed during immunsuppression due to transplantation, cancer chemotherapy, or human immunodeficiency virus (HIV) infection and stresses the importance of an intact host immunologic response for recovery from viral infections.

Although the occurrence of drug-resistant viruses is observed rarely during short-term treatment with antivirals, their appearance is quite common when therapy has to be continued for several months, as is the case in HIV-infected individuals. The development of resistance results from mutations within the viral genome, and the presence of selective drug pressure leads to the emergence of a resistant virus population. In the meantime, specific mutations resulting in critical amino acid substitutions in a target protein could be correlated with the resistance of viruses against defined substances. This made it possible to develop novel diagnostic tests by which the existence of resistant variants could be recognized rapidly.

At present, antivirals with documented prophylactic or therapeutic efficacy are available for the treatment of infections with herpesviruses, human immunodeficiency viruses, and specific orthomyxoviruses, paramyxoviruses, and arenaviruses. These antiviral agents can be categorized as nucleoside and nucleotide analogues, nonnucleoside reverse-transcriptase inhibitors (NNRTIs), pyrophosphate analogues, derivatives of amantadine, and protease inhibitors. In addition, immunomodulatory substances such as interferon-α have been used successfully in the treatment of chronic hepatitis caused by hepatitis B or C viruses.

INFECTIONS WITH HERPESVIRUSES

Disease presentation

The family of herpesviruses contains at present eight members that can be isolated from humans and, in some instances, are responsible for life-threatening infections. These are the herpes simplex virus types 1 and 2 (HSV-1 and HSV-2), varicella-zoster virus (VZV), human cytomegalovirus (HCMV), human herpesvirus type 6 (HHV-6), human herpesvirus type 7 (HHV-7), Epstein-Barr virus (EBV), and human herpesvirus type 8 (HHV-

8), which is also known as *Kaposi's sarcoma-associated herpesvirus* (KSHV). Most herpesviruses are ubiquitous agents that infect a considerable proportion of the normal population and usually cause relatively mild but troublesome disease. One characteristic of herpesviruses is their ability to persist after primary infection in a latent state and to cause recurrent infections. This is of paramount importance under conditions of immunosuppression, where reactivation occurs frequently and can lead to fatal or devastating disease.

The target protein for chemotherapy of herpesviral infections is the virally encoded DNA polymerase that is essential for the synthesis of viral progeny DNA. Most antiherpesviral drugs belong to the class of nucleoside analogues that need to be converted to the triphosphate form in order to be active. In most cases this is catalyzed by a virus-specific kinase. Thus, the specificity of the available agents not only is determined by the sensitivity of the respective DNA polymerase but also depends on the affinity to the kinase encoded by the respective virus. Therefore, at least two factors contribute to the specificity of action of nucleoside analogues. The following drugs or prodrugs have proven to be effective for prophylaxis and therapy of herpesviral infections: acyclovir and its prodrug valaciclovir, penciclovir and its prodrug famciclovir, brivudine, ganciclovir, vidarabine, idoxuridine, and trifluridine. In addition to these nucleoside analogues, cidofovir, a phosphorylated nucleoside (nucleotide), and foscarnet, a pyrophosphate analogue, are able to inhibit herpesviral DNA polymerases without a prior modification by virus-encoded enzymes (Tab. 40.1).

HSV INFECTIONS

Disease presentation

The herpes simplex viruses types 1 and 2 are mainly responsible for causing mucocutaneous lesions that are preferentially located either in the orofacial region or in the genital region and are characterized by vesicles that rapidly ulcerate. Usually, primary infection is associated with more severe symptoms than recurrent infection. In oropharyngeal and orofacial infections, the spectrum of severity ranges from the trivial, involving the buccal and gingival mucosa, to severe, painful ulcerations of the mouth, gingivae, and fauces. Ocular infection, leading most commonly to a characteristic dendritic corneal ulcer, ultimately can result in blindness. Primary infection of the genital tract is often a severe clinical entity. The illness usually lasts about 3 weeks and can be associated with fever, dysuria with urethritis and/or cystitis, localized inguinal adenopathy, malaise, and pain, which may be a prominent feature. In comparison with primary infection, recurrent genital herpes is a mild but troublesome disease with the appearance of a limited number of vesicles and a localized irritation. The mean healing time in recurrent genital herpes is 15 days, compared with 7.5 days in recurrent oral disease.

In immunosuppressed patients and patients with atopic eczema, both primary and recurrent infection can cause severe mucocutaneous infection with a further cutaneous dissemination that may be indistinguishable clinically from varicella. Progression to severe generalized infection involving several visceral organs (e.g., liver and lung) also can occur and is a life-threatening condition.

Herpes simplex encephalitis most commonly presents as a focal encephalopathic process with signs and symptoms that localize to the frontotemporal and parietal areas of the brain. Without prompt initiation of antiviral chemotherapy, necrotizing HSV encephalitis is associated with a high mortality (70-90% in the absence of specific therapy). This is also true for neonatal herpes infections, which can manifest in a predominantly encephalitic, mucocutaneous, or generalized form involving several visceral organs.

Treatment

The most common disease presentation with herpes simplex viruses is the recurrent form of oropharyngeal or genital HSV infection, which is a mild and self-limiting disease in the immunocompetent patient. Because of the short duration of symptoms, trials to treat recurrent HSV infections with both topical and oral acyclovir revealed only modest clinical effects. Studies on the use of valaciclovir (2×1000 mg per day) or famciclovir (3×125 mg per day) in recurrent genital HSV infections suggest an advantage over acyclovir when oral therapy is initiated early. However, in general, the relative effectiveness of antiviral chemotherapy in treating noncomplicated, recurrent HSV infections is rather limited. In patients with frequently recurring genital herpes, chronic oral acyclovir (400 mg bid) has been demonstrated to reduce the frequency of recurrences by about 90%. The same protective effect was found for valaciclovir with the advantage that the dosage of this drug can be reduced to 500 mg qd. Thus, frequent episodes of HSV recurrencies can be effectively suppressed by either chronic oral acyclovir or valaciclovir treatment, which has proven to be a safe procedure. For treatment of primary genital HSV infection, oral acyclovir (200 mg 5 times daily for 5-10 days) should be initiated as early as possible. Recent studies indicate that valaciclovir (3×1 g per day), due to its higher oral bioavailability, may be superior for this indication. HSV keratitis also should be treated immediately. Ophthalmic formulations of acyclovir or trifluridine for topical treatment appear to be most suitable for ocular involvement.

In immunosuppressed patients, acyclovir and valaciclovir can both be used for the prevention and treatment of mucocutaneous HSV infections. Again, for oral treatment, valaciclovir has the advantage of producing higher plasma concentrations. In severe infections, iv acyclovir (10 mg/kg q8h) is currently the treatment of choice. This is also true for HSV encephalitis and neonatal HSV infection, where treatment should be initiated as early as possible, even without a firm virologic diagnosis. Prolonged use of acyclovir can result in the development of drug-resistant strains of HSV. This is seen only in occasional patients, mainly immunosuppressed patients undergoing long-term acyclovir prophylaxis or therapy. Most acyclovir-resistant strains remain sensitive to foscarnet, which should be the first-choice alternative in problem cases (Tab. 40.1).

VZV INFECTIONS

Primary infection with VZV is the cause of chickenpox (varicella), a disease that is seen most commonly in children. The illness usually begins with the appearance of a rash, but prodromal symptoms such as fever also may occur. The skin lesions progress through the stages of macules and papules to vesicles that ulcerate rapidly with crust formation. Patients with VZV infection are considered to be infectious from a couple of days before the rash until all vesicles have crusted. In children, the general constitutional symptoms of the illness typically are mild; however, complications such as bacterial superinfection, primary viral pneumonia, and viral encephalitis can occur. Infections in adult patients are

Table 40.1 Drugs for antiherpesviral therapy

Drug	Substance class	Main indications interaction	Main toxicity/
Acyclovir	Nucleoside analogue	1. HSV encephalitis (iv) 2. Neonatal HSV infections (iv) 3. Severe HSV and VZV infections in immunosuppressed patients (iv) 4. Primary herpes genitalis (oral) 5. Prophylaxis of HSV recurrencies (oral) 6. Varicella in adults (oral) 7. HSV keratitis (topical)	Nausea, diarrhea, rash, headache (< 3%), neurotoxic and nephrotoxic effects (mainly after iv use in association with high acyclovir concentrations)
Valaciclovir	Nucleoside analogue	1. Primary and recurrent herpes genitalis (oral) 2. Prophylaxis of HSV recurrencies (oral) 3. Herpes zoster (oral)	See acyclovir
Penciclovir	Nucleoside analogue	Recurrent herpes labialis (topical)	Burning, hypersensitivity reactions
Famciclovir	Nucleoside analogue	1. Herpes zoster (oral) 2. Recurrent herpes genitalis (oral)	Headache and nausea (in rare cases)
Brivudine	Nucleoside analogue	Herpes zoster, in particular in immunosuppressed patients (oral)	Nausea, vomiting, diarrhea (in rare cases), the concomitant use of antimetabolites (5-fluorouracil) is contraindicated
Ganciclovir	Nucleoside analogue	Treatment of life-or sight-threatening HCMV infections (iv, for maintenance therapy oral treatment possible)	Myelosuppression
Cidofovir	Nucleotide analogue	Treatment of HCMV retinitis in HIV -infected patients (iv)	Nephrotoxicity
Foscarnet	Pyrophosphate analogue	1. Treatment of HCMV retinitis in HIV-infected patients (iv) 2. Treatment of CNS-manifestations of HCMV infections (iv) 3. Management of ganciclovir-resistant HCMV-infections or acyclovir-resistant HSV or VZV infections.	Nephrotoxicity
Vidarabine	Nucleoside analogue	1. HSV keratitis (topical) 2. Supportive treatment of mucocutaneous HSV infections (topical)	Burning, hypersensitivity reactions
Idoxuridine	Nucleoside analogue		
Trifluridine	Nucleoside analogue		

usually more severe than those in children. In immuno-suppressed patients, primary VZV infection is a dreaded disease with a high mortality rate mainly due to a fulmi-nating course of viral pneumonia. In addition, primary infections with VZV in pregnancy can lead to malforma-tions or to neonatal infection depending on the time point of infection.

The recurrent form of VZV infection leads to a sec-ond disease, known as *herpes zoster,* or *shingles.* This disease is the result of viruses reactivating in a single sensory ganglion and then proceeding peripherally to infect the skin supplied by that nerve. Therefore, herpes zoster typically affects one single dermatome of the skin. The trigeminal ganglion is also a common site for reactivation, which can lead to involvement of the eye. Skin eruptions usually are preceded by paresthesia and/or burning or shooting pain. The most common and important complication of herpes zoster is postherpetic neuralgia, which develops in up to 10% of patients and is characterized by a severe, disabling pain that persists for months. Moreover, immunocompromised patients are in danger of experiencing a severe, disseminated form of herpes zoster.

Treatment

Noncomplicated varicella in immunocompetent children should not be treated with antivirals on a routine basis because the disease is usually mild and self-limiting. However, varicella in the adult patient can be considered an indication for treatment, which is due to the higher rate of complications seen in this patient group. Several studies demonstrated a positive effect of oral acyclovir on the course of the disease when therapy was initiated within the first 24 hours after appearance of lesions. Compared with HSV infections, higher concentrations of acyclovir (5×800 mg for 7 days) have to be used because the DNA polymerase of VZV is less sensitive. Although not thoroughly documented by studies, one can assume that the newer drugs valaciclovir and famci-clovir are at least as effective as oral acyclovir for this indication and have the advantage of a more convenient dosing (3×1 g per day for valaciclovir and 3×250 mg per day for famciclovir). Severe complications (e.g., pneumonia, encephalitis) should be treated with intra-venous acyclovir (10 mg/kg q8h). Postexposure prophy-laxis with oral acyclovir (40-80 mg/kg per day), valaci-clovir, or famciclovir beginning 1 week after exposure may reduce the risk of varicella in household contacts. Alternatively, a hyperimmune serum is available that also can be used for postexposure prophylaxis of vari-cella. In particular, this is indicated after exposure of a seronegative pregnant woman in order to prevent a pri-mary VZV infection.

For treatment of herpes zoster in immunocompetent patients, antiviral chemotherapy should be initiated within 72 hours of rash onset. While no influence of high-dose oral acyclovir (5×800 mg per day for 7 days) on the development of postherpetic neuralgia has been observed, both famciclovir and valaciclovir were able to reduce the duration of postherpetic neuralgia. Therefore, they are currently the agents of choice for treatment of herpes zoster in immunocompetent patients.

In immunocompromised patients, iv acyclovir (10 mg/kg q8h for 7 days) is considered to be the treatment of choice for both varicella and zoster, both localized and disseminated. Alternatively, oral brivudine has been shown to have a comparable effectiveness. However, care should taken to avoid concomitant use of brivudine with 5-fluorouracil, since this has resulted in fatalities. In addition, a live, attenuated viral vaccine (Oka strain) is available for the prevention of varicella, particularly in immunosuppressed patients.

HUMAN CYTOMEGALOVIRUS (HCMV) INFECTIONS

With HCMV infections one has to distinguish between infection of the immunocompetent and infections of individuals with an immature or incompetent immune system. In the immunocompetent patient, primary or recurrent HCMV infection only occasionally leads to severe disease. Some patients may experience a mononucleosis-like syndrome. In rare cases, complica-tions can arise, such as myocarditis, hepatitis, or encephalitis. In addition, an association between HCMV infection and the development of Guillain-Barré syn-drome has been reported.

One major problem with HCMV are congenital infec-tions that occur in approximately 1% of newborns in the United States. In most cases, this is due to a primary infection with HCMV during pregnancy. While a large proportion of children with congenital infection have subclinical, chronic infection, approximately 5% experi-ence severe, generalized cytomegalic inclusion disease (CID). CID of the newborn is characterized by damage to the central nervous system (CNS), including intracra-nial calcifications, ventriculomegaly, microcephaly, and ophthalmic and/or auditory damage, petechiae, hepatosplenomegaly, jaundice, and/or retinitis. Mortality in infants with CID is as high as 30%, and the prospects for normal development are poor in surviving infants, since more than 90% develop significant CNS or percep-tual defects.

The second high-risk group for infections with HCMV are individuals with an incompetent immunity, such as patients with severe combined immunodeficien-cy (SCID), patients with acquired immune-deficiency syndrome (AIDS) due to HIV infection, or immunosup-pressed patients after transplantation or chemotherapy. Both primary and recurrent infections can lead to severe disease in these patients. Symptoms can range from fever, thrombocytopenia, neutropenia, and myalgia to interstitial pneumonia, hepatitis, gastritis, colitis, encephalitis, and retinitis. Whereas retinitis is observed most commonly in AIDS patients, life-threatening inter-stitial pneumonia is a frequent manifestation after bone marrow transplantation. The reason for this differential manifestation of HCMV disease depending on patient groups is not understood but may be attributable to the different modes of immunosuppression.

Treatment

At present, three agents are available for the therapy of HCMV infections: ganciclovir, foscarnet, and cidofovir. All three drugs have severe limitations: Their oral bioavailability is rather poor, and they have a variety of side effects. The principal dose-limiting effect of ganciclovir is bone marrow toxicity, whereas foscarnet and cidofovir are mainly nephrotoxic. Therefore, all three agents are currently approved only for the treatment of patients at risk or with life- or sight-threatening HCMV infections. In addition, treatment should be based on a firm virologic diagnosis. However, one has to consider that only an early initiation of treatment proved to be effective in the prevention of fatalities due to HCMV pneumonia in bone marrow transplant patients. In order to fulfill these criteria, i.e., early initiation of treatment based on a virologic diagnosis, the concept of preemptive therapy is currently practiced for transplant patients. During the first months after transplantation, the occurrence of HCMV in the patient's peripheral blood is monitored weekly by means of polymerase chain reaction (PCR) detection of HCMV DNA or by the antigenemia test (detection of the viral antigen pp65 in leukocytes). In the case of positive results, antiviral therapy is initiated prior to the appearance of symptoms in order to prevent the development of severe disease. For transplant patients, iv ganciclovir (5 mg/kg q12h for 10-21 days) is currently the first-choice drug. Ganciclovir-resistant strains of HCMV, which occasionally develop in transplant patients after prolonged therapy, usually remain susceptible to foscarnet. In addition, CNS manifestations of HCMV infection preferentially should be treated with foscarnet because of its higher concentrations in cerebrospinal fluid.

For AIDS patients, iv foscarnet may be advantageous, and this may be related to foscarnet's intrinsic antiretroviral effects. This has been suggested by a comparative trial with ganciclovir for the treatment of HCMV retinitis that revealed an improved survival in the foscarnet group. In addition, foscarnet can be used in combination with zidovudine. For induction treatment, 60 mg/kg every 8 hours of iv foscarnet should be administered for 14 to 21 days. In contrast to transplant patients, a chronic iv maintenance therapy with foscarnet (90-120 mg/kg per day) is necessary in AIDS patients to delay the progression of HCMV retinitis. Since daily infusions are very inconvenient for those patients, alternatives have been developed: although the oral bioavailability of ganciclovir is low, 1000 mg of oral ganciclovir tid results in plasma concentrations that are effective in maintenance therapy. In addition, ganciclovir pellets for local treatment of HCMV retinitis after implantation into the respective eye have been developed. However, local therapy should always be combined with systemic treatment; otherwise, HCMV disease may occur in the contralateral eye or in other locations. As a second alternative, iv cidofovir can be used. For maintenance therapy, this drug has to be administered only once every 2 weeks, which is related to the extended intracellular half-life of cidofovir metabolites. A novel compound for local treatment of HCMV retinitis is fomivirsen, presently available in the US and other countries. This drug is interesting because of a new mechanism of action: As a phosphorothioate oligonucleotide, it targets an essential viral mRNA via antisense mechanisms.

Unfortunately, the therapeutic options in severe congenital HCMV infection are still rather limited. Although a phase II study of ganciclovir treatment of symptomatic congenital HCMV infection suggested a potentially positive effect, the toxicity of ganciclovir was evident in a significant number of children in this study, resulting in neutropenia, thrombocytopenia, and elevated results of liver function studies. Therefore, no general recommendation for routine use of ganciclovir in symptomatic congenital HCMV infection could be given based on this study. A phase III clinical trial that randomizes children to receive or not receive treatment is currently going on.

INFECTIONS WITH OTHER HERPESVIRUSES

Epstein-Barr virus (EBV) is the causative agent of infectious mononucleosis. In addition, this virus is involved in the development of lymphoproliferative disease in transplant patients and AIDS patients. One particular syndrome in AIDS patients is oral hairy leukoplakia, where lytic replication of EBV can be observed in epithelial cells of the oral cavity. The difficulty in antiviral chemotherapy of EBV infections relates to the fact that EBV is able to establish latency in lymphocytes, thereby triggering a proliferation of the respective cells that are mainly responsible for causing disease. During latency, however, the target of the current antiherpesviral chemotherapy, the herpesviral DNA polymerase, is not expressed, since replication of the viral genome during latency is catalyzed by the cellular DNA polymerase. Therefore, although several antiviral drugs including acyclovir are able to inhibit lytic replication of this virus, latent EBV in B-lymphocytes is currently not amenable to the available drugs. Consistent with this, trials to treat infectious mononucleosis of normal hosts with iv or oral acyclovir revealed a transient suppression of salivary EBV excretion but no important effects on other illness parameters. However, case reports suggest that some cases of severe EBV infection or EBV-related lymphoproliferation appear to respond to antiviral treatment. For this, iv acyclovir should be used (10 mg/kg q8h), since this drug has fewer side effects compared with other drugs such as foscarnet or ganciclovir that may show a comparable effectiveness. Oral hairy leukoplakia, which is due to a lytic replication of EBV, responds well to oral acyclovir treatment.

HHV-6 has been identified as the causative agent of roseola infantum (also known as *exanthema subitum* or *sixth disease*). Moreover, this virus appears to be responsible for a highly febrile disease in children without fulfilling all criteria to be diagnosed as roseola infantum. Severe disease (i.e., encephalitis, hepatosplenomegaly, hepatitis, and bronchopneumonia) also has been associated with HHV-6 seroconversion in children, but a causative role of this virus is difficult to prove. In transplant patients, some case reports suggest a role of HHV-6 in causing encephalitis, hepatitis, and pneumonia. In vitro studies have shown that HHV-6 replication is largely unaffected by acyclovir, but the virus is sensitive to ganciclovir and foscarnet. Thus, it would appear that the antiviral therapy given for treatment of HCMV infections is also the most suitable for treatment of HHV-6 infections.

Since infections with HHV-7 could not be associated with any specific disease in humans up to now, there is no need for antiviral treatment. At present, there is good evidence to indicate that HHV-8 is involved in the development of Kaposi's sarcoma, a tumor of endothelial cells that is seen frequently in AIDS patients. However, similar to EBV infection, the latent form of the virus is mainly involved in causing disease. Thus, although foscarnet is able to inhibit lytic replication, no significant effect of antiviral chemotherapy on Kaposi's sarcoma has been documented up to now. In contrast, systemic interferon-α proved to be useful for treatment of Kaposi's sarcoma in HIV-infected patients with no prior history of opportunistic infections.

Drug classes

ACYCLOVIR AND VALACICLOVIR

Mechanism and spectrum of action

Acyclovir is the prototype of an antiviral drug with selective activity that is due to the inhibition of virus-specific events. It is a deoxyguanosine analogue with an acyclic side chain lacking the 3' hydroxyl group. Intracellular phosphorylation of acyclovir by the virally encoded thymidine kinase is the first step in the activation of this drug that leads to the monophosphate derivative. Cellular enzymes convert the monophosphate to acyclovir triphosphate, which competitively inhibits viral DNA polymerases. Two mechanisms contribute to the inhibitory effect: First, the triphosphate can be incorporated into viral DNA; however, it acts as a chain terminator because the 3' hydroxyl group required for elongation is missing. Second, the DNA polymerase is inactivated in an irreversible manner because of complex formation between the terminated template and the protein. Valaciclovir, the L-valyl ester of acyclovir, is rapidly converted to acyclovir after oral administration and therefore has the same mechanism of action. The DNA polymerases of various HSVs differ in their sensitivity to acyclovir triphosphate. The polymerase of HCMV appears to be especially sensitive; however, HCMV lacks a thymidine kinase. Therefore, the intracellular levels of acyclovir triphosphate in HCMV-infected cells are low compared with HSV- or VZV-infected cells, where the enzymatic activity of the respective thymidine kinase results in 40- to 100-fold higher concentrations in infected compared with uninfected cells. Thus acyclovir is used mainly for the treatment of HSV and VZV infections. Since the DNA polymerase of VZV is less sensitive than the respective enzymes of HSV-1 and HSV-2, higher drug concentrations are required for effective treatment of VZV infections.

Pharmacokinetics/metabolism

Only about 20% of acyclovir is absorbed after oral administration of tablets. Peak plasma concentrations average 0.4 to 0.8 µg/ml after 200-mg oral doses and increase to about 1.6 µg/ml after 800-mg doses. In contrast, the administration of oral valaciclovir results in a 3- to 5-fold greater acyclovir bioavailability, since valaciclovir is absorbed rapidly and is almost completely converted to acyclovir, probably in first-pass intestinal and hepatic metabolism by a newly characterized enzyme, valaciclovir hydrolase. After a 1-hour infusion of 5 mg/kg of acyclovir, peak plasma concentrations of 10 µg/ml could be observed. Percutaneous absorption of acyclovir after topical administration appears to be low.

Acyclovir distributes widely in body fluids, with cerebrospinal fluid (CSF) concentrations reaching about 50% of plasma values. Plasma protein binding ranges from 9 to 33%. The mean plasma elimination half-life of acyclovir is about 3 hours in adults with normal renal function but increases to about 20 hours in anuric patients. Most of the acyclovir is excreted unmetabolized in urine via glomerular filtration and tubular secretion. Acyclovir is readily removed via hemodialysis but not by peritoneal dialysis. Dosage reductions are indicated in patients with creatinine clearances of less than 50 ml/min; for iv treatment, the dosing interval should be increased to 12 hours for patients with a CrCl of between 25 and 50 ml/min and to 24 hours for patients with a CrCl of between 10 and 25 ml/min. In patients with a CrCl of less than 10 ml/min, 50% of the standard dose should be given every 24 hours. For oral treatment, the dosing interval should to increased to 8 or 12 hours in patients with a CrCl of between 10 and 25 ml/min or less than 10 ml/min, respectively.

Dosage/pharmaceutical forms

Acyclovir is available as a cream for the topical treatment of mucocutaneous lesions, and a corresponding formulation for the topical treatment of ophthalmic lesions is also available. Topical acyclovir should be applied five times a day for 5 to 10 days. For oral administration, tablets of 200, 400, and 800 mg are availaible. Dosage depends on the actual infecting herpesvirus: for treatment of HSV infections in adults, 200 mg five times daily is indicated (for 7-10 days); in VZV infections, the dosage has to be increased to 5 × 800 mg. In severe infections, acyclovir should be given iv (5-10 mg/kg). Because of its higher oral bioavailability, valaciclovir has the potential for less frequent administration (3×1 g per day).

Indications

Indications for intravenous treatment include: (1) HSV encephalitis (early initiation of treatment is important), (2) neonatal HSV infections, and (3) mucocutaneous and disseminated HSV or VZV infections in immunosuppressed patients or patients with eczema.

Indications for oral treatment include: (1) primary HSV infection of the genital tract, (2) recurrent HSV infections (higher efficacy of valaciclovir), (3) prophylaxis of frequent recurrences of oral or genital HSV infections, (4) prophylaxis of HSV infections in immunosuppressed patients, (5) VZV infection in adult patients, and (6) herpes zoster in nonimmunosuppressed patients (for valaciclovir, an influence on postherpetic neuralgia has been documented).

Indications for topical treatment include: (1) HSV keratitis, (2) herpes zoster of the cornea, and (3) supportive treatment of herpes genitalis and herpes labialis (low efficacy).

Side effects and interactions

More than 10 years of acyclovir use, has established an excellent safety profile in clinical practice with a relatively low rate of side effects. Topical administration may result in transient burning, especially when applied to genital lesions. Oral acyclovir has been associated infrequently (<3%) with nausea, diarrhea, rash, headache, and rarely, renal insufficiency and neurotoxicity. Valaciclovir has comparable side effects. After iv application, extravasation of the alkaline solution can lead to inflammation and phlebitis at the site of injection. Uncommonly reported side effects include rash, hematuria, hypotension, headache, and nausea. Neurotoxic effects characterized by lethargy, confusion, tremor, myoclonus, hallucinations, delirium, seizures, and/or coma may manifest in approximately 1% of patients. Most of the neurotoxic effects occur in association with high acyclovir concentrations due to renal insufficiency. Another side effect of iv acyclovir may be a reversible renal dysfunction that commonly occurs after rapid infusion and usually resolves with drug cessation and volume expansion.

Nephrotoxicity may be enhanced by the concomitant administration of other nephrotoxic agents such as cyclosporin A. Combinations of acyclovir with zidovudine that are used for therapy of HIV infection may result in severe somnolence and lethargy. Since acyclovir is in part eliminated via active renal secretion, the renal clearance of other drugs using the same pathway (e.g., methotrexate) may be affected.

Contraindications

There is limited experience during pregnancy and lactation. Topical formulations for skin lesions may not be used for the treatment of ophthalmic or genital lesions.

PENCICLOVIR AND FAMCICLOVIR

Similar to acyclovir, penciclovir is an acyclic nucleoside analogue that depends in its activity on the virally encoded thymidine kinase for initial phosphorylation. Famciclovir is the diacetyl ester prodrug of penciclovir, which by itself is inactive but is rapidly converted to penciclovir after oral administration. The selectivity of action of penciclovir is due to the preferential phosphorylation of this drug in herpesvirus-infected cells to penciclovir triphosphate, which is a competitive inhibitor of the virally encoded DNA polymerase. One important difference from acyclovir is the long intracellular half-life of penciclovir triphosphate in infected cells (7-14 h versus 0.8 h for acyclovir triphosphate). It is thought that this results in a persistent inhibition of viral replication that may be advantageous in certain clinical settings such as the treatment of acute herpes zoster. Again, similar to acyclovir, HSV-1 and HSV-2 and VZV show the highest susceptibility to penciclovir.

Pharmacokinetics/metabolism

Penciclovir is only active when administered parenterally because oral absorption is low. Therefore, the prodrug famciclovir has been developed that is well absorbed after oral administration (<70%) and is rapidly converted to penciclovir. Penciclovir is extensively distributed into tissues. The primary route for elimination of penciclovir is renal (unmetabolized) with a mean plasma half-life of 2 hours. In patients with moderately or severely reduced renal function, dose reduction is recommended. For a creatinine clearance of between 30 and 50 ml/min or between 5 and 29 ml/min, the dosing interval of famciclovir should be increased to 12 or 24 hours, respectively.

Dosage/pharmaceutical forms

Famciclovir is available as tablets of 125 and 250 mg. For treatment of herpes zoster in adults, which is the main indication for this drug, 250 mg tid is indicated. Lower doses are required for the treatment of recurrent herpes genitalis (3×125 mg). Penciclovir is available as a cream for topical treatment of recurrent herpes labialis but is not available for iv treatment.

Indications

Indications include herpes zoster in adult patients (oral), treatment of recurrent herpes genitalis (oral), and supportive treatment of recurrent herpes labialis (topical).

Side effects and interactions

Famciclovir is generally well tolerated but may be associated with headache and nausea. Drug interaction studies with several commonly prescribed drugs such as allopurinol, cimetidine, theophylline, and digoxin have not shown any clinically significant interactions with famciclovir. In addition, no significant interaction after coadministration of famciclovir and zidovudine in HIV-infected patients could be observed. Experience in patients younger than 18 years of age, immunosuppressed patients, and patients with complicated HSV and VZV infections is limited at present.

Contraindications

Contraindications include patients younger than 18 years of age (due to limited experience), patients with disseminated and/or visceral herpes zoster, patients with varicella zoster encephalitis, and patients who are pregnant or lactating.

BRIVUDINE

Brivudine is a pyrimidine nucleoside analogue containing a bromovinyl substitution. It has potent inhibitory activity for VZV with an effective concentration (EC$_{50}$) of 1 µg/l on average. It is also effective against HSV-1 but not against HSV-2. This limits the usefulness of this drug for the treatment of HSV infections, since knowledge about the infecting HSV type is required before therapy can be initiated. The compound is phosphorylated by the VZV- and HSV-1-encoded thymidine kinase and then converted to brivudine triphosphate by cellular kinases, which acts as a competitive inhibitor of viral DNA replication with respect to dTTP. Unlike acyclovir triphosphate, it is not incorporated into viral DNA.

Pharmacokinetics/metabolism

Brivudine seems to be well absorbed after oral administration. An oral dosage of 7.5 mg/kg per day results in plasma drug levels of 1 µg/ml, which is far in excess of its minimum inhibitory concentration for HSV-1 and VZV. Plasma protein binding is over 95 %. Brivudine is rapidly metabolized to its inactive metabolite, bromovinyluracil (BVU). Elimination of both metabolized and unmetabolized drug is by renal excretion.

Dosage/pharmaceutical forms

Brivudine is available as tablets of 125 mg. For treatment of HSV-1 and VZV infections in immunocompromised patients, 125 mg four times daily is recommended. In children, the dosage should be reduced to 5 mg/kg of body weight tid.

Indications

Indications include HSV-1 and VZV-infections in immunosuppressed patients.

Side effects and interactions

Oral brivudine is generally well tolerated. During short-term administration in the absence of other drugs, no serious side effects have been recognized. The most frequently reported adverse events are nausea, vomiting, abdominal pain, diarrhea, and headache. Rarely, elevations of hepatic enzyme values have been observed. The most significant interaction occurs during concomitant use of 5-fluorouracil (5-FU); the metabolite of brivudine inhibits the enzyme dihydropyrimidine dehydrogenase, which is required for 5-FU metabolism. Thus, the half-life of 5-FU increases in the presence of brivudine from approximately 20 minutes to 5 hours. This potentiates the toxicity of 5-FU, and fatalities have occurred in oncology patients treated with both drugs. In addition, the high plasma protein binding may compete with the binding of other drugs.

Contraindications

Contraindications include concomitant use of 5-fluorouracil or other antimetabolites, pregnancy and lactation, and renal insufficiency.

GANCICLOVIR

Mechanism and spectrum of action

Ganciclovir, which is a deoxyguanosine analogue, has inhibitory activity against all herpesviruses. However, its unique characteristic is potent inhibition of HCMV replication that cannot be achieved by acyclovir. This is due to the action of an HCMV-encoded protein, the UL97 kinase, which monophosphorylates ganciclovir. This leads to at least 10-fold higher concentrations of ganciclovir monophosphate in HCMV-infected cells compared with noninfected cells. After further modification to ganciclovir triphosphate by cellular enzymes, the viral DNA polymerase is preferentially inhibited in a competitive manner. In addition, the intracellular half-life of ganciclovir triphosphate is rather long with a t$_{1/2}$ exceeding 24 hours. In HSV- and VZV-infected cells, the monophosphorylation of ganciclovir is catalyzed by the herpesviral thymidine kinase.

Pharmacokinetics/metabolism

The oral bioavailability of ganciclovir is low (<10%). However, the administration of 1000 mg every 6 hours results in a peak plasma level of 1.0 µg/ml, which is within the sensitivity range of most HCMV strains. Thus, oral treatment is feasible in certain clinical situations such as maintenance therapy of HIV-infected patients. After iv administration of 5 mg/kg, peak plasma concentrations average 5 to 11 µg/ml. CSF and brain tissue levels are only approximately 30 to 50% of those in plasma. Intravitreal concentrations are even lower (approximately 1.0 µg/ml). Plasma protein binding is only 1 to 2%. Ganciclovir is eliminated mainly unmetabolized by renal excretion. The plasma t$_{1/2}$ averages 2.4 hours in patients with normal renal function but increases with declining creatinine clearance. In patients with a creatinine clearance of less than 50 ml/min, dose reductions are necessary (3 mg/kg at a dosing interval of 12 h for patients with a CrCl of 50-25 ml/min, 3 mg/kg at a dosing interval of 24 h for patients with a CrCl of 25-10 ml/min, and 1.5 mg/kg at a dosing interval of 24 h for patients with a CrCl of <10 ml/min).

Dosage/pharmaceutical forms

For initial treatment of HCMV infections, administration of ganciclovir should be performed iv with 5 mg/kg bid as a 1-hour infusion for 14 days. For maintenance therapy, dose reductions to 5 mg/kg once daily are possible. Alternatively, oral administration of 1000 mg ganciclovir tid is indicated in patients with stable HCMV retinitis. For oral treatment, capsules of 250 mg ganciclovir are available.

Indications

Indications include treatment of patients at risk for or with life- or sight-threatening HCMV disease, in particular in immunosuppressed patients due to transplantation or cancer chemotherapy or in AIDS patients.

Side effects and interactions

Unfortunately, ganciclovir treatment can be associated with severe side effects. The principal dose-limiting toxicity of ganciclovir is myelosuppression, with neutropenia and thrombocytopenia occurring in up to 40% of patients. This is due to the fact that the inhibitory concentrations of ganciclovir for human bone marrow progenitor cells are similar to those for HCMV replication. Immune responses requiring active DNA synthesis also may be suppressed. Ganciclovir-induced neutropenia is observed most commonly during the second week of treatment and resolves promptly after drug cessation. Granulocyte/macrophage colony-stimulating factor (GM-CSF) can be used for treatment of ganciclovir-induced neutropenia. In addition, CNS side effects can occur, including headache, behavioral changes, and even convulsions or coma. Anemia, rash, fever, liver function test abnormalities, nausea, and eosinophilia also have been reported. Results from animal experiments suggest that ganciclovir can have mutagenic and carcinogenic effects. In addition, teratogenicity and embryotoxicity have been observed in animals at ganciclovir doses comparable with those used in humans.

Contraindications

Contraindications include preexisting neutropenia (<500 neutrophils/ml) or thrombocytopenia and pregnancy; owing to a possible teratogenic effect of ganciclovir, contraception is indicated during treatment and for 90 days after treatment has been finished.

CIDOFOVIR

Cidofovir is a phosphorylated nucleoside (nucleotide) that shows in vitro activity against a broad spectrum of viruses including HSV-1, HSV-2, VZV, HCMV, EBV, and human papillomaviruses. In particular, it has been suggested that cidofovir is 100-fold more potent and selective against HCMV than foscarnet. In contrast to acyclovir or ganciclovir, which require intracellular activation by virus-encoded enzymes, cidofovir is already a nucleotide. Conversion to the active antiviral substance, cidofovir diphosphate, is catalyzed by cellular enzymes. Therefore, cidofovir is still active against TK-negative viruses. Analogous to other antiviral nucleoside triphosphates, cidofovir diphosphate inhibits the viral DNA polymerase.

Pharmacokinetics/metabolism

Pharmacokinetic studies in HIV-infected patients showed that serum concentrations of cidofovir following intravenous infusion were dose-proportional over the dose range 1 to 10 mg/kg. Oral bioavailability was low (<5%). Approximately 90% of the iv dose was recovered unchanged in the urine in 24 hours. Active tubular secretion appears to play a significant role in the clearance of cidofovir. The main advantage of cidofovir is the very long intracellular half-life of cidofovir metabolites, resulting in a prolonged antiviral action that lasts for several days or weeks. This allows infrequent dosing (i.e., every week or every 2 weeks), which is of advantage in the maintenance therapy of HIV-infected patients suffering from HCMV retinitis. Data on the pharmacokinetics of topically administered cidofovir indicate that the drug is usually undetectable in blood, even after prolonged administration.

Dosage/pharmaceutical forms

For initial treatment, cidofovir should be applied as an intravenous infusion of 5 mg/kg once a week for a period of 2 weeks. For maintenance therapy, administration of 5 mg/kg cidofovir can be reduced to one infusion every 2 weeks. Infusion of cidofovir is performed over 1 hour with a constant infusion rate. Patients should be sufficiently hydrated. To further reduce the nephrotoxic effects of cidofovir, oral probenicid should be administered concomitantly (4 g total, 2 g probenecid 3 h before the infusion is started, 1 g probenecid 2 and 8 h after completion of the cidofovir application).

Indications

Indications include treatment of HCMV retinitis in HIV-infected patients without renal dysfunction. Because of limited experience, it is recommended to use cidofovir only when other drugs are not appropriate.

Side effects and interactions

The most important side effect of cidofovir relates to the nephrotoxicity of this drug, which can be observed in up to 50% of treated patients and manifests as proteinuria and/or increased creatinine levels. Furthermore, it has been reported that neutropenia, fever, dyspnea, diarrhea, vomiting, exanthema, and alopecia can occur during concomitant administration of cidofovir and probenicid. Cidofovir should not be used in combination with or within 7 days after the use of other nephrotoxic drugs such as amphotericin B or foscarnet. Interactions of cidofovir have been described with several drugs that are frequently used in HIV-infected patients (e.g., zidovudine, acyclovir, cotrimoxazol, didanosine, fluconazol, and aminoglycosides). It should be considered that probenecid interacts with the renal excretion of various drugs (e.g., acyclovir, nonsteroidal anti-inflammatory drugs, and benzodiazepines).

Contraindications

Pregnancy and lactation are contraindications for the use of cidofovir. Furthermore, preexisting renal insufficiency and dehydration are also incompatible with the use of cidofovir. Parameters for renal function always should be determined before the initiation of therapy; a serum creatinine level of more than 1.5 mg/dl, a creatinine clearance of less than 55 ml/min, and a proteinuria of more than 100 mg/dl are contraindications for the use of cidofovir. Great care also should be taken in patients who were treated previously with foscarnet.

FOSCARNET

Foscarnet is an inorganic pyrophosphate analogue that is inhibitory for all herpesviruses as well as for HIV. Unlike nucleoside analogues, foscarnet does not undergo significant intracellular metabolism. It directly inhibits the DNA polymerases of herpesviruses or the HIV reverse transcriptase by blocking the pyrophosphate binding site of the respective enzyme. This inhibits the cleavage of pyrophosphate from dNTP. Thus foscarnet is effective against most ganciclovir-resistant HCMV and acyclovir-resistant HSV and VZV strains. The selectivity of action of foscarnet relates to an approximately 100-fold greater inhibition of herpesvirus DNA polymerases than cellular DNA polymerase-α.

Pharmacokinetics/metabolism

Oral bioavailability of foscarnet is low (<20%). Peak plasma concentrations after an infusion of 90 mg/kg per day are approximately 500 µmol/l. Plasma protein binding is about 15%. CSF concentrations average 70% of plasma concentrations at steady state in HCMV-infected patients. Foscarnet is eliminated via renal mechanisms ($t_{1/2}$ = 4-8 h), with about 80% of the dose being excreted as unmetabolized drug. Plasma clearance decreases proportionally with creatinine clearance, and dose adjustments for induction and maintenance therapy are necessary for even small decreases in renal function according to a dosing table available from the manufacturer. Foscarnet can be removed via hemodialysis, and plasma levels decrease by about 50% with a 3-hour run.

Dosage/pharmaceutical forms

Foscarnet is available as a solution for infusion. For induction therapy, 60 mg/kg of foscarnet is administered as a 2-hour iv infusion q8h for 2 to 3 weeks. Patients should be hydrated sufficiently. For maintenance therapy, when prolonged administration is necessary, dose reductions to 90 mg/kg qd are possible. For topical treatment of mucocutaneous herpesvirus infections, a 2% cream formulation is available.

Indications

The main indication for foscarnet is HCMV retinitis in AIDS patients. Owing to the simultaneous inhibition of both the HCMV DNA polymerase and the HIV reverse transcriptase, a slight advantage of foscarnet versus ganciclovir treatment in HCMV retinitis has been documented. Because of the higher concentration of foscarnet in liquor compared with ganciclovir, CNS manifestations of HCMV infections also should be treated preferentially with foscarnet. Alternate or concomitant administration with ganciclovir also has been reported for this indication. Furthermore, foscarnet is indicated for management of ganciclovir-resistant HCMV infections and acyclovir-resistant HSV or VZV infections.

Side effects and interactions

Nephrotoxicity with azotemia, mild proteinuria, and possibly acute tubular necrosis is the major dose-limiting side effect of foscarnet. Increases in serum creatinine occur in about 30% of patients. High doses, rapid infusions, dehydration, and preexisting renal insufficiency are risk factors for the development of nephrotoxic effects. In addition, metabolic abnormalities are quite common, including hypo- and hypercalcemia, hypo- and hyperphosphatemia, and hypokalemia. This may cause paresthesias, arrhythmias, tetany, seizures, and other CNS disturbances, including headache, which occurs in up to one-fourth of patients. Other reported side effects are fever, gastrointestinal intolerance, elevation of liver enzymes, and painful genital ulcerations that usually resolve after stopping therapy. Animal experiments indicate that foscarnet is mutagenic and teratogenic. Therefore, safety of this drug in pregnancy or during childhood is uncertain. Since foscarnet is less hematotoxic than ganciclovir, it can be used in combination with zidovudine for treatment of HIV-infected patients. Administration of foscarnet with amphotericin B and other nephrotoxic agents may cause enhanced renal toxicity. Furthermore, intravenous pentamidine can increase the risk of symptomatic hypocalcemia. The solution used for infusion must not be combined with other drugs.

Contraindications

Preexisting severe renal insufficiency (CrCl < 0.4 ml/min/kg), pregnancy, and lactation are contraindications for the use of foscarnet. Furthermore, combinations with other nephrotoxic drugs (e.g., amphotericin B) or with intravenous pentamidine have to be avoided.

DRUGS FOR TOPICAL ADMINISTRATION

In addition to topical formulations of acyclovir and foscarnet, at least three further nucleoside analogues are available for exclusive use in topical therapy. These are vidarabine, idoxuridine, and trifluridine. Because of their severe side effects, idoxuridine and trifluridine cannot be used for systemic therapy. One main indication for these drugs is ocular HSV infection (HSV keratitis). Because of its observed higher rate of adverse reactions (e.g., pain, itching, inflammation, and edema), idoxuridine seems to be less suitable for this indication compared with trifluridine and topical formulations of acyclovir. In addition, idoxuridine is also available for topical treatment of mucocutaneous HSV and VZV infections. However, as already discussed for topical acyclovir, the clinical usefulness of this form of treatment appears to be limited.

INFECTIONS WITH INFLUENZA VIRUSES

Disease presentation

Influenza viruses are subclassified into three different genera, termed influenza A, B, and C. While influenza C infection is usually a relatively mild respiratory infection that is rarely diagnosed, influenza A and B viruses can cause severe disease. Following droplet infection from infected individuals, the incubation period is approximately 48 hours. The onset of illness is usually abrupt. Symptoms in adults commonly include a marked fever, headache, photophobia, shivering, a dry cough, malaise, and aching of muscles. In uncomplicated cases, fever classically lasts for 3 days; then the temperature falls and the symptoms abate. Although the infection usually resolves within 7 days, patients commonly complain of feeling unwell for weeks after acute infection. Complications can include bacterial superinfection, primary viral pneumonia, and encephalitis. In particular, elderly patients with concomitant pulmonary or heart disease are at high risk of developing severe disease.

Treatment

Although manifested influenza infections in later stages are still not amenable to antiviral chemotherapy, the drugs amantadine and rimantadine proved to be useful for prophylaxis and early treatment of infections. Effectiveness is limited to infections with influenza A virus strains. However, influenza A viruses are mainly responsible for causing large epidemics. Prophylaxis is particularly useful for prevention and curtailing nosocomial outbreaks of influenza virus infections. Trials comparing 200 mg per day doses of amantadine with 100 mg per day doses of rimantadine found that both drugs were approximately 90% effective in preventing influenza A illness. Seasonal prophylaxis with rimantadine or amantadine also can be used in high-risk patients if influenza vaccine cannot be administered because of allergy. When begun within 1 to 2 days of onset of symptoms, doses of 200 mg per day of amanta-dine or 100 mg per day of rimantadine were able to reduce the duration of fever and systemic complaints. Thus, a therapeutic effect of amantadine and rimantadine can be observed when therapy is initiated early.

Drug classes

AMANTADINE AND RIMANTADINE

Amantadine and rimantadine are symmetric tricyclic amines that are able to inhibit the replication of influenza A viruses but not of influenza B and C viruses. In in vitro assays, rimantadine has a 4- to 10-fold higher inhibitory effect than amantadine. Both drugs share the same mechanism of action. They interfere with the ion-channel function of the viral transmembrane protein M2 and are therefore able to interfere with the uncoating of viruses. In animal experiments, resistant strains of influenza A virus are rapidly selected and appear to preserve their pathogenic phenotype.

Pharmacokinetics/metabolism

Amantadine is well absorbed after oral administration, reaching peak plasma levels after 2 to 4 hours. The same is true for rimantadine; however, absorption appears to be delayed in comparison with amantadine. Amantadine is excreted unmetabolized in the urine through glomerular filtration and probably tubular secretion. The plasma $t_{1/2}$ is about 12 to 18 hours. Because of age-related declines in renal function, $t_{1/2}$ increases up to twofold in the elderly and even more in patients with impaired renal function. Therefore, dose reductions are required in renal insufficiency. In contrast, rimantadine is extensively metabolized following oral administration. Less than 15% of the dose is excreted unchanged in the urine. The plasma $t_{1/2}$ of rimantadine averages 24 to 36 hours. No significant differences in pharmacokinetics are found in patients with chronic liver disease without significant hepatocellular dysfunction. In patients with severe renal failure, the $t_{1/2}$ is about 50% longer. Dose reduction by one-half is suggested for marked hepatic or renal insufficiency.

Dosage/pharmaceutical forms

Amantadine is available as tablets of 100 mg. Oral prophylaxis or therapy of adults under 65 years of age should be performed with 200 mg per day; for older patients, dose reductions to 100 mg per day are indicated. Children under 5 years of age also can be treated with 100 mg per day. Rimantadine (not available in some European countries) is distributed as a 100-mg coated tablet or a syrup.

Indications

Indications are limited to the prevention and treatment (only effective when initiated within the first 48 h after the onset of symptoms) of influenza A virus infections.

Side effects and interactions

The most common side effects related to amantadine ingestion are minor dose-related gastrointestinal and CNS complaints, including nervousness, difficulty in concentrating, insomnia, loss of appetite, and nausea. CNS side effects are quite common in amantadine recipients (approximately 30%) but appear less frequent with rimantadine. The wider therapeutic margin of rimantadine relative to amantadine most probably relates to the differences in pharmacokinetics between the drugs. In the setting of renal insufficiency or high doses, serious neurotoxic reactions, including tremor, seizures or coma, cardiac arrhythmias, and death, may occur. Psychiatric side effects in parkinsonian patients and psychotic exacerbations in schizophrenic patients may occur with amantadine. The CNS effects of amantadine appear to be increased by concomitant use of antihistamines or anticholinergic drugs. Coadministration of cotrimazol or triamterene/hydrochlorothiazide also has been associated with increased CNS toxicity due to a decreased renal clearance. Drug interactions with rimantadine have not been well studied.

Contraindications

Contraindications include a history of psychotic disorders, confusion or excitation, seizures, severe renal insufficiency, and pregnancy and lactation.

HIV INFECTIONS

Disease presentation

Infection with human immunodeficiency viruses (HIV-1 and HIV-2) initiates a chronic disease that is characterized

---

Table 40.2 Drugs for antiretroviral therapy

Drugs	Alternative name	Substance class	Dosage	Main toxicity interactions	Important therapy	Combination
Zidovudine	AZT	Nucleoside analogue	2 x 250 mg	Neutropenia, anemia, nausea	Ganciclovir (myelotoxicity)	ddI*, ddC*, 3TC*, protease inhibitors, nevirapine
Didanosine	ddI	Nucleoside analogue	2 x 200 mg	Peripheral neuropathy, pancreatitis	Ganciclovir, vincristine, INH (neuropathy)	AZT*, d4T, protease inhibitors, nevirapine
Zalcitabine	ddC	Nucleoside	0.75 mg	Peripheral neuropathy, oral ulcerations	Vincristine, INH (neuropathy)	AZT*, protease inhibitors
Stavudine	d4T	Nucleoside analogue	2 x 20-40 mg	Peripheral neuropathy, pancreatitis	Vincristine, INH (neuropathy)	3TC, ddI, protease inhibitors
Lamivudine	3TC	Nucleoside analogue	2 x 140 mg	Headache	–	AZT*, d4T, ddI, protease inhibitors
Nevirapine		NNRTI	2 x 200 mg	Exanthema	Inhibitors of cytochrome P450	Nucleoside analogues, protease inhibitors
Delavirdine		NNRTI	3 x 400 mg	Exanthema	Inhibitors of cytochrome P450	Nucleoside analogues, protease inhibitors
Saquinavir	Ro-31-8959	Protease inhibitor	3 x 600 mg (up to 3 x 2400 mg)	Diarrhoea, nausea	Inhibitors of cytochrome P450 (ritonavir is most potent), interactions with e.g., rifampicin terfenadine, astemizole, cisapride, ergotamine and various other drugs. These interactions are also true for Nelfinavir	Ritonavir (2 x 400 mg), nelfinavir, nucleoside analogues
Ritonavir	ABT-538	Protease inhibitor	2 x 600 mg	Diarrhoea, nausea, hypertriglyceridemia		Saquinavir, nucleoside analogues
Indinavir	MK-639	Protease inhibitor	3 x 800 mg	Nephrolithiasis, hyperbilirubinemia		Nucleoside analogues
Nelfinavir	AG1343	Protease inhibitor	3 x 750 mg	Diarrhoea, nausea		Nucleoside analogues

*Efficacy of combination therapy documented in clinical studies.

mainly by the continuous destruction of CD4$^+$ T-lympho-cytes. After a varying period of time, this ultimately leads to the development of the acquired immune-deficiency syndrome (AIDS). Primary infection with HIV results in an initial acute illness that has been described as mononu-cleosis-like. A typical representation involves the acute onset of fever, lethargy, malaise, headaches, sore throat, lymphadenopathy, and a maculopapular rash. During this phase, the virus disseminates rapidly and widely within the infected organism. This is also reflected by the high levels of virus in peripheral blood that are easily detectable by virus isolation, antigen assays, or the quan-tification of viral RNA during this time period. Coincident with seroconversion (in most cases occurring 4 to 6 weeks after primary infection) one can observe a strong reduction in virus levels in peripheral blood that appears to be due to a vigorous immune response leading to a containment of the virus. In contrast to earlier assumptions, however, HIV by itself is not latent during this phase but replicates exten-sively, resulting in the production of approximately 10^{10} progeny viruses and the destruction of approximately 10^9 CD4$^+$ T-lymphocytes per day. Thus HIV infection is extremely proliferative during all phases of the disease. This has important implications for the time point of initia-tion of antiretroviral therapy. The interval between the pri-mary illness and the appearance of AIDS-related symptoms has been termed the *clinically latent* or *asymptomatic phase* because the development of symptoms is still prevented by an effective immune response against HIV. This phase may be months or years and depends on a number of factors, including route of infection, dose of virus, state of the immune response, and genetic background of the host. Progression to symptomatic disease is associated with signs of an activated immune system such as the appearance of lymphadenopathy. AIDS by itself is defined by the occur-rence of AIDS-associated diseases, which include oppor-tunistic infections (e.g., *Pneumocystis carinii* pneumonia, cytomegalovirus retinitis, and toxoplasmosis) and malig-nancies (e.g., Kaposi's sarcoma and malignant lym-phomas).

Treatment

Although the first results of antiretroviral therapy that were based on monotherapy with zidovudine were discour-aging due to the rapid selection of resistant viral strains, the introduction of several novel drugs during the years 1991-1996 has improved our therapeutic options dramatically for the treatment of HIV infections. At present, 11 drugs are available for antiretroviral therapy; however, a substantial number of additional agents are in clinical trials. Therefore, one has to be aware that the recommendations given in this chapter may be valid only temporarily. Because of the rapid development in this field of antiviral therapy, it is strongly recommended that physicians consult the actual literature in order to determine the optimal treatment for HIV-infect-ed patients. The currently available drugs can be classified into two groups based on the targeted HIV protein: (1) reverse-transcriptase (RT) inhibitors, including several nucleoside analogues (e.g., zidovudine, didanosine, zal-

Table 40.3 Indications for initiation of therapy in HIV infected individuals

Obligatory indications
1. Patients with AIDS
2. Patients with HIV-associated symptoms
3. Patients with a viral load of (>) 30 000 copies/μl
4. Patients with CD4$^+$cells of (<) 350/μl

Facultative indications
1. Patients with a significant increase in viral load (> 1 $\log_{10}$)
2. Patients with a significant decrease of CD4$^+$ cells (> 25%)
3. Patients with a viral load of > 10 000 copies/μl
4. Patients with CD4$^+$ cells of (<) 500/μl
5. Patients with acute HIV disease after primary infection

Experimental indications
1. Patients with a viral load of (<) 10 000 copies/μl
2. Patients with CD4$^+$ cells > 500/μl

citabine, stavudine, and lamivudine) and two nonnucleo-side reverse-transcriptase inhibitors (NNRTIs, e.g., nevirap-ine and delavirdine) and (2) protease inhibitors (e.g., saquinavir, ritonavir, indinavir, and nelfinavir) (Tab. 40.2). In particular, combination therapy with two RT inhibitors together with protease inhibitors is able to drastically reduce viral replication. This can be monitored by quantifi-cation of viral RNA levels in the peripheral blood of HIV-infected individuals. The currently used test systems for this are the b-DNA assay, quantitative RT-PCR, and the NASBA method (present detection limit approximately 200 to 500 copies of HIV RNA/ml).

The main aims of therapy should be (1) to reduce viral replication as far as possible, (2) to prevent the selection of drug-resistant viral strains, and (3) to prevent the progres-sion of HIV disease. This can be achieved by an aggressive combination therapy with several potent antiretroviral drugs. However, before initiating therapy, one has to con-sider that a lifelong combination therapy with drugs that exert various side effects clearly results in a reduction in life quality. In addition, the compliance of the patient is extremely important. Exact time schedules for the uptake of some drugs have to be followed; a failure to do so may result in the rapid selection of resistant viral strains.

Table 40.4 Combinations of antiretroviral drugs with docu-mented efficacy

Nucleoside analogues	Protease inhibitors
Zidovudine + lamivudine	+ indinavir
Zidovudine + didanosine	+ ritonavir
Zidovudine + zalcitabine	+ nelfinavir
Stavudine + lamivudine	+ saquinavir
Stavudine + didanosine	+ saquinavir
	saquinavir + ritonavir

Although from a virologist's point of view therapy should be initiated as soon as possible after detection of HIV infection, current recommendations distinguish between obligatory, facultative, and experimental indications, which are summarized in Table 40.3.

In patients without prior antiretroviral treatment, the initial combination of drugs should be selected carefully based on the patient's prior history and the side effects exerted by the various agents, since a failure of the initial therapy usually reduces the chances for successful treatment. Preferentially, two nucleoside analogues should be combined with one protease inhibitor (see Tab. 40.4 for combinations with documented efficacy).

Alternative but less efficient combinations are two nucleoside analogues together with one NNRTI, two nucleoside analogues, or two protease inhibitors. Because of their high concentrations in CSF either zidovudine or stavudine should be included. Combinations of zidovudine with stavudine, didanosine with zalcitabine, or zalcitabine with stavudine are not recommended either because of an intracellular competition for phosphoryation or because of identical resistance and toxicity profiles. Therapy should be monitored by determination of CD4$^+$ counts and quantification of the viral load in peripheral blood every 3 months. An effective therapy will be able to decrease the viral load to less than 500 copies per milliliter (i.e., below the detection limit of the currently used methods for quantification of viral RNA) after 3 to 6 months of therapy. The main reasons for a failure of therapy are either the selection of drug-resistant viruses or noncompliance of the patient. A significant increase in viral load (>0.5-0.7 $\log_{10}$) or a decrease in CD4$^+$ counts (>30%) may indicate the selection of drug-resistant viral strains. However, one has to consider that infections or vaccinations also may be able to cause a temporary stimulation of viral replication. Determination of resistance-associated mutations within the HIV reverse-transcriptase or the protease gene by molecular methods can help in decisions on whether a modification of viral therapy is necessary. In case of resistant viral strains, all drugs should be changed simultaneously. Another frequent reason for discontinuation of therapy is toxic side effects of drugs. In this case, it is essential to avoid a suboptimal therapy with only one drug because this potently selects for resistant viral strains. Either therapy should be interrupted entirely, or the drug exerting the toxic effects should be substituted by an alternative agent.

Drug classes

NUCLEOSIDE REVERSE-TRANSCRIPTASE INHIBITORS

Zidovudine

Zidovudine (3'-azido-3'-deoxythymidine) is a thymidine analogue with antiviral activity against HIV-1, HIV-2, and human T-cell leukemia/lymphoma virus type I (HTLV-I).

The inhibitory effect can be observed in acute infections of human T-cell lines and peripheral blood lymphocytes but not in chronically infected cells. The mechanism of action of zidovudine is inhibition of the virally encoded reverse transcriptase. This requires a prior modification of zidovudine to the triphosphate form, which is catalyzed by cellular enzymes. Zidovudine triphosphate competitively inhibits the reverse transcriptase with respect to dTTP and acts as a chain terminator of viral DNA synthesis. The antiviral selectivity results from a higher affinity for HIV reverse transcriptase than for human DNA polymerases. However, low concentrations of zidovudine are able to inhibit human myeloid and erythroid progenitor cells, thus explaining the myelotoxic side effects of this drug.

Pharmacokinetics/metabolism

Zidovudine is rapidly absorbed from the gastrointestinal tract (oral bioavailability 60%). Plasma protein binding is about 30%. CSF concentration averages approximately 50% of that in plasma in adults; in children, lower CSF concentrations have been reported (25%). The plasma $t_{1/2}$ is 1 to 1.5 hours. Zidovudine is rapidly metabolized by glucuronidation, which destroys the antiretroviral activity. Both unmetabolized and metabolized zidovudine are excreted via renal clearance. Renal failure can lead to a marked accumulation of zidovudin and its metabolite.

Dosage/pharmaceutical forms

Zidovudine is available in capsules of 100 and 250 mg. Alternatively, a solution containing 10 mg/ml zidovudine is useful for treatment of HIV-infected children. A solution for infusion containing 200 mg zidovudine is also available. For oral treatment, a dosage of 250 mg every 12 hours is recommended in adult patients. In HIV encephalopathy, 5 × 200 mg per day should be used until clinical improvement is evident. Intravenous treatment should be performed with 6 to 12 mg/kg per day.

Indications

Indications include therapy of HIV infection in combination with other antiretroviral drugs. At present, the only indication where monotherapy with zidovudine is recommended is for prevention of maternal-fetal transmission in HIV-infected pregnant women. The optimal time point for initiation of this therapy is not unequivocally defined. Whereas some studies initiate zidovudine therapy (100 mg 5 times daily) during the fourteenth week of pregnancy, others recommend initiation during the thirty-fourth week until delivery. In addition, delivery by Cesarean section also may be able to reduce the risk of maternal-fetal transmission.

Side effects and interactions

The major toxicities of zidovudine are granulocytopenia and anemia, which occur in up to half of recipients at higher doses. Granulocytopenia usually occurs after 6 to 8 weeks of treatment. Administration of GM-CSF may be used to manage granulocytopenia. Anemia is observed most commonly after the first 6 weeks and may require transfusion.

Severe headache, nausea, insomnia, and myalgia occur commonly during initiation of zidovudine therapy, but these symptoms often resolve or diminish. Myopathy with weakness, pain, and in some cases cardiomyopathy have been associated with prolonged use of zidovudine. After drug cessation these symptoms usually resolve slowly. Toxicity increases with concomitant use of nephrotoxic (e.g., amphotericin B, flucytosine) or myelotoxic substances (e.g., pyrimethamine-sulfadiazine, vincristine, doxorubicine, ganciclovir). Neurotoxicity may occur during concomitant use of zidovudine and acyclovir.

Contraindications

Contraindications include neutropenia of less than 750/μl, hemoglobin level of less than 7.5 g/dl, intravenous treatment of children, and patients with severe hepatic or renal insufficiency.

Didanosine

Didanosine (2',3'-dideoxyinosine) is a purine nucleoside analogue that is active against HIV-1 und HIV-2, including zidovudine-resistant isolates. Didanosine is 10- to 100-fold less potent than zidovudine in activated peripheral blood mononuclear cells but exerts more potent activity in quiescent cells and human monocytes/macrophages. Didanosine is converted by 5'-nucleotidase to dd-IMP and further metabolized by additional cellular enzymes to the active derivative ddATP, which functions as a competitive inhibitor of reverse transcriptase and as a chain terminator after incorporation into DNA. In vitro, a synergistic effect of didanosine together with zidovudine has been documented. Most zidovudine-resistant strains of HIV remain susceptible to didanosine.

Pharmacokinetics/metabolism

Didanosine is very acid-labile. Food decreases the absorption by more than 50%. Therefore, oral bioavailability depends on several factors, including gastric acidity, but reaches 35 to 45% when the tablets are taken 1 hour before a meal. CSF concentration is about 20% that in plasma. Plasma protein binding is low. Approximately 40 to 60% of didanosine is excreted unchanged in the urine with a $t_{1/2}$ of 0.6 to 1.5 hours. In addition, nonrenal pathways of excretion are important but not fully characterized. For patients with renal insufficiency (serum creatinine > 1.5 mg/dl), dose adjustments are recommended.

Dosage/pharmaceutical forms

Didanosine is available as tablets of 25, 50, 100, and 150 mg. For more convenient dosing in children, didanosine is also available as a powder. Owing to the acid lability, each dose should be taken at least 1 hour before or 2 hours after a meal. In adults, two of the chewable tablets should be administered in order to provide adequate buffering. Standard therapy in adults (50-75 kg body weight) is with 2 × 200 mg of didanosine per day.

Indications

Indications include therapy of HIV infection in combination with other antiretroviral drugs.

Side effects and interactions

Side effects are dose-dependent and usually occur after 3 to 6 months of treatment. The major dose-limiting toxicities of didanosine are peripheral neuropathy and pancreatitis. Neuropathy begins with paresthesia, numbness, and pain. After cessation of therapy, the symptoms usually resolve. Pancreatitis has been observed in up to 9% of didanosine-treated patients and rarely may be fatal. A prior history of both pancreatitis and neuropathy constitutes risk factors for experiencing these side effects. In addition, diarrhea, related to the citrate buffer of the tablets, and exanthema are observed frequently. Rare side effects include CNS disturbances (e.g., headache, insomnia, and seizures), retinal depigmentation in children, optic neuritis, increased transaminase levels, hepatic failure, and cardiomyopathy. The buffered formulations of didanosine can decrease absorption of various drugs (e.g., ketoconazole, tetracycline, and the quinolones), which should be administered at least 2 hours after the uptake of didanosine. The risk of pancreatitis is increased by exposure to intravenous pentamidine and possibly several other drugs. Agents associated with peripheral neuropathy (e.g., isoniazid, metronidazole, nitrofurantoin, vincristine, and zalcitabine) should be avoided in association with didanosine.

Contraindications

Contraindications include phenylketonuria (tablets contain phenylalanine), previous history of neuropathy or pancreatitis, severe renal insufficiency, pregnancy and lactation, and concomitant use of rifampicin or rifabutin.

Lamivudine

Lamivudine [(−)-beta-2',3'-dideoxy-3'-thiacytidine] (3TC) is a nucleoside analogue with in vitro activity against HIV-1 and HIV-2 that is comparable with zidovudine. Similar to zidovudine, it has to be activated via phosphorylation and serves as a competitive inhibitor of reverse transcriptase. In addition, recent studies demonstrate an inhibitory effect of lamivudine on replication of hepatitis B virus.

Pharmacokinetics/metabolism

The bioavailability of oral lamivudine is approximately 80%. Lamivudine has a prolonged intracellular half-life (10-15 h) that allows for infrequent dosing of this drug. CSF penetration is low (approximately 10%). Most of lamivudine is excreted unmetabolized in the urine. In the case of renal insufficiency, dose reductions are recommended (for a CrCl of 30-49 ml/min, 150 mg qd; for a CrCl of 15-29 ml/min, 150 mg as an initial dose and then 100 mg qd; for a CrCl of

5-14 ml/min, 150 mg as an initial dose and then 50 mg qd; for a CrCl of <5 ml/min, 50 mg as an initial dose and then 25 mg qd).

Dosage/pharmaceutical forms

Lamivudine is available as tablets of 150 mg and as syrup of 10 mg/ml. For combination therapy, 150 mg bid is used in adult patients.

Indications

Indications include therapy of HIV infection in combination with other antiretroviral drugs and therapy of chronic infections with hepatitis B virus.

Side effects and interactions

In comparison with other antiretroviral drugs, lamivudine has an advantageous safety profile with a relatively low rate of side effects in adult patients. In rare cases, lamivudine may be associated with exanthema, nausea, insomnia, headache, fever, diarrhea, and abdominal pain. In addition, neuropathy, vasculitis, neutropenia, and pancreatitis have been reported during therapy with lamivudine. In children, both pancreatitis and peripheral neuropathy are frequent side effects, occurring in approximately 10% of treated patients. The concomitant use of cotrimoxazol may increase the serum levels of lamivudine.

Contraindications

Contraindications include children with a history of pancreatitis and pregnancy and lactation.

Stavudine

Stavudine (2',3'-didehydro-2'-deoxythymidine, d4T) is a thymidine nucleoside analogue with activity against HIV-1 and HIV-2. The rate-limiting step in the intracellular metabolism of stavudine is its initial phosphorylation to stavudine monophosphate. Conversion to the triphosphate is rapid. Stavudine triphosphate has an intracellular $t_{1/2}$ of 3 to 4 hours. It is a competitive inhibitor of reverse transcriptase with respect to dTTP. In addition, it acts as a chain terminator after incorporation into DNA.

Pharmacokinetics/metabolism

Stavudine is efficiently absorbed after oral administration with a bioavailability of approximately 90%. The plasma $t_{1/2}$ averages 1 hour. CSF concentration is approximately 40% of that in plasma. About 40% of stavudine appears unchanged in the urine; additional clearance is by nonrenal mechanisms. In patients with renal insufficiency, dose reductions are required (for a CrCl of 26-50 ml/min, 20 mg bid for adults weighing

more than 60 kg and 15 mg bid for adults weighing less than 60 kg; for a CrCl of 10-25 ml/min, 20 or 15 mg qd).

Dosage/pharmaceutical forms

Stavudine is available in capsules of 15, 20, 30, and 40 mg. Dosage in patients who weigh more than 60 kg is 2×40 mg per day; in adult patients weighing less than 60 kg, the dosage should be reduced to 2×30 mg per day.

Indications

Indications include therapy of HIV infection in combination with other antiretroviral drugs.

Side effects and interactions

The major toxicity of stavudine is painful sensory peripheral neuropathy that is dose-related. At currently used adult doses, neuropathy occurs in approximately 5% of patients. Symptoms are usually reversible after withdrawal of the drug. Pancreatitis also has been observed in association with stavudine (approximately 0.5% of patients). In addition, anemia, exanthema, elevated transaminase values, fever, headache, depression, and gastrointestinal upset may occur rarely. Zidovudine can antagonize the antiviral effect of stavudine by inhibiting its intracellular phosphorylation. Concomitant use of agents associated with peripheral neuropathy (e.g., isoniazid, vincristine, and zalcitabine) should be avoided.

Contraindications

Contraindications include a previous history of neuropathy or pancreatitis and pregnancy.

Zalcitabine

Zalcitabine (2',3'-dideoxycytidine) is a dideoxynucleoside analogue with inhibitory activity against HIV-1 and HIV-2 including virus strains resistant to zidovudine. It requires an initial phosphorylation by deoxycytidine kinase and is then further modified to its active metabolite dideoxycytidine 5'-triphosphate (ddCTP), which acts as an inhibitor of reverse transcriptase. Zalcitabine also inhibits mitochondrial DNA synthesis. This probably contributes to its clinical toxicities. Combinations of zalcitabine and zidovudine exert a synergistic inhibition of HIV replication in vitro and in vivo.

Pharmacokinetics/metabolism

Zalcitabine has a high oral bioavailability of about 80% in adults. In children, oral bioavailability may be lower. In addition, food is able to decrease bioavailability by approximately 15%. $t_{1/2}$ in plasma is 1 to 2 hours. CSF concentration averages about 15 to 20% of that of plasma. Renal excretion is the primary route of elimination. Dose reductions are recommended in patients with renal insufficiency (for a CrCl of 40-10 ml/min, 0.75 mg bid; for a CrCl of <10 ml/min, 0.75 mg bid).

Dosage/pharmaceutical forms

Zalcitabine is available as tablets of 0.375 and 0.75 mg. Dosage in combination therapy of adult patients is 3×0.75 mg per day.

Indications

Indications include therapy of HIV infection in combination with other antiretroviral drugs.

Side effects and interactions

During the first weeks of treatment, rash, fever, ulcerative stomatitis, and headache are common side effects that may resolve despite continued administration. The major side effect of zalcitabine is painful sensorimotor peripheral neuropathy. It usually develops during the second and third month of treatment in up to 30% of patients. Symptoms include pain and paresthesia and usually are reversible on cessation of therapy; in mild cases, dose reductions may be sufficient. Pancreatitis is a rare complication of treatment with zalcitabine that may be fatal. Additional, rare side effects are esophageal ulcerations, cardiomyopathy, and hematopoietic toxicities. Concomitant use of drugs associated with peripheral neuropathy or pancreatitis should be avoided during zalcitabine treatment. Nephrotoxic drugs are able to interfere with renal excretion of zalcitabine. This may increase the risk of neuropathy.

Contraindications

Contraindications include peripheral neuropathy, pancreatitis, pregnancy, and children younger than 13 years of age.

NONNUCLEOSIDE REVERSE-TRANSCRIPTASE INHIBITORS (NNRTIs)

Nonnucleoside inhibitors of reverse transcriptase are a chemically heterogeneous class of agents that potently inhibit HIV-1 replication but are not active against HIV-2.

They bind directly to the virally encoded reverse transcriptase without the need for a prior intracellular modification. The most important compounds of this class that are used at present in clinical studies are nevirapine and delavirdine. Additional agents of this class are loviride, pyridinone, and derivatives of benzodiazepine (TIBO). These agents always must be used in combination with other antiretroviral drugs, since monotherapy leads to a very rapid selection of resistant virus strains (within days).

Pharmacokinetics/metabolism

Both nevirapine and delavirdine have a high oral bioavailability of more than 80%. Maximal plasma concentrations are observed 4 hours after oral administration. The primary route of elimination of nevirapine is renal (>80%), with an extended $t_{1/2}$ of 30 hours. Delavirdine is eliminated via both renal excretion and metabolization in the liver, with a $t_{1/2}$ of approximately 6 hours. Both drugs are able to inhibit cytochrome P450.

Dosage/pharmaceutical forms

Nevirapine is available in capsules of 200 mg. Therapy is initiated with 200 mg qd for 2 weeks. Afterwards, dosage should be increased to 200 mg bid. This lowers the risk of side effects. For delavirdine, tablets of 100 mg are availabe. Dosage in adult patients is 400 mg tid. Tablets may be dissolved in water to aid administration.

Efavirenz, a newly introduced NNRTI, can be given once daily (600 mg qd).

Indications

Indications include therapy of HIV infection in combination with other antiretroviral drugs.

Side effects and interactions

The major side effect of nevirapine and delavirdine is the induction of exanthemas. For nevirapine, exanthema develops in about 10% of patients; delavirdine is able to induce exanthemas in up to 50% of patients, usually during the second or third week of treatment. In noncomplicated cases, symptomatic treatment of exanthemas (e.g., topical steroids) can be used to control this side effect. For severe exanthemas with concomitant systemic manifestations (e.g., fever, conjunctivitis, and arthralgia), treatment should be stopped immediately. Other side effects include elevation of hepatic enzyme levels, fever, nausea, insomnia, and headache. Efavirenz carries the risk of neuropsychiatric side effects. Both nevirapine and delavirdine are inhibitors of cytochrome P450, resulting in interactions with a variety of other drugs. For instance, concomitant use with rifabutin or rifampin should be avoided. In addition, nevirapine is able to decrease the plasma concentrations of indinavir by about 30%. Thus, when nevirapine is combined with indinavir, dosage of indinavir should be increased to 3×1000 mg. This is not necessary for concomitant use with ritonavir.

PROTEASE INHIBITORS

Saquinavir

Saquinavir was the first protease inhibitor used routinely for treatment of HIV infections. Protease inhibitors specifically target the HIV-encoded protease, which is essential for cleavage of the gag-pol polyprotein into the mature functional proteins. This leads to a defect in virus maturation. In contrast to reverse transcriptase inhibitors, protease inhibitors remain active in chronically infected cells that contain the integrated retroviral genome. Saquinavir is able to potently inhibit both HIV-1 and HIV-2. Therapy always should be performed in combination with either reverse-transcriptase inhibitors or other protease inhibitors, since monotherapy rapidly selects for resistant viral strains.

Pharmacokinetics/metabolism

The oral bioavailability of saquinavir is low (4%). It is mandatory to administer saquinavir within 2 hours after a meal, since resorption is reduced by 90% if given prior to a meal. Plasma protein binding is high (>90 %). Saquinavir is metabolized in a cytochrome P450-dependent manner. Only about 1% of saquinavir is excreted in urine, whereas more than 90% is detectable within feces. The $t_{1/2}$ is approximately 10 hours.

Dosage/pharmaceutical forms

Saquinavir is available in capsules of 200 mg. For optimal resorption, saquinavir has to be given within 2 hours after a meal. A dosage of 600 mg tid is recommended.

Indications

Indications include therapy of HIV infection in combination with other antiretroviral drugs.

Side effects and interactions

The most frequent side effect of saquinavir is diarrhea, which leads to a discontinuation of therapy in about 5% of treated patients. Additional side effects are nausea, abdominal pain, and elevation of hepatic enzyme levels. One side effect that is observed with all HIV-1 protease inhibitor treatments is a syndrome of peripheral lipodystrophy, central adiposity, breast hypertrophy in women, hyperlipidemia, and insulin resistance that may lead to type II diabetes. This syndrome may occur in up to 50% of patients after treatment for 10 months and is most probably due to the inhibition of a human protein that regulates lipid metabolism and has approximately 60% homology to the catalytic region of HIV-1 protease. Because of the metabolization of saquinavir via cytochrome P450, various interactions can occur. Whereas the concomitant use of nucleoside analogues has no significant influence on the pharmacokinetics of saquinavir, rifampicin or rifabutin can drastically reduce plasma concentrations of saquinavir. Similar effects are observed in combination also with other enzyme inducers such as carbamazepine, phenytoin, or dexamethasone. In contrast, ritonavir, indinavir, nelfinavir, ketoconazole, and clarithromycin are able to increase plasma concentrations of saquinavir by 2- to 20-fold.

Contraindications

Saquinavir must not be used in combination with midazolam, triazolam, terfenadine, astemizole, cisapride, or derivatives of ergotamine because this can induce prolonged sedation or life-threatening arrhythmias. Experience with saquinavir during pregnancy and lactation is limited.

Ritonavir

Ritonavir is a potent inhibitor of the HIV-1 protease with a chemical structure that is similar to saquinavir and indinavir.

Pharmacokinetics/metabolism

Ritonavir is well absorbed from the gastrointestinal tract. Maximum plasma concentrations are obtained approximately 2 to 4 hours after oral administration. Plasma protein binding is high (>95%). The $t_{1/2}$ is about 3 hours. Ritonavir is preferentially eliminated fecally after P450-mediated metabolism in the liver.

Dosage/pharmaceutical forms

Ritonavir is available in capsules of 100 mg. Dosage in adult patients is 600 mg bid. Since nausea may develop during the first days of treatment, dosage should be increased sequentially during initiation of therapy, with 300 mg bid on the first day of treatment, 400 mg bid for 2 days, 500 mg bid for the following day, and then 600 mg bid.

Indications

Indications include therapy of HIV infection in combination with other antiretroviral drugs.

Side effects and interactions

Frequently observed side effects with ritonavir are diarrhea, nausea, headache, perioral paresthesia, and elevation of hepatic enzyme levels and plasma triglyceride levels. Because of its metabolism via cytochrome P450, ritonavir is able to interact with many other important drugs. This effect can be used therapeutically because ritonavir is able to increase plasma concentrations of saquinavir by 20-fold. In addition, however, ritonavir is able to increase the concentrations of rifabutin, of several sedatives (e.g., diazepam, flurazepam), of antiarrhythmics (e.g., amiodarone, propafenone), analgesics (e.g., piroxicam), β-adrenergic antagonists, calcium antagonists, anticonvulsive drugs (e.g., clonazepam, carbamazepine), and several antibiotics (e.g., clarithromycin, erythromycin). Concomitant use of fluconazole can lead to an increase in ritonavir levels.

Contraindications

Similar to saquinavir, ritonavir must not be used in combination with several drugs such as terfenadine, astemizole, cisapride, amiodarone, bepridil, bupropion, quinidine, clozapine, and piroxicam. Because of the extensive hepatic metabolism of ritonavir, great care should be taken in patients with hepatic insufficiency. Experience with this drug during pregnancy and lactation is limited.

Indinavir

Clinical studies demonstrated that indinavir is also a potent protease inhibitor that significantly reduces the viral load when given in combination with two nucleoside analogues.

Pharmacokinetics/metabolism

In general, indinavir is rapidly absorbed from the gastrointestinal tract. Maximal plasma concentrations are observed approximately 1 hour after administration. Fatty and protein-rich foods significantly reduce the oral bioavailability of this drug. The $t_{1/2}$ is 1.8 hours. Indinavir is eliminated via renal mechanisms. However, similar to the other protease inhibitors, indinavir is also metabolized via the cytochrome P450 system.

Dosage/pharmaceutical forms

Indinavir is available in capsules of 200 and 400 mg. Dosage is 800 mg tid. In patients with minor hepatic insufficiency, dose reductions to 600 mg tid are indicated. Since food reduces the oral bioavailability of indinavir, administration should be at least 2 hours after or prior to a meal, respectively.

Indications

Indications include therapy of HIV infection in combination with other antiretroviral drugs.

Side effects and interactions

One major side effect of indinavir is the induction of nephrolithiasis, occurring in about 5% of patients. Therefore, patients should be sufficiently hydrated so as to prevent crystalluria. The most frequently observed side effect is hyperbilirubinemia, which can be seen in up to 15% of patients during the first 4 weeks of therapy. In severe cases (>5 mg/dl), indinavir treatment should be discontinued. However, most cases of hyperbilirubinemia resolve despite continued therapy. In addition, nausea, diarrhea, headache, insomnia, pharyngitis, and exanthema have been reported in indinavir-treated patients. Since indinavir is an inhibitor of cytochrome P450, the metabolism of various drugs can be affected. In particular, indinavir should not be combined with calcium antagonists, β-adrenergic antagonists, and antiarrhythmics. Concomitant use of ketoconazole can increase indinavir plasma concentrations by 40%. Vice versa, indinavir is able to increase plasma concentrations of rifabutin, nelfinavir, and saquinavir. Gastrointestinal absorption of indinavir is negatively affected by didanosine. Therefore, if both drugs are used in combination, didanosine should be administered at least 1 hour after indinavir.

Contraindications

Great care should be taken in patients with a preexisting nephrolithiasis or hyperuricemia. Experience with this drug during pregnancy and lactation is limited.

Nelfinavir

Nelfinavir was the fourth protease inhibitor to be approved, and it is also highly potent. Results of clinical trials demonstrate that the combination of nelfinavir with either zidovudine/lamivudine or stavudine results in significant reductions in viral burden and rises in CD4$^+$ cell count.

Pharmacokinetics/metabolism

Oral bioavailability may vary between 20 and 80%. Food is able to increase the gastrointestinal absorption of nelfinavir. The $t_{1/2}$ is 3.5 to 5 hours. Nelfinavir is metabolized in a cytochrome P450-dependent manner.

Dosage/pharmaceutical forms

Nelfinavir is available in capsules of 250 mg. Dosage in adult patients is 750 mg tid. Administration should be with a meal.

Side effects and interactions

Nelfinavir is well tolerated. The most frequently observed side effect is mild diarrhea, which often can be controlled by loperamide. Additional, rarely observed side effects are the induction of hyperglycemia and diabetes as well as symptoms of fat redistribution (e.g., round facies, protease paunch). Inhibition of cytochrome P450 is less than observed with ritonavir, but several important interactions can occur. Rifampin and rifabutin are able to decrease nelfinavir levels. Ketoconazol, saquinavir, indinavir, and ritonavir increase the plasma concentrations of nelfinavir. As described for other protease inhibitors, the concomitant use of drugs with a narrow therapeutic window that are metabolized via cytochrome P450 should be avoided.

Contraindications

Concomitant use of carbamazepine, phenobarbital, astemizole, terfenadine, rifampin, quinidine, midazolam, triazolam, cisapride, amiodarone, and ergot alkaloids is contraindicated. There is no experience with this drug during pregnancy and lactation.

RESPIRATORY SYNCYTIAL VIRUS INFECTIONS

Disease presentation

Respiratory syncytial virus (RSV), a member of the paramyxoviruses, is an important respiratory pathogen of young children, with life-threatening illness occurring most frequently in the first few months of life. Whereas older children and adults mainly suffer from tracheobronchitis and upper respiratory tract infections, infants are prone to develop pneumonia and bronchiolitis during RSV infections. It has been reported in various studies that RSV is responsible for 5 to 40% of the pneumonias and bronchitis in young children, as well as for 50 to 90% of the cases of bronchiolitis. The initial manifestations of RSV infection are usually those of a febrile upper respiratory tract infection. Lower respiratory tract involvement commonly becomes manifest within several days. The infant may even be afebrile by the time the lower tract disease becomes prominent. As the disease progresses, tachypnea and dyspnea may develop. In bronchiolitis, the respiratory rate may be strikingly elevated, and wheezing and hyperinflation can occur. In particular, infants with underlying pulmonary disease, especially bronchopulmonary dysplasia, appear to be at risk of developing prolonged and complicated infections with RSV. This is also the case with immunosuppressed children or those with a congenital immunodeficiency disease. Diagnosis of RSV infection can be made by detection of viral antigen or by isolation of the virus in tissue culture. Nasal washings or tracheal secretions are generally the best specimens for virus detection.

Treatment

In most cases, no specific treatment of RSV infections is required. In the more severely affected infants with lower respiratory tract disease, oxygen may be required due to hypoxemia. In addition, the antiviral agent ribavirin has been approved for specific treatment of RSV infection. For hospitalized infants with lower respiratory tract disease, ribavirin should be administered by small-particle aerosol into an oxygen tent, in an oxygen hood, or via a ventilator for 12 or more hours per day for an average of 3 to 5 days. In several controlled studies, ribavirin aerosol has been shown to have a beneficial effect on the clinical course of RSV bronchiolitis and pneumonia not only in severely ill infants but also in infants that were moderately ill. No major toxicity has been associated with ribavirin aerosol treatment, but administration of the drug requires hospitalization. Therapy, therefore, should be aimed primarily at children most at risk of severe or complicated RSV lower respiratory tract disease (children with cardiac, pulmonary, immunocompromising, or neurologic diseases).

Ribavirin

Ribavirin (1-b-D-ribofuranosyl-1,2,4-thiazole-3-carboxamide), which is a guanosine analogue, inhibits the in vitro replication of a broad spectrum of viruses, including myxo-, paramyxo-, arena-, bunya-, herpes-, adeno-, pox-, and retroviruses. However, for some viruses, high concentrations (30-50 μg/ml) of the agent are necessary to observe an effect on replication. Since ribavirin is able to reversibly inhibit macromolecular synthesis and the proliferation of rapidly dividing, noninfected cells at concentrations of 1 to 10 μg/ml, the in vivo application of this drug is at present limited to infections with respiratory syncytial virus, lassa virus, and, in combination with interferon-α, hepatitis C virus. The antiviral mechanism of action of ribavirin is not fully defined. Within cells, ribavirin is phosphorylated by cellular enzymes to the mono-, di-, and triphosphate derivatives. The monophos-

phate derivative inhibits inosine-5'-phosphate dehydrogenase, thus interfering with the synthesis of GTP. In addition, an effect of ribavirin on virally encoded RNA polymerases and on the formation of the cap structure of viral mRNAs has been observed.

Pharmacokinetics/metabolism

Ribavirin is absorbed rapidly following both oral ingestion or inhalation. After oral administration, bioavailability averages approximately 45% in adults and children. CSF level is about 70% of that in plasma. The disposition of ribavirin is complex. After extensive metabolization, the elimination half-life following inhalation and oral and intravenous routes and from erythrocytes is 9.5 hours, 24 hours, and 40 days, respectively. Elimination routes are renal (about 30-55% excreted in urine within 72-80 h) and fecal (about 15% eliminated within 72 h), with the remainder sequestered in erythrocytes for several weeks. Ribavirin and its metabolites accumulate in red blood cells, reaching steady-state levels in about 4 days and gradually declining with an apparent half-life of 40 days.

Dosage/pharmaceutical forms

For aerosol administration, ribavirin is available in vials containing 6 g of sterile, lyophilized powder to be reconstituted in sterile water at 20 mg/ml. In RSV infections, the aerosol should be administered in an oxygen tent for 12 to 18 h per day for 3 to 7 days. Oral solutions and intravenous preparations must be compounded because these dosage forms are not available commercially. For iv treatment, 4×1 g per day should be used over 4 days; then dose reductions to 3×0.5 g per day are possible. For oral treatment, 1 to 2 g per day is recommended.

Indications

Indications include treatment (aerosol administration) of selected hospitalized infants and young children with severe lower respiratory tract infections due to respiratory syncytial virus (RSV) and treatment (intravenous) of infections with arenaviruses (e.g., lassa, junin, machupo). In addition, recent studies suggest a clinically important enhanced benefit from combination therapy with interferon-α (IFN-α) and ribavirin over IFN monotherapy in chronic hepatitis C.

Side effects and interactions

Systemic ribavirin causes dose-related anemia due to hemolysis. In addition, at higher doses, the release of erythroid cells from bone marrow may be suppressed. Increases in serum bilirubin, serum iron, and uric acid concentrations are also frequently observed side effects. Bolus iv infusion may cause rigors. Chronic oral therapy is associated with dose-related lymphopenia and gastrointestinal and CNS complaints (e.g., headache, lethargy, insomnia, and mood alteration). Aerosolized ribavirin is usually well tolerated; however, mild conjunctival irritation, rash, transient wheezing, and reversible deterioration in pulmonary function can occur. Preclinical studies indicate teratogenic, embryotoxic, mutagenic, tumor-promoting, and possibly gonadotoxic effects of ribavirin. Therefore, this drug is contraindicated in pregnancy. Moreover, pregnant women should not directly care for patients receiving ribavirin aerosol.

Contraindications

Ribavirin is contraindicated in patients hypersensitive to the drug and in women who are or may become pregnant.

HEPATITIS VIRUS INFECTIONS

Disease presentation

The term *viral hepatitis* is used generally to describe infections caused by viruses whose primary tissue tropism is the liver. During the acute phase of infection, hepatitis due to these viruses presents clinically in a very similar fashion, although the responsible viruses belong to distinct virus families. Common clinical features include anorexia, nausea, vomiting, right upper quadrant pain, and increases in hepatic enzymes. Asymptomatic infections are also rather frequent. Jaundice is the hallmark of infection, but anicteric cases are common. At present, six hepatitis virus types are known, termed *hepatitis viruses A, B, C, D, E, and G*. Hepatitis A and E viruses do not persist in the liver, and there is no evidence of progression to chronic liver disease. In contrast, hepatitis B virus (HBV), either alone or in combination with hepatitis D virus, and the major agent of parenterally transmitted non-A, non-B hepatitis, hepatitis C virus (HCV), can establish persistent infections leading to chronic and severe liver disease. For hepatitis B virus, a carrier state becomes established in approximately 5 to 10% of infected adults. However, infection of young children may result in a considerably higher rate of persistent infections. HCV infection becomes chronic in more than 60% of infected persons, establishing a disease that is often only mildly symptomatic and slowly progressive; however, approximately 20% of patients develop liver cirrhosis after 20 years of infection. In addition, an association between hepatitis B and C viruses and the development of hepatocellular carcinoma has been documented.

Treatment

At present, no established antiviral treatment is available for therapy of acute infections with hepatitis viruses. Since the nucleoside analogues famciclovir, ganciclovir, and lamivudine are able to inhibit replication of HBV both in vitro and in vivo, these agents may be tried in severe cases of acute HBV infections. However, no data on the efficacy of this procedure are available. In chronic HBV and HCV infections, interferon-α is the only approved and widely used agent for treatment. The main aims of treatment in chronic infection are eradication of the infecting virus and normalization of liver function. These aims, however, are only reached in a variable percentage of treated patients. In chronic HBV infection, response rates of 40 to 50% are observed in patients with low HBV DNA plasma concentrations (<100 pg/ml), active hepatitis (ALT > 150 U/l), and a short duration of chronic HBV infection (<2 years). In contrast, only 15 to 25% of patients with high DNA levels (>100 pg/ml) and a long duration of chronic infection respond to interferon-α. In chronic HCV infections, interferon-α is able to induce a decrease of HCV RNA plasma levels (which can be quantified by the b-DNA assay) and a normalization of hepatic enzyme levels during the phase of treatment in about 50% of patients. However, the rate of long-term responders is low (10-40 %). In summary, the overall efficacy of interferon-α for the treatment of chronic HBV and HCV infections is far from satisfactory. Therefore, the search for more effective agents and optimized treatment strategies is still going on. Promising new drugs for the therapy of HBV infections are the nucleoside analogues lamivudine and famciclovir that were originally developed for the treatment of HIV and herpesvirus infections, respectively. Both agents are potent inhibitors of HBV replication and are currently being tested in advanced clinical trials for the treatment of chronic HBV infection. In chronic HCV infections, several small studies have reported promising results with a combination of interferon-α and ribavirin. Especially among patients with a previous nonresponse to IFN-α alone, a combination with oral ribavirin, at a dose of 1000 to 1200 mg per day, was able to induce a sustained biochemical response in approximately 50% of patients.

Drug classes

Interferons

Interferons (IFN) are proteins that are synthesized in eucaryotic cells in response to various stimuli such as viral infection, double-stranded RNA, bacteria, polyanions, and certain cytokines and growth factors. In turn, interferons can induce biochemical changes in noninfected cells leading to an antiviral state. The principal antiviral interferons, IFN-α and IFN-β, are approximately 30% homologous at the amino acid level. IFN-γ has less specific antiviral activity but more potent immunomodulatory effects. Interferon exposure of cells leads to the production of more than 20 cellular proteins that are involved in inducing an antiviral state. Among IFN-induced proteins is a protein kinase that can inhibit viral protein synthesis in the presence of double-stranded RNA. Other mechanisms of antiviral defense include the induction of a cellular endoribonuclease that cleaves both cellular and viral RNA. The clinical usefulness of interferons is at present mainly limited to the treatment of chronic HBV and HCV infections. In addition, papillomavirus infections (e.g., condylomata acuminata) and Kaposi's sarcoma in AIDS patients also may respond to interferon therapy.

Pharmacokinetics/metabolism

After subcutaneous injection of IFN-α, absorption

exceeds 80%. Plasma levels are dose-related, peaking at 4 to 8 hours and returning to baseline by 18 to 36 hours. An antiviral state in cells can be detected as early as 1 hour after administration and decreases slowly to baseline by 6 days after injection. CSF penetration is low. The clearance of IFN includes inactivation by various body fluids, cellular uptake, and metabolism by various organs.

Dosage/pharmaceutical forms

Interferon-α is available as a solution for subcutaneous (sc) and intramuscular (im) injection. Dosage for treatment of chronic HBV infection is 2.5 to 5 million U/m² sc three times a week for 6 months. In chronic HCV infections, dosage is slightly higher, with 3 to 6 million U/m² sc three times a week for 6 months.

Indications

Indications include treatment of chronic HBV and HCV infections either alone or in combination with additional agents (e.g., ribavirin).

Side effects and interactions

Subcutaneous injections of IFN doses of 1 million units or more are usually associated with an acute influenza-like syndrome including fever, chills, headache, myalgia, arthralgia, nausea, vomiting, and diarrhea. In particular, this can be observed during the first week of therapy. Fever may range over 40°C. In most patients, tolerance develops. Pretreatment with antipyretics also can help to overcome these side effects. Major toxicities that can limit therapy are bone marrow suppression with granulocytopenia and thrombocytopenia. Further severe side effects include neurotoxicity (e.g., somnolence, confusion, electroencephalographic changes, seizures, and coma), reversible neurasthenia, thyroid dysfunction, and cardiotoxicity with arrhythmias and reversible cardiomyopathy. In addition, elevation of liver enzymes and triglyceride levels, alopecia, proteinuria, renal insufficiency, and hepatotoxicity may occur. IFN reduces the metabolism of various drugs by the cytochrome P450 system, leading to an increased plasma $t_{1/2}$ of such drugs as theophylline. The bone marrow toxicity of myelotoxic drugs can be enhanced by IFN.

Contraindications

Contraindications include pregnancy, cardiac disease, preexisting psychiatric or CNS disorders, hepatic or renal insufficiency, patients with bone marrow suppression; children and adolescents under 18 years of age should not be treated with IFN.

Suggested readings

ALRABIAH FA, SACKS SL. New antiherpesvirus agents: their targets and therapeutic potential. Drugs 1996;52:17-32.
BALZARINI J. Suppression of resistance to drugs targeted to the human immunodeficiency virus reverse transcription by combination therapy. Biochem Pharmacol 1999;58:1-27.
BRYSON YJ. Perinatal HIV-1 transmission: recent advances and therapeutic interventions. AIDS 1996;10(suppl 3):S33-42.
CRISP P, CLISSOLD SP. Foscarnet: a review of its antiviral activity, pharmacokinetic properties and therapeutic efficacy in immunocompromised patients with cytomegalovirus retinitis. Drugs 1991;41:104-29.
DORAN CM. New approaches to using antiretroviral therapy for the management of HIV infection. Ann Pharmacother 1997;31:228-36.
DRAKE SM. NNRTIs: a new class of drugs for HIV. J Antimicrob Chemother 2000;45:417-20.
HAMMER SM. Advances in antiretroviral therapy and viral load monitoring. AIDS 1996;10(suppl 3):S1-11.
HOOFNAGLE JH, BISCEGLIE AM. The treatment of chronic viral hepatitis. N Engl J Med 1997;336:347-56.
MCDONALD CK, KURITZKES DR. Human immunodeficiency virus type 1 protease inhibitors. Arch Intern Med 1997;157:951-9.
PATEL R, BODSWORTH NJ, WOOLLEY P, et al, and the International Valaciclovir HSV Study Group. Valaciclovir for the suppression of recurrent genital HSV infection: a placebo-controlled study of once-daily therapy. Genitourin Med 1997;73:105-9.
PERRY C-M, FAULDS D. Lamivudine: A review of its antiviral activity, pharmacokinetic properties and therapeutic efficacy in the management of HIV infection. Drugs 1997;53:657-80.
SACKS SL. Genital herpes simplex virus and its treatment: focus on famciclovir. Semin Dermatol 1996;15:32-6.
TYRING SK. Efficacy of famciclovir in the treatment of herpes zoster. Semin Dermatol 1996;15:27-31.
WUTZLER P, DECLERCQ E, WUTKE K, FÄRBER I. Oral brivudine versus intravenous acyclovir in the treatment of herpes zoster in immunocompromised patients: a randomized double-blind trial. J Med Virol 1995;46:252-7.

41

Fungal infections

Jacques F. G. M. Meis, Ben E. de Pauw

More than 200 000 species of fungi have been described. These organisms, gathered together in the Kingdom Fungi, include macroscopic and microscopic filamentous forms and yeastlike structures. Fungi are found throughout nature, where they play a major role as saprophytes in decomposing organic matter. Most fungi are harmless, but they can become pathogenic in the presence of immunosuppression. There are only about 200 fungi known to cause disease in humans, and the majority of these are true opportunists, with less than 10 species able to cause fungal infections in otherwise normal human beings. The opportunistic nature of fungal infections has become a significant clinical problem as a consequence of increasing numbers of patients with compromised host defenses. The incidence of invasive opportunistic nosocomial infections has doubled in a decade as a result of advances in cancer chemotherapy, treatment successes of bacterial infections, immunosuppression associated with organ transplantation, and most notably, the emergence of AIDS (Tab. 41.1). In particular, the incidence of aspergillosis has increased steadily compared with that of *Candida* infections. In 1984, 80% of candidal bloodstream infections were due to *C. albicans,* whereas in the 1990s, species other than *C. albicans* have been

shown to be responsible for at least half these infections. Both the decrease in the number of candidal infections and the shift toward non-*C. albicans* strains are presumably related to the use of azoles as prophylaxis. After the introduction of fluconazole at a tertiary care center, the infection rate with *C. krusei* and *C. glabrata* increased compared with historic controls.

C. albicans continues to be one of the most frequently isolated species, followed by *C. tropicalis, C. glabrata,* and *C. parapsilosis,* the latter often in association with central venous catheters. Over the last 10 years, new pathogenic species have been recognized, such as the above-mentioned *C. krusei, C. lusitaniae,* and *C. guillermondii.* Other yeasts such as *Trichosporon beigeilli, Saccharomyces cerevisiae, Rhodotorula* spp., and *Malessezia furfur,* the organism responsible for pityriasis versicolor and folliculitis, also have been identified as the cause of septicemia in humans. Histoplasmosis, coccidioidomycosis, blastomycosis, and paracoccidioidomycosis are referred to as the endemic mycoses because they are confined to certain geographic regions. *Penicillium marneffei* typically was seen in Southeast Asia. However, as a result of increased air travel, patients with these infections can now present anywhere. Other examples of newly emerging fungi in the immunocompromised patient are *Scedosporium* spp., *Fusarium* spp., and *Alternaria* spp. These molds constitute an increasing problem in neutropenic patients and bone marrow transplant recipients, just as do the zygomycetes. Many of these infections follow inhalation, but some originate from superficial cutaneous lesions such as infected nails.

In addition to the significant contribution of fungal infections to the morbidity and often mortality of patients with malignancies, an estimated 15% of the world's population has been infected with superficial dermatophytic fungi. There appears to be a rise in the frequency as well as the intensity of these superficial fungal infections because of life-style changes such as the greater use of swimming pools and health spas and crowded conditions in nursing homes, schools, and prisons.

Fungal infections in humans originate, with a few exceptions, exogenously from the environment through skin contact with or without trauma, inhalation, or ingestion of fungal spores. Therefore, the most common

Table 41.1 Reasons for the increased incidence of invasive fungal infections

Fewer early deaths from bacterial infections due to broad-spectrum antibiotics
Disturbance of the commensal flora of the gastrointestinal tract due to broad-spectrum antibiotics
Prolonged neutropenia due to better anticancer agents
Enhanced mucosal damage, malabsorption, and malnutrition
More patients treated for their malignancy
More elderly patients and patients with a history of a fungal infection
Fewer patients dying from their underlying disease
More matched, unrelated bone marrow transplants
More graft-versus-host disease
Increasing corticosteroid use
More extensive abdominal surgery
Increased use of central venous catheters
Increased travel to regions with endemic mycoses
Continuing building activities in hospitals
Better diagnostic possibilities and increased awareness

classification of disease is by site of infection: superficial, subcutaneous, and systemic mycoses. This chapter discusses the risk factors, epidemiology, diagnosis, prevention, and treatment of superficial, subcutaneous, and invasive systemic fungal infections.

SUPERFICIAL FUNGAL INFECTIONS

Dermatophytic fungi and yeasts are the most common causative agents of fungal infections of the skin, hair, and nails. The dermatophytic fungi or ringworm fungi are classified into three genera: *Microsporon, Trichophyton,* and *Epidermophyton* (Tab. 41.2). At present, about 40 species have been described, with 10 being common causes of human infection. When cutaneous fungal infections are caused by yeasts, the species are generally in the genera *Candida* and *Malassezia.* Dermatophytic infections start after contact with an outside source. Geophilic dermatophytes are found in soil; zoophilic dermatophytes are found on animals such as cattle, dogs, and cats; and anthropophilic dermatophytes originate from infected humans. Dermatophytes create inflammation and pruritus, especial-

ly the zoophilic species. They invade generally only the keratin layers of the stratum corneum, the nails, and hair shafts. The most common clinical classification of infection is according to the body region affected: tinea pedis, tinea cruris, and tinea corporis, in addition to infections of the hair shaft in tinea capitis and tinea barbae (Tab. 41.2). Most of these superficial infections are treated topically, but depending on the site and the extent of the infection, systemic agents may be used. Although dermatophytes are the most common causative agents of superficial fungal infections, yeasts may affect skin and nails. Tinea versicolor due to *M. furfur* and cutaneous candidiasis are examples of such infections. Tinea versicolor is a chronic, mostly asymptomatic, noninflammatory skin disease with fine scaling and either hypo- or hyperpigmentation occurring typically on the trunk. It may cause concern to the patient when areas of hypopigmentation do not tan in the sun. Cutaneous candidiasis presents as intertriginous candidiasis or appears in large skin folds such as under a woman's breasts or in abdominal folds of obese persons. Also, paronychium of fingernails may be caused by *Candida.* However, *Candida* more often affects mucosal sites such as the vagina, mouth, and uncircumcised penis. Other superficial infections that are associated with serious cosmetic effects include black and white piedra or tinea nodosa, tinea nigra, and otomycosis.

Table 41.2 Superficial fungal infections

	Clinical presentation	Microorganisms	Treatment
Tinea corporis	Well demarcated pruritic, circular, scaly, erythema lesion	*T. rubrum,* *T. mentagrophytes,* *M. canis, E. floccosum*	Topical: miconazole, clotrimazole, econazole, naftifine, ciclopirox, ketoconazole, terbinafine Systemic (if no response): itraconazole, terbinafine
Tinea cruris	Pruritic, erythematous, scaly lesions of groin and thighs	*E. floccosum,* *T. rubrum,* *T. mentagrophytes*	As above
Tinea pedis	Scaly, vesicular or pustular lesion between toes, often with nail involvement	*T. rubrum,* *E. floccosum,* *T. mentagrophytes*	As above
Tinea unguium	Nails with adjacent skin involvement	*T. rubrum,* *T. mentagrophytes*	Itraconazole Terbinafine (250 mg/day for 3 months)
Tinea capitis	Localized alopecia with erythematous, scaling lesions with broken hairs	*T. tonsurans,* *T. verrucosum,* *T. mentagrophytes,* *M. canis*	Systemic: griseofulvin (8 weeks) Itraconazole Terbinafine
Tinea barbae	Highly inflammatory dermatophyte infections of the beard	*T. mentagrophytes,* *T. verrucosum*	As above
Tinea versicolor	Scaling patchy lesions on thumb and arms; fail to tan	*Malassezia furfur*	Topical: miconazole, clotrimazole, econazole, ketoconazole, naftifine, haloprogin. Systemic: ketoconazole, itraconazole.

The management of fungal infections should start with obtaining specimens, scales, hair, and nails before treatment is initiated, especially when systemic antifungal drugs are to be started. However, the treatment of most superficial mycoses ought to start with the use of topical agents. Various topical preparations are available that generally are safe to use with rare side effects. When disease is extensive, affects hair and nails, or does not respond to topical agents, it is necessary to prescribe systemic agents (e.g., griseofulvin, terbinafine, fluconazole, or itraconazole).

In most fungi there are a limited number of potential targets for drug action. Although during the past several years new antifungal agents have been formulated (Tab. 41.3), there are still far fewer antimycotics available than antibacterials. There are five major classes of prototype

drugs and several miscellaneous other types of antifungal agents: polyenes, imidazoles, triazoles, allylamines, echinocandins, griseofulvin, flucytosine, potassium iodide, and several topical agents such as amorolfine, tolnaftate, ciclopiroxolamine, and haloprogin. These drugs exert a different action on fungi, have a different safety profile and mode of action depending on the species of fungus, are fungistatic or fungicidal, have different pharmacokinetics, and differ in bioavailability. The fungus involved in the infection, the clinical picture, and the site of the body affected by the fungus are important considerations in the choice of treatment.

In addition to the previously mentioned topical compounds, other topical imidazole derivatives and allylamines are available in many formulations for the treatment of

Table 41.3 History of discovery of prototype antifungal compounds

Year	Compound	Mechanism of action
1907	Whitfield's ointment (acetyl /benzoic acid combination)	Keratolysis and fungistatic action
1939	Griseofulvin	Binds to fungal microtubules and thus inhibits cell mitosis; also inhibition of nucleic acid synthesis
1954	Nystatin (polyenes)	Binding to ergosterol with resulting leakage and finally cell death
1956	Amphotericin B	As above
1957	Flucytosine	Interferes with fungal protein synthesis
1967	Clotrimazole (imidazole)	Inhibition of cytochrome P450-dependent 14α- demethylase or other P450-dependent enzymes
1969	Miconazole	As above
1977	Ketoconazole	As above
1981	Amorolfine	Reduces production of fungal ergosterol
1982	Fluconazole	See imidazoles
1984	Itraconazole	As above
1984	Naftifine, terbinafine	Inhibition of fungal ergosterol synthesis by blocking squalene epoxidase
1984-1990	Echinocandins* (lipopeptides)	β-d-glucan synthesis inhibitor, fungicidal
1992	Voriconazole*	See imidazoles
1983-1990	Lipid-based formulations Liposomal amphotericin B Lipid-complexed amphotericin B Colloidal amphotericin B Liposomal nystatin*	See polyenes

(Several classes of drugs have been withdrawn before the end of clinical studies because of unwanted side effects.)
*Under clinical investigation.

Table 41.4 Antifungal drugs for superficial *Candida* infections

Drug	Dose
Nystatin suspension	10^6 units 5 times daily
Amphotericin suspension	200-400 mg 5 times daily
Amphotericin sucking pastilles	10 mg qid
Clotrimazole suspension	5 mg 5 times daily
Miconazole suspension	100 mg qid
Fluconazole	200 mg qd

superficial fungal infections. Topical use of polyenes (nystatin and amphotericin B) is limited to the treatment of superficial candidiasis (Tab. 41.4). Onychomycosis, tinea capitis, and tinea barbae generally need systemic therapy, sometimes in combination with topical application of antifungal agents. In addition to antifungal treatment, elimination of predisposing factors is essential to the success of treating dermatophytic infections. Daily bathing of feet, careful drying of the toes and interdigital spaces, and avoidance of occlusive footwear are recommended. Finally, it is advised to avoid barefoot walking in public shower areas and saunas and to use separate towels to dry the infected area and the rest of the body.

SUBCUTANEOUS FUNGAL INFECTIONS

These infections are the result of traumatic implantation of a fungus from the environment into the skin in most cases. The fungus remains locally confined, spreads slowly to surrounding tissues (mycetoma), invades locally via lymphatics (sporotrichosis), or in very rare instances disseminates hematogenously throughout the body (chromoblastomycosis). The agents involved in subcutaneous mycoses are usually nonpathogenic soil organisms that can readily adapt to host tissues with different disease development. Especially in debilitated patients, the ensuing disease caused by these saprophytes may be severe (phaeohyphomycosis).

The subcutaneous infections consist of the following clinical groupings: (1) mycetoma, (2) chromoblastomycosis, and (3) phaeohyphomycosis, which are caused by several different species, and (4) sporotrichosis, (5) lobomycosis, and (6) rhinosporidiosis, which are caused by *Sporothrix schenkii, Loboa loboi,* and *Rhinosporidium seeberi,* respectively (Tab. 41.5).

Treatment

Antifungal treatment of the subcutaneous mycoses is ineffective and at best disappointing. Only sporotrichosis is amenable to medical treatment with either saturated potassium iodide (4-6 ml tid for 2-4 months) or long-term treat-

ment with itraconazole (200-400 mg qd for 6 months). Surgical excision remains the treatment of choice for all other subcutaneous mycoses. Without radical removal of the lesions, recurrence is common.

DEEP-SEATED (INVASIVE) FUNGAL INFECTIONS

Invasive fungal infections can be divided in two distinct groups: the endemic or dimorphic mycoses caused by true pathogenic fungi such as *Histoplasma, Coccidioides, Blastomyces,* and *Paracoccidioides* and the opportunistic mold and yeast infections. The opportunistic fungi are ubiquitously distributed saprophytes that only invade immunocompromised or otherwise debilitated hosts, causing aspergillosis, candidiasis, cryptococcosis, zygomycosis, and diseases due to several other hyalohyphomycetes and dematiacious fungi.

ENDEMIC MYCOSES

Blastomycosis

Following inhalation of airborne spores, the fungus *B. dermatitidis* may evolve into a lung infection in patients without apparent immunodeficiency. The disease has a geographically restricted occurrence in the Americas, with some sporadic foci in Africa. It has a predilection for people with outdoor occupations or recreational habits. The infection can occur in epidemics and is generally more prevalent in men than in women. Once the lung has been infected, the fungus can spread hematogenously to other organs such as bone, genital organs, brain, meninges, and preferably the skin. The face, arms, neck, and scalp are the primary sites of metastatic infection.

Coccidioidomycosis

Inhalation of airborne arthrospores of the dimorphic fungus *C. immitis* typically causes a transient self-limiting pulmonary infection in normal individuals. However, in fewer than 1% of individuals the infection will progress to a chronic, ultimately fatal pneumonia with or without dissemination, notably in immunosuppressed patients. Most cases are geographically restricted to the western parts of the United States (deserts) and Central and South America. In addition to the pulmonary localization, the fungus can disseminate to skin, bones, joints, central nervous system, liver, spleen, and other internal organs.

Histoplasmosis

Following inhalation of spores, *H. capsulatum* can cause a mild and transient pulmonary infection in individuals with normal host defenses. In a small proportion of patients the fungus develops a chronic localized infection or disseminates throughout the body in persons with immunosuppression. People become infected in specific regions, especially in the central parts of the United States and Central and South America. One should be aware that *Histoplasma* has a global distribution, with small endemic regions in Africa, Australia, India, Malaysia, and certain European countries, where many bat-infested caves can be found. Most people have a transient, often inconspicuous pulmonary infection that subsides without treatment. However, if the amount of inhaled spores is high, an acute symptomatic infection with fever, chills, headache, cough, and pleuritic chest pain can occur after an incubation period of 1 to 3 weeks. Most patients recover, but occasionally a mediastinal fibrosis with enlarged mediastinal nodes may emerge and can lead to development of a progres-

sive, chronic pulmonary illness with fatal outcome. If left untreated, a rapidly fatal disseminated infection may follow in immunosuppressed patients, children, and older individuals. This infection often goes undiagnosed in nonendemic regions, where histoplasmosis is seldom part of the differential diagnosis. A chronic disseminated form of histoplasmosis can become obvious in immunocompe-

---

Table 41.5 Subcutaneous fungal infections

Disease	Causative agent	Clinical presentation	Treatment
Eumycetoma	*Acremonium* spp. *Aspergillus nidulans* *Curvularia* spp. *Exophiala jeansellmei* *Fusarium* spp. *Leptosphaeria* spp. *Madurella* spp. *Pseudallescheria boydii*	Typical geographical distribution in arid (sub)tropical areas, mainly Africa Chronic suppurative infection of subcutaneous and deeper tissues evolving over many years Feet are most common site	Surgical excision Antifungal treatment disappointing Long term treatment with itraconazole sometimes gives improvement Amputation when no response and if bone involved
Chromoblastomycosis	*Fonsecaea* spp. *Phialophora* spp. *Cladosporium* spp. *Exophiala* spp.	Very slow growing; cutaneous nodules or papules, sometimes abscesses appearing on exposed body sites, especially limbs and lower legs	Surgical excision (only with small lesions; risk of local dissemination) Antifungal treatment disappointing and not well extablished. Itraconazole (400-600 mg daily) looks promising
Phaeohyphomycosis	*Exophiala* spp. *Phialophora* spp. *Alternaria* spp. *Aureobasidium* spp. *Bipolaris* spp. *Cladosporium* spp. *Anoclaria* spp. *Dactylaria* spp. *Drechslera* spp. *Exserohilum* spp. And several other dermatogenous fungi	Subcutaneous and cutaneous painless nodule, sometimes with draining sinuses, mostly on the arms and legs. Deep infections in paranasal sinuses and cerebral lesions after direct spread or from hematogenous dissemination	Surgical excision. Antifungal treatment not well established. Amphotericin B and itraconazole (400 mg daily) have been used with variable success
Sporotrichosis	*Sporothrix schenckii*	Most common localized subcutaneous painless lesions; on limbs lymphatic spread leads to satellite lesions Rare: extracutaneous infections of lung, bone and joint meningitis, and endophthalmitis	Saturated KI treatment of choice in developing countries. Itraconazole (200 mg daily) for 6 months in cutaneous infection. Extracutaneous infections can be treated with 400 mg daily
Lobomycosis	*Loboa loboi* (never isolated in culture)	Geographically restricted to tropical forests of South America. Infection starts with symptomless small papules or nodules, gradually expanding to massive tumors	Only radical surgical excision is effective; current antifungals not effective
Rhinosporidiosis	*Rhinosporidium seeberi* (never isolated in culture)	Polyps or wartlike lesions on mucous membranes of nose and conjunctiva. Rare on genital organs	Only radical surgical excision is effective; optimal drug treatment is unknown

tent patients with liver, spleen, and adrenal gland involvement. Mucosal ulcers in mouth, throat, lip, nose, gastrointestinal tract, or anal region are typically present. Other manifestations include meningitis, focal cerebral infections, and endocarditis. Disseminated disease is a serious problem in AIDS patients who reside in endemic regions or have traveled in endemic regions.

Paracoccidioidomycosis

Inhalation of spores of the dimorphic fungus *Paracoccidioides brasiliensis* causes a pulmonary infection, even in immunocompetent persons. The fungus spreads to other organs and causes granulomatous lesions in the gastrointestinal mucosa, skin, and lymph nodes. The disease is found in individuals living in subtropical mountain forests in Central and South America or those who earlier resided there or visited the region. After infection, the clinical symptoms are often nonspecific, such as cough, fever, malaise, night sweats, and weight loss mimicking tuberculosis. Frequently, a long time elapses before the diagnosis is considered. Mucocutaneous disease presents as painful ulcerated lesions in mouth, nose, and lips and on the face. Hematogenous spread of the fungus results in disseminated infections of internal organs, gastrointestinal tract, joints, bones, and central nervous system. Since asymptomatic infection does not occur, all cases should be treated.

OPPORTUNISTIC FUNGAL INFECTIONS

Yeasts and yeastlike fungi are among the most common mycotic infections in humans. The disease presentation is variable and depends to a large extend on the patient's host defenses and presence of risk factors. Almost all yeasts are potentially pathogenic in the setting of a patient using chronic corticosteroids, immunosuppressive agents, anticancer treatment, long-term broad-spectrum antibiotics, and parenteral nutrition. It is sometimes difficult to attribute a pathogenic role to the most frequently encountered yeast species, *C. albicans,* because 25 to 50% of normal individuals carry this species in the gastrointestinal and female genital tract. Under normal circumstances, the intact epithelial surfaces of the gastrointestinal tract will prohibit invasion by microorganisms, and the mucociliary barrier of the respiratory tract prevents aspiration of fungal cells and spores. Many cancer chemotherapeutic agents cause ulceration of the pulmonary and gastrointestinal mucosa, thus facilitating colonization and invasion by molds and yeasts, as is witnessed by a high incidence of invasive fungal infections in bone marrow transplant recipients relative to those who receive conventional cytoreductive chemotherapy. Yeasts are separated into those without known sexual reproduction, the blastomycetes such as the majority of *Candida* species, and those with a known sexual reproduction, the heterobasidiomycetes such as *Cryptococcus* and the hemiascomycetes such as *Saccharomyces*. Identification of yeasts isolated from significant infections to the species level is mandatory because of their different susceptibilities to antifungal drugs.

Invasive *Candida* infections originate most frequently from endogenous reservoirs in patients with lowered host defense. Exogenous infections in hospitalized patients are frequently transmitted via the hands of health care workers. Deep-seated invasive infections tend to occur in two different patient populations: (1) granulocytopenic patients with a hematologic malignancy and (2) nongranulocytopenic intensive care patients after multiple abdominal surgeries, with central venous lines, renal failure, and treatment with broad-spectrum antibiotics (see Tab. 41.1). The boundary between "just colonized with *Candida*" and invasive *Candida* infection is particularly unclear in the febrile, unstable intensive care patient with negative blood cultures and *Candida* cultured from nonsterile body sites. One should realize that about half the patients with a histologically proven invasive candidiasis at autopsy never had a positive blood culture.

Treatment

Endemic mycosis

Blastomycosis Patients with serious, life-threatening infections and meningitis should be treated with amphotericin B (0.6 mg/kg, at least until 6 weeks after complete resolution of symptoms). Patients who do not respond to amphotericin B and those with indolent or chronic infections are candidates for itraconazole (400 mg qd, total of 6 months).

Coccidioidomycosis Since this disease is usually self-limited, treatment should concentrate on those individuals with impaired immune function and a disseminated infection. Amphotericin B should be given in a dose of 1.0 to 1.5 mg/kg per day for at least 6 weeks, which still might be insufficient to prevent relapses. Hence, after improvement, oral therapy with triazoles for periods up to 12 months is recommended (itraconazole 400 mg qd or fluconazole 400 mg qd).

Histoplasmosis Treatment of acute pulmonary infection is rarely necessary. In most cases the patient is already well at home when the diagnosis is confirmed. In patients with mediastinal involvement and after massive exposition, treatment should be instituted with amphotericin B (0.5 mg/kg per day). Patients with disseminated histoplasmosis and AIDS require initial therapy with amphotericin B followed by itraconazole (400 mg qd) to prevent relapses. Patients with AIDS and mild disease have been treated successfully with itraconazole alone.

Paracoccidioidomycosis Antifungal treatment of choice is itraconazole (100 mg qd) or ketoconazole (400 mg qd). Amphotericin B (1 mg/kg qd) combined with sulfadiazine (1000 mg qid) is a second choice when azole absorption is not adequate or when treatment costs should be considered because of limited resources.

Fatal outcomes in proven invasive fungal infections may well exceed 90%, particularly in patients with persisting neutropenia and unremitting underlying disease. To avoid this complication, most specialists prescribe systemic antifungal therapy to neutropenic patients who have continuing unexplained fever despite adequate broad-spectrum antibacterial treatment. Of course, there are patients at high risk of an invasive fungal infection who will benefit from a very early institution of systemic antifungals. This pertains to the same patients who are the principal candidates for antifungal prophylaxis. If empiric treatment was restricted to this category of patients, it would constitute a preemptive rather than empiric or prophylactic approach. Because all empiric studies have enrolled only small numbers of patients, recommendations on the time to start empiric antifungal therapy, the drugs to be used, and the appropriate length of treatment are hard to formulate. Given its broad spectrum of activity, amphotericin B at a dose of 1 mg/kg per day is still the drug of choice for empiric purposes; the lipid preparation should be reserved for patients who cannot tolerate the conventional formulation, and fluconazole should be reserved for patients with a low risk of invasive mold infections.

Deep Candida infections Disseminated candidiasis, including candidemia, is frequently rapidly fatal without antifungal treatment. Since there are few objective parameters, the clinician has to rely on clinical impression and practical experience to decide when to start treatment. Most authorities recommend antifungal therapy for patients with at least one positive blood culture for *Candida.* Amphotericin B with or without flucytosine is considered the standard therapy; 50 to 70% of patients, including those infected with *C. krusei* and *C. glabrata,* will respond to this regimen. Similar response rates with less toxicity can be expected from the lipid formulations of amphotericin B. *C. lusitaniae* and *C. guilliermondii* have been shown to be less susceptible to amphotericin B. Alternatively, an initially susceptible organism may become resistant during the course of therapy. Patients with an invasive infection by a susceptible *C. albicans* isolate may be treated safely with fluconazole, but superinfections by *Aspergillus* species may emerge when fluconazole is given alone during neutropenia. Given the variable susceptibilities of *Candida* species to fluconazole, an intravenous dosage of 800 mg per day may be considered as primary therapy for hematogenous candidiasis. The dose of fluconazole and that of amphotericin B needs to be adjusted in renal impairment. When the results of culture and susceptibility testing are available, the dose can be decreased to 400 mg daily, and fluconazole can be given orally, depending on the clinical response. It has to be realized that fluconazole and itraconazole are not of value in the treatment of a proven or presumed invasive fungal infection if they have been used as prophylactic agents in an adequate dosage, since it must be assumed that the offending pathogen is resistant to these drugs.

The current practice in patients with candidemia is to continue therapy at least until resolution of the granulocy-topenia and fever. In nonneutropenic intensive care patients, therapy should continue until 10 to 14 days after the disappearance of signs and symptoms of infection. While a short duration of therapy may be adequate for low-risk patients with candidemia, extended therapy is required for patients with visceral involvement. Fluconazole and, theoretically, itraconazole provide the opportunity to manage these patients as well as those with chronic disseminated candidiasis in an outpatient setting, which is both convenient and cost-effective.

Retrospective studies in pediatric patients have suggested that removal of the central venous catheter, if present, is important to decrease the complications of candidiasis. Conversely, another prospective study did not show a significantly improved outcome in hematogenous candidiasis if the central venous catheter was removed promptly. However, removal seems justified when a patient fails to respond to antifungal therapy within 96 hours or when candidemia persists for more than 48 hours.

The basis of treatment of *Malassezia* infections is withdrawal of the catheter and, in the absence of rapid improvement, intravenous administration of amphotericin B. Experience with azole derivatives for this purpose is still limited.

Despite occasional resistance, intravenous amphotericin B is the treatment of choice for systemic *T. beigelii* infections; in less acute situations, itraconazole may be considered as an appropriate alternative. If left untreated, 75% of patients will die of this infection. In patients with severe granulocytopenia, the rapid recovery of neutrophils is of utmost importance.

Cryptococcus infections Cryptococcal disease is the most common life-treatening fungal infection in AIDS patients. At the time of diagnosis, 90% of patients will have meningitis or meningoencephalitis. Cryptococcal infection in transplant patients generally occurs 6 months after transplantation and presents as pulmonary disease or as disseminated disease, with the central nervous system and skin the most common affected organs. *Cryptococcus* is less problematic to diagnose than most other invasive fungal infections. The key diagnostic test is antigen detection in the cerebrospinal fluid (CSF) and serum. Apart from establishing the diagnosis, serial antigen detection offers an objective way to monitor response to therapy. All patients except some immunocompetent individuals need antifungal treatment. The first choice of treatment is considered to be combination therapy with amphotericin B (0.6 mg/kg qd) and flucytosine (100 mg/kg qd) for at least 6 weeks. Itraconazole and fluconazole are less toxic alternatives, but experience with these drugs is still limited. Cryptococcosis in AIDS patients seldom responds well to treatment, and relapse within 6 months of successful initial treatment is common. Therefore, long-term maintenance treatment with either fluconazole (400 mg/kg qd) or itraconazole (400 mg/kg qd) is necessary in AIDS patients.

Aspergillus infections Conventional amphotericin B has remained the standard therapy for invasive aspergillosis for over 30 years. The target dose should be between 1 and 1.25 mg/kg per day, ideally already given on the first day, for at least 10 to 14 days. It is seldom possible to administer this high dose to patients on cyclosporine therapy or those with renal impairment. In these patients, the maximum tolerated dose should be explored, and use of a lipid based preparation might be indicated. The majority of patients with invasive aspergillosis are treated initially on a presumptive diagnosis because invasive diagnostic procedures are usually precluded by concomitant thrombocytopenia. For practical purposes, it is generally accepted that isolation of *Aspergillus* species from clinical specimens in the neutropenic patient connotes either invasive infection or a high risk of developing invasive disease in due time. It is important that even after treatment has commenced, a definite diagnosis should be sought and that infections by other pathogens such as *Actinomyces, Mycobacterium, Nocardia,*

and other rare fungi are excluded. A questionable diagnosis will keep nurturing uncertainty among attending physicians about the optimal therapeutic strategy, particularly if the patient is not responding optimally or if serious adverse events occur. A final diagnosis also will have substantial prognostic value as well as implications for long-term treatment. Whereas the response rate of patients with persisting unexplained fever to systemically active antifungals is about 80% if neutropenia resolves, the successful outcome of documented invasive fungal infection may, even under optimal circumstances, not exceed 20%. This figure is greatly influenced by the state of the underlying disease and possible recovery of the granulocytes. Fewer than 10% of bone marrow transplant recipients with invasive aspergillosis have survived, and patients with disseminated disease or those with diffuse pulmonary disease have a dismal prognosis, whereas those with localized disease have a more than 50% chance of cure with antifungal and/or surgical treatment. Therefore, it is particularly important to have adequate prevention programs and investments in early diagnosis with concomitant early therapy.

An arbitrary total dose of amphotericin B such as 1.5 to

Table 41.6 Kinetics and metabolism of antifungals

	Oral bioavailability (%)	Serum concentration (μg/ml) Peak after single dose	CSF conc. (% of serum)	$t_{1/2}$ (h)	Protein binding (%)	Excretion Urinary	Excretion Hepatic	V_d (l/kg)
Amphotericin B (DOC)	Poor	2.0 (after 50 mg iv)	3	Days	> 90	3% of daily dose	< 15% of daily dose	4
Liposomal	Poor	15 (after 2 mg/kg)						
Lipid complex	Poor	"						
Colloidal suspension	Poor	"						
Miconazole	Poor	3.0 (after 600 mg iv) 0.5-1 (after 1 g po)	Poor	20-24	90	20	21	
Ketoconazole 0.36	50-70	1.7-4.5 (after 200 mg po)	<10	6-10	99	4	Extensive	
Fluconazole	80-90	2.0 (after 100 mg po)	80	30	11	70-80	10%	0.7
Itraconazole	55-80 (pH-dependent: better with cyclodextrine oral solution)	0.25-1 (after 200 mg po) higher after steady state and after tid	< 10	34	> 90	< 0,5	Extensive	9
Flucytosine	80-90	45 (after 2 g po)	75	3-5	<10	90	5 - 10	0.6
Griseofulvin	Variable (25-70% micronized; 100% ultramicronized)	1.5 (after 500 mg po)	Poor	24	84	<1	Extensive	2

(DOC = deoxycholate.)

3 g has been recommended, but this is ill-founded. It is essential to observe a clinical and preferably a radiologic response before therapy is discontinued. On the other hand, in those in whom the criteria for commencing treatment was only "fever unresponsive to antibiotics" without microbiologic or radiologic documentation of invasive aspergillosis, treatment can be discontinued when the neutrophil count recovers.

Surgery is indicated for patients in whom localization of the lesions poses a direct threat of invasion of a major vessel, which can result in fatal hemorrhage, or for debridement of dead tissue after a period of antifungal therapy. Most clinicians would reserve lung or lung segment resection for patients with a limited number of persisting shadows confined to one lobe who have to undergo subsequent bone marrow transplantation or more aggressive chemotherapy or those with hemoptysis.

Lipid-based amphotericin B preparations also have been used successfully in the treatment of invasive aspergillosis. However, their therapeutic usefulness in first-line treatment is still difficult to assess because formal randomized comparisons have never been performed. At first glance, the response rates appear superior, but the vast majority of patients studied had been pretreated with amphotericin B deoxycholate. Recovery from neutropenia is the most important factor in a favorable outcome among patients treated with lipid-based amphotericin B. The addition of rifampicin to amphotericin B in poorly responding patients has been suggested because this combination is sometimes synergistic in vitro. However, rifampin induces the activity of cytochrome P450 enzyme system extensively, and in patients taking cyclosporine or corticosteroids, the underlying disease may flare or rejection may occur. Combination of amphotericin B with high-dose terbinafine (750 mg bid) is the subject of current investigation.

The only other registered antifungal agent that can be used for the treatment of invasive aspergillosis is itraconazole. A randomized study in neutropenic patients comparing itraconazole with amphotericin B hinted at equivalence but did not reach a statistical endpoint. In a large open multicenter study of invasive aspergillosis performed by the Mycosis Study Group in the United States, 41% of patients showed a response by the end of therapy. In this study all the patients were treated with a loading dose of 600 mg qd of itraconazole for 4 days, followed by 400 mg qd thereafter. Unfavorable drug interactions led to failure in several patients, and the relapse rate in patients with continuing immunosuppression and a truncated course of therapy was high. Another indication for itraconazole in the treatment of aspergillosis is infection that is resistant to amphotericin B because anecdotal responses of such patients to itraconazole have been described.

Other filamentous fungi Localized zygomycosis is managed by aggressive surgical removal of all infected necrotic tissue, delay of further immunosuppressive therapeutic interventions when possible, and administration of amphotericin B at the maximum daily dose. Disseminated forms of zygomycosis are almost inevitably fatal. Although very scanty data point to a possible usefulness of itraconazole

and voriconazole, the bulk of the literature indicates that, for the time being, these compounds have no place in the treatment of infections caused by the Mucorales. The mainstay of antifungal therapy remains amphotericin B, but the results are very disappointing in persistently neutropenic patients. A limited number of patients have been treated successfully with lipid formulations of amphotericin B or granulocyte transfusions obtained from growth factor-pretreated donors in combination with amphotericin B. Of all available agents, only amphotericin B seems to have marginal activity against *Fusarium,* and even this compound is not effective during neutropenia. There are some anecdotal reports of successes achieved with liposomal amphotericin B, amphotericin B-lipid complex, and voriconazole.

Scedosporium apiospermum and *S. prolificans* are very difficult to treat. In most cases, surgical debridement and excision of necrotic tissue should be performed in combination with prescription of systemically active antifungal agents. These organisms are refractory to amphotericin B, but administration of miconazole, itraconazole, or high-dose terbinafine may be of benefit in some cases. *Alternariosis* may emerge during prophylaxis with fluconazole. Therapy requires surgical excision and intravenous amphotericin B. Intravenous amphotericin B also constitutes the first-line therapy of *P. marneffei*, with itraconazole and, to a far lesser extent, fluconazole as acceptable alternatives. In contrast, for *Geotrichum* infections, itraconazole appears to be the drug of choice in view of the unpredictable susceptibility of this microorganism to amphotericin B.

Drug classes (Tabs. 41.3, 41.4, 41.6) _____

POLYENES

Amphotericin B has the broadest spectrum of activity against fungi and is considered the most effective treatment for systemic fungal infections in severely ill patients. There is no agreement on the therapeutic dose of amphotericin B deoxycholate; in most centers a starting dose of 1.0 mg/kg per day intravenously in a 1- to 4-h infusion is used. In view of the inherent toxicity, higher doses are used only in the treatment of refractory mycoses. Nephrotoxicity, reversible to some degree, is variable from patient to patient and may be ameliorated with salt preloading. In patients with impaired kidney function and in those who receive other possibly nephrotoxic drugs concomitantly, a starting dose of 0.7 mg/kg per day is recommended. If the serum creatinine level exceeds 2.0 mg/dl (or 2 times the baseline in children), treatment should be interrupted for 1 or 2 days to allow for recovery of kidney function. Thereafter, amphotericin B has to be reinstituted at a dose of 0.5 mg/kg per day with daily increases of the dose to the maximally tolerated level under monitoring of the serum creatinine level. Premedication has been suggested to mitigate adverse events related to amphotericin B infusion such as chills, fever, malaise, headache, and nausea. However, the medications typically administered to treat or prevent adverse events such as antipyretics, nonsteroidal anti-inflammatory drugs (NSAIDs), diphenhydramine, meperidine, and hydrocortisone each have their unwanted side effects.

During the last 10 years, research has yielded lipid formulations of amphotericin B as safer alternatives to the standard deoxycholate preparation. The various products: amphotericin B lipid complex, amphotericin B colloidal dispersion, and liposomal amphotericin B have been used in many studies in the past 8 years. These preparations cause amphotericin B to accumulate in the liver and spleen, whereas less is found in the kidney and serum compared with infusion of DOC amphotericin B. Because individual pharmacologic and chemical properties of these preparations are different, data generated by a trial of one of these drugs are not universally applicable. The rate of acute adverse reactions seems to be lowest for liposomal amphotericin B and highest for amphotericin B colloidal dispersion, but all compounds are better tolerated than conventional amphotericin B, which suggests an improved therapeutic index. On the other hand, it is not settled whether higher doses will produce superior results. A recent trial by the EORTC's Invasive Fungal Infection Cooperative Group demonstrated that a 1 mg/kg per day dose of liposomal amphotericin B was as effective as 4 mg/kg per day in treating invasive aspergillosis. However, until further data on other fungal infections are available, the use of dosages as low as 1 mg/kg per day for treatment of acute invasive fungal infections is not recommended because in animal models DOC amphotericin B was more effective than lipid formulations of amphotericin B on a milligram per kilogram basis. Besides, there are limits to the safety because decreases in creatinine clearance in conjunction with increased serum cyclosporine concentrations and low serum potassium levels have been found in transplant recipients. It is of practical value to know that patients are able to receive infusions of amphotericin B over 30 to 60 minutes without discomfort. Although the product information for all amphotericin B preparations recommends administering a test dose of 1 mg, this is of doubtful value in acutely ill patients with invasive infection. Furthermore, this test dose does not necessarily predict the occurrence of allergic reactions or infusion-related adverse events. The high price is a major drawback of lipid-based amphotericin B products and may consume a large part of a hospital's medication budget. Cost-effectiveness studies may include the reduced number of side effects, but this impact is probably marginal.

Intralipid combined with amphotericin B at a dose of 1 to 2 mg/kg per day has been suggested as a cheaper alternative to treat candidemia in neutropenic patients, but

Table 41.7 Drug-drug interactions of azoles

	Fluconazole	Ketoconazole	Itraconazole
Hepatotoxic drugs (alcohol)	–	Increases hepatotoxicity	–
Drugs which increase gastric pH	–	Reduced absorption	Reduced absorption
Oral antidiabetics	Increased plasma levels of hypoglycemic agents	Increased plasma levels of hypoglycemic agents	Increased plasma levels of hypoglycemic agents
Terfenadine, astemizole	–	Combination contraindicated increased levels of antihistamines	Combination contraindicated, increased levels of antihistamines
Cyclosporine	Increased cyclosporine concentration	Increased cyclosporine concentration	Increased cyclosporine concentration
Phenytoin	–	Increased phenytoin concentration	Increased phenytoin concentration
INH, rifampin	Decreased amount of antifungal	Decreased amount of antifungal	Decreased amount of antifungal
Digoxin	–	–	Increased plasma levels of digoxin
Coumarin derivatives	Increased levels of biologically active factors	Increased levels of biologically active factors	Increased levels of biologically active factors
Cisapride	–	Combination contraindicated	Combination contraindicated

clinical experience is limited, and therefore, this approach should not be used at present.

5-FLUCYTOSINE

Flucytosine is a useful drug, probably synergistic in combination with amphotericin B, against *Candida* and *Cryptococcus* spp. The recommended dose, both orally and intravenously, is 100 to 150 mg/kg at 6-h intervals; serum concentrations should not exceed 100 µg/ml. Flucytosine has important limitations: when it is used alone, resistance will ensue rapidly, and the drug is potentially toxic to bone marrow.

AZOLES

The older azoles, clotrimazole and miconazole, are still prescribed for superficial candidiasis (Tab. 41.4). Ketoconazole seemed to be promising in the treatment of yeast infections, but its toxicity and unreliable absorption tempered the initial enthousiasm. Fluconazole constitutes a far better option in the immunocompromised host. Even when used in high doses, it is the safest of all antifungal drugs, and both its oral and intravenous formulations show good bioavailability. Absorption does not depend on the presence of gastric acid, but significant, potentially dangerous interactions with cytochrome P450-associated drugs have been observed (Tab. 41.7). Development of resistance during short-term use is not a problem, but widespread, long-term use of fluconazole may shift the range of infecting species toward less or nonsusceptible fungi. To circumvent this problem, some investigators suggest combining fluconazole with intravenous amphotericin B, but currently there are no data to support this combination.

Itraconazole, in doses of 400 to 600 mg per day, is active against most *Candida* and *Aspergillus* spp., as well as a wide array of other fungal pathogens. Toxicity is common with doses of more than 400 mg per day, although such doses may be more efficacious. Whether an initial loading dose of more than 800 mg per day would be tolerated is unknown. The drug's unreliable absorption makes this compound less suitable in critical circumstances. The new cyclodextrin-based oral solution may obviate this problem, but at present, these formulations have not been tested sufficiently. Other concerns include the possible inhibition of hepatic enzymes by itraconazole (Tab. 41.7) and a propensity to increase intracellular levels of cytotoxic drugs such as vincristine that might enhance their effects. Prior or concurrent use of rifampicin, phenytoin, carbamazepine, and phenobarbital should be avoided, and transplant patients receiving cyclosporin who are to be given itraconazole should have an immediate cyclosporin dose reduction followed by frequent monitoring (Tab. 41.7). There are theoretical considerations for possible antagonism of azoles and polyenes, but sequential use of these agents did not bear out this concern. This opens possibilities for starting treatment with intravenous amphotericin B, which can be followed by oral itraconazole. There are no data on simultaneous administration of itraconazole with amphotericin B.

NEW ANTIFUNGALS

Promising new antifungal agents such as echinocandins, pneumocandins, high-dose terbinafine, the newer azoles, voriconazole and SCH56592, and liposomal nystatin are under clinical investigation. The first phase II study of voriconazole in 141 patients has already been completed with encouraging results, particularly with invasive aspergillosis.

IMMUNOMODULATORS

Growth factors reduce the duration of neutropenia in both myelosuppressive and myeloablative chemotherapy, but their beneficial effect on documented fungal infections remains unproven. The role of interleukins and interferons in the treatment of invasive fungal infections is still uncertain, but results in animal models are hopeful for the future.

Suggested readings _____

BENNETT J, DISMUKES W, DUMA R, et al. A comparison of amphotericin B alone and combined with flucytosine in the treatment of cryptococcal meningitis. N Engl J Med 1979; 301:126-31.

BOUTATI EI, ANAISSIE EJ. *Fusarium,* a significant emerging pathogen in patients with hematologic malignancy: ten years' experience at a cancer center and implications for management. Blood 1997;90:999-1008.

CURFS JHAJ, MEIS JFGM, HOOGKAMP-KORSTANJE JAA. A primer on cytokines: sources, receptors, effects and inducers. Clin Microbiol Rev 1997;10:742-80.

DENNING DW, LEE JY, HOSTETLER JS, et al. NIAID mycosis study group multicenter trial of oral itraconazole therapy for invasive aspergillosis. Am J Med 1994;97:135-44.

DE PAUW BE. Practical modalities for prevention of fungal infections in cancer patients. Eur J Clin Microbiol Infect Dis 1997;16:32-41.

EDWARDS JE, BODEY GP, BOWDEN RA, et al. International conference for the development of a consensus on the management and prevention of severe candidal infections. Clin Infect Dis 1997;25:43-59

GOODMAN JL, WINSTON DJ, GREENFIELD RA, et al. A controlled trial of fluconazole to prevent fungal infections in patients undergoing bone marrow transplantation. N Engl J Med 1992;326:845-51.

GROLL AH, SHAH PM, MENTZEL C, et al. Trends in the postmortem epidemiology of invasive fungal infections at a university hospital. J Infect Dis 1996;33:23-32.

HIEMENZ JW, WALSH TJ. Lipid formulations of amphotericin B: recent progress and future directions. Clin Infect Dis 1996; 22:S133-44.

MESNARD R, LAMY T, DAURIAC C, LE PRISE PY. Lung abscess due to *Pseudallescheria boydii* in the course of acute leukaemia: report of a case and review of the literature. Acta Haematol 1992;87:78-82.

SHEARER C, CHANDRASEKAR PH. Cutaneous alternariosis and regional lymphadenitis during allogeneic BMT. Bone Marrow Transplant 1993;11:497-9.

SUPPARATPINYO K, CHIEWCHANVIT S, HIRUNSRI P, et al. *Penicillium marneffei* infection in patients infected with human immunodeficiency virus. Clin Infect Dis 1992;14: 871-4.

VERWEIJ PE, DENNING DW. Diagnostic and therapeutic strategies for invasive aspergillosis. Semin Respir Crit Care Med 1997;18:203-15.

VERWEIJ PE, DONNELLY JP, DE PAUW BE, MEIS JFGM. Prospects for the early diagnosis of invasive aspergillosis in the immunocompromised patient. Rev Med Microbiol 1996;7:105-13.

WINGARD JR, MERZ WG, RINALDI MG, et al. Increase in *Candida krusei* infection among patients with bone marrow transplantation and neutropenia treated prophylactically with fluconazole. N Engl J Med 1991;325:1274-7.

42

Infections caused by protozoa and worms

Gerd D. Burchard

Human endoparasites predominantly belong to the protozoa and worms. Protozoa can be seen as microparasites, characterized by short generation periods, by high rates of reproduction within a host, and further by the fact of inducing immunity in the host – if the host survives. Consequently, these diseases mainly are of short duration. Worms, however, are macroparasites. They live longer and generally do not reproduce within the host, and as a consequence, severe disease results from multiple infections only.

Antiparasitic chemotherapy helps the host to cope with the parasite. However, advances have been slow compared with other areas of anti-infective therapy. Computer-assisted drug design and high-throughput systems, automated by robotics, to screen compounds are urgently needed. We still do not know enough about the pharmacokinetics of many drugs. The use of drug combinations to delay resistance has been applied seldomly. And most important, multicenter trials and systematic reviews have yet to make a significant impact in antiparasitic therapy.

AMEBIASIS AND OTHER INTESTINAL PROTOZOA

Disease presentation

Amebiasis is an infection with the parasite *Entamoeba histolytica*. Patients are asymptomatic, or they can develop acute amebic colitis, usually presenting with lower abdominal pain and frequent bloody stools over a period of several weeks. Amebic liver abscess is the most common extraintestinal manifestation, with right upper abdominal pain and fever. The most frequent complication of amebic liver abscess is pleuropulmonary involvement.

Giardia lamblia, Balantidium coli, Isospora belli, Cryptosporidium parvum, and *Cyclospora cayetanensis* can lead to a spectrum of disease ranging from asymptomatic carrier status to abdominal discomfort, diarrhea, and/or malabsorption. *C. parvum, I. belli,* and *Microsporidia* can cause opportunistic infections, e.g., in

AIDS patients. The pathogenicity of *Blastocystis hominis* is still a controversial issue.

Treatment

Amebiasis

All patients with invasive amebiasis require treatment, first with a systematically active compound and subsequently with a luminal amebicide in order to eliminate any surviving organism in the colon. In nonendemic areas, all symptomless cyst carriers also should be treated with a luminal amebicide. Such agents protect the patient from invasive disease and reduce the risk of transmission. Amebic colitis and amebic liver abscess are treated with 5-nitroimidazole derivatives. Most studies have been done with metronidazole for 8 to 10 days; other nitroimidazoles do not seem to have essential advantages. Chloroquine is effective in the treatment of amebic hepatic abscess, but no controlled trials have been published comparing metronidazole plus chloroquine with metronidazole alone. Adjunctive treatment with chloroquine therefore is indicated only in severe forms of the disease. Diloxanide is generally the luminal amebicide of choice; paromomycin is an alternative.

Other intestinal protozoa

Drugs and doses are listed in Table 42.1. Every patient with giardiasis should be treated because ongoing infections can result in malabsorption and impaired growth in children. Infections with *B. coli* must be treated because they can lead to severe disease. Infections with *I. belli* and *C. cayetanensis* are self-limited in immunocompetent patients and only have to be treated in cases of severe diarrhea (followed by a secondary prophylaxis in *I. belli* infection in AIDS patients). Some authors recommend treatment of *B. hominis* if the patient is symptomatic and no other pathogens can be found.

A systematic review of the treatment of giardiasis has been performed by the Cochrane Collaboration, showing that a single dose of tinidazole is the most effective treatment with relatively few side effects.

Table 42.1 Treatment of intestinal protozoa

Etiologic agent	Drug	Dose	Duration
Giardia lamblia	Tinidazole or metronidazole or other nitroimidazoles or mepacrine[1]	1 x 2 g 2 x 1 g	1 day 3 days
Cryptosporidium parvum	So far no active drug available[2]		
Cyclospora spp.	Trimethoprim-sulfamethoxazole	4 x 800/160 mg/d	10 days
Isospora belli	Trimethoprim-sulfamethoxazole	4 x 800/160 mg/d	10 days
Blastocystis hominis	Metronidazole	3 x 250 mg/d	Days
Microsporidia	So far no active drug available[3]		

[1]Mepacrine is an acridine derivative formerly used as an antimalarial drug; today it is only used against giardiasis. Because of side effects (dizziness, headache, and gastrointestinal disturbances) and contraindications (psychosis, psoriasis), it is only to be used in treatment failures with other drugs.
[2]In some preliminary studies, treatment with azithromycin plus paromomycin was associated with some clinical improvement.
[3]In some preliminary studies, albendazole has been shown to be effective in *Enterocytozoon bieneusi*-related diarrhea.

Drug classes

METRONIDAZOLE AND OTHER 5-NITROIMIDAZOLES

Metronidazole is supplied as 250-, 400-, and 500-mg tablets and in vials containing 500 mg of lyophilized powder or in 100-ml plastic containers containing a solution of 500 mg/100 ml for parenteral injection.

Dosage

The dosage in amebiasis is 10 mg/kg tid for 8 to 10 days. The dosage in giardiasis is 2 g daily for 3 days. Metronidazole should be administered with or immediately after food, and patients should be warned not to take alcohol during treatment.

Kinetics/metabolism

The oral absorption of metronidazole is excellent, with bioavailability often reported as greater than 90%. Metronidazole distributes well into a variety of tissues and fluids. It is excreted primarily in the bile as the parent drug and in the urine in its various metabolites.

Side effects and interactions

Major side effects are common when the drug is given in high doses for amebiasis, and these include anorexia, nausea, vomiting, diarrhea, and epigastric distress; in addition, a metallic taste in the mouth is often reported. Oral and vaginal overgrowth of yeast cells may occur. Metronidazole should be avoided in the first trimester of pregnancy because, in animals, it has been shown to have mutagenic and carcinogenic potential. Relative contraindications are chronic alcohol dependence, severe liver disease, diseases of the central or peripheral nervous system, and bone marrow diseases.

Metronidazole potentiates the action of oral anticoagulants. Phenobarbital and corticosteroids lower plasma levels of nitroimidazoles; cimetidine raises them.

Tinidazole is another nitroimidazole that is active against intestinal protozoa. It is available as 500- and 1000-mg tablets. For giardiasis, the dose is 2 g for 1 day. The most common side effects include stomach upset, bitter taste, and itching.

DILOXANIDE

Diloxanide furoate is an amebicide that is active only against organisms in the gut lumen. It is marketed in 500-mg tablets.

Dosage

The dosage for adults is 500 mg tid for 10 days; for children, 20 mg/kg is given daily in three divided doses for 10 days. Diloxanide furoate (or another luminal agent) must follow every metronidazole treatment.

Diloxanide furoate is hydrolyzed by intestinal esterases. The hydrolysis product, diloxanide, is absorbed and excreted in the urine with a half-life of approximately 6 hours.

Flatulence leads the list of side effects, and some patients have other mild gastrointestinal complaints. Treatment should be deferred until after the first trimester of pregnancy.

CHLOROQUINE

Dosage in extraintestinal amebiasis

For adults, 600 mg base is given daily for 2 days, followed by 300 mg base daily for at least 2 to 3 weeks. For children, 10 mg/kg is given daily for 2 to 3 weeks (maximum 300 mg base daily).

LEISHMANIASIS

Disease presentation

Protozoa of the *Leishmania* spp. are responsible for at least three clinically distinctive diseases. Cutaneous leishmaniasis with skin ulcers in the Old World is predominantly caused by *L. major* and *L. tropica* and in the Americas predominantly by *L. mexicana, L. braziliensis,* and *L. peruviana.* Mucocutaneous leishmaniasis with skin lesions and later ulcerations of mucous membranes is most frequently caused by *L. braziliensis.* Visceral leishmaniasis (kala-azar), characterized by chronic fever, hepatosplenomegaly, and pancytopenia and opportunistic infections in AIDS patients, is predominantly caused by *L. donovani, L. infantum,* and *L. chagasi.*

Treatment

Cutaneous leishmaniasis

Mild lesions can be left to heal spontaneously within a year. Defacing or multiple lesions should be treated systemically with pentavalent antimonial compounds. Alternatively, defacing single lesions can be treated with antimonials administered locally or with paromomycin ointment (15% paromomycin plus 12% methylbenzethonium chloride in soft white paraffin). Cutaneous leishmaniasis in the Americas always must be treated to prevent subsequent mucocutaneous leishmaniasis.

Mucocutaneous leishmaniasis

All patients must be treated with antimonials. Patients who fail to respond should receive amphotericin B or pentamidine. Plastic surgery may be necessary.

Visceral leishmaniasis

This is usually responsive to the antimonial compounds. However, if there are no monetary constraints, treatment with amphotericin B liposomal/lipid complex (see Chap. 41) should be preferred. AIDS patients with kala-azar should undergo monthly prophylaxis with 4 mg/kg pentamidine.

Drug classes

PENTAVALENT ANTIMONY

Pentavalent antimony compounds (Sb5+) are sodium stibogluconate (1 ml equivalent to 100 mg antimony) and *N*-methylglucamine antimonat (1 ml equivalent to 85 mg antimony).

Dosage

Dosage in cutaneous leishmaniasis is 20 mg Sb5+ per kilogram of body weight intramuscularly daily until a few days after clinical cure (at least 4 weeks in *L. braziliensis* infec-

tions); for single lesions, 1 to 3 ml is injected into the base of the lesion once a week for 4 to 6 weeks or 15 times on alternate days.

Dosage in mucocutaneous and visceral leishmaniasis is 20 mg Sb5+ per kilogram of body weight (maximum 850 mg) intramuscularly daily for a minimum of 20 days; in India, susceptibility seems to be lower, so 40 days of treatment can be recommended .

Electrocardiograms (ECGs) should be monitored every 2 to 3 days because typically, T-wave inversion and prolongation of the QT interval precede serious arrhythmias. Weekly determinations of transaminases, amylase, lipose levels and blood cell counts should be done. Dosage must be reduced if abnormalities occur. Moreover, dosage should be adjusted in the presence of renal failure.

Kinetics/metabolism

These drugs are only poorly absorbed, so they must be administered parenterally or by local injection. More than 80% of a parenteral dose is excreted through the kidneys during the first 6 hours after dosing.

Side effects

These drugs may have cardiotoxic side effects and occasionally produce arthralgia, myalgia, impairment of liver and renal function, skin rashes, and facial edema. Treatment-induced subclinical pancreatitis seems to be common. Safety in pregnancy has not been established, but because visceral leishmaniasis is life-threatening, it must be treated without delay. Contraindications are severe heart, kidney, or liver diseases.

PENTAMIDINE

Pentamidine is an aromatic diamidine compound with antiprotozoal activity. It is supplied in single-dose ampules containing 200 or 300 mg pentamidine isethionate for intravenous or intramuscular administration or as powder for inhalation in the treatment of *P. carinii* pneumonia.

Dosage

Dosage in leishmaniasis is injection of 4 mg/kg three times a week for 5 to 25 weeks or longer, until the lesion is no longer visible in mucocutaneous leishmaniasis or until no more parasites are detectable in two follow-up examinations 14 days apart in visceral leishmaniasis, respectively. Similar doses, for a shorter period of time eventually associated with higher dose cotrimoxazole, may be given in *P. carinii* pneumonia (see below).

Deep intramuscular injection is preferred because intravenous infusion can lead to acute hypotension and syncope. All patients should remain supine and under supervision for at least 30 minutes after each injection. Resuscitation equipment always should be readily available. Blood pressure, blood cell count, and the serum creatinine level should be monitored every few days, and the blood glucose level should be monitored daily.

Kinetics/metabolism

Pentamidine is unreliably absorbed from the gastrointestinal tract, so it must be given by either intramuscular or intravenous injection. The drug is excreted mainly unchanged through the kidneys. The terminal half-life is in the order of days.

Side effects

Major side effects are sterile gluteal abscesses, nausea, vomiting, headache, and acute hypotension, especially after inadvertent intravenous injection. After continuous treatment, pancreatic damage with hypoglycemia due to insulin overrelease and subsequent deficiency may occur, and rarely, hypocalcemia, renal failure, confusion, arrhythmias, thrombocyto- and leukopenia, elevated transaminases, and Stevens-Johnson syndrome may be seen. Use in pregnancy can induce abortion.

AMPHOTERICIN B

This macrocyclic polyene antibiotic with a broad activity against mycetes (see Chap. 41) is also active against *Leishmania* spp. It is used with different drug regimens, e.g., 1 mg/kg given iv every other day for up to 20 injections.

Amphotericin B must be administered by slow infusion, if possible via a central venous line. Infusions are prepared with 5% glucose. Vials must be protected from light. During therapy, a high fluid intake should be maintained. Blood counts, renal parameters, and K levels have to be checked regularly. Potassium supplements may be required. Dosage must be reduced if serum creatinine levels rise by over 50%. Rarely, blood transfusions become necessary.

Three new formulations of amphotericin B have been developed in which deoxycholate has been replaced by other lipids; these formulations are liposomal amphotericin B, amphotericin B colloidal dispersion, and amphotericin B lipid complex (see Chap. 41). These formulations seem to be an effective treatment for visceral leishmaniasis in immunocompetent patients.

MALARIA

Disease presentation

Human malaria is caused by four species of plasmodial parasites: *Plasmodium falciparum* results in the most severe infections and life-threatening diseases, *P. vivax* and *P. ovale* result in tertian malaria, and *P. malariae* causes the

least severe but persistent quartan malaria. Tissue forms (hypnozoites) that persist in the liver are responsible for relapses in *P. vivax* and *P. ovale* infections. Such latent forms are not generated by *P. falciparum* or *P. malariae*.

The clinical response depends both on the species of the parasite and the immunologic status of the patient. Nonimmune travelers to malarious areas risk severe attacks. Symptoms in all forms of malaria include fever, chills, and headache. However, symptoms can be diffuse, and malaria can mimic many other diseases such as gastroenteritis, pneumonia, influenza, hepatitis, etc. Because of synchronization of the parasite cycle, febrile paroxysms can occur every 48 hours in tertian malaria and every 72 hours in quartan malaria. If not treated in time, falciparum malaria can give rise to severe complications such as cerebral malaria with convulsions, stupor and progressive coma, acute renal failure with acidosis, respiratory insufficiency, shock, or massive hemolysis. Chronic or repeated infections may lead to splenomegaly and progressive anemia.

Treatment

Malaria, especially falciparum malaria, has to be considered life-threatening and must be treated as soon as possible. Treatment depends on the likely pattern of susceptibility of the plasmodia and on the severity of the disease.

Likely pattern of susceptibility

Up to the present, all *P. malariae* strains have shown sensitivity to chloroquine. Chloroquine-resistant *P. vivax* strains have emerged during recent years in Southeast Asia and Oceania. Chloroquine-sensitive *P. falciparum* strains are only those from in North Africa, Central America north of the Panama Canal, Haiti, and the Middle East. Mefloquine remains effective against all blood forms of malaria. Although scattered reports of clinical failures have come from other areas, mefloquine resistance is a problem of significant clinical importance only in the Thai-Cambodian and Thai-Myanmar border regions.

Severity of disease

The criteria used to diagnose severe complicated falciparum malaria are impaired consciousness, repeated convulsions, respiratory distress, shock, renal impairment (creatinine > 3 mg/dl), hypoglycemia (blood glucose < 40 mg/dl), acidosis (pH < 7.25, plasma bicarbonate < 15 mmol), elevated transaminases levels (>3 times normal), and high parasitemia (>5% of erythrocytes affected). It has been shown that the percentage of peripheral pigment-containing neutrophils is a measure of severity (>5% = bad prognosis).

Accordingly, before treatment, the following information must be available: (1) history of the patient (country in which infection took place, mode of transmission, and compliance with chemoprophylaxis), (2) parasitology (*Plasmodium* species, parasite number), and (3) major clinical and laboratory findings.

Tertian and quartan malaria are treated with chloroquine. Patients with vivax malaria originating from Southeast Asia or Oceania also can be treated with mefloquine. Following chloroquine (or mefloquine) treatment, patients with tertian malaria must receive primaquine – which kills hypnozoites – for the radical cure of this infection.

Patients with uncomplicated falciparum malaria can be treated with chloroquine when they come from the previously mentioned areas without resistance; otherwise, mefloquine is at present the drug of choice. Possible alternatives for patients with contraindications to the use of mefloquine or with suspected mefloquine resistance are halofantrine, artemisinin compounds, and the combination of atovaquone and proguanil. Because of the need for a rapid response, severe and complicated malaria should be treated by intravenous quinine infusion, possibly together with doxycycline.

In complicated falciparum malaria, a number of ancillary treatment measures are important, and for these, the patient must be transferred to an intensive care unit. Such complications and their treatments include:

- *Hyperpyrexia.* Clothing should be removed, and the patient should be fanned. Paracetamol is a safe antipyretic, although it has been reported to elongate parasite clearance time.
- *Hypoglycemia.* Blood glucose levels should be checked frequently, and the patient can be treated with a continuous infusion of 15% dextrose.
- *Anemia.* Transfusion with packed cells can be considered when the hemoglobin level falls to 8 to 10 g/dl in nonimmune patients.
- *Cerebral malaria.* Dexamethasone has been shown in double-blind placebo-controlled trials to be ineffective or possibly harmful. Seizures should be treated promptly with iv benzodiazepines.
- *Renal failure.* This may require dialysis or hemofiltration. In less severe conditions, a treatment trial with furosemide and dopamine can be started if the creatinine level is less than 5 mg/dl.
- *Metabolic acidosis.* This may improve after successful antiparasitic therapy. Sodium bicarbonate may be given if the arterial pH falls below 7.2, but the value of this treatment remains controversial. It has to be noted that sodium bicarbonate increases intracerebral pH and thus intracranial pressure. In patients with rhabdomyolysis, the urine should be alkalized. Treatment with dichloroacetate to reduce lactic acidosis still has to be considered as experimental.
- *Respiratory distress.* Respiration and circulation must be monitored. Fluid overload must be prevented by maintaining the central venous pressure between 0 and 5 cmH_2O (pulmonary artery occlusion pressure < 15 mmHg). Patients should be ventilated mechanically if pulmonary edema develops.
- *Septicemic shock.* A secondary bacterial infection always should be suspected. Blood and urine should be sent for culture, and broad-spectrum antimicrobial treatment eventually should be started.

Many adjuvant treatment measures have been suggested, but none has been shown unequivocally to affect outcome. For example, there is no evidence from clinical trials showing the effectiveness of exchange transfusion. Heparin treatment is not indicated because heparin has been shown to be associated with serious bleeding.

Drug classes

CHLOROQUINE

Chloroquine is a 4-aminoquinoline with activity against blood forms of susceptible *Plasmodium* strains. It is supplied in tablets of 100, 150, and 300 mg base (150 mg chloroquine base is equivalent to 200 mg chloroquine sulfate or 250 mg chloroquine phosphate), as a syrup, and as a hydrochloride for parenteral injection.

Dosage

At the onset of therapy, 10 mg/kg of chloroquine base is given; 6 hours after the start of treatment, 5 mg/kg of chloroquine base is given; 24 hours after the start of treatment, 5 mg/kg of chloroquine base is given; 48 hours later, 5 mg/kg of chloroquine base is given. Intravenous administration can cause severe hypotension.

Kinetics/metabolism

Absorption is efficient following oral administration; the bioavailability is about 90%, but high interpatient variation has been described. Chloroquine is 60% bound to plasma proteins and equally cleared by the kidney and liver. Both chloroquine and its metabolite desethylchloroquine decline slowly with an elimination half-life of 20 to 60 days.

Side effects

Severe side effects are rare, but itching is common among Africans. Some patients complain of gastrointestinal disturbances. Visual impairment from accumulation of chloroquine in the retina is a complication of long-term, high-dosage therapy. Chloroquine can be administered safely during pregnancy. Relative contraindications are psoriasis, porphyria, and retinal diseases. Cimetidine may increase chloroquine plasma levels. Bioavailability of ampicillin can be lowered by chloroquine.

Therapy of overdose

Symptoms are nausea and vomiting, slurring of speech, pulmonary edema, convulsions, coma, and arrhythmias. Treatment is symptomatic.

PRIMAQUINE

Primaquine is an 8-aminoquinoline active against the intrahepatic forms of malaria, including the hypnozoites of *P. vivax* and *P. ovale*. Dosage in adults is 0.25 mg/kg (up to 15 mg/day) following chloroquine (or mefloquine) therapy.

Primaquine is readily absorbed and has a complete oral bioavailability. It is rapidly metabolized, and only a small amount is excreted unchanged in the liver.

The major side effect is hemolytic anemia in erythrocyte enzyme defects. Glucose-6-phosphate dehydrogenase deficiency must be excluded before treatment, and primaquine should not be administered concurrently with other drugs that may induce hemolysis. Primaquine is contraindicated in pregnancy and conditions that predispose to granulocytopenia, such as rheumatoid arthritis and lupus erythematosus, and for patients under 1 year of age.

MEFLOQUINE

Mefloquine is a 4-aminoquinoline methanol active against blood forms of all malaria parasites. It is supplied in tablets of 250 mg base.

Dosage

Initial dosage in adults is 750 mg mefloquine base; 6 hours later, 250 mg; and 6 hours later (patient > 60 kg), 250 mg. In children (5-45 kg body weight), 15 mg/kg should be given, followed by 10 mg/kg 6 to 8 hours later.

Mefloquine should be used for the prevention and treatment of chloroquine-resistant and multidrug-resistant *P. falciparium*. It is usually started 2 weeks before entering the area and is given once weekly, ending 4 weeks after leaving the area.

Kinetics/metabolism

The oral absorption of mefloquine is relatively rapid, reaching peak concentrations within 24 hours. Metabolism takes place in the liver. Mefloquine is highly bound to plasma proteins. The elimination is slow – plasma concentrations decay with a half-life from 15 to over 30 days (partially dependent on racial origin, e.g., shorter in Thais than in Caucasians) – and mainly by the fecal route.

Side effects

Side effects are dose-related and possibly more frequent in women. Mild reactions include dizziness, nausea and vomiting, diarrhea, and abdominal pain. Neuropsychiatric adverse events have an incidence of about 1 in 200 to 1 in 1200 patients and include vertigo, impaired coordination, affective disorders, anxiety disorders, hallucinations, and sleep disturbances. Cardiovascular events include bradycardia and sinus arrhythmias.

Mefloquine should not be administered within 12 hours of the last dose of quinine. The World Health Organization (WHO) currently advises that mefloquine can be given with confidence during the second and third trimesters of pregnancy. Contraindications are history of epilepsy or severe neuropsychiatric disorders.

HALOFANTRINE

Halofantrine is a phenanthrene methanol active against the blood stages of all malaria parasites. It is supplied as tablets with 250 mg base and a suspension containing 100 mg/5 ml.

Dosage

Dosage in adults and children over 1 year of age is 24 mg/kg in three divided doses at 6-hour intervals. Use should be restricted to treatment in a hospital where the ECG can be monitored. Halofantrine should not be administered with food.

Kinetics/metabolism

Absorption from the gastrointestinal tract is irregular. Halofantrine is almost entirely eliminated by hepatic biotransformation. The principal metabolite is mono-*N*-desbutyl halofantrine, which has marked antimalarial activity.

Side effects and interactions

Side effects include abdominal pain and diarrhea. A reversible increase in the levels of transaminases has been described. First- and second-degree atrioventricular (AV) blocks as well as prolongations of the QTc interval have been found. Ventricular arrhythmias have occurred not only in patients with preexisting (or drug-induced) prolongation of the QTc interval. Dangerous interactions can occur with drugs that may prolong the QT interval, e.g., mefloquine during the preceding 3 weeks, quinine, quinidine, chloroquine, tricyclic antidepressants, neuroleptic drugs and astemizole.

QUININE

Quinine is an alkaloid derived from the bark of the cinchona tree that is effective against all blood forms of malaria parasites. Many different oral and injectable formulations of quinine salts are available.

Dosage

Dosage is 10 mg/kg every 8 hours in adults and every 12 hours in children by slow infusion for 10 days (in combination with doxycycline, 3 mg/kg once daily — of course, not in pregnant women and in children younger than 8 years of age). It is generally recommended to start quinine treatment with a "loading dose" of 7 mg/kg over 30 minutes and then 10 mg/kg over 4 hours; alternatively, 20 mg/kg can be given over the first 4 hours. No loading dose should be given if the patient has received mefloquine within the last 24 hours.

Treatment should be started by slow iv infusion. The dose should be reduced by 30% after the third day of treatment in patients who remain seriously ill. The dose also should be reduced if the QTc interval is prolonged by more than 25% of the baseline value. In renal impairment, the dose must be reduced to half after 2 to 3 days. Oral treatment should be resumed as soon as the patient is able to tolerate it and should be continued for the completion of the course (same dose).

When quinine is not available, therapy can be started with quinidine: the initial loading dose of quinidine should be 10 mg of base per kg infused over 1-2h, the maintenance dose is 0.75 to 1.2 mg base/kg per hour. To avoid cardiotoxicity, patients with severe falciparum malaria receiving quinidine should be monitored for hypotension (related to vasodilatation) and QT prolongation.

Kinetics/metabolism

Quinine is rapidly absorbed when taken orally. Bioavailability is more than 85% in malaria patients. It is metabolized in the liver and subsequently excreted in the urine, mainly as hydroxylated metabolites.

Side effects

Mild signs of cinchonism such as tinnitus, headache, blurred vision, altered auditory acuity, vertigo, and diarrhea do not constitute reasons for withdrawal. A major adverse effect is hyperinsulinemic hypoglycemia, which should be treated with supplementary glucose. Quinine can cause severe hypotension if injected too rapidly. Rarely, quinine may cause hemolysis, severe thrombocytopenia associated with quinine-dependent antiplatelet antibodies, hypersensitivity reactions, or granulomatous hepatitis. Quinine raises digoxin plasma levels. Cimetidine has been reported to reduce the clearance of quinine. There is no evidence of an increased risk of abortion or preterm delivery with use of the standard dosage, and according to the WHO, quinine is safe in pregnancy.

Therapy of overdose

A single dose greater than 3 g can cause a potentially lethal intoxication in adults. Emesis should be induced and gastric lavage undertaken.

ARTEMISININ DERIVATIVES

In the early 1970s, Chinese scientists identified artemisinin, a sesquiterpene lactone peroxide, as the principal active component of the traditional Chinese malaria remedy, the qinghaosu plant (*Artemisia annua*). Artemisinin, dihydroartemisinin, and two derivatives, artesunate and artemether, clear sensitive parasites from the blood more rapidly than other antimalarial drugs. Artesunate is sodium succinyl salt of artemisinin; artemether is a methyl ether derivative.

Dosage

Artesunate is formulated as tablets, suppositories, and a dry powder of artesunic acid for injection. Dosage in uncomplicated malaria in adults and children over 6 months of age is 4 mg/kg orally qd for 3 days, plus mefloquine (15-25 mg/kg) as a single or split dose on the second or third day.

Dosage in complicated malaria is 2.4 mg/kg as an intravenous loading dose on the first day, followed by 1.2 mg/kg iv daily until the patient is able to tolerate oral medication for a maximum of 7 days.

Artemether is formulated as tablets and capsules as well as an oily solution for injection. Dosage in uncomplicated malaria is the same as for artesunate. Dosage in complicated malaria is 3.2 mg/kg as a loading dose by intramuscular injection, followed by 1.6 mg/kg daily until the patient is able to tolerate oral medication for a maximum of 7 days.

When given alone, treatment courses of less than 5 days result in high relapse rates. Therefore, artesunate or artemether always should be combined with mefloquine.

Kinetics/metabolism

Artesunate is rapidly hydrolyzed to its principal active metabolite, dihydroartemisinin, and tightly binds to erythrocyte membranes. Pharmacokinetic data are limited. Artemether and its metabolite dihydroartemisinin have shown large variability in plasma concentrations.

Side effects

Of some concern is the finding that artemisinin and its derivatives cause neurotoxicity in animals. However, to date, there is no clear evidence of neurotoxicity in humans. Possible drug-related adverse effects of artesunate include dizziness, itching, vomiting and other gastrointestinal effects, reduction in neutrophil count, and convulsions. Transient laboratory effects have been reported for artemether, including a decrease in reticulocyte count, an increase in transaminases, and sinus bradycardia. Little experience has been gained with artemisinin derivatives in pregnancy, but they should not be withheld if they are considered lifesaving for the mother.

ATOVAQUONE PLUS PROGUANIL

Atovaquone is a broad-spectrum antiprotozoal drug licensed in many countries for the treatment of *P. carinii* pneumonia. Proguanil is an inhibitor of the plasmodial dihydrofolate reductase and is employed extensively in prophylaxis.

The combination of atovaquone and proguanil is approved in several countries for treatment of uncomplicated falciparum malaria, generally in the fixed combination of 250 mg atovaquone plus 100 mg proguanil.

Dosage

Dosage is atovaquone 1000 mg per day for 3 days plus proguanil 400 mg per day for 3 days.

Kinetics/metabolism

Atovaquone has poor oral bioavailability that varies with dose and diet. The main route of elimination is via the liver. Proguanil is absorbed rapidly and metabolized to active cycloguanil and 4-chlorophenylbiguanide. There is a pronounced intersubject variability in the capacity to metabolize proguanil.

Side effects and interactions

Side effects include abdominal pain, diarrhea, coughing, nausea and vomiting, and sometimes a reversible increase in aminotransferases. Metoclopramide and rifampin can reduce atovaquone concentrations.

Prophylaxis

Prophylaxis is based on exposition prophylaxis (prevention of mosquito bites) and on chemoprophylaxis, since an effective vaccine is not available. In areas without chloroquine resistance, prophylaxis is done by means of chloroquine, whereas in those areas with high malaria infection rates and frequent cases of resistance, mefloquine generally is used; in areas with more or less rare cases of chloroquine resistance, chloroquine and proguanil can be taken. The assignment of countries to one or the other area may change in the course of years. Standby treatment may be given to travelers who are unable to reach medical services for extended periods (Tab. 42.2).

Some experts strongly advise combination therapies to prevent the development of resistance. Some clinical studies are under way, e.g., with co-artemether (artemether + benflumetol), which is already licensed in some countries, or LAPDAP (chlorproguanil + dapsone). Pyronaridine is another blood schizontocide synthezised in China, but the mode of action is unknown. In the long run, the identification of new drugs by results from basic research into the physiology of the parasite seems to be more promising; an example is the development of Na^+/H^+ exchange inhibitors, which are still in the preclinical phase.

Some cytokines correlate with disease severity and outcome. Accordingly, initial studies have been performed. For example, in a double-blind trial in 610 Gambian children with cerebral malaria, a monoclonal antibody to tumor necrosis factor attenuated fever but did not reduce mortality.

TOXOPLASMOSIS

Disease presentation

Toxoplasmosis is the clinical disease caused by *Toxoplasma gondii*, as distinct from *Toxoplasma* infection, and is asymptomatic in the vast majority of immunocompetent patients. People with competent immune systems some-

---

Table 42.2 Malaria prophylaxis

Regional characteristics	Prophylaxis	Countries (selection)
No malaria	No prophylaxis	Africa: Tunisia, Seychelles, Réunion Asia: Israel, Jordan, Kuwait, Brunei, Singapore, Hong Kong, Taiwan America: the Caribbeans (excluding Haiti and the Dominican Republic, Chile, Uruguay)
Low incidence of malaria	No regular prophylaxis (however, in case of fever, test for malaria)	Africa: Marocco, Mauritius Asia: Turkish Riviera, Syria United Arab Emirates America: Paraguay, North Argentina, Dominican Republic
Areas without choroquine resistance	Chloroquine (300 mg chloroquine base per week)	Africa: Egypt during Summer months America: Central America
Areas with chloroquine resistance	Chloroquine + proguanil (300 mg chloroquine-base per week + 200 mg proguanil per day)	Africa: Northern districts of Namibia, Botswana Asia: Indian subcontinent, rural districts in southern China, parts of Indonesia, western Malaysia South America: Pacific Coast
Areas with high rate of chloroquine resistance and high frequency of *Falciparum* malaria	Mefloquine (250 mg per week)	Africa: East, Central, and West Africa Asia: Laos, Cambodia, Vietnam South America: Amazon basin and influx areas

[Start chemoprophylaxis 1 week before departure (2 weeks in case of mefloquine) and continue chemoprophylaxis for 4 weeks after returning home. In the individual case, personal aspects may give way to differing recommendations, e.g., residential stay only in big cities, stay restricted to a few days, prior diseases, drug contraindications, etc.]

times develop mild lymph node enlargement. Reactivation of the chronic infection can occur in severely immunocompromized patients, leading to encephalitits and meningoencephalitis. Primary infection in immunodeficient patients may result in encephalitis, myocarditis, or pneumonitis. Neonatal infection may result from acute maternal infection during pregnancy, sometimes leading to chorioretinitis and other sequelae.

Treatment

Immunocompetent patients with the lymphadenopathic form of infection generally are not treated unless visceral disease is clinically overt. Immunodeficient patients always should be treated when the infection is acute. Pyrimethamine combined with sulfadiazine and folinic acid is the therapy of choice. Alternative regimens include pyrimethamine in combination with clindamycin, azithromycin, atovaquone, or dapsone. Toxoplasmosis in pregnant women can be treated with spiramycin (1 g tid until term). When amniocentesis is done and has provided evidence of infection, alternating 3-week courses of pyrimethamine/sulfadiazine and spiramycin can be administered from the beginning of the second trimester until term.

Drug classes

PYRIMETHAMINE

Pyrimethamine is structurally related to trimethoprim. It inhibits folic acid metabolism and kills *T. gondii* tachyzoites (it is also effective against erythrocytic stages of all four species of malaria). Dosage in immunocompetent patients is 50 mg per day (together with 4 g sulfadiazine per day) for 3 weeks; in immunodeficient patients, 200 mg is given in divided doses for 1 day, followed by 75 to 100 mg daily for at least 6 weeks. Patients should receive folinic acid concurrently.

Pyrimethamine is absorbed rapidly. It is partially metabolized in the liver and ultimately excreted in urine.

Side effects include gastrointestinal symptoms, ataxia, tremors, and seizures. Pyrimethamine is contraindicated during the first trimester of pregnancy.

SULFADIAZINE

Sulfadiazine acts synergistically with pyrimethamine (see above). Sulfadiazine is absorbed rapidly and is excreted in the urine after partial acetylation in the liver.

Side effects are those of the sulfonamides (see Chap. 38), including nausea, vomiting, and diarrhea. Rarely, hypersensitivity reactions including Stevens-Johnson syndrome and toxic epidermal necrolysis can occur. Sulfadiazine is contraindicated during the first trimester of pregnancy. The blood count must be monitored twice weekly to detect signs of bone marrow depression. High urinary output must be maintained to avoid crystal formation.

PNEUMOCYSTIS CARINII PNEUMONIA

Disease presentation

The taxonomic position of *P. carinii* is unclear (sequence analyses of ribosomal RNA plead for classification as a fungus). *P. carinii* pneumonia (PcP) is a frequent opportunistic infection in patients with HIV infection and is characterized by tachypnea, fever, coughing, hypoxemia, and ultimately, respiratory failure.

Treatment

Trimethoprim-sulfamethoxazole (cotrimoxazole) is the drug of choice for the treatment of PcP and extrapulmonary disease because of excellent tissue penetration, rapid clinical response, and satisfactory oral bioavailability comparable with parenteral administration. The main alternative parenteral agent is pentamidine-isetionate. Other alternatives include atovaquone (approved by the U.S. Food and Drug Administration for the treatment of mild to moderately severe PcP), trimetrexate, and clindamycin-primaquine. Adjunctive therapies include corticosteroids and, potentially, colony-stimulating factors.

Adults and adolescents with HIV infection should be administered chemoprophylaxis against PcP if they have a CD4+ T-lymphocyte count of less than 200/µl or if they have a history of PcP. Cotrimoxazole is the preferred prophylactic agent.

Drug classes

COTRIMOXAZOLE

The two components of this combination inhibit different steps in the enzymatic synthesis of tetrahydrofolic acid. Cotrimoxazole is available as tablets, oral suspension, or concentrate for intravenous infusion (see also Chap. 38). Therapy for PcP is initiated with 20 mg trimethoprim plus 100 mg sulfamethoxazole per kg per day in three to four divided doses for 14 to 21 days. The drugs should be administered intravenously if there is uncertainty about gastrointestinal function and marked hypoxemia.

Side effects are generally those of sulfa drug allergy: rash, fever, neutropenia, thrombocytopenia, erythema multiforme exsudativum, toxic hepatitis, and nephrotoxicity. Trimethoprim may induce a megaloblastic anemia. Therapy can be continued despite mild side effects. In renal dysfunction, dosage must be reduced. The risk of sulfonamide crystalluria is decreased by maintaining a urinary output of at least 1.5 liters daily.

PENTAMIDINE ISETIONATE

In PcP, pentamidine isetionate (see above) is given by

slow infusion in 5% glucose as a single dosage of 4 mg/kg/day. Newer pentamidine analogues under development appear to have significantly superior therapeutic and lower toxicity profiles than pentamidine.

TRICHOMONIASIS

Disease presentation

This disease – caused by the parasitic protozoan *Trichomonas vaginalis* – encompasses a broad spectrum of symptoms ranging from vaginal discharge, dysuria, and vulvovaginal itching in women and urethritis in men to a relatively asymptomatic carrier state. Complications associated with trichomoniasis include adnexitis, pyosalpinx, infertility, and cervical erosion.

All patients and all asymptomatic carriers should be treated. Today, the standard treatment of trichomoniasis is metronidazole. However, other 5-nitroimidazole derivatives such as tinidazole, nimorazole, and ornidazole are also highly effective. Known sexual contacts should be treated at the same time. Refractory cases, for which a second standard treatment is not curative, are treated with higher doses of metronidazole.

Treatment

Metronidazole is given for trichomoniasis at a dosage of 250 mg orally tid for 7 days or as single 2-g dose. Infants more than 4 weeks old should receive 5 mg/kg tid for 3 days. During early pregnancy, when metronidazole is contraindicated, symptoms may be relieved by clotrimazole suppositories.

AFRICAN TRYPANOSOMIASIS

Disease presentation

African trypanosomiasis, or sleeping sickness, is a protozoan infection caused by two subspecies of *Trypanosoma brucei* — *T. brucei gambiense* and *T. brucei rhodesiense* — and transmitted by *Glossina* spp. (tsetse flies). Sleeping disease caused by *T. brucei gambiense* is characterized by weakness, wasting, fever, lymphadenopathy (most obvious in the posterior cervical region and known as Winterbottom's sign), and eventual involvement of the central nervous system (CNS). Trypanosomiasis caused by *T. brucei rhodesiense* develops more rapidly, and early death may occur.

Treatment

All patients have to be treated because otherwise the disease usually will have a fatal outcome. In the early stages when the CNS is not involved, suramin is the first-line drug in *T. brucei rhodesiense* infections. In early *T. brucei gambiense* infections, some authors regard suramin as the first-line drug; others use pentamidine. In the meningoencephalic stage, an arsenical compound, melarsoprol, previously was the only drug used to cure infection. Recently, clinical experience has confirmed the effectiveness of eflornithine in the meningoencephalitic stage of *T. brucei gambiense* infection. It is less toxic than melarsoprol, and thus some authors regard it as the first-line drug.

Follow-up

In *T. brucei gambiense* infection, lumbar puncture is performed every 6 months for 2 years; in *T. brucei rhodesiense* infection, lumbar punctures are performed after 3 and 6 months and then every 6 months for 2 years. Demonstration of trypanosomes in the cerebrospinal fluid (CSF), elevated cell counts, or specific IgM antibodies indicate relapse.

Drug classes

SURAMIN

A complex derivative of urea (sulfated naphthylamine) was introduced in the 1920s for the treatment of African trypanosomiasis (it is also active against the adult worm of *Onchocerca volvulus;* see below).

Dosage

Suramin is available in 1-g vials. An escalated dosage should be used. Initially, with testing, 5 mg/kg (first day) should be used, followed by 10 mg/day (third day) and 20 mg/day (1 g maximum) on days 5, 11, 17, 23, and 30. Administration of all doses should be by slow iv injection of the 10% solution in "water for injection." Urine should be tested before each dose; if protein is present, the dose should be reduced. In heavy proteinuria, treatment must be discontinued.

Kinetics/metabolism

The drug is not metabolized. Total-body clearance is low, and plasma protein binding is extremely high. The main route of elimination is renal. The terminal half-life has been estimated to be about 40 days.

Side effects

In about 1 in 20 000 patients, severe reactions occur, with emesis, convulsions, and shock. Renal toxicity is the most common problem. Other toxic effects are exfoliative dermatitis, severe diarrhea, prolonged high fever and prostration, and bone marrow depression. Lesser symptoms include tiredness, anorexia, malaise, polyuria, and neurologic complications (including tenderness of the palms and soles, metallic taste, and headache). Suramin has teratogenic effects in mice. In pregnancy, the benefits must be weighed against toxicity. Contraindications are an anaphylactic reaction following the first injection and severe liver or renal disease. Concomitant onchocerciasis will increase the risk of hypersensitivity reactions with suramin and should be treated first with ivermectin.

MELARSOPROL

Melarsoprol is a trivalent arsenical compound that is active against all stages of *T. brucei gambiense* and *T. brucei rhodesiense* infection. It is available in ampules containing 5 ml of a 3.6% solution in propyleneglycol, corresponding to 180 mg melarsoprol. Treatment regimens may vary, and updated international guidelines should be checked.

Melarsoprol must be administered by slow iv infusion. Propyleneglycol is a powerful tissue irritant, and extravascular leakage should be avoided. Some authors recommend concomitant application of prednisolone (1 mg/kg per day, maximum 40 mg) as long as melarsoprol is given (amebiasis and strongyloidiasis should be excluded by fecal examination).

Melarsoprol is largely metabolized to nontoxic pentavalent compounds and is excreted within 5 days, primarily via the bile and, to a lesser extent, the kidneys.

The most serious side effect is encephalopathy, which is especially frequent in patients with severe disease. Between 1 and 5% of patients die during treatment. Encephalopathy begins 3 to 10 days after the first dose and is characterized by headache, tremor, slurring of speech, and motor excitation progressing into coma and convulsions. Other side effects include albuminuria, exfoliative dermatitis, agranulocytosis, and myocardial damage; hemolytic reactions may be seen in glucose-6-phosphate dehydrogenase deficiency. Melarsoprol should be given only in extreme circumstances during pregnancy. Pregnant women with meningoencephalitic involvement possibly also can be treated with pentamidine and suramin.

EFLORNITHINE

Eflornithine is an ornithine derivative with specific activity against *T. brucei gambiense*. It is available as eflornithine hydrochloride for intravenous injection. Dosage is 100 mg/kg (children: 150 mg/kg) iv every 6 hours for 7 to 14 days. One ampule should be diluted into 400 ml of 0.9% NaCl and then infused over 45 minutes.

The plasma half life is 3 to 3.5 hours, and the drug is excreted mainly via the kidneys. Side effects include abdominal complaints, osmotic diarrhea, thrombocytopenia, and rarely, seizures, alopecia, hearing loss, and skin rashes. Eflornithine is contraindicated during pregnancy and lactation.

AMERICAN TRYPANOSOMIASIS (CHAGAS' DISEASE)

Disease presentation

American trypanosomiasis is a zoonotic infection caused by *Trypanosoma cruzi* and transmitted by triatomine bugs to humans. Acute Chagas' disease, characterized by fever, malaise, lymphadenopathy and hepatomegaly, myocarditis, and meningoencephalitis, may be a life-threatening sequela. If not treated, *T. cruzi* infection may persist and decades later cause chronic Chagas' disease, chiefly notable for severe cardiomyopathy and pathologic dilatation of the esophagus and colon.

Treatment

Acute Chagas' disease must be treated with nifurtimox or benznidazole to prevent progression to chronic Chagas' disease. The efficacy of antiparasitic treatment during the intermediate stage or in chronic Chagas' disease is not proven, but if parasites are still detected, treatment is indicated.

Symptomatic treatment may be necessary in chronic Chagas' disease. Therapy of heart failure is problematic and may lead to transplantation. Treatment of arrhythmias is also problematic because of frequent bundle-branch blocks. Complete or second-degree atrioventricular (AV) block and bradycardia respond to a pacemaker. Megaesophagus and megacolon may require pneumatic dilation or surgical treatment.

Drug classes

NIFURTIMOX

Nifurtimox is available as 30- and 120-mg tablets. Dosage is 8 to 10 mg/kg per day in three doses for 60 to 90 days (children: 15 mg/kg in four doses for 60 to 90 days). Nifurtimox should be given under close medical supervision. Daily dosage should be reduced if weight loss, neurologic disturbances, or other severe side effects occur. Alcohol should be avoided because it may increase the severity of side effects.

Nifurtimox is efficiently absorbed from the gastrointestinal tract. It is almost completely degraded and excreted in the urine. Side effects include anorexia, peripheral polyneuritis, psychosis, gastrointestinal symptoms, and hemolysis in glucose-6-phosphate dehydrogenase deficiency. Safety in pregnancy has not been established.

BENZNIDAZOLE

Benznidazole is a trypanocidal nitroimidazole derivative that is available as 100-mg tablets. Dosage is 5 mg/kg/day in adults and 5 to 10 mg/kg/day in children orally in two divided doses for 60 days. Leukocytes must be monitored throughout treatment. Alcohol should be avoided during treatment.

Absorption is fairly rapid; peak plasma levels are reached after 3 to 4 hours. Benznidazole is partly metabolized, and metabolites are eliminated rapidly in the urine and stools. Side effects include rashes (often photosensitive), nausea, peripheral polyneuritis, and rarely, agranulocytosis. Lymphomas have been described in animals but not in humans. Safety in pregnancy has not been established.

Allopurinol (see Chap. 71) is being studied as an alternative drug for Chagas' disease. Preliminary data support effectiveness of 300 mg bid for 60 to 90 days in adults.

CESTODE INFECTIONS

Disease presentation

Intestinal cestode infections

Several tapeworms are responsible for intestinal infections in humans. Many infected individuals are asymptomatic, but some have abdominal pain and nausea. A few carriers of the fish tapeworm *Diphyllobothrium* develop a macrocytic, megaloblastic anemia.

Cysticercosis

Cysticercosis is infection by the larval stage of the tapeworm *Taenia solium*. Cystic lesions in the CNS system can cause headache, seizures, intracranial hypertension, and hydrocephalus and can lead to death. Cysts in skin, muscle, and other tissues are mostly asymptomatic.

Echinococcosis

The hydatid cysts of *Echinococcus granulosus* tend to form in the liver or lung and, rarely in the brain, heart, or bones. When symptoms do occur, they are due to the mass effect of the enlarging cyst. Alveolar cyst disease caused by *E. multilocularis* is more aggressive; the gradual invasion of adjacent tissues is tumor-like.

Treatment

Intestinal cestode infections

All patients with tapeworm infections should be treated. Treatment of *T. solium* is particularly important because of the risk of cysticercosis. Praziquantel rapidly kills adult tapeworms in the intestine and generally is the drug of choice for treatment. Praziquantel seems to be more effective than the longer-established compound niclosamide, to be regarded as of second choice. Control examinations should be performed 2 to 3 months after the initial treatment. In diphyllobothriasis, hydroxocobalamine injections and folic acid supplements may be required.

Cysticercosis

Antihelminthic therapy generally is considered to be indicated in newly identified active neurocysticercosis. Treatment must be individualized on the basis of cyst location, symptoms, viability of the cysts, and degree of host inflammatory response. Antiparasitic drugs of

choice are praziquantel and albendazole. In comparative studies, no clear-cut advantage of one of the two drugs could be demonstrated. Albendazole, however, is regarded as superior because of shorter treatment time and lower costs. If symptoms worsen under therapy, dexamethasone or anticonvulsants should be administered. Dexamethasone causes an increase in albendazole levels but reduces praziquantel levels. Patients suffering from hydrocephalus or intraventricular cysts should be referred for neurosurgery.

Echinococcosis

Surgery is the treatment of choice for operable cystic disease due to *E. granulosus*. Chemotherapy with one of the benzimidazoles, mebendazole or albendazole, is indicated in inoperable patients but also prior to surgery. In alveolar disease due to *E. multilocularis,* both surgery and long-term treatment with either mebendazole or albendazole are indicated.

In cystic echinococcosis, ultrasound-guided cyst puncture (PAIR = puncture, aspiration, injection, and respiration) offers an alternative for treatment, especially for inoperable cysts and for patients with a high surgical risk.

Drug classes

PRAZIQUANTEL (see below)

Dosages in cestode infections are reported in Table 42.3. For cysticercosis, 50 to 60 mg/kg is given daily in three divided doses for 14 days (in dermal cysticercosis, 6 days of treatment seems to be sufficient). Bioavailability is markedly reduced when praziquantel is given together with antiepileptics or corticosteroids, especially carbamazepine, phenytoin, or dexamethasone. Cimetidine increases plasma concentrations.

ALBENDAZOLE

Albendazole is a benzimidazole antibiotic that is chemically related to metronidazole. It is available in chewable tablets of 200 and 400 mg and in 2% and 4% suspensions for pediatric use.

Cysticercosis

Albendazole is administered at a daily dosage of 15 mg/kg for 30 days (the choice of 30 days is based on treatment experiences in echinococcosis; preliminary data indicate that 8-day courses may be as effective).

Echinococcosis

Adults are treated with 10 to 15 mg/kg daily for 28 days, followed by a treatment-free period ("washout") of 14 days. At least two such courses are necessary in cystic echinococcosis, and at least 2 years (sometimes lifelong) of treatment are necessary in alveolar echinococcosis.

The drug is given with meals. During treatment of

Table 42.3 Intestinal cestode infections: dosages of praziquantel

Taenia saginata (beef tapeworm)	Single dose of 5-10 mg/kg
Taenia solium (pork tapeworm)	Single dose of 5-10 mg/kg
Hymenolepis nana (dwarf tapeworm)	Single dose of 15-25 mg/kg
Hymenolepis deminuta	Single dose of 10-25 mg/kg
Dypilidium caninum (dog tapeworm)	Single dose of 5-10 mg/kg
Diphyllobothrium latum (fish tapeworm)	Single dose of 5-10 mg/kg

echinococcosis, transaminase levels and leukocyte and platelet counts must be monitored regularly.

Although albendazole is very poorly absorbed from the gastrointestinal tract, it reaches higher plasma concentrations than mebendazole. It is metabolized rapidly in the liver to the primary metabolite, albendazole sulfoxide (ALBSO), considered to be directly or indirectly responsible for both toxicity and efficacy outside the gastrointestinal tract. Concentrations of ALBSO are highly variable between individuals, and the half-life is between 6 and 15 hours.

Side effects are rare. Transient epigastric upset and headache are reported by some patients, and reversible increases in transaminases and reversible reductions in leukocyte counts do occur. Severe reactions such as pseudomembranous colitis and aplastic anemia are uncommon. Concomitant administration of dexamethasone or praziquantel increases plasma concentrations of ALBSO. Albendazole should not be administered during the first trimester of pregnancy.

NICLOSAMIDE

Niclosamide acts only against adult intestinal cestodes. It is available as 500-mg tablets. Treatment is with a single dose of 2 g (children < 10 kg: 0.5 g as a single dose; 10 to 35 kg: 1 g as a single dose). *H. nana* infections must be treated for 7 consecutive days (2 g on day 1, followed by 1 g daily for 6 days). In the treatment of *T. solium* infections, an antiemetic before and a laxative 1 to 2 hours after giving niclosamide have been recommended to avoid the risk of cysticercosis.

The drug is not absorbed from the gastrointestinal tract and may cause minor gastrointestinal discomfort. No mutagenic, teratogenic, or embryotoxic effects have been shown.

MEBENDAZOLE (see below)

Mebendazole is used in echinococcosis at daily doses of 50 mg/kg for at least 3 to 6 months (serum drug concentrations should be monitored after 2 and 4 weeks).

INTESTINAL, LIVER, AND LUNG FLUKES

Disease presentation

Patients with intestinal flukes are mostly asymptomatic. Only in heavy infections are gastrointestinal symptoms encountered. Patients with liver flukes also may be asymptomatic; patients with heavy worm loads may suffer from cholangitis. Patients with *Fasciola hepatica* infection may show an early phase characterized by fever and pain in the right upper quadrant. The major clinical manifestations of paragonimiasis are chest complaints.

Treatment

In principle, all infections, including light, asymptomatic ones, should be treated. Virtually all patients (with the exception of those with *F. hepatica* infections) can be cured with praziquantel.

Drug classes

PRAZIQUANTEL (see below)

Dosages in intestinal, liver, and lung fluke infections are reported in Table 42.4.

SCHISTOSOMIASIS

Disease presentation

Schistosomiasis is caused by any of five species of trematode parasites. Infection with *Schistosoma haematobium* (Bilharzia) is associated with urinary tract symptoms, including hematuria, dysuria, or frequency; heavily infected patients can develop obstructive uropathy. *S. mansoni* infection may lead to colonic polyposis and inflammation; however, hepatosplenic involvement is the most frequent cause of morbidity. The clinical manifestations of *S. japonicum, S. mekongi,* and *S. intercalatum* infections are similar to those of *S. mansoni*.

Treatment

All individuals with parasitologically confirmed (or serologically suspected) schistosomiasis should be treated. Praziquantel has been shown to resolve and prevent most forms of clinical morbidity and is the drug of choice against all species of the parasite. Older drugs including metrifonate, active against *S. haematobium,* and oxamniquine, active against *S. mansoni,* are still used in developing countries.

Late complications of schistosomiasis may require surgical treatment (e.g., ureteric reconstruction in bilharzial megaureter, splenectomy in pancytopenia caused by

Table 42.4 Dosages of praziquantel in intestinal, liver, and lung fluke infections according to species

Intestinal flukes

Fasciolopsis buski	Single dose of 25 mg/kg
Echinostoma spp.	Single dose of 25 mg/kg
Gastrodiscoides hominis	Single dose of 25 mg/kg
Heterophyes heterophyes	Single dose of 25 mg/kg
Metagonimus yokogawai	Single dose of 25 mg/kg
Watsonius watsoni	Single dose of 25 mg/kg

Liver flukes

Fasciola hepatica	Triclabendazol[1]
Clonorchis sinensis and *Opisthorchis* spp.	3 x 25 mg/kg for 2 days

Lung flukes

Paragonimus spp.	3 x 25 mg/kg for 2 days

[1]Triclabendazol is only available as a veterinary formulation; contact tropical institute.

hepatosplenic schistosomiasis, and sclerotherapy for esophageal varices).

Although the immune response of the host is an important factor in praziquantel efficacy, persons with HIV infection can be treated effectively for schistosomiasis with this drug.

Drug classes

PRAZIQUANTEL

Praziquantel is a pyrazinoquinoline derivative that is effective against a broad range of trematodes and cestodes. It is available for human use in tablets of 600, 500, and 150 mg.

Dosage

In schistosomiasis, a single dose of 40 mg/kg leads to a cure rate of about 60 to 95% (defined by the complete absence of eggs from the urine or feces 3 to 6 months after treatment). If patients have no liver dysfunction, treatment should be 40 mg/kg daily for 3 days to achieve safe elimination of the worms, although this has not been proven in controlled trials. Tablets should be taken preferably during or after meals. In patients with hepatosplenic schistosomiasis, caution should be taken because drug metabolization in the liver may be reduced. When patients come from areas with endemic human cysticercosis, it is advised to hospitalize them.

Kinetics/metabolism

After oral administration, more than 80% of the drug is absorbed, and peak plasma concentrations are reached after 3 to 4 hours. Praziquantel undergoes extensive first-pass metabolism, and 80% of the dose is excreted as metabolites within 24 hours in the urine.

Side effects and interactions

Praziquantel is well tolerated; only mild and transient side effects (dizziness, abdominal distress, lassitude) have been reported. Concomitant administration of cimetidine can raise plasma concentrations. Concomitant administration of chloroquine can decrease bioavailability of praziquantel. Praziquantel has not been shown to be mutagenic, teratogenic, or embryotoxic. Nevertheless, treatment should be postponed until after delivery unless there is a strong indication for its use. Lactation should be interrupted for 3 days after treatment.

Reports of low praziquantel cure rates have been published recently from a very intense *S. mansoni* focus in northern Senegal, and the suspicion has arisen that praziquantel-resistant/tolerant schistosomes may exist. The two long-known drugs oxamniquine and metrifonate are thus valuable alternatives. Only very few new potential antischistosomal compounds are in the pipeline, e.g., 9-acridanone hydrazone derivatives or the immunosuppressant drug cyclosporin A.

FILARIAL INFECTIONS

Disease presentation

Filarial nematode infections cause the important tropical diseases of lymphatic filariasis, onchocerciasis, and loiasis. In the adult stages, human filarial parasites inhabit the lymphatic system (*Wuchereria bancrofti* and *Brugia malayi,* leading to lymphangitis, hydrocele, and elephantiasis), subcutaneous tissues (*Onchocerca volvulus,* leading to subcutaneous nodules), and deep connective tissues (*Loa loa,* leading to fugitive swellings). Adult females produce microfilariae that are detectable in the peripheral blood or cutaneous tissues depending on species. In onchocerciasis, the microfilariae cause dermatitis, resulting in depigmentation and atrophy of the skin, and ocular lesions, resulting in blindness.

Treatment

Loiasis

All symptomatic patients should be treated. Diethylcarbamazine is effective against microfilariae and immature stages; adult worms are only partially killed.

Lymphatic filariasis

For mass treatments in endemic countries, treatment once a year with diethylcarbamazine (6 mg/kg) plus ivermectin (400 µg/kg) has been recommended. However, in Europe, killing of all adults worms with diethylcarbamazine should be attempted. Coexisting secondary infections also must be treated. Large hydroceles and elephantiasis usually require surgical intervention.

Onchocerciasis

Nodulectomy will remove adult worms, but usually not all nodules can be excised. Suramin kills adult worms but should not be used because of severe side effects. Until a safe and effective macrofilaricide is discovered, radical cure of onchocerciasis will remain impossible. The drug of choice for suppressive treatment of microfilariae is ivermectin. A single annual dose suppresses microfiladermia to a degree that prevents the development of clinical disease. It is adequately tolerated so as to be used in large-scale control campaigns.

Drug classes _____

DIETHYLCARBAMAZINE

Diethylcarbamazine (DEC) is a piperazine derivative that was first reported to have filaricidal effects in 1947. It is available as diethylcarbamazine citrate (100 mg citrate is approximately equivalent to 50 mg base) in 50- and 100-mg tablets and in oral solutions.

Dosage

In loiasis, 2 to 3 mg/kg is given tid up to 600 mg for 21 days. In *W. bancrofti* infections, 6 mg/kg is given daily for 12 days. In *B. malayi* infections, 6 mg/kg is given daily for 6 days. Treatment of loiasis should be done in hospital because of the danger of meningoencephalitits. DEC dosage should be reduced in patients with renal impairment. It has been reported that DEC may provoke relapses in asymptomatic malaria.

Kinetics/metabolism

DEC is almost completely absorbed after oral administration, peak plasma concentrations being reached in 1 to 2 hours. It is rapidly metabolized and excreted primarily via the kidneys. In patients with chronic renal disease, renal excretion is substantially reduced.

Side effects

The adverse effects per se are mild, but antifilarial treatment often results in adverse reactions related to the death of the microfilariae or damage to the adult worms. Immunologic reactions similar to the Mazzotti reaction in onchocerciasis can occur, with fever, headache, dizziness, urticaria, asthma, sometimes reversible proteinuria, and formation of nodules by killed worms along the spermatic cord (in lymphatic filariasis). Neurologic complications resembling encephalitis, frequently with a fatal outcome, typically occur in loiasis patients with high microfilaremia. Pregnant women should not be treated until after delivery.

IVERMECTIN

Dosage

In onchocerciasis, a single annual dose of 150 µg/kg (adults and children over 5 years) suppresses microfila-

dermia. In strongyloidiasis, 200 µg/kg is given for 3 days. No food should be taken for at least 2 hours before and after dosage.

Kinetics/metabolism

Ivermectin is well absorbed and metabolized, and it is excreted in the feces over a period of some 2 weeks.

Side effects

Transient postural hypotension may occur within 12 to 24 hours. Other side effects include rash, myalgia, enlarged lymph nodes, and swelling of the face. Ivermectin should not be used in children under 5 years of age because safety in this age group has not been established. Safety in pregnancy also has not been established. Symptoms of overdose are mydriasis, somnolence, depressed motor activity, tremor, and ataxia. Treatment is symptomatic, including pressor agents if hypotension is present.

NEMATODE INFECTIONS (WITHOUT FILARIAL DISEASES)

Disease presentation_____

Intestinal nematodes

In these infections, adult worms are located in the gut lumen. Intestinal nematodes vary widely in size, development, and disease manifestations. Morbidity and disease in these infections are largely a function of the number of worms harbored in the body.

Clinical presentation includes gastrointestinal discomfort (in all nematode infections), bowel obstruction and hepatobiliary obstruction (in ascariasis), anemia (in hookworm infections), chronic dysentery and rectal prolapse (in trichuriasis), pruritus ani (in enterobiasis), and malabsorption (in strongyloidiasis). Even moderate infections may contribute to malnutrition and diminished work capacity.

Tissue nematodes

Larvae and sometimes adult worms parasitize in different organs leading to a number of symptoms, e.g., *Gnathostoma spinigerum* and *Angiostrongylus cantonensis* as well as *Toxocara* spp. leading to visceral larva migrans and *Ancylostoma braziliense* leading to cutaneous larva migrans. In some cases the parasites are located in the bowel wall and also can be classified as intestinal nematodes (*Angiostrongylus costaricensis, Ancylostoma caninum*). *Trichinella spiralis* shows adult worms in the intestine, causing gastrointestinal symptoms, and larvae penetrating into muscle, causing fever, edema, and muscle pain.

Treatment

Trichuriasis

All infected patients should be treated, including patients with mild infections that lead to growth retardation. Mebendazole and albendazole are both effective.

Enterobiasis

This condition is self-limited within a few weeks if reinfection does not occur. However, all patients should be treated to prevent autoinfection. Drugs of choice are mebendazole and albendazole. Treatment should be repeated after 2 and 4 weeks.

Trichostrongyliasis

Mebendazole and albendazole are effective in dosages used in hookworm infections.

Capillariasis

Albendazole is the drug of choice because it is effective against both adults and larvae.

Ascariasis

All infected patients should be treated because even a single worm can cause severe allergic reactions and hepatobiliary complications. Benzimidazolcarbamate compounds (albendazole and mebendazole) are the drugs of choice. Such complications as bowel obstruction and hepatobiliary disease may require surgical intervention.

Ancylostoma duodenale and Necator americanus infections

All infected patients should be treated. Broad-spectrum antihelminthics are preferred. Albendazole and mebendazole are the drugs of choice.

Strongyloidiasis

All infected patients should be treated. It is especially important that infection is eliminated in patients who are to receive immunosuppressive therapy. Human trials with albendazole have demonstrated rates of parasite eradication ranging from 60 to 90%. Ivermectin also is effective in treating noncomplicated strongyloidiasis.

Angiostrongylus costaricensis infection

No specific therapy is available.

Trichinellosis

In symptomatic patients, therapy with either mebendazole or albendazole for about 2 weeks is advisable. The effect of therapy on encapsulated larvae is not known. In severe infections, adjunctive treatment with corticosteroids may become necessary.

Toxocariasis (visceral larva migrans)

Treatment is primarily symptomatic. The value of an antihelminthic therapy is not established. Prior to treatment, eye involvement should be excluded. Usually, albendazole and diethylcarbamazine are recommended.

Cutaneous larva migrans

Without treatment, migration can persist for several months. In mild infections, topical thiabendazole can be tried (10-15% in an inert ointment, possibly with 3% salicylic acid). In severe infections, oral ivermectin or albendazole can be added.

Gnathostomiasis

Albendazole is the drug of choice and is especially effective in subcutaneous forms. Visible larvae in the eye or skin should be removed surgically.

Angiostrongylus cantonenesis infection

Since the pathology is mainly caused by death of the worms, there is considerable doubt whether to treat with antihelminthics. Marked amelioration of symptoms can be achieved at times with prednisone.

Drug classes

MEBENDAZOLE

Mebendazole is a benzimidazole derivative with a wide range of antihelminthic activity against both cestodes and nematodes, as well as against the tissue stages of the parasites and against gut luminal forms. Mebendazole is available as 100- and 500-mg tablets and as a suspension.

Dosages for adults and children over 2 years

For trichuriasis, 100 mg is given bid for 3 days. A single dose of 500 mg can be given during mass treatments. For enterobiasis, a single dose of 100 mg is given daily and repeated two to four times at 7- to 14-day intervals. For ascariasis, a single dose of 500 mg or 100 mg bid is given for 3 days. For *Ancylostoma duodenale* and *Necator americanus* infections, 100 mg is given bid for 3 days. For trichinellosis, several treatment regimens have been recommended, e.g., 30 to 50 mg/kg daily for 2 weeks. Each dose preferably should be taken between meals. In patients with severe hepatic disease, the drug should be used with caution.

Kinetics/metabolism

Only small amounts are absorbed after oral dosage. Absorption is increased when the drug is taken with a fatty meal. When absorbed, it is rapidly metabolized in the liver and excreted into the bile.

Side effects

Side effects generally are restricted to transitory abdominal pain and diarrhea. The drug is not recommended in the first trimester of pregnancy.

ALBENDAZOLE

Dosages

For trichuriasis, a single dose of 400 mg is given; in heavy infections, 400 mg is given daily for 3 days. For enterobiasis, a single dose of 400 mg is given and is repeated after 2 and 4 weeks. For intestinal capillariasis, 400 to 800 mg is given daily for 10 days. For ascariasis, a single dose of 400 mg is given. For *Ancylostoma duodenale* and *Necator americanus* infections, a single dose of 400 mg is given. For strongyloidiasis, 400 mg is given bid for 3 to 7 days for 60 kg body weight: 15 mg/kg/day divided into two doses). For trichinellosis, several treatment regimens have been recommended, e.g., 400 mg daily for 2 weeks. For gnathostomiasis, several treatment regimens have been recommended, e.g., 400 mg daily for 3 weeks.

Suggested readings _____

ADEN ABDI Y, GUSTAFSON LL, ERICSSON Ö, HELLGREN U. Handbook of drugs for tropical parasitic infections, 2d ed. New York: Taylor and Francis, 1995.

BERMAN JD. Human leishmaniasis: clinical, diagnostic, and chemotherapeutic developments in the last 10 years. Clin Infect Dis 1997; 24:684-703.

CIOLI D. Chemotherapy of schistosomiasis: an update. Parasitol Today 1998;14:418-22.

FISHMAN JA. Treatment of infection due to *Pneumocystis carinii*. Antimicrob Agents Chemother 1998;42:1309-14.

FREEMAN CD, KLUTMAN NE, LAMP KC. Metronidazole: a therapeutic review and update. Drugs 1997;54:679-708.

KRISHNA S, WHITE NJ. Pharmacokinetics of quinine, chloroquine and amodiaquine: clinical implications. Clin Pharmacokinet 1996;30:263-99.

PEPIN J, MILORD F. The treatment of human African trypanosomiasis. Adv Parasitol 1994;33:1-47.

DE SILVA N, GUYATT H, BUNDY D. Anthelminthics: a comparative review of their clinical pharmacology. Drugs 1997; 53:769-88.

WARRELL DA, GREENBERG AE, CAMPBELL CC. Management of severe and complicated malaria. Trans R Soc Trop Med Hyg 1990;49:84-65.

WHITE AC. Neurocysticercosis: a major cause of neurological disease worldwide. Clin Infect Dis 1997;24:101-15.

WHITE NJ. The treatment of malaria. N Engl J Med 1997;335:800-6.

WHO. Guidelines for treatment of cystic and alveolar echinococcosis in humans. Bull WHO 1996;74:231-42.

WHO. Drugs used in Parasitic Diseases, 2d ed. Geneva: WHO, 1995.

WHO. International Travel and Health Vaccination Requirements and Health Advice. Geneva: WHO, updated every year.

New areas of drug development

Harald Labischinski

Within a very short time period historically, bacterial infections appeared to have lost their previous horror for humanity, at least in the developed countries, because of the tremendous progress achieved in prevention and therapy. The hallmarks of this development were the effective implementation of modern hygienic conditions in hospitals and the community and the extraordinary success in the development and therapeutic use of several highly effective antibiotic classes. Although bacterial resistance to antibiotics was recognized almost at the time when antibiotics were introduced into clinical practice, for most of the past 50 years, bacterial resistance was seen more as a scientifically interesting but medically controllable phenomenon, since new antibiotics with improved potency were being developed almost continually and seemed to offer sufficient treatment options. Until relatively recently have scientific funding agencies, national and international public health organizations, and many pharmaceutical companies, in response to the long duration and costly nature of today's drug research and development (R&D) process (10 years and up to US $ 500 million), drastically reduced their efforts in antibiotic research and discovery. Thus, it was only during the last few years that the consequences of these actions have become obvious.

Bacteria are highly adaptable because of their capacity to mutate and exchange genetic material with other microorganisms within very short times, so the spread of resistance to existing antibacterial drugs, depending on the properties of the antibiotic and its prudent use, is almost inevitable. Therefore, approximately 15 years after new class of antibiotics reached the clinic (the last new class introduced was the fluoroquinolones), multiresistant pathogens are seen to emerge. Although resistance is now a problem in gram-negative as well as gram-positive bacteria, the situation is especially difficult with the latter bacteria. An increasing number of vancomycin-resistant enterococci are less amenable to any rational therapy design (this development led to the phrase "return of the pre-antibiotic era"), and the fear that vancomycin resistance eventually also will arise in *Staphylococcus aureus* has become quite realistic, as proven by the detection of *S. aureus* strains in Japan with minimum inhibitory concentration (MIC) values already as high as 8 µg/ml.

Although these strains still fall in the "intermediate susceptibility" range of many national breakpoint definitions, they have been associated with treatment failures, fostering the fear of possibly untreatable multiresistant staphylococci as a potential public health disaster. While these resistance problems occur mainly in the hospital setting, especially in large teaching hospitals, it should be noted that resistance also is becoming an important issue for community-acquired infections, especially, for example, penicillin- , cephalosporin- , and macrolide-resistant pneumococci. Moreover, these trends are compounded by the fact that the patient population has changed considerably (i.e., more elderly population, immunocompromised patients, aggressive chemotherapy, etc.), leading to the emergence of "new" bacterial species not considered important human pathogens in the past, for which the antibiotics available today have never been optimized. Considering all these factors together, it is becoming clear why the death rate from infectious diseases crept up by 58% (22% AIDS-adjusted) from 1980 to 1992 in the United States according to a recent report from the Centers for Disease Control and Prevention (CDC), bringing infectious diseases back to rank as the third leading cause of death.

For all these reasons, there is an urgent need for new antibacterial agents and, consequently, also greatly renewed interest in the pharmaceutical industry to find and develop new antibiotics, preferably with new modes of action and without cross-resistance to currently used antibiotics. Furthermore, there is good reason to believe that there is still potential for optimizing some of the existing classes with respect to efficacy, pathogen spectrum, resistance-induction potential, and other important parameters. In this short review, drugs that have progressed to the later phases of clinical development will be discussed. These drugs have a good chance of reaching the application stage by the readership of this chapter (although it should be stressed that even in late clinical trials there is a considerable chance of failure). Only short mention will be made of the extraordinary progress in early antibiotic discovery research resulting from the revolutionary developments in bacterial genomics and the application of robotics to the search for new antibiotic lead structures. Furthermore, new developments originating from existing drug classes and those from completely new molecular entities have made it clear that the division line is not always obvious.

NEW ANTIBIOTIC DEVELOPMENTS ORIGINATING FROM KNOWN DRUG CLASSES

New quinolones

The 4-fluoro-quinolones can be regarded as the last new class of antibacterial compounds, brought successfully to the arsenals of modern antibiotic therapy in the 1980s. While the structurally related nalidixic acid was limited to the treatment of urinary tract infections, the new compounds, exemplified by the class's most successful member, ciprofloxacin, showed a drastically improved pathogen spectrum and effectiveness, resulting in widespread use in many serious hospital- and community-acquired infectious diseases. In particular, their oral bioavailablity, lack of cross-resistance against other antibacterial classes, spectrum of activity that previously was observed only with certain intravenous antibiotics, and high bactericidal activity and good tolerability made the fluoroquinolones the fastest growing antibiotic class of the late 1980s and 1990s. Based on data suggesting cartilage toxicity in young animals, the fluoroquinolones are not used in pediatric patients. Ciprofloxacin, however, seems to be well tolerated in such patients, so the relevance of the restrictions in pediatric patients has been questioned for the treatment, for example, of recurrent *P. aeruginosa* infections in patients with cystic fibrosis.

Despite these important advantages, the lower inherent activity of the fluoroquinolones against gram-positive bacteria, especially staphylococci, has limited their use in many important clinical and community situations. In addition, contrary to earlier expectations, resistance especially against the notorious resistant strains of *Staphylococcus* and *Pseudomonas* has grown to substantial numbers. In view of this situation, it is logical that several pharmaceutical companies have started R&D programs to develop a new generation of fluoroquinolones with improved gram-positive activity, possible activity against already low-resistant pathogens, and less potential for further development of resistance.

It has become clear that an additional major challenge is to keep or even improve the good tolerability of compounds such as ciprofloxacin. Since this chapter should concentrate on new developments that are just or may be available to the medical community in the near future, I will discuss here only two such well-advanced compounds, namely, trovafloxacin and moxifloxacin. Both compounds show a drastically improved in vitro activity against gram-positive pathogens while retaining the excellent activity against gram-negative bacteria known for the older quinolones with the exception of *P. aeruginosa*. In vitro as well as in vivo data reveal that besides the usual core indications for fluoroquinolones, both new compounds may be especially suitable for community- and hospital-acquired respiratory tract infections because their spectrum of activity targets all important pathogens including streptococci, pneumococci, staphylococci, *Hemophilus influenzae, Moraxella catarrhalis, Mycoplasma pneumoniae, Chlamydia pneumoniae, Klebsiella pneumoniae,* and *Legionella* spp.

It is noteworthy that about 20% of the total prescriptions for respiratory tract infections are written for children. Thus, a scientifically based evaluation of the above-mentioned restrictions on quinolone use in pediatric patients seems especially important in the near future, given the fact that the resistance of common respiratory tract pathogens to β-lactams and macrolides is rising. An interesting difference in in vitro activity between the otherwise very similar microbiologic profiles of trovafloxacin and moxifloxacin is seen in their activity against *C. pneumoniae*. Here, moxifloxacin appears to be more active by a factor of about 4 to 10. *C. pneumoniae* is not only an important pathogen in community-acquired respiratory tract infections but also has been suggested as a potential causative factor in coronary heart diseases; thus, besides macrolides, which are already under consideration for clinical trials in this new area, the new quinolones, which also have good antichlamydial activity, may become useful in this quite unexpected potential antibiotic application. Taking all available in vitro susceptibility data together, it is apparent that both trovafloxacin and moxifloxacin have a broader spectrum of activity and improved potency against gram-positive pathogens than existing quinolones and also should be active against pathogens with intermediate levels of resistance to the existing quinolones.

From the pharmacokinetic data available, it is clear that both these new quinolones can be used once daily (half-lives of 10.5 and 13 hours for trovafloxacin and moxifloxacin, respectively). Both showed linear pharmacokinetics with C_{max} values of 1.5 μg/ml (trovafloxacin) and 0.43 μg/ml (moxifloxacin) after a single oral dose. Protein binding was 70% for trovafloxacin and below 30% for moxifloxacin; urinary excretion was 10 and 20%, respectively. From the clinical trial data, both compounds seemed to be well tolerated and safe. Both quinolones are practically free of phototoxicity, a common problem with some of the existing quinolones. However, after registration and use in larger patient populations, rare but very serious hepatotoxic side effects became obvious for trovafloxacin which led to the cancellation of its registration in Europe and serious use restrictions in the US. Moxifloxacin has now been used in more than a million patients and appears to be a very safe and efficacious drug especially suited for respiratory tract infections. Other new important quinolones which just reached or might reach the market in the near future are gatifloxacin and gemifloxacin.

New members of the macrolide-lincosamide-streptogramin family

The (macrolide-lincosamide-streptogramins, MLS) antibiotics are composed of three well-known groups that have a long tradition mainly against gram-positive pathogens in human as well as veterinary medicine. They all act on bacterial protein biosynthesis, usually in a bacteriostatic manner. Two new drugs in this group appear especially interesting, the streptogramin RP 59500 (Synercid) (see also Chap. 38) and the ketolide (a structurally modified macrolide) HMR 3647 (telithromycin).

Streptogramins are mixtures of two structurally distinct components, A and B, which in case of RP 59500 are quinupristin (B component) and dalfopristin (A component) in a 30:70 ratio. Unlike the macrolides, these mixtures are bactericidal, provided they are present and active at the same time and place. Quinustoprin-dalfopristin represents the first injectable mixture of this class, derived from a derivatization program to enhance the water solubility of the natural poorly water soluble streptogramins. The mixture's in vitro activity spectrum is typical for streptogramins and other MLS antibiotics and consists of most gram-positive cocci (staphylococci, streptococci, pneumococci, *Enterococcus faecium,* but not uniformly *Enterococcus faecalis*) and *Hemophilus influenzae, Moraxella catarrhalis, Legionella* spp., *Mycoplasma pneumoniae, Listeria monocytogenes,* and obligate anaerobes. Synercid is now available for the treatment of life-threatening infections resulting from vancomycin-resistant *E. faecium* in the US and many European countries. However, it should be noted that despite the low use up to the present, descriptions of resistance are beginning to emerge during therapy.

One interesting property of Synercid is its strong bactericidal activity despite the fact that both of its components alone act only in a bacteriostatic manner. Unfortunately, this advantage is lost if for pharmacokinetic reasons both substances are not present at the same time at the desired site of action or if one of the components is not active, e.g., due to the relatively widespread MLS resistance phenotype. Since neither of the two components of Synercid is an inducer of the MLS resistance phenotype, only constitutive strains should be hit by this problem; however, constitutive mutants usually emerge relatively easily. Furthermore, most methicillin-resistant staphylococci (MRSA) do constitutively express the MLS phenotype (due to the *ermA* gene present in Tn*554* found in the associated DNA sequence). Therefore, a separate susceptibility test with both components seems to be desirable to be sure of its bactericidal capacity in the clinical situation. Thus, a complete evaluation of human pharmacokinetics and pharmacodynamics, as well as of the influence of MLS resistance, eventually will determine the extent to which potentially serious gram-positive infections can be treated clinically; in view of increasing problems with vancomycin-resistant *E. faecium,* there is certainly an urgent medical need for new treatment alternatives.

Another new development in the streptogramin area is a new oral streptogramin mixture called *efepristin* (RPR 106732). This antibiotic is presently in phase III clinical studies and seems to share a similar profile with its injectable counterpart described earlier.

The ketolide telithromycin, appears to be the eventual result of an optimization program within this structural class and is presently in late clinical trials (phase III clinical trials have been completed). Ketolides are 14-membered ring macrolides that differ from the classic structure by a keto group at position 3 of the macrolide ring system replacing the L-cladinose moiety, which seems to play an important role in induction of the MLS resistance phenotype. Thus, an important property of this molecule is the missing inducibility of this resistance phenotype. Therefore, although the antimicrobial spectrum of telithromycin is more or less identical to that of existing macrolides such as clarithromycin or azithromycin, it is also active against pathogens displaying inducible MLS resistance. While constitutively resistant staphylococci and enterococci are not hit by the drug, constitutively resistant streptococci are. Together with the fact that available susceptibility data point to lower MIC values for most of the important respiratory pathogens, telithromycin appears to be an attractive new macrolide to overcome the alarming increase in resistance against present-day macrolides in community-acquired infections with respiratory pathogens. Another ketolide in late clinical development is ABT 773.

LY 333328, a new vancomycin-type glycopeptide

Vancomycin and other members of the glycopeptide family belong to the oldest class of antibiotics used, and until recently, they seemed not to be bothered by resistance. This may be due to the fact that the mode of action of these antibiotics is of a physical nature. They bind to the D-alanyl-D-alanine moiety of the cell wall of gram-positive bacteria, thereby blocking the polymerization reactions necessary to build up the essential macromolecular murein network outside the cell. Thus, all pump-based bacterial resistance mechanisms are of no importance, and the complicated structure cannot be modified by any known bacterial enzymatic system. However, for a natural antibiotic, there has to be a natural resistance system, and there are several known examples of naturally resistant species against vancomycin. Nevertheless, the alarming increase in and spread of vancomycin-resistant enterococci, especially of *E. faecium,* in serious hospital-acquired infections in many countries were unexpected. There are hints that the wide use of avoparcin, an animal growth promoter (not to be mistaken for the use of antibiotics in animal health), has contributed to this development. More research in this area is certainly warranted, since despite the ban on avoparcin in animal feed in most countries, there are still two important antibiotic classes for human health in use as animal growth promotion additives in Europe (macrolides and streptogramins).

Vancomycin-resistant enterococci (VRE) comprised the first examples of bacteria not amenable to rational antibiotic therapy, and there is a great fear that resistance could spread to the clinically even more important staphylococci. Although vancomycin-resistant staphylococci with the enterococcal resistant determinants have not been detected in clinics yet, there are increasing reports of coagulase-negative staphylococci and even *S. aureus* strains with diminished susceptibility to this drug class by another mechanism(s).

All these developments have spurred the search for a new generation of glycopeptides that ideally would not be touched by the resistance phenomena discussed. LY 333328 is the most advanced result and is currently in phase II clinical trials. Its antimicrobial spectrum is almost identical to that of vancomycin, with the important exception that it is active against both VRE and, as far as can be judged today, staphylococci as well. Interestingly, while vancomycin acts mainly as a bacteriostatic substance and kills only very slowly, LY 333328 is primarily bactericidal. As a rule, its in vitro activity is better than that of vancomycin and approaches that of teicoplanin. It also displays synergism with aminoglycosides. Further clinical studies are needed to evaluate the future potential of this new developmental drug.

Other new developments from existing antibiotic classes

Numerous other clinical developments are being seen in almost all existing drug classes for which it is either too early to judge (i.e., not enough data are available to even estimate their possible advantages over existing antibiotics of the same class) or no clear-cut advantages can be detected. Many trials to further optimize the various classes of β-lactam antibiotics have been undertaken; although in principle it is easy to write down a profile for a more ideal β-lactam in the various subclasses (e.g., penicillins, cephalosporins, penems, carbapenems, monobactams, etc.), reality presents many difficulties in actually reaching this goal. It has proven to be exceedingly difficult to optimize the desired properties (e.g., MRSA activity, *Pseudomonas* activity, better pharmacokinetics, extended spectrum, stability, etc.) without losing important other ones. Thus only a few compounds will be mentioned here. One attractive goal is to arrive at a β-lactam with the activity of the injectable carbapenems but good oral availability. One of the candidates was sanfetrinem cilexetil, a compound of a carbapenem subclass also designated as trinems. This compound was in late clinical trials (phase III), but clinical development recently was delayed.

Another compound with a potential for reaching this goal soon is CS 834, an oral carbapenem in phase III clinical trials in Japan. CS 834 is a prodrug with compound R 95867 as the active metabolite. This compound has good activity against methicillin-susceptible staphylococci (not MRSA), streptococci (including penicillin-resistant *S. pneumoniae*), *N. gonorrheae, M. catarrhalis,* the family Enterobacteriaceae (except *Serratia marcescens*), *H. influenzae,* and *Bordetella pertussis* (MIC90 values below or equal to 1 µg/ml). It was not drastically affected by class A extended spectrum β-lactamases (ESBLs) and class C β-lactamase-producing strains. No activity against *P. aeruginosa* could be demonstrated. CS 834 shows dose-dependent, linear kinetics up to 400 mg, reaching C_{max} values of up to 2.5 µg/ml, with the typical short half-life of many carbapenems (0.75 h), i.e., requiring tid dosing. Main adverse effects included a decrease in anaerobic gut flora, loose stools, diarrhea, and a moderate rise in some liver enzymes. Thus this compound eventually may show its usefulness in oral treatment, especially for upper respiratory tract infections caused by *S. pneumoniae, H. influenzae,* and *M. catarrhalis.*

One more interesting compound in this area is faropenem daloxate, the oral prodrug of faropenem. In contrast to faropenem sodium, which is already marketed in Japan, it has an extremely good bioavailability (> 80%). This together with the high intrinsic activity of faropenem against the most important respiratory tract pathogens, its stability against penicillin-resistant pneumococci as well as its excellent tolerability and safety profile has led to renewed interest in this compound outside Japan. The compound is, therefore, in phase II clinical trials and might show its usefulness in the oral treatment especially of respiratory tract infections.

The only other β-lactam I will mention here is a compound named L749345, which is in phase II clinical trials as an injectable carbapenem. Its activity and spectrum appear to be similar to those of imipenem, with improved activity against *Morganella morganii, Proteus mirabilis, Proteus vulgaris, Klebsiella pneumoniae,* and *E. coli* but only marginal activity against *P. aeruginosa* and *E. faecalis.* Its already relatively long half-life (about 4 h) is exaggerated by a complex dose-dependent pharmacokinetics partly due to concentration-dependent plasma protein binding resulting in a very long apparent half-life that might even allow once-daily dosing regimens. The agent appears to be generally well tolerated.

Another new development is the so-called glycylcyclines. These are derivatives of tetracyclines characterized by a glycine containing modification at position 9 of the tetracycline ring system. One of those, CL 331928, is in phase II clinical development. Tetracyclines have been of great value because of their very broad antimicrobial spectrum and their oral and parenteral routes of administration, but they probably have suffered the most of all antibiotic classes from diverse and widespread types of resistance. Mechanisms include practically all imaginable variations with the exception of drug modification, i.e., various bacterial efflux pumps to exclude the drug from its target site (the ribosome), protection of the target site itself, and other still not fully understood mechanisms. The easy spread of the various resistance determinants has largely obscured the advantages of this drug class. The structural variations introduced in CL 331928 appear to protect the drug against several, if not most, of these resistance mechanisms, leaving intact broad-spectrum activity against a host of gram-positive, gram-negative, and anaerobic pathogens. Again, it is too early in the clinical testing of this interesting antibiotic to evaluate its real prospects for therapy.

NEW DEVELOPMENTS FROM NEW ANTIBIOTIC CLASSES

From the foregoing discussion it should be obvious that in contrast to what was expected by many critics of the approach, impressive and therapeutically very important progress has been achieved by targeted modification of existing drug classes. Progress has been made not only with respect to general effectiveness and antimicrobial spectrum, pharmacokinetics, and other important parameters but also in terms of the treatment of pathogens resistant to older members of the drug class. As a rule, however, there remains some cross-resistance between older and newer compounds, and some of the highly resistant pathogens may not be reached by the newer representatives. Thus, the need for completely new chemical entities with novel modes of action is obvious, since these compounds ideally will be free from cross-resistance to any known antibiotic class.

Development of bacterial resistance is almost inevitably coupled to its application, even the most prudent one, because of the extraordinary adaptability of bacteria to their environment, and thus this tends to be a continuous challenge to pharmaceutical research. Whether there is a biologic rationale for the belief that new antibiotics will be available in the future will be discussed later. At least it is reassuring that two classes fitting the definition of completely new compounds are in clinical trials today.

Everninomycins

Everninomycins are chemically complex oligosaccharide compounds with molecular weights on the order of that of vancomycin. Being relatively hydrophilic, these compounds cannot penetrate the outer membrane of gram-negative bacteria but are active against all important gram-positive pathogens, including streptococci, staphylococci, enterococci, and *Clostridium difficile*. The remarkable similarity to vancomycin is extended by a similar or slightly superior in vitro and in vivo efficacy in all (animal) models tested, with the important exception that there is uniform sensitivity of all strains tested so far, including, for example, VRE, MRSA, and penicillin-resistant pneumococci (PRP). Everninomycins act mainly as bacteriostatic compounds, and their mode of action involves inhibition of protein synthesis.

Ziracin (SCH 27899) is a derivative of the natural antibiotic everninomycin D and seems to be the first compound of its class with low nephrotoxic potential. Presently, it is undergoing phase III clinical testing as an injectable antibiotic. An effective half-life of approximately 8 hours was observed in humans, and the available data indicate that the drug is safe and generally well tolerated, the most frequently reported adverse effects being mild to moderate injection-site reactions such as pain. Thus, depending on the outcome of the ongoing clinical trials, this compound may be a promising candidate for the treatment of hospital-acquired infections by gram-positive pathogens, including those resistant or multiresistant to commonly used antibiotics.

Oxazolidinones, linezolid (U 100766)

A new class of drugs know as *oxazolidinones* seems to be one of the most promising new antibacterials.

Oxazolidinones are completely synthetic molecules (thus, there will be no preformed resistance mechanism in nature) that are orally available and easily amenable to further chemical modification. It is therefore not surprising that many pharmaceutical companies have started research programs within this class. Oxazolidinones act within a well-validated antibacterial target area – bacterial protein biosynthesis – but they target the translation of ribosomal RNA. They bind the 50 S ribosomal subunit, near the interface with the 30 S subunit, thereby preventing the formation of the 70 initiation complex. Consequently, there is a uniform susceptibility in sensitive bacteria independent of resistance/multiresistance to other antibiotics. As usual in this target area, oxazolidinones act mainly as bacteriostatics. Their activity is directed against all important gram-positive pathogens, including staphylococci, streptococci, and enterococci. It is not yet clear whether the low or missing activity of the presently known compounds against most gram-negative bacteria is due to low outer membrane permeability or to bacterial efflux pumps or a combination of both.

The most advanced compound of this new class is linezolid (U 100766) recently approved for clinical use in the US. The oral absorption of linezolid is rapid and almost complete, with dose-related pharmacokinetics. The elimination half-life is about 4.5 to 5.5 hours (intravenous/oral); based on the observation that linezolid concentrations after dosing of 625 mg were above the MIC90 value of target organisms (4µg/ml) for 10 hours or more, a bid regimen appears feasible for both the oral and the iv formulations. The most frequent adverse effect was coating/discoloration of the tongue after iv or oral dosing. Other events involved the gastrointestinal tract, and in the oral application group there were medical events in the skin category, including a folliculitis-type rash and fungal dermatitis. Based on its uniform activity against all present gram-positive pathogens, linezolid may find its place in the treatment of serious infections due to staphylococci, streptococci, and enterococci, especially those resistant to currently available antibiotics. Based on the novelty of this compound class, its amenability to chemical optimization, and the large research efforts directed toward this class, one can expect to see the emergence of additional compounds of this class in the future.

OUTLOOK: THE SEARCH FOR NEW TARGET SITES IN MICROBES

If one looks at the new developmental compounds currently in clinical trials, it becomes apparent that most of those derive from long-known antibacterial drug classes, the exception being the oxazolidinones and everninomycins; furthermore, even the two new compound classes were detected some time ago by classic microbial susceptibility testing procedures and their molecular targets are still not clearly elucidated in detail. This raises the question of whether there will be chances to discover or develop badly needed new classes of antibiotics in the future at all and, if so, with higher probabilities of success than at present.

The first question is relatively easy to answer in light of recently available information on several complete bacterial genomes and studies on the essentiality of bacterial genomes for bacterial survival. From these studies it follows that of the 2000 or so genes in a bacterium such as *Staphylococcus,* about 10 to 15% are essential in the sense that if they are knocked out, the bacterium is not capable of growing. Many of these genes are broadly conserved in the bacterial world and appear as good target candidates to combat microbial pathogens. Thus, even conservative estimations tell us that at least 100 to 200 essential targets for antimicrobial therapy are reachable, in clear contrast to the 10 to 20 targets covered by presently available antibiotics.

Therefore, the main problem appears to reside in the second question – that of productivity. Again, it is hoped that technologic advancements will overcome this part of the problem. First, the identification and evaluation of possible new targets not covered by existing drug classes have become feasible in a systematic manner using the genomic information mentioned earlier, combined with techniques to prove the essentiality of a given target and to construct screening systems to find inhibitors of the target in question by robotic output screening techniques, i.e., scanning huge libraries comprised of several hundreds of thousands of compounds in a few days. Compared with the techniques in use even a few years ago, these developments should increase our chances enormously of finding new starting compounds for indepth evaluation, although at drastically increased research costs. The same techniques also offer a chance to tailor new antibacterial compounds more rationally toward medical needs, for example, in terms of antibacterial spectrum and probabilities of fast resistance development.

Despite all this progress, it should be kept in mind that a huge collection of distinct properties must come together to result in medical progress in antibacterial therapy. Most of these properties are not covered by the advances in microbial genomics and screening technologies discussed earlier. Combinatorial chemistry capable of delivering unprecedented numbers of analogues of a lead structure for optimization in a short time period will help to overcome some of these problems, as will other approaches with respect to faster optimization of pharmacokinetic properties and safety/tolerability aspects. Nevertheless, each new class of antibiotics and each new member of a known group of antibiotics still does and will in the foreseeable future provide a challenge to a great number of disciplines involved to demonstrate its value to the medical community and eventually to the patient.

Suggested readings

AGOURIDAS C, BONNEFOY A, CHANTOT JF. Antibacterial activity of RU 64004 (HMR 3004), a novel ketolide derivative active against respiratory pathogens. Antimicrob Agents Chemother 1997;41:2149-58.

BRYSKIER A. Novelties in the field of fluoroquinolones. Exp Opin Invest Drugs 1997;6:1227-45.

CHANT C, RYBAK MJ. Quinupristin/dalfopristin (RP59500): A new streptogramin antibiotic. Ann Pharmacother 1995;29:1022-7.

CHOPRA I. *N*-Alkyl-substituted glycopeptide antibiotics. Exp Opin Invest Drugs 1997;6:299-303.

DIEKEMA DI, JONES RN. Oxazolidinones: a review. Drugs 2000;59:7-16.

DOMAGALA JM, SANCHEZ JP. New approaches and agents to overcome bacterial resistance. Ann Reps Med Chem 1997;32:111-20.

HIRAMATSU K, HANAKI H, INO T, et al. Methicillin-resistant *Staphylococcus aureus* with reduced vancomycin susceptibility. J Antimicrob Chemother 1997;40:135-46.

HOOPER DC. Expanding and preserving the utility of quinolone antimicrobials. In: Busse WD, Zeiler H-J, Labischinski H, eds. Antibacterial Therapy: Achievements, Problems and Future Perspectives. Berlin: Springer-Verlag, 1997;27-36.

JORGENSEN JH, MCELMEEL ML. Trippy CW. In vitro activities of the oxazolidinone antibiotics U-100592 and U-100766 against *Staphylococcus aureus* and coagulase negative *Staphylococcus* species. Antimicrob Agents Chemother 1997;41:465-7.

LABISCHINSKI H, JOHANNSEN L. New antibiotics with novel mode of action. In: Hakenbeck, R, ed. Antibiotic resistance: recent developments and future perspectives. Heidelberg: Spektrum Verlag, 1997;59-62.

LEVY SB. Balancing the drug-resistance equation. Trends Microbiol 1994;2:341-2.

MERCIER RC, PENZAK SR, RYBAK MJ. In vitro activities of an investigational quinolone, glycylcycline, glycopeptide, streptogramin, and oxazolidinone tested alone and in combinations against vancomycin-resistant *Enterococcus faecium.* Antimicrob Agents Chemother 1997;41:2573-5.

PINNER RW, TEUTSCH SM, SIMONSEN L, et al. Trends in infectious diseases mortality in the United States. JAMA 1996; 275:189-93.

SUNDELOF JG, HAJDU R, GILL CJ, et al. Pharmacokinetics of L-749,345, a long-acting carbapenem antibiotic, in primates. Antimicrob Agents Chemother 1997;41:1743-8.

WANG E, SIMARD M, BERGERON Y, et al. In vivo activity and pharmacokinetics of Ziracin (SCH27899), a new long-acting everninomycin antibiotic, in a murine model of penicillin susceptible and penicillin resistant pneumococcal pneumonia. Antimicrob Agents Chemother 2000;44:1010-8.

Rheumatic diseases and bone

44

Drugs used in rheumatic and bone diseases

Howard Bird

Up to 150 different conditions can affect the joints. A basic subdivision is between *degenerative* conditions, of which osteoarthritis is the main example, and *inflammatory* conditions, of which rheumatoid arthritis is the most common example. The course of osteoarthritis, however, can be punctuated by episodes of inflammation, sometimes related to crystal shedding within the joints. Rheumatoid arthritis, when in its late burnt-out phase, can be complicated by degenerative arthritis affecting the joint. Rheumatoid arthritis is more common than seronegative spondarthritis, a group of conditions that also involve organs in the body as well as joints but which are distinguished from rheumatoid arthritis by their seronegativity for rheumatoid factor and their greater propensity for familial clustering. Autoimmune diseases of connective tissue, of which systemic lupus erythematosus (or lupus) is a prime example, also affect many organs as well as the joints but are less common than rheumatoid disease in all temperate zones and even in the tropics, with the possible exception of the West Indies.

For some rheumatic conditions, e.g., gout (see Chap. 71), polymyalgia rheumatica (which overlaps with temporal arteritis), and septic arthritis, specific curative drug treatment is available. Rheumatologists are now concerning themselves increasingly with diseases of bone as well as of the joints, and among these, osteoporosis is the most common, causing the greatest morbidity (see Chap. 46), although brief consideration is also given in this chapter to Paget's disease, a local aberration of bone metabolism, for which specific treatment is available.

Drug classes

The many drugs used for the treatment of musculoskeletal conditions can be divided simplistically into analgesics, nonsteroidal anti-inflammatory drugs (NSAIDs), and specific treatments applicable to certain (but not all) rheumatic diseases. The primary care physician is likely to limit prescribing to analgesics and NSAIDs, which between

them relieve symptoms across almost all rheumatic conditions. In general, analgesics are safer and have fewer side effects, particularly in the elderly. NSAIDs are collective inhibitors of prostaglandin synthetase, and since this enzyme has protective functions at certain sites in the body, use of NSAIDs is inevitably associated with side effects, particularly in the elderly. In the prescribing of both types of compounds, attention should be directed to the half-life of the agent, which in turn allows the minimum efficacious dose to be selected, with a consequent reduction in side effects. In general, an analgesic can be prescribed with an NSAID, and certain analgesics may be prescribed together, normally in a particular formulation. There is less benefit, however, to prescribing two NSAIDs simultaneously.

Since all drugs have side effects, it is important for the practitioner to consider whether the prescription of systemically absorbed compounds can be avoided.

When degenerative conditions are precipitated or aggravated by biomechanical factors, rest is usually helpful, and this may be enforced by the use of a splint, molded to shape the joint contour to reduce the amount of movement while giving stability to the joint for lifting of loads, with a resulting decrease in pain and lessened need for analgesics. Correction of leg-length inequality by the provision of a raise to a shoe may reduce pain in the hip and knee. If drug therapy is needed, intraarticular therapy, providing localization of response can be achieved and may be preferable to systemic drug therapy, although opinions differ on the value of topical applications immediately over the painful joint. If systemic therapy is necessary, attention should be paid to the characteristic daily pain pattern for the patient.

The systemic inflammatory conditions, including rheumatoid arthritis, are invariably catabolic, causing muscle wasting and tiredness. Adequate periods of rest, spaced throughout the day and, if necessary, in bed, should be recommended. Attention should be paid to a nutritious diet, and the anemia of chronic disease should be corrected with appropriate hematinics. Obesity, less common in inflammatory arthritis, should be treated by diet. Physiotherapists may relieve acute joint pain by a variety of treatments, including hot packs, ice packs, ultrasound, short-wave diathermy, and hydrotherapy, among others. Occupational therapy can provide appropriate splints and appliances to reduce the workload of inflamed joints. If the disease is localized, localized intraarticular or intralesional steroid therapy may reduce the need for systemic drug therapy. Surgery also may be of value when particular joints are involved, and total joint replacement is especially effective for the hip, knee, and finger joints.

The pain and stiffness of inflammatory arthritis are likely to persist throughout the day and night. Here a greater case can be made for prescription of symptom-relieving drugs with a long half-life or even drugs with a short half-life in sustained-release formulations. Specific disease-modifying drugs may reduce the need for the more toxic NSAIDs.

ANALGESICS

A number of analgesics are available, particularly acetaminophen, but also (in most countries) codeine and dihydrocodeine, although the choice is not so great as for NSAIDs. An analgesic always should be the first choice of drug therapy in degenerative joint disease and normally should be the first choice of drug therapy in patients over age 60 with any arthritis, although if the arthritis is of the inflammatory type, analgesics are less likely to be effective when used alone. Nevertheless, some studies have shown that careful counseling and selection of drugs will allow 30% of elderly patients taking NSAIDs to discon-

tinue such medication in favor of analgesics alone. For inflammatory arthritis in younger patients, an analgesic alone is unlikely to suffice, although consideration always should be given to prescribing an analgesic in combination with a NSAID to reduce the consumption of the latter drug. Pharmacokinetic parameters of analgesics are given in Table 44.1.

Acetaminophen (paracetamol) This is likely to be the analgesic of first choice in most countries. Taken in a dose of up to 4.0 g per day, with a half-life of about 2 hours, acetaminophen requires dosing qid if adequate plasma concentrations are to be achieved throughout the whole 24 hours; the drug thus lends itself to "as required" prescribing in 500-mg increments. At this dose, mild hepatic side effects are rarely seen. The risk of overdose should not be forgotten if the patient is depressed, although adequate rescue is now normally available from overdose with this compound. However, overdose, with as little as 10 to 15 g (20-30 tablets), can cause severe hepatocellular necrosis and, less frequently, renal tubular necrosis. Nausea and vomiting are early features; liver damage is maximum at 3 to 4 days. The antidotes, acetylcysteine and methionine, protect the liver if given within 10 to 12 hours of ingestion. A graph of plasma acetaminophen concentrations against time predicts those at risk of severe tissue damage, who should be treated accordingly. The initial dose of acetylcysteine, given by iv infusion, is 150 mg/kg in 200 ml glucose solution over 15 minutes, followed by 50 mg/kg in 500 ml over 4 hours and then 100 mg/kg in 1000 ml over 16 hours.

Compound analgesic preparations and new molecules Because acetaminophen alone sometimes proves ineffective, small amounts of stronger analgesics are sometimes formulated with acetaminophen to give a compound

Table 44.1 Pharmacokinetic parameters for analgesics

	MW	pK$_a$	Oral absorption (%)	Presystemic metabolism (%)	Plasma half-life h (mean)	Volume of distribution (l/kg)	Plasma protein binding (%)
Acetaminophen (paracetamol)	141.2	9.5	>95	20	1.5-3.0 (2.3)	0.9	<20
Codeine phosphate	406.4	8.2	>90	50	3-4	3.6	7-25
Dihydrocodeine tartrate	451.5	8.8	95-100	Considerable	3.4-4.5	1.1	–
Dextropropoxyphene (HCl)	375.9	6.3	>95	60	8-24 (15)	(16)	70-80
Meptazinol	269.8	8.7	100	92	1.5-6 (1.9)	3.1	27
Pentazocine (HCl)	321.9	8.7	95	7.1	2	250-550	48-75
Tramadol	263	8.3	68	Variable (CYP2D6)	6		20

preparation. Theoretically, this reduces the side effects from both compounds because smaller amounts of each are formulated in the effective tablet. Anxiety about compound preparations containing drugs with two different half-lives and the theoretical risk of accumulation if patients respond to only one of the two drugs contained in the mixture has been allayed by the facts that dosing is invariably chronic (where differential half-lives have less importance) and that the half-lives of most compounds in this group are similar.

The drugs used most commonly for admixture are dextropropoxyphene, codeine, and dihydrocodeine. Dextropropoxyphene sometimes causes the central nervous system (CNS) side effect of euphoria, although this is often an advantage in patients with chronic arthritis. Codeine causes constipation. Dihydrocodeine causes both constipation and CNS system side effects and thus represents the third choice in this group.

A number of additional analgesics, most introduced recently and therefore more expensive, are also available for the treatment of arthritic pain (see Chap. 9). These

Table 44.2 NSAIDs by chemical structure

Carboxylic acid
  Salicylic acids and esters
    Acetylsalicylic acid
    Diflunisal
    Benorylate
  Acetic acids
    Phenylacetic acid
    Diclofenac
    Alclofenac
    Fenclofenac
  Carbo- and heterocyclic acid
    Etodolac
    Indomethacin
    Sulindac
    Tolmetin
  Propionic acids
    Carprofen
    Fenbufen
    Flurbiprofen
    Ketoprofen
    Oxaprozin
    Suprofen
    Tiaprofenic acid
    Ibuprofen
    Naproxen
    Fenoprofen
  Fenamic acids
    Flufenamic
    Mefenamic
    Meclofenamic

Enolic acids
  Pyrazolones
    Oxyphenbutazone
    Phenylbutazone

Oxicams
  Piroxicam
  Sudoxicam
  Tenoxicam

Nonacidic compounds
  Nabumetone

Table 44.3 Mean plasma half-lives of some commonly used NSAIDs

NSAID	Half-life (h)	Typical dosage
Propionic acid derivatives		
Ibuprofen	2	400 mg qid
Naproxen	14	500 mg bid
Ketoprofen	2	100 mg bid
Flurbiprofen	3-4	50 mg tid
Fenbufen	10-17	300 mg mane 600 mg hs
Fenoprofen	3	600 mg tid
Tiaprofenic acid	1.5-2	200 mg tid
Phenylacetic acid derivatives		
Diclofenac	1-2	50 mg tid
Indoles and related drugs		
Indomethacin	4-5	50 mg tid
Acemetacin[1]	4-5	60 mg bid
Sulindac[2]	16	200 mg bid
Benzotriazines		
Azapropazone	12-14	600 mg bid (maximum in the elderly 300 mg bid)
Oxicams		
Piroxicam	45	20 mg qd
Tenoxicam	72	20 mg qd
Fenamic acids		
Mefenamic acid	2-4	500 mg tid
Tolmetin	5	500 mg tid
Nonacid compounds		
Nabumetone[3]	24	1 g qd hs
Pyranocarboxylates		
Etodolac	7	300 mg bid

(bid = twice daily; hs = at bedtime; mane = in the morning; qd = once daily; qid = 4 times daily; tid = 3 times daily.)
[1] Mainly metabolized to indomethacin.
[2] Active sulfide metabolite.
[3] Active metabolite.

include meptazinol, pentazocine, and tramadol. In the case of tramadol, because P450 2D6 is involved in the formation of the active metabolite, the compound can be ineffective in poor metabolizers. This may account for the idiosyncratic response of many rheumatic patients to this and other opioid-like analgesics. More potent opioid analgesics are not prescribed routinely in the management of arthritis.

NONSTEROIDAL ANTI-INFLAMMATORY DRUGS (NSAIDs)

Although almost all NSAIDs are acidic compounds ultimately derived from acetylsalicylic acid (aspirin), a wider selection is available than for analgesics, in part as a result of the competitive market for the prescription of such compounds. All NSAIDs also share a complex mechanism of action that involves inhibition of prostaglandin synthetase. Since prostaglandins are protective at certain sites, particularly the gastrointestinal tract and the kidney, these drugs are associated with gastric irritation and a small but consistent and reversible fall in creatinine clearance as the prostaglandin-mediated effect of renal vasodilation is blocked. In practice, the gastric side effects are the limiting factor in prescription of these compounds, and because peptic ulceration and its attendant risk of hemorrhage and perforation is associated with increased morbidity and mortality in persons over the age of 60 years, NSAIDs should be prescribed with extreme caution and at a reduced dose in the elderly.

NSAIDs can be classified by chemical structure (Tab. 44.1), which not only is of developmental interest but also has some bearing on side effects, or by half-life (Tab. 44.2), which is a more practical classification. In general, the longest established drugs are likely to be the safest, in that all possible side effects will have emerged and will have been quantified so that patients know what they are getting. Generic formulations are now available for many of the 25 commercially available NSAIDs, and the reduced cost of these, coupled with the long history of their use, makes this group a logical first choice. Fewer of these drugs are available in the United States. Table 44.3 illustrates the mean plasma half-life of the range of such compounds, and more detailed pharmacokinetic data on NSAIDs generically available in the United Kingdom are presented in Table 44.4.

Classification by structure

Aspirin, the prototype, still has some devotees, although the many side effects of this drug, particularly its propensity to cause gastric erosion, mean that only modern and more expensive derivatives of aspirin are realistically prescribed. The next two drugs to be synthesized were indomethacin and phenylbutazone. Next came the propionic acids, of which ibuprofen was the prototype, soon followed by naproxen and ketoprofen. Subsequent remodeling of the molecule produced the related families of the arylacetic acids (e.g., diclofenac, although this also has a distant resemblance to indomethacin) and the oxicams

(e.g., piroxicam). All these NSAIDs share the side effects of gastrotoxicity and a slight impairment in renal function, but each group may display additional side effects. Thus, aspirin and its derivatives are associated with tinnitus, occasional angioneurotic edema, and a greater propensity to drug-induced asthma than the others. Indomethacin is associated with the CNS side effects and a little fluid retention. The propionic acids may cause less gastrointestinal toxicity, but they are associated more frequently with skin rash, although this is not a significant problem. As a group, the parent compounds, rather than their derivatives, nowadays provide the treatment of first choice, and chemical modification within the acidic molecule gives diversity of half-life.

Pharmacokinetics

Considering that all NSAIDs have the same basic mechanism of action, there is an unusual diversity of half-life among them, ranging from 0.5 hour for the compound with the shortest half-life (i.e., tolmetin) to 72 hours for the longest (i.e., phenylbutazone). In general, a drug with a half-life of 4 hours or less needs to be given four times a day to keep up adequate plasma levels to maintain relief from inflammation throughout the full 24 hours. Drugs with half-lives between 6 and 12 hours can be given twice a day. Drugs with half-lives of over 12 hours can be given once a day.

Table 44.3 illustrates the way in which a small group of long-established NSAIDs provides diversity in both half-life and, to some extent, chemical structure. Most practitioners would accept ibuprofen as a first choice, although some might prefer naproxen with its ring structure and longer half-life. Ketoprofen provides only a little novelty over ibuprofen, so the more distant relatives diclofenac and piroxicam may be preferred. Some practitioners will have anxiety about the particularly long half-life of piroxicam, although there is no evidence that this much longer half-life confers a greater toxicity. Indomethacin, which most feel is the most toxic drug of all, as well as being, arguably, the most effective, probably should be kept in reserve for patients who have failed to respond to the earlier alternatives.

The oral route of administration is the most conventional and invariably the least expensive. Even though the

---

Table 44.4 Pharmacokinetic parameters for NSAIDs

	MW	pK$_a$	Oral absorption (%)	Presystemic metabolism (%)	Plasma half-life h (mean)	Volume of distribution (l/kg)	Plasma protein binding (%)
Ibuprofen	206	4.4	>95	Low	2	0.1	99
Indomethacin	357	4.5	100	Low	1-16 (4)	1.0	90-99
Diclofenac	318	4.0	>90	40	1-2	0.12	99.5
Ketoprofen	254	4.55	>90	Minimal	1-3	0.1	95
Piroxicam	331	6.3	~100	–	30-60	0.1	99
Acetylsalicylic acid	180	3.5	>80	High	15-20 min	0.2	Variable

oral route is inevitably associated with gastrointestinal side effects, these are not necessarily prevented if other, more expensive routes of delivery are selected. Several preparations are available in suppository formulation for rectal administration. The drug is absorbed reliably from the rectal mucosa, and adequate plasma levels are obtained, often with a more gradual buildup, which tends to extend the period of action. However, gastrointestinal side effects are only reduced by a factor of about 30% following rectal administration. NSAIDs also can be given systemically by the im route. Absorption is more rapid and relief of symptoms faster, although the intramuscular route is often impractical and usually used only when patients are vomiting. The risk of gastrointestinal side effects is only reduced by a factor of about 30%, again indicating that most such side effects arise from concentrations of circulating metabolites rather than from local irritation.

Several NSAIDs are formulated in topical preparations that can be applied to the skin over the affected joints. Although tissue concentrations are a little higher under the area of application, they are not markedly so, and the drug, after slightly delayed but reliable absorption through the skin, passes to all other parts of the body via the bloodstream. Nevertheless, plasma levels are usually lower, so side effects sometimes are not so intense. In addition, there may be a strong placebo effect resulting from local application, some patients strongly favoring this and others finding it time-consuming and messy. Invariably these preparations are more expensive than the equivalent dose of the same drug given by mouth.

Side effects

The gastric toxicity of NSAIDs has lead to various attempts at gastroprotection. Prescription of NSAIDs should be avoided in the elderly whenever possible because the elderly are most at risk for gastrointestinal irritation. Moreover, NSAIDs probably should not be prescribed in patients with a previous history of peptic ulcer

disease. In some countries, gastroprotective agents are invariably prescribed in parallel, particularly for those at additional risk. In others, the gastroprotective agent may be kept in reserve until symptoms develop.

Misoprostol (see Chap. 33) was developed as a specific prostaglandin analogue to fill this particular niche, although its use is associated with an unacceptably high frequency of diarrhea. Many practitioners therefore prefer H_2 blockers such as cimetidine or ranitidine or protein pump inhibitors such as omeprazole and lansoprazole. The extent to which these various preparations are licensed for the prophylactic treatment of either gastric or duodenal ulcers alongside concomitant NSAID therapy varies from country to country. Recent evidence suggests that omeprazole prevents and heals NSAID-induced ulcers better than ranitidine.

A recent development has been the marketing of a formulation containing an NSAID plus a gastroprotective agent, such as diclofenac plus misoprostol. The pharmacologic justification for such polypharmacy, in fixed ratios of dose within the same tablet, is uncertain. A non promising approach is that of COX-2 inhibitors (see Chap. 48).

Local treatment of arthritis

A number of local treatments are available, and they are used particularly when arthritis is confined to one or a small number of joints. The obvious example is the use of intraarticular or intralesional steroids. In some countries, radioactive synovectomy is also employed.

The number of steroids theoretically available for intraarticular use is actually quite large (Tab. 44.5). In general, the least potent (and normally least expensive) is associated with the fewest side effects. As we climb the developmental ladder, the drugs become more potent but carry a greater risk of side effects. A major problem is localization

Table 44.5 Duration of action and solubility of commonly used intraarticular steroid preparations

Preparation	Relative doses required to provide equivalent pharmacologic effect	Average duration of pain relief (days)	Solubility[1]
Hydrocortisone acetate	×6.25	6.0	0.0018
Hydrocortisone t-butyl acetate	×6.25	12.1	–
Prednisolone acetate	×5	7.8	–
Prednisolone t-butyl acetate	×5	14.5	<0.0010
6-Methylprednisolone acetate	×5	8.2	0.0014
Dexamethasone acetate	1	7.6	–
Dexamethasone t-butyl acetate	1	14.9	–
Triamcinolone diacetonide	×5	7.7	0.0056
Triamcinolone acetonide	×5	14.2	0.0040
Triamcinolone hexacetonide	×5	21.2	0.0004

[1]Percentage by w/v in H_2O at 25 °C.

within the joint. Here, the evidence strongly suggests that the least soluble molecules have the longest effect.

Hydrocortisone is the parent physiologic compound, available commercially, but the least effective. Prednisolone is a synthetic compound that can be rendered less soluble, as in prednisolone *t*-butylacetate, the least soluble salt that is the most efficacious of the prednisolone derivatives available. Additional activity is conferred on the steroid molecule by adding a methyl group (methylprednisolone) and even more by halogenating it with a fluorine atom (triamcinolone).

The primary care physician, while encouraged to attempt intraarticular or intralesional injections (e.g., at the epicondyle in tennis elbow), is advised to restrict the practice to the use of hydrocortisone or prednisolone, perhaps with methylprednisolone for joints. Triamcinolone normally should only be injected intraarticularly by a trained rheumatologist who is competent in this procedure.

Radioactive synovectomy has largely replaced chemical synovectomy with agents such as osmium tetroxide for the local treatment of proliferative synovitis. Several isotopes are available, varying according to their molecular weight and particle emitted. Radioactive yttrium is the isotope of choice for injection of the knee joint. Radioactive erbium is probably the isotope of choice for injection of finger joints. Administration of the radioactive substance requires substantial precautions. Partly because of this, and partly because controlled trials have shown little additional benefit from radioactive synovectomy compared with intraarticular injection of high-dose corticosteroids, radioactive synovectomy has tended to fall into disrepute. Nevertheless, it may be useful when repeated steroid injections have failed and has a specific indication in the precancerous synovial proliferation found in pigmented villonodular synovitis.

Chondroprotective agents   In German-speaking countries, these compounds are generally available and normally are given by the intraarticular route. It has been claimed that long-term regular injections with these agents prevents the progression of very early osteoarthritis. Three compounds (dona-200S, glycosaminoglycan polysulfate,

and glycosaminoglycan peptide complex) are particularly favored. Side effects of these compounds, which are derived from crustaceans or cattle, include antigenicity and a heparin-like action that occasionally may result in hemorrhage. Ultimately, these compounds may be replaced by artificial lubricants currently under trial or by hyaluronic acid, which is available in some European countries.

SYSTEMIC STEROIDS

Controversy exists over whether systemic steroids are an acceptable therapy for inflammatory polyarthritis. The severe side effects that occur as a result of their use became apparent a few years later and restricted their popularity. Prednisolone is used at a dose of 5 mg per day or less, since fewer side effects occur at this dose, but this is not always adequate to control the proliferative synovitis of rheumatoid disease (Tab. 44.6). The effect of corticosteroids on reducing the total body collagen causes particular anxiety in the treatment of rheumatoid arthritis, already a destructive disease. There is a strong anecdotal impression that patients treated with steroids develop more lax joints as a result of the weakened collagen than their non-steroid-treated counterparts; therefore, they are more susceptible to subluxation and perhaps even to compression neuropathy. The second anxiety specific to rheumatoid arthritis is the osteoporotic effect of steroids, particularly at the spine, since these patients are not afforded the protection normally provided by adequate exercise. Rheumatologists may deceive themselves in their frequent preference for intraarticular steroid use. Measurement of endogenous corticosteroid levels confirms that suppression of the hypothalamic-pituitary-adrenal axis (HPA) occurs whenever intraarticular steroids are given. Some practitioners advocate regular im injections of methylprednisolone to produce remission. The evidence that this spares the patient the side effects associated with systemic steroids is not great, although this technique may be of value for the production of rapid clinical remission if methylprednisolone is then followed by the introduction of a specific disease-modifying drug for rheumatoid arthritis.

It has been suggested recently that low-dose steroid therapy given early in rheumatoid arthritis may have a particularly beneficial effect, although the long-term consequences of this use of steroids still requires evaluation.

DISEASE-MODIFYING DRUGS FOR RHEUMATOID ARTHRITIS

All the treatments described so far can relieve symptoms but will not reduce or eradicate disease progression in systemic inflammatory polyarthritis such as rheumatoid arthritis. The agents known as *disease-modifying antirheumatic drugs* (DMARD) will reduce both a raised erythrocyte sedimentation rate (ESR) and an acute-phase response. They may reduce the titer of circulating rheumatoid factor and slow down the progression of rheumatoid erosions, monitored by X-ray. The patient,

Table 44.6 Approximate relative activity of oral steroid preparations

	Daily dose (mg) above which HPA axis suppression possible	Plasma half-life (min)	Biologic half-life (h)
Cortisol	20-30	90	8-12
Prednisone	7.5-10	200 or more	18-36
Prednisolone	7.5-10	200 or more	18-36
Betamethasone	1-1.5	300 or more	36-54

over a period of weeks (or, for the slower-acting compounds, months), will experience a gradual improvement in overall disease activity with fewer exacerbations and of a lesser severity when it does occur. Stabilization will allow a reduction in the consumption of NSAIDs and possibly of analgesics, although all drugs should be continued in unaltered doses as the disease-modifying drug is introduced and would only be reduced as the drug begins to take effect. These disease-modifying drugs also reduce the need for systemic steroids. Unfortunately, a large number of patients have to discontinue these drugs, and it is not uncommon for patients to try five or six of these drugs in turn over a 15-year period of their disease.

Ten years ago, the choice of a disease-modifying drug would have been restricted to injectable gold, an antimalarial, D-penicillamine, and azathioprine, some European countries favoring alternative immunosuppressive agents such as busulfan. The last decade has seen a proliferation of interest in sulfasalazine in Europe and low-dose methotrexate in the United States such that these two compounds have, in the last few years, become the initial treatment of choice. The current trend is to start with sulfasalazine in Europe, moving to methotrexate if this is ineffective, but to start with methotrexate in the US, probably adding sulfasalazine to recapture response if this is lost. Gold tends to be held in reserve, and D-penicillamine and hydroxychloroquine are waning in popularity.

The last decade also has seen a plethora of new disease-modifying drugs for rheumatoid arthritis such that a selection of up to 20 may now be available in specialist centers, even if most of these are used infrequently. The pharmacokinetic parameters of these drugs that are not described elsewhere in this book are listed in Table 44.7.

Sodium aurothiomalate is the most commonly prescribed gold salt, but other injectable gold salts exist and are used in some parts of Europe. It is probable that it is a thiol group rather than the gold atom that is the active moiety. Auranofin, an oral gold preparation, is also available, but it has not gained general acceptance mainly because of its poor efficacy and the side effect of diarrhea. D-Penicillamine was the best of a number of analogues, some are still prescribed, and one, bucillamine, is very popular in Japan. Sulfasalazine is not the only sulfonamide with disease-modifying activity.

Sulfapyridine is effective but has too many side effects.

Minocycline, probably acting as an anticollagenase compound (since it is the only tetracycline to possess the activity and the only tetracycline effective as a disease-modifying drug in rheumatoid arthritis), most likely is underutilized. Retinoic acids, also effective, are too toxic, particular for women. Of the newly synthesized commercial compounds, cyclosporine is the most recent arrival, but its use is associated with the side effects of hypertension and impaired renal function.

In parallel, immunologists have developed and championed such biologic agents as monoclonal antibodies and tumor necrosis factor-alpha (TNF-α) competitor agonists and antagonists. In general, these compounds have to be given systemically, often by the intravenous route. They sometimes cause local sensitization, and increasing doses tend to be required to maintain benefit. Pharmacokinetic analyses leading to selection of an optimal dose and an optimal dosing frequency often are minimal compared with compounds that come from the drug industry.

Sulfasalazine   The enteric-coated formulation should be prescribed. The normal maintenance dose is 2.0 g per day, reached over 2 to 4 weeks in 500-mg increments. Some patients need to climb to 3.0 g per day. The main side effect is gastrointestinal, intolerance restricting its use in about 30% of patients. Sometimes it is possible to desensitize patients by dropping the dose and reintroducing the drug more slowly. A regular complete blood count (CBC) is recommended as the patient builds up the dose because neutropenia can be a particular problem. In the long term, there is a reversible reduction in sperm count in males and folate-sensitive macrocytic anemia in either sex.

Methotrexate   This drug was used originally in cancer therapy in much higher doses than those currently used in rheumatoid arthritis. It is borrowed from psoriasis treatment and was first used in psoriatic arthritis, where it become apparent that a small weekly dose, by intramuscular injection, kept psoriatic arthritis at bay. Subsequently, a series of controlled trials in rheumatoid

Table 44.7 Pharmacokinetic parameters of selective disease-modifying drugs

	MW	pK$_a$	Oral absorption (%)	Presystemic metabolism (%)	Plasma half-life h (mean)	Volume of distribution (l/kg)	Plasma protein binding (%)
Hydroxychloroquine	433	–	<90	–	18 days	–	50
Auranofin	678	–	13-33	Nil	17-25 days	–	60
Aurothiomalate	390	3.2	Oral, nil	Extensive	Initial 5.5 days		
					Term 250 days	0.1	95
Penicillamine	149	7.9	40	–	1-6	0.8	85
Prednisolone	360	Not ionizable	Rapid	3-20	2.1-3.5 (2.8)	30-40	70-90

(Other disease-modifying drugs are described elsewhere in this book.)

Table 44.8 Interactions of some drugs used in the treatment of rheumatic diseases

Acetaminophen (Paracetamol)
Anion-exchange resins: Cholestyramine reduces absorption.
Anticoagulants: Prolonged regular use of acetaminophen possibly enhances warfarin activity.
Metoclopramide and domperidone: Metoclopramide accelerates absorption of acetaminophen (enhanced effect).

Opioid analgesics
Alcohol: Enhanced sedative and hypotensive effect.
Antibacterials: Rifampicin accelerates metabolism of methadone (reduced effect); erythromycin increases plasma concentration of alfentanil; manufacturer of ciprofloxacin advises avoidance of premedication with opioid analgesics (reduced plasma-ciprofloxacin concentration).
Anticoagulants: Propoxyphene may enhance effect of coumarins and warfarin.
Antidepressants: CNS excitation or depression (hypertension or hypotension) if pethidine and possibly other opioid analgesics are given to patients receiving MAO inhibitors (including moclobemide)-avoid concomitant use and for 2 weeks after MAO inhibitor discontinued; tramadol possibly increases risk of convulsions with SSRIs and tricyclics.
Antiepileptics: Propoxyphene enhances effect of carbamazepine; effect of tramadol decreased by carbamazepine; phenytoin accelerates methadone metabolism (reduced effect and risk of withdrawal effects).
Antifungals: Metabolism of alfentanil inhibited by ketoconazole (risk of prolonged or delayed respiratory depression).
Antipsychotics: Enhanced sedative and hypotensive effect.
Antivirals: Methadone possibly increases plasma concentration of zidovudine.
Anxiolytics and hypnotics: Enhanced sedative effect.
Cisapride: Possible antagonism of gastrointestinal effect.
Dopaminergics: Hyperpyrexia and CNS toxicity reported with selegiline.
Metoclopramide and domperidone: Antagonism of gastrointestinal effects.
Ulcer-healing drugs: Cimetidine inhibits metabolism of opioid analgesics, notably pethidine (increased plasma concentration).

Nonsteroidal anti-inflammatory drugs
Interactions do not generally apply to topical NSAIDs.
ACE inhibitors: Antagonism of hypotensive effect; increased risk of renal damage and increased risk of hyperkalemia on administration with indomethacin, ketorolac, and possibly other NSAIDs.
Other analgesics: Avoid concomitant administration of two or more NSAIDs, including aspirin (increased side effects).
Anion-exchange resins: Cholestyramine reduces absorption of phenylbutazone.
Antacids and adsorbents: Antacids reduce absorption of diflunisal.
Antibacterials: NSAIDs possibly increase risk of convulsions with quinolones.
Anticoagulants: Anticoagulant effect of coumarins and warfarin seriously enhanced by azapropazone and phenylbutazone (avoid concomitant use), and possibly enhanced by diclofenac, diflunisal, flurbiprofen, mefenamic acid, piroxicam, sulindac, and other NSAIDs; increased risk of hemorrhage with parenteral diclofenac and ketorolac and all anticoagulants, including low-dose heparin (avoid concomitant use).
Antidepressants: Moclobemide enhances effect of ibuprofen and possibly other NSAIDs.
Antiepileptics: Effect of phenytoin enhanced by azapropazone (avoid concomitant use), phenylbutazone and possibly other NSAIDs.
Antihypertensives: Antagonism of hypotensive effect.
Antipsychotics: Severe drowsiness possible if indomethacin given with haloperidol.
Beta-blockers: Antagonism of hypotensive effect.
Bisphosphonates: Bioavailability of tiludronic acid increased by indomethacin; alendronic acid possibly increases gastrointestinal side effects of NSAIDs.
Cardiac glycosides: NSAIDs may exacerbate heart failure, reduce GFR, and increase plasma-cardiac glycoside concentration.
Corticosteroids: Increased risk of gastrointestinal bleeding and ulceration.
Cyclosporine: Increased risk of nephrotoxicity; cyclosporine increases plasma concentration of diclofenac (halve diclofenac dose).
Cytotoxics: Excretion of methotrexate reduced by aspirin, azapropazone (avoid concomitant use) diclofenac, indomethacin, ketoprofen, naproxen, phenylbutazone, and probably other NSAIDs (increased risk of toxicity).
Desmopressin: Effect potentiated by indomethacin.
Diuretics: Risk of nephrotoxicity of NSAIDs increased; NSAIDs, notably indomethacin and ketorolac, antagonize diuretic effect; indomethacin and possibly other NSAIDs increase risk of hyperkalemia with potassium-sparing diuretics; occasional reports of decreased renal function when indomethacin is given with triamterene.
Lithium: Excretion of lithium reduced by azapropazone, diclofenac, ibuprofen, indomethacin, ketorolac (avoid concomitant use), mefenamic acid, naproxen, phenylbutazone, piroxicam, and probably other NSAIDS (risk of toxicity).
Mifepristone: Manufacturer recommends avoiding aspirin and NSAIDs until 8-12 days after mifepristone administration.
Muscle relaxants: Ibuprofen and possibly other NSAIDs reduce excretion of baclofen (increased risk of toxicity).
Tacrolimus: Ibuprofen increases risk of nephrotoxicity.
Thyroxine: False low total plasma thyroxine concentration with phenylbutazone.
Ulcer-healing drugs: Plasma concentration of azapropazone possibly increased by cimetidine; risk of CNS toxicity with phenylbutazone increased by misoprostol.
Uricosurics: Probenecid delays excretion of indomethacin, ketoprofen, ketorolac (avoid concomitant use), and naproxen and increased by misoprostol.
Vasodilators: Risk of ketorolac-associated bleeding increased by oxpentifylline (avoid concomitant use).

Chloroquine and hydroxychloroquine
Antacids: Reduced absorption.
Antiarrhythmics: Chloroquine increases risk of ventricular arrhythmias with amiodarone (avoid concomitant use).
Antiepileptics: Antagonism of anticonvulsant effect.
Other antimalarials: Increased risk of convulsions with mefloquine; increased risk of arrhythmias with halofantrine (see also Halofantrine, Chap. 42).

(continued)

Table 44.8 (continued)

Cardiac glycosides: Hydroxychloroquine and possibly chloroquine increase plasma concentrations of digoxin.
Cyclosporine: Chloroquine increases plasma cyclosporine concentration (increased risk of toxicity).
Parasympathomimetics: Chloroquine and hydroxychloroquine have potential to increase symptoms of myasthenia gravis and thus diminish effect of neostigmine and pyridostigmine.
Ulcer-healing drugs: Cimetidine inhibits metabolism of chloroquine (increased plasma concentration).

Injectable gold
Increased risk of toxicity with other nephrotoxic and myelosuppressive drugs.

Penicillamine
Antacids: Reduced absorption of penicillamine.
Iron: Reduced absorption of penicillamine.
Zinc: Reduced absorption of penicillamine.

arthritis led to increasingly low doses being adopted as effective. It has been realized that a certain proportion of patients escape on this low dose, necessitating a climb to 20 or even 30 mg per week in some patients. The drug can cause serious bone marrow depression, and regular CBCs are essential. The drug also can cause hepatic toxicity and a climb in ALT or AST supported by a climb in γ-glutamyl transpeptidase. This is more significant than a raised alkaline phosphatase level, which is often disease-related. Regular liver biopsy is no longer necessary. The drug also occasionally may cause a fibrosing alveolitis in the lungs. More frequent but lesser side effects include buccal ulceration. This may be circumvented by the use of folic acid tablets, which also guard against the development of macrocytic anemia.

Antimalarials Hydroxychloroquine, although more expensive than chloroquine, is probably the treatment of choice. It is normally given in a dose of 400 mg per day, but if this can be reduced to 200 mg, the risk of high toxicity is substantially less. For shorter periods, doses as high as 600 mg per day may be required. Regular eye examinations are mandatory, although there is controversy over the best examination approach and whether the need for examination can be avoided if the dose is kept below a certain cumulative level.

Injectable gold As mentioned earlier, sodium aurothiomalate is the salt prescribed most frequently. After an intramuscular test dose of 5 mg (to guard against a hypersensitivity reaction or the rare exfoliative dermatitis) and additional test doses of 10 and 20 mg (to check that the platelet count is not falling), therapy is started at 50 mg im every week. Each injection is preceded by a CBC and urine test for protein. The other common complication is skin rash, which normally is preceded by itching and resembles psoriasis once present. Treatment continues with weekly injections until response is obtained or until the patient has reached a total of 1000 mg. Whenever either of these occurs, the dose is then dropped to 50 mg im every month, although a recent innovation has been to titrate the dose against clinical activity in the region of 50 mg every second week to 50 mg every sixth week. The therapeutic-toxicity ratio for this compound is particularly narrow.

D-Penicillamine Prescribed orally, normal maintenance therapy with D-penicillamine, once regarded as up to 2.0 g per day, is now established at 500 mg per day, although in some patients a climb in 250-mg increments is required up to 1000 mg per day. Maintenance levels should be reached over about 4 weeks. The side effects are almost identical to those of gold (suggesting that the active moiety for this compound is also its thiol group), although they are less severe when they occur and sometimes slower in onset. Regular CBCs and urine testing for protein are mandatory. Patients occasionally develop a loss of taste or a metallic taste as the dose is increased. Myasthenia gravis is a rare side effect.

Azathioprine Taken orally, maintenance therapy with azathioprine is normally 1.5 mg/kg per day in divided doses rounded up to the nearest 50 mg. The drug causes bone marrow suppression, hepatotoxicity, and skin rash. Appropriate precautions therefore are required.

Cyclosporine A Maintenance therapy with cyclosporine A is normally in the region of 300 mg per day or less. Side effects include hypertension and impaired renal function. Precautions include the regular monitoring of blood pressure and of serum creatinine, although recent evidence suggests that plasma cyclosporine determinations are not essential. They are used occasionally to monitor erratic absorption, compliance, or toxicity. However, if the creatinine level increases by 30% above baseline at the start of treatment, the dose of cyclosporine should be reduced by 0.5 to 1.0 mg/kg per day.

Seronegative spondarthritis

This group of inflammatory systemic conditions is different from rheumatoid arthritis on several counts. The distribution of joint involvement differs, often with early involvement of the sacroiliac joint, a site virtually never affected in rheumatoid arthritis. Patients are negative for circulating rheumatoid factor, and although organ involvement occurs, the organ distribution is different from that in rheumatoid arthritis. In the eye, for example, seronegative disease is associated with anterior uveitis, whereas rheumatoid arthritis characteristically causes scleritis and Sjögren's syndrome. The marker of genetic susceptibility has been identified as the antigen HLA-B27, found in 10% of normal European populations but 90% of patients with some of these conditions. Involvement of the enthesis may represent the primary pathologic abnormality. Several conditions cluster to form this group. The diseases comprise ankylosing spondylitis, psoriatic arthritis, colitic arthritis, reactive arthritis, and Reiter's syndrome.

Initial management is again with analgesics and NSAIDs. Disease-modifying drugs also may be required, particularly if the C-reactive protein level and ESR or plasma viscosity are raised. The efficacy of the standard disease-modifying drugs for rheumatoid arthritis is different in these conditions, however.

Sulfasalazine is particularly effective, also guarding against the onset of colitis. Methotrexate is effective, as is azathioprine. Penicillamine and hydroxychloroquine are ineffective. There is controversy about the use of injectable gold. Although the balance of the literature is in favor of efficacy, psoriasis may be exacerbated by its use.

Connective tissue disorders

In this group of conditions, immunologic abnormalities are more widespread throughout the body. Joint involvement is less marked, although it still occurs in systemic lupus erythematosus, the most common member of this group. However, the joint involvement is often milder than in rheumatoid arthritis, sometimes characterized by arthralgia alone. Lupus related syndromes include polymyositis, dermatomyositis, polyarteritis nodosa, and scleroderma, now reclassified into systemic sclerosis, the CREST syndrome, and localized morphea.

Management of joint symptoms can be achieved initially with NSAIDs and/or analgesics. Steroids play a greater role in this group of conditions, and when vasculitis predominates, cyclophosphamide can be invaluable. Other immunosuppressive agents are used, including methotrexate and azathioprine. The antimalarials are effective for mild lupus.

Polymyalgia rheumatica/temporal arteritis

Polymyalgia rheumatica is a disease of the elderly characterized by bilateral shoulder girdle stiffness or pelvic girdle stiffness in a smaller proportion of patients, tiredness, general malaise, and sometimes depression; it is also associated with a very high ESR or plasma viscosity and C-reactive protein. A characteristic that distinguishes it from rheumatoid arthritis in the elderly and the pain of bilateral osteoarthritis of the shoulder is an almost instantaneous onset of symptoms, normally easily recollected by the patient. A number of patients also describe symptoms attributable to temporal arteritis, and for the last 30 years, the two conditions have been regarded as opposite ends of the same disease spectrum. Those presenting with temporal arteritis complain of intense throbbing headaches over the temporal region, leading to visual disturbance and even blindness. For both conditions, the specific treatment of systemic steroids is indicated. For polymyalgia rheumatica alone, the normal starting dose is 20 mg prednisolone qd. For polymyalgia rheumatica associated with temporal headache, this normally would be increased to around 30 mg qd, and for visual symptoms associated with temporal arteritis, 40 or 60 mg prednisolone is required. If blindness has occurred recently, rescue sometimes can be achieved by a large dose of iv hydrocortisone.

On the introduction of prednisolone, relief is dramatic and normally occurs within 1 or 2 days, providing a useful diagnostic test, since apart from temporal artery biopsy when the temporal artery is involved, there are no specific markers for this condition, which remains a clinical diagnosis. The raised ESR also falls quickly, providing original confirmation of diagnosis. Historic evidence from the pre-steroid era suggested that the mean duration of the disease was 2 years, with a range of 6 months to 10 years. For this reason, patients are maintained on minimum doses of steroids to keep symptoms at bay and the ESR down for a period of 2 years, at which point a cautious weaning of steroids using 1 mg pediatric prednisolone, normally over a period of 3 to 6 months, is attempted. About 50% of patients are able to remain off steroids as a result, although in about 10 to 15% the condition will recur, necessitating reintroduction of steroids. If the weaning proves impossible, the steroid should be reinstated and continued for perhaps up to 5 months, when a weaning once again should be attempted.

Septic arthritis

An infection in a joint is a rheumatologic emergency. Patients with inflammatory polyarthritis such as rheumatoid arthritis are more susceptible to joint infection (and infection elsewhere) than others, possibly because of disordered immunity. In addition, joint prostheses may act as a focus for infection, either in the period immediately after operation or later if mechanical loosening or metal sensitivity occurs. At present, however, antibiotic prophylaxis to cover dental treatment in patients who have joint prostheses is not recommended, so small is the risk.

Septic arthritis should be suspected whenever a single joint becomes acutely swollen and erythematous without obvious cause. The differential diagnosis includes gout, classically confined to the big toe or knee. Patients with rheumatoid disease are particularly at risk. Here, suspicion is aroused when one joint is disproportionately involved in relation to the others. Normally, there is systemic upset with high swinging fever and sometimes septicemia. Hospital referral is mandatory to allow early bacteriologic diagnosis. At this stage, a diagnosis of gonococcal arthritis should be based on sexual contact; skin lesions, a milder flitting arthritis, relative lack of pus on aspiration, and no organism identified in the joint culture, although the organism sometimes can be isolated from the bloodstream.

In the clinical absence of gonacoccal arthritis, antibiotic treatment should be based on identification of the organism (most likely *Staphylococcus* but may be *Streptococcus* and occasionally *Hemophilus*) and sensitivity. Local osteomyelitis may occur, and a longer rather than shorter duration of treatment is recommended. Regular aspiration of the joint to dryness, normally daily in the first instance, and/or surgical drainage may be required. The most popular antibiotic option is clindamycin alone or flucloxacillin plus fusidic acid. If *H. influenzae* is identified, amoxicillin or cefuroxime should be given (see Chap. 38). Typically, the acute disease is treated for 6 weeks, and a chronic infection with osteomyelitis proven on radiograph is treated for at least 12 weeks.

Paget's disease

This localized disorder of bone is associated with remodeling. The process is initiated by an increase in osteoclast-mediated bone absorption with subsequent compensatory increases in new bone formation leading to a disorganised structure of woven and lamella bone at widespread and varied skeletal sites. The condition presents with pain. At a later stage, bone deformity may occur. A high alkaline phosphatase level (bony origin) alerts suspicion. Patients are invariable elderly. Seventy percent of lesions are asymptomatic.

In a majority of patients, symptoms can be controlled by analgesics alone. If the alkaline phosphatase level continues to rise, or if deformity becomes prominent or pain is unrelieved by analgesics, calcitonin or bisphosphonates can be used (see Chap. 46). Calcitonin, given by injection, was the original treatment. However, a disadvantage of calcitonin is its plateau phenomenon, and for reasons that are unclear, up to 50% of patients failed to respond. A nasal spray may reduce unpleasant side effects. With erythromycin too toxic to provide an alternative, attentions were directed toward bisphosphonates, and the second-generation bisphosphonates are likely to become increasingly the treatment of choice for this condition. Remission from bisphosphonates can last for years compared with calcitonin. Disodium etidronate, disodium pamidronate, and alendronic acid are all available. The serum alkaline phosphatase level should be monitored from time to time while the drug is being used.

Fibromyalgia

Until recently, there has been dispute about whether this syndrome actually exists. A group of patients with musculoskeletal pain, typically involving the muscles rather than the joints and of diffuse character, in whom other demonstrable arthritis was excluded, have been labeled as having fibromyalgia. Some have suggested that there is a histrionic component. Certainly the discomfort normally is described in graphic detail with the use of adjectives that are not normally applied to arthritis localized to the joints.

Recent research has suggested an association between fibromyalgia and sleep disturbance, and specific tender pressure points have been claimed to be of diagnostic value. Whatever the etiology, management with analgesics and/or NSAIDs is often unsatisfactory.

A recent innovation has been the use of tricyclic antidepressants in a relatively small dose at night to relieve symptoms. Until recently, amitriptyline has been the drug of first choice, but early indications suggest that alternatives that have fewer side effects, such as dothiepin, may be equally effective.

Suggested readings _____

AHERN M. Methotrexate. In: van de Putte LBA, Furst DE, Williams HJ, van Riel PLCM, eds. Therapy of the systemic rheumatic diseases. New York: Marcel Dekker, 1998:183-206.

BIRD HA. A modified release of NSAIDs for rheumatic complaints. Prescriber 1997;8:57-63.

BIRD HA. Intraarticular and intralesional therapy. In: Kippel JH, Dieppe PA, eds. Rheumatology, 2nd ed. London: Mosby, 1998.

BURKHARD D, GHOSH P. Laboratory evaluation of antiarthritic drugs as potential chondroprotective agents. Semin Arthritis Rheum 1987;17(suppl 1):3-34.

COCH M, DEZI M, FERRARIO M, CAPURSO L. Prevention of nonsteroidal anti-inflammatory drug-induced gastrointestinal mucosal injury. Arch Intern Med 1996;156:2321-31.

DOUGADOS M. Sulfasalazine. In: van de Putte LBA, Furst DE, Williams HJ, van Riel PLCM, eds. Therapy of the Systemic Rheumatic Diseases. New York: Marcel Dekker, 1998:165-82.

GOLDENBERG DL. Fibromyalgia and related syndromes. In: Klippel JH, Dieppe PA, eds. Rheumatology, 2nd ed. London: Mosby, 1998, sec 4, chap 15, 1-12.

HAZLEMAN BL. Polymyalgia rheumatica and giant cell arteritis. In: Klippel JH, Dieppe PA, eds. Rheumatology, 2nd ed. London: Mosby, 1998, sec 7, chap 21, 1-8.

HUSKISSON EC, DUDLEY HART F. Joint disease: all the arthropathies. Bristol, England: Wright, 1987.

KIRWIN JR, Arthritis & Rheumatism Council, Low Dose Glucocorticoid Study Group. The effect of glucocorticoids on joint destruction in rheumatoid arthritis. N Engl J Med 1995;333:142-6.

MCENTEGART A, CAPELL HA. Gold therapy. In: van de Putte LBA, Furst DE, Williams HJ, van Riel PLCM, eds. Therapy of the systemic rheumatic diseases. New York: Marcel Dekker, 1998:143-63.

PERKINS F, DRAY A. Novel pharmacological strategies for analgesia. Ann Rheum Dis 1996;55:715-22.

WALKER JF, SHEATHER-REID RB, CARMODY JJ, et al. Nonsteroidal anti-inflammatory drugs in rheumatoid arthritis and osteoarthritis. Arthritis Rheum 1997;40:1944-54.

YEOMANS ND, TULLASSAY Z, JUHASZ L, et al. A comparison of omeprazole with ranitidine for ulcers associated with nonsteroidal anti-inflammatory drugs. N Engl J Med 1998;338:719-25.

Rheumatoid arthritis and osteoarthritis: management strategies

Haiko Sprott, Gerold Stucki

RHEUMATOID ARTHRITIS

Rheumatoid arthritis (RA) is characterized by a progressive destruction of joints accompanied by synovial hyperplasia, inflammation, and autoimmune phenomena. The understanding of the pathogenesis of RA has advanced dramatically in recent years. Management of RA is important for the disease course, progression of destruction, and primary and secondary health care costs. From a quality perspective, one distinguishes outcomes, processes, and structure.

RA has a major impact on function and quality of life and frequently affects patients in their most productive years, causing major economic loss. Studies show that patients with active polyarticular rheumatoid-factor-positive RA have a 70% probability of developing joint damage or erosions within 2 years of the onset of disease. Other studies suggest that early aggressive treatment may alter the disease course, reduce morbidity, maintain function, prolong life, and reduce health care costs. There are a wide range of treatments for RA (see Chap. 44). Moreover, exercise programs reduce pain and improve function for RA patients. Also, patient education programs and psychoeducational interventions improve function and quality of life, reduce physician visits by 40%, and decrease health care costs.

Who to treat and when to start treatment

The initiation of disease-modifying antirheumatic drug (DMARD) therapy should not be delayed for more than 3 months for any patient with an established diagnosis who, despite of adequate treatment with nonsteroidal anti-inflammatory drugs (NSAIDs), has ongoing joint pain, significant morning stiffness or fatigue, active synovitis, or persistent elevation of the erythrocyte sedimentation rate (ESR) or C-reactive protein (CRP) levels.

To identify the risk of unnecessary treatment, we need to know the rate of remission. The *rate of spontaneous remission* has been defined as "no arthritis on examination in a patient who has not taken second-line drugs or steroids in the preceding 3 months". The rate of natural remission described in a large community-based study was only 25% and was reflected by the relatively low prevalence of rheumatoid factor positivity, indicating less severe disease in patients with inflammatory polyarthritis after 2 years. Furthermore, only 9% of patients were in "sustained remission" both at 1 and 2 years. Rates of remission in treated patients found in a similar study did not differ. While 25% of patients fulfilled the criteria for remission at least once during the study period, only 15% fulfilled the criteria at two consecutive visits. Visits in which patients are in remission may not always be consecutive. Remission may thus be best understood as being often a temporary state at the lower end on the stability of systemic inflammation or disease activity.

Treatment strategies

Therapeutic strategies for RA have been evolving from the traditional "pyramid" approach toward one based on early and sustained use of DMARDs (see Chap.44). The faster mode of action of methotrexate (MTX) and sulfasalazine, two effective drugs with good "survival" curves, compared with gold and D-penicillamine in combination with the use of measurement-improvement systems has made it possible to virtually "titrate" disease activity.

A major problem with the currently used single-drug therapy is the discontinuation of treatment. In a study of 152 RA patients taking MTX, the 10-year maintenance of treatment (survival) was 30%. Another study of 629 patients estimated median drug survival periods of 51 months for MTX, 39.9 months for azathioprine, 34.9 months for gold salts, and 16.4 months for D-penicillamine. Lack of efficacy and toxicity are the two main reasons for the discontinuation of DMARDs. Other reasons, including costs, noncompliance, improvement or remission, nonmedical factors, psychologic factors, misunderstanding, and expired prescriptions, may each account for less than 25% of treatment failures. The reasons seem to vary strongly across the settings. Toxicity has been singled out as the most important reason (53.3%), whereas lack of efficacy led to discontinuation in only 6.4% of the patients taking MTX. In contrast, lack of response to therapy was the single most important reason for treatment failure in other studies, for all drugs except D-penicillamine, where toxicity was most important.

Because of the problems with efficacy and toxicity associated with the use of single-drug regimens, there has been an increasing interest in combination therapy. The concept of combination therapy has been used successfully in oncology with excellent results in terms of efficacy and toxicity when treating lymphoproliferative diseases with multiple cytotoxic drugs. The theoretical arguments for combining DMARDs in the treatment of RA are summarized in Table 45.1, which indicates the specific advantages and disadvantages of strategies used in clinical trials in terms of time. Because of the lack of theoretical knowledge about mode of action, experimental studies comparing single therapy with combination therapy and different combination regimens are needed in order to find effective treatment protocols for increasing favorable long-term outcomes. There is increasing evidence that some combination-therapy regimens are superior in terms of efficacy and toxicity.

Comprehensive overviews of the most important studies of combination therapies with DMARDs are widely available (Tabs. 45.1 and 45.2).

New drugs such as leflunomide have been developed. This is a novel isoxazol drug with disease-modifying properties for the treatment of RA that has promising features, e.g., high tolerability and efficacy in patients with advanced RA. The drug was tested in many multicenter, randomized, double-blind, controlled trials that included as active comparators MTX and sulfasalazine. Once-daily administration of leflunomide appears to be effective in patients with active RA.

Optimized treatment control

Once initiated, the importance of optimal adjustment of DMARDs to control disease activity cannot be overemphasized. Because untreated or insufficiently treated disease activity is associated with joint destruction and deteriorating health outcomes, it is necessary to use sufficient doses in DMARD therapy. Because disease activity is suppressed with potentially toxic drugs, it is critical to find the minimally effective dose as precisely as possible. Since there are only a few drugs available and DMARD therapy may take up to 6 months before being effective, much is lost if an efficacious but overdosed DMARD causes intolerable side effects and needs to be stopped.

Control of disease activity in RA is a measurement-improvement process with the goal of reducing clinical symptoms (e.g., swollen and tender joint counts, acute-phase reactants), pain, and patient-perceived disease activity in the short term and damage and consequent disability in the long term.

Ideally, the physician should rely on standardized, reliable, valid, sensitive, and easily interpretable measures with clear-cut decision rules for each dimension of the measurement-improvement process. With the development of psychometrically sound patient questionnaires, e.g., the Health Assessment Questionnaire (HAQ) for the assessment of disability and the Rheumatoid Arthritis Disease Activity Index (RADAI) for the assessment of self-perceived disease activity, it is now possible to measure the patient's perspective according to these requirements. For the measurement of clinical disease activity, the Disease Activity Score (DAS), which calculates the number of swollen, tender joints and the sedimentation rate, is the only empirically and statistically derived and extensively tested algorithm currently available:

$$DAS28 = 0.28 \times \text{number of swollen joints} + 0.56 \times \text{number of tender joints} + 0.7 \times \ln(\text{sedimentation rate}) + 0.16$$

The DAS28 is based on 28 joint counts for the number of both swollen and tender joints and is more efficient as well as more valid than the DAS44, which is based on 44 joints. The DAS is superior to individual articular index scores (e.g., the Ritchie score). It places disease activity on a continuum from 0 to 10. The DAS is advantageous because it provides a more reliable estimate than each individual measure. The precision is approximately 0.6; that is, a change of greater than 0.6 is unlikely to be by chance. For patients with mild disease activity, a change of 0.6 represents a clinically relevant change. With more pronounced disease activity, a larger response of 1.2 is required to be of clinical relevance. In a group analysis, a DAS of 3.1 or less (using the 28-joint version of the DAS) was shown to be associated with halted X-ray progression. By gauging the DAS according to the American College of Rheumatology (ACR) criteria for remission, which include the same variables as used in the DAS but in addition include pain, fatigue, and morning stiffness, i.e., primary patient-oriented health outcomes, the cutoff for remission in terms of the DAS was 2.4 (with the 28-joint version of the DAS). The cutoff for avoidance of damage in terms of X-ray progression together with remission is the most useful guideline in clinical practice. The goal should be the permanent reduction of disease activity to below 3.1 or ideally 2.4. While these cutoffs are valid for the original version of the DAS, other cutoffs apply for the DAS based on reduced joint counts using only 28 swollen and tender joints, which may be preferable in clinical practice. In the short term (6 months), the DAS and RADAI allow for best possible adjustment of anti-inflammatory and immunosuppressive treatment.

RA diagnosis is frequently delayed for several months after onset of symptoms, largely because of a delay in diagnosis by the physician. Early treatment requires accurate and timely diagnosis. However, diagnosis of RA may be difficult in the early stages of the disease because of the relatively low prevalence of patients with RA and relatively low prevalence of DMARD-treated patients, and primary care physicians lack sufficient experience with these drugs. Improving health services provisions with educational programs thus may be as important as optimizing management.

OSTEOARTHRITIS

Osteoarthritis (OA) is a degenerative condition of the joints and is the most prevalent rheumatic disease. Thus efficient and cost-effective management strategies will be

of ever-increasing importance. Pain is the major symptom that leads patients to consult their physicians for treatment. Pain can have multiple causes. These include cartilage fragments, meniscal tears or degeneration, synovial effusions, osteophytes, and periarticular sources (such as tendons, bursae, and muscles), among others. Therefore, effective pain control is an important goal in the management of OA besides education of the patient and his or her family about the disease and its therapy. The histologic hallmark of OA is damaged articular cartilage. Two main hypotheses have been formulated: (1) OA is viewed as either a failure of the chondrocyte to maintain normal bio-

Table 45.1 Strategies in combination therapy

Strategies	Potential advantages	Potential disadvantages
1. Parallel	Fast response when it is most beneficial High response rate Less side effects with use of relatively low initial doses Less loss of efficacy (e.g., drug tolerance)	Difficulty to attribute side effects to individual drugs Overtreatment with unnecessarily high doses and unnecessarily continued combination therapy Undertreatment and delayed response with too low initial doses Unclear which drug to reduce first
2. Step-down	Fast response when it is most beneficial High response rate Fewer side effects with use of relatively low initial doses Less loss of efficacy (e.g., drug tolerance) Combination therapy necessary only until response is achieved	Difficulty to attribute side effects to individual drugs Overtreatment with unnecessarily initial doses Unclear which drug to drop first
3. Step-up	Avoidance of toxicity of the first drug by adding a second Reduced risk of overtreatment Attribution of side effects to individual drugs and doses	Delayed response A possibly ineffective first drug is unnecessarily continued
4. Overlap and switch	Identification of an additive/synergistic effect and the need for continued combination therapy May be used sequentially to identify best combinations Prevention of flare when substituting an insufficiently effective drug A possibly ineffective first drug is not unnecessarily continued	Delayed response
5. Cyclic or intermittent	A well- tolerated but (intermittently) insufficient therapy can be maintained Combination therapy only when needed Fewer side effects Rationale approach to combine conventional DMARDs and biologic agents Time schedule adjustment possible	Cyclic drug must be fast acting Intensive cooperation of physician and patient required to ensure compliance More lab controls

1. Two or more drugs applicable.
2. In the parallel setting, two DMARDs are given at the same time, as early as possible in the disease course.
3. In the step-up setting, an additional drug is added when the single-drug therapy is insufficient.
4. In the step-down setting, two or more DMARDs are given initially. With control of disease activity, one drug after the other is tapered.
5. In the intermittent setting, an additional DMARD is given for a limited period of time when disease activity is not sufficiently controlled during disease flares; in the cyclic setting, a fast-acting DMARD is added to a given drug in a cyclic way.

Table 45.2 The most recent combination therapies
MTX alone
MTX in combination with sulfasalazine and hydroxychloroquine
MTX in combination with sulfasalazine or hydroxychloroquine
Combination with MTX and azathioprine versus single DMARDs
MTX in combination with cyclosporine A
MTX in combination with hydroxychloroquine and cyclosporine A
Initial combination of MTX, sulfasalazine, and prednisone in early RA
Combination of MTX with anti-CD4 antibodies

chemical homeostasis, or (2) OA is viewed as a biochemical failure of cartilage and/or subchondral bone secondary to physical stress.

The disease course can, however, be punctuated by episodes of inflammation. Biomechanical factors play a major role in the development of OA.

Obesity, an important risk factor for hip and knee damage in both sexes, should be treated by diet. Specific dietary therapy and other unproven therapies are not recommended in the management of patients with OA. Rest is usually helpful, sometimes by the use of a splint to reduce the amount of (pathologic) movement of the joint and giving stability. Occupational trauma (especially repetitive motion, trauma, and bending) also may contribute to the development of OA. Symptomatic therapy is directed primarily at relief from pain. The approach should combine physical measures, medicinal measures, psychologic approaches, and judicious use of surgical interventions.

Physical measures include exercise, supportive devices and orthotics, and thermal modalities. Physiotherapy can alleviate joint pain through the use of cold and hot packs, ultrasound, short-wave diathermy, hydrotherapy, etc. Most patients with OA prefer heat. Heat can decrease joint stiffness, reduce pain, relieve muscle spasm, and help prevent contractures. Cold applications may relieve muscle spasm, decrease swelling in acute trauma, and relieve pain from inflammation. Daily living activities should be appropriately modified. Motion exercises (to prevent contractures) and strengthening exercises are mandatory. A supervised program of fitness walking and education has been shown to improve functional status. Swimming is a particularly good exercise, especially for knee and hip joints.

Supportive devices and orthotics can be effective in management. Canes can take the weight off an affected hip by as much as 60%. Orthotics, such as shoe inserts, can be of help in OA affecting the metatarsal joints. Knee braces can be useful for those with lateral instability. Orthotics play an important role in helping to reduce or eliminate pain in OA. In a controlled study, 64 patients with OA wearing orthoses only for relief of pain had a statistically significant longer period of pain relief than those on NSAIDs. Fifty-five percent of the subjects using orthoses and NSAIDs also had a statistically significant longer period of pain relief than those receiving NSAID therapy only.

Medication-based therapy can be subdivided into NSAIDs, analgesics, narcotics, antispasmodics, antidepressants, and intraarticular agents. Traditionally, NSAIDs have been the agents of choice for the treatment of pain in patients with OA. Recently, however, because of concerns about possible deleterious effects of NSAIDs on articular cartilage metabolism, questions have been raised about the role of synovial inflammation in the natural progression of OA, the greater risk of toxicity from prolonged NSAID therapy in elderly patients with OA, and the central role of NSAIDs in the treatment of OA patients. Nonopioid analgesic drugs are recommended as the drugs of choice for systemic treatment of symptomatic OA. Opioid analgesics may be helpful for the treatment of acute exacerbations of pain. If the patient fails to respond to these oral analgesics, the use of an NSAID is indicated. Indomethacin, however, may be associated with accelerated joint destruction in patients with OA and probably should not be used for long-term therapy. The intensity of pain in patients with OA may vary from day to day as well as within a single day, so the use of short-half-life NSAIDs on an "as needed" basis is preferable if they offer adequate pain relief (see Chap. 44).

Opinions as to the value of topical therapy over the painful joint differ. If drug therapy is needed, intraarticular application may be preferable to systemic therapy. The use of intraarticular glucocorticoids is recommended not to exceed three to four injections per joint per year. Systemic glucocorticoids should not be used. The understanding that OA is not a passive "wear and tear" phenomenon but an active process that may be potentially modified has led to a rising interest in "chondroprotective" agents. Chondroprotective agents, such as glycosaminoglycans and proteoglycans, should be able to prevent the progression of very early OA. In general, they have been reported to reduce pain for prolonged periods of time (months) and potentially to improve mobility. The mechanisms of action are not known but there is evidence for an anti-inflammatory effect (particularly at high molecular weight), a short-term lubricant effect, an analgesic effect caused by direct buffering of synovial nerve endings, and a stimulating effect on synovial lining cells to produce normal hyaluronic acid. More advanced chondroprotective agents or disease-modifying drugs for OA have been studied in several animal models and may be available in the future for use in humans.

Pharmacotherapy should play an adjunctive role to nonpharmacologic measures in the overall management of patients with OA symptoms. Patients should be instructed on how to rest or unload involved joints, to protect them through appropriate manipulation of their environment and appropriate methods of lifting and bending, and to maintain and improve muscle strength and flexibility to ensure joint stability and prevent contractures.

Surgery may be of value when particular joints are

involved. These interventions include arthroscopic surgery, osteotomies, and joint replacement. Patients with severe symptomatic OA of the hip require an aggressive approach to decrease pain, increase mobility, and improve function. Such patients may benefit from orthopedic consultation and evaluation for osteotomy or total-joint arthroplasty. Arthroscopy enables the direct observation of cartilage and other joint structures and also can serve as a way to repair meniscal tears, remove loose bodies, or shave articular cartilage or synovium. Total-joint replacement is especially effective for the hip, knee, shoulder, and finger joints.

Obesity, multiple medical problems, and inability to endure a rehabilitation program are relative contraindications. An untreated systemic or joint infection is an absolute contraindication.

In conclusion, treatment of patients with OA should be individualized and tailored to the severity of symptoms. In individuals with mild symptomatic disease, treatment may be limited to patient education, physical and occupational therapy, other nonpharmacologic modalities, and drug therapy with nonopioid oral and topical analgesics. In the majority of patients, simple analgesics are probably as effective as NSAIDs. In patients who are unresponsive to this treatment regimen, use of an NSAID in addition to nonpharmacologic therapy is appropriate unless it is medically contraindicated. Judicious use of intraarticular steroid injections has a role either as monotherapy or as an adjunct to systemic therapy. Many alternative strategies of pain management such as local drug applications, intraar-ticular steroid injections, acupuncture, radiosynovectomy, transcutaneous nerve stimulation, and antidepressants may be effective, but their precise place in the armamentarium has not been fully established. Patients with severe symptomatic OA require an aggressive approach to decreasing pain, increasing mobility, and improving function; such patients may benefit from orthopedic consultation and evaluation for osteotomy or total-joint arthroplasty.

The management of OA has been limited to symptomatic treatment to decrease pain and improve function without modifying the underlying disease process. New insights into the structure, physiology, and function of cartilage, however, have led to the development of promising approaches that ultimately may modify the underlying disease process. Transplantation of chondrocytes or mesenchymal stem cells to repair and/or regenerate cartilage has become possible in humans. If this is found to be practical, it will radically alter the management of OA in selected patients.

Proposed guidelines for the management of RA and OA should identify aspects of current guidelines directly related to outcome; educate clinicians in the aspects of care; ensure guidelines are introduced into practice and the outcome of care subsequently improves; regularly update the guidelines to reflect current opinion.

Suggested readings

ALARCÓN GS, TRACY IC, STRAND GM, et al. Survival of drug discontinuation analysis in a large cohort of methotrexate treated rheumatoid arthritis patients. Ann Rheum Dis 1995;54:708-12.

BJELLE A. Primary care and rheumatology in musculoskeletal disorders: bridging the gap. J Rheumatol 1996;23:205-6.

BORIGINI MJ, PAULUS HE. Combination therapy. Baillières Clin Rheumatol 1995;9:689-710.

HARRISON BJ, SYMMONS DPM, BRENNAN P, et al. Natural remission in inflammatory polyarthritis: issues of definition and prediction. Br J Rheumatol 1996;35:1096-100.

MORELAND LW, PRATT PW, MAYES MD, et al. Double-blind, placebo-controlled multicenter trial using chimeric monoclonal anti-CD4 antibody, cM-T412, in rheumatoid arthritis patients receiving concomitant methotrexate. Arthritis Rheum 1995;38:1581-8.

O'DELL J, HAIRE CE, ERIKSON N, et al. Treatment of rheumatoid arthritis with methotrexate alone, sulfasalazine and hydroxychloroquine, or a combination of all three medications. N Engl J Med 1996;334:1287-91.

PLANT MJ, SAKLATVALA J, BORG AA, et al. Measurements and prediction of radiological progression in early rheumatoid arthritis. J Rheumatol 1994;21:1808-13.

PREVOO MLL, VAN GESTEL AM, VAN'T HOF MA, et al. Remission in a prospective study of patients with rheumatoid arthritis: American Rheumatism Association preliminary remission criteria in relation to the Disease Activity Score. Br J Rheumatol 1996;35:1101-5.

SALAFFI F, CAROTTI M, CERVINI C. Combination therapy of cyclosporine A with methotrexate or hydroxychloroquine in refractory rheumatoid arthritis. Scand J Rheumatol 1996;25:16-23.

STUCKI G. Specialist management: needs and benefits. Baillières Clin Rheumatol 1997;11:97-106.

STUCKI G, SANGHA O. Clinical quality management: putting the pieces together. Arthritis Care Res 1996;9:405-12.

STUCKI G, LIANG MH, STUCKI S, et al. A self-administered Rheumatoid Arthritis Disease Activity Index (RADAI) for epidemiological research: psychometric properties and correlation with parameters of disease activity. Arthritis Rheum 1995;6:795-8.

VAN DER HEIDE A, JACOBS JW, BIJLSMA JW, et al. The effectiveness of early treatment with "second line" antirheumatic drugs: a randomized, controlled trial. Ann Intern Med 1996;124:699-707.

VAN GESTEL AM, PREVOO MLL, VAN'T HOF MA, et al. Development and validation of the European League Against Rheumatism response criteria for rheumatoid arthritis. Arthritis Rheum 1996;39:34-40.

WILLKENS RF, SHARP JT, STABLEIN D, et al. Comparison of azathioprine, methotrexate, and the combination of the two in the treatment of rheumatoid arthritis. Arthritis Rheum 1995;38:1799-806.

Osteoporosis

Bernard Bannwarth

Osteoporosis is a systemic skeletal disease characterized by low bone mass and loss of microarchitectural integrity resulting in an increased risk of fractures. Since bone mass is a major determinant of bone strength and may be assessed by several techniques, especially dual-energy X-ray absorptiometry, the diagnosis of osteoporosis is at present based on densitometric criteria. As such, bone density values are expressed in relation to reference data as standard deviation (SD) scores: a T score representing the number of standard deviations above or below the reference values for young adults. Accordingly, osteoporosis is defined as a T score below −2.5, and established (or severe) osteoporosis denotes a T score below −2.5 in the presence of one or more fragility fractures. Osteopenia is defined as a T score between −1 and −2.5. A reduction in bone density of 1 standard deviation is associated with a 1.5- to 3-fold rise in fracture risk. Therapeutic intervention may vary according to the severity of bone loss as well as the pathophysiologic status and gender of the patient.

Disease presentation

Bone mass increases throughout childhood and adolescence, reaching a peak between the ages of 20 and 25 years. However, bone undergoes continual turnover throughout life. Bone remodeling proceeds in cycles in which the resorption of old bone by osteoclasts is followed by formation of osteoid by osteoblasts. Osteoid tissue may be mineralized secondarily. This process replaces old bone matrix with new at an annual turnover rate of about 25% in cancellous (trabecular) bone and 2 to 3% in cortical bone. During adulthood, osteoclast activity slightly exceeds that of osteoblasts, so each cycle leads to a small loss of bone. Age-related bone loss is on the order of 0.5 to 1% per year in both sexes. Superimposed on the effect of aging is menopause, which induces a dramatic increase in bone turnover, with osteoclastic activity predominating. Thus, the annual rate of loss accelerates to between 3 and 6% for 5 to 10 years after cessation of ovarian function. In this case, the rate of loss of trabecular bone exceeds that of cortical bone because of the high surface-to-volume ratio of cancellous bone. A further con-

sequence of postmenopausal bone loss is trabecular disconnection, which contributes to skeletal fragility. This fact accounts for the discrepancy between the variations in bone mass and those in bone strength.

Risk factors for osteoporosis relate first to low bone mineral density as a result of low peak bone mass or subsequent excessive bone loss or both. Risk factors for low peak bone mass include low dietary calcium intake, physical inactivity, and smoking. However, the role of these factors is probably incidental because peak bone mass is largely under genetic control. In this respect, white and Asian people and people with a familial history of osteoporosis are prone to lower peak bone mass. Furthermore, loss of ovarian function due to menopause, oophorectomy, athletic or stress-related amenorrhea, hyperprolactinemia or anorexia nervosa, and hypogonadism in males, as well as primary hyperparathyroidism, hyperthyroidism, alcoholism, and several drugs (e.g., glucocorticoids, anticonvulsivants, and thyroxine), are associated with increased bone loss.

Treatment

Treatments of general use in the disease

A logical approach to the prevention of bone weakness and the management of established osteoporosis is first to minimize risk factors where possible. In this respect, alterations in life-style such as reducing smoking, avoiding heavy alcohol consumption, engaging in regular moderate weight-bearing exercises, and improving nutrition are advisable at all ages. In fact, adequate amounts of calcium are recommended throughout life (Tab. 46.1). Adequate amounts of vitamin D are also necessary for optimal calcium absorption and bone health; a daily intake of 400 to 800 IU (10-20 mg) is considered to be sufficient in most countries to prevent the development of rickets in children and to inhibit seasonal increases in parathyroid hormone secretion in adults, including postmenopausal women. It is also essential to titrate medications inducing bone loss to maintain disease control while minimizing adverse effect on the skeleton. Since trauma is a major determinant of fracture, preventing falls is of primary importance in osteoporotic patients. Caution

Table 46.1 Optimal elemental calcium requirements recommended by the 1994 National Institutes of Health consensus panel

Age group	Recommended intake (mg/day)
Infants	
Birth-6 months	400
6 months-1 year	600
Children	
1-5 years	800
5-10 years	800-1200
Adolescent/young adults	
11-24 years	1200-1500
Women	
25-50 years	1000
Pregnant and nursing	1200
Postmenopausal (>50 years)	
On estrogens	1000
Not on estrogens	1500
Men	
25-65 years	1000
Elderly (>65 years)	1500

should be exercised in the prescription of any drug with sedative effects, especially long-acting psychotropics.

Established osteoporosis may be regarded as an indication for pharmacologic intervention. Drug therapy also may be proposed to prevent osteoporosis, especially at the time of menopause and in patients at high risk, such as those receiving long-term corticosteroids. The compounds used generally are classified as antiresorptive or anabolic, most falling into the former category (Tab. 46.2). The main effect of antiresorptive drugs is to slow down the rate of bone loss, although small increases in bone mass may occur as a result of infilling of the remodeling space and secondary mineralization. By contrast, anabolic drugs have the potential to increase bone density in a substantial manner.

Since estrogen deficiency is the major determinant of postmenopausal osteoporosis, hormone replacement therapy (HRT) appears to be the preventive treatment of first choice. In fact, postmenopausal HRT rapidly normalizes both bone resorption and bone formation, leading to a reestablishment of a positive or a balanced outcome of

Table 46.2 Drugs currently used in the prevention and treatment of osteoporosis

Antiresorptive drugs	Anabolic drugs
Estrogen	Fluoride
Bisphosphonates	Anabolic steroids
Calcitonin	
Calcium-vitamin D	
Vitamin D metabolites and analogues	

bone turnover in all areas. The decrease in overall mortality and incidence of ischemic heart diseases and possibly stroke is a major extraskeletal beneficial effect of HRT (see Chap. 67).

Other antiresorptive agents may be alternatives to estrogen for prevention of osteoporosis in women who are unwilling to undergo HRT or in whom HRT is unsuitable. Calcitonin and bisphosphonates were shown to prevent bone loss in early postmenopausal women, at least in the first years of treatment. The effect of calcium supplementation alone is more controversial. Overall, protective effects of these agents against fractures have not been definitively demonstrated, and non-HRT methods of prevention are clearly devoid of extraskeletal benefits.

Stimulators of bone formation in theory may be appropriate in osteoporotic patients. However, fluoride appears to have a poor risk-benefit ratio, whereas studies on other anabolic agents are still in progress. Thus antiresorptive agents, especially estrogens and bisphosphonates, are presently the most widely used agents in the treatment of osteoporosis. Calcitonin also may preserve bone mass in established disease. Whether this effect is associated with a significant reduction in fracture risk, however, is uncertain. Finally, dietary supplementation with vitamin D and calcium may reduce the risk of nonvertebral fractures substantially among elderly patients in residential care.

Osteoporotic fractures are a major cause of morbidity and mortality in the elderly populations in developed countries. The mortality rates of women from osteoporotic fractures appear to be greater than the combined mortality rates from breast cancer and ovarian cancer. In the United States, the remaining risk for any fragility fracture in 50-year-old Caucasian women and men has been estimated at 40 and 13%, respectively. In Great Britain, the remaining lifetime risk of osteoporotic fracture in a 50-year-old Caucasian women is 14% for the hip, 13% for the wrist, and 11% for the spine. The corresponding figures are slightly higher in North American women. The economic burden of osteoporosis is directly related to the cost of fractures, especially hip fractures.

Drug classes

ESTROGENS

Historically, conjugated equine estrogen was the most common agent for postmenopausal use. Now, a more popular agent is 17β-estradiol, the potent, naturally occurring hormone, which is available for various routes of administration. However, estradiol is seldom used orally because it undergoes extensive metabolism within the intestinal mucosa and liver. Estradiol may be delivered systemically by means of cutaneous application of a gel or transdermal patches. Long-lasting pellets may be implanted subcutaneously; however, there are wide differences in the rate of decline in plasma estradiol concentrations.

Various esters of estrogens are also employed for hormone replacement therapy (HRT) (see Chap. 67). In this respect, estradiol valerate is a synthetic derivative used largely in Europe in oral form. Conjugated estrogens, particularly the sulfate esters of estrone, equilin, and other native compounds, are still used widely by the oral route in the United States. Oily preparations of aryl and alkyl esters of estradiol are intended for intramuscular administration.

It is worthy of note that the dose of estrogen used for postmenopausal HRT is substantially less than that used in oral contraception. Accordingly, ethinyl estradiol is unsuited for HRT.

The protective effect of HRT on bone is well established. When given at a minimal effective dose of 0.625 mg per day of conjugated estrogen or its equivalent, HRT preserves bone density in all areas of the skeleton, and this effect is virtually maintained for as long as HRT is given. Furthermore, the risk of osteoporotic fractures of both wrist and hip is reduced by approximately 50% in women who begin HRT within the first 3 years of menopause and continue it for 6 to 9 years. Vertebral fractures are also significantly reduced. Interestingly, the effectiveness of combined HRT in preventing fractures appears to be similar to that of unopposed estrogen therapy. Consequently, all women at high risk for osteoporosis – and coronary artery disease – should be offered long-term HRT, unless contraindicated. Women without risk factors should be allowed to make their own informed decision based on knowledge of the benefits and risks of HRT.

The optimal timing and duration of HRT for osteoporosis are uncertain. The rationale for starting treatment at menopause is that the skeleton will be preserved before significant bone loss has occurred. At this time, the beneficial effects of HRT on postmenopausal symptoms may improve compliance. It is generally admitted that HRT should be continued for at least 7 to 10 years beyond menopause for satisfactory bone protection. Since discontinuation of estrogens is followed by immediate resumption of bone loss, longer-term or even lifelong use has been advocated. Recent evidence suggests that long-term HRT initiated many years after menopause is also effective in preserving bone mass. Thus, HRT has been approved for both prevention and treatment of osteoporosis in several countries, including the United States.

Pharmacokinetics

Whatever the route of administration, absorption of estrogens is generally good in accordance with their lipophilicity. However, transdermal patches not only avoid the first-pass metabolic effect but also provide more constant plasma levels than are obtained with oral doses. Ester derivatives are rapidly hydrolyzed by a variety of esterases, thereby producing the active compound. Estradiol undergoes primarily extensive biotransformation to estrone, which is converted to estriol.

In summary, due largely to differences in metabolism, the potencies of various estrogen preparations differ widely. In this respect, comparable bone responses are obtained from daily administration of 0.625 mg oral conjugated estrogens, 2 mg oral estradiol, 0.05 mg transdermal estradiol, and 1.5 g percutaneous gel (containing 1.5 mg estradiol).

Mode of use

All forms of estrogens are effective in the prevention of bone loss, provided that an adequate plasma concentration is obtained. Unopposed estrogen therapy should be considered only in women who have had a hysterectomy. Various progestogens may be used, including medroxyprogesterone acetate 5 to 10 mg and norethindrone 0.35 to 0.7 mg. The former is used more commonly.

Estrogens may be administered continuously or in 28-day or 1-month cycles consisting of 21 or 25 days of treatment followed by a 1-week or 5-day treatment-free interval. As stated earlier, the inclusion of a progestogen for 12 to 14 consecutive days of each month is recommended. This will result in regular withdrawal bleeding in 50 to 80% of women. Withdrawal bleeding is a major reason for noncompliance in women over age 65. Therefore, continuous combined therapy should be considered for these patients (see Chap. 67).

Side effects

Early adverse effects of HRT include typical dose-related estrogenic effects such as upper gastrointestinal symptoms (e.g., nausea, vomiting), breast tenderness, headaches, fluid retention, vaginal spotting or bleeding. HRT also may reactivate endometriosis. Transdermal patches may cause local skin reactions that consist usually of mild erythema and itching. Estrogens have various metabolic effects. Besides improvement in the lipid profile, oral estrogens may slightly alter carbohydrate metabolism and increase the biliary cholesterol saturation index and plasma levels of renin and some clotting factors. These effects are virtually abolished by transdermal administration of 17β-estradiol.

The primary danger of HRT relates to malignancies. Unopposed estrogen therapy is associated with an increased risk of endometrial cancer depending on dose and duration of use. With 5 or more years of use, there is at least a fivefold increase in risk of endometrial carcinoma. This risk is prevented in a duration-dependent fashion by the addition of cyclic progestogen therapy.

The most controversial issue is that of breast cancer risk. A recent collaborative reanalysis of the worldwide data on this topic confirmed that breast cancer risk depends on the duration of HRT. The relative risk of having breast cancer was 1.35 (95% confidence interval, 1.21-1.49) for women who had undergone HRT for 5 years or longer. It appeared to be greater for women of lower rather than higher weight or body-mass index. These cancers are less advanced clinically than those diagnosed in never-users of HRT. However, it is unknown whether HRT affects mortality from breast cancer. Finally, the risk of breast cancer associated with HRT decreases after cessation of use of estrogens and has largely, if not wholly, disappeared after 5 years.

Contraindications

Absolute contraindications to HRT are breast cancer, active liver disease or vascular thrombosis, and a history of unexplained vaginal bleeding. Caution is warranted and low initial dosages of estrogens are preferred in the following conditions: migraine, chronic hepatic dysfunction, uterine leiomyomas, history of uterine cancer, thromboembolism and endometriosis, gallbladder disease, familial hypertriglyceridemia, and strong family history of breast cancer. Moreover, low doses of estrogen should be used at the beginning of HRT in women over age 65.

BISPHOSPHONATES

Bisphosphonates are carbon-substituted analogues of pyrophosphate, an endogenous inhibitor of tissue calcification that has a strong affinity for bone. Unlike pyrophosphate, bisphosphonates are resistant to enzymatic hydrolysis owing to their phosphate-carbon-phosphate (P_i–C–P_i) bond. Their major effects are to inhibit skeletal or extraskeletal calcifications and osteoclast-mediated bone resorption. The inhibition of mineralization appears to be linked to their P_i–C–P_i structure, whereas the side chain seems to play a role in their antiresorptive potency.

As a class, bisphosphonates are capable of increasing the bone mineral density in postmenopausal patients with established osteoporosis. This increase is modest (2-10% depending on the skeletal site measured and the drug used) and may level off after 2 to 3 years of therapy. Etidronate and alendronate are both widely employed for the management of osteoporosis.

The license of etidronate is based on two randomized, double-blind studies suggesting that intermittent cyclic etidronate (400 mg per day for 2 weeks followed by 11-13 weeks of calcium supplementation alone) over 2 to 3 years may offer protection against new vertebral fractures, especially in women with severe osteoporosis (high initial number of fractures and low bone mass) and possibly accelerated bone loss. Neither study had adequate statistical power to detect changes in overall vertebral fracture rate. Furthermore, the effect of etidronate on the nonvertebral fracture rate is not established. Subsequently, etidronate was approved only for the treatment of vertebral osteoporosis with preexisting fragility fractures (in France) and/or bone-density criteria for osteoporosis (in Canada).

A large 3-year placebo-controlled trial of women with postmenopausal osteoporosis showed that alendronate given at the optimal daily dose of 10 mg resulted in a 48% reduction in the proportion of patients with new vertebral fractures. Similarly, 4 years of alendronate therapy in osteoporotic women without preexisting vertebral fractures decreased the incidence of vertebral fractures by 44% compared with placebo. A metaanalysis of clinical trials indicates that alendronate reduced the risk of nonvertebral fractures in postmenopausal women with osteoporosis. Thus, the estimated cumulative nonvertebral fracture rate after 3 years was 12.6% in the placebo group and 9% in the alendronate group. Consistent with these findings, alendronate is licensed in many countries for treatment of both vertebral and nonvertebral postmenopausal osteoporosis.

Bisphosphonates also may be beneficial in preventing bone loss in early postmenopausal women who are not undergoing HRT and may be useful in the management of different forms of secondary osteoporosis. For instance, cyclic etidronate as well as alendronate and risedronate were reported to reverse partially or prevent bone loss induced by glucocorticoids.

Major molecules

Sodium etidronate is the prototype and most potent mineralization inhibitor in this class of drugs. This property led to its use in heterotopic calcification following hip surgery or paraplegia. However, inhibition of mineralization occurs at close to the dose effective in inhibiting bone resorption, so long-term administration of etidronate may result in osteomalacia. Second- and third-generation bisphosphonates are characterized by greater potency than etidronate for the inhibition of bone resorption without increased effects on mineralization.

Clodronate and tiludronate show a 10-fold greater potency than etidronate. All three have received approval in different countries for the treatment of Paget's disease and/or hypercalcaemia of malignancy. Pamidronate is 100 times more potent than etidronate. Since it is available primarily for parenteral administration, it is approved for management of hypercalcaemia and adjunctive treatment in patients with multiple myeloma. Alendronate, risedronate, and ibandronate have at least a 500- to 1000-fold greater antiresorptive potency than etidronate.

Pharmacokinetics

The absorption of orally administered bisphosphonates is very poor, ranging from 0.6 to 5% of the dose, and decreases even further in the presence of calcium-containing foods or other divalent cations that chelate these drugs. The plasma elimination half-life of bisphosphonates is short (0.3-2 hours), in part related to rapid skeletal uptake. Between 20 and 60% of the absorbed dose is taken up by the skeleton, the remainder being excreted unchanged in the urine. The elimination of bisphosphonates from the skeleton is extremely slow, occurring only during active bone resorption. This accounts for the prolonged skeletal effects of these drugs.

Mode of use

Etidronate must be given in a cyclic, intermittent regimen, 400 mg per day for 2 weeks every 3 months. Calcium supplementation (500 mg per day), exclusive of dietary calcium, is given during the rest of the 3-month cycle. Conversely, alendronate is given continuously as a daily dose of 10 mg; calcium is not included in the formulation but is recommended in patients with a low dietary calcium intake. Patients should be advised to take bisphosphonates in an empty stomach, at least 30 minutes before the next meal. Furthermore, alendronate must be taken with a minimum of 200 ml of water after rising in the morning, and patients are instructed not to lie down for 30 minutes afterwards and until they have eaten their breakfast.

The duration of treatment is an unresolved clinical issue. Although etidronate and alendronate are licensed for a treatment period of 3 years only in some countries, no maximum treatment period is stipulated in other countries.

Side effects

The bisphosphonates are generally well tolerated. The most frequently reported side effects are gastrointestinal symptoms such as abdominal pain, nausea, dyspepsia, and diarrhea. Alendronate may have adverse effects on the esophagus, including chemical esophagitis that justifies specific administration instructions. Transient altered taste or asymptomatic decreases in the serum calcium level and, rarely, hypersensitivity reactions, including pruritus, urticaria, and other rashes, and angioedema also have been reported in osteoporotic patients receiving bisphosphonates.

During long-term therapy with bisphosphonates, two major clinical issues need to be considered. The first concerns the quality of newly formed bone. Continuous administration of etidronate leads to inhibition of mineralization, resulting in osteomalacia. This side effect is virtually abolished by the cyclic regimen used in osteoporosis. Newer, more potent bisphosphonates do not show such osteomalacic potential, so continuous use is conceivable. The second issue concerns the possible suppression of bone turnover to a degree that may impair the ability of bone to remodel. Since remodeling is the principal method for self-repair of fatigue damage and response to changes in stress, this may give rise to skeletal failure and spontaneous fractures. Fortunately, there is no evidence that bisphosphonates compromise the biomechanical competence of bone.

Contraindications

Bisphosphonates are contraindicated in the following circumstances: hypersensitivity to these drugs, hypocalcaemia, and advanced renal failure. In addition, alendronate is contraindicated in patients with any disorder that affects esophageal emptying, such as stricture or achalasia, and in patients who are unable to stand or sit upright for at least 30 minutes. Finally, alendronate should be used with caution in women with dyspepsia, dysphagia, or other active gastrointestinal disease.

CALCITONIN

Calcitonin is a single-chain peptide hormone of 32 amino acid residues that possesses specific receptors on the osteoclasts. Its inhibitory effect on osteoclastic activity is used in diseases characterized by excessive bone resorption, such as Paget's disease, hypercalcemia, or algodystrophy. The place of calcitonin in the management of osteoporosis is much debated.

There have been few well-designed clinical trials with injectable calcitonins. Present evidence suggests that salmon calcitonin given daily or every other day at 50 or 100 IU along with calcium supplements may maintain bone density or produce a small increase in spinal bone mass in osteoporotic patients. However, there are no prospective data con-

firming a reduction of fracture rates in established osteoporosis. Conversely, nasal salmon calcitonin (50-200 IU per day) combined with calcium supplements (500 mg per day) may produce a slight dose-dependent increase in mineral bone density of the spine and reduce the overall rate of fractures in elderly women treated for 2 years.

Several short-term studies suggest that all forms of calcitonin may be effective in preventing bone loss in the early postmenopausal period. However, the effect on cortical bone is equivocal. Furthermore, there is inconsistency in the data regarding the preventive effect of nasal calcitonin, the optimal dose and regimen for which are far from clear. Overall, there is some concern that resistance to calcitonin may develop with time, and it is not proven that the apparent benefits of the drug are sustained beyond 2 years of therapy.

The approval status of calcitonin varies greatly among countries. Both parenteral and nasal preparations of calcitonin are approved for the treatment of postmenopausal osteoporosis in the United States, whereas in France parenteral forms only are approved for the management of pain due to osteoporotic vertebral fractures. The last indication is based on the analgesic properties of calcitonin, distinct from its antiosteoclastic effects. The consensus is that calcitonin is not a first-line agent but rather an alternative to other treatments of osteoporosis or conventional analgesics, respectively. It is fair to add that calcitonin is far more expensive than HRT and bisphosphonates.

Pharmaceutical forms

Apart from porcine calcitonin, extracted the from the pig thyroid gland, the available calcitonins are synthetic. These include salmon, human, and a derivative of eel calcitonin. There are interspecies differences in the amino acid composition of the calcitonins, and these differences are associated with different potencies. Both fish calcitonins are more potent than human calcitonin and act over a longer period.

The traditional route of calcitonin administration has been via sc or im injection. Considering the drawbacks to parenteral formulations, alternative delivery forms, especially nasal preparations, have been developed. A nasal spray of salmon calcitonin is presently available in various countries, including some European countries, Japan, and the United States.

Pharmacokinetics

Calcitonin is absorbed rapidly after either parenteral or nasal application. Peak plasma concentrations appear within 30 minutes. Absorption of intranasal calcitonin, however, is erratic. The biologic effects obtained after nasal administration of 200 IU are comparable with those of approximately 50 to 100 IU given parenterally. The plasma elimination half-life of the drug is less than 1 hour.

Mode of use

The usually recommended daily dose of calcitonin for the treatment of osteoporosis is 50 to 100 IU sc or 200 IU intranasally in alternating nostrils. In addition, patients should ensure adequate calcium and vitamin D intake. Similar doses of intranasal and parenteral formulations usually are given on a daily or alternate-day basis over a period of a few weeks for the treatment of acute pain associated to vertebral crush fractures.

Side effects

Unpleasant reactions are very common in patients receiving im or sc calcitonin such that up to a third of treated people discontinue therapy. The most frequent adverse effects are gastrointestinal symptoms (e.g., anorexia, nausea, vomiting, diarrhea, or a metallic taste) and vascular phenomena (e.g., flushing of the extremities, headache) followed by dermatologic changes (e.g., generalized or local rash at the injection site, pruritus). True allergic reactions, including urticaria and anaphylaxis, are rare but contraindicate further use of the compound. Most adverse effects are dose related and decrease in severity with duration of use. Nasal administration minimizes the systemic side effects of calcitonin and improves patient compliance. However, rhinitis and other nasal symptoms may occur.

CALCIUM

Optimal mineral accretion in the growing skeleton and subsequent maintenance of bone health depend partly on an adequate supply of calcium (Tab. 46.1). To ensure optimal bone health, adequate amounts of calcium should be consumed throughout life. There is general agreement that the best form of calcium is food sources. Thus the use of calcium supplements should be considered in subjects who do not meet their calcium requirements through dietary sources. Calcium supplements were shown to have beneficial effects on bone mass in women at least 3 years postmenopause. They are less effective in the years during or immediately after menopause. At present, there is no definitive evidence that calcium therapy alone reduces the risk of osteoporotic fractures. Finally, calcium supplementation is used mainly as an adjunct to other therapies of osteoporosis.

Pharmaceutical forms

Calcium supplements are available as different salts whose elemental calcium content is highly variable. Calcium carbonate contains 40% elemental calcium by weight, whereas calcium phosphate contains 31%, calcium citrate 24%, calcium lactate 13%, and calcium gluconate 9%. These exist in various forms (e.g., powder, liquid, tablets, chewable forms, and dissolvable tablets).

Pharmacokinetics

There are small, insignificant differences in the bioavailability of calcium among most proprietary preparations.

Since calcium citrate does not require gastric acid for optimal absorption, it has been suggested to consider use of this salt in older individuals with reduced gastric acid production. However, this does not matter if calcium supplements are taken with a meal. It is more important to divide the daily dose because the absorption of calcium salts is most efficient at individual doses of 500 mg or less. Overall, adequate vitamin D is essential for optimal absorption of calcium.

Side effects

Calcium salt preparations are usually well tolerated but may cause indigestion and constipation, especially at high doses. The chance of developing hypercalcemia or nephrolithiasis is virtually absent with doses up to 1.5 to 2 g elemental calcium daily. However, these problems may arise if the patient is receiving concomitantly vitamin D. Furthermore, caution should be exercised in supplementing patients who have a history of kidney stones because high calcium intakes may result in hypercalciuria. In addition, iron absorption can be decreased by many forms of calcium supplementation. Interestingly, though, calcium citrate may enhance iron absorption. Finally, calcium may interfere with absorption of certain medications such as tetracyclines, bisphosphonates, and fluoride.

VITAMIN D, ITS METABOLITES, AND ANALOGUES

Vitamin D is the name applied to two related lipid-soluble compounds, cholecalciferol (vitamin D_3) and ergocalciferol (vitamin D_2). The former is derived from the diet and from the skin by ultraviolet irradiation of 7-dehydrocholesterol, the principal provitamin found in animal tissues. The latter is derived from the ultraviolet irradiation of plant sterols, namely, ergosterol. There is no practical difference between vitamins D_3 and D_2 with respect to their metabolism and actions in humans.

Both dietary vitamin D and intrinsically synthesized vitamin D require a series of hydroxylations to become biologically active. The first step in the activation involves its conversion in the liver to a 25-hydroxylated derivative (25-hydroxycholecalciferol, or 25-OH-D_3, or alfacalcidiol). This is the major circulating vitamin D metabolite, which is commonly measured clinically to provide an index of vitamin D nutritional status. Its normal steady-state concentration is 15 to 50 ng/ml. The second step occurs mainly in the kidney. It involves further hydroxylation to either 24,25- or 1,25-dihydroxy derivatives. The 1α-hydroxylase is subject to tight regulatory control, such as the calcium and phosphate status of the individual. The primary active metabolite is 1,25-dihydroxycholecalciferol [1,25-(OH)2-D_3, or calcitriol]. It can be considered the hormonal form of vitamin D.

Calcitriol plays a major role in the regulation of calcium and phosphate homeostasis. Specifically, it facilitates their absorption from the small intestine and their reabsorption from the distal renal tubule as well as their mobilization from bone. This latter function requires the presence of parathyroid hormone. Furthermore, calcitriol plays a pivotal role in mineralization of the skeleton. It acts either directly (osteoblasts) or indirectly (osteoclasts) on cells that are involved in bone remodeling. Overall, by stimulating events in both bone formation and bone resorption, calcitriol serves to maintain the dynamic nature of bone, which contributes to keeping it healthy.

The mechanism of action of calcitriol resembles that of steroid hormones. It crosses the plasma membrane and interacts with a specific DNA-binding, zinc finger protein known as the *vitamin-D receptor* within the target cells. This ligand-receptor complex binds to a specific vitamin D–responsive element, thereby influencing gene transcription. For instance, calcitriol stimulates intestinal absorption of calcium through induction of calcium-transporting proteins.

The major therapeutic uses of vitamin D are the prevention and cure of nutritional and metabolic rickets or osteomalacia, the treatment of hypoparathyroidism, and the management of osteoporosis. In this respect, aging was found to be associated with a negative calcium balance, resulting in increased parathyroid hormone secretion and increased bone resorption. Thus, it was suggested to correct the calcium imbalance in the elderly by vitamin D supplementation. Annual injections of ergocalciferol (150000-300000 units) were shown to reduce fracture risk in the elderly, whereas daily doses of 400 IU cholecalciferol did not. Hip fractures and total nonvertebral fractures were reduced by 43 and 32%, respectively, compared with placebo in institutionalized elderly women receiving 800 IU vitamin D_3 and 1.2 g calcium supplements daily over 18 months. Finally, there is enough evidence for an effective public health approach to the prevention of osteoporotic fractures by supplementing elderly nursing home residents with calcium and vitamin D. Whether healthy ambulatory old people also may benefit from such supplementation is less clear.

Alfacalcidiol (calcifediol) and calcitriol were reported to have beneficial effects on bone mass in women with postmenopausal osteoporosis. Alfacalcidiol (0.5-1 mg per day) was shown to have a beneficial impact on vertebral fracture rates, spinal bone densities, and cortical thickness at least in Japanese patients (whose calcium consumption is quite low compared with other people). Accordingly, alfacalcidiol is approved for the treatment of osteoporosis in Japan. Calcitriol may have a modest effect in increasing bone mass, but it appears to have efficacy in preventing vertebral fractures in postmenopausal women with established osteoporosis. A daily dose of 0.5 mg or more is required for antifracture effects. Given the potential for hypercalcemia and hypercalciuria, calcitriol should be reserved for specialist use, possibly in patients with renal impairment, in whom parent vitamin D may not be as effective or there is intolerance to bisphosphonates.

Many preparations containing various doses of parent vitamin D are marketed for oral or intramuscular administration. Oral preparations combining 400 IU vitamin D_3 with 500 mg calcium are very popular in some European countries.

Alfacalcidiol (1α-OH-D_3) is a synthetic derivative that is readily converted to calcitriol in the liver. Therefore, it was introduced as a substitute for the latter compound. Dihydrotachysterol is the pure crystalline compound obtained by reducing vitamin D_2. Like alfacalcidiol, it is metabolized in the liver to the active form 25-OH-dihydrotachysterol. Calcifediol (25-OH-D_3) has also been launched. It bypasses hepatic hydroxylation and may be transformed into calcitriol in the kidney. Finally, calcitriol is available for oral use or injection.

Pharmacokinetics

Vitamin D_2 and D_3 usually are given by mouth. Bile is essential for their adequate absorption from the small intestine. Vitamin D and its metabolites are present in the blood complexed to vitamin D-binding protein, a specific α-globulin. The parent compound disappears from plasma with a half-life of about 24 hours, but it is stored in fat depots for prolonged periods. The main route of vitamin D excretion is the bile; only a small fraction is recovered in the urine. Vitamin D and its metabolites undergo extensive enterohepatic recirculation. Overall, the 25-OH derivative has a biologic half-life of 19 days. The plasma elimination half-life of calcitriol is short (5-8 hours), but its action may persist over 2 to 4 days.

Side effects

The major adverse event of vitamin D therapy is hypervitaminosis D, whose initial signs and symptoms are those associated with hypercalcemia. Prolonged hypercalcemia or hypercalciuria may contribute to the development of nephrolithiasis or nephrocalcinosis and consequent decreases in renal function. Prolonged vitamin D intoxication also may induce osteoporosis. In fact, low doses of vitamin D (400-800 IU per day) are generally well tolerated. Conversely, the 1α-hydroxylated derivatives (i.e., calcitriol, alfacalcidiol, and dihydrotachysterol) have relatively narrow therapeutic windows, so the plasma calcium level and renal function should be checked regularly, especially after a change in dose and in patients with a high calcium intake or concomitant thiazide diuretic use.

FLUORIDE

Fluoride markedly stimulates osteoblastic bone formation. This leads to defective bone mineralization that may be prevented by concurrent calcium and vitamin D administration. Although fluoride has been approved by regulatory agencies in several European countries, its status as a therapy for osteoporosis is controversial. Fluoride induces a dose-dependent increase in cancellous bone mass. Effects at the spine are dramatic, as shown by an increase in lumbar spine bone density of about 5% per year in postmenopausal women receiving a 50-mg daily dose of sodium fluoride. However, up to 40% of patients are unresponsive to fluoride. The major concern is that the increase in bone density does not correlate with an increase in bone strength. Continuous use of 50-mg daily doses of sodium fluoride or its equivalent along with calcium (and sometimes vitamin D) for 2 to 4 years was not shown clearly to reduce the fracture rates in postmenopausal osteoporotic women. Conversely, a recent study suggests that an intermittent regimen of slow-release sodium fluoride (50 mg per day) in conjunction with continuous calcium intake for 4 years may be safe and effective in inhibiting new vertebral fractures in established postmenopausal osteoporosis.

Pharmaceutical forms

Preparations of fluoride include sodium fluoride as a tablet and enteric-coated or sustained-release formulations. Disodium monofluorophosphate is available in some European countries. A dose of 100 mg is equivalent to 13.2 mg fluoride ion and about 30 mg sodium fluoride.

Pharmacokinetics

Sodium fluoride solutions are almost completely absorbed. The use of enteric-coated and sustained-release formulations leads to decreased bioavailability and greater intersubject variability in absorption. With the exception of monofluorophosphate salts, bioavailability is significantly reduced in the presence of food, calcium, and antacids. Fluoride is primarily deposited in bone, especially in sites with great metabolic activity. The resulting patchy distribution of fluoride within the skeleton may account for the heterogeneity of clinical response and for the induction of stress fractures. Fluoride is mainly excreted via the kidneys.

Mode of use

Although the optimal treatment schedule needs to be determined, fluoride is usually approved for the treatment of established postmenopausal osteoporosis at a continuous regimen of 50 mg sodium fluoride or 200 mg disodium monofluorophosphate daily for a few years together with calcium supplements (1 g per day) and even physiologic doses of vitamin D.

Side effects

A syndrome of lower extremity periarticular pain is common in fluoride-treated patients. Its incidence is dose-dependent, and it resolves usually within 4 to 8 weeks on withdrawal of fluoride. It is often related to microfractures or even stress fractures. The latter are likely due to high focal concentrations of fluoride that inhibit the repair of microfractures. Other side effects include gastrointestinal irritation that is markedly reduced by use of enteric-coated and sustained-release formulations of sodium fluoride as well as monofluorophosphate salt preparations.

Contraindications

Fluoride is contraindicated in patients with renal failure. The presence of osteomalacia must be excluded before fluoride therapy is started.

New areas of drug development

Other therapies are currently used in some countries for the treatment of postmenopausal osteoporosis, such as ipriflavone, a synthetic isoflavonoid derivative that inhibits bone resorption. Anabolic steroids, especially transdermal testosterone, are useful in the management of osteoporosis in men with hypogonadism.

New therapeutic approaches to osteoporosis are currently in development. There is increasing interest in developing compounds with estrogen agonist/antagonist effects like tamoxifen. These tissue-specific estrogens such as raloxifene are currently referred to as selective "estrogen-receptor modulators" (SERM). They should preserve bone mineral density without adversely affecting breast or uterine tissue. Raloxifene, a drug with this type of profile, has recently entered the US market. Direct inhibitors of osteoclasts are also being investigated. Strontium salts may both decrease the number of active osteoclasts and promote bone formation. Other stimulators of bone formation are at various stages of preclinical and clinical testing: parathyroid hormone peptides and analogues, bone growth factors, and silicon derivatives. These, together with improved formulations or regimens of existing therapies, should lead to improvements in the prevention and management of osteoporosis in the near future.

Suggested readings

Bannwarth B, Schaeverbeke T, Dehais J. Calcitonin and osteoporosis: Fact and fiction. Rev Rheumatol Engl Ed 1995;62:3-6.

Belchetz PE. Hormonal treatment of postmenopausal women. N Engl J Med 1994;330:1062-71.

Briançon D. Fluoride and osteoporosis: an overview. Rev Rheumatol Engl Ed 1997;64:78-81.

Chapuy MC, Meunier PJ. Prevention and treatment of osteoporosis. Aging (Milano) 1995;7:164-73.

Collaborative Group on Hormonal Factors in Breast Cancer. Breast cancer and hormone replacement therapy: collaborative reanalysis of data from 51 epidemiodogical studies of 52,705 women with breast cancer and 108,411 women without breast cancer. Lancet 1997;350:1047-59.

Compston JE. Prevention and management of osteoporosis: current trends and future prospects. Drugs 1997;53:727-35.

Hardman JG, Limbird LE, Molinoff PB, et al. Goodman and Gilman's The pharmacological basis of therapeutics, 9th ed. New York, McGraw-Hill, 1996.

Jeal W, Barradell LB, McTavish D. Alendronate: a review of its pharmacological properties and therapeutic efficacy in postmenopausal osteoporosis. Drugs 1997;53:415-34.

Jones G, Hogan DB, Yendt E, Hanley DA. Vitamin D

metabolites and analogues in the treatment of osteoporosis. Can Med Assoc J 1996;155:955-61.

KANIS JA. Osteoporosis, Oxford: Blackwell, 1994.

KARPF DB, SHAPIRO DR, SEEMAN E, et al. Prevention of non-vertebral fractures by alendronate: a metaanalysis. JAMA 1997;277:1159-64.

MURRAY TM, STE-MARIE LG. Fluoride therapy for osteoporosis. Can Med Assoc J 1996;155:949-54.

PATEL S. Current and potential future drug treatments for osteo-porosis. Ann Rheum Dis 1996;55:700-14.

SCIENTIFIC ADVISORY BOARD, OSTEOPOROSIS SOCIETY OF CANADA. Clinical practice guidelines for the diagnosis and management of osteoporosis. Can Med Assoc J 1996;155:1113-33.

SILVERMAN SL. Calcitonin. Am J Med Sci 1997;313:13-16.

47

Lupus and autoimmune disorders

Reinhold E. Schmidt, Torsten Witte

Systemic lupus erythematosus (SLE) is still the prototypical model of autoimmune diseases. The diseas presents with a variety of different signs and symptoms and may affect every organ system, ranging from superficial cutaneous manifestations to deep organ involvement (e.g., pleuritis, pneumonia, pericarditis, and nephritis) and to central nervous system affections (e.g., change in consciousness, seizures, and strokes). Diagnosis and treatment of SLE still remain a challenge even for experienced clinicians.

Disease presentation

Skin manifestations in SLE, i.e., malar rash, discoid lupus, photosensitivity, and aphthous ulceration, represent four of the eleven American Rheumatism Association (ARA) classification criteria of SLE. Since four criteria are sufficient to make the diagnosis of SLE, this points to their importance.

The so-called malar or butterfly rash is the classic cutaneous symptom of lupus and is described as fixed erythema, flat or bulging, over malar eminences, tending to spare the perinasal and labial areas. Macular rashes of the disease may extend to other areas of the skin, especially those which are sun exposed. The so-called discoid lupus may appear anywhere on the skin. The aphthous ulceration is characterized as oral or nasopharyngeal ulceration, usually "painless". Another manifestation in the skin of lupus patients is subacute cutaneous lupus (SCLE), occurring in about 9% of patients. Additional presentations are alopecia or livedo reticularis. Livedo reticularis is a characteristic manifestation associated with antiphospholipid antibodies that may occur in patients with and without SLE. Other symptoms in patients with antiphospholipid antibodies are acrocyanosis, capillaritis, superficial thrombophlebitis, and Raynaud's phenomenon.

Polyarthralgia or polyarthritis is one of the most common features in SLE and occurs in about 90% of patients. Similar to rheumatoid arthritis, the small joints of the hands are involved, but in addition, muscle involvement also can be found, with myalgia and myositis. Additional musculoskeletal manifestations may present as tenosynovitis or tendon ruptures.

A renal disorder by the ARA criteria is defined by persistent proteinuria of more than 0.5 g per day or by cellular casts — red cell, hemoglobin, granular, tubular, or mixed. Renal manifestations occur in about 50% of the patients and represent a severe organ involvement.

A most frequent manifestation of SLE is pleurisy, which may occur with or without pleural effusion. Another presentation is lupus pneumonitis. However, acute pneumonitis can lead to chronic interstitial lung disease, and other pulmonary manifestations are bronchiolitis obliterans, pulmonary emboli, and pulmonary hypertension. Pericarditis occurs in 25% of SLE patients and is found in more than 60% of patients at autopsy. Another frequent cardiac manifestation is valvular disease, most often involving the mitral valve.

According to the ARA criteria, major central nervous system (CNS) manifestations include seizures and psychosis. The long list of CNS manifestations due to lupus also includes organic brain syndrome, visual scotomata, retinopathy, cranial neuropathy, lupus headache, stroke mononeuritis multiplex, transverse myelitis, peripheral neuropathy, chorea meningitis, and cognitive impairment. Seizures are a very frequent symptom. They have been reported in more than half of patients. Psychosis is a rare event, occurring mostly during the first year of active SLE. All other symptoms are very difficult to discriminate from those of demyelinating diseases such as multiple sclerosis.

Hematologic symptoms are defined by hemolytic anemia, leukopenia, and lymphopenia, as well as by thrombocytopenia. Anemia can be found in more than 50% of patients and usually is due to chronic inflammatory disease. It also can be caused by hypersplenomegaly or autoimmune hemolytic anemia. Thrombocytopenia can be found in 15 to 50% of patients and usually is due to reduced platelet survival, i.e., autoimmune thrombocytopenic purpura. Lymphopenia is a characteristic feature of SLE; erythrocytopenia is a rarer event.

Diagnostic criteria

The American College of Rheumatology (ACR) criteria for SLE include:
1. Butterfly exanthema
2. Discoid lesions of the skin
3. Photosensitivity
4. Oral ulcerations
5. Arthritis and arthralgia
6. Serositis
7. Renal involvement
8. Neurologic involvement
9. Hematologic disturbance
10. Immunologic disturbance
    a. dsDNA antibody
    b. SM antibody
    c. Phospholipid antibodies
11. Antinuclear antibody

Four of these eleven criteria should be present to establish a diagnosis of SLE.

For the treatment of SLE, determination of the type of organ involvement or measurement of disease activity is critical. A number of measurements to evaluate disease activity have been developed. Examples include the SLEDAI, SLAM, and ELAM scores. Other criteria for disease activity include determination of clinical fluctuations and/or laboratory parameters such as complement levels, plasma complement split products, or anti-double stranded DNA antibodies.

Treatment

Treatments of general use in the disease

Drug therapy in SLE is based on three principles: anti-inflammatory agents, antimalarial agents, and immunosuppressive drugs. Nonsteroidal anti-inflammatory drugs (NSAIDs) are still the main form of treatment for lupus arthritis, fever, and serositis. Antimalarial drugs, particularly chloroquine and hydroxychloroquine, are reserved for long-term treatment. They are particularly recommended for SLE patients with skin manifestations, and they also are used as part of therapy for organic forms of the disease such as arthritis and arthralgia, as well as for serositis. In a recent double-blind, randomized study, patients taking hydroxychloroquine were found to have a lower incidence of flares and a low risk of disease exacerbation.

The cornerstone of SLE therapy is still systemic corticosteroid therapy. Steroids are always used at the beginning of SLE therapy, as well as to control life-threatening complications. Dosage should be adjusted according to the activity and duration of the disease.

Steroids are very effective in eliminating the inflammatory symptoms of SLE. However, for long-term immunosuppression, as well as for stopping disease progression, such immunosuppressants as azathioprine, cyclophosphamide, or methotrexate are necessary. These agents also help to control the activity and frequency of flare-ups in SLE.

Basic principles and aims of treatment

If the major clinical manifestation is fever, it is very critical to rule out an infection or drug fever. Therapy should be started with NSAIDs, and only when infection has been ruled out should low-dose prednisone be added. In patients with weight loss, gastrointestinal lupus or malignancy should be excluded. In the presence of general fatigue, depression and myalgia should be ruled out.

Drug classes

FIRST-CHOICE DRUGS

Nonsteroidal anti-inflammatory drugs (NSAIDs)

There are usually two situations in which the SLE patient is adequately treated with NSAIDs. Most frequently, one of the first symptoms with which patients present is arthralgia. Since the diagnosis usually has not yet been made, NSAIDs such as diclofenac, ibuprofen, aspirin, or piroxicam are prescribed (see Chap. 44). These drugs are no longer indicated if a patient is receiving more than 30 mg prednisone per day, when the ulcerogenic potential may exceed the benefit. NSAIDs also may be useful for small flare-ups of arthralgia when the patient is on a small daily dosage of prednisone.

Corticosteroids

Introduction of high-dose systemic steroid treatment has dramatically improved the prognosis of SLE. Initiation of steroids, particularly in major active flare-ups, is always necessary when an infectious agent has been excluded. The mode of application, as well as the dose, of steroid medication depends on the severity of clinical symptoms. In minor flare-ups, e.g. skin manifestations, muscle or skeletal system involvement, serositis, or Raynaud's phenomenon, initial doses of 25 to 50 mg of prednisone are usually sufficient.

In severe, life-threatening flare-ups, including lupus nephritis, CNS involvement, pleuropericarditis, or necrotizing vasculitis, treatment usually begins with doses around 1 to 2 mg/kg of body weight. Low doses should be given once in the morning; higher doses can be divided into two doses. Alternatively, high-dose methylprednisolone (500-1000 mg) can be given iv on three subsequent days. However, the efficacy of this high-dose steroid regimen has not yet been proven in large trials.

Usually there is a rapid response to steroid treatment, allowing a reduction in prednisone doses. A good rule of thumb is to halve the dose over double time, e.g., 200 mg for 3 days, 100 mg for 6 days, 50 mg for 12 days, etc. The lower the dose, the more slowly a reduction should be carried out. In patients with severe organ involvement, additional immunosuppressive therapy should be started to keep the response under control.

Antimalarial drugs

Two forms of antimalarials are used in lupus therapy:

chloroquine and hydroxychloroquine (see Chap. 42). Antimalarials are mandatory in patients with cutaneous lupus and in those with systemic disease with predominant skin and joint involvement; they are also used to spare the patient from long-term steroids. Chloroquine is started at 250 mg orally bid and is then reduced to 250 mg per day after 2 weeks.

Antimalarials are usually well tolerated. Side effects include changes in blood counts, liver toxicity, and allergic reactions. Every 4 months, ophthalmologic examination should be performed to detect the deposition of chloroquine in the cornea and retina. If this rare side effect is observed, chloroquine should be discontinued; the deposits will disappear shortly. Antimalarials can be given up to a total dose of 100 g. This is approximately equivalent to 2 years of treatment with one tablet daily.

IMMUNOSUPPRESSIVE DRUGS

Antimetabolites

The purine analogue azathioprine derivative of 6-mercaptopurine is the most widely used immunosuppressant (see Chap. 75). This drug usually is indicated after steroids have induced a good response in light to moderately severe cases. The main indication is to lower the dose of steroids without risking a new flare-up. The general daily dose recommendation is 2 to 4 mg/kg of body weight orally. Generally, 50 mg of azathioprine is given three times daily in addition to prednisone treatment. Efficacy of azathioprine is seen only after 3 to 4 weeks of treatment. Thereafter, a reduction in steroid doses may be considered. Azathioprine can be administered for many years without any problems. Frequently, steroids can be discontinued completely.

Azathioprine should be stopped if there is no steroid-sparing effect, when relapses occur during treatment, in the presence of bone marrow or liver toxicity, and when pregnancy is planned or is ongoing.

In general azathioprine is a well-tolerated immunosuppressant. Toxic allergic reactions are seen in only 5% of SLE patients and include hepatitis, fever, stomach ache, exanthema, and cholestasis. No teratogenic side effects have been observed, even though many children have been born under azathioprine treatment. Only a slightly increased incidence of non-Hodgkin's lymphoma during azathioprine therapy has been observed.

Methotrexate

Methotrexate has achieved a well-recognized place in the treatment of rheumatoid arthritis (see Chap. 44). In SLE, there are still no controlled studies on the initiation of methotrexate prior to azathioprine. Usually, methotrexate or cyclophosphamide is used only after failure of one or the other drug. Dosing is in the range of 15 to 25 mg of methotrexate per week. It can be given orally or intravenously.

The most severe side effects of methotrexate are bone marrow toxicity, mucositis, diarrhea, allergic skin rashes, and liver toxicity. In addition, interstitial pneumonitis is a well-described side effect. A problem for SLE treatment is that many of the disease symptoms are similar to the side effects of methotrexate. Therefore, use of this drug in SLE must be considered carefully. Methotrexate is not indicated during pregnancy.

ALKYLATING DRUGS

Cyclophosphamide

For a long time it was unclear whether the use of alkylating drugs is at all justified in the treatment of autoimmune diseases. Early on, Austin et al. observed that only alkylating drugs can really stop the progression of active lupus nephritis. As a result, many controlled studies subsequently have clearly proved the efficacy of cyclophosphamide.

Cyclophosphamide (see Chap. 49) is given orally in daily doses of 2 to 3 mg/kg of body weight, and intravenous doses of 500 to 1000 mg/m^2 are given once every 2 to 4 weeks. In life-threatening situations, iv treatment is far superior in terms of efficacy and incidence of side effects such as infectious complications, suppression of hematopoesis, etc. An intravenous bolus of 500 to 1000 mg/m^2 is a well-accepted standard form of treatment. Drug therapy should be combined with adequate liquid volume and protected by intravenous application of MESNA. Twenty percent of the dose of cyclophosphamide should be given at 0, 4, and 8 hours after the start of cyclophosphamide. Usually, a frequency of 3 to 6 applications of cyclophosphamide is sufficient to control lupus nephritis.

Suggested readings _____

AUSTIN HA, KLIPPEL JH, BALOW JE, et al. Therapy of lupus nephritis: controlled trial of prednisone and cytotoxic drugs. N Engl J Med 1986;314:614-9.

AUSTIN HA, MUENZ LR, JOYCE KM, et al. Prognostic factors in lupus nephritis: contribution of renal histologic data. Am J Med 1983;75:382-91.

HOCHBERG MC. Updating the American College of Rheumatology revised criteria for the classification of systemic lupus erythematosus. Arthritis Rheum 1997; 40:1725.

48

New areas of drug development

Dirk O. Stichtenoth, Jürgen C. Frölich

Rheumatic diseases, i.e., inflammatory and noninflammatory affections of the joints, bones, muscles, tendons, and connective tissues, constitute a wide field for drug development. However, most efforts have been spent in the autoimmune rheumatic disorders, for which rheumatoid arthritis (RA) serves as a paradigm. The care of primarily noninflammatory rheumatic diseases is in the domain of physical and orthopedic treatments. Thus, new drug development generally has not been impressive.

In recent years, three promising lines in the development of new treatments for rheumatic diseases have been emerged:

• *New nonsteroidal anti-inflammatory drugs (NSAIDs): Selective COX-2 inhibitors.* The development of NSAIDs with selectivity for inducible cyclooxygenase (COX-2; see below) will provide drugs with no better efficacy but much fewer side effects compared with conventional NSAIDs. This is of great clinical and epidemiologic importance because NSAIDs are the most often prescribed drugs (and also are available without prescription) for the treatment of a wide variety of rheumatic diseases and pain. It is estimated that up to 80% of fatal gastric ulcer complications and 3% of acute and 30% of chronic renal failures are caused by NSAIDs. In a retrospective epidemiologic study in Finland, 3% of the overall mortality in RA patients was attributable to antirheumatic medications, and nearly two-thirds of these drug-induced deaths were caused by NSAID treatment.

• *New disease-modifying drugs (DMARDs).* There is a plethora of potentially useful agents for disease-modifying therapy. In particular, the following approaches are noteworthy: anticytokine therapy, inhibition of metalloproteinases, leflunomide, and nondepleting T-cell antibodies. Most promising, anticytokine treatment directed against interleukin 1 or tumor necrosis factor alpha has now reached the clinic. We wonder whether advances in the rapidly growing field of molecular biology and pharmacology will give us a new armamentarium for the treatment of chronic inflammatory joint diseases.

• *New treatment strategies for RA using currently available DMARDs.* In contrast to the traditional pyramidal approach, which has proven insufficient in the control of

disease progression, new strategies such as the "sawtooth strategy" or the "step-down bridge" (see Table 45.1) propose an earlier initiation of DMARDs, a more aggressive use of DMARDs, together with glucocorticoids or NSAIDs and the combination of two or more DMARDs. So far experience with these new strategies reveals better control of the disease with a tolerable increase in adverse effects. However, RA progresses in one-fourth of patients despite more intensive treatment. The major obstacle to controlling RA is the delay between onset of the disease, diagnosis, and institution of effective drugs. Thus the overall management of RA needs improvement. Since this chapter focuses on new drugs, we will not discuss the new treatment strategies in detail.

From the point of view of a clinical pharmacologist evaluation of in vitro testing, animal experiments and even phase II studies provide only hints about the possible clinical usefulness of a new treatment modality, which must be proven in large-scale, double-blind, controlled, randomized studies with head-to-head comparisons with established DMARDs. The use of validated study parameters for efficacy is a major requirement. For example, tenidap and γ-interferon emerged in early studies as useful drugs for the treatment of the RA. Following phase III trials, however, γ-interferon was not further investigated because of poor efficacy; moreover, the launching of tenidap was stopped because of concerns about its risk-benefit ratio. The same pattern was seen in trials with depleting anti-CD4 antibodies: open pilot studies resulted in positive clinical benefit, whereas double-blind trials showed no benefit. Thus, in the following detailed analysis of new treatment strategies, it is necessary not to misinterpret positive results in early studies as proof of clinical usefulness.

NONSTEROIDAL ANTI-INFLAMMATORY DRUGS (NSAIDs): SELECTIVE COX-2 INHIBITORS

In 1971 it was discovered that NSAIDs exert their major therapeutic and adverse effects by inhibition of cyclooxygenase (COX). COX is a key enzyme of prostanoid synthesis, catalyzing the reaction from arachidonic acid to the cyclic endoperoxide prostaglandin G_2 and in a second step to prostaglandin H_2, which is further metabolized to various prostaglandins, prostacyclin (PGI_2) and thromboxane A_2 (TXA_2). As autacoids, these prostanoids are involved in many physiologic and pathophysiologic mechanisms. For example, in the gastrointestinal tract, prostaglandin E_2 (PGE_2) and PGI_2 maintain mucosal blood flow and bicarbonate and mucus secretion for the integrity of the mucosa. In the kidney, PGE_2 and PGI_2 are essential to maintain renal blood flow and glomerular filtration rate, in particular in patients with impaired renal function and in those with disorders characterized by a low effective plasma volume. Furthermore, prostanoids are potent antagonists of antidiuretic hormone action; they directly inhibit tubular sodium reabsorption, and they mediate renin release in the macula densa. In the cardiovascular system, prostanoids regulate the tone of arteries and veins. In pathophysiologic conditions, prostanoids are mediators of inflammation and fever, and they sensitize pain receptors. Thus, inhibition of prostanoid synthesis by NSAIDs leads to the desired analgesic, antipyretic, and anti-inflammatory effects but also leads to a disturbance of homeostatic prostanoid production, causing the typical NSAID side effects of gastrointestinal ulceration, deterioration of renal function, and inhibition of platelet aggregation. In addition, aspirin-induced asthma is linked to inhibition of COX, but the exact mechanism is not known. Furthermore, the interactions of NSAIDs with lithium and antihypertensive drugs are the result of COX inhibition.

Much effort has been expended on the avoidance of NSAID side effects. So far this work has been unsuccessful or only partially successful. Thus, comedication with misoprostol is an effective approach for prevention of NSAID-induced ulcer, but it provides no protection against NSAID side effects on kidney, platelet aggregation, and regulation of blood flow. A new and promising pharmacologic strategy is the selective inhibition of the inducible COX (Fig. 48.1). This strategy is based on the discovery of two isoforms of the COX enzyme: a constitutive form, called *COX-1,* and an inducible isoenzyme, called *COX-2,* that is expressed after stimulation by cytokines or endotoxins. COX-2 is mainly localized to inflamed tissue. The human COX-1 and COX-2 genes are localized on chromosomes 9 and 1, respectively, and cover approximately 22 and 8 kilobases of DNA, respectively. The amino acid sequences of COX-1 and COX-2, both with a molecular weight of approximately 70 kDa, are only 60% homologous, but the residues lining the enzymatically active regions are highly conserved. Sequence homology between mammalian species is greater than 80%. The three-dimensional structures of COX-1 and COX-2, determined by X-ray crystallography, show a long hydrophobic channel where the sites for peroxidase and cyclooxygenase activity are adjacent. Compared with COX-1, in COX-2 this channel is much larger and has a side pocket and two topographically important changes in the amino acid sequence. These differences have profound implications for the design of

isoenzyme-selective NSAIDs; it is thus possible to produce compounds that can reach the active sites of COX-2 but not those of COX-1.

Whereas COX-1 is responsible for physiologic prostanoid synthesis, mucosal protection, platelet aggregation, maintenance of renal function, and regulation of blood flow, in contrast, COX-2 is the source of the enhanced synthesis of prostanoids in pathophysiologic conditions that contribute to the process and clinical signs of inflammation. A drug with selectivity for COX-2 thus would inhibit proinflammatory prostanoid synthesis while sparing physiologic prostanoid synthesis. Such a drug therefore would be anti-inflammatory with fewer or no typical NSAID adverse effects (Fig. 48.1).

The hypothesis that selective COX-2 inhibition is a promising strategy for the avoidance of NSAID side effects is supported by the following findings: first, studies on the gastrointestinal effects of various NSAIDs clearly show that the risk for ulceration, perforation, and bleeding is highest with piroxicam, acetylsalicylic acid, and indomethacin but less with ibuprofen, nabumetone, or diclofenac. These results correlate well with the selectivities of these drugs for the COX isoenzymes. Piroxicam, acetylsalicylic acid, and indomethacin preferably inhibit COX-1, whereas ibuprofen, nabumetone, and diclofenac inhibit both COX isoenzymes to a similar degree. Second, nonacetylated salicylates are selective COX-2 inhibitors. They possess an equipotent anti-inflammatory efficacy but do not inhibit platelet aggregation and seldom cause deterioration of renal function. The superficial injury of the gastric mucosa by salicylic acid is due to its local action and is not caused by COX inhibition. If this local effect is circumvented by use of the prodrug salsalate, which is cleaved in the body into two molecules of salicylic acid, nonacetylated salicylates seldom lead to gastrointestinal erosions or ulceration. Third, glucocorticoids are potent suppressors of COX-2 expression but without inhibitory activity on preformed COX. Despite their impressive anti-inflammatory actions, glucocorticoids alone are poorly ulcerogenic, and they do not impair renal function or platelet aggregation.

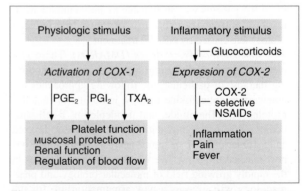

Figure 48.1 Strategy of selective COX-2 inhibition. Cyclooxygenase pathways and the effects of glucocorticoids and selective COX-2 inhibitors are depicted. (COX-1 = constitutive cyclooxygenase; COX-2 = inducible cyclooxygenase; PGE_2 = prostaglandin E_2; PGI_2 = prostacyclin; TXA_2 = thromboxane A_2.)

However, there are some issues concerning the strategy of selective COX-2 inhibition that need to be adressed to elucidate the COX pathways in health and disease:

- It is possible that COX-1 contributes to the proinflammatory prostanoid synthesis and vice versa that COX-2 contributes to the production of protective prostanoids. Crofford and coworkers showed that COX-1 is also induced by cytokines, suggesting a role for COX-1 in the inflammatory process. On the other hand, COX-2 was found in sizable quantities in almost every tissue, especially in the lung and prostate. In the kidneys, an immunohistologic study localized COX-2 immunoreactive protein to endothelial and smooth muscle cells of blood vessels and intraglomerularly in podocytes. Thus, it could be speculated that COX-2 may be involved to some degree in the regulation of renal perfusion and glomerular hemodynamics. Recently, we found in healthy volunteers that COX-2–selective meloxicam inhibits furosemide-stimulated plasma renin activity, suggesting that the COX isoenzyme responsible for renin release in humans is COX-2.
- In an animal model of transmural colitis induced by trinitrobenzene sulfonic acid, COX-2 expression in the inflamed area is markedly increased. Surprisingly, the highest increase in lethality due to gut perforation was seen after treatment with the highly selective COX-2 inhibitor L-745,337. The increase of lethality was less with COX-nonselective NSAIDs and not different from that with vehicle and acetylsalicylic acid. The results of this study suggest that enhanced COX-2 expression plays a protective role in this model of mucosal damage.
- Studies with mice that are genetically free of COX-2 (COX-2 knock-out mice) pointed out as yet unknown risks of COX-2 inhibition: these mice showed renal malformations and were susceptible to peritonitis. In addition, most of the animals died by the sixteenth week of age. However, in humans, COX-2 is detectable only at the end stage of renal development and is apparently not involved in organogenesis. Overall, this animal model is very helpful for pharmacologic studies but is far removed from the therapeutic situation.
- COX-2 is expressed in the pregnant uterus and may be the most important source of prostanoids.
- The in vitro testing of the COX selectivity of NSAIDs sometimes yielded discrepant results. For example, Gierse and coworkers found a more than 30-fold selectivity of naproxen for the COX-1, whereas the results of Mitchell and coworkers showed comparable inhibition of both COX isoenzymes by this NSAID. These discrepancies are caused by different in vitro test systems. Isolated enzymes, cell membranes, and whole cells from various tissues and species are used. In the in vivo situation, the high plasma protein binding and the pharmacokinetics, particulary the penetration of NSAIDs into the target cells, must be considered. Thus, the human whole-blood assay is a useful approach to measure inhibition of COX isoenzymes by NSAIDs in vitro and is used by most investigators. However, all in vitro results should be confirmed by animal experiments and finally in human studies. For assessment of the in vivo

synthesis of prostanoids, several index parameters are validated. Platelet aggregation and platelet thromboxane B_2 (TXB_2) formation in response to arachidonic acid are exclusively dependent on COX-1 and reflect activity of this COX isoenzyme. Urinary PGE-M and PGE_2 excretion rates are the index parameters of total-body and renal PGE_2 production, respectively. An appropriate study design with the use of gas chromatography-tandem mass spectrometry for prostanoid analysis is a requirement to obtain meaningful results.

NEW CLASSIFICATION OF NSAIDs

Since the usual chemical classification of NSAIDs does not consider their clinically relevant COX isoenzyme selectivity, a new classification of NSAIDs on the basis of their inhibitory activity on COX-1 and COX-2 is suggested: (1) *Selective COX-1 inhibitors.* This category comprises only low-dose acetylsalicylic acid, which inhibits selectively COX-1 in platelets. (2) *Nonselective COX inhibitors.* Most of the current NSAIDs inhibit both COX isoenzymes; they also impair platelet aggregation and cause significant gastrointestinal and renal side effects. A subclass of drugs with preference for COX-1, e.g., piroxicam or indomethacin, could be separated, and these have a higher risk of such adverse effects. (3) *Selective COX-2 inhibitors,* including nonacetylated salicylates and meloxicam. These drugs inhibit proinflammatory more than physiologic prostanoid synthesis. Thus, they have fewer adverse effects than nonselective COX inhibitors in equivalent anti-inflammatory dosages. (4) *Highly selective COX-2 inhibitors.* The experimental substances belonging to this category are expected to have none to minimal typical NSAID side effects. However, it is possible that complete COX-2 inhibition carries as yet unknown risks, and it is reasonable to consider that some COX-1 inhibition is needed for full anti-inflammatory efficacy.

Selective COX-2 inhibitors

The first NSAID, salicylic acid, is a selective COX-2 inhibitor. In vitro, nonacetylated salicylates are weak inhibitors of both isoenzymes. In a rat model of inflammatory exudate, sodium salicylate in a dose causing significant inhibition of prostaglandin synthesis in the inflamed tissue failed to inhibit COX activity in the gastric mucosa. In contrast, acetylsalicylic acid, indomethacin, naproxen, and flurbiprofen inhibited proinflammatory as well as protective prostaglandin synthesis and induced gastric erosions. Convincingly in humans, sodium salicylate in the anti-inflammatory dose of 53 mg/kg of body weight did not inhibit platelet aggregation, total body production of PGE_2 and PGI_2, and renal PGE_2 synthesis; the equivalent dose of acetylsalicylic acid markedly decreased all these parameters. In clinical studies, salsalate, the prodrug of salicylic acid, is equipotent in its anti-inflammatory, analgesic, and antipyretic efficacy as compared with other NSAIDs but causes fewer typical NSAID side effects. Furthermore, patients with aspirin-sensitive asthma can take salsalate safely.

Meloxicam is a new NSAID approved in many European countries. The ratio of the ID_{50} values for inhibition of COX-2/COX-1 by meloxicam depends on the experimental model and ranges between 0.013 (human recombinant enzymes) and 0.09 (human whole blood), thus showing an approximately 75-fold selectivity for COX-2. We have demonstrated in healthy volunteers that 7.5 mg per day of meloxicam in contrast with indomethacin in the anti-inflammatory equivalent dose of 25 mg tid had no effect on platelet aggregation and platelet thromboxane formation. In addition, renal PGE_2 synthesis remained unaffected by meloxicam but was markedly inhibited by indomethacin. These results clearly show that meloxicam in a dose of 7.5 mg per day is COX-1 sparing in humans.

Clinical studies prove that these findings could translate in a favorable risk-benefit ratio. In patients suffering from osteoarthritis and RA, 7.5 mg per day of meloxicam was shown to be as therapeutically effective as 100 mg per day of diclofenac or 750 mg per day of naproxen; the incidence of adverse effects, especially gastrointestinal damage, was significantly lower with meloxicam treatment in comparison with the other NSAIDs. In 25 patients with mild renal impairment, who are at increased risk for NSAID-induced renal failure, meloxicam at the maximum recommended dose of 15 mg per day for 28 days did not cause further deterioration of renal function. Recently, the results of two large-scale, double-blind, randomized, prospective trials comparing 7.5 mg meloxicam with 100 mg diclofenac and 20 mg piroxicam, respectively, in patients with osteoarthritis, were presented. While meloxicam was equivalent with respect to clinical efficacy, gastrointestinal and renal toxicity of meloxicam was significantly less compared with the two nonselective COX inhibitors diclofenac and piroxicam.

Highly selective COX-2 inhibitors

The selective COX-2 inhibitors approved so far show at best a 100-fold selectivity. Thus, at therapeutic doses they can exert clinically relevant COX-1 inhibition. Compounds with an up to 1000-fold selectivity for COX-2 are in development. Some members of this new generation of NSAIDs have failed in animal or early clinical trials, whereas rofecoxib and celecoxib are now approved in the US. Rofecoxib possesses a long half-life, allowing a once-daily dosage schedule. The gastrointestinal tolerability of rofecoxib at 250 mg per day for 1 week was tested in a gastroscopic study in healthy volunteers. In this study, the incidence of erosions by rofecoxib was 15%; i.e., it was not different from placebo. In contrast, treatment with 2.4 g per day of ibuprofen or 2.6 g per day of acetylsalicylic acid produced erosions in 80 and 95%, respectively, of the volunteers. In addition, platelet aggregation was not inhibited by rofecoxib in doses up to 1 g

per day. For therapeutic efficacy, a small fraction of the aforementioned dosage is needed. In 209 patients with osteoarthritis, rofecoxib in daily doses of 25 and 125 mg, respectively, was compared with placebo. Only 25 mg rofecoxib was sufficient for therapeutic efficacy, and there was no difference between the two doses of rofecoxib. In dental pain, 50 mg rofecoxib was as effective as 500 mg rofecoxib, again showing a ceiling for the effect of rofecoxib on pain and inflammation. Based on these results, the recommended dose of rofecoxib for ongoing trials is 25 to 50 mg per day.

The other currently leading compound for highly selective COX-2 inhibition is celecoxib. With a half-life of 8 hours, it must be given twice daily. As for rofecoxib, gastroscopic studies in healthy volunteers showed that celecoxib, even in supratherapeutic doses, does not produce more erosions than placebo. Moreover, platelet aggregation and thromboxane B_2 production were not inhibited by celecoxib in the high dose of 600 mg bid. Double-blind, placebo-controlled trials in patients with osteoarthritis and RA, respectively, demonstrate that celecoxib is effective for the symptomatic treatment of inflammation and pain with no gastrointestinal side effects. For subsequent studies, doses of 100 to 200 mg bid for osteoarthritis and pain and 200 to 400 mg bid for RA are recommended.

DEVELOPMENT OF NEW DISEASE-MODIFYING DRUGS (DMARDs)

There are many new potential disease-modifying therapies for chronic inflammatory joint diseases, and these are summarized in Table 48.1. Not listed are cyclosporin A, which is now approved as a DMARD, and substances such as tacrolimus and mycophenolate mofetil, with a similar mode of action as established DMARDs (cyclosporin A and azathioprine, respectively). The most promising approaches will be discussed in the following section.

ANTICYTOKINE THERAPY

Cytokines play a key role in the network of immunologic actions that produce the chronic inflammatory synovial pannus, cartilage, and bone destruction. In RA, interleukin 1 (IL-1) and tumor necrosis factor alpha (TNFα), mainly produced by macrophages, are the predominant cytokines in the inflamed joints and systemically. They lead to secretion of other cytokines, enhanced proliferation of synoviocytes and lymphocytes, and increased production of prostanoids, metalloproteinases, and nitric oxide (NO), the effectors of the destructive inflammatory process. Metalloproteinases and NO are also direct targets for disease-modifying therapy. However, only inhibition of metalloproteinases reached the clinic, as below described. Inhibition of proinflammatory NO synthesis is exclusively experimental because so far there are no suitable drugs for chronic use in humans.

In contrast, lymphocyte-derived IL-2, IL-3, and interferon-γ are sparse. This points to the concept of invasive pannocytes as pathologic mechanism of RA. Convincingly, previous treatment strategies directed against lymphocyte-derived IL-2 or the T-helper cells themselves failed. Thus, current anticytokine therapy focuses on IL-1 and TNFα (Tab. 48.1). Other possible candidates are anti-IL-6 receptor antibodies and treatment with anti-inflammatory cytokines IL-4, IL-10, and IL-13 (Tab. 48.1).

Anti-TNFα therapy   Some clinical studies show that anti-TNFα antibodies suppress clinical and laboratory disease activity. These studies were carried out with monoclonal chimeric antibodies, i.e., antibodies consisting of a murine variable region and a human constant region. Chimeric antibodies are less immunogenic than strictly murine antibodies, but further attempts to decrease immunogenicity have resulted in construction of humanized antibodies, which contain only the hypervariable regions of the murine antibodies. Humanized anti-TNFα antibodies are now being used in clinical trials. Another approach to anti-TNFα therapy is the use of soluble TNFα receptors, which bind to TNFα, thus preventing its action on the membrane-bound receptors. These truncated versions of the membrane-bound TNFα receptor are the naturally occurring inhibitors of TNFα activity. Most recently, a double-blind, placebo-controlled, randomized trial in 180 patients with RA who received for 3 months TNFR:Fc, a recombinant fusion protein that consists of the soluble TNF receptor p75 linked to the Fc portion of human IgG$_1$, indicated a dose-dependent significant improvement in clinical disease activity, biochemical markers, and quality of life. After cessation of TNFR:Fc, parameters of disease activity moved toward baseline levels. As adverse events, mild injection-site reactions and infections of the upper respiratory tract were noted. Remarkably, there were no dose-limiting toxic effects, and no antibodies to TNFR:Fc were detected. These results encourage investigation efficacy, particulary in terms of disease progression, and safety of long-term treatment with TNFR:Fc.

Anti-IL-1 therapy   As far as anti IL-1 therapy is concerned, only a few clinical studies have been published. In a double-blind, randomized study of 175 patients with active RA, 7-week treatments with different dosage schedules of a recombinant IL-1 receptor antagonist (IL-1Ra) were carried out. Results showed that 70 mg IL-1Ra daily appeared optimal, with significant improvement in painful and swollen joint count and overall assessment of disease activity. However, a definite conclusion on the efficacy of IL-1Ra was not possible because of the lack of placebo controls. Injection-site reactions led to dicontinuation in 5% of patients, and four infections were rated as adverse events. More information will be available when an ongoing, large-scale study with daily injections of 30, 75, and 150 mg of IL-1Ra is reported. An intermediate analysis of this study, prolonged from 6 weeks to 12 months, showed significant improvement, in 43% of the 150 mg IL-1Ra

Table 48.1 New disease-modifying drugs in development

Target	Agent
Anticytokine therapy	
TNFα	Soluble TNFα receptor Anti-TNFα antibody
IL-1	IL-1 receptor antagonist Soluble IL-1 receptor type I
TNFα and IL-1	Signal transduction inhibitors Transcription factor inhibitors
IL-6	Anti-IL-6 receptor antibody Soluble IL-6 receptor
Anti-inflammatory cytokines	IL-4 IL-10 IL-13
Cellular targets	
T- and B-lymphocytes	Leflunomide
T-helper cells	Nondepleting anti-CD4 antibodies
T-lymphocytes	Vaccination with autoreactive T-cells T-cell receptor-derived peptides Induction of oral tolerance
Adhesion molecules	Anti-ICAM-1 antibody Antisense oligonucleotide against ICAM-1 LFA-3 blocking protein Anti-LFA-1b antibody
Antigen-presenting cells	Antibodies to MHC class II antigens Vaccination with allogeneic mononuclear cells Blockade of antigen presentation by specific peptides
Synovial cells	Induction of apoptosis by anti-Fas (CD95) antibodies
Miscellaneous approaches	
Metalloproteinases	Minocycline, doxycycline Tetracycline derivatives without antibiotic activity Tissue inhibitors of metallo-proteinases
TNFα? Macrophages?	Thalidomide
Genes (gene products like soluble TNFα receptors, IL-1 receptor antagonist protein, tumor growth factor β)	Gene therapy

(IL = interleukin; TNFα = tumor necrosis factor alpha; ICAM = intercellular adhesion molecule; LFA = leukocyte function-associated antigen; MHC = major histocompatibility complex.)

group compared with 27% of the placebo group at 24 weeks. As for the anti-TNFα treatment described earlier, another approach for anti-IL-1 therapy is the use of soluble IL-1 receptors. In a phase I study, the efficacy, safety, and pharmacokinetics of a recombinant soluble IL-1 receptor (rhu IL-1R) administered intraarticularly were determined. In comparison with placebo rhu IL-1R led to a significant reduction in joint circumference. No severe adverse events occurred. However, studies with systemic application of rhu IL-1R did not show improvement in clinical disease activity. This could be explained by the biologic properties of the two distinct IL-1 receptors, classified as type I and II: the soluble IL-1 receptors used so far were derived from the type I receptor, which binds more avidly to the IL-1Ra than to IL-1. Thus, for anti-IL-1 therapy, the soluble IL-1 receptor type II (binding more avidly to IL-1) promises to be more efficacious.

One of the open questions is whether anti-IL-1 and anti-TNFα treatment must be combined to suppress both the inflammatory and invasive components of RA, which some workers suggest are mediated by distinct mechanisms. From animal studies it is known that TNFα mediates mainly the inflammatory component, whereas IL-1 is responsible for the destructive process.

INHIBITION OF METALLOPROTEINASES

In arthritic diseases, metalloproteinases, such as collagenase and stromelysin, play an important role in the process of irreparable degradation of the extracellular matrix. Thus, inhibition of enzyme activity or enzyme synthesis, the latter by glucocorticoids or D-penicillamine, is a reasonable attempt to interrupt the pathogenic mechanisms of joint destruction (Tab. 48.1). Tetracyclines are potent inhibitors of metalloproteinases, which inhibit collagenolytic activity of synovial tissue in vitro and in vivo. In two double-blind, placebo-controlled studies, 160 and 219 patients, respectively, with active RA were randomly assigned to receive 100 mg minocycline bid or placebo for 26 and 48 weeks, respectively. In both studies, minocycline significantly improved clinical and laboratory parameters of disease activity. The major adverse effect was dizziness, leading to 3 and 10% dropouts, respectively. In a smaller but equally well designed study, minocycline clearly showed efficacy for the treatment of early RA. In the face of these results, further efforts in this treatment strategy are reasonable.

LEFLUNOMIDE

Leflunomide is a novel isoxazole drug that inhibits T- and B-cell proliferation and function. The mechanism of action is not fully understood, but inhibitions of pyrimidine synthesis and tyrosine kinase activity are the leading hypotheses for the mode of action of A771726, the active metabolite of leflunomide. Leflunomide is effective in a daily dose of 10 mg in active RA, as shown by a placebo-controlled, double-blind trial in 402 patients. Improved efficacy with a dose of 25 mg daily was associated with a higher incidence of adverse effects, mainly gastrointestinal symptoms and reversible alopecia. Remarkably, there were no differences in the incidence of infections between the treatment and placebo groups, and no opportunistic infections were seen. Thus leflunomide is one of the promising new substances, and further trials in comparison with established DMARDs are under way.

NONDEPLETING ANTI-CD4 ANTIBODIES

Previous studies with depleting anti-CD4 antibodies failed, similar to the case of agents targeting other T-cell-specific antigens, such as anti-CD4, anti-CD5, anti-CD7, CD52 antibodies, and IL-2 toxin. As mentioned earlier, this may reflect a minor role for T-cells in established RA. Another possible explanation is that the use of depleting anti-T-cell antibodies is limited by severe immune suppression before T-cells in the synovium are reduced. To circumvent this problem, which was accompanied by allergic reactions and neutralizing antibodies when murine antibodies were used, now nondepleting, humanized or primatized anti-CD4 antibodies are in development. The results so far demonstrate efficacy and much fewer side effects compared with the first-generation T-cell antibodies when monoclonal antibody technology was just starting. Thus the renaissance of anti-T-helper-cell therapy may prove to be a useful approach.

Suggested readings _____

CAMPION GV, LEBSACK ME, LOOKABAUGH J, GORDON G, CATALANO M and The IL-1Ra Arthritis Study Group. Dose-range and dose-frequency study of recombinant human interleukin-1 receptor antagonist in patients with rheumatoid arthritis. Arthritis Rheum 1996;39:1092-101

CROFFORD LJ, WILDER RL, RISTIMÄKI AP, REMMERS EF, EPPS HR. Cyclooxygenase-1 and -2 expression in rheumatoid synovial tissues: effects of interleukin-1β, phorbol ester, and corticosteroids. J Clin Invest 1994;93:1095-101.

DREVLOW BE, LOVIS R, HAAG MA et al. Recombinant human interleukin-1 receptor type I in the treatment of patients with active rheumatoid arthritis. Arthritis Rheum 1996;39:257-65.

ELLIOT MJ, MAINI R, FELDMANN M ET AL. Randomised double-blind comparison of chimeric monoclonal antibody to tumour necrosis factor alpha (cA2) versus placebo in rheumatoid arthritis. Lancet 1994;344:1105-10.

FIRESTEIN GS, ZVAIFLER NJ. Anticytokine therapy in rheumatoid arthritis. N Engl J Med 1997;337:195-7.

FORD-HUTCHINSON AW. New highly selective COX-2 inhibitors. In Vane J, Botting J, eds. Selective COX-2 Inhibitors: pharmacology, clinical effects and therapeutic potential. Dordrecht: Kluwer Academic Publishers, 1998;117-25.

FRÖLICH JC. A classification of NSAIDs according to the relative inhibition of cyclooxygenase isozymes. Trends Pharmacol Sci 1997;18: 30-4.

FRÖLICH JC, STICHTENOTH DO. NSAID: can renal side effects be avoided? In: Vane JR, Botting JH, Botting RM eds: Improved nonsteroid anti-inflammatory drugs: COX-2 enzyme inhibitors. Dordrecht: Kluwer Academic Publishers, 1996;203-28.

HAWKEY CJ. Cox-2 inhibitors. Lancet 1999;353:307-14.

HUMMEL KM, GAY RE, GAY S. Novel strategies for the therapy of rheumatoid arthritis. Br J Rheumatol 1997;36:265-7.

ISAKSON P, ZWEIFEL B, MASFERRER J. Specific COX-2 inhibitors. From bench to bedside. In: Vane J, Botting J eds. Selective COX-2 inhibitors: pharmacology, clinical effects and therapeutic potential. Dordrecht: Kluwer Academic Publishers, 1998;127-33.

MLADENOVIC V, DOMLJAN Z, ROZMAN B, et al. Safety and effectiveness of leflunomide in the treatment of patients with active rheumatoid arthritis. Arthritis Rheum 1995;38:1595-603.

MORELAND LW, HECK LW, KOOPMAN WJ. Biologic agents for treating rheumatoid arthritis. Arthritis Rheum 1997;40:397-409.

STICHTENOTH DO, FRÖLICH JC. Nitric oxide and inflammatory joint diseases. Brit J Rheumatol 1998;37:246-57.

STICHTENOTH DO, WAGNER B, FRÖLICH JC. Effects of meloxicam and indomethacin on cyclooxygenase pathways in healthy volunteers. J Invest Med 1997;45:44-9.

TAK PP, TAYLOR PC, BREEDVELD FC, et al. Decrease in cellularity and expression of adhesion molecules by anti-tumor necrosis factor alpha monoclonal antibody treatment in patients with rheumatoid arthritis. Arthritis Rheum 1996;39:1077-81.

TILLEY BC, ALARCON GS, HEYSE SP, et al. Minocycline in rheumatoid arthritis: A 48-week, double-blind, placebo-controlled trial. Ann Intern Med 1995;122:81-9.

VANE JR. Towards a better aspirin. Nature 1994;367:215-6.

VINCENTI MP, CLARK IM, BRINCKERHOFF CE. Using inhibitors of metalloproteinases to treat arthritis? Arthritis Rheum 1994;37:1115-26.

SECTION

9

Antitumorals

Section editor: Boris Labar

49

Drugs used
in cancer treatment

Cesare R. Sirtori, Franco Pazzucconi

Antitumoral chemotherapeutic agents generally are classified according to three major characteristics: (1) specificity or nonspecificity for phases of the cell cycle; (2) mechanism of action; (3) chemical structure.

The cell cycle may be summarized schematically as follows: (1) phase preceding DNA synthesis (G_1); (2) synthesis of DNA (S); (3) premitotic interval between the end of DNA synthesis and mitosis, also called the *postsynthetic phase* (G_2); (4) mitosis (M).

Cells in the G_2 phase contain a double complement of DNA and may be divided into two daughter cells; those in phase G_1 may start the reproductive cycle again or remain in a nonproliferative stage, called G_0. Cells from specialized tissues (e.g., brain, hormonal tissue, smooth muscle cells in arteries, etc.) may differentiate into functional or nonfunctional stages, but unless pathologic events occur, they do not divide. In contrast, cells from slow-growth tumors, for example, may remain in the G_0 phase for prolonged periods and enter the cell cycle only after some time.

Drugs used for the treatment of tumors may affect processes such as the synthesis of DNA (S) or of the mitotic spindle (M). Others may affect the synthesis of DNA precursors or damage the integrity of DNA itself. Most antitumor drugs are effective against cells in the proliferating phase. Agents not specifically affecting any of the steps in the cell cycle are called *phase aspecific* (in the past *cycle specific*). These agents, particularly the ansamycins (e.g., doxorubicin, epirubicin, etc.), are currently used in most combination drug protocols because they are additive in their effect to the phase-specific agents. Among these latter agents, some alter cells during S phase (e.g., cytosine arabinoside and methotrexate) or during mitosis (e.g., taxol, *Vinca* alkaloids) and do not kill quiescent cells.

Damaged cells going from G_1 to S phase undergo *apoptosis*, or programmed cell death, if gene p53 is intact and exerts its normal control function. If gene p53 is mutated and apoptosis does not occur, damaged cells, potentially mutated, may go past S phase, thus leading to a cell population that is resistant to drugs.

Drug classes

The following drug classes are identified as expressing the major chemical types and actual mechanisms among antitumoral agents (Tab. 49.1).

ALKYLATING AGENTS

Alkylating agents are a heterogeneous group of highly reactive chemical compounds that substitute alkyl groups onto active moieties in DNA or RNA (sulphydril, imidazole, carboxylic, phosphate, and amine). Their major mode of antitumor activity is, however, exerted by alkylation of the reactive N residue of guanine.

The consequences of the alkylating process for replication and transcription of DNA are numerous and can explain the biological effects of these drugs: cytotoxicity, mutagenesis, teratogenesis, and carcinogenicity. Many of the effects attributed to alkylating agents share considerable similarities with those of ionizing radiation, thus leading to the suggestion of grouping these drugs under the general term *radiomimetic drugs*.

Alkylation occurs in both proliferating and quiescent cells. The most sensitive cells, however, are those in the S and advanced G_1 phases, and these cells are significantly more damaged by alkylating drugs compared with cells in the G_2, M, and early G_1 phases. Resistance to alkylating agents has considerable clinical significance, since the degree of cross-resistance among the different drugs in the clinic is highly variable. It is thus possible that a patient resistant to a regimen containing an alkylating drug may still respond to a different drug from the same class.

At least five different classes are recognized among classical alkylating agents: (1) nitrogen mustards (e.g., mechloretamine, cyclophosphamide, iphosphamide, chlorambucil, and melphalan); (2) busulfan; (3) ethyleneimines (e.g., thiotepa and altretamine); (4) nitrosoureas (e.g., BCNU, CCNU, carmustine, semustine, nimustine, fotemustine and streptozotocin), (5) triazenes (e.g., dacarbazine).

All these drugs, while chemically quite heterogeneous, share the same complex mechanism of action described above. However, they have differences in reactivity, chemical stability, kinetics, toxicology, and clinical indications. The choice of one agent versus another therefore depends on the pattern of clinical activity and, in some cases, is wholly empirical.

The most severe risk in the use of alkylating agents, in addition to those proper of all major antitumor drugs (e.g., marrow toxicity and others), is that of developing acute leukemias. This major side effect is proportional to the administered dosage and may reach 10% in patients with

Table 49.1 Antitumoral drugs of most common use: doses, mechanisms, toxicities, pharmacokinetis and indications

Agent	Dosage	Category and action	Common toxicities	Other toxicities
Altretamine (Hexamethyl-melamine)	260 mg/m²/day (divide qid) x 14-21 days per 28 day cycle	Unknown, possibly reactive intermediates of the drug selectively inhibit the incorporation of radioactive thymidine and uridine into DNA and RNA, by inhibiting DNA and RNA synthesis	Leukopenia, thrombocytopenia, nausea, vomiting, anorexia	Nephrotoxicity, neurotoxicity
Amsacrine	Adult doses 75 to 120 mg/m²/day iv, pediatric doses 125 to 150 mg/m²/day iv	Intercalates with the DNA molecule and inhibits topoisomerase II	Myelosuppression, nausea, vomiting, diarrhea, stomatitis, phlebitis, transient liver function abnormalities	Cardiac ischemia, atrial, ventricular arrhythmias, leukopenia, thrombocytopenia
Asparaginase	1000-20000 IU/m² iv or im daily for 1-40 days	Enzyme. Depletion of nonessential amino acid L-asparagine; inhibition of protein synthesis	Nausea, vomiting, fever, chills; inhibition of protein synthesis (albumin, insulin, clotting factors); disorientation, coma, seizures; liver function abnormalities	Hypersensitivity (urticaria, bronchospasm, hypotension), pancreatitis
Azacytidine	150-300 mg/m² iv daily for 3-5 days	Antimetabolite. Substrate for RNA synthetase, incorporated into RNA	Myelosuppression, nausea, vomiting	Liver function abnormalities, fever, rash myalgias
Bleomycin	5-15 units/m² iv, or sc weekly	Antibiotic. DNA strand breakage	Pneumonitis, pulmonary fibrosis; skin erythema, peeling, hyperpigmentation	Hypertension, fever, hypersensitivity, hyperbilirubinemia
Busulfan	0.05-0.2 mg/kg po daily continuously	Alkylating agent. Alkylation of DNA	Myelosuppression	Pulmonary fibrosis, addis onian state (skin pigmen tation, weakness)
Carboplatin	200-400 mg/m² iv every 28 days	Alkylating agent. DNA binding	Myelosuppression, nausea, vomiting	Myelosuppression, nausea, vomiting
Carmustine: See Nitrosoureas				
Chlorambucil	0.05-0.2 mg/kg po daily continuously	Alkylating agent. Alkylation of DNA	Myelosuppression	Acute leukemia
Cisplatin	30-120 mg/m² iv every 3-4 weeks	Alkylating agent. DNA binding	Renal toxicity, hypomagne semia, nausea, vomiting, myselosuppression (platelets and leukocytes)	Peripheral neuropathy, hypersensitivity, ototoxicity
Cyclophosph-amide	500-1500 mg/m² iv every 3-4 weeks; 60-100 mg/m² po daily for 1-14 days	Alkylating agent. Alkylation of DNA	Myelosuppression, nausea, vomiting, alopecia, immunosuppression, sterility	Hemorrhagic cystitis, renal tubular water retention, acute leukemia, pulmonary fibrosis, myocardial necrosis

Kinetics	Active metabolites	Metabolism	Indication
$t_{1/2}$: 13 h	Tri- di- mono-methyl-melamine	Extensively metabolized in the liver and excreted in urines (<15% unmodified)	Ovarian cancer, uterine cervix cancer, pancreatic cancer, prostatic carcinoma
$t_{1/2}$: 5 h V_d: 1.67 l/kg	No	Primarily by hepatic extraction and metabolism	Adult and childhood acute leukemias
$t_{1/2}$: iv: 8-30 h; im: > 49 h V_d: 63 ml/kg	No	Unclear; trace excretion in urine	Childhood acute leukemia
$t_{1/2}$: 3.5 h (iv), 4.2 h (sc)	No	Unclear; rapidly removed from plasma	Adult nonlymphocytic leukemia
$t_{1/2}$: 2 h (bolus iv), 89 h (infusion) V_d: 0.22 l/kg	No	Renal excretion, drug unchanged	Testicular cancer, malignant pleural effusions, Hodgkin an non-Hodgkin lymphoma
$t_{1/2}$: 2-3 h V_d: 0.99±0.23 l/kg	No	Renal excretion of metabolite	Chronic myelogenous leukemia, preparative regiments for bone marrowtransplantation
$t_{1/2}$: 3-6 h >5 days (platinum) V_d: 0.24 l/kg	No	Renal excretion	Advanced ovarian cancer, testicular cancer
$t_{1/2}$: 1.5 h; 2.5 h active metabolite V_d: 0.14-0.24 l/kg	Phenylacetic acid mustard	Metabolic transformation	Chronic lymphocytic leukemia, low-grade non-Hodgkin lymphoma
$t_{1/2}$: 25-49 min; 58-73 h (platinum) V_d: 11-12 l/m^2	No	Renal excretion of native drug and metabolites	Advanced ovarian cancer, advanced bladder cancer, testicular cancer, small cell lung cancer, advanced non-small cell lung cancer, head and neck cancer, advanced esophageal carcinoma, advanced gynecologic cancer
$t_{1/2}$: iv: 8 h; oral: 4 h V_d: iv 0.71 l/kg; oral: 0.48 l/kg	4-Hydroxy cyclophosphamide, aldophosphamide, phosphoramide mustard, acrolein	Unclear: metabolism of drug to active agents by the liver	Breast cancer, soft tissue sarcoma, plasma cell myeloma, small cell lung cancer, advanced non-small-cell lung cancer, non-Hodgkin lymphoma, childhood solid tumors

(continued)

Table 49.1 (continued)

Agent	Dosage	Category and action	Common toxicities	Other toxicities
Cytarabine	100 mg/m² iv or sc every 12 hours or continuous infusion for 7-12 days; 2-3 g/m² iv every 12 hours for 3-4 days	Antimetabolite	Myelosuppression, nausea, vomiting, diarrhea, gastrointestinal mucositis, hepatotoxicity	Seizures with intrathecal use
Dacarbazine (DTIC)	150-250 mg/m² iv daily for 5 days every 28 days	Alkylating agent. Alkylation of DNA	Nausea, vomiting, myelosuppression	Flu syndrome, toxic synergy with doxorubicin
Dactinomycin	0.5 mg/m² iv daily for 5 days	Antibiotic. DNA intercalation, standard breakage	Myelosuppression, gastrointestinal mucositis, alopecia, skin toxicity	Increased inflammations and pigmentation in areas previously or concomitantly subjected to x-rays
Daunorubicin	30-60 mg/m² iv for 1-3 days every 3-4 weeks	Antibiotic	Myelosuppression, oral mucositis, alopecia, skin damage with extravasation, cardiac toxicity (acute and chronic)	X-ray toxicity synergy
Dexrazoxane	Dosage ratio of dexrazoxane to doxorubicin is 10 to 1	Cardioprotective agent by virtue of its antioxidant and chelating effects	Myelosuppression	Elevated prothrombin and partial thromboplastin times and decreased plasma levels of fibrinogen and clotting factors.
Doxorubicin (adriamicin)	25-90 mg/m² iv every 3-4 weeks	Antibiotic. DNA intercalation; DNA strand breakage	Myelosuppression, oral mucositis, alopecia, skin damage with extravasation, cardiac toxicity (acute and chronic)	X-ray toxicity synergy
Epirubicin	70 to 90 mg/m²	Antibiotic. DNA intercalation, DNA strand breakage	Myelosuppression (particularly leukopenia), vomiting, stomatitis, alopecia, congestive heart failure	Phlebitis, peripheral neuropathy, nausea, vomiting
Etoposide (Vepesid, VP16)	50-150 mg/m² iv daily for 1-5 days; 200-250 mg/m² iv weekly	Plant alkaloid. Action unknown; perhaps inhibition of DNA synthesis	Leukopenia, thrombocytopenia, nausea, vomiting, mild peripheral neuropathy	–
Fluorouracil	7-15 mg/kg iv daily for 5 days or once weekly	Antimetabolite. Inhibition of thymidylate synthetase and synthesis of DNA	Oral and gastrointestinal mucositis, myelosuppression (mild)	Cerebellar ataxia, myocardial necrosis syndrome, conjunctivitis, tear duct stenosis, phlebitis with protracted infusion, dermatitis
Fotemustine	100-125 mg/m²	See Nitrosoureas	Thrombocytopenia, protracted nausea/vomiting and ototoxicity. Renal toxicity	Deep vein thrombosis
Gemcitabine	1000 mg/m²	Antimetabolite	Myelosuppression, flu-like symptoms, fatigue, fever, peripheral edema, proteinuria, cutaneous reactions, and gastrointestinal effects	–

Kinetics	Active metabolites	Metabolism	Indication
$t_{1/2}$: 1-3 h V_d: 32-40 l	Phosphocytarabine	Hepatic metabolism	Acute non-lymphocytic leukemia, meningeal cancers, non-Hodgkin lymphoma
$t_{1/2}$: 5 h V_d: 1.5 l/kg	5-aminoimidazole-4-carboxamide (AIC)	Hepatic activation; excretion unclear	Malignant melanoma, Hodgkin lymphoma, soft tissue sarcoma
$t_{1/2}$: 36 h	No	Bile and urinary excretion, drug unchanged	Ewing's sarcoma, embryonal rhabdomyosarcoma, Wilms' tumor, gestational trophoblastic tumor, Hodgkin lymphoma
$t_{1/2}$: 18.5 h; 26.7 h active metabolite V_d: 39 l/kg	Daunorubicinol	Hepatic metabolism; biliary and renal excretion of metabolites	Acute nonlymphocytic leukemia
$t_{1/2}$: 2-3 h V_d: 1.3 l/kg	No	40% to 60% of a dose is excreted in the urine within 24 hours	Amelioration of ansamycin induced cardiotoxicity
$t_{1/2}$: 12-28 h V_d: 25.4 l/m^2	Doxorubicinol	Hepatic metabolism; biliary and renal excretion of metabolites	Breast cancer, small-cell lung cancer, advanced non-small-cell lung cancer, Hodgkin disease and non-Hodgkin lymphoma, soft tissue sarcoma, plasma cell myeloma, gastric cancer, acute nonlymphocytic leukemia, neuroblastoma, , advanced ovarian cancer, embryonal rhabdomyosarcoma, thyroid cancer, bladder cancer, hepatocellular carcinoma
$t_{1/2}$: 30-38 h V_d: 1400 l/m^2	Epirubicinol	Liver metabolism, excreted primarily via the bile	Advanced breast cancer, lung cancer, ovarian carcinoma, and soft-tissue sarcomas
$t_{1/2}$: 3-19 h V_d: 7-17 l/m^2		Metabolic degradation; 45% excreted in urine as native drug and metabolites	Small-cancer lung cancer, testicular cancer
$t_{1/2}$: 5-10 min V_d: 0.25 l/kg	5-Fluorouridine monophosphate, floxuridine monophosphate (5-FUMP, 5-FdUMP)	Hepatic metabolism to 5-dihydrofluorouracil	Breast cancer, gastrointestinal cancer, head and neck cancer, hepatocellular carcinoma
$t_{1/2} = 25.8 \pm 11.5$ min	Diethyl (1-isocyanatoethyl) phosphonate	Mostly hepatic, glutathione conjugated metabolites 17-32% excreted in urine	Malignant melanoma, gastric cancer, brain primary tumors and metastases, non-small cell lung cancer
$t_{1/2}$: 32-639 min V_d: 18-257 l	Gemcitabine-5'-triphosphate	Liver metabolism; 92% to 98% excreted in urine 95% as 2',2'-difluorodeoxyuridine	Breast cancer, non-small-cell lung cancer, pancreatic carcinoma, and ovarian carcinoma

(continued)

Table 49.1 (continued)

Agent	Dosage	Category and action	Common toxicities	Other toxicities
Hydroxyurea	25 mg/kg po daily continuously	Antimetabolite. Inhibition of nucleotide reductase and DNA synthesis	Myelosuppression, nausea, vomiting, oral mucositis, skin rash	Convulsions
Idarubicin	12 mg/m²/day for 3 days	Antibiotic; see doxoru-bicin	Myelosuppression, particularly leukopenia, nausea, vomiting, alopecia, and stomatitis	Congestive heart failure and hepatic dysfunction
Ifosfamide	0.8-1.2 g/m² iv daily for 5 days; 3-4 g/m² iv every 3 weeks	Alkylating agent; alkylates DNA, produces strand breaks	Bone marrow suppression, hemorrhagic cystis (must be coadministered with MESNA), alopecia	Nephrotoxicity, confusion, hepatotoxicity, nausea, vomiting
Interferon-α 2a	3 million IU given im or sc daily or 3 times weekly (up to 30 million IU or more for investiga-tional use)	Biological agent. Direct anti-tumor activity and immunologic modulation	Fever, chills, flulike symp-toms, myalgias, headache, anorexia, nausea, leukope-nia, thrombocytopenia, ane-mia, AST elevation	Diarrhea, vomiting, dizzi-ness, central nervous sys-tem abnormalities
Irinotecan	100 mg/m²	Topoisomerase I inhibitor: inhibitor of DNA and RNA synthesis	Neutropenia, eosinophilia, diar-rhea, hemorrhagic cystitis	–
Lomustine: See Nitrosoureas				
Mechloretha-mine	6 mg/m² iv on days 1 and 8 every 4 weeks	Alkylating agent. Alkylation of DNA, RNA, protein	Myelosuppression, nausea, vomiting, skin necrosis with extravasation, alopecia	Dermatitis, sterility
Melphalan	0.05-0.2 mg/kg po daily for 5 days	Alkylating agent. Alkylation of DNA	Myelosuppression, alopecia, nausea, vomiting	
Mercapto-purine	1-2 mg/kg po daily for 5 days	Antimetabolite. Inhibition of de novo purine synthesis; incorporation into DNA	Myelosuppression, hepatotoxi-city, gastrointestinal mucosi-tis, inhibition of cell-mediated immunity, increased toxicity with allopurinol	Dermatitis, fever, Budd-Chiari syndrome
Methotrexate	20-100 mg/m² iv, im, po by a variety of schedules; 3-12 g/m² iv with leucov-orin	Antimetabolite. Inhibition of formation of tetrahy-drofolate by dihydrofo-late reductase	Myelosuppression, gastroin-testinal mucositis, nausea, vomiting, alopecia, dermati-tis	Renal tubular necrosis, pul-monary fibrosis, cirrhosis, osteoporosis, transverse myelitis and microcalcific leukoencephalopathy with radiation fever
MESNA (sodi-um-2-mecap-to-ethane-sulphonate)	20% of dose of com-bined alkylating agent per 3	Protective against toxicity of alkilating agents (par-ticularly bladder toxicity)	Exhaustion, diarrhea, abdom-inal pains, tachycardia and transient hypertension after iv injection	Subjective poor tolerability (unpleasant taste)
Mitomycin	10-20 mg/m² iv every 6-8 weeks	Antibiotic. Alkylation of DNA and inter-and intrastrand cross-link-ages	Myelosuppression (cumula-tive), nausea, vomiting, cuta-neous necrosis, alopecia, oral mucositis, skin rash	Pulmonary fibrosis, renal failure, microangiopathic hemolytic, anemia, car-diomyopathy
Mitotane	2-10 g po daily con-tinuously	Adrenal cytotoxic agent. Adrenocortical atrophy; inhibition of mitochondria	Nausea, vomiting, diarrhea, lethargy, somnolence, skin rash	Leukopenia, hepatic toxicity
Mitoxantrone	10-14 mg/m² iv every 3-4 weeks	Antibiotic. Action unclear; may cause DNA breaks	Myelosuppression, skin necro-sis with extravasation	Nausea, vomiting, car-diotoxicity, alopecia

Kinetics	Active metabolites	Metabolism	Indication
$t_{1/2}$: 2-3 h	No	Hepatic metabolism	Chronic myelogenous leukemia, preparative regimens for bone marrow transplantation
$t_{1/2}$: 14-35 h V_d: 64 l/kg	Idarubicinol	Liver metabolism, urine excretion	Acute nonlymphocytic leukemia and acute lymphocytic leukemia; advanced breast cancer
$t_{1/2}$: 7-15 h V_d: 37-49 l/m^2	No	Activation by liver; catalysis in liver and kidneys	Advanced testicular cancer, soft tissue sarcoma
$t_{1/2}$:5-7 h V_d: 31 l/m^2	No	Renal clearance and renal tubular degradation	Hairy cell leukemia, renal cell carcinoma, malignant melanoma, Kaposi's sarcoma, refractory Hodgkin and non-Hodgkin lymphoma
$t_{1/2}$: 8 h V_d: 136 l/m^2	7-ethyl-10-hydroxycamptothecin (SN-38)	Plasma metabolism, bile excretion	Lung cancer, colorectal carcinoma, ovarian carcinoma, non-Hodgkin lymphoma, heavily pretreated small-cell lung cancer
$t_{/2}$: 15 h	No	Rapid tissue binding and inactivation; metabolites excreted in urine	Hodgkin lymphoma
$t_{1/2}$: 38-71 min V_d: 0.5-0.6 l/kg	No	Metabolism in plasma; <15% excreted in urine	Advanced ovarian cancer, plasma cell myeloma, breast cancer
$t_{1/2}$: 10-90 min iv, 1.2-2. 4 h po V_d: 0.9±0.8 l/kg	Several nucleotides	Metabolism in liver to inactive thiopurine	Adult acute non-lymphocytic leukemia
$T_{1/2}$: 3-10 h po; 8-15 h iv V_d: 0.6-0.9 l/kg	No	Renal excretion, drug unchanged	Osteogenic sarcoma, breast cancer, non-Hodgkin lymphoma, head and neck cancer, meningeal cancers, bladder cancer, adult leukemia, gestational trophoblastic cancer, ovarian cancer
$t_{1/2}$: iv: MESNA: 20 min; dimesna 70 min; oral: same bioavailability: 50% V_d: 0.65 l/kg	No	To dimesna (inactive)	Antagonism to the toxicity of alkylating agents
$t_{1/2}$: 23-78 min V_d: 2-48 l/m^2	No	Metabolism in liver and other tissues; minor renal excretion	Gastrointestinal cancers, non-small-cell lung cancer
$t_{1/2}$:18-159 days	o,p'-DDE	Hepatic and renal metabolism; excretion of metabolites in urine	Cancer of the adrenal cortex
$t_{1/2}$: 9-12 h days (mean 75 h) V_d: 1000 l/m^2 (14 l/kg)	No	None	Acute nonlymphocytic leukemia, breast cancer, ovarian cancer, non-Hodgkin lymphoma

(continued)

Table 49.1 (continued)

Agent	Dosage	Category and action	Common toxicities	Other toxicities
Nimustine (ACNU)	2-3 mg/kg intrathecal or 80-200 mg/m^2 iv	Alkylating agents. DNA strand breakage and cross-linkages	Bone marrow suppression, especially thrombocytopenia, nausea and vomiting, convulsions, facial weakness, fecal incontinence, meningitis, hemiparesis, leukoencephalopathy	Paralytic ileus
Nitrosoureas: Carmustine (BCNU), Lomustine (CCNU), Semustine (methyl-CCNU)	100-200 mg/m^2 every 6-8 weeks	Alkylating agents. DNA strand breakage and cross-linkages	Myelosuppression (delayed), alopecia, nausea, vomiting, oral mucositis, pain with intravenous injection (carmustine)	Bone marrow aplasia, acute leukemia, pulmonary fibrosis, renal toxicity (semustine), central nervous system and peripheral nerve toxicities
Oxaliplatin	130 mg/m^2	See Cisplatin	Reversible peripheral sensory neuropathy	Mild hematologic and gastrointestinal toxicities
Pegaspargase	2500 IU/m^2 im	See Asparaginase	Low serum fibrinogen levels and antithrombin III activity	Nausea, vomiting, loss of appetite, abdominal pain, and diarrhea
Plicamycin	0.025-0.05 mg/kg iv daily for 1-3 days, or iv every other day to toxicity	Antibiotic. Inhibits DNA-directed RNA synthesis	Nausea, vomiting, thrombocytopenia, prolonged prothrombin time, hemorrhage, renal toxicity, liver toxicity	Fever, myalgias thrombosis
Porfimer	2 mg/kg	Photosensitizing agent, followed by light application to the tumor	Photosensitivity, anemia, leukopenia and thrombocytopenia	Allergic reactions, liver function test abnormalities, and constipation
Procarbazine	100-200 mg/m^2 po daily continuously or for 14 days	Radiomimetic with alkylating ability. Alkylation of DNA	Myelosuppression (delayed), nausea, vomiting, flulike syndrome, lethargy, oral mucositis, diarrhea	Peripheral neuropathy dermatitis, radiation sensitizer, MAO inhibition and medication interactions
Raltitrexed (tomudex)	2-3.5 mg/m^2	Antimetabolite: folate-based thymidylate synthase inhibitor	Myelosuppression, nausea/vomiting, diarrhea, asthenia and transient asymptomatic increases in liver transaminases	See Methotrexate
Semustine: See Nitrosoureas				
Streptozocin	0.5-1.5 g/m^2 iv daily for 5 days or weekly for 6 weeks	Nitrosourea; inhibition of DNA synthesis; damage to pancreatic B cell	Nausea, vomiting, nephrotoxicity (hypophosphatemia, renal tubular defects)	Mild myelosuppression, liver toxicity, alteration of glucose metabolism, burning of vein
Taxol (Paclitaxel)	135 mg/m^2 iv 24-h infusion	Plant alkaloid. Stabilizes tubulin polymerization	Leukopenia, alopecia, anaphylaxis	Cardiac arrhythmias, peripheral neuropathy oral mucositis
Taxotere (Docetaxel)	60 to 100 mg/m^2	See Taxol	Neutropenia, hypersensitivity reactions, asthenia, nausea, vomiting, diarrhea, alopecia	Sensory neuropathy, mucositis, cutaneous reactions, fluid-retention syndrome
Teniposide	165 mg/m^2	See Etoposide	Leukopenia, thrombocytopenia, or pancytopenia	Nausea, vomiting, diarrhea, mucositis, and phlebitis

Kinetics	Active metabolites	Metabolism	Indication
$t_{1/2}$: < 1 h	No	Mostly hepatic, urine excretion	Malignant melanoma, glioma, myeloid leukemia, disseminated brain tumors
$t_{1/2}$: <20min (carmustine) 1.3-2.9 h (metab) 16-48 h (lomustine and semustine) V_d: 3.3 l/kg (carmustine)	No	Spontaneous decompensation to active intermediates in aqueous solution; urinary excretion	Primary brain cancer, non-Hodgkin lymphoma, gastrointestinal cancers, malignant melanoma, metastatic brain cancer, plasma cell eloma
$t_{1/2}$: 31.3 h	Yes, unknown		Advanced colorectal cancer, ovarian cancers, non-small cell lung cancer, metastatic kidney cancer
$t_{1/2}$: 2 to 3 weeks V_d: 2.1 l/m^2	No	Serum proteases	Serum proteases
		Unknown	Testicular cancer, chronic myelogenous leukemia in blast crisis, Malignant hypercalcemia
$t_{1/2}$: 250 ± 285 h V_d: 0.49 ± 0.28 l/kg	No	Slow photodestruction (photo-bleaching)	Esophageal cancer, lung cancer, and bladder cancer
$t_{1/2}$:10 min	Hydroxyl radical, hydrogen peroxide	Liver metabolism and renal excretion of inactive metabolites	Hodgkin and non-Hodgkin lymphoma
$t_{1/2}$: 2-4 h V_d: 548 l	No	40-50 % unchanged in urine, 10% fecal	Advanced colorectal cancer, head and neck cancer, hormone-resistant prostate cancer, pediatric and adult leukaemias, small-cell lung cancer
$t_{1/2}$: 35 min	No	Rapid biotransformation after intravenous injection; renal excretion of 15% of total dose	Pancreatic islet cell tumors, pancreatic carcinoma, carcinoid tumors
$t_{1/2}$: 1-9 h V_d: 67 -182 l/m^2	No	Unknown, probably hepatic metabolism	Ovarian cancer, breast cancer
$t_{1/2}$:10-18 h V_d: 80-90 l/m^2	No	Metabolized to some degree in the liver, biliary excretion	Metastatic breast cancer, ovarian and non-small cell lung cancer
$t_{1/2}$: 10-38 h V_d: 28% of body weight	No	Metabolized extensively in the liver (86% of a dose) 50% urinary excretion	Refractory acute childhood lymphoblastic leukemia, neuroblastoma, retinoblastoma, lymphoma

(continued)

Table 49.1 (continued)

Agent	Dosage	Category and action	Common toxicities	Other toxicities
Thioguanine	100 mg/m² iv daily for 5 days	Antimetabolite. Inhibition of de novo purine synthesis; incorporation into DNA	Myelosuppression, nausea, vomiting	Hepatotoxicity, inhibition of cell-mediated immunity
Thiotepa	0.2-0.5 mg/kg iv or im daily for 5 days or once weekly	Alkylating agent. Alkylation of DNA	Myelosuppression, nausea, vomiting	–
Topotecan	1.5-2.5 mg/m²/d for 5 d cycle (0.4 mg/m²/d x 21 d)	Topoisomerase I inhibitor: inhibitor of DNA and RNA synthesis	Myelosuppression, GI toxicity (nausea, vomiting, diarrhea)	Nephrotoxicity, lung toxicity
Vinblastine	1.5-2 mg/m² iv daily for 5 days; 4-6 mg/m² iv weekly	Plant alkaloid. Binding of tubulin; mitotic arrest	Leukopenia, constipation, skin necrosis with extravasation, alopecia, peripheral neuropathy (loss of reflex, nerve palsies, muscle wasting, paresthsias)	Nausea, vomiting
Vincristine	0.5-2 mg/m² iv weekly	Plant alkaloid. Binding of tubulin; mitotic arrest	Peripheral neuropathy (see Vinblastine), leukopenia, constipation, skin necrosis with extravasation	Alopecia, nausea, vomiting
Vindesine	2-3 mg/m² iv weekly	Plant alkaloid. Binding of tubulin; mitotic arrest	Peripheral neuropathy, leukopenia, skin necrosis with extravasation	Thrombocytosis, alopecia, nausea, vomiting
Vinorelbine	30 mg/m²	See Vinblastine	Neutropenia, anemia, thrombocytopenia, neurotoxic effects	Nausea, vomiting, diarrhea, stomatitis, alopecia, local injection-related complications, hypersensitivity reactions

ovarian carcinomas who have been treated intensively with one or more of these drugs for more than 10 years.

Local toxicity, e. g., hemorrhagic cystitis after cyclophosphamide can be effectively prevented by the concomitant administration of MESNA (see Tab. 49.1 and Chap. 59).

ANTIMETABOLITES

Antimetabolites are characterized by a chemical structure similar to those of natural substances such as vitamins, nucleosides, or amino acids. They have all been designed on theoretical grounds, with the goal of inhibiting critical metabolic pathways, usually leading to a blockade of DNA or RNA synthesis in a more or less direct manner. Generally, antimetabolites interact with cell enzymes in one of the following ways:

• They may substitute for a natural metabolite normally incorporated into a biological molecule, e.g., DNA or RNA, thus altering function.

• They may compete with a natural substrate by occupying the catalytic site of a key enzyme.

Classically, antimetabolites are divided into three groups: (1) folate antagonists (e.g., methotrexate and other antifolates); (2) pyrimidine analogues (e.g., 5-fluo-

rouracil, cytosine arabinoside, raltitrexed, gemcitabine and others); (3) purine analogues (e.g., 6-mercaptopurine, azathioprine, thioguanine, pentostatin, and others).

ANTIBIOTICS

To this drug class belong a number of natural products mainly derived from the culture media of different fungal species (Streptomycetes). Some of the antibiotics are among the drugs most widely used in clinical oncology.

All antitumor antibiotics bind to DNA, most often by intercalating between a couple of bases. The resulting alteration is an "uncoiling" of the double helix, thus severely altering DNA function and not allowing it to act as a template for the synthesis of new DNA or RNA. A second mechanism of action of this drug class is the damage to DNA exerted by the free radicals formed inside the cells following administration of the antibiotic.

In general, antitumor antibiotics exert different effects on the cell-cycle phases. However, the kinetics of their cytotoxic activity is typical of phase-aspecific agents. This is the major reason why antitumor antibiotics are used most commonly in drug combinations for solid-

Kinetics	Active metabolites	Metabolism	Indication
$t_{1/2}$: 25 min - 8 h	Thioguanosine 5'-phosphate (thioguanine ribose phosphate)	Hepatic metabolism; renal excretion	Adult acute non-lymphocytic leukemia
$t_{1/2}$: 2.4 h; TEPA 17.6 h (active metabolite)	TEPA	Renal excretion unchanged drug and metabolic	Breast cancer, malignant effusions, superficial bladder cancer
$t_{1/2}$: 3.31 h (3-14 min for the lactone form) V_d: 132 l	Active lactone and form and inactive open-ring hydroxyacid	Minor pathway to N-demethylated metabolite	Recurrent ovarian cancer, small and non small cell lung cancer
$t_{1/2}$: 25 h V_d: 27.3 l/kg	Desacetylvinblastine	Hepatic metabolism and biliary excretion	Testicular cancer, Kaposi's sarcoma, Hodgkin and non-Hodgkin lymphoma, non-small-cell lung cancer
$t_{1/2}$: 85 h V_d: 165±105 l/m²	No	Hepatic metabolism and biliary excretion	Acute lymphocytic leukemia, acute non-lymphocytic leukemia, plasma cell myeloma, Hodgkin and non-Hodgkin lymphoma, Wilms' tumor
$t_{1/2}$: 24 h V_d: 8.1 l/kg	No	Hepatic metabolism and biliary excretion	Non-small-cell lung cancer
$t_{1/2}$: 43 h V_d: 75 l/kg	Dexacetylvinorelbine	Liver metabolism, urinary excretion	Advanced breast cancer, non-small cell lung cancer, Hodgkin and non-Hodgkin lymphoma, ovarian carcinoma

tumor chemotherapy. The major components of these drug classes are the ansamycins (e.g., doxorubicin, idarubicin, epirubicin, daunorubicin, and mithoxantrone), whose therapeutic use is aided by the administration of desrazoxane, a specific inhibitor of ansamycin cardiotoxicity; bleomycin, mitomycin C, and actinomycin D.

PLANT DERIVATIVES

Plants release a variety of substances with well-known toxic properties. Among these chemicals, a large number have been shown to possess a pharmacologic activity that antagonizes cell multiplication. Some agents, such as the *Vinca* alkaloids, have been known for a number of years. Others, such as epipodophyllotoxin and extracts from the bark of the Pacific yew tree (i.e., taxol and derivatives), have just entered clinical therapy. Inside this drug class, the single agents have different patterns of activity, but curiously, among plant derivatives, drugs belonging to one group are cross-resistant with agents belonging to the other groups.

Among the *Vinca* alkaloids, vincristine, vinblastine, and vindesine are the most widely used. They block the mitotic spindle in metaphase. They are thus also called *antimitotic* and are specific to M phase.

Epipodophyllotoxins, such as etoposide and teniposide, and the alkaloids from *Camptotheca acuminata*, such as topotecan and irinotecan instead inhibit topoisomerase II. This enzyme promotes the uncoiling of DNA from a double helix to a single helix, thus allowing the synthesis of new DNA. In the absence of this enzyme, nucleic acids undergo fragmentation. Finally, the Pacific yew tree extracts taxol and taxotere bind tubulin, impairing polymerization and the consequent stabilization of microtubules.

HORMONES FOR CANCER THERAPY

Treatment with hormones is an important therapeutic modality in some so-called hormone-dependent tumors, in which progression is controlled by hormones. Major examples of such tumors are breast cancer, endometrial carcinoma, and prostate carcinoma. Hormone-responsive patients achieve therapeutic results equivalent to those obtained with other therapeutic modalities at lower cost, both economic and in terms of toxicity.

Hormonal therapy may be medical or surgical (generally castration), this latter with fewer and fewer indications. Indications for hormonal therapy are dictated by (1) the age of the patient; (2) the site of metastasis; (3) the extent of disease; (4) the lethality and complications from rapid expansion of the disease

Surprisingly, the mechanism of action of these drugs is mostly unknown. Some of the major findings in hormonal therapy are, in fact, contradictory. For example, in breast cancer, response to hormone therapy depends on the presence of so-called estrogen and/or progestogen receptors. However, in other hormone-responsive tumors, there is no correlation between response and presence or absence of receptors. It is as yet unclear why breast cancer can respond to estrogen antagonists or to estrogens themselves at pharmacologic doses; hormone therapy is generally linked to a cytostatic, not a cytotoxic effect. In line with this concept, hormone therapy frequently is used with palliative goals. However, recently, hormone therapy also has been used successfully as adjuvant treatment, thus suggesting a cytotoxic effect.

The various forms of pharmacologic therapy with hormones can be divided into three groups:

- *Additive:* Use of natural or synthetic hormones acting in the same way as endogenous hormones: estrogens (e.g., dethylstilbestrol, conjugated estrogens), progestins (e.g., medroxyprogesterone acetate; megestrol acetate), androgens (e.g., testosterone propionate and enanthate), corticosteroids;
- *Competitive:* Blockade of the action of endogenous hormones on target tissues: antiestrogens (e.g., tamoxifen), antiandrogens (e.g., flutamide, finasteride, cyproterone acetate);
- *Inhibitory:* Drugs inhibiting key enzymes or releasing hormones affecting target tissues: aromatase inhibitors (e.g., aminogluthetimide, astrozole, letrozole), OH-androstenedione, gonadotropin-releasing hormone analogues (e.g., buserelin, goserelin, leuprolide), inhibitors of biosynthesis (e.g., ketoconazole).

OTHER AGENTS

Chemically different compounds display a mechanism of action not strictly corresponding to those of the other drug classes. Such is certainly the case with the enzyme asparaginase, which leads to the depletion of asparagine, a key amino acid for leukemic cell growth. However, the drugs cisplatin, carboplatin (see Chap. 59), and oxaliplatin as well as procarbazine, act, to some extent, as alkylating agents. Hydroxyurea acts in a similar way as an antimetabolite, and amsacrine as an inhibitor of topoisomerase II. Porfimer acts, instead, as a photosensitizing agent, followed by light application to the tumor. Finally, interferons, in particular IF α-2a, have specific roles especially in tumors of the lymphatic and hemopoietic tissues. The drugs belonging to this last group have been known for a long time and are used widely in daily cancer chemotherapy.

50

Basis for antitumoral therapy and rationale for multimodality therapy

Riccardo Rosso, Catia Angiolini

Research in biochemistry, immunology, and molecular biology has yielded profound insight into the causes and pathogenesis of many forms of cancer and offers hope for the development of specific and selective new cancer treatments. Major breakthroughs, however, have yet to have an impact on the clinical approach to the treatment of neoplastic disease. The mechanisms of action of most current anticancer drugs are not selective but target vital macromolecules (e.g., nucleic acids) or metabolic pathways that are critical to malignant and to normal cells. Moreover, the clinical development and use of cancer chemotherapy are fundamentally empirical. Despite these limitations, the introduction of chemotherapy has resulted in the development of curative therapeutic interventions for patients with several types of solid and hematopoietic neoplasms.

The first attempt at the cure of cancer with drugs, carried out at Yale–New Haven Medical Center in 1943, was based on the observation that alkylating agents, products of the secret war gas program in world wars, caused marrow and lymphoid hypoplasia. At the beginning of 1960s, the first success in the treatment of leukemias and malignant lymphomas with combination chemotherapy proved that human cancers, even in their advanced stages, could be cured by drugs.

Although only a relatively small number of malignancies are effectively cured by chemotherapy, drugs are used at some point during the treatment of most cancers. Many tumors can be cured by surgical resection; chemotherapy is used primarily to treat advanced cancers, and although few forms of metastatic cancer can be cured, chemotherapy is now increasingly effective as a component in the multimodal management of apparently localized cancers. Chemotherapy can in fact be used with different aims: (1) as primary treatment, for patients presenting with advanced disease for which no alternative treatment exists (induction chemotherapy), (2) as an adjuvant to another treatment modality (adjuvant chemotherapy), (3) as initial treatment (primary chemotherapy), indicated for patients with localized advanced disease for which the reduction of the neoplastic mass enables more conservative surgery or for patients with neoplasms in which chemotherapy is the primary therapeutic modality, and (4) as local treatment, administered into the spinal fluid or into pleural, pericardial, or peritoneal spaces or by site-directed perfusion of specific regions of the body affected by cancer.

SCIENTIFIC BASIS OF CANCER CHEMOTHERAPY AND MODELS OF CELL GROWTH

Cancer is a clonal disease. A single cell becomes uninhibited in its growth and continues to divide, leading to the formation of a tumor. Cellular division generally takes place over quite a long time; for example, breast cancer cells generally divide every 100 days. In both animal models and human tumors, growth occurs according to Gompertzian kinetics. The growth rate of malignant cells is exponential, and most tumor cells traverse the complete cell cycle. As the tumor burden grows larger, the fraction of cells traversing the cell cycle decreases, more cells remain in a G0 phase (resting phase), and in the later stages of tumor development the growth rate of neoplastic cells becomes less rapid.

Most chemotherapeutic drugs attack cells during the synthesis of DNA. Is it unclear whether any current chemotherapeutic agents are effective in killing cells in the G0 phase.

The first major conceptual model of neoplastic growth and pattern of response to chemotherapy was the log-kill model developed by Skipper and Schabel in 1964. The *Skipper model* is based on observations using L1210 mouse leukemia cells, which undergo exponential growth and are in cycle and dividing, with no cells in G0 phase, so that the cell number doubles at a tumor-specific rate. The first of Skipper's laws is that the doubling time of proliferating cells is constant, forming a straight line on a semilog plot. The second law is that cell kill by drugs follows first-order kinetics; i.e., the percentage of cells killed at a given drug dosage in a given cancer is constant, regardless of the tumor cell burden. For example, the dose of chemotherapy able to kill two logs of cells (log kill = 2) can equally reduce the number of tumor cells from 10^{10} to 10^8 or from 10^6 to 10^4. The Skipper model considers the tumor cured only if the number of surviving cells is equal to or lower than 10^4. This model explains why chemotherapy is not effective in most advanced cancers. The tumor is curable only if the number of cells surviving chemotherapy is very small; i.e., an inverse relationship exists between the initial tumor mass and the curability of the tumor.

The Skipper model applies to some forms of neoplastic disease. In breast cancer, colon cancer, and osteosarcoma, the same chemotherapy can lead to cure in cases of micrometastatic spread (adjuvant chemotherapy) but only to transient responses in cases of metastatic disease. In ovarian carcinoma, the probability of survival after chemotherapy is related to the extent of residual disease after surgery.

Skipper's laws apply only to the proliferating compartment of the tumor, i.e., the fraction of cells actively growing within the tumor. The concept of *tumor growth fraction*, first introduced by Mendelsohn, suggested instead that each tumor harbors a subpopulation of cells equivalent to the stem cells present in normal tissues, whose proliferation accounts for all tumor growth. This population is therefore the target for antineoplastic agents.

The fact that proliferating cells are distinct from the nonproliferating population is responsible for the therapeutic refractoriness of human tumors. Human tumors, in fact, show a pattern that differs from the straight-line growth seen by Skipper in mouse leukemia; human tumors, instead, follow a Gompertzian growth curve that describes a population of cells that increases as a result of cell birth and decreases as a result of cell death. Experimental tumor cell populations approximate this curve because in addition to proliferating cells, there are subpopulations that have ceased to proliferate and cells that have died. As cells proliferate into a smaller and smaller mass, the diffusion process by which oxygen reaches the tumor is insufficient to supply cells in a central site. Expanding solid tumors regularly outgrow their blood supply, leading to anoxia, slowing of the cell cycle, exit of some cells into the nonproliferating compartment, and cell death and necrosis. As some cells exit from the proliferative compartment and enter the G0 resting phase, Skipper's laws of cell kill no longer apply. Quiescent cells in G0 phase become, in fact, temporarily resistant to chemotherapy; they are less sensitive to antineoplastic agents in part perhaps because they have time to repair DNA damage. The underlying rationale for fractioning radiation therapy has always been that tumor shrinkage allows the improvement of circulation during therapy. Thus, resting cells enter the proliferating radiation-sensitive pool. The Gompertzian growth curve is sigmoid-shaped; cell number grows slowly at the beginning because the number of dividing cells is small, and a rapid accumulation of cells then follows, reaching a maximum growth rate at about one-third of maximum tumor volume. There ensues a gradual slowing of growth, almost to a plateau, as the tumor approaches the volume necessary to kill the host.

Tumor growth has been put into a variety of model curves, but it is likely that no single model describes all malignant growths. A sigmoid-shaped growth curve approximating Gompertzian growth has been seen in almost all malignancies studied. Small tumors have a larger growth fraction than large tumors, presumably because their supply of nutrients and oxygen is optimal. But since total cell number is small, even a large growth fraction yields only a small increase in tumor cell number. Therefore, the success of chemotherapy is often highly dependent on the cellular kinetics of the tumor at the time the drugs are given.

Since the 1980s, research on tumor responsiveness to chemotherapy has been substantially conditioned by Goldie and Coldman's model. Tumor cell progression is dominated by a mutational process, and the evolution of human tumors is allowed by the natural selection of those mutations which predispose to malignant growth. Tumor cells have an inherently greater mutation rate than do normal cells, and this rate increases in progressing tumor cells. It is therefore reasonable to assume that genetic resistance to chemotherapeutic agents, in addition to other alterations in phenotypic behavior, occurs in mutant clones.

Goldie and Coldman developed a mathematical model for relating the drug sensitivity of tumors to their spontaneous mutation rate. Because mutation is a random event, the number of drug resistant clones increases as a direct function of tumor size and length of time it has been present. More precisely, the number of resistant clones is a direct function of the number of cell divisions that have occurred in the tumor, i.e., its mutation rate. In most human cancers, the size of the primary tumor is directly related to the incidence of distant metastases and survival, since resistance to chemotherapy is a major cause of treatment failure. An important consequence of drug resistance as tumors progress is that at diagnosis most tumors harbor resistant clones.

As a consequence of Goldie and Coldman's hypothesis, alternating sequences of chemotherapy regimens (using drugs with different mechanisms of action) have been conceived and developed both to lower the odds of encountering cross-resistance and to obtain additive or synergistic effects. Ideally, drugs with different dose-limiting toxicities should be combined. This approach allows each drug to be given at or near full therapeutic doses. Unfortunately, most chemotherapeutic agents have a significant overlap in toxic effects, with almost all having myelosuppression as their dose-limiting toxicity. As a result, dose reductions are common in combination chemotherapy. Moreover, alternating sequences of chemotherapeutic regimens in the treatment of either Hodgkin's disease or small cell lung cancer have not demonstrated unequivocal advantages. The study conducted at the Milan National Cancer Institute to evaluate the efficacy of the alternating MOPP/ABVD regimen (MOPP = mechlorethamine, vincristine, procarbazine, prednisone; ABVD = doxorubicin, bleomycin, vinblastin, dacarbazine; see Chap. 63) versus the MOPP regimen alone demonstrated a significant advantage of the alternating regimen. However, more recently, evaluation in a three-arm randomized trial of the efficacy of alternating MOPP/ABVD versus MOPP versus ABVD reported the superiority of the two arms containing ABVD versus MOPP alone. The superiority of the alternating MOPP/ABVD regimen therefore had to be ascribed not to the alternating regimen but to the superiority of the ABVD regimen. In one of the earliest prospective, randomized trials evaluating alternating chemotherapy, patients with advanced small cell lung cancer received either six cycles of CAV (cyclophosphamide, doxorubicin, vincristine) or CAV alternating with EP (etoposide, cisplatin) (see Chap. 56). The patients in the alternating arm showed higher response rates and improved progression-free survival. It was concluded that the alternating regimen was better than CAV alone. Other trials using an etoposide-based regimen also proved to benefit patients with either limited or extensive disease. However, it was not clear if this advantage was due to the alternating strategy or to the superiority of the EP regimen.

The other major conclusion of the Goldie-Coldman model was that adjuvant treatment should be instituted as soon as possible after surgery. The failure of cure is assumed to be a consequence of the presence of drug-resistant cells arising by random somatic mutation before or during treatment. The ideal strategy to ensure the greatest likelihood of cure would entail reducing as much and as quickly as possible the total number of malignant cells so as to minimize the probability of resistance emerging in the residual cells.

In 1986, Day reanalyzed the Goldie-Coldman model, suggesting a different approach to sequencing combination chemotherapy. Because in many instances no two combination regimens are likely to be strictly non-cross-resistant or have equal cell-killing capacity, Day formulated the *worst-drug rule*. This theory refers to any strategy entailing the administration of more or earlier doses of a treatment that is the less effective of two available regimens in order to prevent the overgrowth of those cells resistant to the best chemotherapy regimen, possibly eliminated by the weaker regimen.

Although the various models used to describe the cytotoxic effects of chemotherapy have been useful to the understanding of general phenomena, they are not sufficient to describe the complexity of the behavior of human cancers during chemotherapy in the clinical setting. Chemotherapy is planned on the basis of observed differences between normal and tumor cells in response to antitumor agents used both singly and in combination. Part of the difference between normal and tumor cells can be explained by consideration of proliferative characteristics. However, cell kinetics cannot explain all the consequences of tumor cell exposure to a drug, since these are also dependent on pharmacokinetics, biochemistry, and tumor biology.

COMBINATION CHEMOTHERAPY

The use of antineoplastic drugs in combination regimens has been established in the treatment of most types of cancer. In fact, with the sole exception of choriocarcinoma, single-agent chemotherapy rarely allows cure, whereas the use of drug combinations significantly increases both the percentage of patients achieving complete remission and the duration of their remissions.

The overriding rationale for the use of combination chemotherapy is to overcome drug resistance to individual agents. Because it is not feasible to predict whether a particular tumor will respond to a given drug, administering anticancer drugs in combination ensures a greater chance of achieving a response. Combination chemotherapy also may prevent or delay the development of acquired resistance in initially responsive tumors and may as well provide additive or synergistic cytotoxic effects if agents with different mechanisms of action are selected.

A thorough knowledge of the clinical pharmacology of individual anticancer drugs is required to design effective combination chemotherapy regimens. Traditionally, combination chemotherapy regimens contain drugs with demonstrated single-agent activity against the type of tumor being treated, with preference given to agents that produce complete responses in patients with advanced or recurrent disease. A combination regimen normally includes drugs that are non cross-resistant to overlap drug-resistant subpopulations of tumor cells, drugs with nonantagonistic and preferably additive or synergistic mechanisms of action, and drugs with nonoverlapping toxicity profiles, allowing each agent to be administered at its optimal dose and schedule.

Drug combinations also have been designed to take advantage of biochemical interactions (synergism). The active folate leucovorin does not have inherent antitumor activity, but when administered with 5-fluorouracil (5-FU), it can markedly increase the cytotoxic effect of 5-FU by enhancing the binding of an active intracellular metabolite of 5-FU to its target enzyme, thymidylate synthase. The combination of leucovorin and 5-FU has demonstrated a higher response rate than 5-FU alone against a variety of epithelial tumors, principally colorectal cancer.

Scheduling

Chemotherapy is usually administered every 3 to 4 weeks, primarily to alleviate the toxicities induced by many chemotherapeutic agents. Since most drugs are not tumor-specific, those cells in the body which are normally in active division and replication can be severely affected by chemotherapy. The organ most frequently and adversely affected by chemotherapy is the bone marrow, followed by peripheral blood cells. Myelosuppression (including leukopenia, neutropenia, and rarely, thrombocytopenia and anemia) induced by chemotherapeutic agents is generally reversible. The nadir of neutrophils and platelets usually occurs between the tenth and fourteenth days after the administration of chemotherapy; for only few drugs, such as melphalan and nitrosoureas, is the nadir delayed until the third or fourth week.

Because of differences in the peripheral blood half-life of leukocytes and platelets, myelosuppression first takes the form of leukopenia, followed by thrombocytopenia. Generally, the leukopenia is more severe than the thrombocytopenia. Platelets represent the cell line that is the slowest to recover after bone marrow suppression.

The subsequent cycle of chemotherapy is administered only after recovery to normal hematologic levels is achieved. It is presumed that stem cells, actively proliferating during the cycle, are more prone to damage by chemotherapeutic agents. Nevertheless, regardless of hematologic levels, many schedules adopt the administration of drugs at days 1 and 8, in the belief that during the first week proliferating activity in the bone marrow is low and stem cells are in the resting phase.

For some tumors, such as leukemias and lymphomas, the proliferating activity of tumor cells is so high that those cells surviving chemotherapy are able to proliferate before the subsequent cycle of chemotherapy. In these malignancies, chemotherapy is scheduled with the weekly administration of drugs, with alternating myelotoxic and nonmyelotoxic agents.

Very few anticancer drugs are truly nonmyelosuppressive. The only agents known to be completely nontoxic to normal bone marrow are steroidal hormones (the only exception being tamoxifen, which rarely induces leukopenia and thrombocytopenia). However, agents such as bleomycin, vincristine, and L-asparaginase do not usually cause bone marrow suppression.

Dosing

For drug-sensitive cancers, the limiting factor for effective therapy is often proper dosing. The dose-response curve in biologic systems is usually sigmoidal in shape, with a threshold, a lag phase, a linear phase, and a plateau phase. For radiation therapy and chemotherapy, it is the difference between dose-response curves of normal and tumor tissues that must be used during treatment. Because anticancer drugs are toxic, it is often necessary to avoid acute but non-life-threatening toxicity by diminishing the dose or increasing the intervals between treatment cycles. Several experimental studies have demonstrated the importance of administration of the maximum dose, since a reduction in dose resulted in decreased therapeutic effect. Empiric adjustment of dosing is a major reason for treatment failure in patients with drug-sensitive cancers.

A major area of evaluation in oncology regards the concept of *dose intensity*, i.e., dose per unit time. In the adjuvant treatment of operable breast cancer, retrospective studies suggest that increased dose intensity within the conventional range of cytotoxic drug dosage could have a marked effect on outcome. This hypothesis of increasing overall and disease-free survival with an increase in dose per unit time is based on experimental data demonstrating a logarithmic increase in cytotoxicity with a linear increase in dose. Moreover, the use of high dose levels of chemotherapy may reduce selection of resistant cells.

DRUG RESISTANCE AND ITS MECHANISMS

Failures after chemotherapy are definitely due to drug resistance. Different mechanisms may account for drug resistance: an increased DNA repair activity, a reduced intracellular drug concentration, the presence of different metabolic pathways that allow an increased drug catabolism, and/or a decreased drug activation. Finally, one of the most relevant factors is the cellular phase of the neoplastic cell at the time of chemotherapy. In fact, sensitive cells are temporarily resistant to chemotherapy when nonproliferating. The capacity of certain cancers to resist the cytotoxic effects of cancer chemotherapy may be more closely related to a loss of regulation of cell cycle control genes than to the mechanisms of resistance to each agent. Rapidity of growth may induce resistance but not sensitivity to a cancer cell population. Although normal tissue never develops resistance to chemotherapy, one of the most remarkable features of both radiation therapy and chemotherapy, when used for sensitive tumors, is that the toxic effect of these agents may be greater initially in the neoplastic cells than in the two most sensitive tissues of the body (namely, the hematopoietic system and the gastrointestinal tract). In other words, doses that will eradicate some sensitive tumors will not ablate the bone marrow or destroy the capacity of the gastrointestinal mucosa to regenerate. The explanation for this phenomenon (therapeutic index) has a molecular basis, and it appears to be related to mechanisms that allow normal renewal of cell populations (like bone marrow and gastrointestinal precursors), to monitor and repair damaged DNA or to destroy cells with irreparable DNA damages rather than allow damaged cells to proceed through the cell cycle and potentially replicate their damaged DNA. Normal cells can almost always recover from exposure to DNA-damaging anticancer agents. Initially, sensitive cancer cells can be destroyed by effective chemotherapy, but if not eradicated, they develop resistance to further treatment, perhaps in part because of drug-induced DNA mutations. This resistance may be linked to the dysregulation of the same gene pathways that control entry into the cell cycle.

P53 is the protein responsible for causing the arrest of the G1 phase of the cell cycle when cells are exposed to DNA damage-causing agents. P53 also mediates the activation of programmed cell death, or apoptosis, within a cell in which DNA damage has occurred. In a normal cell, apoptosis can occur following exposure to radiation or chemotherapy that has caused significant DNA damage. Apoptosis induced by chemotherapy or irradiation in experimental systems occurs to a lesser degree in tumor cells that lack the p53 gene.

The acquisition of changes within the p53 gene should be very common in neoplasms that are often resistant to chemotherapy because a loss of functional p53 would prevent DNA damage–induced apoptosis in the DNA synthetic phase of the cell cycle. In fact, one of the most commonly encountered secondary mutations in most cancer cells is point mutational changes in the p53 protein, which is correlated with resistance to chemotherapy in many solid tumors. Although it was initially thought that drug-curable tumors in general were less often found to have p53 mutations, this is not always the case. In addition, there are p53-dependent and p53-independent mechanisms of apoptosis. Generally speaking, the presence of identifiable p53 abnormalities has been correlated with a poor prognosis, even in curable tumors. Insertion of normal p53 genes in some tumors by a gene therapy approach is being attempted.

ADJUVANT CHEMOTHERAPY

Chemotherapy appears to be most effective when administered in the adjuvant setting to patients who show no evidence of residual disease after local therapy (surgery and/or radiation) but who are at high risk of relapse at metastatic sites. The aim of adjuvant chemotherapy is to prevent metastatic recurrence by eliminating micrometastatic tumor deposits in the lungs, bone, bone marrow, lymph nodes, or other sites at the time of diagnosis. Adjuvant chemotherapy has been demonstrated to be efficacious for most common adult cancers, such as breast, colon, and ovarian cancer. In the pediatric age group, adjuvant chemotherapy is used effectively in most neoplasms, including Wilms' tumor, Ewing's sarcoma, and osteosarcoma.

Clinical considerations and experimental evidence support the use of adjuvant chemotherapy. Microscopic foci of tumor should be more chemosensitive on a cell kinetic basis because a larger fraction of the cells are actively proliferating and potentially susceptible to the cytotoxic effects of drugs. The smaller burden of tumor cells also implies a lower probability that drug-resistant cells are present. The experiments of Goldie and Coldman predict that the chance for cure is maximized if all available active drugs are given simultaneously in the adjuvant setting, when there is minimal residual disease and the probability is low that drug-resistant cells are present. Clinical experience well supported a correlation between low tumor burden and the efficacy of chemotherapy.

Numerous breast cancer trials have shown the ability of systemic chemotherapy to enhance the cure rate over standard surgical resection alone (see Chap. 61), and chemotherapy has been shown to improve survival in both node-positive and node-negative patients with early breast cancer. In patients with colon cancer, surgery followed by adjuvant chemotherapy with 5-FU plus levamisole has shown advantages over surgery alone and has become standard treatment.

The selection of appropriate drugs and the optimal timing of drug therapy related to the definitive local therapy are important considerations in the design of successful adjuvant chemotherapy regimens. Traditionally, drugs have been selected on the basis of their activity in advanced disease. Animal models and clinical experience have shown

that regimens producing the most dramatic responses in metastatic or recurrent disease have the greatest likelihood of being curative in the adjuvant setting.

Adjuvant chemotherapy should begin as soon as possible after definitive local therapy. A delay to allow for recovery from surgery or radiation therapy may compromise the chance of curing the patient. One strategy to avoid delays caused by potential adverse interactions between chemotherapy and surgery or irradiation is the administration of drug therapy before definitive local therapy. This approach, known as *primary* or *neoadjuvant chemotherapy,* also may improve local control of the primary tumor and provide earlier therapy for micrometastases.

MULTIMODALITY THERAPY

Many cancer patients require a multimodality approach involving either surgery or radiotherapy, or both, in order to obtain local control of the disease and systemic chemotherapy to control possible micrometastatic cancer foci. Local therapies, such as surgery and radiotherapy, can be combined optimally with chemotherapy (Tab. 50.1).

Chemotherapy and radiation therapy

The past two decades have witnessed a growing interest in combining chemotherapy with radiation therapy in the treatment of most human cancers. The main objectives of this

---

Table 50.1 Multimodality therapy in oncology

Chemotherapy - radiotherapy combinations
Radiation therapy improves local control, while chemotherapy treats sistemically. Some chemotherapeutic agents sensitize neoplastic cells to the effect of radiations (e.g., Cisplatin, Gemcitabine, 5-Fluorouracil)

Examples: small cell lung cancer, advanced head-neck cancer, lymphomas, esophageal cancer, advanced cervical cancer

Chemotherapy - surgery combinations
Surgery is a local modality, while chemotherapy is a systemic modality; their enhanced effect forms the rationale for adjuvant chemotherapy in common cancer, as colon cancer and breast cancer. Chemotherapy could be used preoperatively (neoadjuvant chemotherapy), reducing tumor size and improving surgical results

Examples: early or locally advanced breast cancer, colon cancer head-neck cancer, ovarian cancer

Chemotherapy - surgery - radiotherapy combinations
Sequencing of these modalities are highly variable. All three treatment modalities are being employed in the treatment of most malignancies with different aims: local control (surgery), regional control (radiotherapy), or systemic control (chemotherapy)

Examples: locally advanced or inflammatory breast cancer, rectal carcinoma, esophageal cancer, Wilms' tumour, rhabdomyosarcoma

approach are to increase local tumor control, decrease distant metastasis, and improve survival.

A theoretical benefit for the combination of chemotherapy and radiotherapy is provided by the hypothesis of Goldie and Coldman. This assumes that drug-resistant or radioresistant cell populations arise spontaneously at a frequency that depends on the total number of clonogenic cells and on their mutation frequency. This model assumes that cells eventually resistant to both chemotherapy and radiotherapy are more likely to occur than would be expected considering the simple product of the individual mutation rates. Assuming that the kinetic behavior of resistant cells is similar to that of the parental clone, the Goldie-Coldman model predicts that the use of noncross-resistant modalities of treatment, combined as closely as possible, would be the optimal strategy.

The ultimate goal of multimodality therapy is to improve the therapeutic ratio. Ideally, when chemotherapy is combined with radiotherapy, it is hoped that the combined treatment will result in an enhancement of supra-additive effects in tumors but not in normal tissues.

Four major combination strategies have evolved:

1. *Spatial cooperation (adjuvant chemotherapy)*. The concept of spatial cooperation was first used by Steel to describe the mechanism whereby chemotherapy and radiotherapy act on diseases at different sites to achieve an improved therapeutic effect. In this case, there is no interaction between chemotherapy and radiotherapy, and scheduling strategies entail an attempt at administering full doses of both. This strategy is usually employed when there is high likelihood of disease outside the radiation field, such as in the combination of adjuvant chemotherapy and radiotherapy in breast-conserving surgery, or there is a limited area of expected chemotherapy failure, such as the sanctuary sites of testes and central nervous system in acute lymphocytic leukemia and osteosarcoma.

2. *Neoadjuvant chemotherapy*. In this case, chemotherapy is given as initial cytoreductive treatment and is followed by definitive locoregional radiotherapy, with or without surgery. It is an appropriate approach when the aim is to increase local tumor control while also treating potential micrometastases. Since the risk of drug-resistance increases with the increase of the tumor mass, it is theoretically useful to apply neoadjuvant chemotherapy as early as possible. This approach is used especially in patients with locally advanced breast cancer, lung cancer, and head and neck cancer. The underlying assumption of neoadjuvant chemotherapy is that by combining partially effective, noninteracting treatments with different toxicities, each can be given at full doses.

3. *Simultaneous radiation/chemotherapy*. In this approach, chemotherapy is administered during the radiotherapy course, usually during the initial few days of treatment. Often radiotherapy is given in a split-course fashion, each course being started with concomitant chemotherapy. This approach has yielded encouraging clinical results for patients with head and neck, esophageal, anal, and cervical cancer. Chemotherapy regimens usually contain drugs known to have radiosensitizing effects, such as gemcitabine, 5-FU, cisplatin. The drug given in this simultaneous strategy could have a systemic adjuvant effect as well as a direct interactive effect with radiation on the primary tumor.

4. *Alternating radiation/chemotherapy*. This approach uses a repetitive sequence of a short course of chemotherapy followed by a short course of radiation until the tolerance doses of each are reached. The best example is the use of combined-modality therapy for patients with stage III Hodgkin's disease, for which chemotherapy and radiotherapy are delivered in an alternating manner in order to avoid compromising either one. There are strong theoretical bases for this approach: a delay in delivering chemotherapy can increase the probability that a resistant clone of cells will develop in the local tumor and/or will result in the spread and growth of micrometastic disease. Delaying radiotherapy, especially if tumor response is not good, could decrease the possibility of achieving tumor control and cure. In this way, as theorized by Goldie and Coldman, radiotherapy can be considered as the non-cross-resistant treatment in combination chemotherapy.

The combination of chemotherapy and radiotherapy has produced clinically relevant results in many forms of cancer (head and neck, lymphomas, cervix, esophagus, and lung). In some of these malignancies, randomized, controlled trials have demonstrated that the combined-modality strategy is superior to radiotherapy or chemotherapy alone. In this field it seems extremely relevant to select drugs with spectra of toxicity different from that of radiotherapy.

Chemotherapy and surgery

The rationale for combining chemotherapy and surgery is quite similar to that for the use of chemotherapy and radiation therapy: a local approach (surgery) is used together with a systemic modality (chemotherapy) to enhance the curability of disease that cannot be treated by either modality alone.

The use of adjuvant chemotherapy has already been discussed. The use of neoadjuvant chemotherapy is the subject of increased attention for a variety of solid tumors. In patients with locally advanced breast cancer, preoperative chemotherapy can decrease tumor mass, thus permitting better surgical resection; in these patients, radiation therapy is given as definitive treatment to sterilize locoregional sites. In localized breast cancer for patients whose tumors are too large for a conservative surgical approach, neoadjuvant chemotherapy can reduce tumor size so that a lumpectomy can be performed with satisfactory results.

Although considerably good results have been obtained with the integration of surgery, chemotherapy, and radiation therapy modalities, much work on the optimization of the integration of these treatment modalities remains to be done. The advent of new biologic therapies poses future challenges for the combination of various modalities of treatment and offers new hopes of cure for cancer patients.

DAY RS. Treatment sequencing, asymmetry and uncertainty: protocol strategies for combination chemotherapy. Cancer Res 1986;46:3876-85.

DEVITA VT. The James Ewing lecture. The relationship between tumor mass and resistance to treatment of cancer. Cancer 1983;51:1209-20.

DEVITA VT. Principles of cancer management: chemotherapy. In: DeVita VT, Helman S, Rosenberg SA, eds. Cancer. Principles & practice of oncology. 5th ed., Philadelphia: Lippincott-Raven, 1997; chap 17, p 333, 1997.

FAN U, JOHNSON KR, MILLER MC. In vitro evaluation of combination chemotherapy against human tumor cells. Oncology Rep 1998;5:1035-62.

GOLDIE JH, COLDMAN AJ. A mathematic model for relating the drug sensitivity of tumors to the spontaneous mutation rate. Cancer Treat Rep 1979;63:1727-33.

GOLDIE JH, COLDMAN AJ. The genetic origin of drug resistance in neoplasms: implication for systemic therapy. Cancer Res 1984;44:3643-53.

GOLDIE JH. Scientific basis for adjuvant and primary (neoadjuvant) chemotheraphy. Semin Oncol 1987;14:1-7.

LOWE SW, BODIS S, MCCLATCHEY A, et al. P53 status and the efficacy of cancer therapy in vivo. Science 1994;266:807-10.

MENDELSOHN ML. Autoradiographic analysis of cell proliferation in spontaneous breast cancer in CH3 mice. III. The growth fraction. J Natl Cancer Inst 1962;28:1015-29.

NORTON LA. A Gompertzian model of human breast cancer growth. Cancer Res 1988;48:767-71.

SKIPPER HE, SCHABEL FM, WILCOX WS. Experimental evaluation of potential anti-cancer agents. XII. On the criteria and kinetics associated with "curability" of experimental leukemia. Cancer Chemother Rep 1964;35:1-11.

Biologic therapy and hematopoietic growth factors

Heinz Zwierzina

The potential to influence malignant processes with biologic approaches provides preclinical and clinical scientists with a fascinating new challenge and is expected to revolutionize cancer therapy. Biologic therapy of cancer encompasses cytokines and hematopoietic growth factors (HGFs), as well as treatment strategies using (humanized) antibodies, vaccines, and various gene therapy approaches. The spectrum of in vivo effects of biologics covers modulation of immune response, stimulation/inhibition of hematopoiesis, direct regulation of cellular growth and differentiation, and modulation of tumor vascularization. Rapid progress toward an understanding of the mechanisms of action and evaluation of the clinical relevance of this broad range of agents is requiring new research strategies with close collaboration between preclinical and clinical scientists.

Compared with cytotoxic agents, a number of differences exist not only in the principles of preclinical investigation but also in the in vivo application of biologics. Treatment frequently leads to modulation of a cascade of events that cannot be foreseen from experimental animal studies. Modulation of complex networks means that unexpected effects including unwelcome side effects can occur that must be monitored carefully. To further aggravate the dilemma, induction of secondary effects may be variable and related to the timing of application as well as to the dose.

The problem of dosage is a major difficulty and a potential pitfall in the setup of clinical trials with biologic. In biologic therapy, the aim is usually less the definition of the maximally tolerated dose (MTD) but much more the definition of the optimal immunomodulatory dose (OID), the minimal dose resulting in significant augmentation of effector cell activity correlated with therapeutic response. An example of the possible pitfalls of dosage is represented by interferon-γ (IFN-γ), where a bell-shaped curve of activity has been shown in vitro and confirmed in vivo, suggesting that too high a dose may suppress a desired response and too low a dose may fail to invoke it. From this example it can be seen that the dose of a biologic

response modifier (BRM) may be independent of the MTD and that in vivo more is not necessarily better.

The therapeutic value of biologic agents in cancer therapy lies more in the prolongation of complete or partial remission achieved after surgery, chemotherapy, and/or radiotherapy, when the tumor load has been reduced to a level where the body is able to destroy minimal residual disease by means of its own immunosurveillance. Instead of regression, stable disease may occur that is essential in the palliative setting, provided life quality is maintained.

Drug classes

INTERFERON-α (IFN-α)

The interferons are a group of proteins produced by a variety of cells and have manifold biologic activities. Some of them have potential antitumor characteristics such as antiproliferative effects, immunomodulation, promotion of differentiation, and inhibition of oncogene activation and angiogenesis. The mechanisms of action are not clearly understood but appear to involve binding of the IFN molecule to its receptors on the cell membrane, which in turn initiates a second message to synthesize new proteins by gene activation.

IFN-α has been studied most extensively in human diseases and has been approved for clinical use in various malignant disorders (Tab. 51.1) such as chronic myelogenous leukemia (CML) and hairy cell leukemia (HCL). However, IFN-α has little or no activity against such common cancers as breast, lung, or colon cancer. Side effects of IFN-α therapy are dose-dependent and consist of constitutional complaints such as fever, chills, myalgia, headache, nausea, anorexia, and weight loss (so-called flulike syndrome). Although this flulike syndrome is self-limited, it is the most common dose-limiting side effect. Myelosuppression may occur but is reversible within 1 to 3 days after discontinuation of therapy. A

Table 51.1 Therapeutic schedules of interferon-α in different tumors

Disease	Therapy	Dose	Schedule	Duration
Melanoma				
Adjuvant therapy	Induction: IFN-α2b	20 MU/m² iv	5 d/week	4 weeks
	Maintenance therapy: IFN-α2b	10 MU/m² sc	3 times per week	48 weeks
Palliative therapy	Induction: IFN-α	10 MU/m² sc	Daily	4 weeks
	Maintenance therapy: IFN-α	3-5 MU/m² sc	3 times per week	Individually
Renal cell carcinoma	IFN-α	6-18 MU/m² im, sc	3 times per week	Individually
AIDS-related Kaposi's sarcoma (AIDS-KS)	IFN-α	3, 9, 18 MU when tolerated: up to 36 MU	Daily: 3 days each	Until CR or progression under highest possible dose
	IFN-α + zidovudine (AZT)	9-18 MU, 600 mg/d sc	Daily	Until CR or progression
Carcinoid tumors	IFN-α	3-5 MU sc	3-5 times per week	At least 3 months
Hairy cell leukemia	IFN-α	3-5 MU sc	3-5 times per week	At least 3 months
Chronic myeloid leukemia	IFN-α	5 MU sc	Daily	At least 12 weeks
Essential thrombocythemia	IFN-α	3 MU sc	Daily	At least 12 weeks
Multiple myeloma	IFN-α	3-5 MU sc	3 times per week	At least 12 weeks as maintenance therapy
Non-Hodgkin's lymphoma (centroblastic-centrocytic)	IFN-α	5 MU sc	3 times per week	Until relapse

(MU = million units; CR = complete response.)
Note: When only α is indicated, either α2a or α2b may be used.

modest elevation of liver enzymes is common and without clinical significance. Rare complications include interstitial nephritis, confusion, coma, arrhythmia, and hypotension.

The commercially available doses are 3, 4.5, 6, 9, and 18 million units for IFN-α2a and 1, 3, 5, and 10 million units IFN-α2b.

Melanoma

In malignant melanoma, the adjuvant use of high-dose IFN-α2b for 1 year significantly prolonged disease-free survival as well as complete survival compared with the observation arm of the study in patients with stage IIb or III melanoma after operation. The study included patients with primary tumors that were 4 mm or more in size. Adjuvant IFN-α increased the median overall survival to 3.8 years in the treatment group compared with 2.8 years in the observation group and yielded a 5-year survival rate of 46 versus 37%. The response to therapy was greatest among patients with clinical evidence of nodal metastasis. The toxicity associated with this regimen was substantial, however. Almost 80% of IFN-α-treated patients experienced grade 3 or greater toxicity, and dose modifications were required in almost 40% of patients.

Numerous clinical trials have been reported for treatment of metastatic melanoma in the palliative setting. With various schedules, response rates of 15 to 20% were demonstrated [complete response (CR): 5%; partial response (PR): 10-15%], and preferentially, a subgroup of patients with lung or soft tissue metastases responded best to therapy with IFN-α. The duration of therapy must be defined on the basis of the response.

Renal cell carcinoma

For renal cell carcinoma, no proven value has been reported for IFN-α therapy in the adjuvant setting. For palliative treatment, the duration of therapy depends on the response. Published studies demonstrate a response rate around 15% (CR + PR) with doses ranging from 1 million units three times per week to 36 million units daily. Analysis of published trials shows no clear dose-response relationship, but it has been demonstrated that doses below 3 million units per day lead to lower response rates than higher dosages. The side effects of IFN-α can be considerable, but the addition of corticosteroids may substantially block the major toxicities without attenuating response. Patients with pulmonary metastases have the highest response rate.

AIDS-related Kaposi's sarcoma (AIDS-KS)

The optimal therapy for patients with AIDS-KS has not been determined. Treatment is directed at palliation of disease-related symptoms because no therapy has been proven unequivocally to influence survival. IFN-α is useful mainly in patients with mucocutaneous disease or asymptomatic visceral involvement. A close correlation exists between baseline values of CD4+ (helper) T-lymphocytes and response to IFN-α treatment. While the overall response rate ranges between 30 and 40%, patients with greater than 200/mm^2 CD4+ T-lymphocytes demonstrate a significantly better response rate of more than 45%, with 30 to 40% pathology-proven CR.

Carcinoid tumors

Treatment with IFN-α leads to responses in 15 to 20% of patients, with a further 40% demonstrating stable disease. Even more patients report a decrease in clinical symptoms, and a median duration of response between 12 and 20 months can be expected. No dose-response relationship is apparent, but a threshold dose of 3 million units given suncutaneously three times weekly is essential, whereas a further increase of dose seems to have no impact.

Hairy cell leukemia (HCL)

Improvement in blood count usually has been demonstrated after 2 months of treatment. Partial remissions are achieved in more than 80% of patients, but complete disappearance of hairy cells in bone marrow is rare. IFN-α has lost much of its role in the treatment of HCL because 2-chlorodeoxyadenosine has proven superior as a first-line therapy.

Chronic myelogenous leukemia (CML)

Clinical effectiveness has been proven in several reports, with complete remissions occurring in about 30% of patients and partial remissions in a further 50% (see Chap. 63). Hematologic remission may occur within only a few weeks and is less important for survival than cytogenetic remission, which occurs later in only 10 to 20% of patients.

Essential thrombocythemia

In essential thrombocythemia, platelet counts are significantly decreased within 2 to 3 weeks, and frequency of thrombotic or hemorrhagic complications is reduced. The response rate (CR + PR) lies around 90%.

Multiple myeloma

In multiple myeloma, IFN-α may prolong progression-free survival after chemotherapy, but overall survival is not influenced.

Non-Hodgkin's lymphoma (centroblastic-centrocytic)

IFN-α finally may have a role in centroblastic-centrocytic lymphoma (NHL cb/cc) for maintenance therapy after chemotherapy. Clinical trials have proven that maintenance therapy with IFN-α leads to a significant prolongation of disease-free survival.

INTERLEUKIN 2 (IL-2)

IL-2 is a glycoprotein produced by mature T-lymphocytes during an immune response after the lymphocyte has received a signal from an antigen-presenting cell. The interaction of IL-2 with its receptor finally stimulates proliferation of the antigen-reactive T-cell clone and gives rise to the specific effector cells that mediate helper, suppressor, and cytotoxic T-cell functions. In terms of stimulation of the antitumor activity of lymphocytes, recombinant human IL-2 expressed in *Escherichia coli* exerts an identical biologic activity as the naturally occurring glycoprotein. The antitumor activity of IL-2 is thought to result mainly from activation and expansion of lymphokine-activated killer (LAK) cells that can kill the tumor cells directly. IL-2 alone at high doses or in combination with LAK cells or tumor-infiltrating lymphocytes (TILs) has been used to treat a variety of cancers (Tab. 51.2).

The side effects of IL-2 administration include fever, chills, rash, arthralgia, hypotension, weight gain with edema, oliguria, pulmonary edema, congestive heart failure, and central nervous system (CNS) toxicities. Most of

Table 51.2 Therapeutic schedules of interleukin-2 in different tumors

Disease		Dose	Schedule	Duration
Melanoma	Bolus intravenous application: IL-2	600 000 IU/kg	5 days	Cycle repeated after ~10 days
	Continuous infusion: IL-2	16-24 × 10^6 IU/m^2/d	3-5 days	Weekly for ≥8 weeks
Renal cell carcinoma	Continuous infusion: IL-2	18 × 10^6 IU/m^2/d	5 days	Cycle repeated after 7 days
	Subcutaneous application: IL-2	18 x 10^6 IU/d	Days 1-5	Week 1
		9 x 10^6 IU/d	Days 1-5	Weeks 2-3

the cardiovascular, renal, and CNS complications can be explained by a capillary leak syndrome caused by peripheral vasodilatation and the increased demand of cardiac output and oliguria. The side effects of IL-2 depend on the dose and schedule of administration. IL-2 is available for clinical use in vials containing 18 million units (MU).

Melanoma

Various clinical trials using different dosages have been reported. In general, the number of cycles applied depended on toxicity and response in individual patients. Remissions in 15 to 20% of patients are seen with high-dose iv IL-2 application but are associated with considerable toxicity.

Renal cell carcinoma

For renal cell carcinoma, palliative treatment can result in response rates of 15 to 20%. A significant minority of patients may have major tumor regressions, and some of these responses (5-7% of all treated patients) are complete responses, capable of being sustained for years in the absence of any ongoing therapy.

HEMATOPOIETIC GROWTH FACTORS (HGFs)

The HGFs represent a subgroup of cytokines with well-defined effects on the hematopoietic system. Until now, three factors have been registered for clinical application: the myeloid growth factors granulocyte and granulocyte/macrophage colony-stimulating factor (G- and GM-CSF) and erythropoietin, the main regulator of erythroid growth. In addition, thrombopoietin has been cloned and tested clinically.

When given in the recommended dose, HGFs are relatively safe drugs with limited toxicities and can be injected subcutaneously by the patient himself or herself. However, HGFs are also expensive drugs, and noncritical application must be avoided.

Erythropoietin

Erythropoietin is produced in the kidney and exerts its maximal activity at the level of the more differentiated erythroid precursor cells (see Chap. 73). It is registered in many countries for the treatment of renal anemia. In more recent years, it also has been demonstrated convincingly that the majority of patients suffering from anemia due to malignant disease may benefit from treatment.

Erythropoietin is available for clinical use in vials containing between 1000 and 10000 units. In anemia due to malignant disease and chemotherapy-related anemia, doses of 150 to 300 units/kg subcutaneously three to five times per week, of a duration depending on response, can stimulate erythropoiesis in 50 to 70% of patients. Furthermore, erythropoietin is effective in improving the functional sta-

tus and quality of life in anemic cancer patients receiving chemotherapy, as well as in increasing hemoglobin levels and decreasing transfusion requirements. In order to predict response as soon as possible, the individual endogenous erythropoietin level should be determined before therapy. If after 2 weeks of therapy the hemoglobin value has increased by 0.5 g/dl or more, with initial endogenous erythropoietin levels under 100 milliunits/ml, 95% of patients will respond. In patients who respond, the dose can be reduced and adapted according to requirements.

Myeloid growth factors

Myeloid growth factors significantly shorten the duration of neutropenia following chemotherapy, whereas the nadir usually remains unaffected. One major indication for use of the myeloid growth factors G-CSF (filgrastim and lenograstim) and GM-CSF (molgramostim) is prophylaxis of neutropenic fever in patients treated with chemotherapeutic regimens that are likely to produce this complication (primary prophylaxis). The time until neutrophil recovery can be shortened and the incidence of febrile neutropenia reduced by use of myeloid growth factors, whereas infection-related mortality and patient survival remain unaffected. The use of myeloid growth factors is justified when the risk of febrile neutropenia exceeds 40% or when a patient is expected to have poor bone marrow tolerance.

The recurrence of neutropenic fever can be prevented in patients who developed an infection after a previous cycle of chemotherapy and in whom dose reduction would be inappropriate (secondary prophylaxis). Secondary prophylaxis therefore is recommended mainly in the curative setting when a dose reduction would lead to a decrease in expected long-term success rates and the continuation of full-dose treatment could expose the patient to life-threatening complications.

The toxicity profile of myeloid growth factors is quite favorable, and G-CSF is particularly well-tolerated, with bone pain the only relevant side effect. The pattern of toxicity of GM-CSF is more typical of that which has been reported for the administration of other cytokines, with fever and/or chills occurring in some patients.

The vials available for clinical application contain filgrastim 300 µg (30 million units) or 480 µg (48 million units), lenograstim 263 µg (34 million units), or molgramostim 150, 300, or 400 µg (Tab. 51.3).

Neutrophil granulocyte count increases under therapy with G- or GM-CSF in 70 to 80% of myelodysplastic patients but without any increase in survival. Therefore, application of a myeloid growth factor is only indicated in patients with severe neutropenia in combination with an increased incidence of infections.

NEW CONCEPTS OF BIOLOGIC THERAPY

Monoclonal antibodies (MABs)

MABs are in the process of becoming an integral component of medical cancer therapy. Because of their specific antigen binding, MABs represent a potentially extremely

Table 51.3 Treatment schedules of myeloid growth factors for major indications

Indication		Dose	Schedule and duration
Febrile neutropenia	G-CSF	5 µg/kg/d sc	Beginning 24-72 h after chemotherapy
	GM-CSF	250 µg/m²/d sc	until neutrophil count for 3 days > 1000/µl
Myelodysplastic syndromes (MDS)	G-CSF	1-3 µg/kg/d sc	
	GM-CSF	100 µg/m²/d sc	

effective form of cancer treatment without causing the classic cytotoxic side effects (fever, flulike symptoms, etc.). "Humanized" antibodies produced by genetic engineering have the advantage of remaining in the body for long periods of time. Therapeutic MABs act on tumor-associated surface structures in a manner similar to the immune response induced by antitumor vaccines. Binding of the antibody to the cell surface recruits cytotoxic effector cells such as lymphocytes and macrophages while also activating the complement system. In parallel, most therapeutically effective antibodies use a transmembrane transfer of signals into the neoplastic cell and induce mechanisms that can cause programmed cell death (apoptosis).

The *murine monoclonal antibody 17-1A* recognizes a glycoprotein that occurs mainly on the surface of adenocarcinomas. The mode of action of the 17-1A antibody is complex and mediated by inducing antibody- as well as the complement-dependent cell-mediated cytotoxicity, thus making the immunologic effector cells aware of the colorectal carcinoma. As an additional mode of action, it is assumed that the antibody leads to the production of so-called anti-idiotypic antibodies that bind to certain structures of the 17-A1 antibody. In the ensuing cascade, immunoglobulins against the anti-idiotypic antibodies are formed that possess a cross-reacting antitumor activity, thus further enhancing the 17-A1 antibody effect.

In a randomized clinical phase III study in patients with locally advanced colorectal carcinoma after radical surgery, one group of patients received 500 mg of the 17-1A antibody iv 2 weeks after surgery for the first time and four times thereafter (100 mg intravenously at 4-week intervals). Patients in the antibody group had a significant reduction in relapse rate and disease-induced mortality at 5 years compared with a control group without antibody therapy.

The first "humanized" antibody, directed at the CD20 surface structure on B-lymphocytes, has been approved for administration to patients with non-Hodgkin's lymphoma (NHL). The *CD20 antigen* is expressed on the surface of mature B-lymphocytes and by the majority of malignant lymphomas derived from B-cells. In contrast, the CD20 antigen is not expressed by hematopoietic stem cells or very early B-cells and T-cells. Clinical studies involving the intravenous administration of this CD20 antibody (Rituximab) in patients with low-grade NHL,

most of whom had previously undergone chemotherapy, showed enhanced removal of B-cells expressing CD20, with an overall response rate of approximately 40%. Unfortunately, recent reports indicate the occurrence of a "cytokine syndrome" in some Rituximab-treated patients. A radioactive formulation of this MAB (Bexxar) is in advanced clinical development.

Another MAB recently approved for human therapy is a *"humanized" anti-HER-2 antibody* (Trastuzumab). The interaction between epidermal growth factor (EGF) and its receptor (EGFR) correlates with proliferation and prognosis in several types of cancer. About 25 to 30% of breast and ovarian carcinomas express a mutated form of EGFR, the so-called HER-2, that is activated without ligand binding and which indicates poor prognosis. Clinical phase II and III trials performed to date show that Herceptin induces durable objective tumor responses as single agent, and when added to chemotherapy, it can significantly increase response rate and progression-free survival in HER-2+ metastatic breast cancer (see Chap. 61).

Anticancer vaccines

The identification of a variety of tumor-associated or tumor-specific antigens presents a unique opportunity to induce antitumor immunologic responses in vivo. Therefore, numerous early clinical trials have been initiated on potential cancer vaccines. Although the relative antitumor efficacy of antibody versus cell-mediated immune responses is not yet known, the vast majority of cancer vaccines entering into clinical trials have been designed to induce cell-mediated immune responses. Antigens recognized by T-cells are peptide fragments of intracellular proteins bound to major histocompatability complex (MHC) molecules and then expressed on the cell surface.

Antitumor vaccines are based on three concepts: peptide vaccination, vaccination with genetically modified organisms (GMOs), and application of autologous tumor cells that may be genetically modified. Peptide vaccination implies the possibility to produce a tumor-associated antigen by means of gene technology and apply it as a drug subcutaneously. Clinical trials are under way mainly in cancers such as melanoma, where the tumor-associated antigenic structures on the cell surface are well defined. Although the first results seem encouraging, vaccination with peptides has the potential disadvantage of requiring a more or less intact immune system, a supposition that is often not fulfilled in advanced stages of cancer. Another important problem is the antigen restriction by the MHC. The MHC comprises a number of genes coding for membrane-bound proteins that play an important role in T-cell activation. For specific recognition of a foreign cell by a T-lymphocyte, not only is antigen expression of the cell important, but also antigen presentation by the respective MHC molecule is necessary. Therefore, immune responses underlie the control of MHC-coded membrane-bound proteins, and a successful peptide vaccination is restricted by the fact that cytotoxic T-lymphocytes can only recognize the respective tumor-associated antigen (TAA) in patients with the correct HLA phenotype.

Another approach using the vaccination strategy focuses on the application of genetically modified organisms (GMOs). A GMO usually is represented by a virus transfected with the genetic information to code for a tumor-associated antigen. The advantage of GMO vaccination is that MHC restriction may be avoided because proteins expressed by the virus in human cells can be processed by the immune system and expressed on the cell surface without underlying the diversity of the MHC.

Finally, interest has been raised by the possibility that cytokine genes can be introduced into cancer cells to modulate immunogenicity. Techniques of somatic gene therapy allow the generation of immunogenic cancer vaccines from the patient's own tumor and seek to locally alter the immunologic environment of the tumor. In particular, genes that express cytokines such as IL-2 or GM-CSF are already being used in clinical trials. Cytokine gene-transduced tumor cells produce cytokines at very high concentrations local to the tumor. Since systemic concentrations of cytokines are usually very low, this paracrine physiology much more closely mimics the natural biology of cytokine action than does systemic application.

Suggested readings

CREAGAN ET, AHMANN DL, FRYTAK S, et al. Three consecutive phase II studies of recombinant interferon-alpha-2a in advanced malignant melanoma. Cancer 1987;59:638-40.

CREAGAN ET, LOPRIZI CL, AHMANN DL, et al. A phase I-II trial of the combination of recombinant leukocyte A interferon and recombinant human interferon-gamma in patients with metastatic malignant melanoma. Cancer 1988;62:2472-4.

DORVAL T, FRIDMAN WH, MATHIOT C, et al. Treatment of metastatic malignant melanoma with interleukin-2. Bull Cancer 1992;79:781-7.

EVANS LM, ITRI LM, CAMPION M, et al. Interferon-alpha-2a in the treatment of acquired immunodeficiency syndrome-related Kaposi's sarcoma. J Immunother 1991;10:39-50.

THE ITALIAN COOPERATIVE STUDY GROUP ON CML. Interferon-α-2a as compared with conventional chemotherapy for the treatment of chronic myeloid leukemia. N Engl J Med 1994;330:820-5.

KIRKWOOD M, STRAWDERMAN MH, ERNSTOFF, et al. Interferon-alpha-2b adjuvant therapy of high-risk resected cutaneous melanoma: The Eastern Cooperative Oncology Group trial EST 1684. J Clin Oncol 1996;14:7-17.

LUDWIG H, FRITZ E, LEITGEB C, et al. Prediction of response to erythropoietin treatment in chronic anemia of cancer. Blood 1994;84:1056-63.

MALONEY DG, GRILLO-LOPEZ AJ, WHITE CA, et al. IDEC-C2B8 (Rituximab) anti-CD20 monoclonal antibody therapy in patients with relapsed low-grade non-Hodgkin's lymphoma. Blood 1997;90:2188-95.

NEGRIN RS, HAEUBER DH, NAGLER A, et al. Maintenance treatment of patients with myelodysplastic syndromes using recombinant human granulocyte colony-stimulating factor. Blood 1990;76:36-43.

PARKINSON DR, ABRAMS JS, WIERNIK PH, et al. Interleukin-2 therapy in patients with metastatic malignant melanoma: a phase II study. J Clin Oncol 1990;8:1650-6.

RIETHMÜLLER G, SCHNEIDER-GÄDICKE E, SCHLIMOK , et al. Randomized trials of monoclonal antibody for adjuvant therapy of resected Dukes' C colorectal carcinoma. Lancet 1994;343:1177-83.

SPIELBERGER RT, MICK R, RATAIN MJ, GOLOMB H. Interferon treatment for hairy cell leukemia: an update on a cohort of 69 patients treated from 1983-86. Leukemia Lymphoma 1994;14:89-93.

UMEDA T, NIJAMA N. Phase II study of alpha interferon on renal cell carcinoma: summary of three collaborative trials. Cancer 1986;58:1231-5.

WEST WH, TAUER KW, YANNELLI JR, et al. Constant-infusion recombinant interleukin-2 in adoptive immunotherapy of advanced cancer. N Engl J Med 1987;316:898-905.

ZWIERZINA H. Practical aspects of cytokine therapy. Stem Cells 1993;11:144-53.

Stem cell transplantation

Boris Labar

Stem cell transplantation has been employed increasingly for a wide variety of malignant diseases. Table 52.1 summarizes the indications, types of transplants administered, and sources of stem cells used for transplants in different malignant tumors.

ALLOGENEIC STEM CELL TRANSPLANTATION

Allogeneic stem cell transplantation is the grafting of stem cells from a donor into a recipient who is not genetically identical. Histocompatibility in humans is determined by the HLA system, and the prerequisite for treatment is a genotypically matched patient and donor. HLA incompatibility is associated with an increased risk of rejection and increased incidence of graft-versus-host disease (GvHD).

Stem cells for transplantation usually are obtained from bone marrow by multiple aspirations from the posterior iliac crest. In adult patients, a volume of 700 to 1000 ml with a total of 2 to 3×10^9 nucleated cells per kilogram of patient body weight usually is enough for engraftment. In the recent years, stem cells increasingly have been collected from the blood after mobilization procedures. In mobilization, granulocyte colony-stimulating factor (G-CSF) at a dose of 5 to 10 mg/kg of donor body weight frequently is administered. In most donors, G-CSF can be given safely with only mild to moderate bone pain. Stem cells are infused intravenously into the recipient if the donor and

---

Table 52.1 Indications, timing, and stem cell sources for transplantation

Disease	Ideal timing	Stem cell sources	
		first choice	alternatives
AML	CR1	Sibling HLA-matched	ABMT, MUD
ALL			
Adults	CR1	Sibling HLA-matched	ABMT
Children	CR2		MUD
CML	Chronic phase (within 1 year)	Sibling HLA-matched	MUD
			PBSC
MDS	RAEB, RAEBt, CMML	Sibling HLA-matched	ABMT
			MUD
Lymphoma	CR2, PR	APBSC	ABMT
			Sibling HLA-matched
Myeloma	Aggressive disease	APBSC	Sibling HLA-matched
Solid tumors	CR, PR	APBSC	ABMT
Neuroblastoma			Sibling HLA-matched
Breast cancer			
Ovarian carcinoma			
Germ cell cancer			
Lung cancer			

(ABMT=autologous bone marrow transplantation; ALL=acute lymphoblatic leukemia; AML= acute myeloblastic leukemia; APBSC=autologous, peripheral blood stem cell; CML=chronic myeloid leukemia; CMML=chronic myelomonocytic leukemia; CR=complete remission; MDS=myelodysplastic syndrome; MUD=matched unrelated donor; PR=partial remission; RAEB= refractory anemia with excess of blasts; RAEBt= refractory anemia with excess of blasts in transformation.)

recipient are ABO compatible. In the event of major ABO incompatibility, the graft must be depleted of red blood cells by sedimentation methods, or the antibody in the donor blood has to be decreased significantly by two to three plasma exchange procedures before stem cell infusion. Another source of stem cells is human umbilical cord blood, which is rich in early and committed progenitor cells.

The use of unrelated matched donors for allogeneic transplantation is still controversial. According to recent results, transplants from unrelated matched donors can be performed in younger patients with acute leukemia and chronic myelogenous leukemia.

Before transplantation, patients received intensive preparative regimens. The main goal of such regimens is to eradicate tumor cells in the recipient. The preparative regimens also decrease or remove host resistance to grafting. Host immune cells such as T-cells and natural killer (NK) cells that are capable of rejecting the graft have to be eliminated. The conditioning regimen is also important for creating the "space" for donor marrow, which will replace the host hematopoietic system. The most frequently used preparative regimens are summarized in Table 52.2.

The donor cells enter the recipient's circulation and repopulate the recipient's hematopoietic cells. The cells that possess the donor characteristics are peripheral blood cells, osteoclasts, Kupffer cells of the liver, Langerhans' cells of the skin, alveolar macrophages, and microglial cells of the brain. Circulating progenitor donor cells bind selectively to the marrow stroma. The receptor membrane-binding proteins mediate this so-called homing process. After binding to stromal cells, progenitor cells divide and proliferate. With maturation, homing receptors are diluted and lost. Mature cells do not possess homing receptors and can be released into the circulation. After the infusion of stem cells, the patient is severely pancytopenic. The first sign of engraftment can be detected in the bone marrow at the beginning of the second week after grafting. The main criterion for engraftment is defined by the number of granulocytes. More than 0.5×10^9/liter of granulocyte is the main criteria for engraftment. The speed of engraftment varies from 12 to 35 days and mainly depends on the underlying disease, previous chemoradiotherapy, preparative regimen, and type of transplantation, as well as the drugs used for GvHD prophylaxis. The immune reconstitution takes a longer period of time. Most recipients require at least 3 to 4 months to reach normal T- and B-cell numbers and a year until the ratio of CD4 to CD8 cells has returned to normal. Allogeneic stem cell transplantation, when indicated, is the treatment of choice for acute leukemia, myelodysplastic syndrome, and chronic myelogenous leukemia (see Chap. 63).

Table 52.2 Common intensive preparative regimens

Regimen	Agent	Disease
Cyclophosphamide + TBI Melphalan + TBI Busulfan + cyclophosphamide		Acute leukemia, CML, lymphoma, multiple myeloma, AML AML, CML
CBV	Cyclophosphamide Carmustine Etoposide	HD
BEAC	Carmustine Etoposide Cytarabine Cyclophosphamide	HD
BEAM	Carmustine Etoposide Cytarabine Melphalan	NHL, HD
BACT	Carmustine Cytarabine Cyclophosphamide Thioguanine	Lymphoma, leukemia
VICE	Etoposide Ifosfamide Carboplatin Cytarabine	Breast cancer
Cyclophosphamide, thiotepa, carboplatin		Breast cancer

(ALL= acute lymphoblastic leukemia; AML=acute myeloid leukemia; CML=chronic myeloid leukemia; HD=Hodgkin's disease; NHL=non-Hodgkin's lymphoma; TBI=total body irradiation.)

Table 52.3 Major problems with stem cell transplantation

Early toxicity of chemoradiotherapy
  Reversible side effects
  Nausea and vomiting
  Mucositis
  Diarrhea
  Hemorrhagic cystitis
  Marrow aplasia (infections, bleeding complications)
  Alopecia
  Proctitis

Life-threatening side effects
  Interstitial pneumonitis
  Hepatic venoocclusive disease
  Cardiomyopathy

Late toxicity of chemoradiotherapy
  Gonadal insufficiency (sterility)
  Growth disturbancies in children
  Cataracts
  Secondary malignancies

Graft rejection

Graft-versus-host disease

Relapse of malignant tumor

Graft failure is relatively rare in patients with malignant tumors (<2%). The possible mechanism could be destruction of the stromal cells and more frequently relapse of the original tumor.

Infection and GvHD are the most frequent complications after allogeneic stem cell transplantation (Tab. 52.3). In the first months after transplantation, during the period of aplasia and severe pancytopenia with breakdown of skin and mucosal barriers, bacterial and fungal infections predominate. During this period, patients must reside in reverse isolation rooms or laminar airflow rooms. The main effort is to prevent infections by administering oral nonabsorbable antibiotics for selective gastrointestinal decontamination. The incidence of fungal infection is decreased by the administration of fluconazole or low-dose amphotericin B. Patients are at risk for both gram-positive and gram-negative infections. Because of selective intestinal decontamination and indwelling central venous catheters, in the recent years, gram-positive bacteremia, predominantly from methicillin-resistant *Staphylococcus* spp., increasingly has been documented. A febrile neutropenic patient often is treated with a combination of broad-spectrum antibiotics, and further treatment depends on clinical response, signs of localized infection, and culture results. If fever persists despite broad-spectrum antibiotics, a fungal infection should be suspected, and treatment with amphotericin B or lipid-formulated amphotericin B must be instituted. In selected patients, fluconazole also may be of benefit. For herpes simplex infection, intravenous acyclovir is effective.

After neutrophil recovery, the main problem is prolonged immunosuppression, especially in patients with GvHD. In about 15 to 20% of patients, cytomegalovirus (CMV) interstitial pneumonitis usually occurs 2 to 3 months following stem cell transplantation. Interstitial pneumonitis is a consequence of the direct cytopathic effect of viral replication and host-dependent immunopathologic mechanisms. In seropositive patients, the infection develops secondary to reactivation of latent virus, whereas in seronegative patients, the infection is transmitted from seropositive grafted stem cells or blood products as a primary infection. In seronegative patients who received seronegative grafts, CMV infection can be prevented effectively with transfusion of seronegative blood products. Until recently, the mortality rate of interstitial pneumonitis was over 95%. The combination of ganciclovir and high-dose intravenous immunoglobulins has resulted in survival rates of about 50 to 60%. Interstitial pneumonitis caused by *Pneumocystis carinii* is almost completely eliminated by prophylactic administration of co-trimoxazole.

GvHD, an immunologic reaction of donor T-lymphocytes against the recipient's tissues, is the most serious complication of allogeneic stem cell transplantation. Acute GvHD develops during the first 100 days following allografting. Acute GvHD affects the skin (from maculopapular rash to erythroderma and bullae formation), gut (from vomiting and diarrhea to abdominal cramping pain, ileus, and gut perforation) and liver (elevated bilirubin and alkaline phosphatase levels that may progress to liver failure). Clinically, GvHD is graded on a scale of 1 to 4 based on the severity of organ involvement. Moderate to severe acute GvHD that clinically represents grades 2 to 4 has a significant mortality rate. The most important predictive factor for the incidence and severity of GvHD is HLA incompatibility between donor and recipient. However, this complication also develops in about 40% of recipients who receive stem cells from HLA-identical sibling donors even when prophylactic therapy is given.

Two main approaches to the prevention of GvHD are currently used. For prophylactic immunosuppressive therapy, methotrexate, cyclosporine, and prednisone alone or in combination are given. Methotrexate and cyclosporine given as a single agent are associated with moderate to severe acute GvHD in approximately 60% of patients. A combination of these drugs is superior to either agent given alone, reducing the incidence to approximately 30%. The combination of prednisone with methotrexate and cyclosporine gives the best results. The incidence of grades 2 to 4 acute GvHD in the triple combination is less than 10%. Another prophylactic approach is the removal of T-lymphocytes from the graft. Many methods have been used for T-cell depletion, such as monoclonal antibodies alone or in combination with complement, monoclonal antibodies linked to toxins, and physical separation methods such as counterflow centrifugation, soybean lectin agglutination, and E-rosette depletion. T-cell depletion is a very effective approach that completely eliminates moderate to severe acute GvHD. Recurrence of the underlying malignant tumor depends primarily on the remission status of the patient at the time of transplantation. Chronic GvHD develops in 30 to 40% of patients who survive more than 100 days following allografting. The syndrome resembles autoimmune disorders such as scleroderma. Chronic GvHD is characterized as limited (localized skin and liver involvement) or extensive (generalized skin or multiorgan involvement). Treatment includes cyclosporine or azathioprine and thalidomide in combination with prednisone. Allogeneic stem cell recipients with moderate to severe acute GvHD were found to have a significantly lower relapse rate compared with allogeneic recipients with mild or no GvHD or with syngeneic stem cell recipients. Chronic GvHD also decreases the relapse rate. The graft-versus-tumor effect of GvHD is mediated by T-cells. Attempts to modulate GvHD in order to increase the graft-versus-tumor reaction have not been successful to date.

Other complications associated with allografting are venoocclusive disease, neurologic disorders, and late complications such as cataracts, endocrine disorders (e.g., gynecologic abnormalities, infertility, hypothyroidism, and growth and developmental abnormalities), and rarely, secondary malignancies (Epstein-Barr virus-associated B-cell lymphoproliferative disorders and solid tumors).

AUTOLOGOUS STEM CELL TRANSPLANTATION

Autologous stem cell transplantation is the grafting of patients with their own stem cells. The rationale for autologous stem cell transplantation is intensification of chemotherapy that might eliminate malignant cells and cure the patient. The main limitation of dose escalation is severe myelotoxicity and very prolonged hematopoietic recovery. This problem is overcome by infusing into the patient his/her own stem cells previously harvested and cryopreserved. A good treatment efficacy has been obtained for malignancies with a steep dose-response

relationship. In such tumors, a small increase in dose results in large increases in tumor kill. Table 52.4 summarizes dose escalation for some agents used in stem cell transplantation.

The sources of stem cells in autografting are bone marrow and peripheral blood. At the beginning, blood cells were used as an alternative source for stem cells in patients whose bone marrow was contaminated with malignant cells and in patients with marrow damaged by intensive chemoradiotherapy. The procedure involved in harvesting a sufficient number of nucleated cells and colony-forming unit granulocyte/macrophage (CFU-GM) progenitor cells was cumbersome and time-consuming. Therefore, peripheral blood stem cell transfusion (PBSCT) was used relatively seldom. After observations that the number of circulating peripheral blood stem cells could be vastly enhanced by exposure to chemotherapy and hematopoietic growth factors, interest in PBSCT has grown exponentially.

The number of progenitor cells in peripheral blood may be significantly increased by using a combination of cytotoxic agents and hematopoietic growth factors. Cyclophosphamide and etoposide are the most popular cytotoxic drugs because they do not posses major stem cell toxicity. In high doses, these drugs are very effective mobilizing agents. Drugs with substantial stem cell toxicity such as melphalan and carboplatin are also effective mobilizers. Intensive regimens with profound myelosuppression are more effective in mobilizing stem cells. It was speculated that with more intensive chemotherapy, hematopoietic insult might induce greater secondary productions of cytokines by the bone marrow stroma. Administration of myelosuppressive chemotherapy produces a maximum mobilization effect approximately 19 days later, when recovery of neutropenia induced by chemotherapy begins. This effect lasts only a few days. The optimal mobilization technique of progenitor cells with chemotherapy has not been established yet. Growth factors also were shown to increase progenitor cells in peripheral blood. Most of the data are based on granulocyte/macrophage colony-stimulating factor (GM-CSF) and G-CSF administration. Cytokine-induced mobiliza-

Table 52.4 Dose escalation of single agents

Agent	Usual conventional dose	Maximun dose with SCT	Limited extramedullary toxicity
Cyclophosphamide (mg/kg)	50	200	Cardiac, bladder
Carmustine (mg/m^2)	200	1200	Pulmonary, hepatic
Melphalan (mg/m^2)	40	200	Gastrointestinal, hepatic
Etoposide (mg/m^2)	360	2400	Gastrointestinal
Ifosfamide (mg/m^2)	5000	18,000	Renal, bladder
Thiotepa (mg/m^2)	50	1135	CNS, gastrointestinal
Carboplatin (mg/m^2)	400	2000	Hepatic, renal
TBI (Gy)	3.5[1]	12-14	Pulmonary, hepatic

(SCT=stem cell transplantation; TBI= total body irradiation.)
[1]Maximum dose without stem cell transplantation.

tion differs from chemotherapy-induced mobilization in that cytokine administration does not induce neutropenia. The maximum mobilization effect occurs within the first 5 days of growth factor administration, and the effect seems to persist as long as administration of growth factors continues. Growth factor administration can be associated with a number of side effects, including flulike symptoms such as headache, vomiting, dyspnea, fever, and bone pain. The combination of growth factors and chemotherapy seems to be the most powerful mobilization procedure. High-dose cyclophosphamide and GM-CSF increase the number of progenitor cells up to 1000 times. The combined approach results in a maximum mobilization effect that occurs approximately 5 days earlier, i.e., 14 days after administration of the cytotoxic drug, as compared with chemotherapy-induced mobilization. The major mobilization effect lasts a few days and apparently cannot be prolonged to any degree by continued administration of cytokine. Neutropenia is often abrogated to some degree by growth factor administration. The patient is at risk for the side effects of cytokine administration and neutropenia. Peripheral progenitor cells could be expanded in culture by using stem cell factor (SCF), interleukin 1b (IL-1b), IL-3, IL-6, and erythropoietin. At days 12 to 14 of culture, up to a 115-fold increase in progenitor cells was found.

PBSCT shortens the duration of myelosuppression, especially thrombocytopenia. Many clinical reports indicated a reduction in the number of units of blood and platelets transfused, antibiotic therapy, and duration of hospitalization for patients receiving PBSCT compared with marrow transplantation.

The number of blood stem cells necessary to produce engraftment has not been defined precisely. Traditional assessments of blood stem cell content and capability of transplant cells to engraft have relied on the number of nucleated cells and the CFU-GM cloning assay. It seems that collection of more than 2×10^8 nucleated cells per kilogram of body weight and collection of 15 to 50×10^4 CFU-GM per kilogram of body weight is sufficient to produce sustained engraftment. Human stem cells express the cell surface marker CD34. Flow cytometric determination of CD34$^+$ cells in the circulation is used currently as a more effective method of monitoring the engraftment capacity of collected cells. More than 2×10^6 CD34$^+$ cells per kilogram of body weight collected is sufficient for engraftment.

PBSCTs seem to be less frequently contaminated with tumor cells than bone marrow transplants. This is true for lymphoma, myeloma, and some solid tumors such as breast cancer. In Hodgkin's lymphoma, peripheral blood is more frequently contaminated with Hodgkin's cells. With mobilization techniques, malignant cells are also mobilized, and increased numbers are found in peripheral blood. In multiple myeloma, circulating myeloma and B cells belonging to the malignant clone have been detected in peripheral blood even in the early stages of the disease. The number of circulating myeloma cells is further increased in apheresis collections following high-dose chemotherapy with hematopoietic growth factor support. In breast cancer, malignant cell recruitment and contami-

nation of peripheral blood stem cell collections can occur in patients with and without bone marrow involvement. Peripheral blood appears to be significantly less frequently contaminated than bone marrow. The potential to reinfuse viable clonogenic tumor cells is a potential disadvantage of autologous bone marrow or blood stem cell transplantation. By using a variety of purging methods, an attempt is made to remove tumor cells from the graft. For acute leukemia and some solid tumors, pharmacologic agents such as mafosfamide and 4-hydroperoxycyclophosphamide are effective purging agents. Monoclonal antibodies directed against lymphoid and myeloid markers plus complement have been able to remove 99% of tumor cells. This is so-called negative selection. Alternatively, hematopoietic stem cells may be concentrated and isolated and then removed from the graft (positive selection). Human hematopoietic stem cells express marker CD34 and another antigen, Thy-1, but do not express lineage-specific markers. Positive selection of CD34$^+$ cells with monoclonal antibodies results in a 1 to 4 log reduction in tumor cells in apheresis products, but whether this time-consuming technique improves survival is currently under investigation. Autologous stem cell transplantation, when indicated, is the treatment of choice for lymphoma, multiple myeloma, and solid tumors (see Chaps. 51 and 63).

The main problem with autologous stem cell transplantation is still the high tumor relapse rate. The lack of graft-versus-tumor effect described in allografting may be responsible for this. Recently, several attempts have been made to induce an autologous immune antitumor effect. Administration of IL-2, and cyclosporine activates in vitro NK cells and subpopulations of T-cells and induces the release of interferon-γ and tumor necrosis factor. The immune antitumor effect has not yet been proven in clinical trials.

Stem cells are ideal for gene engineering and therapy. Recently, a gene transfer technique was used mostly to mark hematopoietic progenitor cells prior to transplantation so that their subsequent fate could be tracked in vivo. The goal was preferentially to improve the process of PBSCT. Gene marking also was used to determine whether harvested progenitor cells in marrow or blood were contaminated with malignant cells and whether attempts to remove such cells were successful.

It has to be stated that peripheral blood progenitor cells allow the implementation of a new strategy for the evaluation of new anticancer drugs. In this setting, drugs may be evaluated up to their dose-limiting nonhematologic toxicities, with a somewhat lower limit imposed solely by hematologic clearance. Ex vivo stem cell expansion techniques may provide cleansed products to support high-dose chemotherapies and may be able to eliminate the hematologic toxicities of cytotoxic therapy altogether. New methods of gene transfer by using peripheral progenitor cells are a promising tool of anticancer therapy. All these developments imply that stem cell transplantation is a very promising approach for the development of novel therapeutic initiatives.

Suggested readings

ARMITAGE S, HARGREAVES R, SAMSON D, et al. CD34 counts to predict the adequate collection of peripheral blood progenitor cells. Bone Marrow Transplant 1997;20:587-91.

BRENNER MK, RILL DR, MOEN RC, et al. Gene marking to trace origin of relapse after autologous bone marrow transplantation. Lancet 1993;341:85-6.

BRUGGER W, BROSS K, GLATT M, et al. Mobilization of tumor cells and hematopoietic progenitor cells into peripheral blood of patients with solid tumors. Blood 1994;3:636-40.

CAIRO MS, WAGNER JE. Placental and/or umbilical cord blood: An alternative source of hematopoietic stem cells for transplantation. Blood 1997;90:4665-78.

GRATWOHL A, HERMANS J, BALDOMERO H. Blood and marrow transplantation activity in Europe 1995. Bone Marrow Transplant 1997;19:407-19.

DEEG HJ, LIN D, et al. Cyclosporine or cyclosporine plus methotrexate for prophylaxis of graft-versus-host disease: a prospective randomized trial. Blood 1997;89:3880-7.

EMERSON SG. Ex vivo expansion of hematopoietic precursors, progenitors and stem cells: the next generation of cellular therapeutics. Blood 1996;87:3082-8.

FIELDING AK, WATTS MJ, GOLDSTONE AH. Peripheral blood progenitor cells versus bone marrow. J Hematother 1994;3:299-304.

GRUEN JR, WEISSMAN SM. Review: evolving views of the major histocompatibility complex. Blood 1997;90:4252-65.

KEATING A. Autologous bone marrow transplantation. In: Armitage JO, Antman KH, eds. High-dose cancer therapy, 2nd ed. Baltimore: Williams & Wilkins, 1995.

KESSINGER A, ARMITAGE JO. The evolving role of autologous peripheral stem cell transplantation following high-dose therapy for malignancies. Blood 1991;77:211-3.

MOLINEUX G, POJDA Z, HAMPSON IN, et al. Transplantation potential of peripheral blood stem cells induced by granulocyte colony-stimulating factor. Blood 1990;76:2163-9.

ROCHA M, UMANSKY V, LEE KH, et al. Differences between graft-versus-leukemia and graft-versus-host reactivity: I. Interaction of donor immune T cells with tumor and/or host cells. Blood 1997;89:2189-202.

SPANGRUDE GJ. Biological and clinical aspects of hematopoietic stem cells. Annu Rev Med 1994;45:93-104.

THOMAS ED, STORB R, CLIFT RA. Bone marrow transplantation. N Engl J Med 1985;292:832-95.

TO LB, HAYLOCK DN, SIMMONS PJ, JUTTNER CA. Review: the biology and clinical uses of blood stem cells. Blood 1997;89:2233-58.

CHAPTER

53

Central nervous system

Erhard Suess, Christoph C. Zielinski

Complex therapeutic approaches are necessary to deliver sufficient support to patients suffering from primary or secondary neoplasms of the central nervous system (CNS). CNS malignancies frequently are accompanied by severe neurologic deficits that necessitate differentiated symptomatic therapy. Epileptic seizures, increased intracranial pressure (ICP), and hemi- or paraparesis of limbs or spasticity are common clinical symptoms. Maintenance of quality of life is a primary criterion for therapeutic decisions.

Consequently, the extent of surgical resection often is limited owing to involvement of functional brain areas by the tumor. Likewise, the total cumulative dose of radiotherapy delivered to brain tumors is limited by long-term adverse effects, including leukencephalopathy and induction of necrosis.

Promising progress has been made in the therapy of CNS tumors during the last decade. The combination of surgery, radiotherapy, and chemotherapy was found to be most effective in CNS tumors in most early studies, but some newer protocols applying combined cytoreductive agents have produced superior results. Combination chemotherapy given for primary brain tumors of oligodendroglial origin administered following surgery was found to be superior to chemotherapy following surgery and radiotherapy. Moreover, grade IV oligodendroglioma presented with a much better response than de novo glioblastoma.

Most chemotherapeutic drugs used in patients with brain tumors are given systemically via either the iv or oral route. Because of the presence of the blood-brain barrier, pharmacokinetics differ significantly in brain tumors as compared with other organ tissues, and permeability may vary extremely even within single tumors. Moreover, tumor margins often show reduced regional cerebral blood flow. Therefore, insufficient concentrations of even highly lipophilic agents may be reached in the target tumor. Hydrophilic chemotherapeutic agents including methotrexate, cytarabine (Ara-C), and at times steroids also can be applied intrathecally with the help of lumbar puncture or intraventricularly via, for example, the Omaya reservoir. Major side effects specifically linked to these modes of application are aseptic menin-

gits, myelitis, leukencephalopathy, and cerebral seizures.

When surgery is performed, local chemotherapy with instillation of cytotoxic agents into the resection cave can be applied with consecutive installations via a reservoir.

CENTRAL NERVOUS SYSTEM TUMORS SENSITIVE TO CYTOREDUCTIVE CHEMOTHERAPY

Treatment options for malignant neoplasms that have been shown to be sensitive to cytotoxic chemotherapy are presented in Table 53.1.

Gliomas represent about 30 to 40% of intracerebral tumors. The group of gliomas includes astrocytic tumors, glioblastomas, oligodendroglial tumors, and ependymomas. The pilocytic astrocytoma of childhood and adolescence is classified as World Health Organization (WHO) grade I astrocytoma; WHO grade II astrocytomas and oligodendrogliomas are highly differentiated and show a low potential for proliferation and no criteria of malignancy; WHO grade III anaplastic astrocytomas and oligodendrogliomas histologically fulfill the criteria of malignancy by frequently exhibiting mitosis, polymorphism of nuclei, neovascularization, and a high tendency to proliferation; WHO grade IV astrocytomas and oligodendrogliomas are classified as glioblastomas that are histologically identical to grade III but additionally present with necrosis.

Ependymomas originate from the ependymal tissue of the ventricular system or from disseminated ependymal cells of the terminal filum. They are the most common intramedullary tumors. About 50% of all gliomas are glioblastomas, and about 20 to 30% are astrocytomas (grades I-III). Oligodendrogliomas occur in about 3 to 8%, but only 2 to 6% of primary brain tumors are ependymomas.

World Health Organisation grade III anaplastic astrocytomas, glioblastomas, grade III anaplastic oligodendrogliomas, and grade IV oligodendrogliomas are partially sensitive to cytotoxic chemotherapy. In ependymomas, chemotherapy still has an experimental status. In contrast, chemotherapy is not recommended in low-grade astrocy-

Table 53.1 Chemotherapy protocols

Anaplastic astrocytoma III, glioblastoma

ACNU	100 mg/m^2	Single dosage	Interval: 6 weeks
or			
BCNU	80-130 mg/m^2	Single dosage	Interval: 6-8 weeks
or			
Fotemustine	100 mg/m^2	Days 1+21	Interval: 3 weeks
or			
Carboplatin	250 mg/m^2	Days 1+2	Interval: 4 weeks
+Vepeside	150 mg/m^2	Days 1-3	

Anaplastic oligodendroglioma III, glioblastoma of oligodendroglial origin (PCV therapy)

Procarbazine	60 mg/m^2	Days 1-21	Interval: 6 weeks
CCNU	100 mg/m^2	Day 1	
Vincristine	2 mg absolute	Days 8+21	

PNET, medulloblastoma, pineal blastoma (adults)
Modified HIT 91

MTX	5000 mg/m^2	Day 1 (24 h)	3 cycles, interval: 3-4 weeks
Ifosfamide	1500 mg/m^2	Days 1-3	3 cycles, 4 weeks + G-CSF days 5-10
Cisplatin	20 mg/m^2	Days 1-3	
Vepeside	100 mg/m^2	Days 1-3	

Modified EIP

Ifosfamide	1500 mg/m^2	Days 1-3	Interval: 3-4 weeks
Cisplatin	20 mg/m^2	Days 1-3	
Vepesid	100 mg/m^2	Days 1-3	

Primary cerebral lymphoma (NHL)
CHOP-BLEO

Cyclophosphamide	750 mg/m^2	Day 1	Interval: 21 days
Doxorubicin	50 mg/m^2	Day 1	Cumulative dosage: 550 mg/m^2
Vincristine	2 mg absolute	Days 1+5	
Bleomycin	15 units/day	Days 1+5	
Prednisolone	100 mg/day	Days 1-5	

Intraarterial chemotherapy following blood-brain barrier disruption

MTX	2500 mg ia	Days 1+2	Interval: >28 days performed consecutively over 1 year
Cyclophosphamide	15 mg/kg iv	Days 1+2	
Etoposide	150 mg/m^2 iv	Days 1+2	

Systemic monotherapy with MTX

MTX	1000-8000 mg/m^2	Single dosage	Interval: 4 weeks

(continued)

Table 53.1 (continued)

Intrathecal chemotherapy in meningeal carcinomatosis and leukosis

MTX	12.5 mg (Omaya reservoir) 15 mg (by lumbar puncture)	Single dosage	2-3 x per week or once a month over 12 months
Dexamethasone	4 mg it	Single dosage	
Leucovorin	4 x 5 mg po		
Ara-C	30 mg it	Single dosage	Alternating with MTX

Chemotherapy of cerebral metastases
Systemic chemotherapy of metastases from breast cancer

Cyclophosphamide	100 mg/m^2 po	Days 1-14	Interval: 4 weeks
MTX	40 mg/m^2 iv	Days 1 + 8	8 consecutive cycles
Fluorouracil	600 mg/m^2 iv	Days 1 + 8	

Systemic chemotherapy of metastases from malignant melanoma

Fotemustine	100 mg/m^2	Once weekly	3 consecutive weeks, followed by interval: 6 weeks
Fotemustine	100 mg/m^2	Once weekly	

(MTX = methotrexate; ACNU = nimustine; BCNU = carmustine; CCNU = lomustine; CSF = cerebro spinal fluid; EIP = ifosfamide cisplatin, etoposide; CHOP-BLEO = combined iv chemotherapies.); it=intrathecal; ia=intracranial.

tomas (grades I-II) as well as in highly differentiated grade II oligodendrogliomas.

Anaplastic astrocytomas (grade III) predominantly occur in the fourth and fifth decades of life. These tumors are located most frequently in the cerebral hemispheres as well as in the basal ganglia. Infratentorially located anaplastic astrocytomas are rare. Typical histologic findings are polymorphism of nuclei, neovascularization, a high number of mitoses, but an absence of necrosis. Using computed tomography (CT) as well as magnetic resonance imaging (MRI), anaplastic astrocytomas can be distinguished from grade II astrocytomas by the presence of perifocal edema and heterogeneous contrast enhancement. T_1-weighted MRI images show hyperintense lesions.

Initial clinical features vary, and cerebral seizures, focal neurologic deficits, signs of increased ICP, and psychoorganic syndromes all may constitute first signs. Mean survival time after diagnosis is 3 to 4 years. Major prognostic factors for a longer survival period are young age of the patient, good clinical condition, cerebral seizure as initial symptom, early diagnosis after initial symptoms, and small tumor burden after surgery.

A combination of surgical tumor resection followed by radio- and cytotoxic therapy constitutes the established therapeutic protocol in these tumors. The extent of surgical reduction of tumor mass is of critical importance to the duration of recurrence-free and progression-free intervals. Since 90% of tumor recurrences occur within tumor margins, focal radiotherapy has been shown to be superior to whole-brain radiotherapy. Single fractions of 1.8 to 2 Gy up to a total dose of 40 Gy are applied to the tumor and to adjacent brain tissue, and this is followed by the application of 20 Gy to the tumor bed. Alternative radiation techniques including BNCT, stereotactic focal radiation (Gamma-knife), hyperfractionated radiation, and the use of radiosensitizers (e.g., hydroxyurea, bromodeoxyuridine) have to be considered as experimental at present. Several studies have shown that anaplastic astrocytomas respond differently to chemotherapy than glioblastomas, in that a chemotherapy-associated prolongation of the mean survival time of about 10 to 15% was obtained. Following radiotherapy, polychemotherapy using, procarbazine, CCNU vincristine (PCV) has been shown to be of best efficacy.

Glioblastomas

Glioblastomas represent about 50% of glial tumors. They either develop from lower-grade astrocytomas (grade II) due to malignant transformation or occur primarily and de novo as glioblastomas. Although glioblastomas also may occur in childhood, the highest incidence is observed in the fifth and sixth decades of life. Mean survival time is about 9 months.

The most common localization is either in one hemisphere or multicentrically in both hemispheres, and some tumors cross the midline across the callosum, thus forming a so-called butterfly glioma. Tumors often contain cystic compartments. Metastatic dissemination may occur as a consequence of a connection with cerebrospinal fluid (CSF), whereas extracerebral migration was found only in rare cases. Histologic findings are identical to those of anaplastic astrocytoma but show additional necrosis. Variations of glioblastomas include giant cell glioblastomas, gliosarcomas, and glioblastoma with oligodendrocytic elements.

Initial clinical symptoms frequently are the result of increased ICP, focal neurologic deficits, hemianopsia, or apraxia. Cerebral seizures are rare as initial symptoms. Radiologic investigation often reveals a circular contrast-enhaced lesion with central hypodensity and perifocal edema on CT. Magnetic resonance imaging shows a hyperintense, inhomogeneously enhanced structure with extended edema in T_2-weighted images.

Surgery is performed with the intention to reduce tumor mass and to verify diagnosis. The extent of the tumor burden following surgery correlates with the duration of the recurrence-free interval. Some clinical centers practice consecutive tumor resections in recurrent glioblastomas. However, surgery is not indicated in the presence of tumor multicentricity or a low Karnofsky performance status of the patient.

The established therapeutic regimen includes surgery and percutaneous radiotherapy with a total dose of 55 to 60 Gy, and this has been shown to significantly prolong

survival time (mean after sugery alone 17.5 weeks, mean after surgery and adjuvant radiotherapy 37.5 weeks). Additional chemotherapy with BCNU following combination treatment with surgery and radiotherapy has been shown to prolong mean survival time significantly to 51 weeks in randomized trials. However, given that glioblastomas as well as grade II anaplastic astrocytomas and about 5% of oligocytic tumors were included in these studies, the results must be viewed with caution. Furthermore, only 20 to 25% of patients were true long-term survivors, whereas the majority of other patients did not show significant responses. Because of the unfavorable side effect profile of BCNU, including the induction of pulmonary fibrosis, ACNU is now recommended as first-line therapy in this setting. Of major importance is histologic discrimination from oligodendroglial tumors, which have a high likelihood of response to PCV therapy.

In recurrent gliomas, the clinical condition of the patient has a major influence on the modality of further treatment: thus, in some cases, palliative surgical resection may be appropriate, but in other cases local installation of BCNU has been proven to be effective, leading to a prolongation of lifespan from 23 to 31 weeks.

Oligodendrogliomas

About 2% of all intracerebral tumors are oligodendrogliomas, and about 5 to 8% of gliomas are of oligodendroglial origin. Anaplastic oligodendrogliomas are classified as WHO grade III, and those containing necrotic areas are classified as glioblastomas. They are located most frequently (50%) in the frontal lobe; some are found in the temporal or parietal lobe, and some occur rarely in regions of the occipital lobe. Lower-grade oligodendrogliomas mainly appear in young adults, most frequently in the fourth decade of life. Higher-grade oligodendrogliomas predominantly occur in recurrent tumors due to malignant progression. Initial clinical symptoms in 70 to 80% of patients are epileptic seizures, increased ICP, focal neurologic deficits, and psychoorganic syndromes.

Computed tomography is essential for diagnosis: Usually, a tumor with variable density, no or inhomogeneous contrast enhancement, and typical focal calcifications present in about 50% of its mass is seen. Perifocal edema is common in higher-grade oligodendrogliomas.

World Health Organisation grade III anaplastic oligodendrogliomas histologically are characterized by neovascularization and polymorphism. Necrotic areas indicate a grade IV oligodendroglioma. Malignant tumors of this type may disseminate metastases to the fourth ventricle by means of the cerebrospinal fluid.

First-line therapy consists of surgical tumor resection followed by radiotherapy (55-60 Gy). Malignant oligodendrogliomas are sensitive to consecutive cytotoxic chemotherapy and are considered to be a good example of chemosensitive brain tumors. Polychemotherapy with PCV has proven to be most effective, reaching responses in more than 70% of patients. Complete and partial remissions last for 18 to 60 months. Likewise, glioblastomas of oligodendroglial origin also respond to PCV therapy, with about 30% of patients showing a 50% reduction in tumor mass on CT following chemotherapy.

Medulloblastomas represent about 20% of brain tumors in children up to 5 years of age. The 5-year survival rate is 50%. The predominant location is close to the midline with consecutive extension to the fourth ventricle, the cerebellar hemispheres, and via the CSF to the spinal cord. Spinal and cerebral dissemination are found in about 10 to 40% of patients. Major clinical symptoms are headache, nausea, and vomiting. Ataxia, diplopia, and palsy of the cranial nerves may reflect invasion of the brainstem.

Magnetic resonance imaging reveals both cerebral and spinal manifestations. Radical surgical resection – though not curative – is prognostically relevant. Following surgery, radiotherapy along the entire craniospinal axis is indicated. Five-year survival without tumor recurrence can be reached in 43% by this strategy. Additional chemotherapy with a combination of vincristine, CCNU, and prednisone (HIT 91 protocol) improved this result drastically, resulting in a 2-year survival of 90% and a 5-year survival of 80%.

Primitive neuroectodermal tumors (PNETs)

About 5% of brain tumors in children are of primitive neuroectodermal origin (PNETs). Compared with medulloblastomas, tumors of this group are located predominantly in the forebrain, the temporal lobes, and the pineal gland. They grow rapidly and frequently involve craniospinal dissemination. Two-year survival is poor.

Magnetic resonance imaging of the brain and spinal cord reveals inhomogeneous tumors that include cystic as well as necrotic areas and focal calcifications. Since the use of radiotherapy is restricted in young children because of developing neural structures, surgery is followed by chemotherapy. Using a combination of carboplatin, VP-16, and thiotepa, a remission-free interval of 2 years was achieved in 42% of patients. Because of the relatively high therapy-related mortality of 10%, this treatment is restricted to specialized pediatric centers.

Primary CNS lymphoma

About 1 to 2% of primary cerebral neoplasms are malignant non-Hodgkin's lymphomas, mainly of B-cell origin. Secondary cerebral manifestations of extraneuronal malignant non-Hodgkin's lymphomas are rare but may result in leptomeningeal invasion in an advanced state of the disease. These lymphomas may arise at any age in adults, with the highest incidence in the sixth and seventh decades of life. Premorbidity from ataxia teleangiectasia, Wiskott-Aldrich syndrome, acquired immune-deficiency syndrome (AIDS), and previous prolonged treatment with immunosupressive drugs increases the risk of development of CNS lymphomas.

Primary multifocal cerebral manifestation is most common, whereas primary intramedullar localization is rare.

Rarely, visual impairment due to infiltration of the optic bulb is a leading symptom, sometimes preceding cerebral manifestations by some years. More than 50% of patients show focal neurologic deficits or psychoorganic alterations initially. Clinical diagnosis involves CT, MRI, and examination of the CSF. With CT, isodense or hyperdense leasions with strong contrast enhancement are seen with periventricular or intraventricular localization. Magnetic resonance imaging shows a similar image with contrast-enhanced hyperintense intra- and/or periventricular lesions.

Neurosurgical tumor resection has no positive influence on the course of the disease. External whole-brain radiotherapy (30-55 Gy) carries an increased risk for the development of leukencephalopathy, which is more likely when the radiotherapy is administered to elderly patients or combined with chemotherapy.

Lymphomas are sensitive to chemotherapy with methotrexate (MTX). Thus, high-dose MTX treatment ($3.5-8$ g/m^2) prolongs mean survival time from 3 to 5 months in untreated controls to more than 40 months in treated patients. At present, several therapeutic protocols use coadministration of MTX and Ara-C with good results. In addition, intraventricular administration of 12 mg MTX twice weekly is recommended. As an alternative, combined intravenous chemotherapies (CHOP-BLEO) as well as intraarterial application of MTX following blood-brain barrier disruption can be performed. Complete remissions of up to 70% for several years have been reported.

Cerebral metastases

Cerebral metastases originate most frequently from lung cancer (40-60%), breast cancer (20%), malignant melanoma (10-15%), urogenital tract neoplasms (5%), and gastrointestinal tract neoplasms (5%). Intracerebral manifestation of the tumor is the first clinical symptom in about 10 to 15% of patients, but in about 5% the primary tumor cannot be identified. Initial clinical symptoms are often cerebral seizures, focal neurologic deficits, or psychoorganic alterations due to increased ICP. Magnetic resonance imaging has a major impact on the detection and identification of cerebral metastases. In general, either single or multiple well-defined lesions with hyperintense margins and perifocal edema are seen. Differential diagnosis consists of primary cerebral tumors, vascular malformations, specific granulomas, or an abscess. Stereotactic surgery may help to identify the primary carcinoma. Mean survival time without therapy is 1 to 2 months.

About a third of all patients suffering from breast cancer develop cerebral metastases. Whereas 40% of patients have singular cerebral metastases, leptomingeal structures are affected in approximately 50% of patients who suffer from cerebral metastases. About 40% of cerebral metastases originating from breast cancer are sensitive to chemotherapy, which leads to the combined use of cyclophosphamide, MTX, and 5-fluorouracil (CMF) in eight consecutive cycles as an established procedure. In the case of estrogen-receptor-positive metastases, therapy with tamoxifen (3 x 10-20 mg/d) is indicated, as this reaches a significantly higher concentration in the tumor than in the surrounding normal neuronal tissue and may reduce tumor size significantly.

About half the patients with cerebral metastases suffer from lung cancer. In both subgroups of lung cancer, small cell and non-small cell lung cancer, the combination of surgery and radiotherapy (whole-brain radiotherapy with 30-40 Gy) constitutes first-line treatment. Small cell lung cancer is also sensitive to chemotherapy, including anthracyclines, cyclophosphamide, MTX, procarbazine, etoposide, ifosfamide, cisplatin, and the *Vinca* alkaloids. Respose rates of 76% in primary manifestations and 42% in metastases recurring after radiotherapy are reported.

Cerebral metastases occur in 16 to 75% of patients with malignant melanoma. Only about 10% develop neurologic symptoms. About 10% of patients with cerebral metastases also show leptomingeal involvement. In 20 to 30% of cerebral metastases, imaging reveals typical central hemorrhage. Standard therapeutic regimens include surgery and radiotherapy, although whole-brain radiotherapy with 20 to 50 Gy is only palliative. Response to systemic chemotherapy using fotemustine is reportedly 17 to 47%. This chemotherapy is recommended for recurrent cerebral manifestations following the standard procedure.

Therapy of increased intracranial pressure

Brain edema causing increased intracranical pressure with conseguent herniation can represent a terminal complication of brain tumors. Therefore, an early diagnosis and treatment of cerebral edema are essential, as cerebral edema can present clinically with focal signs, seizures, and psychoorganic distubances. Imaging with CT or MRI regularly reveals the extent of edema and the resulting compression of brain tissue.

The standard therapeutic procedure uses either steroids (4 x 4 mg dexamethasone orally or 40 mg as an iv bolus) or 20% mannitol iv. Alternatively, acetazolamide may be administered. In addition, forced diuresis using furosemide may be necessary. As the maximal therapeutic approach, barbiturate anesthesia and external respiratory support via tracheal tube can be initiated. Electroencephalographic monitoring is necessary in such cases due to burst suppression.

Suggested readings

BALMACEDA C, HELLER G, ROSENBLUM M, et al. Chemotherapy without irradiation – A novel approach for newly diagnosed CNS germ cell tumors: Results of an international cooperative trial. J Clin Oncol 1996;14:2908-15.

BESELL EM, GRAUS F, PUNT JAG, et al. Primary non-Hodgkin's lymphoma of the CNS treated with BVAM or CHOD/BVAM chemotherapy before radiotherapy. J Clin Oncol 1996;14:945-54.

BOOGERT W, DALESIO O, BAIS EM, et al. Response of brain metastases from breast cancer to systemic chemotherapy. Cancer 1992;69:972-80.

BROWN MT, FRIEDMANN HS, OAKES WJ, et al. Chemotherapy for pilocytic astrocytomas. Cancer 1993;71:3165-72.

CAIRNCROSS G, MACDONALD D, LUDWIN S, et al. Chemotherapy for anaplastic oligodendroglioma. J Clin Oncol 1994;12:2013-21.

FINE HA. The basis for current treatment recommendations for malignant gliomas. J Neurooncol 1994;20:111-20.

GLASS J, GRUBER ML, CHER L, et al. Preirradiation methotrexate chemotherapy of primary central nervous system lymphoma: Long-term outcome. J Neurosurg 1994;81:188-95.

KHAYAT D, GIROUX B, BERILLE L, et al. Fotemustine in the treatment of brain primary tumors and metastases. Cancer 1994;72:414-20.

KRISTENSEN CA, KRISTJANSEN PE, HANSEN HH. Systemic chemotherapy of brain metastases from small-cell lung cancer: A review. J Clin Oncol 1992;10:1498-502.

LEVIN VA, WARA WM, DAVIS RL, et al. Phase III comparison of BCNU and the combination of procarbazine, CCNU and vincristine administered after radiotherapy with hydroxyurea for malignant gliomas. J Neurosurg 1985;63:218-23.

NEURWELT E, GOLDMAN DL, DAHLBORG SA, et al. Primary CNS lymphoma treated with osmotic blood-brain barrier disruption: Prolonged survival and preservation of cognitive function. J Clin Oncol 1991;9:1580-90.

PACKER RJ, SUTTON LN, ELTERMANN R, et al. Outcome for children with medulloblastoma treated with radiation and cisplatin, CCNU and vincristine chemotherapy. J Neurosurg 1994;81:690-8.

SPOSTO R, ERTEL IJ, JENKIN RD, et al. The effectiveness of chemotherapy for treatment of high-grade astrocytoma in children. Results of a randomized trial. J Neurooncol 1989;7:165-77.

YUNG WKA, MECHTLER L, GLEASON MJ. Intravenous carboplatin for reccurent malignant glioma: A phase II study. J Clin Oncol 1991;9 :860-4.

Head and neck

Gabriela V. Kornek, Christoph C. Zielinski

The incidence of squamous cell carcinomas of the head and neck (HNSCC), localized in the upper airway or digestive tract, amounts worldwide to approximately 4%. HNSCC is more common in men (male-female ratio = 4:1). The incidence and mortality increase with age, and HNSCC patients typically are older than 50 years. Approximately 90% of HNSCCs occur after exposure to tobacco (whether inhaled or chewed), alcohol use, or the combination of tobacco and alcohol. Nutritional deficiency and suboptimal oral hygiene are also generally implicated in a great proportion of patients suffering from HNSCC and are frequent social concomitants of alcoholism. Improvements in dental and oral hygiene, as well as lower alcohol and cigarette consumption, have led to a falling incidence except for tumors of the oral cavity and oropharynx, in which the frequency among younger patients is rising. Other etiologic factors besides tobacco and alcohol are viruses (e.g., Epstein-Barr, herpes simplex, human papillomavirus), genetic predisposition, occupation (e.g., wood dust, nickel, petroleum), radiation exposure, and diet.

Pathology and staging

More than 90% of head and neck cancers are squamous cell carcinomas. Other less common tumor types include mucoepidermoid carcinoma, adenoid cystic carcinoma and adenocarcinoma, neuroendocrine and small cell carcinomas, lymphomas, melanomas, sarcomas, and extramedullary myelomas. The histologic grading of HNSCC is based on the amount of keratinization: A well-differentiated tumor is characterized by greater than 75% keratinization, a moderately differentiated tumor by 25 to 50%, and a poorly differentiated tumor by less than 25%. Better differentiated carcinomas are thought to be less likely to metastasize.

The TNM staging system is the most commonly used classification. Prognosis correlates strongly with stage at diagnosis. The presence of regional lymph node metastases is the most important determinant of prognosis in HNSCC and is associated with a 50% decrease in overall survival rates compared with patients without lymph node involvement.

Since the extent of disease at the time of diagnosis is the most important prognostic factor of HNSCC, identification and treatment of early cancers correlate with excellent survival rates. Symptoms such as dysarthria, hoarseness, dysphagia, odynophagia, globus sensation, unilateral pain, stridor, and dyspnea demand visualization of the involved areas by laryngoscopy. Any suspicious neck mass in adult patients should be viewed as malignant until proven otherwise. The physical examination should include rigorous inspection of all visible oral mucosa, bimanual palpation of the floor of the mouth and the tongue, careful assessment of cranial nerves, and systematic examination of the neck. Endoscopic evaluation should include all regions of the pharynx, larynx, and esophagus. Multiple biopsy specimens of suspect lesions or random biopsies of all sites are indicated to define the extent of primary disease and identify possible synchronous sites of second primary tumors.

Diagnostic imaging is employed to assess the extent of disease and the presence of lymph node involvement and include computed tomographic (CT) scan and/or magnetic resonance imaging (MRI) of the head and neck, sonography of the cervical lymph nodes, barium swallow, and chest radiography

Laboratory tests are performed as baseline assessment of the patient´s general medical condition. There are no specific screening markers, but carcinoembryonic antigen (CEA) and Epstein-Barr virus (EBV) antibody titer can be useful in the follow-up.

If a thorough search for a primary tumor has been completed and the primary tumor was not detected, a fine-needle aspiration should be performed. The accuracy of cytologic interpretation depends on the physician´s skill, but false-negative rates are below 10%.

Treatment

In contrast to malignancies of other origin, HNSCC does not tend to disseminate, and patients die as a result of complications of the advanced primary tumors or local failure. Therefore, standard therapy is focused on locoregional treatment modalities, including surgery and/or radiation therapy. Possible exceptions are combined chemotherapy and irradiation for laryngeal and nasopharyngeal carcinomas. For small tumors (stages I and II), radical surgical resection or curative radiation is recommended. The prognosis of patients with locally advanced tumors (stage III or IV) is much worse, and only one-third of them can be cured by extensive surgery plus radiation therapy. The general principle in treating patients with HNSCC is to offer cure at the lowest cost in terms of functional and cosmetic morbidity. Early rehabilitation (voice and swallowing), reconstructive surgery, and social/psychologic support are also essential in treating HNSCC patients and require the interaction of a multidisciplinary team.

Surgery or radiation therapy

Patients with stage I or II disease undergo either surgery or radiation therapy alone with curative intent. The locoregional control rates of early-stage tumors with single-modality therapy are 80 to 90%. The prognosis of stage III or IV disease is much worse, and patients undergo extensive surgery and radiation therapy. The cure rates for these patients are less than 30%. Radiation therapy can be given either pre- or postoperatively. Preoperative radiation therapy is used to shrink tumor size and to sterilize microscopic disease at the site of resection. The dose of preoperative irradiation is 45 to 50 Gy given over 5 weeks. Postoperative radiation therapy reduces the incidence of locoregional failures in stage III and IV disease after radical surgical resection. Because of alteration in the blood supply after surgery, the dose of postoperative radiation therapy is as high as curative radiation given as monotherapy (60-70 Gy over 7 weeks). Decisions regarding the extent of resection, necessary for optimal therapy, should be handled by experienced surgeons and must be seen in relation to overall cancer control. Reconstruction, both cosmetic and functional, is an integral component of surgical management of HNSCC.

The surgical treatment of the neck is standardized, but controversy exists as to the value of elective neck dissection in node-negative disease. To plan an optimal treatment approach of advanced tumors, it is essential to separate management of the primary tumor and the neck dissection, especially in patients with small primary tumors and lymph node involvement (N2,3). Small primary lesions can be treated with radiation therapy alone, whereas neck involvement should receive radiation therapy plus dissection.

Chemotherapy

Despite optimal local therapy, more than half the patients with HNSCC will develop local recurrence or distant metastases. The median survival of these patients is 6 to 10 months, and only 20% of patients are alive at 1 year. The use of chemotherapy, considered standard practice, is palliative at best and without long-term benefit. Consequently, patients with recurrent or metastatic HNSCC are candidates for phase I and II trials of new agents and new combination regimens (Tab. 54.1).

Single agents The most active agents in HNSCC are methotrexate, bleomycin, cisplatin, carboplatin, ifosfamide, and the taxanes-paclitaxel (taxol) and docetaxel. The response rates of single agents vary between 15 and 35%, with remission durations of 3 to 5 months. The taxanes are the most active single agents, with overall response rates of 40% in pretreated patients with HNSCC (Tab. 54.1). These agents act by stabilizing microtubules and inhibiting tumor cell mitotic division. Several trials conducted in the United States and Europe evaluated paclitaxel in recurrent or metastatic HNSCC and reported an overall response rate of 30 to 40%. The recommended dose of paclitaxel for patients with moderate and poor performance status is 135 mg/m^2, whereas a dose of 200 mg/m^2 is reserved for patients with excellent performance status.

Combination chemotherapy Combination chemotherapy has demonstrated higher response rates than single agents, but this has not resulted in prolonged survival. In the early 1980s, several authors reported response rates greater than 70% with complete remissions (CRs) in about one-fourth of all patients suffering from advanced HNSCC using cisplatin (100 mg/m^2, day 1) and infusional 5-fluorouracil (5-FU, 1000 mg/m^2, days 1-5), repeated every 21 days (Tab. 54.2).

Several treatment strategies have been studied to improve the activity of systemic chemotherapy. One strategy to increase CR rates has been the biochemical modulation of the cisplatin/5-FU regimen. Preclinical and clinical studies have shown that the cytotoxic effects of 5-FU can be enhanced by folinic acid. In the neoadjuvant setting, the combination of leucovorin and cisplatin/5-FU has achieved an 80% overall response rate with 66% CRs after three courses.

Adjuvant (postoperative) chemotherapy Despite more than two decades of experience with cytotoxic chemotherapy in HNSCC, the role of adjuvant chemotherapy after curative surgery and/or radiation therapy remains unclear.

Table 54.1 Single agents in recurrent or metastatic HNSCC

Drug	No. of patients	Response rate
Methotrexate	1612	31%
Bleomycin	347	21%
Cisplatin	543	27%
5-Fluorouracil	201	15%
Carboplatin	169	22%
Cyclophosphamide	77	36%
Ifosfamide	99	26%
Paclitaxel	107	40%
Docetaxel	74	31%
Gemcitabine	61	13%
Topotecan	26	14%
Navelbine	41	11%

Table 54.2 Combination chemotherapy for head and neck cancer

INDUCTION CHEMOTHERAPY: FOLLOWED BY RADIATION THERAPY ± SURGERY

CDDP/5-FU

Cisplatin	100 mg/m^2	90 min iv	Day 1	Every 21 days
5-Fluorouracil	1000 mg/m^2	24 h iv	Day 1-5	Every 21 days

After 3 cycles: assessment of response
Responder → Radiation therapy → Follow-up
Nonresponder → Surgery →   Radiation therapy →   Follow-up

Experimental

CDDP/5-FU/IFNα/LV → 5-FU/HU

Cisplatin	100 mg/m^2	6 h iv	Day 1	Every 21
5-Fluorouracil	640 mg/m^2	24 h iv	Days 1-5	days, 3
L-Leucovorin	300 mg/m^2	24 h iv	Days 1-5.5	courses
IFN-γ	2 MU/m^2	sc	Days 0-5	
5-Fluorouracil	800 mg/m^2	24 h iv	Days 1-5	Every 14
Hydroxyurea	1 g	q12h po	Days 1-5	days, 7
Radiation therapy	2 Gy/d		Days 1-5	courses

Taxotere/CDDP/5-FU/LV

Taxotere	60 mg/m^2	1 h iv	Day 1	
Cisplatin	25 mg/m^2	24 h iv	Days 1-5	Every 28 days
Leucovorin	500 mg/m^2	24 h iv	Days 1-5	
5-Fluorouracil	700 mg/m^2	24 h iv	Days 2-5	
G-CSF	30 MU/d	sc[1]		

COMBINATION CHEMOTHERAPY: FOR PALLIATIVE USE

CDDP/5-FU

Cisplatin	100 mg/m^2	90 min iv	Day 1	Every 21 days
5-Fluorouracil	1000 mg/m^2	24 h iv	Days 1-5	

CDDP/LV/5-FU

Cisplatin	100 mg/m^2	90 min iv	Day 1	Every 21-28 days
Leucovorin	100 mg	q4h po	Days 1-5	
5-Fluorouracil	1000 mg/m^2	24 h iv	Days 1-5	

Carbo/5-FU

Carboplatin	300 mg/m^2	15 min iv	Day 1	Every 21 days
5-Fluorouracil	1000 mg/m^2	24 h iv	Days 1-4	

Experimental

Taxol/carbo

Taxol[2]	230 mg/m^2	3 h iv	Day 1	Every 21 days
Carboplatin	AUC = 7.5[3]	1 h iv	Day 1	

Taxol/ifosfamide/CDDP

Taxol[2]	175 mg/m^2	3 h iv	Day 1	Every 21-22 days
Ifosfamide[4]	1000 mg/m^2	2 h iv	Days 1-3	
Cisplatin	60 mg/m^2	90 min iv	Day 1	

Taxotere/CDDP

Taxotere[2]	75 mg/m^2	1 h iv	Day 1	Every 21 days
Cisplatin	75 mg/m^2	90 min iv	Day 1	

Nav/CDDP/5-FU

Cisplatin	80 mg/m^2	90 min iv	Day 1	
5-Fluorouracil	600 mg/m^2	4 h iv	Days 2-5	Every 28 days
Navelbine	25 mg/m^2	bolus iv	Days 2 + 8	

Ifosfamide/CDDP

Ifosfamide[4]	1500 mg/m^2	1h iv	Days 1-5	Every 28 days
Cisplatin	10 mg/m^2	90 min iv	Days 1-5	

MU = million units.
[1]Day 6 until neutrophil count >1000/ml
[2]Premedication with dexamethasone, cimetidine, diphenhydramine.
[3]Carboplatin dose (mg) = AUC × (GFR + 25).
[4]Uroprotective MESNA 600-mg iv bolus at 0, 4, and 8 h after.

The major goals of adjuvant chemotherapy are to decrease the incidence of distant failures by eliminating circulating micrometastases and to improve disease-free and overall survival. Initially, several promising uncontrolled trials have indicated that adjuvant chemotherapy may improve the outcome of high-risk patients with HNSCC. More recently published trials, however, have failed to reproduce the positive effect of additional adjuvant or systemic chemotherapy but have reported an increased treatment toxicity, especially mucositis.

Combined treatment modalities in locally advanced HNSCC Surgery followed by definitive radiation therapy is the accepted standard for patients with locally advanced but resectable tumors, and radiation therapy alone is reserved for unresectable carcinomas. Survival rates for locally advanced HNSCC after standard therapy with surgery and/or radiation therapy remain poor, primarily due to the high locoregional failure rates and secondly due to distant metastases and second primary tumors.

The rationale for induction chemotherapy in patients with advanced HNSCC is the high sensitivity to several cytotoxic drugs, particularly to the combination of cisplatin and infusional 5-FU. Sufficient reduction of tumor size after chemotherapy renders the tumors more radioresponsive and may circumvent extensive surgical resection. Induction chemotherapy results in significant tumor regression in approximately 70 to 100% of patients, with CRs in up to 50% of patients with locally advanced HNSCC. Although patients who achieve complete tumor regression have a much better survival than those who do not respond (or respond partially), overall survival has not been improved significantly by neoadjuvant

chemotherapy. Induction chemotherapy followed by definitive radiation therapy, however, is an effective strategy to achieve organ preservation in patients with laryngeal and hypopharyngeal cancer without compromising overall survival or enhancing treatment toxicity (Fig. 54.1). The combination of cisplatin and infusional 5-FU is considered a standard cytotoxic regimen, but induction chemotherapy remains an excellent tool to investigate new drugs or combinations with or without biochemical modulation (Tab. 54.2).

The rationale for concurrent chemoradiation is the potentially enhanced activity of radiotherapy by several cytotoxic agents inhibiting sublethal damage repair, sensitizing hypoxic cells, synchronizing the cell cycle, and thus improving outcome in patients by achieving better local control. Early administration of cytotoxic drugs may help to eradicate circulating micrometastases when given at adequate dosages. Recent published trials show that concurrent chemoradiation has resulted in higher complete response rates, better 5-year overall survival, and better 5-year locoregional relapse-free survival compared with patients who received radiation therapy alone.

Chemoprevention Agents with proven chemopreventive activity in oral premalignancies are α-tocopherol, β-carotene, selenium, and the retinoids. Several randomized trials have demonstrated positive results with high rates of reversal of dysplasia. Toxicity for patients receiving high-dose retinoids (2 mg/kg per day) was unacceptable; cheilitis, facial erythema, skin dryness, and conjunctivitis occurred in 70 to 85% of patients. The reduced dose of retinoids (1 mg/kg per day) showed similar response rates and an acceptable toxicity. The results of chemoprevention in patients with a history of HNSCC are promising, but large randomized trials are ongoing to investigate not only the efficacy but also the tolerability of long-term therapy.

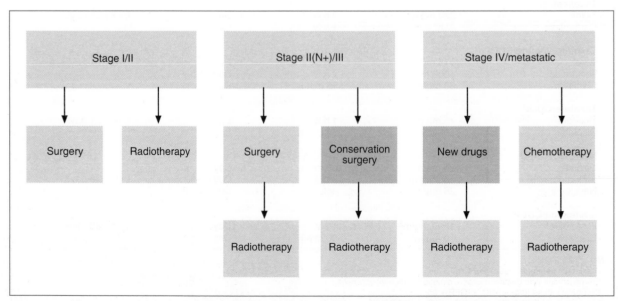

Figure 54.1 Treatment modalities/options for patients with head and neck squamous cell carcinomas.

DIMERY IW, HONG WK. Overview of combined modality therapies for head and neck cancer. J Natl Cancer Inst 1993; 85:95-111.

EL-SAYED S, NELSON N. Adjuvant and adjunctive chemotherapy in the management of squamous cell carcinoma of the head and neck region: A meta-analysis of prospective and randomized trials. J Clin Oncol 1996;14:838-47.

HEERMAN R, LENARZ T, SCHMOLL HJ. Lippen-, Mundhöhlen- und Oropharynx-Tumoren. In: Schmoll HJ, Höffken K, Possinger K, eds. Kompendium internistische Onkologie, Vol 2. Berlin: Springer-Verlag, 1997.

LEFEBVRE JL, BONNETERRE J. Current status of larynx preservation trials. Curr Opin Oncol 1996;8:209-14.

SCHANTZ SP, HARRISON LB, FORASTIERE AA. Tumors of the nasal cavity and paranasal sinuses, nasopharynx, oral cavity and oropharynx. In: De Vita V, Hellman S, Rosenberg SA, eds. Cancer. New York: Lippincott-Raven, 1997.

VOKES EE, WEICHSELBAUM RR, LIPPMAN SM, et al. Head and neck cancer. N Engl J Med 1993;21:184-194.

Cutaneous
melanoma

Branko Malenica

The incidence of malignant melanoma has increased at an alarming rate over the past few decades. In 1935, only 1 in 1500 individuals developed a melanoma. By 1980 this ratio had dropped dramatically to 1 in 250 and by 1987 to 1 in 135. The reasons for the increased incidence are unclear but may relate to a combination of (1) increased recreational exposure to sunlight, (2) increased amount of ultraviolet B (UVB) irradiation from sunlight that reaches the earth's surface, and (3) early detection. Fortunately, most new cases of melanoma are diagnosed early in the clinical course of the disease, when it usually can be cured by simple excision, but nevertheless, it is fatal in about one-fifth of cases. Because of the often capricious biologic behavior of melanoma, it is important to identify the dominant prognostic variables that help in the design of treatment modalities involving adjuvant therapy as well as surgery.

Disease presentation

A convenient way to categorize melanoma is by the growth pattern. Different growth patterns represent distinct pathologic entities and have unique clinical features and different prognoses. Histologic confirmation and staging are essential before any definitive treatment plans are made. The four major growth patterns are *superficial spreading melanoma, nodular melanoma, lentigo maligna melanoma* and *acral lentiginous melanoma*. Patients with superficial spreading melanoma and lentigo maligna melanoma have the best survival rate, whereas those with nodular melanomas have the worst. It is not clear whether the acral lentiginous melanoma subtype is associated with a worse prognosis.

A standardized and uniformly accepted melanoma staging system is an essential and fundamental requirement to enable meaningful comparisons across patients populations. Histologic microstaging of primary melanoma is now an integral part of the staging and clinical management of melanoma. Two methods have been used: the Breslow thickness determination and Clark's levels. In the *Breslow method*, the thickness of the lesion is measured with an ocular micrometer to determine the total vertical height (not just the depth) of the melanoma from the granular layer to the area of deepest penetration. Numerous

studies have confirmed a good relationship of melanoma thickness in millimeters to metastasis and patient survival. The *Clark microstaging method* categorizes different levels of invasion that reflect increasing depth of penetration into the dermal layers of the subcutaneous fat. *Clark's level I* is defined as confinement of melanoma cells to the intraepidermal compartment (melanoma in situ). *Clark's level II* is defined as melanoma cells that have extended into the papillary dermis, whereas *Clark's level III* melanoma cells fill the papillary dermis. In *Clark's level IV*, tumor cells extend into the reticular dermis, and in *Clark's level V*, there is involvement of the subcutaneous fat. The Clark level of invasion also shows good correlation with metastases and patient survival. The original and most widely used classification is the *three-stages system* (stage I, localized melanoma; stage II, regional metastasis; and stage III, distant metastasis). The system is simple and easy to recall but does not incorporate disease criteria such as tumor thickness for more accurate staging. A major limitation is that 85% or more of melanoma patients now have clinically localized disease (stage I). The *new staging system* proposed by the American Joint Committee on Cancer (AJCC) represents the first formal integration of

---

Table 55.1 The 1992 AJCC/UICC TNM staging system for melanoma

Stage	Criteria
IA	Primary melanoma < 0.75 mm thick and/or Clark level II (T1N0M0)
IB	Primary melanoma 0.76-1.5 mm thick and/or Clark level III (T2N0M0)
IIA	Primary melanoma 1.51-4.00 mm thick and/or Clark level IV (T3N0M0)
IIB	Primary melanoma > 4.00 mm thick and/or Clark level V (T4N0M0)
III	Regional lymph node or in-transit metastases (any TN1M0)
IV	Systemic metastases (any T any NM1)

(T = tumor; N = lymph node; M = metastasis.)

microstaging into the staging criteria. Four stages are described (Tab. 55.1).

Basically, the system divides clinically localized melanomas into groups according to microstaging criteria, with the result that the metastatic risk categories are more evenly grouped among four stages. Recent data support changes in the AJCC staging system to comply with controversial areas such as (1) the relevance of the level of invasion compared with tumor thickness, (2) the importance of ulceration, (3) satellites versus in-transit metastases, (4) microsatellites versus macrosatellites, (5) satellites versus local recurrence, (6) number of positive nodes versus the size of the nodal mass, (7) importance of nodal metastases in more than one nodal basion, and (8) prognostic significance of distant metastases.

Treatment

Surgical management

Surgical excision remains the mainstay of treatment for skin melanoma. Early detection, while the lesion is still thin (<1 mm), and appropriate excision offer the best chance for cure. It seems that radical margins of excision are not required to cure melanoma. When conservation of normal tissue is important or significant subclinical spread is anticipated, Mohs' micrographic surgery is the treatment of choice. Elective lymph node dissections are no longer indicated in management. The standard of care for patients with lesions greater than 1 mm thick is to perform a sentinel node biopsy, and if the sentinel node is found to contain melanoma cells, an appropriate node

dissection has to be performed.

Adjuvant immunotherapy

The prognosis for localized, surgically curable melanoma depends on the depth of the primary lesion and the presence of involved regional lymph nodes. The majority of primary melanomas with a depth of less than 1.5 mm (stage I) can be cured by wide local excision alone. Patients with stage IIB (depth > 4.0 mm) have an estimated 5- and 10-year survival rate of 47.9 to 69.3% and 35.5 to 54.5%, respectively, depending on other prognostic indicators such as ulceration. Patients with stage III melanoma (regional lymph node involvement) have an estimated 5-year survival of 10 to 46% depending on the number of involved nodes. Consequently, clinical trials investigating the possible benefit of systemic adjuvant immunotherapy (biotherapy) or immunotherapy combined with chemotherapy (biochemotherapy) have focused on this group of patients.

Many agents have been evaluated as postoperative adjuvant immunotherapy in a number of randomized clinical trials. Adjuvant administration of bacille Calmette-Guérin (BCG), C. parvum, and levamisole failed to demonstrate any benefit in prolonging either disease-free or overall survival. During the last decade, much interest has been focused on the use of interferons (IFNs), both α and γ, in the adjuvant therapy of surgically resected high-risk melanoma. Results from a few randomized clinical trials (Tab. 55.2) show that only patients who receive initial high-dose intravenous therapy (20 million units/m²/day 5 days weekly for 4 weeks followed by 10 million units/m² subcutaneously three times weekly for a further 11 months) had a significantly prolongation of disease-free survival (1.7

Table 55.2 Adjuvant immunotherapy of IFNs in stage II and III melanoma

Treatment	Dose and schedule	No. of patients	Stage of disease	Disease-free survival	Overall survival
IFN-α2b	20 MU/m²/d iv or 5 per wk (48 weeks)	287	IIB-III	Prolongation ($p = 0.002$)	Prolongation ($p = 0.02$)
		249	III	($p = 0.0006$)	($p = 0.006$)
IFN-α2b	1 MU/d sc or 3 per wk (1 year)	850	II-III	NS	NS
IFN-α2a	20 MU/m² im or 3 per wk (12 weeks)	262	II-III	NS	NS
IFN-α2a	3 MU/m² sc or 3 per wk (36 months)	444	III	NS	NS
IFN-γ	0.2 mg/m² sc daily (1 year)	284	II-III	NS	NS

(NS = not significant; MU = million units.)

versus 1.0 year) and overall survival (3.8 versus 2.8 years) The significance of the impact on relapse-free interval and overall survival was most consistent and pronounced among the stage III than stage IIB patients. Unfortunately, this treatment regimen had substantial toxicity. Dose modification or delays were required at least once in 50% of patients during the intravenous induction phase and in 48% of patients during the subcutaneous maintenance phase. The adverse effects of IFN include flulike symptoms of fever, chills, headache, myalgia, arthralgia, fatigue, and anorexia, usually seen in the initial phases of treatment (see also Chap. 51). The symptoms can be managed successfully, and with continued treatment patients usually experience a decrease in symptoms. However, high-dose therapy may lead to hematologic side effects, including

anemia, leukopenia, and thrombocytopenia, as well as gastrointestinal side effects. Abnormal liver function test results also can be seen as an adverse effect.

Given the significant and durable benefits (37% of patients continuously disease-free at 5 years with treatment as opposed to 26% in the observation group), this therapy has been adopted rapidly as the "standard" adjuvant therapy for resected high-risk melanomas. However, dosage, duration, and regimen of IFN administration are still under investigation. Current approaches focus on refinement of dose and duration of treatment with IFN (comparison of the preceding high dose with a lower dose of IFN given for a longer period of time, namely, 3 mil-

Table 55.3 Results of immunotherapy and biochemotherapy with IFNs in patients with metastatic melanoma

Treatment	Dose regimen	No. of patients	CR	PR	RR (%)
IFN-α2a	3-50 MU/d im or 3 per wk	189	9	15	13 (6-23)
IFN-α2b	10-30 MU/d im or sc or 3 per wk	106	9	15	22 (14-27)
IFN-γ	0.003-4.0 mg/d iv	150	2	7	6 (0-13)
IFN-γ + IFN-α	0.01-0.2 mg/d im 2-10 MU/d im or sc or 3 per wk	53	0	1	2 (0-5)
IFN-α2a + cimetidine	4-50 MU im 3 per wk or 50-250 mg im	66	6	11	26 (22-30)
IFN-α2b + cimetidine	10-100 MU sc 3 per wk 300 mg im	45	0	2	4 (0-6)
IFN-α2a + DTIC	3-18 MU/d sc, 200-800 mg iv	175	13	32	26 (20-35)
IFN-α2b + DTIC	9-15 MU/d sc, 200-800 mg iv	102	16	19	34 (26-53)
IFN-α2b + cisplatin	5-10 MU/d sc, 5-50 mg iv	31	1	7	25 (9-35)
IFN-α2a + IL-2 + cisplatin	9 MU/d sc, 18 MU iv, 100 mg iv	39	5	16	54
IFN-α2a + IL+2 polychem.[1]	5 MU/d 9 MU/d CVD/d	149	23	62	57 (54-62)

(MU = million units; RR = response rate; CR = complete response; PR = partial response.)
[1]FN-α2a on days 1-5, 7, 9, 13; IL-2 on days 1-4; CVD: cisplatin 20 mg/m^2 on days 1-4, vinblastine 1.2-1.6 mg/m^2 on days 1-4 or 5, DTIC 800 mg/m^2 on day 1.

Table 55.4 Results of immunotherapy and biochemotherapy with interleukin-2 in patients with metastatic melanoma

Treatment	Dose	No. of patients	CR	PR	RR (%)
IL-2	600 000 U/kg iv (bolus)	208	2	26	15 (5-26)
IL-2	720 000 U/kg iv (bolus)	182	12	15	15
IL-2	3-72 MU/m²/d iv (continuous)	144	0	16	11 (0-22)
IL-2 + IFN-α2a	1-18 MU/m² iv, 3-12 MU/m² im or sc	281	12	50	18 (4-41)
IL-2 + CYC	2-36 MU/m² iv (bolus), 25-300 mg iv	114	1	23	21 (4-43)
IL-2 + DTIC	2-25 MU/m² iv, 200-1200 mg	114	9	21	26 (22-35)
IL-2 + DTIC + CDDP	3-24 MU/m² iv (bolus), 750 mg/m² iv, 100-1000 mg/m² iv (bolus)	131	24	45	53 (33-83)

(RR = response rate; CR = complete response; PR = partial response; CYC= cyclophosphamide.)

lion units sc three times weekly for 2 years) and potential interactions with and comparison with active specific immunotherapy with vaccines.

Immunotherapy of metastatic disease

Prognosis for patients with distant metastatic disease remains dismal, with a median survival of around 6 months. Less than 10% of patients are alive 5 years after the diagnosis. At present, systemic chemotherapy for the treatment of disseminated disease still remains unsatisfactory. Mainly for this reason, therapeutic strategies for metastatic disease include a few immunotherapeutic possibilities and their combination with chemotherapy.

"Classic" immunostimulation using BCG, MER (methanol extractable residue from BCG), and some other biologic response modifiers (BRM) is completely disappointing. Recently, much interest has focused on the possible role of various cytokines in the treatment of metastatic melanoma. Recombinant IFN-α and interleukin 2 (IL-2) have been studied extensively. IFN-α was the first recombinant cytokine to be investigated clinically in metastatic melanoma. Aggregate results of reported clinical trials show that IFN-α has activity in disseminated disease (Tab. 55.3). Objective response rates average between 13 and 22%. Responses generally have been partial and short-lived and have occurred mainly in skin, subcutaneous tissue, lymph nodes, and lung. Occasional long-term complete responses also have been observed. The effective dose has ranged from 10 million units/m²

per day to 50 million units/m² three times per week, with uninterrupted treatment being significantly more effective then cyclic interrupted schedules. Toxicity is manifested mainly by flulike symptoms, myalgia, chills, and fever, with an accompanying drop in performance status during treatment with high doses. Continued treatment generally is associated with a decrease in side effects. Responses to IFN-α could be observed as late as 6 months after initiation of therapy. IFN-α is currently being evaluated in combination with other cytokines (IL-2, IFN-γ) and cytotoxic agents. Combined treatment data with IFN-γ, cimetidine, DTIC, and cisplatin shows no significantly higher response rates in comparison with IFN-α alone (Tab. 55.3). However, this treatment modality yields high toxicity. More encouraging results have been observed with sequential biochemotherapy [cisplatin or CVD (cisplatin, vinblastine, DTIC) plus IL-2 and IFN-α]. Cumulative data show a response rate of 54 and 57%, with 14 to 15% complete responses, and median survival of about 11 to 12 months. About 10% of all patients appear to be disease-free at greater than 2 years. In contrast to chemotherapy or immunotherapy alone, responses were seen in all diseases sites with equal frequency. Treatment activity appeared greatest when the chemotherapy was administered first. Unfortunately, these regimens involved extensive inpatient treatment and substantial toxicity.

Many clinical trials also have shown that IL-2 alone or in combination with IFN-α or chemotherapy has antitumor activity in metastatic melanoma (Tab. 55.4).

Compiled data show that high-dose bolus recombinant IL-2 (600 000-720 000 IU/kg iv every 8 hours on days 1 to 5 and 15 to 19, maximum 28 doses per course) either alone or in combination with lymphokine-activated killer (LAK) cells produced overall responses in 15% of patients, with complete responses observed in about 6%. Long-term follow-up of patients treated on early high-dose IL-2 trials confirms that IL-2 produces significant clinical benefit for a minority of patients. In a retrospective analysis (266 patients), the median response duration was reported to be 6.5 months (range 4-96 months), with 60% of complete responders remaining progression-free at 5 years. Unfortunately, the utility of high-dose IL-2 has been limited by extensive multiorgan toxicity. Side effects include varying degrees of hypotension, cardiac arrhythmias, pulmonary edema, increased capillary permeability, anemia, thrombocytopenia, leukopenia, nausea, vomiting, diarrhea, transient renal insufficiency, catheter-related sepsis, and rarely, death. For a given dose, continuous infusion of IL-2 (over 24 hours) is more toxic than the same dose given by bolus infusion. Most side effects resolve within 2 to 3 days of IL-2 discontinuation. A number of toxicity dissociation approaches (antibiotic prophylaxis, addition of dexamethasone) have been tried with limited success. Although no randomized studies have been performed, in general, the overall response rate and the quality and duration of response have been superior with high-dose IL-2 than with either lower doses of IL-2 or alternative administration schedules or routes. The extensive toxicity of this regimen has limited its use to patients with excellent organ function treated by experienced clinicians in specialized programs capable of providing intensive care. None of the treatment combinations have been shown to be more effective than treatment with IL-2 alone, except combination with polychemotherapy (see Tab. 55.4). Cumulative data show a response rate of

53% and median survival of about 8 months. Other cytokines, such as tumor necrosis factor (TNF), IL-4, IFN-γ, and IL-6 have been evaluated extensively in patients with metastatic melanoma, and they are essentially inactive. Interestingly, both TNF and IFN-γ have shown potential utility in isolated limb perfusion of locoregionally recurrent extremity melanomas. It was shown that administration of IFN-γ and TNF and high-dose melphalan limb perfusion give up to 100% overall response and 90% complete responses. Randomized trials aimed at determining the role of TNF and IFN-γ in isolated limb perfusion are under way.

The use of IL-2 to generate in vitro autologous cells with antitumor activity opened the way for the successful use of adoptive immunotherapy in melanoma. The first studies of adoptive transfer of antitumor effector cells were conducted with lymphokine-activated killer (LAK) cells. LAK cells are lymphocytes with the ability to lyse fresh tumor but not fresh normal cells after incubation with high doses of IL-2. These cells are reinfused into patients with metastatic disease with high doses of IL-2. About 15% of patients respond to this treatment (Tab. 55.5). Some complete responses of long duration were observed. Unfortunately, the combined LAK cell plus IL-2 therapy produced considerable toxic effects, predominantly severe hypotension, often requiring inotropic support, and renal dysfunction. The side effects are reversible and quickly resolve once IL-2 administration is discontinued. Later prospective, randomized trials have shown that LAK plus IL-2 treatment does not provide significantly higher response rates than IL-2 alone. Adoptive transfer of tumor-infiltrating lymphocytes (TILs), which are specific and

Table 55.5 Adoptive immunotherapy in patients with metastatic melanoma

Treatment	No. of patients[1]	CR	PR	RR (%)
IL-2+LAK	32	1	5	19
	33	0	1	3
	50	1	6	14
	48	4	6	21
IL-2+LAK	85	10	14	28
IL-2 alone	79	3	13	20
IL-2+TIL	13	1	3	31
	21	1	4	24
IL-2+TIL	86	5	24	34
Prior IL-2	28	1	8	32
No prior IL-2	58	4	16	34
DC (Ag-pulsed in vitro)	16	2	3	31

[1] Cumulative data adapted from different references.
(CR=complete response; PR=partial response; RR=objective response rate; LAK=lymphokine activated killer cells; TIL=tumor infiltrating lymphocytes; DC=dendritic cells.)

more effective in their in vitro antitumor reactivity, provides a response rate of from 24 to 34% in melanoma patients. Objective responses also were observed in 32% of patients, many of whom had experienced tumor progression following prior IL-2 therapy. The modification of TILs with transfection of genes for IL-2, IFN-γ, and TNF is currently being explored. Adoptive transfer of autologous antigen-presenting cells such as dendritic cells (DCs) pulsed in vitro with immunogenic tumor-specific peptides is a new adoptive immunotherapeutic strategy in metastatic melanoma. Results of the pilot study show 31% response to treatment (Tab. 55.5). The treatment was well tolerated. No physical signs of autoimmunity were detected in any of the patients. DC transfer (vaccination) induced a delayed-type hypersensitivity reaction (DTH) in the majority of patients. However, the precise role of TILs and DCs in the treatment of melanoma patients remains to be defined.

New areas of drug development

Vaccination therapy of patients with metastatic disease with a variety of melanoma cell preparations has been pursued for the past several decades. A large number of clinical trials of vaccines made of allogeneic whole melanoma cells, tumor cell lysates, shed melanoma antigens, and autologous melanoma cells modified by hapten conjugation have been published, and most of them are still ongoing. Only a few studies have shown potential benefit in prolonging relapse-free and overall survival (relative to historical control) of patients developing an immune response to the vaccine. The lack of a control arm and the crude nature of these vaccines make it difficult to determine the true benefit of these agents. With the recent advances in molecular biology and understanding of immunologic recognition of tumor-specific antigens, greater emphasis has been placed on studying melanoma vaccines using defined antigens such as GM2 ganglioside, MAGE-1, and gp100. Results of phase I/II clinical trials show some objective responses after immunization with these antigens in adjuvants. Prospective, randomized clinical trials are necessary to evaluate the effects of vaccines on the clinical course of melanoma.

An alternative approach to active specific immunotherapy is gene therapy. This is focused primarily on injecting genes that will enhance the immunogenicity of melanoma cells. Clinical trials using vaccinations with autologous melanoma cells transfected with IL-2, IL-4, IL-6, IL-7, IL-12, INF-γ, GM-CSF, B7, HLA-B7, MART-1, and gp100 genes are under way. It is unclear, however, whether these may offer any advantages over the various nonspecific immune adjuvants mentioned previously.

Suggested readings

BALCH CM. Cutaneous melanoma: prognosis and treatment results wolrdwide. Semin Surg Oncol 1992;8:400-15.

BALCH MC, HOUGHTON A, PETERS L. Cutaneous melanoma. In: DeVita TV Jr, Hellman S, Rosenberg AS, eds. Cancer: principles and practice of oncology. Philadelphia: Lippincott, 1989,1499-542.

DEVITA VT JR, HELLMAN S, ROSENBERG AS, eds. Biologic therapy of cancer. Philadelphia: Lippincott, 1995.

GUTZMER R, GUERRY D. Gene therapy for melanoma in humans. Hematol Oncol Clin North Am 1998;12:519-38.

KOH KH (ed). Melanoma. Hematol Oncol Clin North Am 1998;12:68-934.

MORTON DL, BARTH A. Local therapy with biologic agents: Intralesional therapy. In: DeVita TV Jr, Hellman S, Rosenberg AS, eds. Biologic therapy of cancer. Philadelphia: Lippincott, 1995, pp 691-704.

NESTLE OF, ALIJAGIC S, GILLIET M, et al. Vaccination of melanoma patients with peptide or tumor lysate-pulsed dendritic cells. Nature Med 1998;3:328-332.

OETTGEN FH, OLD JL. The history of cancer immunotherapy. In: DeVita TV Jr, Hellman S, Rosenberg AS, eds. Biologic therapy of cancer. Philadelphia: Lippincott, 1991, pp 87-119.

OETTGEN FH, OLD JL, LIVINGSTON OP. Immunotherapy by active specific immunization: Melanoma. In: DeVita TV Jr, Hellman S, Rosenberg AS, eds. Biologic therapy of cancer. Philadelphia: Lippincott, 1995, pp 682-701.

PARMIANI G, COLOMBO MP, MELANI C, ARIENTI F. Cytokine gene transduction in the immunotherapy of cancer. Adv Pharmacol 1997; 40:259-307.

ROSENBERG AS, KAWAKAMI Y, ROBBINS FP, WANG RF. Identification of the genes encoding cancer antigens: Implications for cancer immunotherapy. Adv Immunol 1996;62:145-77.

ROSENBERG AS, YANG JC, WHITE DE, STEINBERG SM. Durability of complete responses in patients with metastatic cancer treated with high-dose interleukin-2: Identification of the antigens mediating response. Ann Surg 1998;228:307-19.

ROTH AJ, CRISTIANO JR. Gene therapy of cancer: What have we done and where are we going? J Natl Cancer Inst 1997;89:21-39.

WALLACK MR, SIVANANDHAN M, BALCH CM, et al. Surgical adjuvant active specific immunotherapy for patients with stage III melanoma: The final analysis of data from a phase III, randomized double-blind multicenter vaccinia melanoma oncolysate trial. J Am College Surg 1998;187:69-77.

56

Lung cancer

Bernd Weidmann, Norbert Niederle

Lung cancer ranges among the leading causes of cancer death in the developed world. While mortality rates are currently reaching a plateau in the white male population of the industrialized countries, the incidence is rising in developing countries as well as in women and nonwhite males. In western Europe, Canada, and the United States, lung cancer comes first or second in the list of cancer fatalities. Since approximately 80% of malignant lung tumors can be attributed to smoking habits, it is one of the few preventable malignancies and therefore requires major attention by health care workers, teachers, and politicians. Although surgical and medical treatments have been improved substantially during recent decades, the overall 5-year survival rates are low and do not exceed 20%.

Therapy of lung cancer is based mainly on the histologic subtype and on the tumor stage, i.e., on the extent of local and systemic spread.

Etiopathogenesis

Cigarette smoking can be regarded as the most important etiologic factor in lung cancer. The lifetime risk of developing lung cancer is 10 to 20% for smokers. The currently available data concerning passive smoking support the hypothesis of a slightly increased risk (relative risk = 1.35). Additional risk factors include air pollution, occupational hazards (particularly arsenic and asbestos), exposure to occupational and environmental radioactivity (radon), a family history of lung cancer or genetic diseases with increased susceptibility to cancer (e.g., Li-Fraumeni syndrome and familial retinoblastoma), and probably dietary factors.

The role of genetic factors has not been entirely elucidated to date. There are data supporting a genetic predisposition, e.g., a mutation of the P450IA1 gene (see Chap. 3). According to our current knowledge, genetic factors make, if at all, only a minor contribution to the individual risk of lung cancer. However, since fewer than 20% of smokers develop lung cancer during their lives, there have to exist other environmental or genetic factors that modify the effects of tobacco.

The most important means of primary prevention is a reduction in tobacco use, particularly in adolescents.

Large studies focusing on vitamin supplementation as a preventive measure yielded conflicting results, as did studies aimed at early diagnosis by X-ray and sputum cytology screening. Therefore, reducing tobacco consumption and, to a far lesser extent, reducing indoor radon exposure in high-risk areas remain the cornerstones of lung cancer prevention.

Histologic classification and staging

For therapeutic and prognostic reasons, lung cancers are classified as small cell or non-small cell lung cancer (SCLC or NSCLC). The subclassification within these two main entities is less important and underwent several changes. Mixed types are rather frequent (up to one-third) and contribute to treatment failures. Between 20 and 25% of lung cancers are SCLCs, whereas 75% are NSCLCs, with approximately 45% squamous cell carcinomas, 40% adenocarcinomas, and 9% large cell carcinomas, respectively. The distribution of histologic subtypes varies among institutions. Adenocarcinomas seem to increase more rapidly than the other histologic subtypes.

Lung cancers are staged according to the TNM classification. For prognostic and therapeutic reasons, in patients with SCLC, *limited disease* (LD) – tumor confined to one hemithorax-is distinguished from *extensive disease* (ED) – tumor either confined to the thorax (ED I) or with distant spread (ED II).

Disease presentation

Patients with lung cancer usually present with symptoms caused by locally advanced disease, mainly cough or hemoptysis, dysphagea, hoarseness, or dyspnea. Others – particularly patients with SCLC – may experience symptoms from early metastatic spread, e.g., bone pain, palpable lymph nodes, abdominal pain from liver or retroperitoneal metastases, or focal neurologic signs. Ten percent of SCLCs are associated with clinically apparent paraneoplastic symptoms, caused predominantly by ectopic production of normal and abnormal hormones or by the induction of autoantibodies. The most common paraneoplastic syndromes are summarized in Table 56.1.

Table 56.1 Common paraneoplastic syndromes occuring in small cell lung center and their management

---

Syndrome of inappropriate secretion of antidiuretic hormone (SIADH)
Cause: secretion of ADH by tumor cells with water intoxication and hyponatremia
Symptoms: fatigue, confusion, headache, seizures, coma
Treatment *: fluid restriction, in severe cases hypertonic saline (raising serum sodium less than 12 mmol/l daily to avoid central pontine myelinolysis), occasionally demethylchlortetracycline 600-1200 mg/d

Cushing's syndrome
Cause: secretion of ACTH by tumor cells
Symptoms: hypertension, truncal obesity, moon facies, hirsutism, hypokalemia, hyperglycemia
Treatment *: ketoconazole 400-1200 mg/d, octreotide, metyrapone 500-4000 mg/d, bilateral adrenalectomy

Hypercalcemia
Cause: secretion of, e.g., parathyroid hormone-related peptide (PTH-rP)
Symptoms: polydipsia, fatigue, lethargy, weakness, polyuria, renal insufficiency, constipation
Treatment*: fluid replacement (isotonic saline), furosemide, prednisolone, bisphosphonates, calcitonin

Eaton-Lambert myasthenic syndrome
Cause: antibodies to calcium channels in presynaptic nerve terminals
Symptoms: dysphagia, muscle weakness (predominantly proximal)
Treatment *: 3,4-diaminopyridine, guanidine hydrochloride, plasmapheresis immunosuppressive drugs

---

* Mainstay in the treatment of any paraneoplastic syndrome is the effective control of the underlying malignant disease.

Diagnostic procedures aim at establishing the diagnosis and histologic classification of lung cancer, staging and resectability, evaluating prognostic parameters, and examining the patient's general health and operability. Tumor markers, although not helpful in establishing the diagnosis of lung cancer, can be useful for monitoring the response to therapy. Among the numerous parameters, carcinoembryonic antigen (CEA) and neuron-specific enolase (NSE) are widely used and seem to correlate with tumour burden and response to therapy at least to a certain extent. In patients with paraneoplastic syndromes, additional serologic parameters have to be determined. All diagnostic procedures should be restricted to the amount needed for therapeutical decisions. For example, once distant spread of SCLC has been established, there is no need to submit the patient to frequent imaging studies or to bone biopsy.

Treatment

Treatment of lung cancer always requires an interdisciplinary approach. Therapeutic strategies depend primarily on the histologic type, followed by tumor stage. Because of their different biologic behavior, SCLC and NSCLC are covered separately. While limited stages of NSCLC may be cured surgically, SCLC has to be regarded as a rapidly proliferating disease with early spread to distant sites. It is considerably more sensitive to cytotoxic drugs than NSCLC. It is therefore imperative to establish the correct histologic diagnosis before starting therapy.

Small cell lung cancer (SCLC)

Small cell lung cancer is characterized by rapid tumor cell proliferation, short tumor doubling time, early hematogenous metastatic dissemination, and a high sensitivity to cytotoxic drugs with almost regular development of secondary resistance. At the time of diagnosis, approximately 60% of patients have extensive disease. The median survival time of untreated patients is 3 to 5 months. Therapy extends median survival to 12 to 16 months in patients with LD and to approximately 10 months in those with ED. Less than 5% of patients with ED and 15% with LD may survive 5 years.

Therapy of SCLC has to apply a *multimodal approach,* assuming occult or overt systemic spread. *Indications for surgery* are confined to small peripheral tumors (T1-2, NO-1), usually performed to establish the diagnosis in a patient with a suspect pulmonary lesion. All other patients are primarily submitted to *chemotherapy* with the aim of complete remission (CR). The high rate of local recurrence even after CR (more than 50%) and the incidence of inducing clinically apparent cerebral involvement can be reduced by additional *irradiation* of the chest and brain, both of which are indicated only in a subset of patients with a comparatively good prognosis.

Limited disease At least in patients with LD, first-line therapy has a *curative intention.* Patients with unresected tumors as well as patients after initial tumor resection receive cytostatic chemotherapy with concomitant or subsequent chest irradiation. Prophylactic cranial irradiation is added in patients with CR.

Extensive disease There is no indication for surgery as the primary treatment. All patients receive chemotherapy. Currently, there is no unequivocal evidence supporting additional irradiation. Patients with disease confined to the thorax, however, who reach a partial or complete remission probably derive benefit from radiotherapy to the chest. Patients with distant tumor spread or recurrent disease have a very poor prognosis, making individually chosen treatment modalities considering quality of life necessary.

Virtually every patient with SCLC should receive *chemotherapy.* Even patients with poor performance status or concomitant diseases experience symptomatic improvement and prolongation of life. Combination chemotherapy yields significantly higher response rates than single-agent therapy. At present, there are no clear indications for single-agent therapy in first-line treatment of SCLC; however, it may have a role in far-advanced disease or in patients with a poor performance status, especially in ED.

Standard combinations are ACO (adriamycin, cyclophosphamide, vincristine), EpiCO (epirubicin, cyclophosphamide, vincristine), ACE (adriamycin,

Table 56.2 Anthracycline- and alkylating-agents-based regimens in small cell lung cancer

Adriamycin/cyclophosphamide/vincristine			ACO(CAV)
Adriamycin	60 mg/m²	iv	Day 1
Cyclophosphamide	750 mg/m²	iv	Days 1, 2
Vincristine	1,5 mg	iv	Days 1, 8, 15

q 21 days
(Vincristine max. 1 mg in patients >65)

Epirubicin/cyclophosphamide/vincristine			EpiCO
Epirubicin	40 mg/m²	iv	Days 1, 2
Cyclophosphamide	750 mg/m²	iv	Days 1, 2
Vincristine	1,5 mg	iv	Days 1, 8, 15

q 21 days
(Vincristine max. 1 mg in patients >65)

Adriamycin/cyclophosphamide/etoposide			ACE
Adriamycin	45 mg/m²	iv	Day 1
Cyclophosphamide	1000 mg/m²	iv	Day 1
Etoposide	50 mg/m²	iv	Days 1-5

q 21 days

Ifosfamide/etoposide			
Ifosfamide	1500 mg/m²	iv	Days 1-5
Etoposide	120 mg/m²	iv	Days 3-5

q 21 or 28 days

cyclophosphamide, etoposide), PE (cisplatin, etoposide), and CEV (carboplatin, etoposide, vincristine) (Tabs. 56.2 and 56.3). Incorporating ifosfamide instead of cyclophosphamide appears promising yet more toxic (CEIV= carboplatin, etoposide, ifosfamide, vincristine). The role of newer agents such as paclitaxel, docetaxel, gemcitabine, or navelbine, all of them showing response rates of more than 20%, has not been fully established.

All the preceding regimens result in objective response rates of up to 90% in patients with LD (40-60% CR) and 80% in patients with ED (15-30% CR). There is no clear superiority of one regimen in terms of overall survival. ACO (CAV), EpiCO, and ACE are well tolerated and easy to administer but have the disadvantage of enhancing toxicity of radiotherapy. These regimens can be recommended as first-line therapy for patients not intended to undergo irradiation, mainly those with extensive disease. Patients with limited disease are more frequently treated with platinum compounds, particularly carboplatin, in combination with etoposide, especially since there is little interference with concomitant or subsequent radiotherapy. Carboplatin-etoposide regimens have a reduced emetogenic potential, but they display significant hematologic toxicity. Cisplatin is less myelosuppressive but is rarely applied in a palliative approach, being emetogenic and potentially nephrotoxic.

Tumor response has to be evaluated after two cycles of chemotherapy. If there is no remission after two cycles, therapy can be switched to an alternative regimen. In patients with partial or complete remissions, it is continued for a total of four to six cycles, followed by radiotherapy to the chest in patients with LD or ED I disease. Recent data

support simultaneous or alternating chemoradiotherapy rather than sequential schedules. However, these approaches add significant toxicity to the lungs, mediastinum, and spinal cord. Cranial irradiation should be given to all LD patients with complete remission after chemotherapy or irradiation.

Second-line therapy for recurrent or progressive disease has to be chosen on an individual basis. Crossover from anthracycline-alkylating agent combinations to platinum-etoposide regimens can induce second, however short-lasting, tumor responses. On the other hand, single-agent therapy with etoposide, ifosfamide, or anthracyclines is possible, as is the application of newer agents, e.g., topotecan, paclitaxel, docetaxel, irinotecan, gemcitabine or bendamantine.

Adequate *dosing* adhering to the schedule is crucial for achieving optimal remission rates. Except for patients with underlying chronic diseases or poor performance status, there is no indication for a "mild", i.e., underdosed, treatment. On the other hand, there are no convincing data supporting extensive dose escalation yet. High-dose chemotherapy with the support of growth factors or either autologous bone marrow or peripheral stem cells did not result in longer overall survival.

Long-term *maintenance therapy* may prolong progression-free but not overall survival. Studies using interfer-

Table 56.3 Platinum-based and single-agent etoposide regimens in small cell lung cancer

Cisplatin/etoposide			PE
Cisplatin	50 mg/m²	iv	Days 1, 7
Etoposide	170 mg/m²	iv	Days 3, 4, 5

q 21-28 days

Carboplatin/etoposide/vincristine			CEV
Carboplatin	300 mg/m²	iv	Day 1
Etoposide	140 mg/m²	iv	Days 1, 2, 3
Vincristine	1,5 mg	iv	Days 1, 8, 15

q 28 days

Cyclophosphamide/cisplatin/adriamycin/etoposide			
Cyclophosphamide	225 mg/m²	iv	Days 2-5
Cisplatin	80 mg/m²	iv	Day 2
Adriamycin	40 mg/m²	iv	Day 2
Etoposide	50 mg/m²	iv	Days 1-3

q 27-32 days (radiotherapy after cycles 2, 3, and 4); cyclophosphamide 300 mg/m² and cisplatin 100 mg/m² during thr first cycle

Etoposide intravenously			
Etoposide	170 mg/m²	iv	Days 1, 3, 5

q 21-28 days (dose escalation according to toxicity)

Etoposide orally			
Etoposide	2 x 50 mg/m²	po	Days 1-10 (or 1-14)

q 21 days

on-alpha (IFN-α) seem promising but await further confirmation. So far there is no established indication for extended induction or for maintenance therapy.

Non-small cell lung cancer (NSCLC)

Non-small cell lung cancer (NSCLC) differs in its biologic behavior from SCLC. Tumor doubling time is longer, hematogenous spread occurs later in the course of disease, and the sensitivity to cytotoxic drugs is low. Therefore, surgical resection is the mainstay of therapy. At the time of diagnosis, approximately 30% of patients have resectable tumors. While 10% of all patients survive 5 years, the prognosis of patients with stage I or II tumors is much better (40-60 and 30% 5-year survival, respectively) than in advanced stages. Percutaneous radiotherapy is indicated as an adjuvant or palliative modality in stage III disease, as well as in all patients with progressive or symptomatic unresectable carcinomas. The role of chemotherapy is less well defined than in SCLC. In patients with stage III tumors, multimodal approaches involving neoadjuvant (preoperative) or adjuvant chemoradiotherapy are increasingly studied in order to improve resectability as well as survival. With the development of new drugs and drug combinations, a changing and more pronounced role of cytotoxic chemotherapy can be expected for the next years.

Stage I/II All patients in these early stages should undergo surgery if there are no contraindications. If the tumor stage is confirmed intraoperatively, there is no indication for adjuvant irradiation or chemotherapy. Within clinical trials, however, adjuvant chemotherapy in stage II disease is studied. Patients not receiving surgery receive radiotherapy to the chest or combined-modality approaches.

Stage IIIA For therapeutic reasons, stage IIIA tumors have to be divided into those with (T1–3N2) and without (T3N1) ipsilateral mediastinal involvement. The latter should have surgical resection, eventually followed by adjuvant radiotherapy. Pancoast tumors are irradiated pre- and postoperatively. The treatment of patients with advanced (more than one location) ipsilateral mediastinal lymph nodes (N2) is currently investigated in prospective, randomized trials. The main problems are the poor local tumor control with conventional approaches and the high incidence of distant recurrences. The most promising results have been obtained with preoperative (neoadjuvant) chemotherapy or chemoradiotherapy, followed by surgical resection and adjuvant or additive radiotherapy. Patients with stage IIIA NSCLC should be included in clinical trials whenever possible.

Stage IIIB Stage IIIB tumors are usually not resectable. Some patients are able to undergo surgery after preoperative chemotherapy or chemoradiotherapy. All other patients are usually treated by radiotherapy alone or chemotherapy followed by consolidating irradiation.

Table 56.4 Platinum-based chemotherapy regimens for non-small cell lung cancer

Cisplatin/etoposide			PE
Cisplatin	60 mg/m²	iv	Days 1, 7
Etoposide	130 mg/m²	iv	Days 3, 4, 5
q 21-28 days			
Mitomycin/cisplatin/vindesine			**MVP**
Mitomycin	10 mg/m²	iv	Day 1
Cisplatin	50 mg/m²	iv	Days 1, 22
Vindesine	3 mg/m²	iv	Days 1, 22
q 42 days			
Cyclophosphamide/adriamycin/cisplatin			**CAP**
Cyclophosphamide	400 mg/m²	iv	Day 1
Adriamycin	40 mg/m²	iv	Day 1
Cisplatin	40 mg/m²	iv	Days 1, 2, 3, 4
q 28 days			
Paclitaxel/cisplatin			
Paclitaxel	135 mg/m²	iv	Day 1
Cisplatin	75 mg/m²	iv	Day 2
q 21 days			
Cisplatin/gemcitabine			
Cisplatin	100 mg/m²	iv	Day 2
Gemcitabine	1000 mg/m²	iv	Days 1, 8, 15
q 28 days			

Table 56.5 Single-agent and non-platinum-based regimens for non-small cell lung cancer

Mitomycin/vindesine			MV
Mitomycin	10 mg/m²	iv	Day 1
Vindesine	3 mg/m²	iv	Days 1, 8
q 21days			
Paclitaxel			
Paclitaxel	175-225 mg/m²	iv	Day 1
q 22-29 days			

Stage IV For a long time, patients with disseminated disease usually were treated with supportive care only, including radiotherapy to bone metastases or to the primary tumor, if symptoms or complications (such as poststenotic pneumonia) occurred. Intrabronchial therapy (e.g., laser therapy, brachytherapy, stents) can alleviate symptoms as well. However, systemic chemotherapy has gained much attention. It can improve symptoms in many patients and yields a moderate yet statistically significant prolongation of survival, and has a positive impact on the quality of life.

Moderate single-agent activities in NSCLC are shown by cisplatin, carboplatin, ifosfamide, mitomycin, vindesine, vinblastine, vinorelbine, etoposide, paclitaxel, docetaxel, gemcitabine, and irinotecan. Single-agent therapy is indicated only in a palliative setting in stage IV patients (e.g., paclitaxel, gemcitabine, or vinorelbine). Moreover, there are some promising data using single-agent cisplatin or paclitaxel for radiosenzitation. Combination therapy is superior to the application of single agents. Remission rates, however, do not exceed 40 to 50% with only a few complete remissions.

Most of the currently used standard combinations (Tabs. 56.4 and 56.5) are cisplatin-based, such as MVP (mitomycin, cisplatin, vindesine) and MIC (mitomycin, ifosfamide, cisplatin) or PE (cisplatin, etoposide). The combinations of cisplatin-paclitaxel or cisplatin-gemctabine seem to be superior to the "standard combination" of cisplatin-etoposide; these data require further confirmation.

In *second-line therapy* for recurrent or progressive disease after initial treatment, careful attention has to be given to toxicity and quality of life. In general, a significant prolongation of survival is rather rare. At present, there are neither indications for *high-dose chemotherapy* involving growth factors or hematopoietic stem cell support, nor data supporting *maintenance therapy*. Studies aimed at secondary prevention using vitamins or other drugs are under way.

Suggested readings

ARRIAGADA R, LE CHEVALIER TH, BORIE F, et al. Prophylactic cranial irradiation for patients with small cell lung cancer in complete remission. J Natl Cancer Inst 1995;87:183-90.

BROWN MM, CAPORASO NE, PAGE WF, HOOVER RN. Genetic component of lung cancer: cohort study of twins. Lancet 1994;344:440-3.

DANCEY J, LE CHEVALIER T. Non-small cell lung cancer: An overview of current management. Eur J Cancer 1997; 33(suppl 1):S2-7.

CRINÒ L, SCAGLIOTTI G, MARANGOLO M, et al. Cisplatin-gemcitabine combination in advanced non-small-cell lung cancer: a phase II study. J Clin Oncol 1997;15:297-303.

EBERHARDT W, WILKE HJ, STAMATIS G, et al. Preoperative chemotherapy followed by concurrent chemoradiation therapy based on hyperfractionated accelerated radiotherapy and definitive surgery in locally advanced non-small-cell lung cancer: mature results of a phase II trial. J Clin Oncol 1998; 16:622-34.

EDELMAN MJ, GANDARA DR, ROACH M III, BENFIELD JR. Multimodality therapy in stage III non-small cell lung cancer. Ann Thorac Surg 1996;61:1564-72.

FETSCHER S, BRUGGER W, ENGELHARDT R, et al. Dose-intense therapy with etoposide, ifosfamide, cisplatin, and epirubicin (VIP-E) in 100 consecutive patients with limited- and extensive-disease small-cell lung cancer. Ann Oncol 1997;8:49-56.

JOHNSON DH. Small cell lung cancer in the elderly patient. Semin Oncol 1997;24:484-91.

LASSEN UN, HIRSCH FR, ØSTERLIND K, et al. Outcome of combination chemotherapy in extensive stage small-cell cancer: any treatment related progress? Lung Cancer 1998;20:151-160.

LILENBAUM RC, LANGENBERG P, DICKERSIN K. Single-agent versus combination chemotherapy in patients with advanced nonsmall cell lung carcinoma: a meta-analysis of response, toxicity, and survival. Cancer 1998;82:116-6.

NIEDERLE N, SCHÜTTE J, SCHMIDT CG, SEEBER S. Treatment of recurrent small cell lung carcinoma with vindesine and cisplatin. Cancer Treat Rep 1984;68:791-2.

PORT META-ANALYSIS TRIALISTS GROUP. Postoperative radiotherapy in non-small-cell lung cancer: systematic review and meta-analysis of individual patient data from nine randomised controlled trials. Lancet 1998;352:257-63.

STEWARD WP, VON PAWEL J, GATZEMEIER U, et al. Effects of granulocyte-macrophage colony-stimulating factor and dose intensification of V-ICE chemotherapy in small cell lung cancer: a prospective, randomized study of 300 patients. J Clin Oncol 1998;16:642-50.

VANSTEENKISTE JF, DE LEYN PR, DENEFFE GJ, et al. Vindesine-ifosfamide-platinum (VIP) induction chemotherapy in surgically staged IIIA-N2 non-small-cell lung cancer: a prospective study. Leuven Lung Cancer Group. Ann Oncol 1998; 9:261-7.

VOKES EE, LEOPOLD KA, HERNDON J, GREEN MR. Investigations of new drugs in combination with cisplatin in stage III non-small cell lung cancer. Semin Oncol 1997;24(suppl 8):42-5.

Gastrointestinal tumors

Salvatore Siena

Gastrointestinal tumors comprise a wide variety of malignant tumors affecting major digestive and metabolic organs; foremost among these are tumors of the esophagus, stomach, large bowel, liver, and pancreas. For some of these tumors, a multidisciplinary approach including surgery, radiation, and chemotherapy has provided strikingly beneficial results, whereas for others, e.g., primary pancreatic cancer, biliary tract cancer, and metastatic liver tumors, prognosis remains dismal.

ESOPHAGEAL CANCER

Esophageal cancer is the ninth most common malignancy worldwide. It occurs rarely in persons under 25 years of age, and incidence and mortality rise with advancing age. In western countries, the median age of occurrence is 67 years. These tumors generally occur much more frequently among men (two to four times more than among women). Rates of squamous cell carcinomas are nearly six times higher among black men than among white men, whereas adenocarcinomas occur at a frequency three times greater in whites. The incidence of squamous cell carcinomas, however, is declining.

The primary causes of squamous cell esophageal cancer in the western world are tobacco and alcohol consumption, although other nutritional factors also may contribute, with a high intake of fresh fruits and vegetables consistently associated with reduced risk. Smoking also is a risk factor for adenocarcinomas, and obesity has been documented as an important element of risk.

Among the most frequent causes of esophageal cancer is the presence of Barrett's esophagus, i.e., a condition characterized by columnar metaplasia, which develops as a complication in 10 to 20% of patients with chronic gastroesophageal reflux disease (GERD; see also Chap. 33) and predisposes to the development of adenocarcinoma. Since the 1970s, the incidence of Barrett's-associated adenocarcinoma has been increasing rapidly in the western world. Detection of Barrett's esophagus, particularly in high-risk populations, relies on repeated biopsies and may prevent a considerable number of carcinomas.

Treatment

Treatment approaches consist of endoscopic palliative techniques, single modalities (e.g., surgery, chemotherapy, or radiation), and combination therapy.

Endoscopic therapy The purpose of various endoscopic techniques is palliative i.e., to stent a malignant obstructing esophageal lesion. Esophageal intubation, endoscopic recannulation with laser therapy, and electrofulguration are currently used to restore esophageal continuity. Complications include esophageal perforation, hemorrhage, and aspiration pneumonia.

Surgery Surgical therapy is still the best approach for local tumor control and durable relief of dysphagia. Morbidity and mortality largely depend on the location of the lesion, being highest in the upper esophagous and lowest in the lower esophagous. Thus, it is not always possible to resect the segment of esophagus and reconstruct it with an end-to-end esophagogastrostomy.

Radiation therapy The effectiveness of radiation therapy depends greatly on the bulk of lesion. Tumors that are less than 5 cm in length and nonobstructing can be treated with good local control and 5-year survival is 15 to 20% of patients. Radiation as a curative treatment also can be used for localized resectable disease in patients with associate medical illnesses that make the risks of surgery unacceptable.

Chemotherapy Chemotherapy was used originally as palliation for advanced disease (i.e., metastatic and recurrent carcinoma). Treatment response was transient and had no impact on survival. Currently, chemotherapy is an integral part of the primary management of patients with locally confined disease. Of the single agents tested to date, cisplatin and mitomycin appear to be most active. However, some new agents, namely, the *Vinca* alkaloids vindesine and vinorelbine, paclitaxel, and docetaxel, appear to be very active. Response rates range between 20 and 35%. The response rate of combination therapy with cisplatin and bleomycin tested in patients with advanced disease is 25 to 40%, with a mean dura-

Table 57.1 Esophageal carcinoma: list of major chemotherapy protocols

Cisplatin + 5-Fluorouracil*

Cisplatin	75-100 mg/m^2 iv	Day 1
5-Fluorouracil	1000 mg/m^2/day iv (continuous infusion)	Days 1-4

*To be repeated every 3 weeks.
Predominantly used in the preoperative setting concurrently with radiotherapy

CBV*

Cisplatin	50 mg/m^2 iv	Day 1
Bleomycin	10 mg/m^2 single iv bolus 10 mg/m^2 iv (24 h continuous infusion)	Day 1 and days 1-4
Vindesine	3 mg/m^2 iv	Day 1

*To be repeated every 6-8 weeks

ECF

Epirubicin	50 mg/m^2 iv	Day 1*
Cisplatin 200	60 mg/m^2/day	Day 1*
5-Fluorouracil	200 mg/m^2/day (continuous infusion)	for 21 days*

*To be repeated every 21 days

PCF

Paclitaxel	175 mg/m^2 iv (3-h infusion)	Day 1
Cisplatin	15-20 mg/m^2 iv	Days 1-4*
5-Fluorouracil	750-1000 mg/m^2 (continuous infusion)	Days 1-4

* To be repeated every 4 weeks

tion of 6 months. Similar responses have been obtained with a combination of cisplatin and 5-fluorouracil (5-FU). Some authors have reported a 53% incidence of partial responses. Major protocols of chemotherapeutic combinations for esophageal cancer are listed in Table 57.1.

Combined-modality therapy Four treatment approaches have been evaluated. Combination of surgery and radiation therapy is not better than surgery alone. The response rate to preoperative chemotherapy was 40 to 60%. Most trials used cisplatin in combination with 5-FU or vindesine/vinblastine and bleomycin/mitoguanone. Chemoradiotherapy after nonradical surgery is associated with a 25 to 30% response rate with a median of 12 to 18 months. In this approach, agents with radiosensitizing potential (cisplatin, 5-FU, and mitomycin) were used. In most trials, the radiation dose was 30 Gy. Similar agents with radiotherapy were administered as an alternative to surgery. Patients received combination chemotherapy with cisplatin (75-100 mg/m^2) and 5-FU (1000 mg/m^2, 2-4 cycles) followed by radiotherapy (40-60 Gy).

Surgery alone or surgery following preoperative cisplatin-based chemotherapy should be considered for all patients with local and locoregional esophageal cancer. For inoperable patients secondary to local tumor invasion, optimal treatment includes endoscopic therapy along with radiation or combined chemoradiation therapy.

STOMACH CANCER

Cancer of the stomach is responsible for approximately three-quarters to a million deaths globally each year. The insidious nature of the onset of symptoms and their similarity in the early stages to benign causes of dyspepsia can make diagnosis difficult or delayed without a high index of suspicion. Without early diagnosis and surgical treatment, the prognosis remains poor.

There are wide variations in the prevalence rates of gastric cancer throughout the world. In Japan, it is the most common cause of cancer-related death, whereas in the United States and Sri Lanka, it is relatively rare.

An increase in carcinoma of the proximal stomach relative to the antrum has been reported. The importance of environment is clearly seen in studies of Japanese families who migrated to Hawaii and to the Bay Area in California. In one generation, gastric cancer rates were halved in siblings, and rates for other cancers, such as carcinoma of the colon, increased. Dietary factors play a very important role in specific countries and exert positive protective effects where vitamin C intake is high, but in others countries, dietary factors have a negative effect, such as in Japan with its high salt diet.

Gastric cancer begins in the mucosa with a long latency period of possibly up to 15 to 20 years from initial gastritis to subsequent carcinoma development. The changes underlying the multistage process often begin either in childhood or in the early teenage years.

Treatment _____

Surgical excision of the gastric and nodal components of the disease remains the primary therapy for all potentially curable stomach cancers. The procedure of extended lymphadenectomy will not benefit most patients with locally extensive stomach cancer. Most of these patients (except

Table 57.2 Results of adjuvant chemotherapy for stomach cancer

No. of patients	Year	Regimen	Statististical significance
42 40 41	1980	Mitomycin C Mitomycin C/5-FU/Ara-C Control	Positive
73 76 74	1984	Mitomycin C/5-FU/Ara-C/5-FU po Mitomycin C/Ftorafur Ara-C/5-FU po Control	Positive
133 148	1990	FAM* Control	Negative
33 37	1991	Mitomycin C Control	Positive

*5-fluorouracil, doxorubicin, mitomycin.

Table 57.3 Gastric carcinoma: list of major chemotherapy protocols

ECF

Epirubicin	50 mg/m² iv	Day 1*
Cisplatin	60 mg/m² iv	Day 1*
5-Fluorouracil	200 mg/m² iv (continuous infusion)	For 21 days

* To be repeated every 21 day

FAMTX

Methotrexate *1 hour later*	1000-1500 mg/m² iv	Day 1*
5-Fluorouracil	1500 mg/m² iv	Day 1*
Doxorubicin	30 mg/m² iv	Day 15
Folinic acid	15 mg/m² po	Every 6 hours, total of 12 doses, starting 24 h after methotrexate dose

* To be repeated after 4 weeks at the earliest

ELF

Etoposide	120 mg/m² iv (60 min infusion)	Days 1-3*
Folinic acid	150 mg/m² iv (15 min infusion)	Days 1-3*
5-Fluorouracil	500 mg/m² iv (15 min infusion)	Days 1-3*

*To be repeated every 3-4 weeks

those with lesions confined to mucosa or submucosa) potentially would benefit from adjuvant locoregional or systemic treatment. Response rates of 50% or more are reported for a number of drug combinations, but only a minority of randomized trials have proved the benefit of adjuvant chemotherapy. Table 57.2 summarizes some of the major adjuvant chemotherapy randomized trials.

Adjuvant irradiation and chemotherapy are reasonably well tolerated, decrease locoregional involvement, and may improve survival. Single-institution studies have documented some efficacy for neoadjuvant (preoperative) chemotherapy with or without irradiation. A clinical

response of 68% (15% of pathologic complete remissions) is achieved with preoperative chemotherapy with etoposide, adriamycin, and prednisone (EAP). About half the treated patients with resectable lesions show a good clinical response after adjuvant chemotherapy with 5-FU and cisplatin. For patients with metastatic disease, a better response was documented for those receiving combination chemotherapy versus single agents, with a survival advantage. Single agents with 20% short-term response (36 months) include doxorubicin, cisplatin, 5-FU, etoposide, and mitomycin C. The response rates with combination chemotherapy range between 25 and 50%. Combination chemotherapy regimens are reported in Table 57.3.

COLORECTAL CANCER

Colorectal cancer is the fourth most common malignancy worldwide. According to the World Health Organization, approximately 800000 new cases are diagnosed every year. The highest incidence occurs in developed countries-United States, Canada, Western Europe, Australia, and New Zealand-but the incidence in developing countries is rising. Colorectal cancer is equally distributed between men and women.

About one-third of the tumors in the large bowel are located in the rectum; two-thirds are found in the colon, with the majority of those in the left colon. Cancer of the sigmoid colon represents about 25% of all cancers in the large bowel, and those of the descending colon represent 5 to 10%. The incidence of tumors in the right colon relative to tumors in the left colon has been slowly increasing, probably due to an aging population, and now represent about 25% of all colorectal cancers. Most colorectal cancers are adenocarcinomas. Rarely, anal carcinomas, carcinoids, and melanoma are found.

Approximately 70% of all patients with a colorectal cancer can be operated on with curative intent. In 10% of patients, the tumor cannot be resected owing to advanced

Table 57.4 Staging and 5-year survival for colorectal cancer (see text)

Stage	Dukes/Astler-Coller	TNM criteria	Description	5-year survival
0		TIS, NO, MO	Carcinoma in situ	100%
I	A/A or B1	T1-2, NO,MO	Tumor limited to muscularis propria	85-100%
II	B/B2 or B3	T3-4, NO, MO	Primary tumor has infiltrated beyond muscularis propria	50-80%
III	C/C1, C2 or C3	T1-4, N1-3, MO	Regional lymph nodes infiltrated by cancer	30-60%
IV	D	T1-4, NO-3, M1	Distant metastasis	<5%

(From Pahlman L. Colorectal cancer. In: Bianchi Porro G, Cremer M, Krejs G, et al, eds. Gastroenteroloy and hepatology. London: McGraw-Hill, 1999;354.)

Table 57.5 Colorectal and anal carcinoma: list of major chemotherapy protocols

COLORECTAL CANCER

5-Fluorouracil as monotherapy
A1. *Bolus administration*

5-Fluorouracil	500-1000 mg/m^2 iv	Days 1-5
To be repeated every 4 weeks		

A2. *Continuous infusion*

5-Fluorouracil	300 mg/m^2/day iv (continuous infusion)	
(up to 12 weeks)	for 4 weeks or more	

Note: in the event of significant toxicity, the infusion should be interrupted until resolution of the toxicity and then restarted at 50 mg/mq/day reductions following each interruption

5-Fluorouracil + folinic acid
B1. *Monthly schedules*

5-Fluorouracil	425 mg/m^2	Days 1-5 given after
Folinic acid	20 mg/m^2	Days 1-5

To be repeated every 4-5 weeks
Note: high-doses folinic acid, i.e., 200 mg/m^2/day, was not better

or

5-Fluorouracil	370 mg/m^2 iv	Days 1-5
Folinic acid	500 mg/m^2 iv (30-min infusion, 1 h before 5-FU)	Days 1-5

To be repeated every 4 weeks (6 cycles adjuvant therapy for patients with Dukes' B/C colon cancer)

B2. *Weekly schedules*

5-Fluorouracil	500 mg/m^2 iv, administered via bolus 1 hour after	Weekly 6
Folinic acid	20 or 500 mg/m^2 iv (2-h infusion)	Weekly 6

Also as adjuvant therapy for patients with Dukes' B/C colon cancer

or

5-Fluorouracil	2600 mg/m^2 iv (24-h infusion)	Weekly 6
Folinic acid	500 mg/m^2 iv (30-min infusion)	Weekly 6
To be repeated on day 56		

5-Fluorouracil + radiotherapy
NCI recommendation for adjuvant treatment of high-risk rectal cancer, stage II and III, Dukes' B2 and C

5-Fluorouracil	500 mg/m^2 iv	Days 1-3, at weeks
	450 mg/m^2 iv	1, 5, 9 and
		Days 1-5 at weeks 3, 17, 21
Radiation (45 Gy followed by boost of 5.4 Gy in 3 fractions to the tumor bed)		Over 6 weeks

Ralitrexed (Tomudex)

Ralitrexed	3 mg/m^2 iv	Day 1
To be repeated every 3 weeks		

Irinotecan (CPT-11)
(as first- or second-line treatment)

Irinotecan	125 mg/m^2 iv (90-min infusion)	Weekly 4
To be repeated every 6 weeks		

or

Irinotecan	300-350 mg/m^2 iv (90-min infusion)	Day 1
To be repeated every 3 weeks		

Oxaliplatin
(as first- or second-line treatment)

Oxaliplatin	130 mg/m^2 iv (2-h infusion)	Day 1
To be repeated every 3 weeks		

UFT
(combination of ftorafur with uracil at a molar ratio of 1:4, 100 mg ftorafur + 224 mg uracil). UFT has been administered as a single agent or biomodulated by folinic acid daily in split doses for periods up to 28 days, e.g.,

UFT	100 mg/m^2 po	Days 1-28
Folinic acid	150 mg po	

To be repeated every 6 weeks
Monoclonal antibody 17-1A (Edrecolomab)
For adjuvant immunotherapy of colonic carcinoma

Edrecolomab		Day 1
	500 mg iv (2-h infusion)	
	100 mg iv (2-h infusion)	Days 29, 57, 85, 113

(continued)

Table 57.5 (continued)

Nonresecable liver metastases

Hepatic arterial infusion of fluoropyrimidines may achieve higher response rates than systemic chemotherapy

5-Fluoro-2-deoxyuridine	0.3 mg/kg ia	Days 1-14

To be repeated every 4 weeks

ANAL CARCINOMA

Concomitant radiochemotherapy

5-Fluorouracil	750 mg/m^2 iv (continuous infusion)	Days 1-5 or
	1000 mg/m^2 iv (continuous infusion)	Days 1-4
Mitomycin	10-15 mg/m^2 iv	Day 1

To be repeated at 4 weeks

Concomitant with radiation therapy 45 Gy (1.8 Gy/d 5 per week for 5 weeks)

or

Mitomycin	5 mg/m^2 iv	Day 1
5-Fluorouracil	1000 mg/m^2 iv (22-h infusion)	Days 1-4 (weeks 1 + 5)
Radiotherapy	2 Gy/d	Days 1-5 (weeks 1–3)

Followed by

5-Fluorouracil	1000 mg/m^2 iv (22-h infusion)	Days 1-4 (weeks 10, 14, 18)
Cisplatin	100 mg/m^2 iv (1-h infusion)	Day 1 (weeks 10, 14, 18)

local growth, and in another 20%, distant spread has already occurred at the time of diagnosis, making curative surgery impossible.

Dukes' classification

The most widely used system for classifying colorectal tumors after histopathologic examination of the specimen is the Dukes' system, which considers the depth of tumor penetration in the bowel wall and the occurrence of locoregional lymph node deposits. Stage A defines tumor growing into but not through the bowel wall, i.e., the muscularis. Stage B defines a tumor growing through the muscularis propria, and stage C defines a tumor with regional lymph node metastases. Patients with distal metastases are classified as Dukes' stage D. The Astler-Coller classification subdivides stages A and C into different substages. The more classic TNM classification criteria, recently applied, may allow more complete staging and also prediction of 5-year survival (Tab. 57.4).

Treatment

The principles of surgical en bloc resection with in-continuity lymph node resection have been the hallmark of surgical therapy. Local management of rectal tumors includes snare excision of malignant polyps as well as transanal, transsphincteric, and parasacral excisions. Current criteria for such treatment include well-differentiated tumors less than 4 cm in size.

Radiotherapy In patients with rectal cancer, radiotherapy is used (1) to eradicate micrometastases that were impossible to resect at surgery and (2) to reduce the size of large tumors, with the aim of making the tumor resectable. Based on tumor biology and experience from numbers of adjuvant trials, it is generally accepted that the minimum dose required to treat micrometastases is about 45 to 50 Gy given in fractionated doses of 1.8 to 2.0 Gy daily. Also, the literature supports the idea that preoperative treatment is more dose-effective than postoperative radiotherapy. It has been demonstrated that the local recurrence rate after surgery can be reduced by approximately 60% if irradiation is given at a high dose level preoperatively compared with about 30 to 40% if the treatment is given at the same or even higher dose levels postoperatively.

Chemotherapy Postoperative adjuvant chemotherapy of colorectal cancer is aimed at reducing the risk of relapse by preventing growth of micrometastatic disease. A number of clinical trials have clearly shown that adjuvant chemotherapy is indicated in Dukes' stage C disease and results in an increased 5-year survival of approximately 10 to 20%. Although this may sound like a minor increase, the potential impact worldwide is enormous. However, no further data exist to support the concept that patients with Dukes' stage B disease also should have adjuvant chemotherapy. Recent data demonstrated that patients with Dukes' stage B2 cancer represent the group most likely to take advantage of adjuvant chemotherapy, especially if the tumor expresses adverse prognostic features such as G3 histology, high growth rate, and high serum carcinoembryonic antigen (CEA) levels.

Drug combinations effective in colorectal cancer are mainly based on 5-FU and folinic acid in European countries and 5-FU and levamisole in the United States. More recently, therapeutic combinations have been enriched with raltitrexed, a new thymidylate synthase inhibitor, and oxaliplatin, whereas results from the administration of monoclonal antibodies (Panorex) are still pending. Table 57.5 reports major drug combinations for the treatment of colorectal and anal cancer. The list includes some novel therapeutic strategies such as irinote-can, folate-based thymidylate synthase inhibitors (raltitrexed) being evaluated in phase III trials, and oxali-platin, which already has shown significant efficacy in prolonging survival, as well as protocol combinations with monoclonal antibodies and radiotherapy.

PRIMARY HEPATIC CANCERS

Hepatocellular carcinoma accounts for more than 90% of primary hepatic malignancies and is one of most common malignant tumors worldwide, with a rising incidence. Estimated worldwide incidence of hepatocellular carcino-mas is 1 million per year, with more than 250 000 deaths per year. Hepatocellular carcinoma ranks as the seventh most common cancer in men and the ninth most common in women. The most important risk factors are liver cir-rhosis of any etiology and chronic hepatitis B and C infections. There are no special clinical symptoms associ-ated with liver carcinoma. Most patients are either asymptomatic or present with signs of liver insufficiency or abdominal pain.

Nutritional factors that raise the risk of hepatocellular carcinoma are alcohol intake (about 30% of hepatocellu-lar carcinoma patients have relevant chronic alcohol intake) and toxins (e.g., aflatoxin, derived from *Aspergillus flavus*), found mainly in tropical countries in contaminated food. The prognosis of hepatocellular carci-noma depends on tumor stage and degree of liver cirrho-sis but generally is dismal, with a mean survival of 2 to 6 months in untreated patients.

Treatment

Resection and transplantation are the only potentially curative treatment options in hepatocellular carcinoma, but more than 80% of patients do not qualify for either. Percutaneous ethanol injection may offer one of the best palliative opportunities, being contraindicated in patients with a bleeding diathesis, prothrombin activity of less than 40%, and severe ascites. Alcoholization leads to 70 to 90% tumor cell necrosis without evident damage to the sur-rounding liver. Treatment effects can be assessed by visual-ization of the necrotic tumor parts by computed tomo-graphic (CT) scan or magnetic resonance imaging (MRI), revealing changes to hypointensity on T2-weighted images. The 5-year survival rate in Child class A patients is report-ed to be 41% in those with single tumors less than 5 cm in size and 33% in those with multiple tumors. Results in Child class C patients are disappointing.

Chemoembolization (i.e., injection of vasoocclusive material into tumor feeding vessels) is generally carried out with Lipiodol, an iodinated ethyl ester of the fatty acid of poppyseed oil. This is retained in hepatocellular carcinoma after intra-arterial application for up to a year. So-called lipiodolization achieves a more target-specific

and longer-lasting activity than systemic application. Studies report partial responses in 10 to 60% of patients treated with lipiodol and cisplatin. Mild side effects occur in 60% of patients, and severe side effects are seen in 25%. A recent prospective, randomized trial of adjuvant intraarterial ^{131}I-labeled Lipiodol in resectable hepatocel-lular carcinoma indicated a significant 3-year survival benefit (86.4% versus 46.3% in the control group). Microwave coagulation therapy, which works by inducing local tissue necrosis, can be applied through laparotomy or laparoscopy. Early studies from Japan report good tol-erance, even in cirrhotic patients. However, complete tumor necrosis cannot always be achieved when tumors up to 9 cm in diameter are treated.

A number of approaches, including systemic and intra-arterial chemotherapy with drugs such as 5-FU, mitoxantrone, cisplatin, etoposide, neocarzinostatin, and epirubicin, show no advantage over doxorubicin in response rate or toxicity. This last drug at currently rec-ommended doses (see Chap. 49) therefore can be regard-ed as the single-agent standard therapy for hepatocellular carcinoma. The average response rate is 20%, and medi-an survival is 4 months. Toxicity, because of the under-lying cirrhosis, is substantial. Administration of estrogen receptor-blocking agents such as tamoxifen has yielded conflicting results. Most extensive trials found no differ-ence between such drugs and placebo. Radiation therapy with doses below 20 and 35 Gy with a target delivery induces partial remission in up to 55% of patients. Success is limited by severe side effects and early tumor progression and metastasis.

Finally, surgical treatment may be attempted in tumors less than 5 cm in size in patients in good clinical condition. Eventually, in patients with nonresectable tumors, orthotopic liver transplantation can be attempt-ed. Present results, however, have shown clearly that tumor may recur after transplantation, mostly in the liver, lungs, or bones. Hepatitis B–induced cirrhosis seems to be an adverse prognostic factor.

PANCREATIC CARCINOMA

Pancreatic carcinoma is the twelfth most common cancer in the western world, but it is the fifth most common cause of cancer death. It is an insidious malignancy that causes late symptoms and hence late diagnosis, so cure is uncommon. In the rare instances when an early diag-nosis is made, surgical pancreaticoduodenectomy with curative intent may be attempted by physicians skilled and experienced in the performance of this challenging procedure. Although operative mortality rates are much improved, survival is only slightly improved.

Adjuvant chemoradiation therapy has prolonged survival in some trials and not in others. Toxicity of the combined-modality therapy is severe. Active drugs (response rate 10% or better) include 5-FU, mito-mycin, streptozotocin, ifosfamide, and doxorubicin. Gemcitabine appears to have relevant activity and has been approved by the Food and Drug

Administration (FDA) in the United States for this indication. Although several combinations have been reported to have activity greater than single agents, this has not been demonstrated in prospective clinical trials. In fact, FAM (fluorouracil, doxorubicin,

and mitomycin) was no more effective than 5-FU alone or mitomycin alone

Suggested readings

ANONYMOUS. Tamoxifen in treatment of hepatocellular carcinoma: a randomised controlled trial. TRIP Group (Cancer of the Liver Italian Programme). Lancet 1998;352:17-20.

BIANCHI PORRO G, CREMER M, KREJS G, et al. Gastroenterology and hepatology. London: McGraw-Hill, 1999.

BJARNASON GA, CRIPPS C, GOEL R, et al. Phase I-II study of 5-fluorouracil, leucovorin, doxorubicin, methotrexate, and long-term oral etoposide (FLAME) in unresectable or metastatic gastric cancer. Am J Clin Oncol 1998;21:537-42.

CARMICHAEL J. Clinical response benefit in patients with advanced pancreatic cancer: role of gemcitabine. Digestion 1997;58:503-7.

CASCINU S, GRAZIANO F, CATALANO G. Chemotherapy for advanced pancreatic cancer: It may no longer be ignored. Ann Oncol 1999;10:105-9.

CASCINU S, LABIANCA R, GRAZIANO F. Intensive weekly chemotherapy for locally advanced gastric cancer using 5-fluorouracil, cisplatin, epidoxorubicin, 6S-leucovorin, glutathione and filgrastim: A report from the Italian Group for the Study of Digestive Tract Cancer (GISCAD). Br J Cancer 1998;78:390-3.

DE GRAMONT A, LOUVET C, ANDRE T, et al. A review of GERCOD trials of bimonthly leucovorin plus 5-fluorouracil 48-h continuous infusion in advanced colorectal cancer: evolution of a regimen. Groupe d'Etude et de la Recherche sur les Cancers de l'Ovaire et Digestifs (GERCOD). Eur J Cancer 1998;34:619-26.

GUNASEKARA NS, FAULDS D. Raltitrexed: a review of its pharmacological properties and clinical efficacy in the management of advanced colorectal cancer. Drugs 1998;55:423-35.

KOK TC. Chemotherapy in oesophageal cancer. Cancer Treat Rev 1997;23:65-85.

LAU WY, LEUNG TWT, HO SKW, et al. Adjuvant intra-arterial iodine-131-labelled lipiodol for resectable hepatocellular carcinoma: a prospective randomised trial. Lancet 1999;353:797-801.

MACHOVER D. A comprehensive review of 5-fluorouracil and leucovorin in patients with metastatic colorectal carcinoma. Cancer 1997;80:1179-87.

MOERTEL CG, FLEMING TR, MacDONALD JS, et al. Levamisole and fluorouracil as adjuvant therapy of resected colon carcinoma. N Engl J Med 1990;332:52.

PUNT CJ. New drugs in the treatment of colorectal carcinoma. Cancer 1998;83:679-89.

RADERER M, KORNEK GV, HEJNA MH, et al. Treatment of advanced gastric cancer with oral etoposide, leucovorin and 5-fluorouracil (ELF) regimen. Eur J Cancer 1998;34:1128-30.

VANCUTSEM E, PEETERS M, VERSLYPE C, et al. The medical treatment of colerectal cancer: actual status and new developments. Hepatogastroenterology 1999;46:709.

WILS J J. Treatment of gastric cancer. Curr Opin Oncol 1998;10:357-61.

Urinary tract tumors

J. Alfred Witjes

PROSTATE CANCER

Although the incidence of prostate cancer is rising in all developing countries, risk factors have still not been clearly identified. There is, however, a familiar predisposition, and the first prostate cancer gene has been mapped.

Detection of prostate cancer is done with a combination of digital rectal examination (DRE), serum prostate-specific antigen (PSA) determination, and transrectal ultrasound (TRUS) examination. Since TRUS examination is time-consuming, expensive, and very operator-dependent, and since it does not seem to have a great additional diagnostic value over to the combination of DRE and PSA determination, it is reserved for guiding biopsies to confirm histology. Detection is achieved routinely by the combination of DRE and PSA determination. Sensitivity and specificity of this combination depend on the cut off value of PSA. Refinements in the use of PSA determination, such as age-specific PSA references, PSA velocity, PSA density, and the free to total PSA ratio, are under investigation to improve the value of PSA determination as a screening tool.

Digital rectal examination and transrectal ultrasound give information about the local stage of the tumor: T1 means a nonpalpable or visible tumor detected on transurethral resection or biopsy; T2 means a palpable or visible tumor confined to the prostate; T3 means a tumor that invades the capsula or seminal vesicle; and T4 means a tumor of the bladder or other organs. It is noteworthy that even in very experienced hands, around 50% of clinically staged T2 tumors appear to be T3 tumors and that 10 to 20% of clinically staged T3 tumors are T2 tumors. After histologic confirmation of an adenocarcinoma of the prostate and determination of the grade of differentiation, further screening can be done with a bone scan for bone metastasis and a computed tomographic (CT) scan or magnetic resonance imaging (MRI) for the detection of lymph node metastasis. Several studies have indicated that screening for metastasis as well as a lymph node dissection before definitive treatment can be omitted safely in patients with of a low PSA level and Gleason grade and local tumor less or equal than stage T2 (e.g., PSA < 20 ng/ml, Gleason grade < 3).

Treatment

Treatments for localized prostate cancer

Treatment with a curative intent is considered when the tumor needs treatment and the patient would die of prostate cancer if left untreated. That not all tumors need treatment is clearly demonstrated by the fact that in the case of low-grade and low-stage tumors, a "wait and see" policy gives excellent survival results. On the other hand, if a patient has a life expectancy of less than 10 years (>70-75 years of age) or has significant comorbidity, radical treatment will be overtreatment, and medical treatment could be postponed until complaints arise.

Radical treatments consist mainly of radiotherapy and radical prostatectomy. Cryosurgery and high-intensity focused ultrasound are still investigational. Radiotherapeutic options are external-beam radiation or brachytherapy. Although there are very few randomized comparisons between external-beam radiotherapy and radical surgery, the 10- to 15-year cancer control of external-beam radiotherapy appears lower than that of radical surgery. Whether improvements in computer technology and brachytherapy also will improve the long-term results of radiotherapy remains to be seen. Currently, radical retropubic prostatectomy remains the treatment of choice for localized prostate cancer despite the short- and long-term complications of this operation, namely, anastomotic stricture, incontinence, and erectile dysfunction. The number of patients with a measurable PSA level after radical prostatectomy, however, remains impressively high: 22, 48, and 60% after 5, 10, and 15 years, respectively. This is probably due in part to our limited ability to determine the correct clinical stage. Lymph node dissection gives additional staging information but has no therapeutic value. In the case of positive lymph nodes, systemic disease has to be assumed, and cure is probably impossible.

Drug therapy

Hormonal treatment

All forms of medical treatment aim at lowering the male sex hormones. Castration, for example, reduces the level of circulating testosterone by up to 90%. The remaining

10% is produced in the adrenal glands. The concentration of the active metabolite dihydrotestosterone (DHT), however, is only lowered by 60%. Approximately 75% of patients have a decrease of PSA after castration and a reduction of their prostate size by 20 to 30% in 3 months. Side effects of castration are loss of libido and energy, hot flushes, and gynecomastia.

Drugs with the same effect as surgical castration are estrogens and analogues of luteinizing-hormone releasing hormone (LHRH). Estrogens are cheap, but cardiovascular side effects made them obsolete. The efficacy and side effects of LHRH analogues are similar to the side effects of surgical castration. After an initial flare-up, castration levels of testosterone are reached within 3 weeks. The advantage of LHRH analogues is that their effects are reversible. LHRH analogues are available as depot preparations, active for a period of up to 1 to 3 months (goserelin 3.6 and 10.8 mg, respectively, for 1 and 3 months and buserelin 6.3 mg for 2 months).

To reduce the levels of testosterone and DHT after surgical castration or LHRH analogue treatment, antiandrogens are used. The steroidal antiandrogen cyproterone acetate reduces the excretion of LH and has a progestagenic effect. An advantage of this progestagenic effect is that flare-ups are almost absent and even can be reduced in castrated patients. A combination of cyproterone acetate and castration offers no advantage in cancer control.

Nonsteroidal antiandrogens, such as flutamide, nilutamide, and bicalutamide, are competitors for the DHT receptor. The testosterone level increases because of an interruption of the negative feedback of the testicular-hypothalamic axis. Loss of libido and energy, therefore, are much less frequent than after castration. The efficacy of antiandrogen therapy, however, seems to be less than that of castration. The most frequent side effects are diarrhea and hepatotoxicity (flutamide); disturbed vision, nausea, vomiting, and alcohol intolerance (nilutamide); and gynecomastia and flare-ups (bicalutamide). Long-term therapy with nonsteroidal antiandrogens can cause changes in the receptor of the prostate cancer cell in 30% of patients, resulting in a stimulating instead of an inhibiting effect of these drugs. Withdrawal of these drugs may result in a PSA decrease in these patients.

A combination of castration and nonsteroidal antiandrogens, so-called maximal androgen blockade, reduces the effect of DHT on the prostate cancer cell as compared with castration alone. This leads to an increased time to progression, but whether this results in a higher cancer-specific survival is still not proven. Some large studies indeed have found an advantage of maximal androgen blockade, but a recent meta-analysis could not confirm this. Whether maximal androgen blockade improves cancer-specific survival in patients from a good prognostic subset also remains to be proven. Accepted indications for maximal androgen blockade are prevention of a flare-up due to LHRH treatment in symptomatic patients and neoadjuvant treatment before radiotherapy to reduce the size of the prostate.

A recent development in hormonal therapy is intermittent androgen blockade. This approach might limit the growth possibilities of hormone-insensitive cells, which are thought to be responsible for the final prognosis of a patient. Although this approach is still under investigation, side effects during intermittent treatment are less.

Cytotoxic therapy

The role of cytotoxic therapy is very limited and predominantly palliative. Estramustine has estrogenic and cytotoxic properties, and because of the steroidal structure, it binds selectively with prostate cells. Its efficacy as monotherapy is comparable with that of flutamide or estrogens. Toxicity is mainly nausea, although cardiovascular side effects are possible. Estramustine is used predominantly as second-line treatment, with response rates between 19 and 69%. Mitoxantrone recently was approved by the Food and Drug Administration (FDA) in the United States because of its palliative effects in selected patients with hormone-resistant symptomatic prostate cancer.

CARCINOMAS OF THE URINARY BLADDER

Bladder cancer is the second most common malignancy of the urinary tract and accounts for 2% of all malignancies. In 1993, 52300 cases were registered in the United States; the mortality was 9900. The most important risk factor for the development of transitional cell carcinoma (TCC) of the urinary tract is cigarette smoking. Although the etiology is probably multifactorial, there is a clear relation between cigarette smoking and bladder cancer mortality. Bladder cancer is seen predominantly in the sixth and seventh decades of life. The male-to-female ratio is approximately 4:1. The most frequent presenting symptom is microscopic or macroscopic painless hematuria. After urethrocystoscopy to confirm the presence of a bladder tumor, a transurethral resection (TUR) with or without random mucosal biopsies is the initial step in histologic diagnosis of the tumor and the determination of tumor stage and grade. In most countries, more than 90% of bladder tumors are transitional cell carcinomas. Less than 10% are adenocarcinomas and squamous cell carcinomas. About two-thirds of transitional cell carcinomas will present as superficial [Pta, pT_a, carcinoma in situ (CIS)]. One-third of the tumors are invasive in the detrusor muscle (pT2-4) or disseminated (N^+ or M^+) at initial presentation.

Superficial TCC of the urinary bladder

The recurrence rate of superficial tumors is high and depends on several factors and the period of follow-up. In a review of six historical series with long-term follow-up, the recurrence rates after 5, 10, and 15 years were 65, 81, and 88%, respectively. The actuarial risk of disease progression to muscle-invasive disease is around 10%. Potential prognostic factors to predict recurrence and progression of superficial tumors are tumor grade and especially stage, recurrence rate, multiplicity, size, and localization. Factors under investigation are DNA ploidy, chromosomal abnormalities, and marker chromosomes.

In superficial transitional cell carcinoma of the urinary bladder, intravesical instillations are used to delay or prevent tumor recurrences (prophylaxis), or in the case of an incomplete resection (e.g., carcinoma in situ), instillations are used to eradicate tumor (treatment). In low-risk patients, such as patients with primary solitary low-grade pTa tumors, the need for adjuvant instillations seems low, although the recurrence rate still can be lowered significantly with one immediate chemotherapeutic instillation. In the intermediate-risk group, intravesical chemotherapy may be used to decrease the recurrence rate. In patients with high-risk tumors, such as patients with recurrent and/or multiple pT1 tumors with or without carcinoma in situ, intravesical immunotherapy could be considered.

Treatment

Intravesical chemotherapy

Several drugs have been used, such as thiotepa, adriamycin, ethoglucid, mitomycin-C, and epirubicin. With low-molecular-weight compounds (e.g., thiotepa), the drug is absorbed systemically, and (bone marrow) toxicity may be present. Local side effects such as chemical cystitis are the main adverse effects and are seen in approximately 25% of patients. Severity increases with the number and frequency of instillations and with the dose. With mitomycin-C, allergic reactions can be a limiting, although reversible, side effect. Usually, a course of 6 to 10 weekly instillations is used. The main effect of these drugs is a (modest) reduction in recurrence rate without a proven effect on tumor progression. An advantage of maintenance therapy has not been proved for any of these drugs.

Intravesical immunotherapy

Most immunotherapeutic drugs (e.g., interferon, interleukines, keyhole-limpet hemocyanin, and bropirimine) have been used in limited clinical studies. Intravesical immunotherapy is predominantly done with bacille Calmette-Guérin (BCG). The effector mechanism is a combination of a clear inflammatory effect and a nonspecific and specific immunologic response. The optimal dose seems to be 5×10^8 to 5×10^9 colony-forming units, although similar success rates have been reported with (very) low doses of BCG with less toxicity. The initial schedule is a course of 6 weekly instillations. For some patients (e.g., those with recurrences or carcinoma in situ), a second course of instillations or maintenance therapy can be given. In patients failing a second course, a significantly higher risk for muscle invasion is found, so more aggressive therapy should be considered. Maintenance therapy has more local and systemic toxicity.

Cystitis-like complaints are found in over 90% of patients and increase with the number of instillations. Minor systemic side effects (e.g., fever, malaise, and nausea) generally subside spontaneously. Severe side effects are seen in about 5% of all patients. In these patients, therapy should be stopped, and eventually, antituberculous therapy should be started. Only a few fatal complications have been encountered. They seem to be related to traumatic catheterization. BCG is superior to intravesical chemotherapy, however, at the cost of more side effects. BCG seems to be the only drug that also reduces tumor progression and bladder cancer death. Although at present BCG seems to be the drug of choice for high-risk superficial transitional cell carcinoma, questions about the mechanisms of action, optimal dose, and clinical schedule remain unanswered.

Surgery, and radiotherapy

Radical cystectomy and lymph node dissection remain the treatment of choice for locally advanced bladder cancer. When there is limited lymph node involvement (less than six nodes without extranodal extension), cure can still be achieved with radical surgery. The choice of urinary diversion (e.g., Bricker diversion, continent diversion, or orthotopic bladder substitution) depends on the urologist and the patient. Bladder-sparing procedures such as radical TUR and partial cystectomy, combined with chemotherapy and/or radiotherapy, should be considered only in highly selected patients with close follow-up. Preoperative radiation therapy is no longer performed, and radiotherapy as a curative option is insufficient compared with surgery.

Chemotherapy

The results of neoadjuvant chemotherapy in patients with locally advanced (>pT2) bladder cancer are conflicting. A Nordic study showed a 15% survival advantage after neoadjuvant chemotherapy and cystectomy with a 5-year follow-up. However, a combined MRC/EORTC study in which 975 patients with locally advanced bladder cancer were randomized for no or three cycles of CMV (cisplatin, methotrexate, vinblastine) prior to definite surgical or radiation therapy showed no difference in survival after a median follow-up of 22 months despite clear activity on the primary tumor (33 versus 12% pathologic complete responses after chemotherapy). In general low tumor stage (pT2) and downstaging to pT0 are important prognostic factors for neoadjuvant chemotherapy.

The efficacy of immediate adjuvant chemotherapy for proven locally advanced disease is also not proven. A significant advantage was seen in the treated group for time to progression (p = 0.001) and survival (p = 0.006), but the treated group was small and not uniform. Freiha in another study showed a progression advantage but failed to find a survival advantage.

In patients with metastasized or relapsing bladder cancer, MVAC (A = adriamycin) chemotherapy is often the only possibility. MVAC seems more effective than other combinations or cisplatin monotherapy. Despite promising initial complete response rates, however, the majority of patients will relapse. Toxicity of MVAC remains a major limiting factor. Different grades of myelotoxicity are seen in almost all patients, and subsequent treatment-related deaths due to a nadir sepsis have been reported. Other side effects are mucositis, nausea, vomiting, alopecia, and renal toxicity. Myelotoxicity during MVAC therapy can be prevented or diminished with hematopoietic growth factors.

Radical cystectomy remains the treatment of choice for locally advanced bladder cancer. The choice of the urinary diversion depends on the urologist and patient. Bladder-sparing procedures are still investigational. Radiotherapy as a curative option is insufficient compared with surgery.

The advantage of (neo)adjuvant chemotherapy for non invasive bladder tumors still has to be proven. For metastasized or locally recurrent tumors, the MVAC regimen remains the most effective treatment modality. Initial response rates are between 40 and 70%, but most tumors recur. Moreover, toxicity is considerable and limiting, especially leukopenia and leukopenic sepsis.

RENAL CELL CARCINOMA

The etiology of renal cell carcinoma (RCC) is unknown. There has been a steady rise in the incidence of renal tumors, and this is also seen in the Netherlands. This is probably due in part to the use of routine abdominal ultrasound, which also increased the relative amount of incidentally discovered renal cell carcinoma during the last decade. Reported percentages vary from 14 to nearly 65% of all diagnosed renal cell carcinoma. Moreover, imaging techniques have improved, and there is a greater awareness about the diagnosis renal cell carcinoma. The classic triad (e.g., painless tumor, hematuria, and general malaise) is not seen much any more. The erythrocyte sedimentation rate (ESR) is usually high. The prognosis of these tumors is in general very good. Five-year survival rates are up to 85% for incidental carcinoma versus 61% in symptomatic patients. Abdominal ultrasound gives a correct local diagnosis in the vast majority of patients, since differentiation with renal cysts is very easy with ultrasound. Besides ultrasound, staging of the tumor, nodes, and possible metastasis is done with a contrast-enhanced CT scan of the abdomen and thorax. Intravenous urography (IVU) and arteriography are not mandatory to determine local tumor extent. Magnetic resonance imaging has no additional value over CT scanning. Further screening is done on indication. Vena caval involvement can be seen with CT scanning, but duplex scanning is the best method to determine the extent of a vena caval thrombus, which has consequences for the extent of surgery.

Tumor stage is classified according to the TNM classification system. The most important differentiation is between local and metastized tumors.

Treatment

The only treatment for nonmetastized local renal cell carcinoma is still radical surgery. Whether in all cases the ipsilateral adrenal gland should be removed as well remains an open discussion. Most urologists remove the adrenal gland if there is an upper pole tumor. Although a lymph node dissection can give additional staging information, it has no therapeutic value. The presence of a vena caval thrombus has no adverse prognostic value, as long as the thrombus can be removed radically. Prognosis after radical resection of organ- and specimen-confined tumors is good. Five-year survival in such patients is more than 90%. Nephron-sparing surgery is a feasible and safe approach, advisable in cases of tumor in a monokidney, bilateral tumors, contralateral compromised kidney function, and Von Hippel-Lindau's disease. When nephron-sparing surgery is considered, an arteriography is advised. The risk of tumor recurrence and multifocality (up to 10%) make it not the first choice when there is a normal contralateral kidney. Radiotherapy has only palliative indications, and chemotherapy has no role in renal cell carcinoma.

Immunotherapy

In metastatic renal cell carcinoma, the only rational approach is immunotherapy. There is no indication for chemotherapy, probably because of overexpression of the multidrug resistance gene in metastatic renal cell carcinoma. When there is a solitary metastasis, excision of this lesion may be advisable.

Although a number of immunotherapeutic strategies haven been tested, interferons (IFN) and interleukins (IL) have been used most extensively. The overall objective response rates with IFN-α range from 12 to 18%. Most of the responses are partial, some are temporary complete responses, and only a very small percentage of patients will survive more than 5 years. Other IFNs seem less effective, and combinations of IFNs or IFN-α and chemotherapy give no additional beneficial effect. IL-2 also has been used extensively in metastatic renal cell carcinoma. Intravenous IL-2 has considerable toxicity. Subcutaneous IL-2, however, has been used successfully on an outpatient basis. Although IL-2 monotherapy does not seem to be more effective than IFN-α, combinations with IL-2 are promising. Tumor necrosis factor (TNF) has been used, but it appeared to be relatively toxic. Other biologic response modifiers are currently under investigation. Since traditional therapies are lacking sufficient efficacy, newer strategies should be explored. Gene therapy could become one such successful strategy in the near future.

The etiology of renal cell carcinoma is unknown, although the incidence is rising. The routine use of abdominal ultrasound has increased the percentage of small tumors discovered and therefore has improved overall prognosis. After complete staging, the most important differentiation is between local and metastatic tumors. Local tumors should be resected radically, even in the presence of a vena caval thrombus. Under certain circumstances, renal-sparing surgery can be considered. Lymphadenectomy is diagnostic, not therapeutic. For metastatic or relapsing patients, currently the only possibility is immunotherapy with IFN-α or IL-2. Success rates are around 15%. New approaches are necessary to improve the prognosis of these patients.

Suggested readings

BOCCARDO F. Therapeutic challenges in the medical management of renal cancer. Surg Forum 1991;1:143-56.

BRETHEAU D, LECHEVALLIER E, EGHAZARIAN C. Prognostic signs of incidental renal cell carcinoma. Eur Urol 1995;27:319.

DE WIT R, STOTER G, KAYE SB, et al. The importance of bleomycin in combination chemotherapy for good prognosis testicular non-seminoma: A randomized study of the EORTC genitourinary tract cancer cooperative group. J Clin Oncol 1997;15:1837-43.

FREIHA F, REESE J, TORTI FM. A randomized trial of radical cystectomy versus radical cystectomy plus cisplatin, vinblastine and methotrexate chemotherapy for muscle invasive bladder cancer. J Urol 1996;155:504-5.

HALL RR. Neo-adjuvant CMV chemotherapy and cystectomy or radiotherapy in muscle invasive bladder cancer: First analysis of MRC/EORTC intercontinental trial. Proceedings ASCO 1996. J Clin Oncol 1996;15:244.

JOHANSSON J-E. Expectant management of early prostate cancer: Swedish experience. J Urol 1994;152:1753-56.

LAMM DL, GRIFFITH JG. The place of intravesical chemotherapy as defined by results of prospective randomized studies (substances and treatment schemes). Prog Clin Biol Res 1992;378:43-53.

LOEHRER PJ, JOHNSON DH, ELSON P, et al. Importance of bleomycin in favorable prognosis disseminated germ cell tumors: An Eastern Cooperative Oncology Group trial. J Clin Oncol 1995;13:470-6.

MALMSTROM PU, RINTALA E, WAHLQVIST R, et al. Five-year follow-up of a prospective trial of radical cystectomy and neoadjuvant chemotherpy: Nordic cystectomy trial I. J Urol 1996;155:1903-6.

MEAD GM, STENNING SP. Prognostic factors for metastatic germ cell cancer treated with platinum based chemotherapy: The International Germ Cell Cancer Collaborative Group (IGCC-CG) project to standardize criteria. Prog Am Soc Clin Oncol 1994;13:251.

OOSTERLINCK W, KURTH KH, SCHRODER F, et al. A prospective European Organisation for Research and Treatment of Cancer Genitourinary group randomized trial comparing transurethral resection followed by a single intravesical instillation of epirubicin or water in single Ta, T1 papillary carcinoma of the bladder. J Urol 1993;149:749-52.

PROSTATE CANCER TRIALISTS' COLLABORATIVE GROUP. Maximum androgen blockade in advanced prostate cancer: An overview of 22 randomised trials with 3283 deaths in 5710 patients. Lancet 1995;346:295-9.

SKINNER DG, DANIELS JR, RUSSEL CA, et al. The role of adjuvant chemotherapy following cystectomy for invasive bladder cancer: A prospective comparative trial. J Urol 1991;145:459-67.

SMITH JR, FREIJE D, CARPTEN JD, et al. Major susceptibility locus for prostate cancer on chromosome 1 suggested by a genome-wide search. Science 1996;274:1371-4.

ZINCKE H, OESTERLING JE, BLUTE ML, et al. Long-term (15 years) results after radical prostatectomy for clinically localized (stage T2c or lower) prostate cancer. J Urol 1994;152:1850-7.

Tumors of gonadal tissue

José-Luis Pico, Luca Castagna, Andres Avila Garavito

Tumors of gonadal tissue, or *germ cell tumors,* can be either seminomatous or nonseminomatous. The vast majority of these tumors are of testicular origin, but extragonadal forms also exist. Even when disseminated, this tumor type can be cured in a very high proportion of patients. This marked improvement in prognosis has been achieved through the use of adapted surgery, chemotherapy including platinum salts, and better defined therapeutic strategies based on prognostic factors (mainly tumor volume and biologic markers). Radiotherapy, however, remains the treatment of choice for seminomas. Germ cell tumors alone represent 90% of all testicular cancers. Non-germ cell tumors, such as Leydig's tumors, gonadoblastoma, sarcoma, and lymphoma, are extremely rare and are not dealt with in this chapter.

Testicular cancer is infrequent (2 cases per 100000 men per year), but it is the most frequent malignancy in men aged between 20 and 34 years and is in fourth position among urogenital tumors. Testicular cancer has a bimodal age distribution. The first peak occurs at between 25 and 29 years and corresponds to nonseminomatous germ cell tumors. The second peak occurs at between 35 and 39 years and corresponds to seminomas. The incidence is higher in Europeans and white Americans and lower in blacks and Asians. Cryptorchidism is a well-established risk factor, since it increases the risk of germ cell tumors 10- to 15-fold, even in patients who undergo late orchidopexy (>7 years); 8 to 10% of patients with testicular tumors have a history of cryptorchidism. Other factors such as trauma, mumps orchitis, and infertility have been implicated but not proven.

The pathologic classification of testicular tumors has undergone many modifications. The current trend is to divide these tumors into seminomatous and nonseminomatous forms. Approximately half of all nonseminomatous tumors have only one histologic component (Tab. 59.1). In practice, with the exception of seminomas, germ cell tumors are considered as a single group, independent of histologic type, since their diagnosis and treatment are identical. One exception is pure choriocarcinomas, rare tumors that carry a grim prognosis.

Classically, high levels of serum human chorionic gonadotropin (hCG) have been found in choriocarcinoma tumors, together with an increase in alpha-fetoprotein

Table 59.1 Histologic classification

Seminomas

Nonseminomas
   Embryonic carcinoma
   Teratoma
   Yolk-sac tumor
   Choriocarcinoma

Combinations of different components
   Embryonic carcinoma and teratoma (teratocarcinoma)
   Choriocarcinoma and all other tumor types

Other combinations

(AFP) levels in yolk sac tumors. Pure seminomas are not associated with a rise in a serum tumor marker, but in 10% of patients the mixture of syncytiotrophoblastic cells may be accompanied by high hCG levels (hCG-positive seminomas). A cytogenetic analysis of tumor cells in germ cell tumors has shown a recurrent anomaly on the short arm of isochromosome 12. Interestingly, this cytogenetic abnormality is also present in leukemic cells when mediastinal nonseminomatous germ cell tumors are associated with acute myeloid leukemia, strongly pointing to a common precursor cell.

Disease presentation

Rare patients initially may develop acute respiratory failure linked to multiple pulmonary metastases. Brain metastases generally occur late but also can be present at diagnosis (6% of poor prognosis forms). Germ cell tumors sometimes occur in extragonadal sites. These forms are infrequent (5-10%) and are distributed similarly between the mediastinal and retroperitoneal regions. They carry a very poor prognosis (especially mediastinal forms). The differential diagnosis of initially testicular forms includes epididymitis, hydrocele, varicocele, spermatocele, and hematoma.

Table 59.2 Use of imaging methods

Initial workup
  Node involvement
  Distant involvement

Follow-up
  Response to treatment
  Early detection of node relapse
  Detection of metastases

Testicular and abdominal ultrasound scans constitute a simple, noninvasive examination with a sensitivity approaching 100% for distinguishing between malignancies and other masses. Testicular tumors as small as 2 to 3 mm can be detected by ultrasound. Retroperitoneal extension and liver metastases also can be identified with this method. The diagnosis is confirmed histologically. Radical orchidectomy by the upper inguinal approach is the key diagnostic and therapeutic technique. A testicular prosthesis can be inserted during the same operation. Transscrotal biopsy can cause local relapses and inguinal node metastases and therefore should be avoided.

Given the frequency of pulmonary involvement and the value of mediastinal investigations, a standard pulmonary radiogram should be obtained, and this always should be backed up by a thoracic computed tomographic (CT) scan, which can detect about 15% more thoracic lesions than standard radiography. A cerebral CT scan should be part of the initial workup for patients with factors suggesting a poor prognosis. The strategy for imaging studies is reported in Table 59.2.

Determination of tumor markers (AFP and hGC) is an essential tool because they are elevated in 80 to 90% of patients, and serious consequences can ensue if they are not assayed. They help with the diagnosis, but most important, they are well-established prognostic markers. They also reflect therapeutic efficacy and can be used to detect a relapse before the onset of clinical signs. They must be assayed both before and after orchidectomy.

hCG is secreted by syncytiotrophoblastic cells. This hormone is a dimer composed of an alpha and a beta subunit. Current assays with modern techniques based on monoclonal antibodies are totally specific; some are also highly sensitive, detecting concentrations in the nanogram per milliliter range. Increases in hCG are not specific to testicular cancer but also can be found in gastric, pancreatic, ovarian, mammary, and lung cancers and hepatocellular carcinoma.

AFP is secreted by yolk-sac components as well as by parenchymal cells of the liver and gastrointestinal tract, which explains its lack of specificity. AFP levels can be high in cancer of the stomach and pancreas and especially hepatocellular carcinoma. Note that AFP levels also can be elevated in benign conditions (e.g., hepatitis) as well as in healthy heavy smokers; this must be borne in mind to avoid a false diagnosis of relapse.

When interpreting the results of these assays, it is crucial to take into account the plasma half-lives of hCG and AFP (24 h and 5 days, respectively). For example, orchidectomy performed for embryonic carcinoma located in the testicles and secreting AFP (levels of 100-200 ng/ml) will only normalize the plasma AFP level after five half-lives, i.e., about a month. In addition, markers can identify hCG-positive seminomas that have the same histologic appearance as seminomas without other components but are associated with a rise in tumor markers (hCG). They represent approximately 10% of all seminomas. Markers also can be precious tools when assessing extension. For example, a patient with apparently localized testicular cancer whose marker values do not normalize after orchidectomy must be considered as having more extensive disease. Plasma lactate dehydrogenase (LDH) values can be of help when assessing the prognostic group.

Retroperitoneal lymph node dissection is now rarely used as part of the extension workup because of the accuracy of paraclinical tests and efficacy of chemotherapy. In addition, it is followed by ejaculatory problems in more than 50% of patients when done bilaterally and when techniques protecting the ejaculatory nerves are not used. In contrast, it is a key examination for assessing residual lesions after chemotherapy (Tab. 59.3).

Staging and prognostic factors

Staging is still useful for seminomas but less so for nonseminomatous tumors. The current trend with nonseminomatous tumors is to classify them using different prognostic factors. There is considerable controversy over prognostic factors, and this explains the different classifications proposed for nonseminomatous germ cell tumors. They are based on tumor volume, organ invasion, and marker levels. This has led to the identification, independent of stage, of a population with a good prognosis (cure rate between 90 and 100%) and a population with a poor prognosis (long-term survival rate of 35 to 60% according to the protocol). The lack of consensus on prognostic criteria is explained by the use of different protocols in each center. Some teams use only clinical and radiologic criteria such as a palpable abdominal mass and metastatic spread (Indiana). Others

---

Table 59.3 Guidelines for the management of testicular tumors

First step
  Testicular and abdominal ultrasound scan
  Markers research (hCG and AFP)
  Chest radiograph

Second step
  Orchidectomy by the upper approach
  Imaging screening (thoracoabdominal
  with or without cerebral CT scan)
  Markers research
  Sperm banking

Third step
  Classification and prognostic factors
  Choice of therapeutic strategy

use nonspecific markers such as LDH (Memorial Sloan-Kettering Cancer Center). The most widely used classification is Boden's three-stage system. Table 59.3 presents guidelines for management of testicular tumors.

Recently, the International Germ Cell Cancer Collaborative Group (IGCCCG) developed a consensus classification for metastatic germ cell tumors (Tab. 59.4). In this study, the analysis was based on more than 5 000 patients from different multicenter study groups. The overall 5-year progression-free survival (PFS) for all the patients was 75%, and the 5-year overall survival (OS) was 80%. In a multivariate analysis, the most important prognostic factors for PFS and OS in nonseminomatous germ cell tumors were the primary site (gonadal and nonmediastinal extragonadal versus mediastinal), presence of nonpulmonary visceral metastases, and serum markers levels. In seminoma, the best factor predicting PFS and OS was the presence of nonpulmonary visceral metastases. Combined use of these variables separated nonseminomatous germ cell tumors into three prognostic groups. The 5-year PFS and OS were 88 and 91% in the good-prognosis group, 75 and 79% in the intermediate group, and 41 and 48% in the poor-risk group, respectively. Two groups of seminoma patients were defined, with 5-year PFS and OS of 82 and 88% in the good-prognosis group and 67 and 72% in the intermediate group, respectively (IGCCCG) (Tab. 59.4).

Treatment

The classification of patients into different prognostic groups has allowed the use of more finely tailored therapy and has helped to reduce toxicity while preserving efficacy.

Seminomas

Seminomas are radiosensitive. Surgery is limited to orchidectomy. Chemotherapy is indicated for stage IIC (nodes >10 cm) and stage III disease. The position of complementary radiotherapy or chemotherapy for residual lesions is controversial:
- *Stage I:* iliolumbar irradiation, 20 to 30 Gy with conventional fractionated radiotherapy;
- *Stage IIA and IIB:* same lumbar irradiation at a higher dose (30-40 Gy);
- *Stage IIC:* chemotherapy (usually the same protocol as for good-prognosis nonseminomatous germ cell tumors, i.e., BEP or EP; Tab. 59.5);
- *Stage III:* chemotherapy (usually the same protocol as for good-prognosis nonseminomatous germ cell tumors, i.e., BEP or EP; Tab. 59.5).

Table 59.4 IGCCCG consensus classification of metastatic germ cell tumors

	Nonseminomatous germ cell tumors	Seminoma
Good	Testis/retroperitoneal tumor and no nonpulmonary visceral metastases and AFP < 1000 ng/ml and hGC < 5000 IU/l or 1000 ng/ml and LDH < 1.5 x N	Any primary site and no nonpulmonary visceral metastases and normal AFP and no hGC and no LDH
	56% of patients	90% of patients
	5-year progression free survival = 89% 5-year overall survival = 92%	5-year progression free survival = 82% 5-year overall survival = 86%
Intermediate	Testis/retroperitoneal tumor and no nonpulmonary visceral metastases and AFP ≥1000 ng/ml and ≤10 000 ng/ml and hGC ≥5000 IU/l and ≤50 000 IU/liter and LDH ≥1,5 x N and ≤10 x N	Any primary site and nonpulmonary visceral metastases and normal AFP and no hGC and no LDH
	28% of patients	10% of patients
	5-year progression free survival = 75% 5-year overall survival = 80%	5-year progression free survival = 67% 5-year overall survival = 72%
Poor	Mediastinal primary or nonpulmonary visceral metastases or AFP ≥10 000 ng/ml and hCG ≥50000 IU/l and LDH ≥10 x N	No patients classified in this group
	16% of patients	
	5-year progression free survival = 41% 5-year overall survival = 48%	

(N=normal levels.)

For advanced disease (stage IIC and stage III), chemotherapy is indicated. Patients must be offered sperm banking before starting chemotherapy. However, only 10 to 25% of these patients enter complete remission after chemotherapy, and surgical intervention is thus required. Histologic examination shows a viable tumor in 10 to 20% of patients. Some studies have shown that the size of the residual mass may be predictive of the presence of residual tumor cells.

Seminoma patients with limited disease have a very good survival rate (99%), whereas in patients with extensive disease, the cure rate is more than 80%.

hCG-positive seminoma Histologically pure seminomas accompanied by a moderate rise in hCG usually are treated in the same way as those accompanied by normal hCG values. Patients with stage IIB or greater tumors and a rise in hCG to more than 100 μIU/ml or a rise in AFP (whatever the value) are treated in the same way as patients with non-seminomatous germ cell tumors.

Nonseminomatous germ cell tumors

Treatment is based on chemotherapy after orchidectomy.

Forms with a good prognosis The reference chemotherapy protocol is three courses of BEP or four courses of EP (Tab. 59.5). The results are good, in that 85 to 95% of patients have long-term survival in remission.

Forms with a poor prognosis Recent trials have mainly focused on PVB, BEP, and protocols comprising double-dose cisplatin (Tab. 59.5). Currently, four courses of BEP remains the standard treatment, but experimental protocols are still warranted because the cure rate is no more than 50 to 70%.

The use of high-dose chemotherapy followed by autologous hematopoietic stem cell transplantation has been explored in recent years and has shown promising results with a high response rate for poor-prognosis patients and even some refractory patients (10-20%), with no evidence of disease in the long-term.

Place of surgery after chemotherapy After chemotherapy, responders belong to two categories: patients in complete biologic and radiologic remission, who require no further treatment, and patients in complete biologic remission but who have residual lesions. These lesions must be excised routinely, since this will determine subsequent management and can itself have a therapeutic effect. In such cases, pathologic examination reveals fibrosis, mature teratoma, or active tumor tissue. Further chemotherapy has to be given if active tumor tissue is found. In the case of mature teratoma, surgical excision is required to prevent malignant transformation (adenocarcinoma or sarcoma). No further treatment is required in the two cases in which active tumor tissue is not found (fibrosis and teratoma); monitoring alone is sufficient, and the cure rate is about 70%.

Elevated tumor marker levels after chemotherapy show

Table 59.5 Testicular cancer list of protocols

BEP	VP16 100 mg/m^2/d, d 1-5 Cisplatin 20 mg/m^2/d, d 1-5. Every 3 weeks, 4 courses Bleomycin 30 mg iv/week (12 weeks)
EP	VP16 100 mg/m^2/d, d 1-5 Cisplatin 20 mg/m^2/d, d 1-5. Every 3 weeks, 4 courses
PVB	Vinblastine 0,15 mg/kg, d 1, 2 Cisplatin 20 mg/m^2/d, d 1-5. Every 3 weeks, 4 courses Bleomycin 30 mg iv/week (12 weeks)
VAB6	Cyclophosphamide 600 mg/m^2, d 1 Actinomycin 1 mg/m^2, d 1 Vinblastine 4 mg/m^2, d 1 Bleomycin 30 mg iv, d 1; then 20 mg/d, continuous infusion d 1-4 Cisplatin 120 mg/m^2, d 4, every 3-4 weeks, 3-4 courses (only the first 3 courses include bleomycin)
VIP	VP16 75 mg/m^2/d, d 1-5
or	
VeIP	Vinblastine 0.11 mg/kg, d 1-2 Ifosfamide 1.2 g/m^2/d, d 1-5 (with MESNA) Cisplatin 20 mg/m^2/d, d 1-5, every 3 weeks, 4 courses

that the tumor tissue has not been eradicated; excision is not warranted in such cases because relapse is almost inevitable. Salvage chemotherapy is indicated, including high-dose chemotherapy with hematopoietic stem cell autografting.

Place of radiotherapy In contrast with seminomas, radiotherapy for nonseminomatous germ cell tumors is limited to the treatment of residual nodes or to analgesia (back pain related to retroperitoneal masses).

Specific cases **Stage I** When orchidectomy leads to marker normalization, two approaches have been recommended: (1) retroperitoneal lymph node dissection (if the histology is negative, simple monitoring suffices; if the histology is positive, the patient is considered to be in stage II and chemotherapy is indicated), and (2) close monitoring, necessitating perfect cooperation by the patient given the frequent examinations required over a period of approximately 2 years. This approach is becoming increasingly popular because it avoids chemotherapy and the associated toxicity. In cases of relapse (17-42%, generally during the first year), these forms are practically always sensitive to further chemotherapy, and almost all the patients are cured.

Relapse and nonremission after first-line chemotherapy Patients who never enter remission have a very poor prognosis and little chance of cure. Patients who relapse after a first complete remission can again enter complete remission 30 to 50% of the time, but no more than 20% are long-term survivors.

The reference protocol is VIP or VeIP (Tab. 59.5), according to the first-line protocol. The mediocre results of these protocols explain the development of new salvage regimens, mainly based on high-dose chemotherapy followed by peripheral blood precursor cell autografting and/or hematopoietic growth factor administration.

Brain metastases Initially, curative radiotherapy (40 Gy) applied to the skull in toto is attempted with superimposition on the lesion over 4 weeks; a noteworthy percentage of patients can be cured if the systemic disease enters prolonged remission. During follow-up, only palliative radiotherapy is recommended, because the onset of brain metastases during treatment reflects a failure to control the systemic disease. One exception is isolated cerebral relapse, in which case surgery is indicated. In initially severe forms (renal failure, acute respiratory failure, etc.), patients require intensive care with all the appropriate resuscitation measures (e.g., prevention of tumor lysis, correction of metabolic disorders, mechanical ventilation, dialysis, etc.). These forms generally carry a grim prognosis.

Modes of drug use

Cisplatin

Cisplatin is administered iv, diluted in 250 ml of 0.9% saline solution, as a continuous infusion over 2 h, together with intravenous hyperhydration (3 liters/m^2) and 20% mannitol hyperdiuresis.

The most troublesome toxic effects of cisplatin include renal dysfunction, nausea and vomiting, peripheral neuropathy, and auditory impairment cumulative and only partially reversible with discontinuation of therapy. The renal toxicity has been attributed to drug-protein interactions and the inactivation of specific renal brush border enzymes. Cisplatin-induced peripheral neuropathy virtually always occurs in a "stocking and glove" distribution and clinically resembles the neuropathy of vitamin B$_{12}$ deficiency. Cisplatin-induced ototoxicity seems to be related to the loss of outer hair cells in the basal turns of the cochlea and is histologically similar to aminoglycoside-induced ototoxicity. A high-tone-frequency loss is found in about one-third of patients.

Carboplatin

Carboplatin produces dose-limiting myelosuppression; in patients with normal renal function, doses of up to 600 mg/m^2 are well tolerated, but the dose must be reduced in patients with renal dysfunction because up to 90% of the drug is eliminated by the kidneys. Doses of carboplatin at the start of high-dose chemotherapy cycles should be administered according to effective EDTA clearance.

Carboplatin is administered iv, diluted in 1000 ml of 5% dextrose solution, as a continuous infusion over 2 h.

Etoposide (VP16)

Etoposide is the second drug (together with platinum derivatives) capable of inducing continuous and complete remission.

Etoposide is administered iv, diluted in 9% saline at a concentration of 0.5 to 1 mg (to avoid precipitation), as a continuous infusion over 2 h.

Common adverse effects include myelosuppression, nausea and vomiting, and alopecia. Myelosuppression is the dose-limiting toxic effect of etoposide. This drug is currently used in most high-dose protocols because of its clear dose-efficacy relationship and only moderate nonhematologic toxicity. At these very high doses with bone marrow rescue, the dose-limiting toxic effect is mucositis.

Vinblastine

Vinblastine is administered iv, diluted in 5% dextrose solution at a concentration of 1 mg/ml of 5% dextrose, administered in a push.

Myelosuppression, particularly neutropenia, is the principal hematologic toxicity. Peripheral neurotoxicity is much less common than with vincristine and vincristine is usually noted in patients receiving protacted therapy, sensory dysfunction and loss of deep tendon reflexes being the most common manifestations. Hypertension is the most common cardiovascular effect. Mild hair loss is common. Like vincristine, vinblastine is a vesicant, and drug extravasation should be avoided.

Ifosfamide

This alkylating agent at doses below 3.8 g/m^2, has a similar rate of metabolism as cyclophosphamide , but a lower proportion of ifosfamide is converted into alkylating and biologically active metabolites. Hemorrhagic cystitis is the main toxic effect and may range from mild cystitis to severe bladder damage with massive hemorrhage. Acrolein may be responsible for cyclophosphamide-induced cystitis. The incidence and severity of the complication can be lessened by adequate hydration and frequent bladder emptying. The most effective agent for preventing oxazaphophorin cystitis is 2-mercatoethane sulfonate (MESNA), which dimerizes to an inactive metabolite in plasma but hydrolyzes in urine to yield the active parent compound that conjugates with alkylating species and prevents cystitis. About 40% of patients develop neurologic adverse effects, and about 5% die. Methylene blue (50 mg qid iv) must be administered promptly.

Ifosfamide is administered iv, diluted in 250 ml of 5% dextrose, as a continuous infusion over 1 h, combined with intravenous hyperhydration (3 l/m^2) and MESNA. The total dose of MESNA is 100% of the ifosfamide dose; 20% of the total MESNA dose is administered in push prior to ifosfamide infusion, and 25% is given every 6 h after ifosfamide infusion.

Bleomycin

In the standard regimen for testicular cancer, bleomycin is given in doses of 30 units per week, and the incidence of fatal pulmonary toxicity in this low-risk population of young male patients is approximately 2%. Various factors have been shown to increase the pulmonary toxicity of bleomycin, such as prior irradiation of the lung parenchyma, administration of high fractional inspired oxygen concentration, the total dose of bleomycin (>400 units), and the age of the patient. There is no specific therapy for patients with bleomycin lung toxicity. The value of corticosteroids in promoting recovery from bleomycin lung toxicity remains controversial, although beneficial effects have been described in isolated patient studies. A more common but less serious toxic effect of bleomycin is cutaneous reactions. Approximately 50% of patients treated with conventional once- or twice-daily doses of this agent develop erythema, induration, hyperkeratosis, and peeling of the skin that may progress to frank ulceration. Hyperpigmentation, hair loss, and nail changes also occur. The most common vascular toxic effect of bleomycin is Raynaud's disease.

Bleomycin is administered iv, diluted in 100 ml of 9% saline, over 30 min.

General side effects of therapy

Patients with testicular cancer have significantly reduced fertility. It is generally assumed that erectile function, libido, and orgasm remain unchanged after treatment. Thorough information on these aspects of response to treatment, given by the physician before, during, and after treatment, seems to reduce these problems. Chemotherapy leads to a reduction in sperm counts. Following orchidectomy, 75 to 80% patients have insufficient sperm counts or abnormal sperm motility. Subnormal Leydig cell function also has been found, and many patients have elevated gonadotrophin levels. About 40 to 60% of patients who wish to have children are thought to do so successfully after standard chemotherapy. Children fathered by men treated for germ cell tumors do not appear to be at an increased risk of birth defects. The analysis of pre-cisplatin-based chemotherapy sperm count together with details of planned treatment can be used to predict recovery of spermatogenesis following treatment. These data can be used to advise individual patients on pretreatment sperm banking.

Psychologic effects Despite clearly measurable effects on several organs, the overall well-being and function of successfully treated patients are very good. However, overtreated relapsing patients often have psychosocial problems, with a greater prevalence of side effects such as anxiety, insomnia, irritability, and depression. Detailed studies are lacking on the long-term psychosocial effects of the diagnosis and therapy of germ cell tumors.

Second nongerm cell malignancies An increased risk of second nongerm cell malignancies has been described following treatment of germ cell tumors, particularly secondary leukemia; the relative risk of leukemia was 1.7 in one analysis. On the basis of currently available data, which cannot be regarded as definitive because of a rather short follow-up, there is no firm evidence that chemotherapy significantly elevates the risk of secondary solid cancers.

Suggested readings

BOKEMEYER C, SCHMOLL H. Treatment of testicular cancer and the development of secondary malignancies. J Clin Oncol 1995;13:283-92.

BOSL GJ, MOTZER RJ. Testicular germ-cell cancer. N Engl J Med 1997;337:242-53.

BOSL GJ, ILSON DH, RODRIGUEZ E, et al. Clinical relevance of the i(12p) marker chromosome in germ cell tumors. J Natl Cancer Inst 1994;86:349-55.

BOYER M, RAGHAVAN D. Toxicity of treatment of germ cell tumors. Semin Oncol 1992;19:128-42.

CULINE S, KRAMAR A, BIRON P, DROZ JP. Chemotherapy in adult germ cell tumors. Crit Rev Oncol Hematol 1996;22:229-63.

DEVESA SS, BLOT WJ, STONE BJ, et al. Recent cancer trends in the United States. J Natl Cancer Inst 1995;87:175-82.

DROZ JP, VAN OOSTEROM AT. Treatment options in clinical stage I nonseminomatous germ cell tumors of the testis: A wager on the future? A review. Eur J Cancer 1993;29A:1038-44.

EINHORN LH. Salvage therapy for germ cell tumors. Semin Oncol 1994; 21(suppl 7):47-51.

GERL A, CLEMM C, SCHMELLER N, et al. Late relapse of germ cell tumors after cisplatin-based chemotherapy. Ann Oncol 1997;8:41-7.

INTERNATIONAL GERM CELL CANCER COLLABORATIVE GROUP. International germ cell consensus classification: A prognostic factor-based staging system for metastatic germ cell cancers. J Clin Oncol 1997;15:594-603.

LAMPE H, HORWICH A, NORMAN A, et al. Fertility after chemotherapy for testicular germ cell cancers. J Clin Oncol 1997;15:239-45.

MOSTOFI FK, SESTERHENN IA. Revised international classification of testicular tumors. In: Jones WG, Harnden P, Appleyard I, eds. Germ cell tumors III, Vol 91 of Advances in the Biosciences. Oxford: Pergamon Press, 1994; 153-8.

MENCEL PJ, MOTZER RJ, MAZUMDAR M, et al. Advanced seminoma: Treatment results, survival, and prognostic factors in 142 patients. J Clin Oncol 1994;12:120-6.

PICO JL, FADEL E, IBRAHIM A, et al. High-dose chemotherapy followed by hematological support: Experience in the treatment of germ cell tumors. Bull Cancer 1995;82(suppl 1):56s-60s.

PONT J, ALBRECHT W, POSTNER G, et al. Adjuvant chemotherapy for high-risk clinical stage I nonseminomatous testicular germ cell cancer: long-term results of a prospective trial. J Clin Oncol 1996;14:441-8.

60

Tumors of female genital tract

Andrea Maneo, Maria Grazia Cantù, Costantino Mangioni

VULVAR CARCINOMA

Vulvar carcinoma represents only 3 to 5% of female genital cancers and occurs in elderly patients (seventh to eighth decades). The human papillomavirus is the suggested etiologic agent. The vast majority of malignancies of the vulva are squamous (85%), 5% are melanomas, and 10% are made up of rare histotypes (e.g., adenocarcinoma, sarcoma, and lymphoma). Overall 5-year survival ranges from 80 to 90% for stage I patients with no node metastasis to 30 to 50% in patients with locally advanced lesions and/or lymph node involvement.

Treatment

Surgery is the accepted primary treatment modality. Postoperative radiotherapy can be delivered in patients with lymph node metastasis or neoplastic involvement of the vulvar resection margins. Radiotherapy was investigated as a preoperative reductive agent in patients who were not fit for surgery; inoperable patients can be rendered operable. Randomized studies comparing chemoradiotherapy followed by surgery versus surgery plus radiotherapy in locally advanced disease are under way. There is at present no single agent or combination chemotherapeutic regimen available to effectively treat carcinoma of the vulva. A phase 2 EORTC study with bleomycin, methotrexate, and lomustine (BMC) (Tab. 60.1) in patients who had not received prior chemo- or radiotherapy showed a response rate of 64%, yet one-third of patients were deemed inoperable even after the BMC treatment.

CARCINOMA OF THE UTERINE CERVIX

Carcinoma of the uterine cervix is the most frequent malignancy of women after carcinoma of the breast, colon-rectum, and endometrium, representing 6% of all female neoplasias. The incidence is 15 cases per 100 000 women per year in western countries, but it rises to 20 to 30 cases per 100 000 in developing areas. The main histologic type is squamous cell carcinoma (80%), with adenocarcinoma and adenosquamous cell types accounting for 15 to 20% of cases; other histotypes (e.g., sarcoma, lymphoma, and carcinoid) are anecdotal. While carcinoma in situ (CIN) is more frequent in the second and third decades of life, invasive cervical carcinoma affects principally women over 45 years of age.

Clinical findings

Staging is assessed on the basis of clinical examination and ancillary investigations: chest X-ray, intravenous pyelogram (to assess renal function and exclude ureteric obstruction), cystoscopy, and rectosigmoidoscopy (when extracervical spread is suspected). Lymphangiogram can demonstrate small metastases not detected by computed tomographic (CT) scanning or magnetic resonance imaging (MRI), although microscopic metastases cannot be excluded.

Treatment

Management is defined by the extent of disease according to the clinical stage. For early-stage disease (stage Ib or IIa), there may be a choice in treatment between surgery, in the form of radical hysterectomy with pelvic lymphadenectomy, or radiotherapy; both exhibit 5-year survival rates ranging from 70 to 90%. Radiotherapy is also the treatment of choice for locoregionally advanced disease confined to the pelvis (stages IIb, III, and IVa). Squamous cell cervical carcinoma is considered to be a chemosensitive disease, but it becomes rapidly resistant after radio- or chemotherapy. Response to chemotherapy is correlated with the amount of pretreatment and is confined to nonirradiated areas. Traditionally, chemotherapy has been reserved as adjuvant treatment or as salvage therapy of metastatic or recurrent disease, radiotherapy and/or surgery being the preferred first choices.

The platinum compounds are the most studied cytotoxic drugs with demonstrated activity against cervical cancer. Cisplatin is regarded as the single agent of choice in the treatment of advanced disease. Various doses and schedules have been explored, and no differences have been observed between 50 and 100 mg/m² per course and between bolus versus continuous infusion administration, with a response rate of 17 to 50% in previously untreated patients. Cisplatin appears to be the preferred drug for the treatment of carcinoma of the cervix compared with other platinum compounds such as carboplatin (15% response rate) and iproplatin (11%), and it is active in both squamous and adenocarcinomatous histotypes.

The second drug of choice is ifosfamide, with a response rate of 29 to 40%. Cisplatin-based combination regimens containing ifosfamide showed a response rate ranging from 67 to 80%.

Other active cytotoxic agents are doxorubicin and epirubicin (response rate 17-20% in adenocarcinoma), 5-fluorouracil (20%), bleomycin (20%), methotrexate (18%), and vincristine and vindesine (18-24%). A drug of interest is dibromodulcitol (also called mitolactol), a halogenated sugar that offers a relatively high order of activity in squamous cell cervical carcinoma (29%).

Since experience with dose escalation of cisplatin has

been disappointing up to the present, efforts have been directed at finding an optimal combination of non-cross-resistant drugs without increasing toxicity. The tested schemes generally contain cisplatin (P) at the dose of 50 to 75 mg/m² combined with either bleomycin (B), vincristine (V), vindesine (E), ifosamide (I), epirubicin (E), or methotrexate (M) with various schedules, administered weekly (e.g., PVB, EP) or every 3 weeks (e.g., BIP, BEMP) (Tab. 60.1). The response rates for PVB and BIP in recurrent cervical cancer are 66 to 69%. The combination of cisplatin plus 5-fluorouracil has been discarded because of disappointing results in uncontrolled trials, whereas they were employed in previous and current trials largely as radiosensitizing agent.

Nowadays, chemotherapy is integrated into the primary treatment of locally advanced tumors (i.e., neoadjuvant chemotherapy), followed by radical surgery; clinical response rates in stage Ib and IIa bulky squamous cell tumors are high (75-100%), and recent trials show a correlation between residual tumor in the surgical specimen after preoperative chemotherapy (pathologic response) and prognosis.

Combined-modality regimens consisting of concurrent chemotherapy and irradiation have been developed to

Table 60.1 Commonly used combination chemotherapeutic regimens in vulvar, vaginal, and cervical cancer

Regimen	Setting	Drugs and dose	Interval

BMC	Vulvar carcinoma	Bleomycin 5 mg im d 1-5
		Lomustine 40 mg po d 5-7
		Methotrexate 15 mg po d 1, 4
		(Methotrexate is administered for
		  the first week only)
			Continuous
			  administration for 6 weeks

POB (or PVB)	SCC Vaginal carcinoma	Cisplatin 50 mg/m² d 1 Vincristine 1 mg/m² d 1 Bleomycin 30 mg d 1	Weekly
BIP	SCC	Bleomycin 30 mg d 1 Cisplatin 50 mg/m² d 2 Ifosfamide 5 g/m² d 2 MESNA 5 g/m² d 2 MESNA 3 g/m² d 3	3 weeks
BEMP	Vulvar carcinoma SCC	Vindesine 3 mg/m² d 1, 8 Cisplatin 50 mg/m² d 1 Bleomycin 15 mg d 2-4 Mitomycin C 8 mg/m² d 2-4	3 weeks
TIP	SCC Vaginal carcinoma Epithelial OC	Paclitaxel 175 mg/m² d 1 Cisplatin 75 mg/m² d 2 Ifosfamide 5 g/m² d 2 infusion 24 h MESNA 5 g/m² d 2 infusion 24 h MESNA 3 g/m² d 3 Infusion 12 h	3 weeks
TEP	Cervical adenocarcinoma Vaginal adenocarcinoma Endometrial carcinoma Epithelial OC	Epirubicin 80 mg/m² d 1 Paclitaxel 175 mg/m² d 1 Cisplatin 75 mg/m² d 2	3 weeks
EP	Cervical adenocarcinoma Vaginal adenocarcinoma Endometrial carcinoma	Epirubicin 80 mg/m² d 1 Cisplatin 50 mg/m² d 1-8-15	Cisplatin weekly, epirubicin every 3 weeks

(All drugs should be administrated as an intravenous bolus if not specified.)
(SCC = squamous cervical carcinoma; OC = ovarian cancer.)

improve the local control of disease, since the pelvis is the most frequent site of relapse after exclusive radiotherapy. The most promising results have been obtained with the concomitant use of continuous-infusion 5-fluorouracil, either alone or in combination with mitomycin C, carboplatin, or cisplatin, and the concomitant use of hydroxyurea. Two randomized studies of the Gynecologic Oncology Group support the evidence of better pelvic control with the hydroxyurea regimen. Other authors suggest that 5-fluorouracil can act as a radiosensitizer even as a single agent, with or without other drugs, and some have started phase 3 trials to determine whether the addition of concomitant 5-fluorouracil to continuous hyperfractionated pelvic radiotherapy improves pelvic control.

Recent phase 2 trials with paclitaxel as a single agent suggest the possible activity of this molecule with a response rate of 17% at a dosage of 170 mg/m^2 every 3 weeks. Its clinical noncross-resistance with the platinum compounds and the alkylating agents in other solid tumors marks this agent as an active drug of particular interest. Randomized trials of cisplatin with or without paclitaxel are under way.

ENDOMETRIAL CARCINOMA

Endometrial carcinoma is the most common invasive neoplasia of the female genital tract, with an incidence of 15 cases per 100 000 women per year in western countries; this is twice the rate of cervical carcinoma and three times that of epithelial ovarian cancer. Management choices are influenced by some of the characteristics of the disease. It occurs during the peri- and postmenopausal ages, so these patients belong largely to the older group. It is significantly associated with obesity, diabetes, and hypertension, which have an effect on therapeutic options. Since the diagnosis of endometrial carcinoma usually occurs at an early stage, most patients can be cured by surgical resection alone or resection followed by radiotherapy, and only a small proportion are candidates for systemic therapy. Thus, current knowledge about the role of chemotherapy is limited.

Most patients are diagnosed in stage I (tumor confined to the uterine corpus) or stage II (cervical spreading) and are classified as low risk or high risk on the basis of histologic grade and myometrial invasion. Five-year survival for early-stage patients treated with surgical resection alone is 85% or better.

Extrauterine neoplastic spreading and lymph node involvement (stage III) are more often diagnosed postoperatively; postoperative radiation and/or chemotherapy should be given depending on the extent of tumor dissemination.

Stage IV disease (e.g., bladder or rectum involvement, distant metastasis) should be treated initially by radiotherapy if confined to the pelvis, with or without adjuvant chemotherapy. Chemotherapy is recommended as a first approach in patients with extrapelvic metastases.

Treatment

Some cytotoxic drugs known to be active in carcinoma of the endometrium have been evaluated in patients with recurrent disease. Doxorubicin is the most extensively studied drug, with a response rate ranging from 24 to 38% when used as a single agent. Another anthracycline, epirubicin, offers a response rate of 26%. The platinum compounds also appear to be effective. Cisplatin at doses of 50 to 100 mg/m^2 show response rates of 21 to 25%. Carboplatin at doses of 300 to 400 mg/m^2 yields a response rate of 29%. Other active agents (e.g., melphalan, 5-fluorouracil, and cyclophosphamide) showed no advantages when combined with doxorubicin as compared with doxorubicin alone. Only the combination of doxorubicin plus cisplatin seems to represent a regimen capable of yielding better responses than single-agent schedules, even in terms of progression-free survival. The PAC scheme (i.e., cisplatin, doxorubicin, and cyclophosphamide; Tab. 60.2) was used in an EORTC study to treat 26 patients with recurrent endometrial cancer and showed a response rate of 60%.

Steroid hormones and endometrial carcinoma have been interrelated both etiologically and therapeutically. Oral progesterone for the palliative cure of recurrent endometrial cancer can be given indefinitely in the case of an objective response with little or no side effects. The response rate varies from 17 to 22% and does not depend on the route of administration (i.e., oral versus im), the dosage (i.e., standard versus high dose), or the type of progestin. However, a recent randomized study on the effect of postoperative medroxyprogesterone acetate on stage I patients does not show any benefit in survival.

Tamoxifen (see Chap. 61) also has been used to treat recurrent endometrial carcinoma. Responses can be achieved mainly in patients previously responding to progestins, and the administration can be continued for as long as the response is observed. The tamoxifen dose ranges from 20 to 40 mg daily, with no apparent advantage to the higher doses.

Finally, paclitaxel recently has claimed a response rate of 35% with 250 mg/m^2 every 3 weeks. As for other solid tumors (e.g., of the ovary, cervix, or breast), paclitaxel is of great potential value because of the evidence of noncross-resistance to platinum compounds and the significant activity level.

UTERINE SARCOMAS

Uterine sarcomas account for 3% of uterine cancers and include a heterogeneous group of lesions. Therefore, treatment protocols are not standardized, and individual experience is limited.

The only treatment of proven curative value for uterine sarcomas is surgical excision, consisting of total abdominal hysterectomy and bilateral salpingo-oophorectomy. Because of the propensity for early hematogenous metas-

Table 60.2 Commonly used combination chemotherapeutic regimens in endometrial and epithelial ovarian carcinomas

Regimen	Setting	Drugs and dose	Interval
PAC	Epithelial OC Endometrial carcinoma Cervical adenocarcinoma Vaginal adenocarcinoma	Cisplatin 50 mg/m^2 d 1 Doxorubicin 50 mg/m^2 d 1 Cyclophosphamide 600 mg/m^2 d 1	3-4 weeks
PEC	Epithelial OC Endometrial carcinoma	Cisplatin 50 mg/m^2 d 1 Epirubicin 70 mg/m^2 d 1 Cyclophosphamide 600 mg/m^2 d 1	3 weeks
CP	Epithelial OC	Cyclophosphamide 600-750 mg/m^2 d 1 Cisplatin 75 mg/m^2 d 1	3 weeks
PT	Epithelial OC	Cisplatin 75 mg/m^2 d 1 Paclitaxel 175 mg/m^2 d 1	3 weeks
CT	Epithelial OC	Carboplatin 400 mg/m^2 or *AUC* 5 d 1 Paclitaxel 175 mg/m^2 d 1	3 weeks
Tax/5-FU	Salvage therapy of epithelial OC and endometrial carcinoma	Paclitaxel 175 mg/m^2 d 1 5-Fluorouracil 750 mg/m^2 d 1-4 continuous infusion	3 weeks
IM	Salvage therapy of epithelial OC	Mitoxantrone 10 mg/m^2 d 1 Ifosfamide 5 g/m^2 d 1 infusion 24 h MESNA 5 g/m^2 d 1 infusion 24 h MESNA 3 g/m^2 d 2 infusion 12 h	3 weeks

(*AUC* = area under curve; OC = ovarian carcinoma. See also Tab. 54.2)

tasis, postoperative chemotherapy is justified for stage Ic or greater tumors and for high malignancy sarcomas. The most important chemotherapeutic agents active against uterine sarcomas are cisplatin, doxorubicin, and ifosfamide. Dacarbazine also has activity in soft tissue adult sarcoma; although there are experimental data to suggest an addictive effect between doxorubicin and dacarbazine, this does not appear to be translated into response rates in the clinical situation. The same applies to cyclophosphamide.

With cisplatin alone (50 mg/m^2 every 3 weeks), the Gynecologic Oncology Group reported an objective response rate of 19% in previously untreated patients with advanced or recurrent mixed mesodermal tumors. Even better results were obtained when cisplatin was administered at the dose of 100 mg/m^2 every 3 weeks.

Leiomyosarcoma appears to be more responsive to doxorubicin at doses of 50 to 90 mg/m^2 every 3 weeks (25% response rate), and ifosfamide has good activity against both histotypes (31 and 17% response rates, respectively). The unexpectedly high actuarial 5-year survival rate of 75% reported in a nonrandomized trial of 17 high-risk patients treated with cisplatin and doxorubicin after surgery suggests a possible activity of the systemic treatment to prevent local and distant failures. A feasible scheme that is currently used involves doxorubicin and ifosfamide every 3 weeks for 6 postoperative courses. CYVADIC (i.e., cyclophosphamide, vin-

cristine, doxorubicin, and DTIC) offered a response rate of 11 to 52% in the treatment of advanced soft tissue sarcoma and can be suggested as second-line chemotherapy as well as VAC (i.e., vincristine, actinomycin D, and cyclophosphamide).

For carcinosarcoma, cisplatin and ifosfamide are active single agents; whereas the response to single-agent doxorubicin seems to be lower. However, superior response rates and increased survival were achieved with cisplatin and doxorubicin-based chemotherapy.

EPITHELIAL OVARIAN CARCINOMA

Epithelial ovarian cancer is third in incidence among gynecologic malignancies, after cancer of the endometrium and cervix, but it carries the highest mortality rate (57%). The interest generated during the past 20 years is related to its responsiveness to chemotherapy and to its occurrence in women at the peak of their productivity (age range 40-70 years).

No method of screening proved useful and cost-effective for ovarian cancer. The CA125 serum assay is positive in 80% of epithelial ovarian tumors, in 6% of patients with benign lesions, and in 1% of persons in the normal population, accounting for a sensitivity of 75% and a specificity of 90%; women of premenopausal age show a lower specificity due to the presence of benign conditions (e.g., endometriosis, pelvic inflammatory disease, and fibroids) associated with abnormal levels of CA125. Furthermore, only half the patients with stage I ovarian carcinoma show elevated levels of CA125. The association of CA125 assay and pelvic ultrasound is recommended in women with a familial history of ovarian carcinoma.

Treatment

The current curative strategies for advanced ovarian cancer are far from optimal as regards long-term survival. In fact, only a minority of tumors (less than 25%) are diagnosed in early stage (stages I-II). Most advanced tumors show an initial gratifying response to chemotherapy, but resistant cell clones emerge within 2 to 3 years of the last treatment. Long-term survival in the drug-resistant population is a rare event.

Primary surgery remains the cornerstone of ovarian cancer staging and therapy. The maximum effort should be made to remove the genital apparatus and the bulky masses. The postoperative residual tumor has a direct relationship with the final outcome.

Single agents active in ovarian cancer include platinum compounds (e.g., cisplatin and carboplatin), alkylating agents (e.g., ifosfamide and cyclophosphamide), anthracyclines (e.g., doxorubicin, epirubicin, and mitoxantrone), taxoids (e.g., paclitaxel and docetaxel), etoposide, hexamethylmelamine, 5-fluorouracil, and camptothecins (e.g., topotecan and irinotecan).

The precise definition of the subsets of patients with stage I ovarian carcinoma who can benefit from adjuvant treatment is under discussion. Women with stage Ia and Ib, grade 1 ovarian cancers do not appear to require postoperative chemotherapy. Conversely, women with poorly differentiated tumors and/or stage Ic lesions are candidates to receive some form of adjunctive treatment. An Italian study evaluated the adjuvant administration of intravenous cisplatin versus intraperitoneal chromic 32 phosphate (^{32}P) for stage Ic ovarian carcinoma and showed a 5-year disease-free survival of 82 and 70%, respectively. Currently, ^{32}P is not recommended as postoperative treatment of early-stage ovarian cancer.

The recommended postoperative treatment for patients with advanced ovarian cancer consists of six courses of platinum-based chemotherapy. It is recognized that chemotherapy is most effective in patients who undergo maximal cytoreductive surgery. The most appropriate combination is still a matter of debate. Platinum compounds are usually associated with cyclophosphamide or cyclophosphamide and doxorubicin (schemes CP and PAC; Tab. 60.2). The platinum compounds are probably more important in generating a response than the alkylating agents and anthracyclines. The routine use of hematopoietic growth factors is not recommended. Some European investigators argue that single-agent cisplatin or carboplatin is just as effective as platinum-based combinations; this thesis is supported by data regarding patients with suboptimal reduction or stage IV disease, but a meta-analysis of more than 8 000 patients suggested very strongly that the combinations are superior to cisplatin alone.

Many studies suggest that carboplatin can be substituted for cisplatin in combination regimens with equivalent activity. Carboplatin does not require hydration and is devoid of renal and neurologic effects, although it causes myelosuppression more frequently than cisplatin and must be managed with caution when combined with myelosuppressive drugs (e.g., alkylating agents and anthracyclines). Objective responses in advanced disease are demonstrated in 60 to 90% of patients with advanced disease, and 20 to 40% will have a pathologic complete response at "second look" laparotomy after induction chemotherapy. About 20% of laparotomies actually hide microscopic persistence of neoplasia, undetectable with standard surgical biopsies. The most evident limit of current chemotherapeutic strategies is the difficulty to control the minimal neoplastic residue. Long-term survival is disappointing: 10 to 20% 5-year survival for suboptimally debulked patients and 30 to 60% for patients with small-volume disease. There is a continuing risk of relapse even in the most mature series.

The role of intraperitoneal chemotherapy has been thoroughly evaluated. One of the largest randomized studies (645 patients) was able to demonstrate a slight advantage to cisplatin given ip rather than iv for patients with small-volume disease, so the optimal route of administration of cytotoxic agents to this subset of patients is being reconsidered in clinical practice.

The recent introduction of taxanes, first for treating recurrent disease and eventually as part of first-line chemotherapy, has produced new hope for better survival. A study comparing standard CP therapy with the combination TP (e.g., tamoxifen and cisplatin; Tab. 60.2) in 385 suboptimally debulked patients showed a significant advantage for the TP scheme, with response rates of 64 and 77%, respectively, and median progression-free survival of 12.9 versus 18 months.

Drug resistance, de novo or acquired after exposure to the agents used in induction chemotherapy, represents a major challenge in the medical treatment of ovarian carcinoma. The response to subsequent treatments is predicted by the platinum sensitivity or resistance of the primary tumor.

When considerng patients with a poor response to therapy, only a few agents can produce objective responses, and in no more than 15 to 25% of patients. When platinum-resistant patients are evaluated, the response range is lower, i.e., 12 to 15% with a brief duration and questionable impact on survival.

NONEPITHELIAL OVARIAN CANCER

Germ cell tumors (e.g., dysgerminoma, teratoma, endodermal sinus tumor, embryonal carcinoma, and nongestational choriocarcinoma) and gonadal stromal tumors (e.g., granulosa cell tumor, thecoma-fibroma, Sertoli-Leydig cell tumor, gynandroblastoma, and sex cord tumor with annular tubules) are commonly grouped as nonepithelial ovarian tumors. They represent 15 and 6% of all ovarian malignancies, respectively.

Germ cell tumors may arise especially in childhood and adolescence in females, presenting as fast-growing adnexal masses, occasionally with pain and abdominal hemorrhage.

The surgical approach and staging procedures are similar to those for epithelial ovarian carcinoma.

Table 60.3 Commonly used combination chemotherapeutic regimens in nonepithelial ovarian cancer and persistent trophoblastic disease

Regimen	Setting	Drugs and dose	Interval
PVB	Germ cell OC	Cisplatin 100 mg/m² d 1 or 20 mg/m² d 1-5 Vinblastine 0.15 mg/kg d 1, 2 Bleomycin 10-15 mg d 1-5	3 weeks
PEB	Germ cell OC	Cisplatin 100 mg/m² d 1 or 20 mg/m² d 1-5 Etoposide 100 mg/m² d 1-5 Bleomycin 30 mg d 1 (infusion 12 h)	3 weeks
VAC	Salvage therapy of germ cell OC	Vincristine 1.5 mg/m² d 1 Actinomycin D 0.5 mg d 1-5 Cyclophosphamide 5-7 mg/kg d 1-5	Monthly
DEC	Salvage therapy of germ cell OC	Doxorubicin 40 mg/m² Cyclophosphamide 500 mg/m² Etoposide 100 mg/m²	Monthly

ADM-Ifo	Uterine sarcomas	Doxorubicin 30 mg/m² d 1, 2, 3
		Ifosfamide 2 g/m² d 1, 2, 3
		  (infusion 24 h)
		MESNA 2 g/m² d 1, 2, 3, 4
		  (infusion 24 h)
			3 weeks

PAI	Mesodermal mixed sarcoma	Cisplatin 50 mg/m² d 1 Doxorubicin 45 mg/m² d 1 Ifosfamide 5 g/m² d 1 (infusion 24 h) MESNA 5 g/m² d 1 (infusion 24 h) MESNA 5 g/m² d 2 (infusion 12 h)	

POMB-ACE	Uterine sarcomas
	Nonepithelial OC
		POMB: Vincristine 1 mg/m² d 1
		  MTX 100 mg/m² d 1
		  MTX¹ 200 mg/m² d 1
		  (infusion 12 h)
		  Cisplatin 40 mg d 2-6
		  Bleomycin 15 mg d 2, 3
		  (infusion 24 h)
		ACE: Actinomycin D 0.5 mg d 1, 2
		  Cyclophosphamide 500 mg/m² d 1
		  Etoposide 100 mg/m² d 1-3
			POMB alternates with ACE every 1.0 days

Methotrexate (MTX)	Low-risk PTD	MTX 50 mg im d 1, 3, 5, 7 Calcium folinate 6 mg im d 2, 4, 6, 8 (30 h after MTX)	Weekly

EHMMA	Medium-risk PTD	(a) Etoposide 100 mg/m² d 1-5
		(b) Hydroxyurea 500 mg po × 2 d 1
		  MTX¹ 50 mg d 2, 4, 6, 8
		  Mercaptopurine 75 mg po d 3, 5, 7, 9
		(c) Actinomycin D 0.5 mg d 1-5
			The courses alternate with the scheme abcbabc

EMA-CO	High-risk PTD, chemoresistant low and medium-risk PTD	EMA: Etoposide 100 mg/m² d 1
		  Actinomycin D 0.5 mg d 1
		  MTX 100 mg/m² d 1 bolus
		  MTX 200 mg/m² d 1
		  (infusion 12 h)
		  Etoposide 100 mg/m² d 2
		  Actinomycin D 0.5 mg d 2
		CO: Cyclophosphamide 1 mg/m² d 1
		  Vincristine 600 mg/m² d 1
			EMA and CO alternate weekly

¹Calcium folinate 30 h after administration of methotrexate.

Currently, there is evidence that stage I pure dysgerminoma can be treated safely with surgery alone. Chemotherapy is advisable for stage Ib dysgerminoma treated with conservative surgery but is mandatory for all dysgerminomas with extragonadal metastases or positive peritoneal cytology and for all nondysgerminomatous tumors (any stage). As for immature teratomas, primary surgery is an adequate therapy for stage I, grade 1; adjuvant chemotherapy is advisable for stage I, grades 2 to 3 and strongly recommended for all patients with peritoneal implants.

Many drugs prove active against these tumors: cisplatin, *Vinca* alkaloids, actinomycin D, bleomycin, etoposide, methotrexate, and cyclophosphamide. The regimens including cisplatin, bleomycin, vinblastine, or etoposide (i.e., PVB and PEB; Tab. 60.3) appear to have a prominent role. Recent reports show excellent 5-year survival rates for both dysgerminomas (95%) and nondysgerminomas (85-90%) treated with PEB or PVB. The addition of etoposide to these schemes is responsible for the improved results over the last decade, so nowadays PEB is considered the therapy of choice after surgery. The recommended duration of chemotherapy for responders is between three and six cycles, with two more optional cycles once the serum marker level has returned to normal (if expressed by the tumor).

Treatment of patients in the category of high-risk recurrent tumors remains a problem, just as in male patients with germ cell tumors (see Chap. 50). Patients recurring after responding to initial cisplatin-based chemotherapy can be rechallenged with cisplatin combination therapy, even when the relapse appears within months. Patients who fail to respond to initial cisplatin combination regimens can be treated with the VAC scheme (i.e., vincristine, actinomycin D, and cyclophosphamide; Tab. 60.3) widely used in the 1970s and early 1980s as postoperative treatment for nondysgerminomatous tumors with a high cure rate (81% in stage I, 49% in stages III and IV). Radiotherapy is effective for the cure of recurrent dysgerminoma, whereas it was abandoned as postoperative treatment.

Gonadal stromal tumors are mostly represented by the granulosa cell tumor (70%). Most histotypes are characterized by indolent growth, rare extrapelvic metastases, and possible endocrine activity (e.g., hyperestrogenism and virilization). Most patients are diagnosed in stage I (no extragonadic metastases), and the prognosis is favorable.

TROPHOBLASTIC DISEASE

Gestational trophoblastic tumors arise from the placental site of an ongoing or recent pregnancy and include hydatidiform mole (complete or incomplete), invasive mole, gestational choriocarcinoma, and placental site trophoblastic tumor. Diagnosis and therapy are based on obstetric history, imaging diagnostics, and serial assays of serum beta human chorionic gonadotropin (β-hCG). Hydatidiform mole may undergo spontaneous abortion or require evacuation. The incidence of persistent trophoblastic disease (PTD) after uterine evacuation is 11 to 14%; prophylaxis with methotrexate is not effective in reducing this rate. Negative assay of serum β-hCG within 60 days from the initial diagnosis and persistence of normal β-hCG after 6 months signify that no further therapy is required. Chemotherapeutic treatment is required in patients with elevated β-hCG levels for a prolonged time after evacuation, persistent uterine bleeding, histology of choriocarcinoma, and the presence of metastases.

PTD patients can be classified as low risk, middle risk, and high risk. The regimen used for the low-risk group consists of methotrexate plus calcium folinate. Toxicity is infrequent. In about 75% of patients the tumor will be eradicated by this treatment alone, but 25% need to change to the medium- or high-risk regimen. The regimen for the medium-risk group consists of alternating courses of etoposide, hydroxyurea, methotrexate, mercaptopurine, and actinomycin D (i.e., EHMMA; Tab. 60.3). Methotrexate can be omitted for low-risk patients switching to the medium-risk regimen if it is clear that β-hCG levels are rising during methotrexate therapy. Complete response can be observed in almost 100% of patients. High-risk patients are at risk for death from drug resistance; therefore, the aim is to give combination chemotherapy with the highest dosages as rapidly as possible. The EMA-CO schedule was found effective in 88% of patients. In all classes of risk, the treatment is prolonged for 6 to 10 weeks after a complete fall in the β-hCG level. Response to chemotherapy is evaluated by the rate of fall of β-hCG, which normally should fall by half a log with each cycle; slower rates of fall are acceptable only in the late phases of the treatment. Stable or progressive disease can be removed surgically, if feasible, or treated with cisplatin and etoposide (EMA-EP).

Expected 5-year survival rates for the low-, medium-, and high-risk groups are respectively 100, 98, and 93% (74% for chemoresistant patients), respectively.

Suggested readings _____

ALBERTS DS, LIU PY, HANNIGAN EV, et al. Intraperitoneal cisplatin plus intravenous cyclophosphamide versus intravenous cisplatin plus intravenous cyclophosphamide for stage III ovarian cancer. N Engl J Med 1996;335:1950-5.

BOLIS G, COLOMBO N, PECORELLI S, et al. Adjuvant treatment for early epithelial ovarian cancer: Results of two randomised clinical trials comparing cisplatin to no further treatment or

chromic phosphate (^{32}P). GICOG: Gruppo Interregionale Collaborativo in Ginecologia Oncologica. Ann Oncol 1995; 6:887-93.

BURKE TW, GERSHENSON DM, MORRIS M, et al. Postoperative adjuvant cisplatin, doxorubicin and cyclophosphamide (PAC) chemotherapy in women with high-risk endometrial carcinoma. Gynecol Oncol 1994;55:47-50.

DE PALO G, MANGIONI C, PERITI P, et al. Treatment of FIGO (1971) stage I endometrial carcinoma with intensive surgery, radiotherapy and hormonotherapy according to pathological prognostic groups: Long-term results of a randomised multicentre study. Eur J Cancer 1993;29A:1133-40.

DURRANT KR, MANGIONI C, LACAVE AJ, et al. Bleomycin, methotrexate and CCNU in advanced inoperable squamous cell carcinoma of the vulva: a phase II study of the EORTC Gynaecological Cancer Cooperative Group (GCCG). Gynecol Oncol 1990;37:359-62.

HARPER P. ICON 2 and ICON 3 data in previously untreated ovarian cancer: results to date. Semin Oncol 1997;24(suppl 15):23-5.

LANDONI F, MANEO A, COLOMBO A, et al. Randomised study of radical surgery versus radiotherapy for stage Ib-IIa cervical cancer. Lancet 1997;350:535-40.

LISSONI A, ZANETTA G, LOSA G, et al. Phase II study of paclitaxel as salvage treatment in advanced endometrial cancer. Ann Oncol 1996;7(8):861-3.

McGUIRE WP, BLESSING JA, MOORE D, et al. Paclitaxel has moderate activity in squamous cervix cancer: a Gynecologic Oncology Group Study. J Clin Oncol 1996;14:792-5.

McGUIRE WP, NEUGUT AI, ARIKIAN S, et al. Analysis of the cost-effectiveness of paclitaxel as alternative combination therapy for advanced ovarian cancer. J Clin Oncol 1997; 15:640-5.

NODA K, SASAKI H, YAKAMOTO K, et al. Phase II trial of topotecan for cervical cancer of the uterus. Proc Am Soc Clin Oncol 1996;15:280.

PETERS WA III, RIVKIN SE, SMITH MR, et al. Cisplatin and adriamycin combination chemotherapy for uterine stromal sarcomas and mixed mesodermal tumors. Gynecol Oncol 1989;34:323-7.

SUTTON GP, BLESSING JA, HOMESLEY HD, et al. A phase II trial of ifosfamide and mesna in patients with advanced or recurrent mixed mesodermal tumors of the ovary previously treated with platinum-based chemotherapy: a Gynecologic Oncology Group study. Gynecol Oncol 1994;53:24-6.

TEN BOKKEL HUININK W, GORE M, CARMICHAEL J, et al. Topotecan versus paclitaxel for the treatment of recurrent epithelial ovarian cancer. J Clin Oncol 1997;15:2183-93.

THIGPEN T, LAMBUTH B, VANCE R. Ifosfamide in the management of gynecologic cancers. Semin Oncol 1990;17:11-8.

61

Breast cancer

Giovanni Rosti, Anna Cariello

The term *breast cancer* usually indicates two different diseases: ductal and lobular carcinoma, each with an in situ counterpart. However, within these morphologic patterns, various neoplastic entities are included that evidence extreme variability in terms of clinical features, biochemical and biological characteristics, endocrinologic correlations, and response to medical treatment. In the past few years, a new opening was provided by the description of a possible genetic predisposition in some women bearing mutated genes (BRCA1 and BRCA2), thus leading to a widely reviewed concept of the origin of this disease, at least in a minority (up to now) of patients.

Pathophysiology

It is well known from physiology that several organs are integrated in a complex network of interactions and endocrine structures. From the pituitary (under the control of upper centers in the hypothalamus), several trophines are produced that act on target organs, e.g., thyroid-stimulating hormone (TSH) on thyroid, follicle-stimulating hormone (FSH) and luteinizing hormone (LH) on testes and ovaries, prolactin on breast, and growth hormone (GH) on bones. The vast majority of target organs respond to stimulation by secreting specific hormones; this is the case for thyroxine from the thyroid gland, testosterone from the testes, and estrogens and progestative hormones from the ovaries.

Breast tissues do not produce any specific endocrine substances but are rather sensitive to stimulation from molecules produced elsewhere; this is the case for molecules with estroprogestinic activity. An easy example is given by the events the occur at the time of menarche or menopause. Furthermore, estrogens are produced by adrenal glands, and this production lasts for the whole lifetime, thus leading to a continuous stimulation of breast tissue. The situation can, in fact, be even more complex. Other substances may act on breast cells, controlling their proliferation; e.g., insulin, prolactin, and epidermal growth factor (EGF) exert a proliferative activity, whereas mammostatin and mammary-derived growth inhibitor (MDGI) exert an inhibitory activity. The scenario is not complete if we do not take into consideration other mole-

cules produced by the stromal cells (transforming growth factor α and transforming growth factor ß) that have opposite effects on normal and neoplastic breast cells (the former acting on proliferation and the latter as an inhibitor).

Hormone receptors

It has been clear for a long time that significant correlations exist between hormonal manipulation and clinical response in certain breast cancer patients. The therapeutic choice, however, was based on semiempirical clinical characteristics, such as the age of onset (e.g., older age = hormone-responsive tumors), free interval between mastectomy and the onset of metastatic disease (e.g., the shortest interval = the highest the chance for the tumor to be sensitive to endocrine treatments), and so on, but it was only after the discovery of estrogen and progesterone receptors that endocrine therapy of breast cancer began to be based on a more scientific basis.

Receptors are dimeric gene-regulatory proteins located within normal breast cells (100% of normal breast cells contain estrogen receptors) and in many breast cancer cells as well (it should be kept in mind that similar receptors also have been detected in colon and kidney tumors). Benign breast tumors contain estrogen receptors (ERs) in 38% of the cases, with a higher frequency in fibroadenomas (55%)

There is a difference in terms of ER positivity based on age or menopausal status. Sixty percent of the breast tumors occurring in premenopausal women are ER positive, whereas this percentage increases to 70% or more in postmenopausal women. Progesterone receptors (PgRs) are found less frequently, around 45%, with no particular difference related to menopausal status.

More important than the presence of receptors per se is the level of positivity (usually expressed in femtomoles per milligram). For clinical purposes, the concomitant expression of both receptors is considered to offer the optimal possibility of obtaining a response to endocrine manipulations.

Both ERs and PgRs are standard receptor proteins, following the general rules of endocrine physiology: they are specific receptors for specific hormones able to distinguish among several stimuli and to transmit a well-defined message to the nuclei. Estrogens enter breast cancer cells via simple diffusion through the cell membrane and bind to receptors, thus forming a complex that is then transferred to the nucleus. The next step is the production of specific RNAs that leave the nucleus for the ribosomes to start the synthesis of specific proteins, also favoring cell proliferation.

The percentage of receptor-positive tumors (ER+ PgR+, ER+ PgR−) is around 60 to 80%; a discordance has been reported frequently between primary tumors and metastatic sites even in the same patient. In naive cases, the level of discordance has been estimated to be around 30%, whereas after medical treatment (e.g., chemotherapy or endocrinotherapy or combined modalities), this difference increases. During the course of disease, the level of PgRs declines, and this event has been found to carry a worse prognosis.

Treatment

Nonpharmacologic treatment

Oophorectomy

Surgical oophorectomy was introduced during the last century based on the observation in 1889 that young women underwent breast atrophy after ovarian removal. Beatson in 1896 reported that endocrine ablation via ovariectomy resulted in regression of skin metastases in breast cancer patients. In 1922, radiation-induced ovarian ablation also was introduced. The overall response rate was in the range of 30%, whereas castration as adjuvant treatment for high-risk breast cancer was introduced in the 1950s, resulting in better survival compared with non-additional therapy after surgery. The use of oophorectomy today seems to be rather limited due to the widespread use of luteinizing hormone–releasing hormone (LH-RH) agonists, as detailed later, but from a clinical point of view, both strategies are comparable, with a slight advantage for ovariectomy.

Other surgical modalities

More than 40 years ago, bilateral adrenalectomy was found to induce impressive results in postmenopausal women, and for some years after the discovery of synthetic cortisone, it was a widely used therapeutic modality for advanced breast cancer, with an overall response rate around 30%. Today, adrenalectomy has been universally abandoned.

The third experimental endocrine ablation method was *hypophysectomy*, introduced in the 1950s. A complex substitutive therapy was mandatory with glucocorticoid, mineralocorticoid, and thyroid hormones. Again, the response rate was around 30 to 35%.

Drug therapy

Estrogens and androgens

In the 1940s, estrogens provided the first endocrine treatment for metastatic breast carcinoma; diethylstilbestrol (DES) was the most commonly used drug at high doses, with a response rate of nearly 25%. There is an apparent paradox regarding the use of estrogens in this disease. In fact, while at minimal or physiologic doses these substances stimulate the growth of breast cancer, at high doses the result is inhibition due to the prolonged cell cycle, reduction in phase S cells, and prolongation of the duration of all cell cycle phases. Prolonged use of pharmacologic doses of estrogens may cause severe complications, e.g., thromboembolism, fluid retention, stress incontinence, and so on. Today, the use of DES in advanced breast cancer patients also has been practically abandoned because of the development of the much less toxic tamoxifen (see below).

Androgens were tested in the 1960s and generally were considered to be less active than estrogens (response rate around 20%). Major side effects, e.g., increased libido, virilization, cholestasis, and so on, led to their abandonment.

DRUGS USED IN THE TREATMENT OF BREAST CANCER TODAY

Tamoxifen

This molecule was discovered in the early 1960s and became available a decade later as an anticancer compound. Today it is the most frequently used drug in the adjuvant setting of breast cancer treatment and represents the first choice for advanced disease with hormonal responsiveness. Tamoxifen (available only in tablets) is metabolized predominantly to *N*-desmethyltamoxifen, further converted to 4-hydroxytamoxifen, which retains high affinity for the ER. The parental drug has a terminal half-life of 7 days (twice that of the metabolite), and excretion occurs after enterohepatic circulation. Tamoxifen has a very mild toxicity profile; the most prominent side effect is hot flushes, which affect nearly half the women using the drug; drug withdrawal, however, is a very rare event.

Tamoxifen has estrogenic properties as well as an antiestrogenic effect, the former being a reduction in total cholesterol, with a suggested reduction in cardiovascular disease risk, and a longer preservation of bone density in postmenopausal women. Rarely, tamoxifen may predispose some individuals to thromboembolic events, and this effect seems to be more frequent if the drug is associated with cytotoxic chemotherapy; the reasons for this are not well understood at this time.

There have been some rumors in the last few years regarding a possible carcinogenic activity of tamoxifen on the endometrium. From a recent overview of some randomized trails of adjuvant tamoxifen it has been suggested that there may be a small but significant increase in the risk of endometrial cancer. Such an increase has not been observed in all studies of chronic tamoxifen therapy, and it may be linked to some unknown elements. Laboratory studies have demonstrated that tamoxifen is hepatocarcinogenic in laboratory rats but not in other species, e.g., humans.

Tamoxifen acts as an antiestrogen, binding to ERs in tumor cells and altering transcriptional and posttranscriptional events mediated by the receptor itself. Accepted daily doses are 20 to 30 mg, but it seems that higher doses are not more effective than 20 mg. In metastatic disease, when tamoxifen is used as first-line treatment, response rates (complete and partial remissions) are in the range of 40 to 60% or better, especially in tumors expressing both receptors at high levels. The reason why endocrine therapies (including tamoxifen) are more active in postmenopausal women lies in the higher receptor content at higher ages. In patients with receptor-negative tumors, tamoxifen (and all other endocrine therapies) is not the drug of choice; however, in particular patient subsets (e.g., elderly patients not suitable for chemotherapy or in the presence of serious comorbidities that contraindicate a cytotoxic therapy), tamoxifen may be tested despite the absence of ERs and/or PgRs; a small minority of such receptor-negative patients (10-15%) will respond to this compound.

Tamoxifen as an adjuvant therapy

A huge amount of data exists on the role of postoperative tamoxifen administration or tamoxifen as an adjuvant therapy. In a recent meta-analysis conducted on more than 30 000 women treated with tamoxifen versus no tamoxifen, the drug was able to reduce the annual risk of recurrence or death by 25% and the risk of death alone by 17%. In this study, the benefit from tamoxifen was clear in postmenopausal women (using age 50 as a surrogate for menopausal status), whose tumors were rich or very rich in ERs. This overview gave less conclusive results about the benefit of tamoxifen in patients with receptor-negative disease and in premenopausal patients. Hence, chemotherapy alone is the first choice of adjuvant therapy in premenopausal patients, whereas tamoxifen alone is a reasonable second choice if the tumor is rich in hormone receptors. Recently, some studies addressed the question of the duration of tamoxifen treatment. A study on 3 887 postmenopausal women with operable node-positive or node-negative invasive breast cancer, comparing 2 and 5 years of tamoxifen administration, showed that at a median follow-up of more than 5 years there was a significant improvement in the event-free and overall survival among patients allocated to 5 years of treatment. The benefit of a longer treatment was restricted to those with ER+ tumors.

Combination of adjuvant chemotherapy with tamoxifen

A recent report from the International Breast Cancer Study Group on patients with node-positive disease randomly allocated to treatment with tamoxifen alone for 5 years or tamoxifen plus CMF (cyclophosphamide, methotrexate, and 5-fluorouracil) (see Tab 61.1) for three courses given on months 1, 2, and 3, tamoxifen plus three delayed courses of CMF on months 9, 12, and 15, or tamoxifen and early and delayed CMF (months 1, 2, and 3 and then 9, 12, and 15) indicated better results with the combination of tamoxifen with cytotoxic chemotherapy (either early or delayed) compared with tamoxifen alone. From the same study there was a detrimental effect on disease-free survival for ER– patients receiving tamoxifen before delayed CMF.

Tamoxifen alone also was compared with CMF plus tamoxifen or MF (methotrexate and 5-flourouracil) plus tamoxifen in patients with lymph node-negative, ER+ breast cancer. Compared with tamoxifen alone. chemohormonal adjuvant therapy reduced the risk of ipsilateral breast tumor recurrence after lumpectomy as well as the risk of recurrence at other local, regional, and distant sites. The reduction was greater in patients aged 49 years or less but still statistically significant. The only subgroup of patients in whom clear conclusions cannot be drawn includes patients with very small tumors (<1 cm in diameter).

Other antiestrogens

Toremifene is structurally and pharmacologically related to tamoxifen, with a similar estrogenic activity and absence of hepatocarcinogenicity in rats. The response rate is similar for both compounds. From the clinical data we have so far, and since toremifene is solely indicated in metastatic disease, no conclusion may be drawn for the role of this new molecule in developing endometrial cancer. Both drugs produce similar increases in endometrial thickness in postmenopausal patients. Toremifene is not likely to be used as second-line therapy after tamoxifen failure owing to cross-resistance. Its ultimate place in advanced breast cancer remains to be determined.

With regard to new investigational agents, e.g., raloxifene, droloxifene, and idoxifene, we do not have conclusive data in terms of breast cancer therapy. Droloxifene seems to have a high affinity for ERs. Raloxifene has high affinity for the receptors but has only a weak estrogenicity for the uterus. It prevents rat mammary tumorigenesis and maintains bone density. It is used at the present time in the treatment of osteoporosis (see Chap. 46). In a recent report, 704 postmenopausal patients up to 80 years of age who had osteoporosis and no history of breast or endometrial carcinoma were randomly assigned to receive raloxifene 60 or 120 mg per day or a matching placebo. At a median follow-up of nearly 30 months, 32 cases of breast cancer were observed, 11 in women assigned to raloxifene and 21 in the placebo group. The risk was similar at each dose level of raloxifene.

Aromatase inhibitors

Aromatase is a key enzyme regulator of the conversion of androstenedione to estrone (E1) through cytochrome P450 19A1. In premenopausal women, aromatase activity is located in ovarian tissues, under the control of follicle-stimulating hormone (FSH), whereas testosterone synthesis is controlled by luteinizing hormone (LH). After menopause, other tissues and organs are the main sources of estrogen produced through the activity of aromatase, e.g., fat, liver, and muscle. Androstenedione is produced mainly by the adrenal glands, even if more recently aromatase activity also has been detected in breast cancer. Inhibition of aromatase causes a decrease in estrogen synthesis, and this is the main reason for the clinical activity of aromatase inhibitors in breast cancer.

Aminoglutethimide was the first clinically effective aromatase inhibitor. First known as an antiepilectic drug, in the 1960s it was subsequently tested as an inducer of what was called "medical adrenalectomy" with a nearly 30% response rate in advanced breast cancer. The concomitant use of steroids to avoid cortisol inhibition and secondary rebound of adrenocorticotropic hormone (ACTH) was at first considered mandatory; subsequently, it became clear that the major action of aminoglutethimide is inhibition of androstenedione aromatization. As for other endocrine treatments available for breast carcinoma, the main prognostic indicator of response is the presence of hormone receptors within the tumor. Standard daily doses are in the range of 500 to 1000 mg, but there are basically no reasons to prefer the latter. Some studies seem to indicate a slightly lower activity when aminoglutethimide is used at 250 mg daily. Today, newer aromatase inhibitors are used instead of aminoglutethimide because of a number of side effects, such as rash, orthostatic hypotension, nausea, drowsiness, and lethargy that may lead to drug withdrawal, but patients with a favorable response to aminoglutethimide are advised not to switch to other aromatase inhibitors.

4-Hydroxyandrostenedione was the first second-generation aromatase inhibitor to become available; it is used every 2 weeks im at the dose of 250 mg, and it is several times more potent than aminoglutethimide. It binds to aromatase, thus acting as a "suicide substrate" inhibitor. Local reaction at the site of injection and hot flashes and somnolence, rarely with transient lethargy, are major side effects. Other available drugs are anastrozole, letrozole, and vorozole. These new selective competitive aromatase inhibitors are a hundred times more active that aminoglutethimide in both animals and humans. They are all taken orally at daily doses, respectively, of 1.0, 2.5, and 2.5 mg (one tablet). They do not need concomitant hydrocortisone administration, and side effects are extremely rare and mild (e.g., muscoloskeletal pain, arthralgia, headache, fatigue, and vaginal bleeding). Recent studies seem to highlight the role of intratumoral levels of aromatase as a predictor of antineoplastic activity. When compared with aminoglutethimide or megestrol (see below), these third-generation drugs often show a therapeutic advantage. Their current indication is metastatic disease in patients failing tamoxifen therapy; at the present time, they are not indicated in the adjuvant setting, until comparative trials with tamoxifen have been performed.

Medroxyprogesterone and megestrol

These compounds are 17-OH progesterone derivatives differing in the double bond position. Their main activities are on tumor cells (direct action) and on estrogen suppression (indirect action). They bind to PgRs, and a cascade of biochemical events follows, including blockade of ER synthesis, thus leading to tumor cell insensitivity to circulating estrogens. The complete spectrum of action of these molecules, however, is not totally understood: suppression of plasma estrone sulfate formation, *P*-glycoprotein (a molecule that plays a crucial role in the mechanisms of multiple-drug resistance) inhibition, and so on. Standard daily doses of megestrol are 160 mg po. For medroxyprogesterone the dose varies between 400 mg per week and 500 mg per day (so-called high doses) po, but an im preparation is available. Megestrol is used more commonly in the United States, whereas in Europe medroxyprogesterone seems to be preferred. Both drugs share a satisfactory activity on advanced breast carcinomas, with a 20 to 25% response rate. Both progestative agents may be used in cancer-related anorexia-cachexia, even if this indication is not approved in some European countries. In non-cachectic patients they may lead to increased body weight, hypertension, and hyperglycemia. Many authors have reported an increased risk of thromboembolic phenomena (e.g., pulmonary embolism and deep venous thrombosis), apparently increasing with the concomitant use of cytotoxic chemotherapy. Megestrol and medroxyprogesterone compete with aromatase inhibitors as second-line therapy in metastatic breast carcinoma after antiestrogen failure.

Gonadotropin-releasing hormone analogues

This new family of drugs leads to "medical orchidectomy" in men and androgen ablation in metastatic prostate cancer. Gonadotropin-releasing hormone analogues can cause tumor regression in metastatic breast cancer as a result of "medical ovariectomy".

Goserelin, decapeptyl, and leuprolide (see Chap. 59) are used as depot im or sc injections on a monthly basis (doses are 3.6 mg for goserelin, 3.75 mg for decapeptyl, and 7.5 mg for leuprolide). Buserelin is given at 0.5 mg three times for the first week and then 0.2 mg daily; it also may be delivered as a nasal spray. Recently, new longer-acting preparations have been made available with the advantage of a single injection every 3 months. Chemically, these agents are analogues of luteinizing hormone-releasing hormone (LH-RH); they bind to LH-RH receptors in the pituitary gland causing a decrease in estrogens to castration levels. This is a multiple-step pathway; in fact, after an initial stimulation of the secretion of FSH and LH with increased adrenal steroidogenesis, an inhibition of gonadotropin release takes place, leading to gonadal suppression. Responses in the range of 30 to 45% have been reported in premenopausal advanced breast carcinoma patients (ER+ patients respond better than ER− patients), with minor activity (around 10%) also in postmenopausal patients. The apparently paradoxical effect in postmenopausal patients seems to be related to the inhibitory effects on the secretion of "weak" androgens

Table 61.1 Adjuvant chemotherapy schedules

Regimen	Drugs	Doses	Delivery	Courses
CMF	Cyclophosphamide	600 mg/m^2	Days 1 and 8	6 q 4 weeks
	Methotrexate	40 mg/m^2	Days 1 and 8	
	5-Fluorouracil	600 mg/m^2	Days 1 and 8	
FEC	5-Fluorouracil	500 mg/m^2	Days 1 and 8	6 q 4 weeks
	Epirubicin	75 mg/m^2	Day 1	
	Cyclophosphamide	500 mg/m^2	Day 1	
AC	Adriamycin	60 mg/m^2	Day 1	4-6 q 3 weeks
	Cyclophosphamide	600 mg/m^2	Day 1	
EPI ⟶ CMF	Epidoxorubicin	120 mg/m^2 followed by CMF x 6 courses	Day 1	3 q 3 weeks

(subsequently converted into estrogens) from the ovaries. Apart from the unavoidable symptoms of castration, treatment with LH-RH agonists is well tolerated. In premenopausal women these analogues usually are administered with tamoxifen to induce a nearly total "hormonal blockade". Side effects include injection site reactions, tumor flare, hot flushes, and loss of libido.

Adjuvant chemotherapy   One of the major successes in cancer treatment is postoperative chemotherapy for high-risk operable breast carcinoma. The early trials started in the mid-1970s using alkylating agents combined with phase-specific drugs, i.e., methotrexate and 5-fuorouracil. CMF (cyclophosphamide, methotrexate, and 5-fluorouracil) was employed initially by the National Cancer Institute in Milan; updated results show a significant difference compared with the control arm in terms of overall and disease-free survival in node-positive patients. Taking into account all CMF trials with adequate follow-up, adjuvant chemotherapy causes a significant 28% annual reduction in the risk of recurrence and a 17% reduction in the risk of death. These results are even better for the group of premenopausal women, whereas no data seem to support a benefit of adjuvant chemotherapy in patients over 70 years of age. The parameter on which the choice for adjuvant chemotherapy was based for more than a decade was the presence of positive axillary nodes. But the results were better for patients at low risk, e.g., those in whom the number of positive nodes was less than 10; in fact, no patient in the group with 10 or more positive nodes remained disease-free after CMF. Newer combinations, e.g., the sequence doxorubicin (three courses) and CMF (six courses), have been tested recently. At present, CMF is the treatment of choice for patients with up to 3 positive nodes, whereas in the presence of more than 3 positive nodes, ansamycin combinations should be used. For very high-risk patients (e.g., those with 10 or more positive nodes), new strategies are warranted because of the lack of

efficacy of standard-dose combinations (20-40% disease-free survival), and several investigators are now developing high-dose chemotherapy programs supported with hematopoietic stem cells. Early results are promising, with 50 to 70% disease-free patients at 5 years. Node-negative patients have a better outcome than those with positive nodes, some biologic and clinical parameters being important in the selection of node-negative women for adjuvant trials: ER−, overexpression of c-*erb*-B2, high percentage of cells in S phase, tumor diameter greater than 2 cm, and poorly differentated histologic pattern. For patients with c-*erb*-B2 overexpression, a monoclonal antibody trastuzumab, (Herceptin) has been made available in the U.S. and is presently being distributed world-wide. At the present time, node-negative patients should be treated only within clinical trials, but clinical results, in appropriately selected patients, have been impressive. Table 61.1 shows the most frequently employed adjuvant schedules.

Combined treatment

Chemotherapy sometimes is delivered with endocrine treatment both in the adjuvant setting and in metastatic disease; the basis of this strategy lies in the possible coexistence of different cell populations within the same tumor. From the available data in the literature, only a few studies have shown a clear benefit for the combined-treatment modality in advanced breast carcinoma. Some trials indicated that there may be a role for the association of diethylstilbestrol, as a recruiting agent, and cytotoxic chemotherapy. The other possibility is to combine tamoxifen with chemotherapy, but results are conflicting. In general, the best results have been achieved with the association of diethylstilbestrol, whereas in many studies the addition of tamoxifen seems to provide the best strategy to start chemotherapy. More extensive studies are under way to improve the field of combined-treatment modalities.

Suggested readings _____

BONADONNA G, VALAGUSSA P, BRAMBILLA C, et al. Adjuvant and neoadjuvant treatment of breast cancer with chemotherapy and/or endocrine therapy. Semin Oncol 1991;18:515-24.

BUZDAR U, HORTOBAGYI GN. Tamoxifen and toremifene in breast cancer: comparison of safety and efficacy. J Clin Oncol 1998;16:348-53.

COSTANTINO JP, KULLER LH, IVES DG, et al. Coronary heart disease mortality and adjuvant tamoxifen therapy. J Natl Cancer Inst 1997;89:776-82.

EARLY BREAST CANCER TRIALIST'S COLLABORATIVE STUDY GROUP. Systemic treatment of early breast cancer by hormonal. cytotoxic or immune treatment. Lancet 1992;339:1-15.

FORBES JF. The control of breast cancer: The role of tamoxifen. Semin Oncol 1997;24(suppl 1):S1-19.

INGLE JN, AHMANN DL, GREEN SJ, et al. Randomized clinical trial of diethylstilbestrol versus tamoxifen in postmenopausal women with advanced breast cancer. N Engl J Med 1981; 304:16-21.

MARTTUNEN MB, HIETANEN P, TIITINEN A, YLOKORKALA O. Comparison of effects of tamoxifen and toremifene on bone biochemistry and bone mineral density in postmenopausal women. J Endocrinol Metab 1998;83:1158-62.

MIKI Y, SWENSEN J, SHATTUK-EIDERS D, et al. Isolation of BRCA1, the 17q-linked breast and ovarian cancer susceptibility gene. Science 1994;166:66-71.

OSBORNE CK. Heterogeneity in hormone receptor status in primary and metastatic breast cancer. Semin Oncol 1985; 12:317-26.

STEARNS V, GELMANN EP. Does tamoxifen cause cancer in humans. J Clin Oncol 1998;16:779-92.

SUNDERLAND MC, OSBORNE CK. Tamoxifen in premenopausal women with metastatic breast cancer. J Clin Oncol 1991; 9:1283-97.

TAYLOR CW, GREEN S, DALTON WS, et al. Multicenter randomised clinical trial of goserelin versus surgical ovariectomy in premenopausal patients with receptor-positive metastatic breast cancer: An intergroup study. J Clin Oncol 1998; 16:994-9.

WOOSTER R, BIGNELL G, LANCASTER J, et al. Identification of the breast cancer susceptibility gene BRCA 2. Nature 1995;789-92.

Soft tissue and bone sarcoma

Andres Avila Garavito, Philippe Nacacche, José-Luis Pico

SOFT TISSUE SARCOMAS

Soft tissues sarcomas are rare, complex tumors of mesenchymal origin, and as a consequence, they are among the most difficult malignancies to treat. These tumors encompass a wide variety of histologic types, often with distinct incidence patterns and risk factors. Although most patients present with apparently localized disease, which can be controlled relatively well, about 50% die of subsequent metastases. Treatment management of soft tissue sarcomas remains fragmented and shared among the many disciplines and specialities of oncology. Surgery and radiotherapy continue to be the treatments of choice for local tumors. The notable chemosensitivity of bone sarcomas contrasts sharply with the comparative initial chemoresistance of soft tissue sarcomas. Recent advances in molecular biology and the systemic treatment of sarcomas must be sustained and rendered applicable so that soft tissue sarcomas are not refractory to better multidisciplinary strategies and further advances in treatment.

Disease presentation

Soft tissue sarcomas are rare tumors (1% of all cancers). The incidence is on the increase and is underestimated. For example, approximately two-thirds of Kaposi's sarcoma cases are designated as malignancies of the skin. Approximately 6000 new cases occur annually in the United States. The male-to-female ratio is also increasing. Soft tissue sarcomas do not have a predilection in any particular age group. Epidemiologic variations suggest heterogeneous etiologic factors that appear to be specific to subsite and cell type.

Soft tissue sarcomas are categorized according to the normal tissues they mimic. Recent discoveries in molecular and oncogene biology provide new insights into the clinical classification of these tumors. During the past decade, an expanding list of immunohistochemical and molecular markers linked to the histopathologic grading of these tumors has been identified with prognostic and/or therapeutic implications. The differential diagnosis of a soft tissue mass includes a number of benign lesions, as well as primary or metastatic carcinoma, lymphoma, and melanoma (Tab. 62.1).

Malignant soft tissue sarcomas often present as very large local masses. Growth is relatively slow in most patients, with tumors very seldom causing early symptoms. These tumors therefore are often discovered only when the mass has become very large. Plain radiographs are useful to determine whether or not there is primary bone disease. Imaging studies such as magnetic resonance imaging (MRI) and computed tomographic (CT) scanning will show clearly the tumor extent in soft tissue. In most cases it is possible to do CT-guided core biopsies of the lesion to obtain adequate tissue for diagnosis. In other cases, however, an open biopsy is necessary. Fine-needle aspiration cytology (FNAC) usually is employed to confirm recurrent disease. Patients with soft tissue sarcomas frequently are managed initially by general surgeons. Inappropriate surgical procedures must be avoided, however, and patients with malignant lesions should be referred to other surgical specialists so that the initial approach can be centralized, thus ensuring that the patients are treated within standardized cooperative protocol structures.

Table 62.1 World Health Organization (WHO) pathologic classification of soft tissue sarcomas

World Health Organization (WHO) categories
Fibrous
Fibrohistiocytic
Lipomatous
Skeletal muscle
Smooth muscle
Blood and lymphatic vessel
Perivascular
Synovial
Mesothelial
Neural
Paraganglionic
Extraskeletal chondroid and osseous tumors
Pluripotential
Miscellaneous
Unclassified tumors

A staging system based on the TNM system was developed by the American Joint Committee on Cancer, and a G category, representing tumor grade, was added. This clinicopathologic staging system is extremely useful and reproducible. The most important prognostic factors for overall survival and the occurrence of metastases are tumor size, site, histologic type, and grade. For local recurrences, the critical factor is the quality of the initial resection; resection is considered suboptimal if the margin is less than 1 cm from the tumor (aponeurosis excluded). Failure to use radiotherapy and/or adjuvant chemotherapy can increase the risk of local recurrence.

Treatment

Soft tissue sarcomas diagnosed at an early stage are highly curable.

Nonpharmacologic treatment

Surgery

Surgery is an essential component of the multidisciplinary treatment of soft tissue sarcomas. There is no standardized surgical procedure that varies according to the anatomic location of the primary tumor. Completed en bloc excision is necessary with histologic analysis of tumor-free margins. Mutilating surgery can be avoided in approximately 90% of patients with extremity soft tissue sarcomas. Reoperation of local recurrences is possible with more complete surgical excision. Resections of lung metastases has been performed for many years when the primary disease has been controlled, the disease-free interval exceeds a year, and there is no pleural effusion or hilar adenopathy.

Radiotherapy

The optimal use of radiation therapy is controversial. Postoperative radiotherapy has demonstrated its efficacy, allowing more conservative surgery and its corollary, reduced functional sequelae. Brachytherapy permits the delivery of higher doses to the tumor bed while sparing the neighboring healthy tissue. Preoperative placement of radioactive sources allows a better definition of the target volume, including the tumor bed and a margin of a few centimeters. Unfortunately, postoperative complications of preoperative radiotherapy are frequent.

Drug therapy

Adjuvant chemotherapy

The variety and complexity of soft tissue sarcomas have rendered patient recruitment difficult, with accrual falling short of expectations and requirements. The reported activity of doxorubicin in this cancer has led to considerable research on the use of doxorubicin-based adjuvant chemotherapy. A recent meta-analysis of adjuvant chemotherapy for localized, resectable soft tissue sarcoma in adults, having identified 1568 patients from 14 randomized trials with a median follow-up of 9.4 years, showed that the efficacy of adjuvant chemotherapy in terms of survival was best in patients with sarcomas of the extremities, with significant improvement seen in the time to local and distant recurrences and overall recurrence-free survival; in addition, there was a trend toward improved overall survival: 70% at 5 years. Future trials should contain a doxorubicin-based chemotherapy control arm. Few studies have been reported on preoperative chemotherapy (systemic and intraarterial). The perfusion of excluded limbs with tumor necrosis factor and melphalan via extracorporeal circulation, with or without hyperthermia, although a cumbersome technique, does yield excellent results.

Doxorubicin   This is considered the most efficient drug for soft tissue sarcomas although less toxic analogues such as epirubicin are being evaluated. Single-agent doxorubicin is preferred in elderly patients because it is less toxic than combination regimens and yields a reasonable response rate, even when given alone.

Ifosfamide   In soft tissue sarcomas, ifosfamide, at a dose of 5 g/m^2, has been demonstrated to be more effective than cyclophosphamide given at myelosuppressive (1.5 g/m^2) doses. As a single agent, ifosfamide has yielded response rates of 8 to 38% and is currently one of the salvage agents.

Dacarbazine   As single-agent, dacarbazine has obtained a response rate of 18%.

Combination chemotherapy   Combination chemother-

Table 62.2 Soft tissue sarcomas: list of protocols

AI
Doxorubicin 60-90 mg/m^2 day 1, bolus or infusion (or epirubicin 60 mg/m^2) days 1 and 2, 5 cycles
Ifosfamide (+ MESNA) 1.8 g/m^2 days 1 to 5, every 21 days
G - CSF upon necessity

CyVADIC
Cyclosphosphamide 500 mg/m^2 4 cycles
Vincristine 1.5 mg/m^2 days 1 and 5, every 21 days
Doxorubicin 50 mg/m^2
Dacarbazine 250 mg/m^2 days 1 to 5

MAID
Doxorubicin 60 mg/m^2 4 cycles
Ifosfamide (+ MESNA) 2-2.5 g/m^2 days 1 to 5, every 21-28 days
Dacarbazine 900-1000 mg/m^2

AD
Doxorubicin 60 mg/m^2 5 cycles
Dacarbazine 750-1000 mg/m^2, every 21 days

apy may include drugs, e.g., vincristine, that are rather ineffective as single-agent therapy. Combination chemotherapy achieves higher response rates; overall survival rates in randomized trials range from of 16 to 35%. New drugs and more finely tuned modulations of older drugs continue to be introduced. Better hematopoietic supportive measures and growth factors have allowed the administration of higher, more effective doses of antineoplastic drugs. All these measures are causes for optimism (Tab. 62.2).

BONE SARCOMAS

Management of osteogenic sarcomas is a paradigm of multidisciplinary collaboration. Orthopedic surgeons, working together with medical and pediatric oncologists, have improved disease-free survival and limb-salvage rates and limb function. Close communication among members of the care team is crucial. Advances in orthopedics, bioengineering, imaging techniques, chemotherapy, and radiotherapy have contributed to safer limb-sparing procedures and the types of surgical reconstructions. Nonmetastatic osteogenic sarcoma is curable in approximately 70% of patients. Ewing's sarcoma is the second most common bone tumor after osteogenic sarcoma, representing 3% of pediatric cancers. It has a common histogenesis with peripheral neuroepithelioma. They belong to a family of tumors that range from poorly differentiated (Ewing's sarcoma) to well differentiated (primitive neuroectodermal tumors) lesions and are not dealt with in this chapter.

Disease presentation

Osteogenic sarcoma represents 60% of all pedriatric bone sarcomas. It is the most frequent bone cancer in children. The mean incidence is 2 per 1 million individuals per year, with a male-to-female ratio of 1.5:1. Osteogenic sarcoma shows a peak incidence between 10 and 29 years of age. The mean age in children is 14 years. The etiology of these tumors is unknown. Tumors that have developed on a flat bone or on a preexisting lesion such as Paget's disease in adults pose very different therapeutic problems. Abnormal bone growth, as in the case of Ollier's dyschondroplasia, hereditary multiple exostosis, and Albright's syndrome, may confer a predisposition to osteogenic sarcoma. Ionizing radiation also can be a risk factor for osteogenic sarcoma. Deletions and rearrangements of some suppressor genes such as p53 on 17p or of the RB-1 (retinoblastoma) gene on 13q may be instrumental in the development of osteogenic sarcoma. There are also cases of familial osteogenic sarcoma that may or may not enter into the Li Fraumeni syndrome.

The role of the pathologist is crucial for the diagnosis and then for the determination of the efficacy of chemotherapy. Osteogenic sarcoma is a high-grade malignant spindle cell tumor arising in a bone. The histopathologic response to initial chemotherapy is the major independent prognostic factor. Classification of bone tumors is based on the cell type and recognized proliferating cell

products. Each tumor must be considered as a separate clinicopathologic entity (Tab. 62.3).

The Surgical Staging System incorporates the following prognostic factors: tumor grade, compartment, and the presence of metastatic disease. A good response to induction chemotherapy (more than 90% of tumor necrosis) is an independent prognostic factor. Other favorable factors include wide surgical margins, prolonged duration of preoperative chemotherapy, low-grade histology, osteosarcoma of the jaw or arising on the surface of long bones, no extrathoracic metastases, and small tumor size. Patients with osteogenic sarcomas originating in the axial skeleton, telangectatic and multicentric osteogenic sarcomas, radioinduced osteosarcoma or associated with Paget's disease, age under 12 years, increased serum lactate dehydrogenase (LDH), and a hyperdiploid cellular DNA content are considered as having a poor prognosis.

Osteogenic sarcomas can occur in any anatomic region and have been reported to affect practically every bone. Although most osteogenic sarcomas are skeletal in origin, extraskeletal osteogenic sarcomas account for about 2%. The most frequent sites of origin are the metaphyseal regions of long bones. More than 50% of cases develop around the knee joint, mostly in the distal femur. With the exception of the serum alkaline phosphatase level, which is elevated in half of the patients, other laboratory findings are not usually helpful. Radiologic parameters (e.g., anatomic site, borders, bone destruction, matrix formation, and periosteal reaction), combined with the clinical history and histologic examination, are essential for an accurate diagnosis. The first clinical sign of disease is pain around the tumor site, often neglected initially or mistaken for trauma. Physical examination usually reveals a firm soft tissue mass fixed to the underlying bone with slight tenderness. The skin temperature at this level is often increased. Systemic symptoms and pathologic fractures are rare. More intense pain linked to the emergence of a swelling leads to bone radiograph. If the radiographs suggest an aggressive or malignant tumor, staging should be performed before biopsy. Bone scintigraphy, angiography, CT scanning, and MRI are important for delineating the

---

Table 62.3 World Health Organization (WHO) pathologic classification of osteosarcomas

Central (medullary) osteogenic sarcomas
Conventional central osteogenic sarcomas
Telangiectatic osteogenic sarcomas
Intraosseous well-differentiated (low-grade) osteogenic sarcomas
Round cell osteogenic sarcomas
Surface osteogenic sarcomas
Parosteal (juxtacortical) osteogenic sarcomas
Periosteal osteogenic sarcomas
High-grade surface osteogenic sarcomas

extent of local involvement and in predicting the response of the osteosarcoma to induction chemotherapy. Metastatic pulmonary disease at diagnosis does not preclude a curative treatment strategy, although the presence of extrathoracic metastases makes cure extremely unlikely.

Treatment

Nonpharmacologic treatment

Surgery

Orthopedic surgeons have managed to centralize most osteogenic sarcomas in the hands of experienced physicians with the support services of a cancer center. Different surgical procedures are employed to remove masses: curettage, marginal, intra- or extracompartmental resection, and radical resection; the global survival is 45 to 65% with surgery alone at 5 years. Limb-salvage surgery is a safe operation for selected patients; more than 80% of osteogenic sarcomas can be treated successfully with this technique. Synchronous or metachronous lung nodules should be resected when feasible. For patients with resectable metastatic pulmonary disease at diagnosis (i.e., usually fewer than 15 pulmonary nodules and a primary tumor of the extremity), the traditional approach is resection of macroscopic disease followed by intensive adjuvant chemotherapy. This aggressive surgical treatment of pulmonary metastases also has been of measurable benefit.

Radiotherapy

Careful planning is mandatory for optimal radiotherapy because large doses are often necessary. A shrinking-field technique is recommended. Local control of the primary tumor while maintaining good function of the affected limb is commonly achieved after radiation therapy. The global survival with associated surgery and radiotherapy is 55 to 75% at 5 years.

Drug therapy

Chemotherapy

Induction chemotherapy dramatically increases overall

Table 62.4 Considerations for preoperative chemotherapy

Advantages

Early institution of systemic therapy against micrometastases

Reduction in tumor size, increasing the chance of limb salvage

Provides time for manufacturing of customized endoprostheses

Individual response to chemotherapy allows selection of different risk groups

Disadvantages

High tumor burden (not optimal for first-order kinetics)

Increased probability of the selection of drug-resistant cells in primary tumor, which may metastasize

Delay in definitive control of bulky disease; increased chance for systemic dissemination

---

responses. The global survival is 60 to 90% at 5 years. Multidrug regimens are now considered essential. Preoperative chemotherapy regimens (intravenous or intraarterial) and postoperative regimens are being evaluated in phase III trials. Restaging after preoperative induction chemotherapy is currently being used (Tab. 62.4).

Preoperatively, tumors that fail to respond have a far less favorable outlook and may benefit from a change in anticancer agents. Doxorubicin and cisplatin in particular have been delivered by prolonged intraarterial infusion to the extremities. Few regimens are highly effective, and complex, constraining, toxic treatments also require long periods of hospitalization. Chemotherapy must be administered by a highly competent team experienced in using aggressive toxic protocols and in a specialized support unit. A few randomized trials are ongoing, evaluating the intensification of active drugs by using growth factor support.

In the T10 regimen and similar protocols, patients are treated preoperatively with hd MTX (high doses of methotrexate), the BCD combination (Bleomycin, Cyclophosphamide, Dactinomycin), and doxorubicin. If patients are good responders, the same therapy is continued postoperatively (more or less 21 additional weeks).

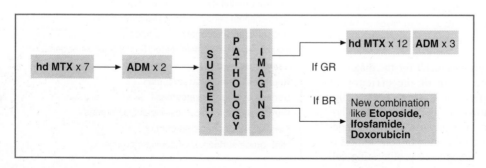

Figure 62.1 Osteosarcoma chemotherapy (protocol example). (hd MTX=methotrexate 12 g/m² per day; ADM=doxorubicin 70 mg/m² per day; GR=good response, >95% tumoral necrosis; BR=bad response, <95% tumoral necrosis).

BIELING P, REHAN N, WINKLER P, et al. Tumor size and prognosis in aggressively treated osteosarcoma. J Clin Oncol 1996; 14:848-58.

BRANWELL V. The role of chemotherapy in the management of non-metastatic operable extremity osteosarcoma. Semin Oncol 1997;24:561-71.

BRULAND, PIHL A. On the current management of osteosarcoma: A critical evaluation and a proposal for a modified treatment strategy. Eur J Cancer 1997;33:1725-31.

COINDRE JM, TERRIER P, BUI NB, et al. Prognostic factors in adult patients with locally controlled soft tissue sarcoma: A study of 546 patients from the French Federation of Cancer Centers Sarcoma Group. J Clin Oncol 1996;14:869-77.

DOME JS, SCHWARTZ CL. Osteosarcoma. Cancer Treat Res 1997;92:215-51.

EGGERMONT AMM, SCHRAFFORDT KOOPS H, KLAUSNER JM, et al. Isolation limb perfusion with tumor necrosis factor alpha and chemotherapy for advanced extremity in soft tissue sarcoma. Semin Oncol 1997;24:547-55.

FLETCHER JA. Cytogenetics of soft tissue tumors. Cancer Treat Res 1997;91:9-29.

GUILLOU L,. COINDRE JM. Prognostic factors in soft tissue sarcomas in the adult. Ann Pathol 1997;17:375-7.

JAFFE N, PATEL SR, BENJAMIN RS. Chemotherapy in osteosarcoma. Hematol Oncol Clin North Am 1995;9:825-40.

LLOMBART-BOSCH A, CONTESSO G, PEYDRO-OLAYA A. Histology, immunohistochemistry, and electron microscopy of small round cell tumors of bone. Semin Diagn Pathol 1996;13:153-70.

REICHARDT P, VERWEIJ J, CROWTHER D. Should high-dose chemotherapy be used in the treatment of soft tissue sarcoma. Eur J Cancer 1997;33:1351-60.

ROSEN G. Pre-operative (neoadjuvant) chemotherapy for osteogenic sarcoma: A ten-year experience. Orthopaedics 1985;8:659-64.

SARCOMA META-ANALYSIS COLLABORATION. Adjuvant chemotherapy for localised resectable soft-tissue sarcoma of adults: Meta-analysis of individual data. Lancet 1997;350:1647-54.

VALLE AA, KRAYBILL WG. Management of soft tissue sarcomas of the extremity in adults. J Surg Oncol 1996;63:271-9.

WHELAN JS. Osteosarcoma. Eur J Cancer 1997;33:1611-8.

Lymphomas and leukemias

Steven Zivko Pavletic, Boris Labar

NON-HODGKIN'S LYMPHOMA

Non-Hodgkin's lymphoma (NHL) is a complex spectrum of malignancies with many different clinical presentations, histologies, and treatment options depending on the histologic type and other prognostic factors. NHL is increasing in incidence at a rapid pace and will be diagnosed in more than 55 000 patients this year in the United States. A number of genetic and acquired factors have been associated with increased risk of developing NHL, including immunodeficiency states, autoimmune disorders, infectious agents, chemicals, and radiation exposure. The standard therapeutic approach to NHL, especially in light of clinicopathologic entities that have been recognized by the Revised European-American Lymphoma (REAL) classification, is discussed in this section.

Considerable progress has been made in the classification of NHL over past 15 years. The successful National Cancer Institute–sponsored international Working Formulation (WF) classification was introduced in 1982 and was meant to be a translation system for other classifications and to serve as a useful tool for practicing physicians. The WF categories include low-, intermediate-, and high-grade lymphoma types based on decreasing survival. However, with the development of newer chemotherapies, the prognosis of NHL changed because of improved cures in the more aggressive categories and stubborn relapse rates and deaths among patients in the so-called favorable categories. In addition, new clinicopathologic entities have been described recently, coincidental with the wider use of immunocytochemistry, cytogenetics, and molecular analysis. These newer entities, among others, include mantle cell, marginal zone, T-cell-rich B-cell, and anaplastic large cell lymphoma. A consensus list of about 20 currently recognizable lymphoid neoplasms has been proposed.

Clinical evaluation of patients suspected of having NHL includes a detailed history and physical examination, with particular attention to B symptoms (see below), skin lesions, and adenopathy, including the Waldeyer's ring. Chest rays and abdominal computed tomographic (CT) scans are essential. Chest CT scans and a gastrointestinal (GI) series are performed if indicated clinically.

Gallium-67 scans are more likely to be positive in evaluating intermediate- and higher-grade lymphomas. In selected patients in whom there is a suspicion of central nervous system (CNS) involvement, CT scans and magnetic resonance imaging (MRI) of the head, as well as spinal fluid analysis, are important. Staging is based on the number of involved lymph nodes, presence of disease above or below the diaphragm, involvement of extranodal sites, and presence or absence of systemic symptoms. Unlike Hodgkin's disease, which spreads to contiguous lymph node groups, NHL spreads unpredictably, and most patients present with diffuse stage III or IV disease.

Prognostic factors

The International Prognostic Index was developed to identify risk groups that may allow more specific risk-directed therapies for NHL. The factors recognized by the International Prognostic Index include age (<60 years versus >60 years), performance status (0.1 versus >2), lactate dehydrogenase (LDH) level (normal versus high), stage (I/II versus III/IV), and number of extranodal sites (<1 versus >1). Through determination of these five pretreatment risk factors, patients can be assigned to one of four risk groups based on the number of presenting risk factors: low risk (0 or 1), low-intermediate risk (2), high-intermediate risk (3), and high risk (4 or 5).

Small lymphocytic lymphoma

Small lymphocytic lymphoma makes up 6% of all NHL. Since this NHL subtype often is a tissue manifestation of chronic lymphocytic leukemia (CLL), if patients who present with predominantly blood and bone marrow involvement are included, the actual incidence would be much higher. The morphology, clinical features, and immunologic phenotype are identical to those of B-cell chronic lymphocytic leukemia (B-CLL); cells with the B phenotype are positive for CD5, typical T-lymphocyte antigen. The therapeutic strategy is similar to that for CLL, and immediate therapy is usually recommended for patients with symptoms, whereas others benefit from a "watch and wait" strategy.

The backbone of chemotherapy has been chlorambucil with or without corticosteroids. This therapy usually produces a response rate in newly diagnosed patients of 40 to 70%; however, complete responses are achieved in less than 5% patients. New drugs such as fludarabine and cladribine, regimens such as CHOP (cyclophosphamide, doxorubicin, vincristine, and prednisone, Tab. 63.1), and high-dose chlo-

rambucil increased complete responses in previously untreated patients up to 30 to 50% and overall response rate up to 80 to 90%. Unfortunately, these improvements in response rates did not result in improvement in survival. Thus, median survival of such patients remains around 5 years, with no indication of a plateau in the survival curve.

Newer promising therapies include humanized anti-CD20 monoclonal antibodies (Rituximab), tumor-specific T-cell therapy, or for younger patients, autologous or allogeneic bone marrow or peripheral blood stem cell transplantation.

Table 63.1 Combination chemotherapeutic regimens for newly diagnosed aggressive non-Hodgkin's lymphoma

	Regimen	Dose (mg/m^2)	Days of administration	Frequency
First-generation				
CHOP	Cyclophosphamide	750 iv	1 q21d	
	Doxorubicin	50 iv	1	
	Vincristine	1.4 iv	1	
	Prednisone	100 po	1-5	
CAP-BOP	Cyclophosphamide	650 iv	1 q21d	
	Doxorubicin	50 iv	1	
	Procarbazine	100 po	1-7	
	Bleomycin	10 sc	15	
	Vincristine	1.4 iv	15	
	Prednisone	100 po	15-21	
Second-generation	Methotrexate	200 iv	8 and 15	q21d
m-BACOD	Bleomycin[1]	4 iv	1	
	Doxorubicin	45 iv	1	
	Cyclophosphamide	600 iv	1	
	Vincristine	1.4 iv	1	
	Dexamethasone	6 po	1-5	
	Leucovorin	10 po	24 h after MTX then q6h for 8 doses	
proMACE-MOPP	Prednisone	60 po	1-15	q28d
	Methotrexate	1500 iv	15	
	Doxorubicin	25 iv	1 and 8	
	Cyclophosphamide	650 iv	1 and 8	
	Etoposide	120 iv	1 and 8	
	Leucovorin	50 iv	24 h after MTX then q6h for doses	
	Standard MOPP		After remission	q28d
Third-generation	Prednisone	60 po	1-14	q28d
proMACE-CytaBOM	Doxorubicin	25 iv	1	
	Cyclophosphamide	650 iv	1	
	Etoposide	120 iv	1	
	Cytarabine	300 iv	8	
	Bleomycin[1]	5 iv	8	
	Vincristine	1.4 iv	8	
	Methotrexate	120 iv	8	
	Leucovorin	25 iv	24 h after MTX then q6h for 5 doses	
MACOP-B	Methotrexate	400 iv	8	q28d x 3
	Doxorubicin	50 iv	1 and 15	
	Cyclophosphamide	350 iv	1 and 15	
	Vincristine	1.4 iv	8 and 22	
	Prednisone fixed dose	75 po	Daily for 12 weeks	
	Bleomycin[1]	10 iv	28	
	Leucovorin	15 po	24 h after MTX then q6h for 6 doses	

[1]Bleomycin dose in units rather than mg/m^2.

Indolent NHL represents approximately 30 to 40% of all lymphoma histologies. Most patients with follicular lymphoma present with disseminated disease including bone marrow involvement (42%). However, many patients can be asymptomatic at the time of diagnosis, and it has been shown that deferral of treatment, the so-called watch and wait strategy, in such patients does not alter survival.

Approximately 10 to 20% of patients who have follicular lymphoma present with localized stage I or II disease. Involved field irradiation almost invariably causes complete clinical regression of follicular lymphoma confined to one or two sites, provided that the lymphadenopathy is not too bulky. A dose-response curve has been reported, with "within field" recurrence following doses greater than 45 Gy being rare. In contrast to the situation for patients with advanced follicular lymphoma, it is customary to recommend radiation therapy (RT) at initial presentation, and disease-free survival after 10 years is on the order of 70%. Trials using the CHOP regimen showed more promising results relative to improved recurrence-free survival in patients with localized follicular NHL as compared with RT only.

Most patients with follicular lymphoma have advanced-stage (III or IV) disease at the time of the diagnosis (67%). Patients who are asymptomatic may be treated with a watch and wait strategy with no documented change in their survival compared with patients treated at initial diagnosis. Single-agent therapy with chlorambucil or oral cyclophosphamide results in responses in 50 to 70% of previously untreated patients with advanced-stage follicular lymphoma. A series of studies evaluating the CVP regimen (cyclophosphamide, vincristine and prednisone) showed a complete response (CR) rate of 57 to 88%. The median duration of remission was 1.5 to 3 years. The use of anthracycline-based regimens in follicular lymphoma also has become popular, although most studies did not show a survival advantage with the addition of an athracycline drug.

Because much of the problem with follicular lymphoma patients, particularly initially in the course of the disease, lies not in attaining remission but in maintaining remission, various maintenance or consolidation therapies have been devised. One popular maintenance therapy has been interferon (IFN) therapy, either combined with combination chemotherapy or used in a maintenance phase. Although some studies demonstrated a survival benefit, IFN has not become a universally accepted part of the standard treatment of follicular NHL.

For advanced disease, recurrence or chemorefractoriness is inevitable, and multiple conventional treatment options are possible. However, none is very effective. Sometimes patients may respond to the same or similar treatments that they received at diagnosis. If after the first cycle or two there is no response, a change to a more intensive regimen may be warranted. In addition, the purine analogues also have been found recently to be active in recurrent follicular NHL. A popular combination is the regimen of fludarabine, mitoxantrone, and dexamethasone, which has been reported to have 47% CR and 47% partial response (PR) rates in patients with recurrent and refractory disease. The median survival after recurrence is around 4.5 years, and no fraction of patients appears to be cured by conventionally available chemotherapies. Overall, the response rates are 78% after first recurrence, with a median duration of second remission of 13 months. Newer approaches, such as use of anti-CD20 monoclonal antibodies, either cold or radiolabeled (Bexxar) also have been found recently to be promising in follicular NHL, with overall response rates ranging from 40 to 60%. However, follow-ups have been short.

In view of poor prognosis of patients with recurrent disease, high-dose therapy followed by autologous or allogeneic stem cell transplantation has been used to treat younger patients with follicular NHL (see Chap. 52).

Marginal zone lymphoma

The term *marginal zone lymphoma* has been proposed to encompass both mucosa-associated lymphoid tissue (MALT) and lymph node-confined monocytoid B-cell (MCBC) lymphoma. These lymphomas are composed of clear cells with reniform or oval nuclei. These two entities have a common immunophenotype that is positive for surface immunoglobulin (Ig), CD19, CD20, and CD22 and negative for CD5 and CD23.

MALT lymphomas discussed here are low-grade NHLs arising most commonly in the stomach, salivary gland, lung, or thyroid tissue and represent a frequent newly recognized subtype of NHL, 5% of all lymphomas. The GI tract, particularly the stomach, is the most frequently involved site. Clinically, patients usually present with nonspecific GI symptoms, including epigastric pain, dyspepsia, loss of appetite, nausea, or GI bleeding. Because the symptoms are so nonspecific, several years often pass from the onset of symptoms to diagnosis. Bacterial infection with the microaerophilic gram-negative rod *Helicobacter pylori* is found in up to 92% of patients with gastric MALT lymphomas. The development of gastric MALT lymphoma is thought to be related to prolonged B-cell proliferation, stimulation, and eventual neoplastic transformation driven by chronic antigenic stimulation from *H. pylori* infection.

Stage I gastric MALT NHL has been shown in several series to be eradicated by a combination of antibiotic therapy and H_2 blocker therapy (see Chap.33). In the two largest reported series, *H. pylori* eradication resulted in complete regression in 67 and 70% of patients with stage IE gastric MALT lymphoma, respectively. Most series recommend a second course of antibiotic and H_2 blocker therapy 3 to 6 months after the first if residual lymphoma is still found.

MALT lymphomas that are localized to areas other than the stomach are often treated successfully with radiation therapy (RT). However, recurrences at other sites may be seen years after the original diagnosis. There is no current evidence that *H. pylori* infection contributes to the MALT lymphomas in other locations. Low-grade MALT lymphomas have one of the highest survivals of any NHL subtype, and even patients with a high International Prognostic Index score have a 5-year survival of 40%.

MCBC is another entity not recognized by the Working Formulation. This lymphoma typically is nodal-based and common in older female patients or in patients who have a history of Sjörgen's syndrome. Such patients typically have an indolent clinical course unless the lymphoma is widely disseminated and in extranodal sites. In patients with high International Prognostic Index score, overall 5-year survival is 50%, but failure-free survival in such patients is 0%. Treatment of MCBC lymphoma is very patient-dependent because it is typically such an indolent lymphoma. If the patient is asymptomatic, a watch and wait strategy may be appropriate because extensive disease is unlikely to be cured with standard conventional-dose chemotherapy. If the patient is symptomatic, single-agent or combination chemotherapy would be appropriate. For more localized disease, irradiation may be warranted.

Mantle cell lymphoma

Mantle cell lymphoma is among the most frequent of the newly recognized subtypes of NHL (6%). Mantle cell lymphomas are characterized histologically by neoplastic expansion of the mantle zone surrounding the lymph node germinal center with a homogeneous population of small lymphoid cells with slightly irregular nuclear outlines, small nucleoli, and scant cytoplasm. As the disease progresses, the germinal centers become effaced by neoplastic infiltrate, generating the diffuse pattern of mantle cell lymphoma. The typical immunophenotype shows the presence of pan B-cell antigens such as CD19, CD20, and CD22, with surface IgM and IgD, in addition to pan T-cell antigen CD5, but CD23 (common in CLL) and CD10 (common in follicular lymphoma) are negative. Patients with mantle cell lymphoma have a striking male predominance, typical median age of the late 50s, usually advanced disease, and one of the worst overall and failure-free survivals among NHL patients.

The median survival time of patients with mantle cell lymphoma has ranged between 2.5 and 4 years in most series. Patients who have the mantle zone variant have a significantly longer median survival when compared with those who have the diffuse variant.

Diffuse aggressive lymphomas

The diffuse aggressive lymphomas of adults are a diverse group of diseases that have in common an aggressive clinical behavior leading to rapid deterioration of the patient and, at the same time, sensitivity to chemotherapeutic agents, rendering them curable in approximately 40 to 50% of cases. In contrast to low-grade lymphomas, the survival curve shows a clear plateau, indicating a long-term, disease-free survival without continuing relapses. This is the most frequent type of NHL.

Patients with stage I and nonbulky stage II disease often can be treated successfully with either localized irradiation or short-course chemotherapy followed by irradiation. Typically, investigators use three courses of CHOP chemotherapy followed by 4000 cGy of irradiation with nearly 100% remission rates and long-term survival of 85%. Following recent randomized therapeutic trials, most centers now recommend short-course chemotherapy with an anthracycline-containing regimen followed by involved-field irradiation for patients with nonbulky stage I or II disease.

The CHOP regimen represented the first major breakthrough in the therapy of advanced aggressive NHL (bulky stage II, stage III, or stage IV). Studies with adequate follow-up have shown that approximately 30 to 40% of patients with advanced disease can have long-term, disease-free survival with CHOP. In an attempt to improve these results, in the 1980s, second- and third-generation regimens were developed including the addition of active agents such as methotrexate, cytarabine, bleomycin, or etoposide (see Tab. 63.2). Agents also sometimes were administered by alternative dosing such as continuous infusion. Single-institution phase II trials appeared promising, showing increased CR rates of 70 to 80% and short-term survival rates of 65 to 70%. Ultimately, a large phase III randomized trial comparing CHOP with methotrexate, calcium leucovorin, bleomycin, doxorubicin, cyclophosphamide, and vincristine (M-BACOD) and with prednisone, methotrexate, calcium leucovorin, doxorubicin, cyclophosphamide, vincristine, prednisone, and bleomycin (MACOP-B) was performed in patients with previously untreated advanced NHL. With a median follow-up of 49 months, there was absolutely no difference with respect to CR rates, time to treatment failure, or overall survival by treatment arm, and overall disease-free survival rates were 43, 44, and 40% at 3 years. In addition, overall survival rates were 54, 50, and 50% per treatment arm ($p = 0.9$). After reports of this trial, many oncologists have returned to using CHOP as their "gold standard" for the treatment of newly diagnosed patients with aggressive NHL.

Patients who do not go into complete remission with initial induction therapy or relapse at a later time need additional therapy for their NHL. If such patients are candidates for high-dose chemotherapy and transplantation, they should be offered such therapy because it has become the "gold standard" as compared with conventional salvage therapy (see Chap. 52).

For patients who are not transplant candidates, a number of different salvage chemotherapy regimens have been reported to have limited results (Tab. 63.3). Most regimens use agents that have some activity against lymphoma but are not as commonly incorporated into front-line regimens. These regimens have shown CR rates of 20 to 40%. However, the long-term failure-free survival rates are only 5 to 15% in most published series.

The use of novel therapies such as monoclonal antibodies for the treatment of relapsed diffuse aggressive NHL has not been as well studied as in the indolent lymphomas. However, a study of ^{131}I-anti-B$_1$ patients with relapsed aggressive NHL showed a 50% CR rate. Such agents, due to their non-cross-resistant mechanism of action, may add an additional or synergistic tumor-killing mechanism to standard chemotherapeutic agents. An alternative therapy that is promising is the development of tumor-specific cytotoxic T-cell clones.

Highly aggressive lymphomas

Highly aggressive lymphomas (Burkitt's and Burkitt-like lymphomas and lymphoblastic lymphoma) are B-cell malignancies in patients who usually present with advanced disease. They are treated with intensive acute lymphoblastic leukemia–like regimens including vigorous CNS prophylaxis. These lymphomas have a high tendency to involve skin, bone marrow, and the CNS and for development of a leukemic phase. With aggressive antileukemic regimens that usually include cyclophosphamide, doxorubicin, prednisone, vincristine, high-dose methotrexate, and intrathecal methotrexate, sometimes with the addition of ifosfamide, etoposide, and high-dose cytarabine, cure rates have been between 57 and 80%. Lymphoblastic lymphoma is a rare (2%), usually a T-cell malignancy, and it is characteristic for its younger median age (28 years) and slightly higher male predominance (64%). Patients with poor prognostic factors such as stage IV disease, bone marrow involvement, or elevated LDH level have only 20% survival, but lower-risk lymphoblastic lymphoma patients can achieve a long-term survival rate of 90%.

HODGKIN'S DISEASE

Hodgkin's disease (HD) is diagnosed approximately in 7500 new patients per year in the United States. The median age is 27 years, and the male-to-female ratio is 1.4:1. There has been a substantial (65%) decrease in mortality as a result of effective treatment. The most common clinical presentation is a young adult discovering an asymptomatic lymph gland swelling, usually nontender and most frequently in the neck region. Another common presentation is the discovery of an anterior mediastinal mass on a routine chest x-ray. A significant proportion of patients with undiscovered HD develop systemic symptoms before or along with the lymphadenopathy (so-called B symptoms), including fever, night sweats, itching, fatigue, and weight loss.

The potential infectious nature of Hodgkin's disease has been a topic of discussion since its earliest description. Suspected agents included *Mycobacterium tuberculosis,* Epstein-Barr virus, and most recently, the HIV virus. The occurrence of geographic variations or even clustering of HD in some areas, besides a possible environmental influence, could represent a contribution of genetics.

HD differs from other known malignancies in its unique cellular composition. A minority of characteristic putative neoplastic cells, Reed-Sternberg cells and their variants, are scattered in an inflammatory background. Two distinct diseases are classified, respectively, as HD: *classic HD,* which consists predominantly of nodular sclerosis and mixed cellularity, and *nodular lymphocyte predominance* (NLPHD), also known as *nodular paragranu-*

Table 63.2 Regimens active in the treatment of Hodgkin's disease

Protocol	Dose (mg/m²)	Days
MOPP		
Mechlorethamine	6	1,8
Vincristine	1.4	1,8
Procarbazine	100	1-14
Prednisone	40	1-14
ChlVPP		
Chlorambucil	6 (total) po	1-14
Vinblastine	6 (max. 10)	1,8
Procarbazine	100	1-14
Prednisone	40	1-14
MOPP/ABV hybrid		
Mechlorethamine	6	1
Vincristine	1.4	1
Procarbazine	100 po	1-7
Prednisone	40 po	1-14
Doxorubicin	35	8
Bleomycin	10 units	8
Vinblastine	6	8
ABVD		
Doxorubicin	25	1, 15
Bleomycin	10 units	1, 15
Vinblastine	6	1, 15
Dacarbazine	375	1, 15
EVA		
Etoposide	100	1, 2, 3
Vinblastine	6	1
Doxorubicin	50	1 q28d

STANFORD V REGIMEN
Doxorubicin: 25 mg/m² iv on days 1 and 15
Vinblastine: 6 mg/m² iv on days 1 and 15
Mechlorethamine: 6 mg/m² iv on day 1
Vincristine: 1.4 mg/m² (maximum 2 mg) on days 8 and 22
Bleomycin: 5 units/m² iv on days 8 and 22
Etoposide: 60 mg/m² iv on days 15 and 16
Prednisone: 40 mg/m² po every other day

Note: Treatment cycle is repeated every 28 days for three cycles. In the third cycle, vinblastine dose is decreased to 4 mg/m² and vincristine to 1 mg/m² for patients 50 years and older. Prednisone is tapered for all patients by 10 mg every other day starting at week 10. All patients receive cotrimoxazole, acyclovir, and ketoconazole as prophylaxis against infection. An H₂ blocker is used to prevent corticosteroid gastritis, and stool softeners prevent constipation from *Vinca* alkaloids. Two weeks after completion of chemotherapy, radiation (3600 cGy) is given to areas of initially bulky disease.

loma. NLPHD differs morphologically, immunophenotypically, and clinically from classic HD and has emerged as a different entity that some investigators believe should be classified among the non-Hodgkin's lymphomas (NHLs).

The generally accepted staging system for HD is a four-stage system, validated with survival data from several centers. There is an increasing proportion of patients with B symptoms as the disease progresses – from 8% in stage I to 68% in stage IV patients. Recommended diagnostic procedures for an adequate staging include adequate surgical biopsy and a competent pathology review, detailed clinical

---

Table 63.3 Some of the commonly used salvage regimens for non-Hodgkin's lymphoma

---

MINE (MESNA-ifosfamide-mitoxantrone-etoposide)

MESNA: 1330 mg/m²/day iv over a 1-hour period on days 1 to 3 and 500 mg orally 4 hours after the ifosfamide dose
Ifosfamide: 1330 mg/m²/day iv over a 1-hour period on days 1 to 3
Mitoxantrone: 8 mg/m² iv on day 1
Etoposide: 65 mg/m²/day iv on days 1 to 3

Note: Repeat every 3-4 weeks

ESHAP (etoposide-methylprednisolone-high-dose cytarabine-cisplatin)

Etoposide: 60 mg/m² iv on days 1 to 4
Methylprednisolone: 500 mg iv on days 1 to 4
High-dose cytarabine: 2000 mg/m² iv over a 2-hour period on day 5 after cisplatin
Cisplatin: 25 mg/m²/day iv on days 1 to 4 by continuous infusion

Note: Repeat every 3-4 weeks

DHAP (cisplatin-cytarabine-dexamethasone)

Cisplatin: 100 mg/m² iv as a continuous infusion for 24 hours on day 1
Cytarabine: 2000 mg/m² on day 2 every 12 hours (two doses for a total of 4000 mg/m²)
Dexamethasone: 40 mg total iv or orally on days 1 to 4

Note: DHAP requires vigorous hydration and adequate antiemetics. Repeat every 3-4 weeks. For patients over 70 years of age, use only 1000 mg/m² cytarabine

---

history, physical examination, complete blood count, chemistry profile and erythrocyte sedimentation rate, bone marrow biopsy, and chest x-ray or chest CT scan if the x-ray is positive. Abdominal and pelvic CT scans, a bipedal lymphogram if the patient presents with inguinal or iliac HD, and a gallium-67 scan are performed, and if these tests are inconclusive, a bone marrow biopsy is done. Staging laparotomy with splenectomy is performed in stage I or II patients only if the change in stage would result in a change of the treatment plan. Note that it is important to immunize patients undergoing splenectomy with pneumococcal, meningococcal, and *Hemophilus* vaccines.

Treatment

The treatment of patients with HD has been one of the most significant successes in oncology. This previously lethal disease is now curable in approximately 75% of patients. In general, the standard treatment of HD depends on the stage of the disease.

Stages I and II

Adult patients who are found to have the most limited disease settings (stages IA and IIA) without unfavorable systemic symptoms and without bulky disease currently are managed with full-dose, extended-field irradiation without chemotherapy. Patients with otherwise favorable disease settings but who have large tumor masses, most frequently in the mediastinum, are best managed with the combined-modality therapy, typically preceding irradiation with combined chemotherapy. Treatment of patients in early stages with systemic symptoms (stages IB and IIB) is surrounded

with more controversy. As a rule, no patient should be presumed to have stage IB or IIB disease and be treated with irradiation only without documentation of the limited extent of the disease by lymphography and staging laparotomy. Because a significant proportion of patients with clinical stage IB and IIB have occult disease in other areas, it is justified in certain groups of clinically staged patients to avoid staging laparotomy and to use combination chemotherapy either alone or in a combined-modality program.

Stages III and IV

The management of patients with clinical or pathologic stage IIIA disease is also controversial. In general, patients with nonbulky disease limited to the upper abdomen, usually defined by staging laparotomy, can achieve 60 to 80% cure rates with radiation alone. Equally good results can be achieved with combination chemotherapy. In some centers, combined-modality programs are used with excellent results. On the other hand, patients with stage IIIA disease who have widespread lymph node involvement in the periaortic and pelvic regions are best treated with combination chemotherapy. There is good general agreement that patients with stage IIIB and IV disease should be treated with a combination chemotherapy programs. Sometimes, additional localized irradiation can be given to sites of initial bulky disease.

Chemotherapy

The history of combination chemotherapy began with the successful MOPP regimen for patients with HD. The wide variety of cytotoxic drugs with activity against HD ultimately has led to a maze of regimens for primary and salvage chemotherapy. The clinician has to choose from a selection of therapeutic regimens, any of which are appropriate for the systemic treatment of advanced disease or high-risk patients with localized disease. The options include single combination chemotherapy given over 6 to 8 months, alternating cycles of two regimens, hybrid regimens such as MOPP/ABV, or intensive weekly regimens of short duration. In the setting of localized disease, the options could include brief courses of an established regimen. Recently, the Stanford V regimen has been developed that intensifies the frequency of chemotherapy with weekly administration of drugs over a relatively short period (Tab. 63.3).

The optimal duration of therapy is uncertain even in patients with advanced disease. The duration of chemotherapy plus irradiation therapy for patients with poor-prognosis stage I/II disease has varied in numerous series from one up to more recently three cycles of chemotherapy followed by irradiation. Use of ABVD for three cycles plus radiation therapy has become more popular for patients with stage I/II disease and unfavorable prognostic factors – without a staging laparotomy. The newer, more intensified 12-week Stanford V regimen appears to be as active as 6 months of ABVD or MOPP/ABV.

Patients who relapse after initial HD therapy have a poorer long-term outcome with conventional second-line chemotherapies. In patients in whom the first remission lasted less than 12 months, 5-year survival is approximately 20%; patients who relapse after more than 12 months of remission do much better.

The principle of residual and dose-dependent drug sensitivity in some patients with relapsing HD is the basis for high-dose therapy regimens followed by autologous bone marrow or peripheral blood stem cell rescue. The presumed dose responses of certain escalatable drugs such as the alkylating agents cyclophosphamide, melphalan, nitrosourea, and etoposide have been the basis for their incorporation into myeloablative regimens. Since a large fraction of patients will have received prior irradiation, radiation-free preparative regimens have been the mainstay of high-dose ablative regimens. In general, high-dose regimens resulted in disease-free survival rates of between 25 and 64% without a clear plateau being achieved in survival curves. At this time, with the tremendously decreased mortality rates for high-dose regimens in HD (now less than 5% transplantation-related mortality), it seems reasonable to recommend high-dose salvage therapy to all HD patients after the first recurrence of their disease.

Prognosis

In general, with standard therapeutic programs that have been in use since the mid-1990s, the 10-year, disease-free survival rates in newly diagnosed HD patients with stage I to IIIA and IIIB to IV disease are around 80 and 70%, respectively, and overall 10-year survival rates are around 95 and 81%, respectively. In almost all series, prognostic factors in advanced-stage disease usually predict the ben-

efits of systemic therapy. Negative prognostic factors identified in various multivariate studies include age older than 40 or 50 years, male sex, lymphocyte count less than 0.75×10^9 per liter, stage III or IV, B symptoms, multiple extranodal sites, reduced hemoglobin levels, low serum albumin level, an increased erythrocyte sedimentation rate, large size of the mediastinal mass, high serum LDH level, and inguinal node involvement.

Acute toxicities of most chemotherapy regimens used to treat HD include myelosuppression, nausea, vomiting, mucositis, and neurologic sequelae of the *Vinca* alkaloids. It has been said that today a physician is more likely to encounter a patient with long-term complications secondary to the prior treatment of HD than a new patient with HD itself. The list of long-term complications includes secondary malignancies, especially secondary myelodysplastic syndromes, and acute myelogenous leukemia. The risk period to develop secondary leukemia is typically within 3 to 8 years after therapy. The risk of developing a secondary breast cancer is not seen until 15 years after treatment and is more increased in girls and young women who have been treated with mantle irradiation. Therefore, these women should have more intensive breast cancer screening at an earlier age. Other more common secondary malignancies after therapy for HD include lung cancer and NHL. Additional long-term toxicities of significance include impaired spermatogenesis and impaired reproductive function in women, especially when using the MOPP regimen. The absence of permanent sterility and secondary myelodysplasia after ABVD regimens and the demonstration of effectiveness equivalent to MOPP have led to more widespread use of ABVD and similar regimens without alkylating agents.

LEUKEMIA

ACUTE LEUKEMIA

Acute leukemia is a clonal malignant disorder of hematopoietic stem cells characterized by the accumulation of immature hematopoietic cells, usually arrested in the blast stage, in the bone marrow. For acute myelogenous leukemia (AML), the diagnosis is made according to the morphologic, cytochemical, immunophenotypic, and cytogenetic and molecular characteristics of leukemic clone. Acute lymphoblastic leukemia (ALL) is also diagnosed on the basis of characteristic morphologic, cytochemical, and cytogenetic properties and subclassified according to the immunophenotypes.

Treatment

The treatment approach in acute leukemia can be divided in remission-induction and postremission therapy. In remission-induction chemotherapy, the objective is to restore normal bone marrow function. Postremission ther-

Table 63.4 Remission-induction and postremission therapy in AML

Drugs dose		Outcome	CR-LFS	Toxicity[1]
Remission-induction therapy				
Ara-C	100 mg/m^2/day in continuous infusion for 7 days	60-80%		Neutropenic typhlitis
DNR	45 mg/m^2/day iv days 1-3			Nausea, vomiting, mucositis
HDAra-C	3 g/m^2 bid for a total of 12 doses	85-90%		Alopecia, myelosuppression Skin rashes (HDAra-C),
DNR	45 mg/m^2/day iv days 1-3			Cerebellar ataxia (HDAra-C)
Ara-C	100 mg/m^2/day in continuous infusion for 7 days	80%		Immunosuppression
IDA	10-13 mg/m^2/per day iv days 1, 3, 5			Cardiac toxicity (dose-dependent-anthracyclines)
Ara-C	100 mg/m^2/day in continuous infusion for 7 days	75-85%		Hepatotoxicity Systemic candidiasis
DNR/IDA/MITO				syndrome
Etoposide	75 mg/m^2/day iv for 7 days			Thrombocytic thrombocytopenic purpura
Postremission therapy				
Standard	Ara-C standard dose plus DNR 2-4 courses		25-30%	Reversible suppression of gonadal function
High-dose consolidation	HDAra-C plus DNR 2-4 courses		30-40%	
Intensive therapy over 3 years	Ara-C plus 6-TG		20-30%	
AlloBMT	Bu/Cy or TBI/Cy		50-55%	
AutoBMT	Bu/Cy or TBI/Cy		40-45%	

[1]All adverse events are characteristics of remission induction and postremission therapy and strongly dependent on the drug dosage. (Ara-C=cytosine arabinoside; Bu=busulfan; CR=complete remission; Cy=cyclophosphamide; DNR=daunorubicin; HDAra-C=high-dose cytosine arabinoside; IDA=idarubicin; LFS=leukemia-free survival; MITO=mitoxantrone; TBI=total-body irradiation; 6-TG=6-thioguanine).

apy is mandatory to decrease or eliminate residual leukemic clones. This therapy has been subdivided into intensification or consolidation with or without stem cell transplantation and prolonged maintenance therapy. In ALL, during remission-induction and postremission therapy, the prophylactic treatment of sanctuary sites such as the CNS is used.

Remission-induction chemotherapy

The most popular remission-induction regimen for AML is cytosine-arabinoside (Ara-C) given over 7 days by continuous infusion and daunorubicin given for 3 days, the so-called 3+7 regimen. Ara-C is the mainstay of AML therapy. It is given in conventional doses (100-200 mg/m^2/per day) by continuous infusion for 7 to 10 days. Daunorubicin is an anthracycline with proven value against AML. It has equivalent efficacy and less toxicity than doxorubicin. In combination with Ara-C, complete remission (CR) can be achieved in 60 to 80% of patients depending on their age.

A new anthracycline, idarubicin, is a more lipophilic analogue of daunorubicin. It has a longer half-life, greater antileukemic activity, and less cardiotoxicity than daunorubicin. It was shown that idarubicin may have greater cytotoxicity than daunorubicin against leukemic cells that express the multi-drug-resistance (MDR) phenotype. A synthetic anthracycline analogue, mitoxantrone, is another cytotoxic drug used in combination with Ara-C. With this combination, a similar CR rate can be achieved. Another agent, amsacrine, is currently under investigation.

To improve the CR rate, a high-dose cytosine-arabinoside (HDAra-C) regimen, i.e., 1000 to 3000 mg/m^2 every 12 hours for 12 doses, alone or in combination with anthracyclines, has been investigated extensively. HDAra-C seems to increase the CR rate to 80 to 90%, but treatment-related toxicity is also increased and overall survival is not clearly improved. Etoposide, a noncross-resistant drug, may improve the CR rate and produce prolonged remission duration when added to the combination of Ara-C and anthracycline. However, no survival improvement was seen. Table 63.4 summarizes the regimens used for remission-induction therapy.

Acute promyelocytic leukemia (APL) is a biologically distinct disease. Disseminated intravascular coagulation, a characteristic clinical feature, results from the release of factors from the promyelocytes' granula that have procoagulant and fibrinolytic activity. Treatment with all-trans retinoic acid (ATRA) has proved to be an efficient remission-induction regimen. ATRA accelerates the terminal differentiation of leukemic promyelocytes to mature cells, leading to apoptosis and CR without marrow hypoplasia and destruction of leukemic cells. No severe bleeding is observed after induction chemotherapy. The effect is a consequence of rearrangement of the *pml/rar-α* oncogene resulting from a chromosomal abnormality at t(15;17). A daily dose of ATRA of 45 mg/m^2 for 6 to 10 weeks alone or in combination with anthracycline produces a CR in 80 to 95% of patients. ATRA toxicity is minor. Headache, dry red skin, and transient elevation of transaminase and bilirubin levels do not limit treatment. Two serious complications are hyperleukocytosis and the so-called ATRA syndrome. Hyperleukocytosis occurs in up to 50% of patients treated with ATRA. It can be explained by the induction of cellular maturation by ATRA. Hyperleukcytosis may be associated with the ATRA syndrome. Hyperleukocytosis may result in leukostasis. The institution of induction chemotherapy or hydroxyurea is efficient in the treatment of leukocytosis. ATRA syndrome develops in the first 3 weeks of the treatment in 20 to 40% of patients. The syndrome is due to tissue infiltration by leukemic promyelocytes and is manifested by fever, hypertension, pulmonary infiltrates and respiratory distress, peripheral edema, and serositis.

For patients with ALL, four drugs are currently used for remission-induction therapy. Vincristine and corticosteroids (prednisone or dexamethasone) with anthracycline (doxorubicin or daunorubicin) and cyclophosphamide are the cornerstone of modern remission-induction therapy. With this combination, CR is achieved in 80 to 85% of patients. Another agent often used in remission-induction chemotherapy is L-aparaginase. Higher CR rates and better disease-free survival with the addition of L-asparaginase to vincristine and prednisone is not proven when daunorubicin is included in the induction regimen.

For patients with AML in first remission who receive no additional therapy, the median disease-free survival is only 4 to 6 months. For patients who received one or two intensive consolidation chemotherapies, disease-free survival at 2 to 3 years is 20 to 30% for younger and middle-aged adults. For this reason, postremission intensive therapy is mandatory for longer survival. In one-third to one-half of younger patients such a treatment approach may even cure AML. Postremission therapy is summarized in Table 63.4.

Most centers are currently using allogeneic or autologous stem cell transplantation as very intensive consolidation therapy during the first remission. Many of the studies performed are nonrandomized and retrospective. Some of the prospective, randomized studies have proven that stem cell transplantation produces a better leukemia-free survival than chemotherapy alone. However, overall survival is not significantly better in transplant arms compared with chemotherapy.

The CNS is frequently involved with leukemic infiltrates in ALL. CNS involvement is common at the time of relapse. For this reason, CNS prophylaxis is an integral part of all currently employed protocols. CNS prophylaxis consists of cranial irradiation and intrathecal methotrexate administration. In recent years, triple intrathecal therapy, with Ara-C and hydrocortisone added to methothrexate, is also used.

Supportive care may influence the outcome of high-intensity and myeloablative treatment in acute leukemia, especially in older patients. Improvements in supportive care, especially platelet and granulocyte transfusions, plus antibiotics and hematopoietic growth factors, have improved the leukemia outcome. Administration of granulocyte-macrophage colony-stimulating factor (GM-CSF) or granulocyte colony-stimulating factor (G-CSF) has resulted in significantly rapid neutrophil recovery, but the incidence of severe infections still remains high.

Elderly patients with acute leukemia

Acute leukemia is very frequent in the elderly, and elderly patients often are omitted from the clinical trials. As yet, therefore, no optimal therapy is available. The main reason for this is that elderly patients are not able to withstand the rigors of intensive chemotherapy and its expected toxicity. They may have a lower bone marrow regenerative capacity, even after successful leukemia cytoreduction. Inability to tolerate long periods of pancytopenia and malnutrition or the nephrotoxicity of aminoglycosides or amphotericin B remains major barriers to successful therapy.

The strategy of using low doses of cytotoxic drugs, such as low-dose Ara-C (10 mg/m^2/12 h for 21 days), is associated with low CR rates but lower toxicity. A CR with orally administered idarubicin in combination with Ara-C and etoposide could be achieved in about 50% of patients, with a median survival of 10 months. Healthy older patients should be treated with curative chemotherapy. A standard regimen is Ara-C (100 mg/m^2/per day for 7 days) and daunorubicin (30 mg/m^2/per day for 3 days). In patients older than 60 years of age, CR is achieved in 50%. Unfortunately, even with postremission consolidation therapy, the overall survival is less than 10% after 4 years. New trials with higher doses of anthracyclines or new anthracyclines and growth factors have reported CR rates of 60%, but the impact on overall survival is not yet known.

Relapsed or refractory acute leukemia

Patients with AML that is resistant to conventional Ara-C regimens are advised to receive HDAra-C. In about 40% of such patients, CR can be achieved with HDAra-C. Similar results were obtained with the combination of etoposide and cyclophosphamide at high dose or mitoxantrone and etoposide. Patients with a long first remission (>1 year) have a 60% second CR rate with the same regimen used for the first induction or with HDAra-C. Patients who have failed all conventional drug protocols may undergo experimental treatment with amsacrine, diazoquone, 5-azacytidine, carboplatin, or interleukin 2 (IL-2). A second allogeneic stem cell transplantation can be suggested for the patients who relapse more than 1 year after the first allotransplant.

Within the first 2 years, half the patients with ALL will relapse. About 20% of relapses will occur in extramedullary sites such as the CNS, lymph nodes, skin, and testes. Patients with localized extramedullary relapses should be treated with systemic chemotherapy because they have a high risk for subsequent bone marrow relapse. HDAra-C alone or in combination with anthracyclines produces CR in about 50% of adult patients. However, the median duration of remission is less than 6 months. The best results for such patients are obtained with allogeneic bone marrow transplantation during the second remission.

MYELODYSPLASTIC SYNDROMES

The myelodysplastic syndromes (MDSs) are clonal malignant disorders of hematopoietic stem cells characterized by peripheral blood cytopenias and hypercellular marrow with characteristic morphologic changes called *dyshematopoiesis*. MDSs are divided in subtypes with different levels of aggressiveness.

Treatment

Chemotherapy for MDSs consists of single-agent and combination chemotherapy. These treatment options are advisable for aggressive subtypes, while for indolent subtypes, symptomatic treatment is suggested. As a single-agent therapy, Ara-C is the most frequently used drug. In patients older than age 60, low-dose Ara-C (10 mg/m^2/per day for 3 weeks) with or without growth factor is recommended. A response rate of 25% was observed. However, the median duration of response was less than 10 months. For patients younger than age 60, HDAra-C was given. CR was achieved in half the patients, but treatment-related mortality because of marrow hypoplasia was high (25% of patients). Combination chemotherapy similar to remission-induction therapy for AML in younger MDS patients is frequently administered. The CR rates obtained with combination chemotherapy range between 40 and 60%, depending on the intensity of the chemotherapy and patient age. Allogeneic stem cell transplantation as postremission therapy is the only curative therapy. Unfortunately, most patients with an MDS are elderly, and only a small fraction of such patients are candidates for this procedure. Long-term disease-free survival is 30 to 40%.

CHRONIC MYELOGENOUS LEUKEMIA

Chronic myelogenous leukemia (CML) is a clonal malignant disease of pluripotent hematopoietic stem cells that is characterized by extreme blood granulocytosis, granulocytic immaturity, and splenomegaly. The leukemic cells contain a cytogenetic marker, the Philadelphia chromosome (Ph^1), described in 1960. The Philadelphia chromosome represents a reciprocal translocation between chromosomes 9 and 22.

Treatment

Effective drugs in the treatment of chronic phase CML are busulfan, hydroxyurea, and interferon-α. Busulfan (4-6 mg/per day orally) may be used until the white blood cell counts fall to about 20 x 10^9/liter. The effect persists for a week. If the leukocyte count starts to increase, maintenance therapy with busulfan 2 mg twice weekly should be started. The chronic use of this drug is associated with skin pigmentation, fever, weakness, pulmonary fibrosis, and a syndrome that simulates adrenal insufficiency. If initial therapy is given for too long, a prolonged and refractory aplasia of the marrow can occur.

Hydroxyurea is now preferred to busulfan. Hydroxyurea is given at 1 to 2 g per day until the total white blood cell counts reaches 15 × 10^9/liter. Afterwards, the dose should be adjusted individually to keep the white blood cell count between 5 and 20 × 10^9/liter. Hydroxyurea acts quickly, and the effect on leukocyte cell counts is less sustained compared with busulfan. There are no serious adverse effects. The major side effect is reversible suppression of hematopoiesis, often with megaloblastic changes.

Interferon-α (IF-α) at a dose of 3 to 9 million units subcutaneously each day produces a normalization of white blood cell count in 75% of patients. One-third of so treated patients have a decrease in Philadelphia chromosome-containing cells after several months, and 10 to 20% of so treated patients have fewer than 5% Ph^1-positive cells. The greater the decrement in Ph^1-positive cells, the longer is the survival of such patients. Patients with at least a 50% decrease in Ph^1-positive cells have a 5-year survival of 90%. The adverse effects of IF-α include fever, fatigue, sweats, anorexia, headache, muscle pain, nausea, and bone pain in about half of patients. Later effects are insomnia, depression, bone pain, apathy, hepatic, renal, and cardiac dysfunction, hypertriglyceridemia and immune-mediated anemia, thrombocytopenia, and hypothyroidism.

Stem cell transplantation is the only curative treatment for patients younger than 55 years of age, with an HLA-identical sibling donor. Long-term disease-free survival according to many reports ranges between 45 to 70%. The risk for leukemia relapse is 15 to 20%.

CHRONIC LYMPHOCYTIC LEUKEMIA

Chronic lymphocytic leukemia (CLL) is the most common form of leukemia. Diagnostic criteria for CLL include (1) a sustained absolute lymphocytosis with a minimal diagnostic threshold of 5×10^9/liter and (2) a majority of lymphocytes reflecting monoclonal B-cell lineage, with a low level of surface membrane immunoglobulins, typically IgM or IgM and IgD, a single immunoglobulin light chain, and expression of one or more B-cell-associated antigens, i.e., CD19, CD20, CD21, or CD24, as well as coexpression of T-cell-associated antigen, i.e., CD5. Using clinically measurable criteria, the Rai and Binet systems of staging separate CLL into three prognostic groups: low-risk patients (stage 0) have lymphocytosis (survival >150 months); intermediate-risk patients (stages I and II) have lymphocytosis and enlarged lymph nodes and enlarged spleen or liver (survival 70-100 months); and high-risk patients (stage III and IV) have lymphocytosis with anemia and/or thrombocytopenia (survival < 24 months).

Treatment

Drug therapy is the most frequent treatment option. Traditionally, the goal of the treatment was palliation. In the recent years, the introduction of new drugs, improvements in supportive measures, and the introduction of stem cell transplantation have changed the goal of treatment, shifting it toward achieving a complete remission (CR) with the hope that it will be long lasting. Drug therapy includes alkylating agents, corticosteroids, nucleoside analogues, and combination chemotherapy. The main problem is when to start therapy. It is usually not necessary to start any therapy immediately after the diagnosis is established. After the period of clinical observation (lasting from a few months to several years), therapy begins with appearance of signs of "active" disease, such as disease-related symptoms (profuse sweets, weight loss, fever, and painfully enlarged lymph nodes), hyperlymphocytosis (especially when leukocyte counts exceed 150 $\times 10^9$/liter), adenopathy and massive splenomegaly, frequent infections, and anemia or thrombocytopenia. Chlorambucil, an alkylating agent, is still a mainstay initial treatment of CLL. It can be given as pulsed-intermittent therapy at 0.8 mg/kg orally for 1 day in intervals of 3 to 4 weeks or a daily dose schedule of 0.08 mg/kg orally. The drug dose is modified according to white blood cell counts and clinical response. Most responses with chlorambucil are partial remissions (in 50-60% of patients). CR is achieved in only 5% of patients. Cyclophosphamide is given orally or iv. The usual oral dose is 1 to 5 mg/kg daily or 10 to 15 mg/kg iv at intervals of 1 to 2 weeks. The treatment outcome is similar to that of chlorambucil. The toxicity of alkylating agents is mainly myelosupression and vomiting and nausea that usually are tolerable. Pulmonary fibrosis, drug fever, hypersensitivity reactions, seizures, and hepatotoxicity have been described less frequently. Cyclophosphamide may cause alopecia, hemorrhagic cystitis, or bladder carcinoma.

The nucleoside analogues fludarabine and cladribine are effective in CLL. Fludarabine is given at a dose of 25 to 30 mg/m^2 per day intravenously for 5 days every 3 to 4 weeks for five or six courses. An overall response was obtained in about 50 to 60% of previously treated and 70 to 90% of previously untreated patients. The CR rate in previously untreated patients is 35 to 40%. The main adverse event is immunosuppression. Fludarabine produces a decrease in the number of T-cells, especially CD4+ T-cells. In these patients, there was an increased incidence of opportunistic infections with *Listeria monocytogenes* and *Pneumocystis carinii*.

Cladribine is a purine analogue that is resistant to adenosine deaminase. Cladribine is given at a dose of 0.14 mg/kg per day in a 2-hour infusion for 5 days. An overall response was reported in 50% of previously treated patients and 85% of previously untreated patients. The CR rate in patients receiving cladribine as a first-line therapy is 10%. The toxicities include thrombocytopenia and, because of immunosuppression, opportunistic infections with *L. monocytogenes, P. carinii,* and *Cryptococcus neoformans.*

Prednisone is the most commonly used corticosteroid. Prednisone is always given in combination with chlorambucil or cyclophosphamide. Initial dose varies from 40 to 60 mg/m^2 per day orally. After 7 to 10 days, the dose is tapered over a period of 2 to 3 weeks and then given in a fixed smaller dose of 20 to 40 mg per day. The toxicities include susceptibility to infection, hyperglycemia, fluid retention, psychotic reactions, cataracts, and osteoporosis. Prednisone is the treatment of choice for CLL complications such as autoimmune hemolytic anemia and immune thrombocytopenia.

Combination chemotherapy includes the well-known COP (cyclophosphamide, vincristine, and prednisone), CHOP (COP with a lower dose of doxorubicin), and CAP (CHOP without vincristine) regimens. With these regimens, the overall response is 70 to 80% (mostly partial responses). High-dose chlorambucil and prednisone give a 30 to 40% CR rate.

Radiation therapy is used as a localized treatment for painful bone lesions, bulky disease, or vital organ compromise. Splenic irradiation is useful in massive painful splenomegaly, especially in patients who are not candidates for surgical splenectomy.

HAIRY CELL LEUKEMIA

Hairy cell leukemia is a rare form of B-CLL. Diagnosis is made when lymphocytes with prominent cytoplasmatic projections in the blood are observed. These are monoclonal B cells that are positive for CD19, CD20 and CD22 but negative for CD5. The cells are positive for tartrate-resistant acid phosphatase (TRAP). Therapy is started when the disease shows laboratory and clinical signs of progression such as painful and massive splenomegaly, cytopenia (hemoglobin < 100 g/liter, platelets < 100 $\times$ 10^2/liter, and neutrophils < 1 $\times$ 10^2/liter), extralymphatic disease, recurrent infections, and autoimmune phenomena. Currently effective therapies include cladribine, pentostatin, and interferon-α. Cladribine is given in a single course, at 0.1 mg/kg per day, by continuous intravenous infusion for 7 days. The incidence of CR ranges from 70 to

85%. It has to be mentioned that more than half of treated patients had received other therapies previously such as IF-α or pentostatin. After a median time of 30 months, 75% of patients were still in CR. The main toxicities include myelosuppression and immunosuppression.

Pentostatin is also very effective in hairy cell leukemia. The dose is 4 mg/m² intravenously every 2 weeks. Most patients responded after 3 to 6 months of therapy. The CR rate is between 60 and 90%. For patients refractory to IF-α, the CR rate is 35 to 40%.

The drug is well tolerated, although myelosuppression and immunosuppression have been observed.

IF-α is given at a dose of 3 million units by subcutaneous injection three times a week. A response is usually reached at between 6 and 9 months. Overall response ranges from 50 to 90%, and CR was observed in less than 25% of patients. The median duration of response is 18 months. The toxicities of IF-α include a flulike syndrome and myelosuppressive effects. In some patients, occult disease could be detected by immunostaining techniques after therapy. Evidence of such minimal disease is not an indication for treatment. The reinstitution of cladribine or other therapy should be considered only after the reappearance of the clinical and laboratory signs listed above.

Suggested readings

ARMITAGE J. Treatment of non-Hodgkin's lymphoma. N Engl J Med 1993;328:1023-30.

ARMITAGE JO, WEISENBURGER DD. New approach to classifying non-Hodgkin's lymphomas: Clinical features of the major histologic subtypes. J Clin Oncol 1998;16:2780-95.

BISHOP JF. Intensified therapy for acute myeloid leukemia. N Engl J Med 1994;331:941-2.

BUCHNER T. Treatment of adult acute leukemia. Curr Opin Oncol 1997;9:18-25.

DEVINE SM, LARSON RA. Acute leukemia in adults: recent developments in diagnosis and treatment. Cancer J Chin 1994;44:326-52.

DE VITA VT, HUBBARD SM. Hodgkin's disease. N Engl J Med 1993;328:560-5.

FISHER RI, GAYNOR ER, DAHLBERG S, et al. Comparison of a standard regimen (CHOP) with three intensive chemotherapy regimens for advanced non-Hodgkin's lymphoma. N Engl J Med 1993;328:1002-6.

HOELZER D. Treatment of acute lymphoblastic leukemia. Semin Hematol 1994;31:1-15.

NON-HODGKIN'S LYMPHOMA CLASSIFICATION PROJECT. A clinical evaluation of the international lymphoma study group classification of non-Hodgkin's lymphoma. Blood 1997;89:3909-18.

PRETTI A, KANTARJIAN HM. Management of adult acute lymphocytic leukemia: present issues and key challenges. J Clin Oncol 1994;12:1312-22.

KALIL N, CHESON B. D. Management of chronic lymphocytic leukaemia. Drugs & Aging 2000;9-28.

URBA W, LONGO D. Hodgkin's disease. N Engl J Med 1992;326:678-85.

VOSE JM. Current approaches to the management of non-Hodgkin's lymphoma. Semin Oncol 1998;25:483-91.

WARRELL RP, DE THE H, WANG Z, DEGOS L. Acute promyelocytic leukemia. N Engl J Med 1993;329:177-89.

ZITTOUN RA, MANDELLI F, WILLEMZE R, et al. Autologous or allogeneic bone marrow transplantation compared with intensive chemotherapy in acute myelogenous leukemia. N Engl J Med 1995;332:217-23.

C H A P T E R

64

New areas of drug development

Nadia Zaffaroni, Rosella Silvestrini

In the last few years, much effort has been devoted to the development of new drugs and new therapeutic modalities to improve the antitumor effect of conventional treatments of human solid tumors. A renewed interest in drugs derived from natural products has led to the identification and development of several active agents, including taxanes, *Vinca* alkaloids, and camptothecins. In addition, other very promising compounds of synthetic origin, such as new antimetabolites, have been added to the therapeutic armamentarium for different types of human cancer.

The dramatic increase in the information on the molecular and cellular processes responsible for carcinogenesis, tumor growth, and metastatic diffusion has led to identification of new and unique targets for innovative therapeutic approaches. Moreover, results obtained from molecular pharmacologic studies have clarified the fine mechanisms of action of old and new compounds, allowing a more rational design of combination therapies. Specifically, progress has been made in the definition of the most active sequences and schedules of drug administration. This chapter describes the different classes of anticancer compounds identified as particularly promising and under development in experimental and clinical settings.

MICROTUBULE-INTERACTING AGENTS

A promising new group of cytotoxic agents is represented by drugs such as the taxanes and *Vinca* alkaloids that interfere with the polymerization of microtubules that form the mitotic spindle. Among the taxanes, the most representative are paclitaxel and docetaxel. Paclitaxel is derived from the bark of the Pacific yew tree (*Taxus brevifolia*), whereas docetaxel is a semisynthetic taxane obtained from the needles of the European yew tree (*Taxus baccata*), which provides a renewable source of the drug.

Taxanes bind specifically and reversibly to the beta subunit of tubulins, promote their assembly, and stabilize the microtubules after spindle formation has occurred. The compounds induce the formation of stable microtubule bundles and, as a consequence, impair reorganization of the microtubular skeleton and induce a block in the G_2M phase of the cell cycle. Experimental evidence has

indicated that cell death induced by taxanes is largely sustained by an apoptotic process, which can occur through p53-dependent as well as p53-independent pathways. Resistance to taxanes appears to be mediated by P-glycoprotein and the multidrug resistance (MDR) phenotype. However, specific alterations in tubulins, which interfere with the mechanism of microtubule stabilization, also may be responsible for taxane resistance.

Preclinical studies have shown that paclitaxel has a broad spectrum of antitumor activity against ovarian, breast, lung, head and neck, and testicular cancers and melanoma. Moreover, experimental evidence indicated that docetaxel is more potent than the parent drug in selected experimental tumor models because of the higher affinity of the former for microtubules and because there is incomplete cross-resistance between the two agents.

Results from clinical studies have shown that paclitaxel is a valuable addition to the therapeutic armamentarium for breast, ovarian, and non-small-cell lung cancers. Docetaxel is currently evaluated for the treatment of anthracycline-resistant breast cancer and is a promising tool in the therapy of non-small-cell lung cancer. Both taxanes are being used in combination with other anticancer agents, such as platinum coordination compounds and anthracyclines, in a variety of different tumor types.

Vinorelbine, a semisynthetic *Vinca* alkaloid, inhibits microtuble assembly and consequently blocks the formation of the mitotic spindle apparatus at metaphase and prevents cell division. The chemical structure of the drug differs from that of the other members of the *Vinca* alkaloid family, such as vincristine and vinblastine, by a substitution on the catharine ring of the molecule instead of the vindoline nucleus. Its structure has been tailored toward inhibition of the nonaxial microtubular system, avoiding neurotoxicity while maintaining antimitotic activity. In fact, one of the most promising aspects of vinorelbine, compared with the parent drug vincristine, is the higher selectivity for nonneuronal microtubules. In tissue culture, vinorelbine is more rapidly taken up and metabolized by isolated human hepatocytes than are other *Vinca* alkaloids. This cellular absorption was found to parallel the lipophilicities of the drugs. The enhanced lipophilicity of vinorelbine has been suggested to account for its difference in pharmacokinetics compared with other *Vinca* alkaloids and its differential effect on microtubules. Like other *Vinca* alkaloids, vinorelbine resistance is presumably mediated by MDR and P-glycoprotein overexpression, which results in enhanced efflux of drug from tumor cells.

Preclinical studies initially indicated a broad spectrum of in vitro antitumor activity of vinorelbine. Successively, clinical trials confirmed its efficacy against a variety of solid tumors, including non-small cell lung, breast, and head and neck cancers and non-Hodgkin's lymphoma.

TOPOISOMERASE INHIBITORS

Topoisomerases are enzymes involved in maintaining DNA structure and function, and recently they have been recognized as important targets for anticancer drugs. A major role for such enzymes appears to be in sensing and relieving the torsional strain that accumulates in DNA during replication and transcription. In humans, two major types of topoisomerases are known: topoisomerase I (topo I) and topoisomerase II (topo II). Moreover, two distinct isoforms of topo II (α and β) have been identified. Topo I creates breaks in single strands of DNA to unwind the molecule ahead of the replication fork and to decrease the torsional strain. Topo II creates double-strand breaks in DNA, allowing strands to pass through one another to control the amount of supercoiling.

Several drugs can interfere with topoisomerase action. Among them are anticancer agents such as doxorubicin, etoposide, amsacrine, and mitoxantrone, which inhibit topo II. Camptothecin and its derivatives are the only known specific topo I inhibitors, and they are being studied extensively in experimental and clinical settings. Camptothecin was isolated from the stemwood of *Camptotheca acuminata,* a tree native to the southern regions of China. Despite its remarkable preclinical potency, the clinical activity of camptothecin was greatly limited by severe toxicity. As a consequence, a great deal of effort has been devoted to the development of analogues with a more favorable toxicity profile, such as topotecan and irinotecan (CPT-11).

When camptothecins form a complex with DNA and topo I, one strand of the DNA helix is cleaved. The drug may stabilize this cleaved complex and produce a potentially lethal lesion if a cleaved complex is encountered by a moving replication fork, which could have the consequence of producing a DNA double-strand break. Resistance to topo I inhibitors mainly results from the inability of tumor cells to stabilize a sufficient amount of topo I-DNA adducts, probably as a consequence of low intracellular levels of the enzyme or mutations in the topo I gene.

Topotecan is a water-soluble camptothecin analogue that has demonstrated a broad antitumor activity in experimental models of different human tumor types including carcinomas and sarcomas. Clinical trials have demonstrated the effectiveness of topotecan in the treatment of metastatic breast and ovarian cancers. Irinotecan is another semisynthetic water-soluble derivative of camptothecin. The drug is rapidly esterified in vivo to SN-38, an active metabolite that contributes significantly to the antitumor activity of irinotecan. Indeed, among camptothecin derivatives, SN-38 has demonstrated the most potent antitumor activity in vitro. In preclinical studies, the drug exhibited a marked activity against a broad range of human tumors, including colorectal, ovarian, and non-small cell lung cancers, as well as mesothelioma. The drug exerts substantial activity in patients with colorectal and non-small-cell lung cancers.

ANTIMETABOLITES

In addition to drugs derived from natural sources, advances in the development of other kinds of compounds also have been made. Antimetabolites, which have been used for almost 40 years, mimic endogenous molecules and bind selectively to cellular constituents, thereby inhibiting the production of molecules essential for cell functions (e.g., enzymes, cofactors, genetic material) and resulting in cellular dysfunction and the eventual death of cells. New antimetabolites such as tomudex, edatrexate, and gemcitabine are under clinical development because they may offer advantages in potency and selectivity over older drugs.

Raltitrexed (tomudex) is a potent, pure inhibitor of thymidylate synthase, the central enzyme in the metabolic pathway responsible for the final step in the de novo synthesis of thymidylate. The drug is an analogue of the folate cofactor and as such uses the reduced folate transmembrane carrier for cellular entry. The rapid intracellular uptake of raltitrexed and its retention in the form of higher-chain-length polyglutamate derivatives contribute to its antitumor activity. Raltitrexed has been shown to induce extensive fragmentation of genomic and newly synthesized DNA. Specifically, DNA double-strand breaks are supposed to be the critical molecular lesions associated with cell arrest and/or death following drug exposure.

Cellular mechanisms of resistance are mainly related to alterations in the target enzyme as well as to reduced intracellular polyglutamation of the drug. Preclinical studies have shown an antitumor activity by the thymidylate synthase inhibitor in experimental models from different human tumor types. Moreover, clinical studies have indicated raltitrexed a very active agent for the treatment of patients with large bowel malignancies.

Edatrexate, 10-ethyl-10-deaza-aminopterin, is a new inhibitor of dihydrofolate reductase, a key enzyme in the maintenance of intracellular levels of folates, such as tetrahydrofolate, playing an essential role in maintaining purine and thymidylate precursors for DNA synthesis. Dihydrofolate reductase inhibition historically has been a popular target for cancer drug therapy, and methotrexate is the most widely used antifolate. This agent inhibits the enzyme via direct competition for the folate binding site. Unfortunately, resistance to methotrexate readily develops through a variety of mechanisms, including impaired drug influx and reduced drug polyglutamation.

Preclinical studies have demonstrated a superior activity of the new analogue edatrexate compared with methotrexate. Edatrexate undergoes extensive polyglutamation within tumor cells but is rapidly eliminated from sensitive host tissues. Clinical studies with this agent are in progress on different human tumor types, including breast and non-small cell lung cancers.

Gemcitabine, 2'2'-difluorodeoxycytidine, is a novel nucleoside analogue structurally similar to cytosine arabinoside. It is a prodrug that needs to be phosphorylated by the enzyme deoxycytidine kinase into its active diphosphate and triphosphate metabolites. Gemcitabine exhibits multiple mechanisms of action, which cause inhibition of the processes required for DNA synthesis and repair through a negative interference with DNA polymerases and ribonucleotide reductase, and also has shown self-potentiating mechanisms that lead to prolonged high intracellular concentration of the active metabolite. Gemcitabine also causes masked DNA chain termination, allowing one additional nucleotide to pair after gemcitabine. In such a way, the fraudulent base is masked and less susceptible to detection by proofreading exonuclease repair.

In preclinical studies, gemcitabine has demonstrated a significant antitumor activity against a variety of experimental human tumor models, including lung, colorectal, pancreatic, and mammary carcinomas. Results obtained from clinical trials have consistently shown an interesting activity against non-small cell lung cancer. Moreover, clinical studies have indicated in this human tumor type a potential additive activity of gemcitabine in combination with cisplatin or carboplatin.

ANTIANGIOGENETIC COMPOUNDS

Angiogenesis, i.e., the proliferation and migration of endothelial cells that results in the formation of new blood vessels, is an essential event in a variety of normal and pathologic processes, including tumor growth. As a consequence, angiogenesis has been identified as a potentially useful target for anticancer drug development. A renewed interest has thus been observed for old, nonantineoplastic drugs (such as minocycline and thalidomide) and metalloproteinase inhibitors (such as batimastat), which have been shown to inhibit tumor angiogenesis in animal models.

Minocycline is an antimicrobial tetracycline whose antiangiogenetic activity seems to be the consequence of collagenase activity inhibition. Recent studies on angiogenesis have highlighted the importance of enzyme-mediated remodeling of extracellular matrix in capillary growth and differentiation. Batimastat, a synthetic inhibitor of matrix metalloproteinase, has been demonstrated to reduce the incidence of lung metastases in different animal models. Moreover, the drug has shown a significant activity on malignant ascites from a human ovarian carcinoma xenotransplanted in a nude mouse model. Batimastat has not shown, however, a significant activity in phase I/II studies and this class of compounds does not appear to have maintained its therapeutic promise.

Thalidomide, well known for its history as a teratogen, recently was shown to be a potent inhibitor of basic fibroblast growth factor β (βFGF)-induced angiogenesis. The drug was successfully tested in multiple myeloma, a poorly drug sensitive tumor, where thalidomide has offered unexpected responses (over 10% complete remission in refractory tumors).

The widely publicized peptide angiogenesis inhibitors, endostatin and angiostatin, are being tested in a variety of human cancers, and results are awaited with interest.

ANTISENSE OLIGONUCLEOTIDES AND RIBOZYMES

New therapies are being developed as a consequence of an increasingly sophisticated understanding of the molecular and cellular processes involved in carcinogenesis and tumor cell growth. In this context, antisense oligonucleotides are a new approach to cancer therapy. This class of compounds has the ability to form complementary double-helix structures with their target mRNAs, thus inhibiting translation and synthesis of specific cellular proteins. If the protein is expressed only by neoplastic cells, with such antisense inhibition it may be possible to selectively eliminate cancer cells while allowing healthy cells to survive.

One of the major problems with antisense strategy is the destruction of oligonucleotides by DNAse, which is ubiquitous in the body. The half-life of oligonucleotides in plasma is short, so chemical modifications to reduce their degradation and increase stability are critical. A common approach is replacement of the phosphodiester backbone of oligonucleotides with phosphorothioate, which greatly increases the half-life of the compound.

Experimental studies have been performed to evaluate the potential of antisense (unmodified, phosphorothioate or methylphosphonate) oligonucleotides to inhibit the expression of the *MDR1* gene, i.e., the gene responsible for the MDR phenotype observed in a large fraction of human tumors. Results from studies, carried out in in vitro and in vivo experimental models of different chemoresistant human tumors, consistently showed that antisense oligonucleotides are capable of significantly and specifically inhibiting the MDR phenotype and suggested that antisense oligonucleotide-mediated therapy could become a useful clinical approach in association with conventional drugs involved in the pleiotropic drug resistance phenomenon.

Ribozymes are small RNA molecules with catalytic activity. A major advantage in their use compared with conventional antisense oligonucleotides to modulate gene expression is their specific catalytic potential. In fact, one molecule of the designed hammerhead ribozyme can cleave several of the chosen mRNAs in *trans* configuration. This implies that, theoretically, lower concentrations are required.

After the cleavage reaction, the substrate is accessible to RNAses, and this step guarantees its permanent inactivation. The advantages of ribozymes in comparison with antisense oligonucleotides have already been confirmed in experimental studies aimed at modulating the expression of genes associated to the MDR phenotype. Specifically, it has been shown that hammerhead ribozymes can induce a specific downregulation of the MDR1 mRNA and, as a consequence, a reduction in the expression of P-glycoprotein, which results in reversal of the MDR phenotype in several in vitro chemoresistant tumor models.

Investigation on the optimal delivery of oligonucleotides and ribozymes to target tissues suggested their entrapment in cationic liposomes. Moreover, receptor ligands or specific antibodies can be incorporated into the complexes to direct them to particular cells. Another possibility is the cloning of ribozymes or oligonucleotides into an expression vector, such as a plasmid or a viral vector, and their delivery to cells by transfection or retroviral infection.

TELOMERASE INHIBITORS

Human telomeres are repeated sequences (TTAGGG) located at the end of chromosomes that are essential for preventing aberrant recombination and exonucleolytic degradation. Evidence indicates that telomeric DNA shortens at every cell division, owing to the end-replication problem, and that the loss of telomeric repeats may be a biologic clock that limits the proliferative life span of somatic cells. In germ line, immortalized, and tumor cells, telomeres are maintained by an RNA-dependent DNA polymerase, called *telomerase,* a ribonucleoprotein containing a short RNA sequence (with an 11-base sequence complementary to the telomere repeat) that serves as a template for the synthesis of telomeric DNA and, as a consequence, for the extension of chromosome ends.

Telomerase has been described as an ideal target for anticancer therapy because it is activated in most tumor cells that concurrently have short telomeres and is not usually expressed in somatic cells. Conversely, human germ cells and stem cells that also express telomerase activity have long telomeres and, therefore, would be affected by telomerase inhibitors later than cancer cells. This would lead to maximal antitumor activity with minimal toxicity.

Nucleoside analogues, such as ziduvidine used in AIDS treatment (see Chap. 75), have been shown to inhibit telomerase in experimental models of immortalized and tumor cells. Specifically, ziduvidine acts as a telomerase substrate and is preferentially incorporated into telomeric DNA sequences. Inhibition of telomerase also has been obtained through the use of phosphorothioate oligonucleotides that mimic the telomeric sequence. The possibility to directly interfere with telomerase activity by using peptide nucleic acids directed against the RNA component of the enzyme also has been proposed. Peptide nucleic acids are one class of modified oligonucletides containing a nonionic backbone in which the deoxyribose linkages have been replaced by N-(2-aminoethyl)glycine units. Such a modification increases the stability of the molecules as well as their affinity and specificity for the substrate. In parallel, other studies performed on human testicular cancer cell lines have suggested a possible antitelomerase activity of conventional drugs such as cisplatin.

Suggested readings

ABRATT RP, BEZWODA WR, FALKSON G, et al. Efficacy and safety profile of gemcitabine in NSCLC: A phase II study. J Clin Oncol 1994;12:1535-40.

ANDERSON KC, ed. Thalidomide therapy for hematologic malignancies. Sem Hematol 2000;37(suppl 3):1-39.

ASKARI FK, MCDONNELL WM. Antisense-oligonucleotide therapy. N Engl J Med 1996;32:2528-33.

BEYERS G, JAVERBERIAN K, LO KM, et al. Effect of angiogenesis inhibitors on multiple carcinogenesis in mice. Science 1999;286:808-12.

BOUFFARD DY, OHKAWA T, KIJIMA H, et al. Oligonucleotide modulation of multidrug resistance. Eur J Cancer 1996;32A:1010-18.

BUDMAN DR. Vinorelbine (Navelbine): a third-generation vinca alkaloid. Cancer Invest 1997;15:475-90.

BURGER AM, DOUBLE JA, NEWELL DR. Inhibition of telomerase activity by cisplatin in human testicular cancer cells. Eur J Cancer 1997;33A:638-44.

HUIZING MT, SEWBERATH MISSER VH, PIETERS RC, et al. Taxanes: A new class of antitumor agents. Cancer Invest 1995;13:381-404.

JACKMAN AL, TAYLOR GA, GIBSON W, et al. ICI DD1694, a quinazoline antifolate thymidylate synthase inhibitor that is a potent inhibitor of L1210 tumor cell growth in vitro and in vivo: a new agent for clinical study. Cancer Res 1991;51:5579-86.

NORTON JC, PIATYSZEK MA, WRIGHT WE, et al. Inhibition of human telomerase activity by peptide nucleic acids. Nature Biotechnol 1996;14:615-19.

POMMIER Y, LETEURTRE F, FESE MR, et al. Cellular determinants of sensitivity and resistance to DNA topoisomerase inhibitors. Cancer Invest 1994;12:530-42.

RAYMOND E, SUN D, CHEN SF, et al. Agents that target telomerase and telomers. Pharm Biotechnol 1996;5:538-91.

ROTH JA, NGUYEN D, LAWRENCE DD, et al. Retrovirus-mediated wild type p53 gene transfer to tumors of patients with lung cancer. Nature Med 1996;2:985-91.

TALBOT DC, BROWN PD. Experimental and clinical studies on the use of metalloproteinase matrix inhibitors for the treatment of cancer. Eur J Cancer 1996;32:2528-33.

VERWEIJ J, CLAVEL M, CHEVALIER B. Paclitaxel (Taxol) and docetaxel (Taxotere): Not simply two of a kind. Ann Oncol 1994;5:495-505.

Endocrine and metabolic diseases

Thyroid

Ulla Feldt-Rasmussen

Enlargement of the thyroid gland (goiter) and dysfunction of the thyroid are very common disorders in any medical practice worldwide. The spectrum of thyroid diseases varies throughout the world depending on the iodine intake of a population. This, as well as some populations having been victims of nuclear disasters, is probably the reason why treatment strategies, especially for thyrotoxicosis, differ widely.

The principal hormones of the thyroid gland are the iodine-containing amino acid derivatives of thyronine, thyroxine (T_4) and triiodothyronine (T_3). Production of the thyroid hormones is controlled by secretion of thyrotropin (thyroid-stimulating hormone, TSH) from the pituitary gland, again controlled by thyrotropin-releasing hormone (TRH) from the hypothalamus. The hypothalamic-pituitary-thyroid axis functions in a feedback-controlled manner. Iodine ingestion is essential for thyroid hormone production, and iodine enters the thyroid gland by an iodine pump, the sodium iodide symporter, with an active transport against a gradient into the gland. The thyroid hormones are stored within the protein thyroglobulin in the colloid of the thyroid follicles, and release of thyroid hormones into the circulation is also controlled by TSH. T_4 is the most abundantly secreted hormone, the majority of T_3 in the circulation arising from peripheral conversion of T_4 by deiodination.

Disease presentation

Goiter

The term *goiter* is a clinical entity to describe a visible and/or palpable enlargement of the thyroid gland. It does not include any description of thyroid function, which may be either normal (as in sporadic or epidemic nontoxic goiters), low (as in Hashimoto's thyroiditis), or high (as in Graves' disease or toxic multinodular goiter).

Nontoxic goiters are more frequent in populations with a low iodine intake and are usually present as diffuse goiters in young persons developing into larger multinodular goiters in older individuals. With time, some of the nodules in such a goiter become more autonomous and may then develop into a multinodular toxic goiter. By far most goiters are benign, but thyroid carcinomas usually also present as a goiter or as a single nodule in an otherwise normal thyroid gland. The annual incidence of thyroid malignancies ranges from 20 to 50 per million inhabitants, and the curative treatment is surgery with or without iodine-131 (^{131}I) ablation. Only a small percentage of the benign goiters need surgery.

Hypothyroidism is a rather common disorder; the spontaneous form in iodine-sufficient areas increases with age, is more prevalent in females, and often is related to autoimmunity (positive antithyroperoxidase, anti-TPO autoantibodies). In severe iodine deficiency, fetal and neonatal development may be compromised. Congenital hypothyroidism, if untreated, may lead to cretinism and is the most common preventable cause of mental retardation in the world. Hypothyroidism can be iatrogenically induced by surgery of the thyroid gland or treatment with radioactive iodine. It also can be induced by various drugs such as amiodarone (an iodine-rich antiarrythmic drug), lithium (used for manic-depressive disorders), and other antithyroid drugs (such as thionamides used for the treatment of hyperthyroidism).

Hypothyroidism often develops very slowly and with very nonspecific symptoms. Most patients may have had the disease for several years, often decades, before diagnosis is made and treatment started. Most cases of hypothyroidism require lifelong treatment, but some reversible forms exist, such as the hypothyroid phases of subacute thyroiditis (a viral infection) or postpartum thyroiditis and silent thyroiditis (both autoimmune disorders), both often preceded by a hyperthyroid phase and often requiring transient treatment in the hypothyroid phase for variable lengths of time. Hypothyroidism is sometimes associated with goiter (as in Hashimoto's thyroiditis, endemic goiter, and subacute thyroidism), but it is often seen without goiter (as in atrophic autoimmune thyroiditis or after removal of the thyroid gland). All the preceding conditions of hypothyroidism represent primary forms; the disease is located in the thyroid gland itself. These are by far the most common, but rare cases of secondary (located in the pituitary) or tertiary (at the hypothalamic level) hypothyroidism exist.

The typical symptoms and signs of hypothyroidism are slow cerebration, cold intolerance, dry skin and hair, constipation, hoarse voice, bradycardia, depression, enlarged tongue, elevated serum cholesterol level, and in severe cases, often angina and even cardiac failure.

Hyperthyroidism is caused by elevated concentrations of circulating free thyroid hormones and is globally a rarer disorder than both nontoxic goiter and hypothyroidism. The worldwide distribution of the various disorders of hyperthyroidism vary substantially mainly due to differences in the iodine intake. The most common cause of hyperthyroidism in iodine-sufficient areas is the autoimmune Graves' disease. The hyperthyroidism in Graves' disease is caused by thyrotropin receptor-stimulating autoantibodies (TRAbs), while the pathogenesis of the underlying autoimmune reaction is not clearly understood. The patients have a genetic predisposition, but other unknown precipitating factors are necessary for manifest disease. Toxic adenomas (a single "hot" nodule) usually account for less than 10% of patients in all populations. Transient forms of hyperthyroidism are seen in the destructive thyroiditides and rarely by exogenous ingestion of thyroid hormone. The thyroiditides include subacute (painful) thyroiditis (a viral infection) and silent or postpartum thyroiditis, the latter occurring in 3 to 10% of postpartum women. The differentiation of the disorders of overproduction of thyroid hormones can be made by a technetium-99m(^{99m}Tc) scintigraphy demonstrating differences in the regional distribution of the radioactivity in the thyroid (diffuse, multinodular, or single nodule). Unlike these forms, patients with destructive thyroiditis have a low uptake on ^{99m}Tc scintigraphy or by a 24-hour radioiodine uptake (RAIU) test due to destruction of the thyroid follicles. Treatment with antithyroid drugs has no influence on the development or course of hyperthyroidism caused by destruction.

As in hypothyroiditis, thyrotoxicosis may or may not be associated with the presence of a goiter (e.g., a toxic adenoma may not be palpable), and approximately one-third of patients with Graves' disease have a normal thyroid gland volume, as do also many patients with postpartum thyroiditis. The signs and symptoms of hyperthyroidism arise from the thyroid hormone-induced excessive heat production, from increased activity of the sympathetic nervous system, and from increased motor activity. The patient thus has flushed, warm, and moist skin, a general heat intolerance and despite increased appetite, often weight loss, increased frequency of bowel movements, increased heart rate, muscular weakness, tremor of hands and muscles, and anxiety. In younger patients the increased heart rate is usually a sinus tachycardia, but in older patients very often other cardiac arrhythmias occur such as atrial fibrillation, and angina and even cardiac failure are frequent events.

Patients with Graves' disease may have associated infiltrative ophthalmopathy (e.g., exophthalmos, thyroid-associated ophthalmopathy), considered to be an autoimmune inflammatory reaction of the extraocular muscles and periorbital connective tissue. It is clinically evident in less than half the patients, but methods such as computed tomography (CT) and magnetic resonance imaging (MRI) or ultrasound of the orbit have revealed some degree of eye muscle involvement in most patients with Graves' disease.

Measurement of thyroid function

In full-blown cases of either hyper- or hypothyroidism with typical clinical features, the diagnosis is confirmed easily by laboratory tests. In many patients, however, symptoms present in a much more subtle way. The thyroid hormones thyroxine and triiodothyronine circulate in the blood bound to thyroid hormone–binding proteins, of which thyroxine-binding globulin (TBG) is the most important. Only a minor portion of the hormones is free, but this part is the active part both in the periphery and in the feedback at the hypothalamic and pituitary levels. Estimation of thyroid function is best done by a combination of measurement of serum thyrotropin (TSH) from the pituitary and an estimate of free T_4 either by using commercial assays directly for this purpose or rather by a combination of measurement of total T_4 concentration together with TBG (or T_3 uptake test) to get a free T_4 index. In thyrotoxicosis, a similar estimate of free T_3 should be made, especially in iodine-deficient areas, where T_3-thyrotoxicosis is often present. The diagnosis of primary hypothyroidism is based on an elevated serum TSH level together with a low serum T_4 concentration. In secondary and tertiary hypothyroidism, the serum TSH concentration is usually normal, and the diagnosis may rest on demonstration of a low serum T_4 concentration in a patient with other pituitary or hypothalamic abnormalities. The diagnosis of hyperthyroidism is based on elevated serum concentrations of T_4 and/or T_3 together with a suppressed serum TSH level.

Very often serum TSH measurements are used for screening of thyroid function, assuming that a normal serum TSH concentration rules out the presence of both hyper- and hypothyroidism. This is in most cases true, but it should be borne in mind that heterophilic antibodies in the serum may cause falsely elevated values, central hypothyroidism may occur with normal TSH concentrations, and measurement in patients in the initial (sometimes also later) phases of treatment of hypo- or hyperthyroidism may not reflect thyroid function (due to a latency of the pituitary).

Treatment

Hypothyroidism

Since hypothyroidism arises from lack of thyroid hormone production from the thyroid gland, the only available treatment is replacement of the lacking hormone(s). No nondrug therapy can be recommended. If left untreated, the disease will slowly progress to a more severe clinical condition, initially increasing the clinical features with bradycardia, depression, progressive heart failure, impaired intellectual function, anemia, cold intolerance, and constipation, but it may eventually lead to the life-threatening condition of myxedema coma. In less severe cases, untreated patients often leave the active workforce early, enter old peoples' home prematurely, or end in psychiatric care with severe depression and dementia.

Thyroxine (levothyroxine sodium) is the hormone of choice for thyroid hormone replacement therapy. Triiodothyronine (liothyronine sodium) may be used occasionally due to its faster onset of action and shorter half-life, such as in myxedema coma and for preparing a patient for ^{131}I therapy in thyroid carcinoma. In chronic replacement therapy, levothyroxine sodium is more desirable due to its longer duration of action and consistent potency. Furthermore, it provides a more physiologic approach because thyroxine is circulating more abundantly in normal situations, most of the serum triiodothyronine arising from peripheral conversion from thyroxine. Liothyronine sodium requires more frequent dosing at higher cost, and the plasma concentration is less stable, with serum T_3 concentrations often rising above the reference range, rendering the patient at risk for cardiac arrhythmias, angina, or even cardiac failure.

The first treatment of hypothyroidism was done by Murray in 1891 by injecting an extract of the thyroid gland, but the following year Howitz, Mackenzie, and Fox independently discovered that oral ingestion of thyroid tissue was fully effective. For decades, desiccated thyroid preparations from whole-animal thyroids have been available, but now they are no longer recommended therapy because of the variable content of thyroxine and triiodothyronine. Recommended drugs are the synthetic preparations of the natural isomers of thyroid hormones.

Levothyroxine sodium (L-T_4) is available in tablets and as a lyophilized powder for injection. Absorption occurs in the small intestine, with only 50 to 80% of the ingested dose absorbed. The absorption is extremely variable, with interference from a variety of drugs such as aluminum hydroxide, magnesium salts, some iron salts, sucralfate, and cholestyramine resin. The mean half-life of ingested levothyroxine sodium is 7 days, the peak effect of a single dose at about 9 days declining to half the maximum in 11 to 15 days. The average adult replacement dose of levothyroxine sodium is 75 to 125 µg. In healthy young individuals with short duration of hypothyroidism, institution of therapy may begin at full replacement dose. In individuals over the age of approximately 50 years with very severe hypothyroidism of long duration and with suspected cardiac disease, institution of a lower daily dose (25 µg per day) of levothyroxine sodium is indicated in order to avoid demasking an undiagnosed cardiac disease. The dose can be increased at approximately 25 µg per day every month or every few months until full replacement dose is achieved (see below). Individuals with preexisting cardiac disease need an even slower initiation (12.5 µg per day), increasing the dose by 12.5 µg daily every 6 weeks to full replacement. Occurrence of angina or arrhythmias during dose increase immediately should lead to a longer period of time on the previous dose level.

Because of the prolonged half-life of levothyroxine sodium, any dose change will not reach steady-state concentration of the hormone until after 4 to 6 weeks. Furthermore, pituitary latency implies a very slow fall in serum TSH concentrations. Increase in dosage thus initially should be guided mainly by the absence of side effects and if necessary – measurement of the serum T_4 concentration every 4 to 6 weeks. The goal of replacement therapy, however, is to achieve a serum TSH concentration within the reference range, but this may take many months. Overtreatment with levothyroxine sodium with suppressed serum TSH may cause a condition similar to subclinical hyperthyroidism with development of osteoporosis (mainly in postmenopausal women) and cardiac dysfunction. Also, due to the long half-life of levothyroxine sodium, therapy may be interrupted for several days (probably up to 7 days) if needed in conjunction with intercurrent illnesses or surgery when oral intake may not be possible.

The indication for treating patients with so-called subclinical hypothyroidism (elevated serum TSH concentration but normal concentrations of T_4 and T_3) is controversial and should be individualized. Patients with subclinical hypothyroidism and one or more of the following features may benefit from treatment: goiter, hypercholesterolemia, symptoms of hypothyroidism, and presence of thyroid autoantibodies (anti-TPO). Pregnant patients with hypothyroidism require special attention, since normal fetal development, particularly of the brain, depends on the thyroid function of the mother, at least in the first trimester. TBG is increasing during pregnancy, induced by estrogen, possibly the reason why women treated with levothyroxine sodium need a higher dose during pregnancy (approximately 30-50% higher than the usual replacement dose). Pregnancy also may induce hypothyroidism in iodine deficiency or in women with thyroid autoantibodies (anti-TPO) and therefore predisposed to autoimmune thyroid disease. The dose of levothyroxine sodium should be adjusted according to concomitant measurement of serum concentrations of TSH and an estimate of serum free thyroxine. In women with thyroid autoantibodies (anti-TPO or thyrotropin receptor–blocking antibodies), the neonate may be transiently affected by hypothyroidism.

Treatment of cretinism has now become more successful as a result of newborn screening for congenital hypothyroidism. Therapy with levothyroxine sodium (initial daily dose 10-15 µg/kg of body weight) should be initiated within the first few weeks of life to obtain normal physical and mental development. In these infants, serum free thyroxine levels should be kept in the upper or elevated range (adjusted for age) and serum TSH concentrations below 20 m/l. The most important assessment of successful treatment is physical growth, motor development, developmental progress, and bone maturation.

Liothyronine sodium (L-T_3) is also available in tablets and in an injectable form. It has a much faster onset of action (4-6 h) than levothyroxine sodium and a shorter half-life (1 day). The absorption is as for levothyroxine sodium from the small intestine and variable. Although less well investigated, the absorption is probably influenced by the same drugs as levothyroxine sodium, and the metabolism is similar, following the physiologic pathways for deiodination of triiodothyronine. The use of liothyronine sodium is limited to a few clinical situations, one of which is in the preparation of patients with thyroid carcinoma for ^{131}I therapy, leaving the patient hypothyroid for a shorter period of time in relation to this therapy (due to shorter drug half-life) and thereby with less side effects/complications to the ^{131}I therapy. Liothyronine often also is used for treatment of myxedema coma, which is a very rare life-threatening condition with a mortality from 50 to 70%, usually precipitated by, for example, pulmonary infection, heart failure, or cerebrovascular accidents. The clinical progression often is facilitated by various drugs (e.g., sedatives, tranquilizers, antidepressants) with a slower metabolism during hypothyroidism and thus perhaps toxic serum concentrations despite usual dosage for a euthyroid person. The clinical features are often difficult to differentiate, and the diagnosis is also in most cases very difficult due to other severe diseases influencing the measurement of thyroid function. Serum TSH is usually very high. The initial treatment is supportive intensive care, with usual treatment of cardiac and respiratory failure, correction of electrolyte disturbances (hyponatremia), and treatment of precipitating disease. The patient may have a coexisting decreased adrenal reserve (5-10% of patients), which is why iv steroid therapy may be indicated. Thyroid replacement is initially given as a loading dose of 200 to 300 μg levothyroxine sodium iv with a subsequent dose of 100 μg given 24 hours later or 20 μg of liothyronine sodium given iv every 8 hours. The dose should be adjusted according to clinical parameters such as cardiac function, electrolytes, and hemodynamic instability.

The side effects of thyroid hormone replacement therapy are mostly due to overtreatment, and the symptoms are thus those of hyperthyroidism. In cases of mild overdosage, the rational approach is reduction of the actual dose. In severe cases of overdosing that may occur accidentally or deliberately (it has been used to obtain weight loss in obesity and in some body builder cultures), the treatment is beta blockade and supportive intensive care. In all cases of initiating thyroid hormone replacement, it must also be borne in mind that the metabolism of a number of other drugs will change; e.g., patients on a stable dose of digoxin in the hypothyroid state will require increased dosage in order to maintain a therapeutic plasma concentration.

Hyperthyroidism

The treatment of thyrotoxicosis depends very much on its cause. In most cases of hyperthyroidism caused by overproduction of thyroid hormones (Graves' disease, uni- and multinodular goiters), the initial treatment is usually antithyroid drug therapy to lower the hormone production, but either as a consequence of relapse after antithyroid drugs in Graves' disease, noncompliance, age, or nodularity of the thyroid gland, the subsequent therapy may be either surgery or radioactive iodine (with ^{131}I). In

Graves' disease, antithyroid drugs often comprise the only therapy, but worldwide discrepancies in treatment strategy exist, Europeans being more in favor of antithyroid drugs in uncomplicated cases but also treating a substantial number of patients with radioactive iodine and few by surgery; in the United States, radioactive iodine is used almost entirely, whereas the Japanese rarely use radioactive iodine and almost entirely use antithyroid drugs, choosing surgery in more complicated cases. The indication for treatment of hyperthyroidism is alleviation of symptoms but also avoidance of long-term effects of untreated hyperthyroidism such as heart failure, mental impairment, severe weight loss, muscular deficiency, and osteoporosis.

Antithyroid drugs A large number of compounds are able to interfere with the synthesis, release, or action of thyroid hormones. The antithyroid compounds that have clinical utility are the thioureylenes, which belong to the family of thionamides. These drugs interfere directly with the synthesis of thyroid hormones. Other thyroid inhibitors exist, such as ionic inhibitors that block the iodide transport mechanism (e.g., perchlorate), high concentrations of iodine itself, and radioactive iodine. Antithyroid drug therapy with thionamide was introduced by Astwood in 1943. The drugs have been used mainly to obtain euthyroidism in patients with chronic hyperthyroidism, whatever the cause, and for long-term medical therapy in Graves' disease. The currently used antithyroid compounds are propylthiouracil (6-*N*-propylthiouracil), methimazole (1-methyl-2-mercaptoimidazole), and carbimazole; this last is a prodrug of methimazole. Thionamides impair the catalytic effect of thyroid peroxidase by completely inhibiting the organification of iodide and hormonogenesis. Both drugs and metabolites appear in the urine. The optimal dose of antithyroid drugs has been discussed extensively, but still no agreement exists. Antithyroid drugs have been used for several decades, but only recently have controlled clinical trials comparing low- and high-dose regimens been carried out. There are in principle two ways to adjust the dose: either by using the so-called block-replace regimen by blocking the thyroid hormone synthesis with a large constant dose of antithyroid drug and adding levothyroxine sodium as replacement or by using a dose-titration of antithyroid drug by monitoring the peripheral thyroid hormones. The advantage of the block-replace regimen is the fact that it is easy and requires few control visits during follow-up; the disadvantage is that higher doses must be used with the risk of more side effects (Tab. 65.1). Furthermore block-replace therapy should not be used during pregnancy, since antithyroid drugs pass the placenta more easily than does levothyroxine sodium, and the fetal thyroid is thus overtreated with antithyroid drugs without replacement.

Propylthiouracil exists in tablets of 100 mg and methimazole/carbimazole in tablets of 5 mg. The usual starting dose of propylthiouracil is 400 mg and of methimazole 20 mg daily in two or three divided doses. With propylthiouracil, the inhibitory effect on thyroid hormone synthesis disappears after less than 24 hours, whereas methimazole has a more prolonged inhibitory effect, still detectable at 24 hours. After 2 to 4 weeks, either levothyroxine (100 mg daily) should be added (block-replace), or the dose should be reduced (titration). The usual long-term titration dose is 2.5 to 10 mg methimazole or 50 to 200 mg propylthiouracil daily. The efficiency with which euthyroidism is restored in a thyrotoxic patient is usually excellent in the initial phase of therapy; failure to obtain euthyroidism is most often due to lack of compliance. The main problem related to medical antithyroid drug therapy is the long-term risk of relapse after discontinuing antithyroid drug therapy – in nodular goiters almost 100% due to autonomic dysfunction and in Graves' disease approximately 40 to 60%. The duration of treatment is controversial, and also in this respect various treatment regimens exist: (1) fixed time of treatment, usually between 6 months and 2 years, and (2) variable length of time using, for example, the disappearance of thyrotropin receptor–stimulating antibodies (TPAbs) as a guideline for stopping therapy. This approach, however, has not been proven very useful in larger studies. Measurement of TPAbs at the end of antithyroid drug therapy also has been used to predict remission or relapse, but too large overlaps between groups diminish its usefulness. Only very high levels of TPAbs seem to be associated with a high relapse rate within 1 to 2 years, and these patients therefore may benefit from a more destructive type of therapy (radioiodine or surgery). In patients with ophthalmopathy, antithyroid drug therapy is usually the treatment of choice, at least in the early stages, since radioactive iodine may worsen or even precipitate the eye condition. Young patients with a large goiter may benefit from near-total thyroidectomy. Patients should be advised to refrain from smoking, which has been demonstrated to be associated with more severe eye signs and progression of the eye condition.

Antithyroid drugs are rapidly absorbed from the gastrointestinal tract and actively concentrated by the thyroid within minutes after administration. Peak serum levels are reached a few hours after drug ingestion, and the half-life of the drugs from serum is short (Tab. 65.2). The pharmacologic action, however, depends rather on the intrathyroidal concentration, which after a single oral dose may be 100 times higher than in plasma. The side effects of

Table 65.1 Percentage of patients with various side effects during treatment with antithyroid drugs

Side effect	Percentage[1]	Relation with dosage
Rash	2-25	Yes
Polyarthralgias	1.6	Yes
Leukopenia	0.4	Yes
Agranulocytosis	0.1-1.2	Yes
Cholestatic jaundice	0.2-0.8	Unknown
Hepatocellular necrosis	0.2	Unknown

[1]Range of percentages taken from the literature.

Table 65.2 Selected pharmacokinetic features of antithyroid drugs

	Propylthiouracil	Methimazole
Plasma protein binding	~ 75%	Nil
Plasma half-life	75 min	~ 4–6 h
Volume of distribution	~ 20 liters	40 liters
Metabolism of drug during illness:		
– severe liver disease	Normal	Decreased
– severe kidney disease	Normal	Normal
Transplacental passage	Low	Increased
Levels in breast milk	Low	Increased

antithyroid drugs are usually mild (e.g., an itching rash), but more serious untoward reactions may occur (Tab. 65.1). Propylthiouracil is associated with more side effects than methimazole, and for propylthiouracil, the side effects are not dose-related as they are for methimazole. The most serious side effect is agranulocytosis, which may occur at any time during treatment but usually during the first few weeks when highest doses are used. Because agranulocytosis may develop rapidly, periodic measurement of white blood cell counts is of little help. Patients should be instructed to report immediately on occurrence of fever, sore throat, rash, and/or arthralgias.

Agranulocytosis – and the other side effects – are reversible; in severe cases, the administration of recombinant human granulocyte colony-stimulating factor (G-CSF) (see Chap. 51) may hasten recovery. Alleviation of the hyperthyroidism (by antithyroid drugs or other means) is associated with changed metabolism of a number of other pharmacologic compounds compared with the hyperthyroid state. Usually doses should be reduced.

Thyrotoxicosis occurs de novo in about 0.2% of pregnancies, most often due to Graves' disease. Women on antithyroid drug therapy are also fertile once euthyroidism is reached, and with a chronic disease liable to relapse, it is often advisable to let the woman become pregnant while on antithyroid drugs in a low dose and after at least 6 months of therapy (to allow the (TPAbs) to decrease and the woman to regain her physical strength and psychological balance). Antithyroid drugs are the treatment of choice, and although propylthiouracil is theoretically more appropriate during pregnancy due to less placental and milk transfer, no adverse reactions or changes in thyroid function has been described in fetuses or neonates when using a low titration dose of either of the drugs.

Radioactive iodine Iodine-131(^{131}I) is used for the treatment of both thyrotoxicosis and nontoxic goiter as well as for ablation in thyroid carcinoma. The radioactive emission includes both gamma rays and beta particles, and it has a half-life of 8 days, over 99% of its radiation being expended within 56 days. ^{131}I is efficiently and rapidly trapped by the thyroid; it is incorporated into the iodoaminoacids and deposited in the colloid of the follicles, from where it is gradually liberated. Cell destruction is done primarily by the beta particles. Small dosages of radioactive iodine have no influence on thyroid function, whereas larger doses do because of necrosis of the follicular cells.

Radioactive iodine is used mainly for treatment of hyperthyroidism, usually after first rendering the patient euthyroid with antithyroid drugs. The indications vary throughout the world but include initial therapy for Graves' disease, therapy for relapse of Graves' disease after an initial course of antithyroid drugs (usually between 6 months and 2 years), and definitive therapy for uni- and multinodular goiters. The cost of radioiodine therapy is low, and the treatment does not require hospitalization.

^{131}I therapy is used at higher doses to ablate the thyroid in thyroid carcinoma, and all these patients end with intended hypothyroidism and lifelong levothyroxine sodium suppression. In recent years, an increasing number of patients with nontoxic benign nodular goiters (and some diffuse goiters) also are being treated with ^{131}I instead of by surgery. This strategy is controversial, however. The dosages used are similar to those used for treatment of hyperthyroidism, and the radiation precautions also are similar. These patients should not be pretreated with antithyroid drugs, but careful follow-up for development of hypothyroidism should be undertaken.

Sodium iodide ^{131}I is carrier-free and available for oral administration either as a solution or in capsules. The effective dose depends primarily on the size of the thyroid, the iodine uptake of the gland, and the release of radioactive iodine subsequent to its deposition in the colloid. Furthermore, patients with nodular goiters with hyperthyroidism require a larger dose than patients with Graves' disease to obtain euthyroidism. There exist several ways of calculating the dose by including one or more of the following: a size measure either by palpation or ultrasound, 24-hour ^{131}I uptake, and the biologic half-life from the thyroid gland. Most centers include a 50% larger dose per gram of tissue in nodular disease compared with diffuse hyperthyroidism (Graves' disease). The optimal dose per gram of tissue thus varies from 80 to 150 mCi; the usual total dose per treatment ranges from 4 to 15 mCi. Owing to the nonpredictability of response to a sophisticated dose calculation, it has been suggested – with success – to simplify the treatment regimen by giving a fixed dose of either 5, 10, or 15 mCi for small, moderate, and large goiters, respectively. Most patients (one-half to two-thirds) are cured by a single dose, one-third to one-fifth require two doses, and the remainder require three doses or more before the hyperthyroidism is relieved. If very high doses are used, hypothyroidism tends to develop within a few months. If an optimal dose is used and the patient is pretreated to euthyroidism with antithyroid drugs in order to prevent exacerbation of

Table 65.3 Examples of commonly used Iodine-containing drugs

Drugs	Iodine content
Oral or local	
Amiodarone	75 mg/tablet
Calcium iodide	26 mg/ml
Iodoquinol	136 mg/tablet
Iodine-containing vitamins	0.15 mg/tablet
Kelp	0.15 mg/tablet
Potassium iodide	145 mg/tablet
Lugol's solution	6.3 mg/drop
Saturated potassium iodide	38 mg/drop
Parenteral preparations	
Sodium iodide, 10% solution	85 mg/ml
Topical antiseptics	
Iodoquinol cream	6 mg/g
Iodine tincture	40 mg/ml
Iodoform gauze	4.8 mg/100 mg
Radiology contrast agents	
Iopanoic acid	333 mg/tablet
Ipodate	308 mg/capsule
Iothalamate	480 mg/ml
Iohexol	463 mg/ml

hyperthyroidism from release of thyroid hormone from the damaged follicles, the disease usually abates over a period of 2 to 3 months, and the antithyroid drugs can be stopped usually after 4 to 6 months.

The only absolute contraindication to radioactive iodine therapy is pregnancy. Most countries have an arbitrary age limit of 35 to 40 years, especially in females with a pregnancy wish. The use of iodine compounds (Tab. 65.3) may preclude treatment with radioactive iodine as well as radioactive imaging of the thyroid gland for many months. Apart from during ongoing pregnancy, the radiation from the therapy is not considered dangerous in relation to future pregnancies or otherwise. The main complications have been associated with worsening of thyroid autoimmunity, i.e., confined to Graves' disease and not nodular goiters or cancer. The main concerns are (1) the massive increase in thyroid-stimulating immunoglobulins (and other thyroid autoantibodies) after radioactive iodine and (2) worsening (or even precipitation) of thyroid-related ophthalmopathy. If radioactive iodine therapy is indicated and chosen over other types of therapy, a 3-month course of glucocorticoid treatment may prevent worsening of the eye disease.

The chief disadvantage of the use of radioactive iodine is the high incidence of delayed hypothyroidism. It is therefore necessary to follow the patient lifelong (or until occurrence of hypothyroidism and institution of relevant therapy) with annual assessments of the thyroid function. The risk of hypothyroidism is higher in Graves' disease, perhaps because of the natural progression of the disease compared with nodular disease, where the nonautonomous thyroid tissue is preserved. A minor disadvantage is the time lapse from giving the patient radioactive iodine to obtaining euthyroidism. While awaiting the full effect, antithyroid drugs can be given (they should be withheld for a few days before and after the therapeutic dose of ^{131}I). Also, beta-blockers such as propranolol are useful to alleviate the symptoms of hyperthyroidism.

Iodide is the oldest substance for control of the signs and symptoms of hyperthyroidism. High concentrations of iodide appear to influence all aspects of iodine metabolism of the thyroid gland, including an acute inhibition of the synthesis of iodothyronines and of the release of thyroid hormones. The response to iodide in patients with hyperthyroidism is very rapid, within 24 hours, reducing the basal metabolic rate dramatically. The maximal effect is obtained after 10 to 15 days, after which the beneficial effect disappears. If treatment is continued, hyperthyroidism often returns to the initial level, or a severe worsening may occur. For this reason, iodide is limited to the treatment of hyperthyroidism in the preoperative period in preparation for thyroidectomy and in conjunction with antithyroid drugs and propranolol in the treatment of thyrotoxic crises. Another use of iodide has been to protect the thyroid from radioactive fallout following a nuclear accident. In Poland this was achieved in 1986 after the accident at the Chernobyl reactor. The dose used is 30 to 100 mg daily.

Several iodine-containing drugs exist (Tab. 65.3). For pretreatment before surgery, often a strong iodine solution (Lugol's solution) is used with 5% iodine and 10% potassium iodide, yielding 6.3 mg per drop. Saturated potassium iodide solution is also available, providing 38 mg per drop. The usual dosage is 3 to 5 drops of Lugol's solution or 1 to 3 drops of saturated potassium iodide 3 times a day. This dosage is by far in excess of the needed amount. A number of other drugs contain iodine that may have implications for developing thyroid disorders or for inducing complications during treatment of hyperthyroidism. This is particularly true for amiodarone (an iodine-rich antiarrhythmic drug), which may induce both hypo- and hyperthyroidism. Treatment of the hyperthyroid condition is very difficult due to blockage of the iodide pump and therefore a reduced access of both antithyroid drugs and radioactive iodine. Two types of hyperthyroidism are seen: overproduction of thyroid hormones or a destructive thyroiditis-like reaction. The former can in severe cases be treated with a combination of antithyroid drugs and perchlorate (which, however, has many side effects); the latter often needs supplementation with glucocorticoids.

Untoward reactions to iodine-containing compounds may be rather severe in some patients and may include angioedema and swelling of the larynx. Most commonly a skin rash is seen. The symptoms subside within a few days after stopping iodine ingestion. The effects on thyroid function, however, remain for several months, maybe even more than a year.

Nontoxic goiter

Most cases of nontoxic goiter do not require any therapy, such as a small or moderate diffuse or nodular goiter without significant symptoms. In some cases of compression symptoms, levothyroxine may be tried as suppressive therapy. The rationale is that by suppressing TSH, the growth-stimulating effect also is reduced. Levothyroxine has its most pronounced effect in diffuse goiter and no effect in cases of autonomy, where TSH is already suppressed. In patients with a single "cold" nodule, surgery is often indicated due to the small risk of the nodule being malignant. The remaining patients with larger diffuse or multinodular goiters can be treated either with radioactive iodine or with surgery. The complications of surgery include damage to the recurrent laryngeal nerve, hypothyroidism, bleeding, and wound infection. Radioactive iodine is simple and only complicated by a risk of hypothyroidism. The effect, however, is slow (months up to 2 years), and in some cases the goiter does not shrink sufficiently. Eventually, most cases of nontoxic goiter in the world may be prevented by iodine prophylaxis of the population (by iodized salt, iodized oil, or otherwise).

Suggested readings

ASTWOOD EB. Treatment of hyperthyroidism with thiourea and thiouracil. JAMA 1943;122:78-89.

BARTALENA L, MARCOCCI C, BOGAZZI F, et al. Relation between therapy for hyperthyroidism and the course of Graves' ophthalmopathy. N Engl J Med 1998;338:73-8.

BRAVERMAN, LE, UTIGER RD (eds). Werner and Ingbar's The Thyroid.. Philadelphia, Lippincott-Raven, 1996.

COOPER DS. Subclinical hypothyroidism. Adv Endocrinol Metab 1991;2:77-89.

DEMERS LM, WARTOFSKY L, KEEFER JH, et al. Standards of laboratory practice symposium on thyroid-function testing. Clin Chem 1996;42:119-92.

FARWELL AP, BRAVERMANN LE. Thyroid and antithyroid drugs. In: Wonsiewics MJ, McCurdy P, eds. Goodman & Gilman's The Pharmacological Basis of Therapeutics, 9th ed. New York: McGraw-Hill, 1996:1383-409.

FELDT-RASMUSSEN U, GLINOER D, ORGIAZZI J. Reassessment of antithyroid drug therapy of Graves' disease. Annu Rev Med 1993;44:323-34.

FELDT-RASMUSSEN U, SCHLEUSENER H, CARAYON P. Meta-analysis evaluation of the impact of thyrotropin receptor antibodies on long-term remission after medical therapy of Graves' disease. J Clin Endocrinol Metab 1994;78:98-102.

GLINOER D. Maternal thyroid function during pregnancy. J Endocrinol Invest 1993;16:374-8.

HAYS MT, NIELSEN KR. Human thyroxine absorption: Age effects and methodological analyses. Thyroid 1994;4:55-64.

WARTOFSKY L, GLINOER D, SOLOMON B, et al. Differences and similarities in the diagnosis and treatment of Graves' disease in Europe, Japan and the United States. Thyroid 1991;1:29-35.

WIERSINGA WM. Amiodarone and the thyroid. In: Weetman AP, Grossman A, eds. Handbook of Experimental Pharmacology, Vol 128: Pharmacotherapeutics of the Thyroid Gland. Berlin: Springer-Verlag, 1997;225-87.

Growth hormone and prolactin

Fabio Celotti, Giuseppe Oppizzi

GROWTH HORMONE DEFICIENCY

At the end of the first month of fetal life, the hypothalamic sulcus is already recognizable, being the first forebrain region to differentiate. Soon after, the median eminence undergoes a rapid differentiation as the specific nuclei and neurotransmitters appear. During the third month, hypothalamic hormones already can be demonstrated, and the relative fiber tracts arise, as well as their terminations close to the capillary loops in the external median eminence. They start to affect pituitary secretion.

Although many neurohormones are produced in several other central nervous system (CNS) areas, as well as in quite distant extracerebral sites such as the exocrine pancreas and gastrointestinal mucosa, the quantitatively most important production location that affects pituitary hormones is concentrated in a small neuronal area within the hypothalamus (Tab. 66.1).

The functional relationships between the hypothalamus and the pituitary can be grouped into three different levels of interactions: (1) the above-mentioned hypothalamic neurosecretions, (2) the feedback effects of circulating pituitary hormones, and (3) paracrine and autocrine effects of the secretions of the pituitary itself.

All three factors interact in a complex way, and the final plasma levels of each pituitary hormone represent in

Table 66.1 Major hypothalamic hypophyseotropic hormones

Neurohormone	Structure	Main site of production	Main activity
Corticotropin-releasing hormone (CRF)	41 aa peptide	Paraventricular nucleus	Synthesis/release of ACTH and POMC[1] derivatives
Growth hormone-releasing hormone (GHRH)	44 aa peptide	Arcuate nucleus, ventromedial	Synthesis and release of GH
Gonadotropin-releasing hormone (GnRH)	10 aa peptide	Arcuate nucleus, lamina terminalis	Synthesis and release of LH and FSH
Thyrotropin-releasing hormone (TRH)	3 aa peptide	Paraventricular nucleus	Synthesis and release of TSH and PRL[2]
Vasoactive intestinal peptide (VIP)	28 aa peptide	Widespread in hypothalams	Release of PRL[2]
Somatotropin-release-inhibiting hormone (SRIH)	14 (28) aa peptide	Periventricular area	Inhibits synthesis and release of GH and TSH
Dopamine	Catecholamine	Arcuate nucleus	Synthesis release of PRL
Arginine vasopressin (AVP)	9 aa peptide	Supraoptic and paraventricular	Release of ACTH

[1]Pro-opiomelanocorticotropin.
[2]Both TRH and VIP release PRL, but are not considered physiological regulators.
[3](PRL= prolactin; aa= aminoacids.)

each instant the result of their interplay on one side and of the degradation pathways on the other. The complex vascularization of the basal hypothalamus and its venous drainage to the pituitary of "arteriolar" blood supply are similar to the liver portal system and are termed the *hypophyseal portal circulation*. Through this blood supply, the neurohormones reach the anterior pituitary to modulate synthesis and secretion of tropic hormones. The whole posterior pituitary lobe (neurohypophysis) is only composed of nerve terminals from the two main nuclei of the anterior hypothalamus, with the function of transporting their neurohormones oxytocin and vasopressin. The two specific hypothalamic neuropeptides, growth hormone-releasing hormone (GHRH) and somatostatin (SRIF), control in opposite ways the release of growth hormone (GH).

Pituitary insufficiency may arise following defects in specific hormone-secreting cells as well as defects in hypothalamic hormones. For example, lack of gonadotropin-releasing hormone (GnRH) may give rise to hypogonadotropic amenorrhea. The availability of neurohormones has allowed development of clinical tests to trace a primitive hypothalamic or pituitary defect.

Among defects of hypothalamic hormone availability, idiopathic GH defects can respond to the GHRH test, and this is postulated as the underlying cause in most patients with growth failure and lack of GH response to classic stimulatory tests.

GROWTH HORMONE-RELEASING HORMONE (GHRH)

Human GHRH is a polypeptide of 44 amino acid residues originating from a 108-amino-acid (aa) precursor. A 40-amino-acid peptide is also present in both the hypothalamus and the pancreas and shows the same activity; synthetic peptides that contain only the first 29 amino acids are fully active and almost as potent as full-length GHRH.

GHRH binds to a G protein-coupled receptor and activates adenylcyclase, thus increasing AMP and cytosolic Ca^{2+} levels in somatotropes. GH synthesis is thus stimulated. When GHRH is given iv to normal subjects (1 μg/kg as a bolus), a marked stimulation of GH release occurs within 15 to 30 minutes. The amplitude of peak plasma levels is an inverse function of the endogenous somatostatin tone (from twice to tenfold or more baseline levels) either between subjects or within the same subject retested. However, when somatostatinergic tone is blocked by giving pyridostigmine (60 mg orally) 60 minutes before GHRH administration, this variability disappears in normal children, a peak of greater than 20 ng/ml is regularly observed, and there is no overlapping with GH-deficient patients (who will not reach 7 ng/ml).

Use of GHRH in the treatment of growth failure

Besides its use as a diagnostic tool, GHRH has been investigated in-depth as a therapeutic agent. In particular, it was first given in a pulsatile pattern by means of a portable minipump (1-3 μg/kg per pulse every 3 h sc), and a marked increase in GH levels, insulin-like growth factor 1 (IGF-1) secretion, and growth rate were recorded during a 6-month treatment course. More than 100 "GH-deficient" children have been studied worldwide during treatment with this neurohormone for periods of up to 30 months. The common results were a high percentage of responsive patients but a progressive decline in growth during prolonged therapy. Surprisingly, GHRH proved effective also when given by continuous subcutaneous infusion and even in a single daily dose (2-18 μg/kg).

The use of this agent as a therapeutic tool has been now abandoned, while its diagnostic use is still being exploited.

GHRH is available for human use as both the 1-29 (sermorelin) and 1-44 aa form, as a water-soluble lyophilized powder containing 50 μg of active principle. An intravenous bolus of 1 μg/kg is the usual recommended dose for the test of GH secretion

GROWTH HORMONE-RELEASING PEPTIDES (GHRPs)

The family of GH-releasing peptides includes very potent analogues such as GHRP-I and hexarelin, with modified structures that render them orally or intranasally absorbed and bioavailable. Moreover, new orally active nonpeptidyl secretagogues (L-163,191 or MK-0677) have been tested and shown effective in normal and GH-deficient children.

GHRPs release GH mainly through specific hypothalamic stimulation, as well as stimulation at the pituitary level, although to a lesser degree. Their specificity for GH release is less clear-cut when compared with GHRH, since they also can stimulate adrenocorticotropic hormone (ACTH), cortisol, and prolactin secretion. At a dose of 1 μg/kg iv, GHRP leads to a higher and more reproducible GH peak than the same dose of GHRH. In humans, the two agents act synergistically, since very low doses of GHRP can greatly potentiate the GHRH-induced GH response. One of the postulated mechanisms of action implies an antagonism of somatostatin activity at the hypothalamic level. Although specific receptors for hexarelin have been identified recently in some tumoral pituitary cells, pointing also to a direct effect, the integrity of the hypothalamic-pituitary unit is essential for GHRP effects.

Preliminary clinical trials with orally active agents, such as MK-0677, clearly indicate their ability to increase GH pulsatility, IGF-1 levels, and growth rate in children. However, GHRP is not yet available for clinical use except in controlled trials. The same applies for the nonpeptide molecules. In the near future, the treatment of children of short stature, adult patients with other GH defects or deficiencies, patients with catabolic conditions, or even the normal elderly certainly will include some of these agents.

GROWTH HORMONE (GH)

The GH secreted by the pituitary is a mixture of peptides that can be distinguished on the basis of size. The principal form is a single polypeptide of 191 aa residues (22 kDa) that has two disulfide bonds and is not glycosylated. From 5 to 10% of circulating GH has a molecular mass of 20 kDa. The physiologic significance of other larger or smaller forms is unclear. The placenta also produces an additional 22-kDa GH variant that is distinguishable from the pituitary product.

GH is the most abundant of the anterior pituitary hormones. It is synthesized and secreted by somatotrophs, which account for about 50% of the hormone-secreting cells of the anterior pituitary. The amount of GH secreted during a 24-hour period is high in children, reaches maximal levels during puberty, and then decreases to its lowest levels during adulthood. Secretion is pulsatile and occurs in discrete but irregular bursts. Between these secretory pulses, the concentration of circulating GH falls to undetectable levels. For these reasons, single determinations of plasma GH levels during the day or over short periods of time are of little value in the diagnosis of GH deficiency. Instead, measurements are done during a 24-hour period or following an acute stimulation test (see below).

This pulsatile release of somatotrophs is regulated by GHRH, which is stimulatory, and by somatostatin, which inhibits GH release. These hypothalamic factors bind to specific receptors on the somatotrophs and activate G proteins, leading to changes in cyclic AMP and intracellular Ca^{2+} concentrations. All the neurotransmitters, drugs, and metabolites stimulating GH secretion act through the hypothalamus, mostly by suppressing somatostatin but in a few cases also by increasing the secretion of GHRH.

When GH deficiency is suspected, one or more provocative tests can be used to assess the capacity of the pituitary to secrete GH. These tests include arginine infusion, insulin hypoglycemia, clonidine, levodopa, etc. All these agents result in a peak of GH release within 30 to 60 minutes. If excessive release of GH is suspected, a suppression test also can be performed by inducing hyperglycemia (oral glucose tolerance test). Although defects can be detected using these tests, they cannot distinguish whether the lesion exists at the level of the hypothalamus or the pituitary.

GH induces in several tissues the production and secretion of the somatomedin IGF-1, the principal mediator of several of the actions of GH, particularly the growth-promoting effect. The IGF-1 receptor is structurally related to the insulin receptor (see Chap. 68) and has intrinsic tyrosine kinase activity, which ultimately is responsible for mediating the hormonal signal and is present in all tissues studied. The liver is the major source of circulating IGF-1, but probably more relevant to the growth effects of GH is on peripheral synthesis at the level of cartilage, where it acts locally as paracrine modulator.

Physiologic effects of GH

GH has direct effects on lipid and glucose metabolism, but its anabolic and growth-promoting effects are mediated by somatomedins (IGF). These physiologic effects can be grouped as direct and indirect:

Direct actions These include stimulated IGF synthesis, hydrolysis of triglycerides in adipose cells, decreased glucose utilization, stimulation of hepatic glucose output (opposite to insulin effect), increased amino acid entry into cells and protein synthesis, and blockade of the activity of receptor-bound insulin. The final metabolic effect is a shift of fuel production from carbohydrates to fat.

Indirect effects (i.e., mediated by IGF) These include anabolic and growth-promoting activity by directly stimulating chondrogenesis, maturation, and growth of bone and soft tissues.

GH preparations

Somatropin indicates a GH molecule with the amino acid sequence identical to native human GH, abbreviated as hGH when derived from human pituitaries or as rhGH when obtained by recombinant DNA technique. *Somatrem* indicates a methionine derivative of recombinant hGH (met-hGH). This latter preparation is more antigenic, but this aspect is considered clinically irrelevant from the points of view of safety and effectiveness.

The potency of available preparations is generally expressed in International Units (International standard WHO rhGH with 1 mg = 3 IU); there is a general tendency in Europe to shift from the older dosing in units to the newer milligram per day units (see below). When GH was extracted from human pituitaries, the range of potency of the products obtained varied according to the extraction and purification methods used. At present, recombinant GH products are essentially equivalent, and this system probably will be changed to in vitro binding assays with GH receptors. The distribution of human-derived GH was stopped in 1985 because of a causal relation between its use and Creutzfeldt-Jacob disease; rhGH was already under clinical investigation and soon became available to replace the human product.

Clinical indications and doses GH is indicated for the treatment of pediatric patients who have growth failure due to inadequate endogenous growth hormone secretion, Turner syndrome with short stature, or chronic renal failure with short stature. In adult patients it is indicated for GH deficiency secondary to pituitary tumors or to their treatment.

In young adults, endogenous GH production rate has been calculated to be 0.25 mg/m^2 of body surface, and about twice this value is attained at puberty. These values formed the basis for a reasonable replacement dose. The dose of the hormone may be tailored to the pubertal stage, age, or peripheral growth factor responses (mainly IGF-1 and its binding protein BP3).

The usual recommended doses in GH-deficient children range from 0.17 to 0.35 mg/kg of body weight per week given in as daily sc administrations. The alternate-day dosing used in the past has been completely replaced by this more effective daily regimen. There is a clear-cut logarithmic relation between the growth response observed and the dose given. Moreover, the younger the patient, the greater is the effect. Children with complete GH deficiency respond better than children with "partial" GH defects.

Intramuscular and sc routes lead to the same growth effects, but the latter is preferred because it is less painful and easier to administer. Maximal plasma concentrations are observed 2 to 4 hours after sc injection, with an apparent terminal half-life of 2 hours. About 40 to 50% of circulating GH is bound to a specific GH-binding protein, ultimately derived from membrane GH receptors. Increased plasma IGF-1 levels appear within 12 hours and peak after 24 hours. Therefore, the biologic effects of a given dose greatly outlast its plasma apparent disappearance.

Clinical effects. Skeletal growth increases due to the action on the epiphyseal plates of the long bones and the increase in IGF-1 that plays a direct role on these tissues. Alkaline phosphatase in serum is also increased during treatment.

In the typical GH-deficient patient, pretreatment growth rates of 3 to 4 cm/year may accelerate up to 10 to 12 cm/year during the first year of therapy; in the second year, the velocity slows to 7 to 9 cm/year; and in subsequent years, a progressive decrease is observed. A more correct parameter frequently used to evaluate and quantify growth changes is the standard deviation score (SDS), which provides more clinically useful information describing the approach of patients to normal height. Patients with a mean pretreatment score lower than –3.6 to –5 SDS (i.e., three or four times the standard deviation lower than mean height for the age) may attain values of –1.5 to –0.7 SDS as final height with therapy.

It is possible to obtain these excellent results only when (1) diagnosis and treatment start early, (2) doses are adjusted frequently on the basis of weight and height changes, (3) attention is paid to compliance, and (4) treatment is continued until bone growth plates close.

The observation that final height is correlated with the height recorded at the onset of puberty in GH-deficient patients corroborates the importance of concentrating every effort on obtaining the maximal prepubertal growth velocity. Some authors also advocate increasing the daily doses in these patients during puberty to imitate the spontaneous GH hypersecretion that is responsible for the growth spurt commonly observed during puberty and lasting for about 2 years. After this huge acceleration in growth, the epiphyseal cartilage almost rules out any further growth potential. The possibility of delaying puberty in these patients with GnRH superagonists, together with increased rhGH regimens, may permit the attainment of greater final heights.

Linear growth is facilitated in part by increased cellular protein synthesis. Nitrogen retention, as demonstrated by decreased urinary nitrogen excretion and serum urea nitrogen level, immediately follows GH administration. The positive nitrogen balance observed is the result of the direct effect of the hormone on amino acid entry into the cells of several different tissues such as muscle, heart, and liver.

Pediatric patients with GH deficiency, and in particular those with multiple pituitary hormone deficiency, frequently experience spontaneous fasting hypoglycemia that improves with treatment with GH. Sometimes large doses of GH can impair glucose tolerance. An increased insulin secretion during prolonged treatment is well documented and is interpreted as a compensatory paraphysiologic consequence of the increased circulating levels of GH, an antagonist of insulin action. Close attention must be paid to the appearance of clinical symptoms of glucose intolerance during prolonged therapy with high doses or concomitant corticosteroid treatment.

GH-deficient patients typically show a greater than normal fat tissue to lean body mass ratio than normal children. GH treatment results in lipid mobilization from fat stores and a consequent increase in plasma levels of free fatty acids. When adult GH-deficient patients are treated with replacement doses of the hormone, these changes are clinically evident and lead to an overall moderate weight loss and a redistribution of body mass with decreased fat tissue and increased muscle mass.

Other indications of GH treatment Chronic renal failure during childhood leads to the loss of growth potential due to various extrapituitary mechanisms including acidosis, accumulation of toxins, loss of urinary proteins, insufficient calorie intake, anemia, etc. Spontaneous GH levels are in the normal to high range, as well as the responses to stimulatory tests. IGF-1, however, is normal to low, and the binding protein BP3 is very low, suggesting a state of acquired partial "resistance" to GH activity. After successful renal transplantation, only about 60% of these children undergo a catch-up growth. GH therapy has been shown to be effective in increasing growth rate; doses should be about twice that used in pure GH deficiency. The decline in GH effect with advancing treatment years seems greater than observed in GH deficiency.

The *adult GH deficiency syndrome* is characterized by lower lean body mass, increased water, increased visceral adipose tissue, decreased bone mass, dyslipidemia, and increased prevalence of atherosclerosis and cardiovascular mortality. The doses of GH for replacement range between 0.05 and 0.1 mg/kg per week, and the maintenance dose can be reached easily by monitoring IGF-1 plasma levels.

New potential indications Because of its anabolic effects, GH is under investigation as an adjunct in the treatment of several catabolic conditions such as burn injuries, surgery, and malabsorption. The positive effects of growth hormone on Ca^{2+} retention and on osteogenesis also may be of use in the treatment of osteoporosis and nonhealing fractures.

The availability of large quantities of recombinant GH has allowed its evaluation in other pathophysiologic conditions. GH administration has been shown to be effective in accelerating the growth rate of children with constitutional growth delay and of short children without GH deficiency. In addition to its questionable use in "enhancing" height in normal children, GH also has a great potential for misuse in adults. Adult athletes may seek GH to increase muscle mass and decrease body fat in a manner that is poorly detectable by current drug abuse testing programs.

Clinical studies with rhGH in adults with childhood-onset GH deficiency have shown a beneficial effect on myocardial wall thickness and cardiac index; moreover, a significant improvement in cardiac function in adults with dilated cardiomyopathy also has been demonstrated. In patients with adult-onset GH deficiency, exercise capacity and diastolic function also have improved. The favorable effect on lipid profile (decrease in low-density lipoprotein and an increase in high-density lipoprotein cholesterol levels) also allows the potential for a positive overall effect on the cardiovascular system.

Contraindications GH should not be used when there is evidence of tumors. Intracranial lesions must be inactive and antitumor therapy completed prior to institution of this treatment. This is of relevance for two main categories of pediatric patients with GH deficiency: (1) those who received cranial radiotherapy as part of the treatment for lymphoproliferative diseases and in whom the GH deficit is the consequence of irradiation on a previously healthy pituitary, and (2) those operated on for craniopharyngioma or other tumors of the hypothalamic-pituitary area.

The large and continuously updated databases concerning GH-deficient children [the National Cooperative Growth Study (NCGS) in the United States and the Kabi International Growth Study (KIGS) in Europe] have not indicated up to the present an increased incidence of tumor recurrence in comparison with non-GH-treated control patients.

Side effects and warnings Pain and discomfort from GH injections are minimal, but sc injections frequently lead to local lipoatrophy if the same site of injection is used continuously. It is therefore recommended that the defined site of injection be changed every day. GH antibodies may form during treatment, a phenomenon more pronounced in the past with human incompletely purified products but also present with met-hGH. The clinical relevance of these antibodies, present in 10 to 20% of treated patients, is modest, and they do not seem to diminish the effectiveness of therapy.

Hypothyroidism may develop during GH treatment, or better, it could be unmasked by this treatment. The thyroid state should be monitored carefully, especially in the first months of GH therapy, by periodic tests, and treatment should be instituted when indicated. Patients with coexisting ACTH deficiency should have their glucocorticoid replacement dose carefully adjusted so as to avoid an inhibitory effect on growth.

GROWTH HORMONE (GH) HYPERSECRETION

Acromegaly and gigantism, the syndromes produced by GH hypersecretion, are due in 99% of the patients to a primary pituitary adenoma, whereas in the remaining patients they may be the result of a hypothalamic or ectopic tumor (e.g., gangliocytoma, bronchial, or pancreatic) that produces GH-releasing hormone (GHRH). Ectopic secretion of GH itself by a pancreatic islet cell tumor also has been described but is a rare event. The prevalence of GH-secreting adenomas is 50 to 80 cases per million.

Somatotropin adenomas are discrete tumors, and the remaining pituitary gland does not show hyperplasia of somatotropic cells. This observation has two relevant implications: with successful tumor removal recurrence is rare, and the etiology is apparently not due to a hypothalamic overstimulation producing hyperplasia. As a matter of fact, a point mutation in a subunit of the Gs protein that constitutively activates adenylcyclase has been identified in several GH-secreting tumors.

Disease presentation

The clinical features of acromegaly develop insidiously and progressively over many years, so they may go unnoticed until complications develop. Manifestations may be due to excessive GH secretion, to the tumor itself (mass effects), to hypopituitarism, to the metabolic consequences of the disease, or to a combination of factors. It suffices to say that acromegaly is a severe systemic disease associated with bony and soft tissue overgrowth (producing progressive disfigurement and osteoarthritis) that shortens life expectancy owing to respiratory, metabolic, and cardiovascular complications and, possibly, to an increased prevalence of malignant disorders of the gastrointestinal tract.

Acromegaly and gigantism (i.e., GH hypersecretion occurring before pubertal epiphysial closure) are generally clinically clear and can be confirmed by measurement of GH plasma levels. However, since secretion of GH is pulsatile, frequent venous sampling every 5 to 20 minutes over 24 hours may be necessary to document the increased GH secretion. However, the diagnosis of acromegaly also can be made easily in outpatients by two simple biochemical tests: the oral glucose tolerance test and measurement of IGF-I (insulin like growth factor I) plasma concentrations. In patients with acromegaly, the normal GH suppression after an oral glucose load does not occur, and a paradoxical GH increase is seen commonly. Moreover, IGF-I concentrations, which are stable and represent a function of the integrated 24-hour GH secretion, are increased. Finally, tumor visualization by CT or MRI scans confirms the diagnosis.

At variance with prolactinomas, at the time of diagnosis 75% of somatotropic adenomas are macroadenomas. GH levels tend to correlate with tumor size.

Treatment

The objectives of therapy are (1) return of GH and IGF-I levels to normal, (2) stabilization or decrease in tumor size, (3) preservation of normal pituitary function, and (4) correction of clinical signs and symptoms.

Variables that still remain controversial are the degree of GH suppression needed to achieve treatment success and what is the best treatment for suppression of GH, IGF-I, or both. Although basal GH values of less than 5 µg/liter formerly were considered to indicate cure, better criteria appear to be a value of less than 2.5 µg/liter (average of at least three to five samples), GH concentrations after suppression with the oral glucose tolerance test less than 2.0 µg/liter, and a normal IGF-I level for age; patients with GH values between 2.5 and 5 µg/liter may have persistent symptoms and increased IGF-I concentrations. Currently available treatment options include surgery, irradiation, and pharmacologic suppression of GH by dopamine agonists or somatostatin analogues. Many patients, particularly those with large adenomas, require more than one type of treatment.

Nonpharmacologic treatment

Surgery by the transphenoidal route has the advantage of producing a rapid therapeutic response, reducing tumor mass and causing immediate improvement in visual abnormalities, headache, and symptoms of excessive GH secretion; it is potentially curative and is the preferred initial treatment. The success of this procedure depends on the completeness of the resection and hence on the size of the tumor and experience of the surgeon. Cure rates vary from 80% for microadenomas to less than 50% for tumors larger than 1 cm in diameter. Surgical mortality is low and complications, such as cerebrospinal fluid (CSF) rhinorrhea, arachnoiditis, and temporary or permanent diabetes insipidus, are rare. Pituitary failure, however, is reported in about 20 to 30% of patients with macroadenomas.

Radiation therapy is currently indicated for patients with contraindications to surgery or with persistent disease after surgery. The main reason is that the response to radiotherapy is slow in producing both a prompt reduction of tumor size and GH hypersecretion; up to 5 years may elapse before a clinically significant decrease in GH is achieved. Moreover, besides rare complications such as optic nerve injury, cranial nerve palsy, impaired memory, lethargy, and local tissue necrosis, radiation damage to the surrounding normal pituitary tissue leads to hypopituitarism in most patients within 10 years.

Drug therapy

Drug therapy is now considered second-line therapy after surgery, but it is possible that the availability of new long-acting formulations of somatostatin analogues will allow reconsideration of this issue in the near future.

At variance with normal individuals, in about 50% of patients with acromegaly, dopamine agonists inhibit GH secretion. Most data have been obtained with bromocriptine. High doses of this compound, up to 20 mg/day, can improve symptoms in about 70% of the patients, but GH levels are reduced to less than 5 µg/liter only in 10 to 20% of patients, and tumor shrinkage occurs in only 10 to 15%. Since high doses are needed, side effects (see above) are commonly a limiting factor. The published evidence does not suggest that any other dopamine agonist has any advantage over bromocriptine.

Somatostatin is a 14-aminoacid (aa) cyclic peptide that represents the physiologic inhibitory controller of GH secretion. When administered parenterally, it suppresses GH secretion in healthy people and acromegalic patients. However, therapeutic use of the native peptide is hampered by its very short half-life (about 3 minutes). Longer-acting synthetic analogues of somatostatin have been developed and used effectively in the treatment of acromegaly. The two 8-aa cyclic peptides that are available clinically in most European countries are octreotide and lanreotide. These compounds maintain the cyclic structure of somatostatin, but introduction of D-aminoacids in key positions in their sequence inhibits the action of the catabolic peptidases; therefore, the half-life of both compounds is about 100 minutes after subcutaneous administration. A single subcutaneous dose of octreotide is able to suppress GH for up to 8 hours in normal and acromegalic patients. Lanreotide is even longer-acting. These compounds exert their antisecretory actions by binding almost exclusively to two of the five somatostatin receptor subtypes, namely, types 2 and 5. The chronic administration of these compounds does not produce tachyphylaxis.

The clinical experience with octreotide is rather extensive. The compound has been administered sc at average dosages of 100 to 200 µg every 8 hours. A combined analysis of 466 patients treated worldwide showed that octreotide administration lowered GH concentrations to less than 5 µg/liter in 49.8% of patients and to 2.5 µg/liter in 29.2%. Normal IGF-I concentrations were present in 39.9%, and tumor shrinkage (>20% decrease in size) was seen in 38.6%. About 90% of patients showed a rapid improvement in disease manifestations.

Side effects were minimal and mainly in the gastrointestinal tract (e.g., steatorrhea, abdominal cramps, nausea, and flatulence). These side effects usually are transient and remit in a few days even when treatment continues. Gallbladder abnormalities (e.g., sediment, sludge, microlithiasis, and gallstones) occur in about 20% of patients and may be due to decreased gallbladder contractility. Usually, however, they are asymptomatic.

Octreotide is 2000 times as potent as somatostatin in inhibiting GH secretion but only 1.5 to 2 times as potent in inhibiting insulin secretion. Although impairment of glucose tolerance or worsening of diabetes mellitus may occur, the GH-lowering effects of the drug may improve glucose tolerance. Inhibition of thyroid-stimulating hormone (TSH) does not result in hypothyroidism.

Depot preparations have been developed to allow injections only once or twice per month and to achieve stable serum concentrations of the drug, good clinical control of symptoms and signs, sustained GH and IGF-I suppression, and good compliance. At present, two depot preparations of long-acting somatostatin analogues are available in several countries. The first is a slow-release form of lanreotide (SR-Lanreotide), and the second is a slow-release form of octreotide incorporated into microspheres of a biodegradable polymer (LAR-Octreotide). SR-Lanreotide usually is given in 30-mg im injections every 10 to 14 days. In a recent study including 57 acromegalic patients evaluated at 12 months, IGF-I was normalized in 35% of patients, and GH levels were less than 5 µg/liter in 54%. Clinical improvement was seen in most patients. Of 33 patients (58%) with normal basal ultrasound examination of the gallbladder, 3 (9%) had developed asymptomatic gallstones or biliary sludge after 12 months. Adverse events generally were mild and transient.

Another study reported the long-term follow-up of a cohort of 22 acromegalic patients treated with SR-Lanreotide for 1 to 3 years. At the 6-month visit, mean GH values were 5 µg/liter or less in 68% and 2.5 µg/liter or less in 27% of patients, and these results remained unchanged during the 1 to 3 years of follow-up. During SR-Lanreotide treatment, the mean IGF-I concentrations remained in the normal range in 63% of patients. No "escape" occurred in any of the patients. A significant decrease in pituitary tumor volume was observed in 3 (13%) patients. The main side effects consisted of minor digestive problems over the 48 hours following each injection reported by 13 patients. Biannual gallbladder echographies revealed the occurrence of gallstones in 4 (18%) patients.

LAR-Octreotide has been administered at a monthly dose of 20 to 30 mg in different series of patients with acromegaly up to a total number of 175 patients. Decreases in GH concentrations below 5 µg/liter were recorded in 86 to 100% and below 2 µg/liter in 39 to 75%. Normal plasma IGF-I concentrations were achieved in 65.3% of patients after the last injection. Tumor shrinkage by more than 20% occurred in 71.8% of patients. The preparation was well tolerated; up to 50% of patients experienced mild to moderate side effects, but they were of short duration and generally subsided with continued drug administration.

The results achieved with the slow-release preparations, although preliminary, are indicative of a comparable efficacy with the standard subcutaneous treatment, but these preparations are probably better tolerated and accepted by patients. Thus, even if surgical resection remains a mainstay of therapy for acromegaly, long-acting formulations provide further advantages for pharmacotherapy, and in the future this therapeutic approach probably will not be limited to patients who have undergone unsuccessful transsphenoidal surgery or who are awaiting the therapeutic effect of external radiation. An issue that should be clarified still is whether the achievement of safe GH concentrations with any treatment improves mortality from cardiorespiratory or neoplastic diseases in acromegalic patients.

HYPERPROLACTINEMIA

Prolactin is the single pituitary hormone that in normal subjects is under inhibitory hypothalamic control exerted mainly by dopamine secretion through the portal circulation. Dopamine reaches the anterior pituitary from the arcuate and paraventricular nuclei of the hypothalamus. Lactotrophs, the pituitary cells that produce prolactin, constitute 15 to 20% of the normal pituitary gland and increase to 70% during pregnancy, under the influence of increased estrogen production, which stimulates growth and replication of these cells and increases prolactin secretion.

Pathophysiology

Hyperprolactinemia is the most common disorder of the anterior pituitary. Its etiology may be related to (1) autonomous production (pituitary adenomas), (2) any process interfering with dopamine synthesis, transport to the pituitary, action at lactotroph dopamine receptors (e.g., hypothalamic diseases or treatments with drugs that block synthesis, release, or action of dopamine, such as neuroleptics, antidepressants, antihypertensives), (3) increased estrogen stimulation, and (4) decreased clearance of prolactin (renal failure).

Microprolactinomas (<10 mm, found in two-thirds of patients) or macroprolactinomas (>10 mm) are the most common causes of hyperprolactinemia not related to drug use. These tumors are found very frequently in autopsy studies, the prevalence of microadenomas varying between 23 and 27%, whereas macroadenomas are less common. The vast majority of individuals bearing a microadenoma have no antemortem evidence of endocrine dysfunction, even if most of these tumors are immunocytochemically positive for prolactin. This indicates that tumor enlargement and/or hypersecretion of prolactin is not a necessary feature of the natural history of the tumor. This should be considered in deciding treatment, in particular when the tumor is incidentally imaged by a computed tomographic (CT) or magnetic resonance imaging (MRI) scan. Hyperprolactinemia due to pituitary adenomas certainly represents the most appropriate indication for medical treatment of prolactin excess and therefore is particularly considered in this chapter.

Disease presentation

The clinical presentation of hyperprolactinemia varies with sex, age, and duration and size of the tumor. Symptoms may be related to the compression produced by the tumor mass (e.g., headache, visual field defects, or cranial nerve involvement) or to the increased prolactin levels (e.g., hypogonadism, disturbance of the menstrual function, decreased libido, impotence, infertility, galactorrhea, or osteoporosis in the long term). Hypogonadism associated with hyperprolactinemia appears to be due to inhibition of hypothalamic release of luteinizing hormone-releasing hormone (LHRH), resulting in defective secretion of luteinizing hormone (LH) and follicle-stimulating hormone (FSH).

A single prolactin measurement may be sufficient to diagnose hyperprolactinemia if values exceed 200 µg/liter (in nonpregnant women), but since secretion of prolactin is pulsatile, at least three measurements are needed if values are lower. Although there is no simple test to distinguish the various causes of hyperprolactinemia, serum prolactin levels above 300 µg/liter are nearly always diagnostic of a prolactinoma; prolactinemia over 150 µg/liter in a nonpregnant patient is usually caused by a pituitary adenoma. Often the size of a prolactinoma correlates with its hormone output; in general, the larger the tumor, the higher are the prolactin levels. Many pharmacologic tests have been devised to distinguish tumoral from nontumoral hyperprolactinemia, but they are no longer in use because of their poor reliability in differential diagnosis. Neuroradiologic studies are mandatory to complete the diagnostic protocol because pituitary macroadenomas and most microadenomas are easily visualized on CT and MRI scans.

The goals of the treatment are to reduce the excessive hormone secretion, inhibit tumor growth, and if possible, to achieve permanent shrinkage of the adenoma.

Treatment

Nonpharmacologic treatment

Surgical removal of prolactinomas with or without pituitary irradiation and primary radiation therapy were the treatments of choice before an effective drug treatment was available. Hypophysectomy, now performed with the less invasive transsphenoidal microsurgical technique, is still the first-line therapy for nonresponding adenomas, but surgery has been replaced progressively by treatments with dopamine agonists in the remaining patients. Although, theoretically, the surgical approach offers the potential for cure, complete cure is actually achieved only in a minority of patients with large tumors, and even in patients with microadenomas the incidence of recurrences is considerable. Transsphenoidal microsurgical resection restores normal prolactin concentrations and eliminates symptoms in 60 to 90% of patients in different series. The results depend largely on the skill and experience of the surgeon. The risks of complications and hypopituitarism are small, but recurrence rates vary substantially among different series (10–50% in 5 years). In patients with macroadenomas, results of surgery are much more disappointing, with a 0 to 40% initial cure rate and recurrence rates between 0 and 90%. Primary radiation therapy prevents further growth of the tumor but is less effective in promoting a prompt decrease in prolactin concentrations. Owing to the high success rate of pharmacotherapy, however, radiotherapy is rarely applied to prolactinomas.

Drug therapy

Since prolactin secretion is inhibited by dopamine, dopamine agonists are the drugs of choice in hyperpro-lactinemia. The semisynthetic ergot alkaloid bromocriptine was the first compound introduced into therapy in 1971 and is still used widely (it is the only such drug available in the United States). Other more recently proposed dopamine agonists include lisuride, terguride, pergolide, metergoline, dihydroergocriptine, quinagolide, and cabergoline (see also Chap. 11). The latter two compounds appear to be of particular relevance because of their good tolerability and sustained activity. All these drugs produce a direct stimulation of dopamine D_2 receptors, inhibiting prolactin synthesis and secretion and decreasing cellular DNA synthesis and tumor growth. In most patients, dopamine agonists correct hyperprolactinemia (but the degree of suppression varies considerably), reduce tumor size, improve visual field and cranial nerve abnormalities, and restore normal gonadal function; however, when the drug is stopped, prolactin levels often return to pretreatment levels, and tumor growth resumes.

A single dose of 2.5 mg bromocriptine can suppress serum prolactin for up to 14 hours, and the biologic effect may persist for 24 hours in individual patients. Restoration of normal prolactin concentrations and tumor shrinkage after bromocriptine administration (2.5–7.5 mg daily, divided in two or three doses) are observed in more than 80% of patients with prolactinomas. In patients who achieve normal prolactin levels, the dose may be reduced progressively; the efficacy of daily therapy has been shown in most patients. Intravaginal administration of bromocriptine also has been tested with partial efficacy. Recently, a depot preparation has been developed that allows monthly im injections of bromocriptine at doses of 50 to 250 mg.

Normalization of prolactin levels usually is followed by the disappearance of clinical symptoms, resumption of the normal gonadal function (i.e., recovery of menses and fertility in women, restoration of normal testosterone levels, libido, and sperm morphology and function in men), and reduction in tumor size. The results achieved do not depend on the patient's sex or on the type of tumor, macroadenomas being equally responsive as microadenomas. Since resumption of ovulatory cycles and recovery of normal fertility occur in 80 to 90% of hyperprolactinemic women during bromocriptine treatment, pregnancy can be expected during therapy. Studies of over 2000 pregnancies indicate no adverse effects on fetal development or pregnancy outcome. It is currently accepted to stop treatment when patients with microprolactinomas realize they are pregnant, whereas in those with macroprolactinomas, treatment may be continued to avoid the risk of estrogen-induced tumor enlargement; alternatively, interrupted treatment can be reinstated if tumor expansion is documented.

Nausea and orthostatic hypotension are the most common side effects and represent the limiting factors in continuation of treatment in 5 to 10% of patients. Less common side effects include headache, dizziness, nasal congestion, abdominal cramping, and constipation. Hallucinations and psychoses also have been reported. Complete or partial resistance to bromocriptine treatment has been observed in about 5% of patients.

Cabergoline and quinagolide are the dopaminergic drugs more recently entered into clinical use. Although experience with these compounds is considerably less than with bromocriptine, they may be considered for patients intolerant or resistant to bromocriptine. Cabergoline is an ergoline derivative with an extremely prolonged duration of action. A single oral dose of 0.6 mg is able to reduce basal prolactin levels for 14 days in normal volunteers. Adequate control of hyperprolactinemia is achieved with 0.25 to 4 mg given once or twice a week. There is evidence that weekly administration of cabergoline is more effective and better tolerated than daily bromocriptine. Moreover, cabergoline treatment at weekly low doses induces substantial tumor shrinkage, and continued suppression of prolactin levels has been shown after drug discontinuation. A depot im injectable preparation of cabergoline also has been developed. This formulation (given at doses of 50-150 mg every 4 weeks) appears to be well tolerated and useful for patients who previously experienced severe side effects from oral therapy.

Quinagolide is a nonergot dopaminergic agonist given orally once daily in a dose range of 75 to 500 µg. Although clinical experience with this drug is limited, it appears effective in normalizing prolactin levels and achieving tumor shrinkage in a high proportion of patients with a better tolerability profile than bromocriptine.

Therapy with dopaminergic agonists should be continued indefinitely. No tachyphylaxis occurs, but the dose can be decreased over the years. In 10 to 20% of patients drug discontinuation does not lead to recurrence of hyperprolactinemia or rapid tumor regrowth. The reason for this is unknown at present (spontaneous tumor infarction?). When the medication is discontinued, patients should be followed closely by frequent determinations of serum prolactin levels so that medical therapy may be restarted if the levels increase.

Suggested readings

CARON P, MORANGE-RAMOS I, COGNE M, JAQUET P. Three year follow-up of acromegalic patients treated with intramuscular slow-release lanreotide. J Clin Endocrinol Metab 1997; 82:18-22.

CHAPMAN IM, PESCOVITZ OH, MURPHY G, et al. Oral administration of growth hormone (GH) releasing peptide-mimetic MK-677 stimulates the GH/insulin-like growth factor-I axis in selected GH-deficient adults. J Clin Endocrinol Metab 1997;82:3455-63.

CICCARELLI E, CAMANNI F. Diagnosis and drug therapy of prolactinoma. Drugs 1996;51:954-65.

COLAO A, LOMBARDI G. Growth-hormone and prolactin excess. Lancet 1998;352:1455-61.

CONSENSUS GUIDELINES FOR THE DIAGNOSIS AND TREATMENT OF ADULTS WITH GH DEFICIENCY. Summary statement of the GH research society workshop on adult GH deficiency. J Clin Endocrinol Metab 1997;83:379-81.

DRUG AND THERAPEUTIC COMMITTEE OF THE LAWSON WILKINS PEDIATRIC ENDOCRINE SOCIETY. Guidelines for the use of growth hormone in children with short stature. J Pediatr 1995;127:857-67.

GILLIS JC, NOBLE S, GOA KL: Octreotide long-acting release (LAR): A review of its pharmacological properties and therapeutic use in the management of acromegaly. Drugs 1997;53:681-99.

GIUSTI M, CICCARELLI E, DALLABONZANA D, et al. Clinical results of long-term slow-release lanreotide treatment of acromegaly. Eur J Clin Invest 1997;27:277-84.

GIUSTINA A, ZALTIERI G, NEGRINI F, WEHRENBERG WB. The pharmacological aspects of the treatment of acromegaly. Pharmacol Res 1996;34:247-68.

MELMED S, JACKSON I, KLEINBERG D, KLIBANSKI A. Current treatment guidelines for acromegaly. J Clin Endocrinol Metab 1998;83:2646-52.

PFEIFER M, VERHOVEC R, ZIZEK B, et al. Growth hormone treatment reverses early atherosclerotic changes in GH deficient adults. J Clin Endocrinol Metab 1999;84:453-7.

THORNER MO, BENGTSSON BA, HO KY. The diagnosis of growth hormone deficiency in adults. J Clin Endocrinol Metab 1995;80:3097-8.

VALCAVI R, GADDI O, ZINI M. Cardiac performance and mass in adults with hypopituitarism: Effects of one year of growth hormone treatment. J Clin Endocrinol Metab 1995;80:659-66.

67

Contraception, sterility treatment, and post-menopausal steroid replacement therapy

Fabio Celotti

FERTILITY REGULATION

Pharmacologic regulation of fertility is a relatively recent achievement because the first estrogen-progesterone contraceptive pill was marketed only in 1960. The availability of an effective, low-cost, easy-to-use family planning method undoubtedly has had a remarkable impact on the life of millions of couples and on the social organization of the industrial societies.

Contraceptive drugs are not used to treat diseases, but they are used in healthy females in a period of years ranging from menarche to menopause, thus possibly for a very long period of time, in a more or less continuous fashion. Consequently, particular attention should be paid to identifying possible untoward effects; either those arising during use of the compounds or those which might appear after discontinuation of use. Recent studies also have shown that oral contraceptives induce positive effects on health not related to contraception, such as, for example, a reduced incidence of ovarian and uterine cancers, of uterine fibroids, of rheumatoid arthritis, etc. These effects should be considered in the overall evaluation of treatment, even if they are not primary in determining whether to start a contraceptive treatment.

Since an appropriate contraceptive treatment is effective and usually devoid of serious risks in healthy women, there are no medical reasons not to use a safe form of contraception in all the subjects willing to do so, starting from the beginning of regular sexual intercourse until the menopause. Absolute or relative contraindications, however, do exist and should be carefully taken into account.

Hormonal contraceptives can be divided into oral and parenteral (long-acting) preparations. The latter are administered im or by silicone implants. Postcoital contraception, an emergency form of contraception, is considered separately.

ORAL CONTRACEPTIVES

Oral contraceptives are among the most widely used drugs in the world and differ in their composition both qualitatively and quantitatively. They can be divided into (1) *combination contraceptives* (CCs), which associate an estrogen and a progestin and are available as fixed combinations or monophasic preparations, biphasic preparations, or triphasic preparations, and (2) *progestin-only contraceptives* (minipill).

Combination oral estrogen-progestogen contraceptives

The first contraceptive preparation, developed by Pincus in 1959, was a fixed-combination product containing an estrogen (mestranol, 150 µg) and a progestin (norethynodrel, 10 mg). Its contraceptive efficacy was virtually complete, but the "pill" contained a huge amount of steroids. After recognition of dose-related untoward effects, thrombosis in particular, and awareness that the contraceptive activity was maintained with much lower amounts of steroids, the doses were gradually reduced. In the 1970s, most preparations contained 50 to 100 µg of ethinyl estradiol (EE) or mestranol (ME) and 2 to 10 mg of a progestin. Nowadays, the estrogen content goes from 20 to 50 µg (30-35 µg in most formulations), and the amount of the progestin does not exceed 1.0 to 1.5 mg. The preparations containing 35 µg or less of estrogen are usually known as "low dose combinations." The amount of progestin is more variable and difficult to compare, since the different synthetic molecules used have a relatively diversified activity profile and variable specific activities. In the continuous attempt to reduce the total amount of steroid administered, of progestins in particular, and to mimic somehow the estrogen-progesterone secretory pattern of the ovarian cycle, biphasic and triphasic preparations were developed.

In biphasic preparations, the amount of progestin added to 35 µg of estrogen in the first 7 to 10 capsules is halved as compared with that present in the fixed-dose preparations. Therefore, a 20 to 22% reduction in the monthly dose is achieved. In triphasic preparations, the progestin is very low in the first phase of the cycle. The initial 6 to 7 tablets contain about one-third the dose present in the monophasic preparations, the following 5 to 7 capsules contain one-half, and only the remaining tablets contain the full dose. In this way a reduction of about 40% is achieved. For example, the total progestin dose in a levonorgestrel (LNG) triphasic preparation is 1.93 mg per cycle, whereas it is 3.15 mg in the corresponding monophasic pill.

Preparations defined as sequential, developed to mimic in some way the cyclic changes of ovarian secretion, were available some years ago. They contained estrogen alone (EE, 50-100 µg) for the first 14 days of the cycle, followed by combination of the same dose of estrogen with a progestin. These products have been removed from the market because they proved to be less effective than the monophasic preparations and because they produced endometrial hyperstimulation in the unopposed estrogenic phase. The bi- and triphasic preparations used today represent the logical development of the sequential concept.

Steroid components

Ethinyl estradiol (EE) and the 3-methylether of EE (ME), are the two semisynthetic estrogens that have been used in CCs since their introduction to the market. Esters of the natural hormone estradiol are used only in the injectable preparations.

Presently, EE is used in virtually all preparations. ME is a prodrug of EE; its metabolic conversion occurs in the gut wall and in the liver. ME bioavalability is about 70% that of EE, but in the woman it appears almost equally active.

EE derives from estradiol by the addition of an ethinyl group in position 17. This change makes the molecule a poor substrate for the 17-estradiol dehydrogenase, a fundamental enzyme in estradiol metabolism, sparing EE from the rapid "first pass" hepatic metabolism and making it orally active. A significant presystemic metabolism still occurs in the gut and liver, primarily to EE-3 sulfate and to a lesser extent to glucuronides, so that the bioavailability of EE in the peripheral circulation is about 40 to 60% of the given dose. The major metabolic pathway of EE appears to be the 2-hydroxylation leading to 2-hydroxy EE, which in turn can be converted to 2-methoxy EE. Hydroxylations in the 6 and 16α positions also occur. The EE metabolites appear to have little estrogenic activity. Small amounts of EE also can be converted to estradiol and estrone.

Peak serum levels of EE occur within 1 to 2 hours of oral intake. The drug circulates largely bound to albumin and minimally to sex hormone-binding globulin (SHBG). About 60% of the dose is excreted in the urine and the rest in the feces, mostly as sulfate or glucuronide conjugates.

EE is cleared from the blood with an elimination half-life of between 9 and 27 hours, 8 hours on average, much longer than estradiol. Plasma levels vary widely, due to marked differences in inter- and intraindividual bioavailability of the compound. Nevertheless, even the low-dose preparations appear to be fully effective as contraceptives. EE exerts its action by binding to the estrogen receptor; in general it has 15 to 20 times the potency of oral estradiol.

Progestins used in combination contraceptive are always synthetic compounds with progestational activity.

Table 67.1 Major biologic characteristics of the principal progestational molecule

Compound	Progestational effects	Androgenic effects	Antiestrogenic effects	Antiandrogenic effects	Ovulation inhibiting dose[1]
Progesterone	+	–	+	–	
Medroxyprogesterone acetate	++	–	+	–	
Chlormadinone acetate	++	–	+	++	1.7
Cyproterone acetate	++	–	+	+++	1
Megestrol acetate	++	–	+	–	
Medrogestone	++	–	+		
Dehydrogesterone	+	–	+		
Demegestone	++	–	+		
Promegestone	+++	–	+		
Nomegestrol acetate	+++	–	+	++	1.25
Norethindrone	++	++	++	–	0.4
Dienogest	+++	–	+/–	++	1
Levonorgestrel	+++	+++	+++	–	0.06
3-Ketodesogestrel[2]	+++	+	++	+/–	0.06
Gestodene	+++	+	++	–	0.04
Norgestimate	+++	+	++	–	0.20

+++, very high activity; ++, high activity; +, moderate activity; –, inactive.
[1] mg/day without estrogens.
[2] 3-Ketodesogestrel is the active metabolite of desogestrel.

Progesterone itself is not active orally owing to extensive "first pass" liver metabolism. Micronized progesterone, which is more bioavailable, is sometimes used in postmenopausal replacement therapy in association with estrogens. The only compounds with the ring structure (pregnane) of the natural steroid used in contraception are medroxyprogesterone acetate (MPA), 17-hydroxyprogesterone caproate, and dihydroprogesterone acetophenide. These are esters of natural progesterone metabolites and are present alone or in combination with estrogens in long-acting injectable contraceptives.

Several compounds, all belonging to the 19-nortestosterone family, are currently employed in CCs. From a structural point of view, they belong to three different groups: those directly derived from 19-nortestosterone, therefore lacking the C-19, C-20, and C-21 carbons of progesterone (e.g., norethindrone or norethisterone, norethynodrel, ethynodiol diacetate, lynestrenol, and the recent dienogest); those, called *gonanes,* derived by the addition of a 13-ethyl group to norethindrone (e.g., norgestrel, LNG, desogestrel, norgestimate, and gestodene); and those derived from 19-norprogesterone (e.g., normegestrol).

Progestins are often grouped in generations according to their biologic activities. The 19-nortestosterone derivatives of the first generation (e.g., norethindrone, norethynodrel, ethynodiol diacetate, and lynestrenol) display primarily progestational effects, since the 19 methyl group, essential for the full expression of the androgenic activity, has been removed. However, the androgenic properties have not been completely eliminated. These steroids are orally active because the presence of a 17-ethinyl group decreases their liver metabolism. The addition of a 13-ethyl group to norethindrone has produced norgestrel (LNG is the active enantiomer of the D,L-racemic mixture), a compound more potent but with a similar selectivity of action. Norgestrel is indicated as a second-generation progestogen.

Even if the residual androgenic and estrogenic activities are clinically insignificant in the low-dose contraceptives, a third generation of progestins has been developed. The new molecules (e.g., desogestrel, norgestimate, gestodene, nomegestrol, and dienogest) possess a lower residual androgenic activity.

There are considerable differences in the pharmacologic, pharmacokinetic, and metabolic characteristics of the individual progestins, as well as in their dose-effect relationships. The ultimate clinical effect might depend on the integration of these characteristics. The recent discovery of two progesterone receptor isoforms (types A and B) with different tissue distribution, control mechanisms, and biologic significance (type A probably acts mainly as repressor of type B-mediated transcription) possibly will help in the future to explain the different behaviors of the progestins. Some of the main biologic activities of the progestational molecules in clinical use are shown in Table 67.1. The evaluation of the properties of the different progestins is based on several tests in animals and on the binding affinity to receptors and should be considered purely indicative. The equivalent doses of some molecules in inducing the secretory transformation of the endometrium in estrogen-treated postmenopausal women are shown in Table 67.2.

A novel progestogen, drospirenone, is now under clinical development. Structurally, the compound is derived from spironolactone, and therefore, it is different from all other derivatives. Its pharmacologic profile is very similar to that of the natural progesterone, it combines a potent progestogenic activity with antimineralcorticoid and antiandrogenic effects.

Finally, it should be recalled that, as in the case of estrogens, serious side effects were more related to the high doses formerly used in the formulations than to the pharmacologic characteristics of the progestins. No major advantage of one molecule over another has been firmly established in contraception.

The chief mechanism of action of CCs is to prevent ovulation by acting on the hypothalamic-pituitary axis to inhibit gonadotropin secretion. Other peripheral mechanisms also may be operative. Changes in the endocervical gland's activity, producing, under the influence of progestins, a scant and viscous cervical mucus impervious to sperm penetration, are surely involved; in addition, endometrial receptivity necessary for implantation is altered by progestins, and tubal motility and function are also possibly affected. These actions might contribute to the global effectiveness of CCs, particularly if the ovarian suppression is not complete, as might happen with the low-dose formulations. It is indeed the multiplicity of their actions that makes these drugs so effective.

The estrogenic component is thought to inhibit mainly follicle-stimulating hormone (FSH) secretion and therefore follicle recruitment, maturation, and selection, whereas progestins mainly inhibit luteinizing hormone (LH) and therefore the ovulatory mechanism.

Hypothalamic actions of the steroids play a major role. A key effect of progestins is to diminish the frequency of the gonadotropin-releasing hormone (GnRH) pulse generator, essential for menstrual cycle progression. The effects of estrogens alone on the pulse generator are less conspic-

Table 67.2 Indicative daily doses of various progestins used in cyclic regimens in postmenopausal hormone replacement therapy to achieve endometrial secretory transformation

Compound	Dose (mg/day)
Progesterone (micronized)	200-300
Medroxyprogesterone acetate	5-10
Chlormadinone acetate	10
Megestrol acetate	5
Dehydrogesterone	10-20
Demegestone	1
Promegestone	0.5
Nomegestrol acetate	0.5
Norethindrone or norethindrone acetate	0.7-1
Dienogest	0.45
Levonorgestrel	0.15
Desogestrel	0.15
Gestodene	0.075
Norgestimate	0.25

uous, but they are known to strengthen the progesterone effects, probably inducing the synthesis of hypothalamic progesterone receptors. The amount of progestin present in the low-dose preparations, particularly of those molecules which display strong peripheral effects, is not always definitely above the ovulation-inhibitory dose of the compound administered alone; in these instances, the combined effect of estrogens appears very important. This is the case, for example, of preparations containing 250 μg norgestimate, an amount only a little higher than the ovulation-inhibiting dose (200 μg).

Multiple effects of the CCs are also exerted at the anterior pituitary level. Globally, the pituitary responsiveness to GnRH appears to be decreased. Estrogens in particular appear effective in suppressing FSH release from the pituitary.

The reduced steroid content of the "pill" has not compromised its efficacy, even if the diminished suppression of circulating FSH may produce substantial residual ovarian activity. Follicle recruitment and growth occur during the pill-free interval and the first week of pill intake or when a substantial number of pills are missed. Nevertheless, follicle growth is usually arrested around the stage of dominant follicle selection, and ovulation does not occur.

The *contraceptive efficacies* of multiphasic preparations, of low-dose (<50 μg) and higher-dose formulations, are entirely comparable. In controlled studies with motivated subjects (method effectiveness), an annual failure rate of 0.1% is achieved. Typical usage is associated with a 3% failure rate during the first year of use. During 1 year of unprotected intercourse, about 85% of women become pregnant.

Pill administration

Monophasic or biphasic preparations or CCs are available in 21-day packs. A pill is taken daily for 21 days, followed by a 7-day "pill-free" period. Some preparations consist of 28 pills, with the last 7 containing the vehicle only.

Contraceptive efficacy starts from the first cycle of use. It is better to take the first pill on day 1 or 2 of the cycle (first or second day of menses), never later than day 5.

Pill omission is a frequent problem. There is no general consensus on the real impact of pill omissions on contraceptive efficacy. It depends on the number of missed pills, on the stage of the cycle, and on individual sensitivity. One is reminded of the difference between the method and the use effectiveness. Missing pills around the pill-free period appear to produce the highest risk.

Pill and lactation

The contraceptive efficacy of lactational amenorrhea is quite variable and unpredictable. The risk of pregnancy during breast-feeding increases with or just before the first postpartum menses. CCs diminish the quantity and quality of milk; therefore, other methods of contraception should be adopted if breast-feeding plays an essential

role, as is the case in developing countries. Nonhormonal methods represent the first choice, but progestin-only contraception also is an effective and safe option.

Side effects

Soon after introduction of the high-dose CCs, reports of adverse events began to appear. The increased risk for cardiovascular side effects (e.g., venous thrombosis, myocardial infarction, and stroke) was the main concern, but also the metabolic effects and the possibly increased incidence of breast, ovarian, and endometrial cancer have been evaluated. There is now a general consensus that the new low-dose formulations have minimal contraindications, provided that specific risk factors are absent. Moreover, these drugs might even exert beneficial health effects not related to contraception.

Cardiovascular side effects **Arterial thrombosis** Myocardial infarction and stroke in CC users appear to be acute estrogen-related events, clearly dose dependent, and not linked to possible alterations (progestogen-induced) of the lipoprotein profile toward a more atherogenic pattern. As a matter of fact, there is no evidence of increased atherosclerotic diseases among the past users of the combined high-dose contraceptives. The highest risk was present in smokers more than 35 years old treated with pills containing more than 50 μg EE. Most of the preliminary epidemiologic data in low-dose CC users are also indicative of a very low risk of myocardial infarction, almost overlapping that of nonusers. However, the relative risk appears slightly increased in some studies; model estimates of incidence of myocardial infarction based on these studies are shown in Table 67.3. It appears that pills containing the third-generation progestins, such as gestodene or desogestrel, are associated with a lower risk (not significantly different from that of nonusers) than those containing second-generation compounds. However, there is general agreement that even with low-dose pills, smokers, particularly if over age 35, still have a definite increased myocardial infarction risk.

The mechanism by which high circulating levels of EE might induce thrombotic events appears to be the dose-related increase of various clotting factors in the blood (factors II, VII, VIII, IX, and X and fibrinogen), as well as the decrease in coagulation inhibitors such as antithrombin III. On the contrary, the low-dose preparations do not have a significant impact on coagulation because the slight increase in thrombin formation observed in some studies is antagonized by an enhanced fibrinolytic activity.

Venous thromboembolism The risk is increased at doses of EE of 50 μg. It is not yet completely clarified whether the low-dose preparations are completely without risk. Recent studies appear to indicate that users of low-dose oral contraceptives containing norgestrel have a risk 3.5 times higher than nonusers. Surprisingly, contraceptives containing the third-generation progestins desogestrel and gestodene, at variance with the myocardial infarction risk, appear to be associated with a higher risk of developing venous thromboembolism (Tab. 67.3). These results are

Table 67.3 Model estimates of myocardial infarction (MI) and venous thromboembolism (VT) in users of low-dose contraceptives (OCs) containing second- and third-generation contraceptives. The incidence is expressed as cases per 100 000 healty women in United States

Age	Non users		OCs, second generation		OCs, third generation	
	MI	VT	MI	VT	MI	VT
15-24	1.3	2.2	4.0	8.1	1.4	16.2
25-34	2.4	4.8	7.4	17.4	2.6	34.7
35-44	14.7	4.7	45.5	17.1	16.1	34.2

difficult to interpret because the hemostatic alterations produced by low-dose contraceptives, including those containing the third-generation progestins, are minor, and the balance between the coagulation and fibrinolytic pathways appears in equilibrium. It has been suggested that third-generation CCs may induce resistance to activated protein C, a natural anticoagulant defense mechanism. However, it cannot be excluded that the results could be due to chance. However, the increase in risk should be evaluated taking into account the low incidence of the idiopathic venous thromboembolism.

Routine laboratory tests do not provide useful information to predict the occurrence of arterial or venous thromboembolic episodes.

Atherosclerosis and lipoprotein metabolism High-density lipoprotein (HDL)-cholesterol was decreased and triglycerides and low density lipoprotein (LDL) -cholesterol were increased during treatment with some CCs containing high amounts of "androgenic" progestins. This change toward an atherogenic lipid profile was one of the main stimuli to develop the new class of progestins with a lower androgenic effect. However, even when plasma lipids are altered by the progestin component, the strong direct effect of EE on the arterial wall appears protective from the formation of atherosclerotic plaques. Moreover, recent studies indicate that the total serum cholesterol level or lipoprotein profile is not changed with the new low-dose formulations and that only limited increases in triglyceride levels are observed.

Hypertension The use of the high-dose CCs was associated with hypertension in 4 to 5% of normotensive subjects and with the worsening of the blood pressure levels in 10 to 15% of women with preexisting hypertension. Small increases in blood pressure can be observed even with the low-dose preparations, particularly with those containing LNG, but the incidence is much lower and the occurrence of clinically significant hypertension has not been reported. The main mechanism of the hypertensive actions of CCs is stimulation of the angiotensinogen synthesis by EE. This induces a small angiotensin II increase with a consequent slight reduction in renal blood flow and a small sodium retention. In susceptible subjects, these changes may produce a rise in blood pressure.

Carbohydrate metabolism With high-dose contraceptives, carbohydrate metabolism was deranged mainly by the progestin component. In particular, impaired glucose tolerance and increased insulin concentrations often were reported in users of preparations containing 75 µg per day of LNG, since progestins with a higher androgenic activity exert a more pronounced effect on glucose metabolism. The impairment of glucose metabolism is once again dose related, and therefore, the low-dose monophasic and multiphasic preparations are considered essentially free of clinically significant effects on carbohydrate metabolism, even if small increases in peripheral insulin resistance have been reported.

Other effects Breakthrough bleeding and spotting are present in a consistent number of women, particularly in the first cycles of use. The incidence varies in different studies, but it might be as high as 20 to 30%; it is then followed by a progressive reduction.

Absence of bleeding in the pill-free period also may occur in 1 to 5% of subjects. It is the expression of endometrial atrophy induced by the progestin dominance. It may be interpreted as a sign of pregnancy.

A transient slight increase in the incidence of *gallbladder disease* has been described in the first 2 years of use. The mechanism could be the estrogen-induced cholesterol saturation of bile and therefore of stone formation in susceptible subjects.

Nausea, breast discomfort, weight gain, headache, and chloasma (a patchy increase of facial pigment) have been reported, but their incidence is smaller than with high-dose CCs.

Acne and hirsutism may occur very rarely, particularly in women using pills with relatively high amounts of 19-nor derivatives. Usually these conditions, when preexisting, are improved by the use of CCs.

Mood changes and reduction of libido have been reported occasionally. An increased incidence of *urinary tract infections* has been reported in some studies. Also, *vaginal candidiasis, cervicitis,* and *chlamydial infections* may be adversely affected by CCs. These proinfectious effects have been observed mainly with high-dose contraceptives, but the low-dose preparations also may influence the recurrence of symptoms of vaginal candidiasis.

The *serum concentration of several proteins,* globulins in particular, is increased by estrogens, which affect their liver synthesis. This phenomenon is often associated with alteration of some laboratory tests (e.g., erythrocyte sedimentation rate, total iron-binding capacity, prothrombin time and partial thromboplastin time, and total but not free plasma levels of thyroid hormones, glucocorticoids, and sex hormones), and it may affect their interpretation.

Teratogenic risk. Claims of an association of human birth defects, in particular of congenital limb-reduction deformities, occasionally have appeared after CC failures. There is now a general consensus that the teratogenic risk is absent in the accidental use of low-dose oral contraceptive in early pregnancy.

Incidence of tumors. The use of CCs and the possible development of cancer has always been a matter of concern. There is now a general agreement that the association between CC use and cancer, if it even exists, is undoubtedly very weak. Actually, CCs may decrease the incidence of some tumors:

• *endometrial cancer:* a protective effect of oral contraception (50% decrease in the risk of developing the disease after 12 months of CC use that lasts at least 15 years after discontinuation) has been shown with low-dose preparations;

• *cancer of the cervix:* some studies appear to indicate an increased risk of cervical cancer in CC users for more than 1 year. However, the incidence of cervical carcinoma is affected by the subject's sexual activity (i.e., number of partners, use of barrier methods, etc.), which changes the exposure to sexually transmitted papillomavirus, a possible etiologic factor of the disease;

• *breast cancer:* late age at menarche, early age at first birth, and a precocious menopause decrease the risk of breast cancer. Thus, length of menstrual life (i.e., the lifetime exposure to ovarian hormones), in particular the fraction occurring before the first full-term pregnancy, is a key component of the total breast cancer risk. There is now a general agreement that the use of CCs does not produce an overall increase in breast cancer risk even after long-term use (i.e., 15 years or more). However, there are data that appear to indicate a slight increase in the risk (1.5) of developing breast cancer before age 45 in women who have had a long duration of use before the first pregnancy (4 years or more).These findings are questionable, and other reports conflict with these conclusions;

• *ovarian cancer:* a 40 to 50% decrease in the risk of developing ovarian cancer after 2 years of use of CCs has been reported. Moreover, the protective effect persists up to 10 to 15 years after discontinuation of the drug;

• *liver tumors:* steroids, both estrogens and androgens, are known to produce benign liver tumors – peliosis and adenomas – that are asymptomatic and may rupture and produce hematoperitoneum. The incidence appears dose dependent, and therefore, the condition is very rare with the low-dose formulations.

Contraindications

Absolute and relative contraindications to the use of low-dose CCs are shown in Table 67.4.

Interactions

Drugs inducing the formation of liver microsomal enzymes may increase steroid metabolism and reduce contraceptive effectiveness. Unwanted pregnancies have occurred with concurrent use of rifampin and anticonvulsants such as phenytoin, phenobarbital, primidone, and carbamazepine. Antibiotics such as ampicillin, tetracycline, chloramphenicol, and even the sulfonamides may alter the intestinal flora and therefore decrease the enterohepatic recycling of conjugated metabolites, reducing contraceptive efficacy. There

Table 67.4 Absolute and relative contraindications to the use of low-dose combined contraceptives

Absolute contraindications	Relative contraindications
Thromboembolic diseases, cerebrovascular disease; ischemic heart disease: disease history or predisposing conditions, e.g., familial hyperlipidemia	Headaches, migraine, benign breast disease
Known or suspected breast carcinoma, carcinoma of the female reproductive tract, or any other steroid-responsive neoplasias	Diabetes
Undiagnosed abnormal vaginal bleeding	Hypertension
Known or suspected pregnancy	Obstructive jaundice in pregnancy
Past or present liver tumors or seriously impaired liver function	Gallbladder disease
Smokers (>15 cigarettes/d) over 35 years of age	Elective surgery, to minimize the risk of thromboembolism after surgery

are reports of unwanted pregnancies during antibiotic therapy, but most are not well documented. Clinical pharmacokinetic studies do not show any consistent effect of antibiotics on the plasma concentration of contraceptive steroids.

Fertility after contraception termination

A delay of at least 1 year, with a greater effect for the high-dose preparations, in recovering normal fertility appears to exist in former users of CCs. However, there is no evidence that infertility is increased after CC use. Moreover, the incidence of postpill amenorrhea is analogous to that of spontaneous secondary amenorrhea (1%). After cessation of oral contraception, 50% of the women conceive by 3 months, and after 2 years, only about 15% of parous and 7% of nulliparous women have not become pregnant. These figures are similar to those reported for spontaneous infertility.

Choice of the preparation

The general rule is to prescribe the effective formulation with the minimal dose of steroids. These are often pills containing 30 to 35 μg of estrogen, but also formulations with 20 μg may be suitable, particularly in low-weight women, provided that breakthrough bleeding does not represent a persistent problem. However, some indication exists that long-term use of 20-μg estrogen preparations may prevent the achievement of peak bone mass when contraception is started early. Multiphasic preparations contain a lower amount of progestins than the corresponding monophasic preparations; thus, they should be preferred theoretically, but the available clinical evidence shows little difference between the two products.

Therapeutic use other than contraception

CCs are very effective in treating dysfunctional uterine bleedings and dysmenorrhea, as well as in the prophylaxis of endometriosis after surgical or GnRH treatments. Moreover, the low-dose CCs can be used in the treatment of acne and hirsutism. Functional ovarian cysts and premenstrual syndrome also may benefit from CC treatment.

Progestin-only oral preparations (minipill)

Minipills (MPs) contain only a progestational agent in doses lower than those present in CCs. The 19-nor derivatives of testosterone (e.g., norethindrone 0.35 mg, LNG 0.03 mg, norgestrel 0.075 mg, lynestrenol 0.5 mg, and ethynodiol diacetate 0.5 mg) are presently used.

Since the doses are lower than those necessary to inhibit ovulation in the absence of the cooperative effect of estrogens, follicle growth and echographic or endocrine evidence of ovulation have been reported in 30 to 60% MP users. The contraceptive mechanism relies more on the peripheral effects on the endometrium and cervical mucus.

Failure rates are a little higher than those reported for the combined preparations: from 1.1 to 9.6% in the first year of use. However, in motivated subjects, the failure rate is not much different from that of CCs (about 3.0% in typical use). Efficacy appears to be lower in younger women compared with those over age 40, in whom fertility is naturally declining. Two factors contribute to the lower efficacy of MPs: first of all, the action depends almost exclusively on peripheral mechanisms (e.g., inhibition of the implant and of mucus penetration by sperm); second, pill-missing has greater consequences for fertility.

Since ovulation is not prevented in a substantial number of cycles, ectopic pregnancies are not impeded to the same extent as uterine pregnancies, even if their overall incidence is not increased. This indicates that the endometrial changes produced by progestins represent an important contribution in the mechanism of action of these preparations. At variance with CCs, the return of fertility occurs immediately after MP discontinuation.

Minipills must be taken daily without any pill-free interval, always at the same time, because the impermeability of the cervical mucus diminishes about 22 hours after administration. Changes in the mucus occur in 2 to 4 hours.

Side effects

Owing to the variable suppression of estrogen production in the face of the continuous effect of the exogenous progestational agent on the endometrium, frequent and irregular menstrual bleedings represent the major problem and the main reason for discontinuation. Because of the low dose of steroid administered, no metabolic effect occurs on carbohydrate or lipid metabolism or on the coagulation system. The incidence of minor side effects (e.g., headache, breast tenderness, nausea, and dizziness)

appears to be increased in some studies, whereas in others it is comparable with that of placebo.

Androgenic side effects (e.g., weight gain, acne, and hirsutism) have been reported, even if rarely, particularly by users of MPs containing LNG. Since follicular development occurs in most of the cycles but is not always followed by ovulation, ovarian cysts develop frequently. Almost all of them are asymptomatic and disappear spontaneously. The available studies have not shown any effect on fetal development associated with the use of oral progestins during pregnancy.

Indications and contraindications

The minipill is specifically suitable when estrogens are contraindicated (see Tab. 67.4), when minor side effects of CCs (e.g., headache, decreased libido, gastrointestinal upset, etc.) make the method not well acceptable, and in lactating women. At variance with CCs, MPs do not produce adverse effects on milk production and quality; on the contrary, there appears to be a small positive impact on lactation. Even if significant amounts of progestins may be present in milk, no adverse effect on the child has been detected so far. Minipills also may be prescribed to assess patient suitability to long-acting progestin preparations.

The absolute contraindications to the use of MPs are known or suspected pregnancy, known or suspected carcinoma of the breast, undiagnosed abnormal genital bleeding, and acute liver disease or liver tumors.

No specific advantage of one preparation over another has been shown. The choice of a progestin with a low androgenic impact may be advisable in women sensitive to androgens.

Interactions

As in the case of CCs, drugs that induce liver microsomal enzymes may increase progestin metabolism and reduce contraceptive efficacy. These include rifampin and anticonvulsants.

PARENTERAL CONTRACEPTIVES

These preparations include implants of capsules or rods of polymers permeable to the steroid molecules and im injections of depot formulations. The continuous release of steroids over a long period of time frees the user from the daily oral dose with a major advantage in compliance. Preparations containing progestins only or an estrogen-progestogen combination may be used in parenteral contraception. The progestin-only systems now in clinical use worldwide are Norplant capsules (set of six silicone capsules) and MPA depot injections. Norplant rods (Norplant-2, consisting in two rods) have been approved recently by the Food and Drug Administration (FDA). Single implants (e.g., Nestorone, 3-keto-desogestrel, and Uniplant) or biodegradable implants releasing LNG or norethindrone. Norethindrone enanthate long-acting injections are under development.

Monthly injectable estrogen-progestogen combinations are available in some countries, particularly in Latin America, China, and India. These formulations have been developed to avoid the major drawback of progestin-only preparations, i.e., menstrual irregularities.

Norplant

Norplant development started about 30 years ago as a Population Council program. Of the several progestins evaluated at that time, LNG appeared to have the best efficacy with the lowest incidence of side effects and a very good stability. The implants were released in the United States at the beginning of 1991; millions of women have used Norplant worldwide.

The Norplant system consists of six medical-grade silicone capsules, each measuring 34 × 2.4 mm, containing 216 mg LNG on the whole. The capsules are inserted subcutaneously in the forearm or upper arm under local anesthesia by means of a no. 10 trocar. Six tubes are necessary to ensure contraceptive levels of the steroid for 5 years.

After initial peak levels of LNG (0.4-0.5 ng/ml), concentrations between 0.35 and 0.25 ng/ml are achieved for the 5-year period. Values below 0.20 ng/ml are associated with increased pregnancy rates. The daily amount of LNG released roughly corresponds to that delivered daily by MPs and to 25 to 50% of the dose delivered by low-dose CCs. There is a significant inverse correlation between body weight and plasma level of LNG. Women weighing more than 70 kg may show circulating levels below 0.2 ng/ml and have an increased risk of pregnancy starting from the third year of use. The weight-related failure increase has been mitigated by the introduction of a more "soft" silastic tubing that contains less inert filter and allows a 15% higher LNG release. All capsules are now manufactured in this way.

The plasma levels of LNG achieved by the implants are not high enough to inhibit ovulation in all subjects, and the number of ovulatory cycles grows with time after insertion. By the fifth year, ovulations documented by ultrasound are about 25 to 35%, and in many more cases luteinized unruptured follicles are produced.

The contraceptive efficacy of Norplant is highest among other hormonal contraceptive methods. The pregnancy rate for the first year of use is 0.2% without a difference between the lowest expected and the typical failure rates. Pregnancy rates in the subsequent years with "soft" silicone implants do not exceed 0.5%. The ectopic pregnancy rate in Norplant users is decreased compared with the noncontraceptors but not completely suppressed. After removal of the implants, most of the circulating steroid is cleared within 4 days, and postremoval conception rates in the first year are comparable with those of women not using contraception.

Side effects

Alteration of the menstrual pattern is the main side effect present in more than 60% of women in the first year of use. Its incidence decreases thereafter. It is also the most frequent reason cited for early discontinuation. Continuation rates range from 76 to 95% in the first year, a figure that is better than that for oral contraceptives or intrauterine devices (IUDs). Menstrual problems include alterations of the rhythm, duration, and volume of bleeding and presence of breakthrough bleeding and spotting. Despite the increased bleeding frequency, hemoglobin concentration usually increases in Norplant users as a result of the decreased amount of menstrual blood loss.

Temporary treatments may be useful, in particular to stop prolonged bleeding episodes. Treatment with oral doses of LNG (30 µg bid for 3 weeks) to achieve a better inhibition of the ovarian activity also has been suggested.

Other side effects reported by Norplant users include headache, acne, weight gain, hirsutism, mood changes, depression, anxiety, ovarian cyst formation, mild hypertension, galactorrhea, and hyperpigmentation over the implants. Not all these side effect have a strong correlation with LNG. Beside menstrual irregularities, the most common side effect is headache: 20% of the discontinuations are due to this problem. Weight gain is mentioned frequently, but studies are contradictory on this issue. Acne is the most frequent skin problem. It is probably due to the residual androgenic activity of LNG unbalanced by an adequate estrogen secretion.

Indications and contraindications

Norplant is highly effective, long-lasting, safe, does not require user compliance, and is rapidly reversible. The system delivers continuously low doses of LNG, avoiding the high initial dose of injectable progestins and the daily hormonal peaks of oral contraception. For these reasons it may be selected as the first-choice contraceptive method. Moreover, only IUDs have a lower overall cost.

As for the other types of progestin-only preparations, it is specifically indicated in all the situations in which CCs are contraindicated (Tab. 67.4).

Interactions

All the drugs that induce microsomal liver enzymes (see interactions of CCs) may increase the risk of pregnancies by reducing the circulating levels of LNG.

Norplant-2

Norplant-2 has been approved recently by the FDA. It consists of two silicone rods (each 43 mm long) in which the steroid is physically mixed with the elastomer in the core. Each rod, in turn, is covered by a thin-walled silicone rubber tubing. The release rate of LNG is higher per surface unit than that of Norplant; therefore, an equal total daily release of steroid is achieved by two rods. Since the total amount of steroid contained in Norplant-2 is 140 mg (versus 216 mg in Norplant), the new formulation has a theoretically shorter duration of contraceptive protection: 3 years. The results of clinical studies after 3 years of use have been published recently. They indicate that the circulating levels of LNG and the clinical performances are comparable between the two formulations. However, Norplant-2 removal appears to be easier than that of the original formulation.

Depo-Provera

Medroxyprogesterone acetate is the 6-methyl derivative of 17-acetoxy progesterone, an ester of the natural progesterone metabolite 17-hydroxyprogesterone. Acetylation of the 17-hydroxy position confers some progestational activity to the inactive parent compound and improves oral absorption; the 6-methyl substitution adds sufficient progestational activity, probably by inhibiting hepatic metabolism. MPA displays a relatively selective progestational activity.

Depo-Provera is a long-acting crystalline aqueous suspension of MPA. The im injection of 150 mg Depo-Provera in the gluteal or deltoid muscle produces effective contraceptive levels lasting 4 months, but injections are repeated every 3 months for safety purposes. Contraceptive serum levels of MPA (>0.5 ng/ml) are reached within 24 hours; then there is a plateau at about 1.0 ng/ml for about 3 months, followed by a gradual decline. Prolonged use of depot MPA every 3 months does not produce drug accumulation. The ideal time to begin depot MPA contraception is within 5 days of the beginning of menses, to ensure that the woman is not already pregnant and to prevent ovulation in the first month of use.

The mechanism of action involves both inhibition of the ovulatory surge of LH, and therefore of the ovulation, and peripheral changes in endometrial receptivity and cervical mucus fluidity. FSH levels, as well as basal LH levels, are not as effectively suppressed as with CCs; therefore, follicular growth is not completely inhibited.

The efficacy of this method is very high: the pregnancy rate is only 0.1% in the first year of use; 0.4% is the cumulative figure after 2 years. After discontinuation, regain of normal menses and return to normal fertility levels are delayed for a variable period of time, on average, about 1 year. The delay does not appear to be related to the number of injections used.

Indications and contraindications

Like other long-term preparations, MPA may be indicated when there are compliance problems. Moreover, it can be used in all situations in which estrogen-containing medications are contraindicated, particularly in subjects with a history of thromboembolic disease. No increased risk of thrombosis has been shown in epidemiologic studies in contraception. On the contrary, thromboembolism has been observed, at much higher doses, when MPA was used in oncology, and for this reason, the history of deep venous thrombosis is a contraindication included in the package insert in some countries (e.g., the United States). MPA is indicated in subjects affected by sickle cell anemia, since it has an inhibitory effect in sickling tests performed in vitro and improves hematologic values during treatment. Moreover, the drug is indicated in epilepsy

because it has been reported to reduce epileptic seizure frequency, and few contraceptive failures have been observed during concomitant treatment with anticonvulsants (known microsomal enzyme inductors).

Side effects

As with the other progestin-only preparations, the major problem is irregular menstrual bleeding, ranging from breakthrough bleeding to amenorrhea. The incidence of irregular bleeding is about 30% in the first year of use and 10% thereafter. Amenorrhea occurs in most women after several injections. Oral estrogen supplementation courses may temporary alleviate the bleeding problems.

Weight gain has been reported frequently, even if well-conducted, controlled studies are lacking. A link between MPA and mood changes or depression has been reported in some case series, but these findings have not been substantiated by specific studies.

Carbohydrate metabolism and coagulation factors show few, if any, changes. A decrease in HDL cholesterol and an increase in total and LDL cholesterol have been described in most, but not all, studies.

Breast tumors were induced in beagle dogs by continuous administration of high doses of MPA. This finding somewhat delayed the use of this steroid in contraception. However, it was shown subsequently that the event was due to the unique capability of beagle dogs to metabolize 17-acetoxy progesterone into estrogens, therefore producing mammary hyperplasia.

A definite protection against endometrial cancer has been shown in MPA users. The relative risk appears to be almost 5 times less than in nonusers. The duration of protection persists for at least 8 years after the last injection.

Estrogen-progestogen long-acting injections

Many once-a-month injectable contraceptives have been studied over the last 30 years, and at least four different formulations are currently in use worldwide, particularly in Latin America and China. Each of these formulations contains an ester of the natural estrogen estradiol and a synthetic progestin.

The major advantage of the combined estrogen-progestogen over the progestin-only injectables is a much lower incidence of menstrual bleeding disturbances and of amenorrhea.

In large clinical trials, the contraceptive efficacy is high, with a failure rate of 0.2 to 0.3% in the first year of use. The discontinuation rates at 1 year appear relatively low: 15 to 20%. Fertility appears to be restored within 60 to 120 days of the last injection.

Progestogen-releasing intrauterine devices (IUDs)

Progesterone- or LNG-releasing IUDs (LNG IUDs) are available. These devices are made of silicone and release progestins in the uterine cavity. LNG IUDs deliver 20 µg of steroid over 24 hours, and their duration is 5 years. Their efficacy is high, 0.1 to 0.3% in the first year of use, a figure comparable with but globally not better than that of copper-T devices. However, data showing a higher efficacy of LNG IUDs as compared with nonmedicated devices in the younger age segment also have been published. The main reason for using a medicated IUD is the 10 times reduced incidence of heavy bleeding, which represents the major cause of IUD removal.

The mechanism of action of LNG IUDs is not the complete inhibition of ovulation. After the first year of use, most of the cycles are ovulatory, as evaluated by the luteal progesterone rise; however, the lower peak LH levels shown in a good percentage of LNG IUD users may be indicative of a reduced rate of follicle rupture and/or of a disturbed corpus luteum function. These effects may account, at least in part, for the device's efficacy.

Even if the dose of LNG delivered is low, the incidence of potentially hormone-related side effects such as depression, acne, headache, weight gain, and breast tenderness is higher than with copper-T devices. The cumulative removal rate for these effects after 12 months is 2.7% for LNG IUDs and 0.1% for nonmedicated devices. No effect on carbohydrate metabolism, serum lipids, blood pressure, liver enzymes, or coagulation parameters could be observed.

At variance with copper-T devices, LNG IUD use appears to be protective of pelvic inflammatory disease (PID) and endometritis to an extent comparable with that observed with CCs. The mechanisms of this protective effect might be changes in cervical mucus composition and strong decreases in the amount and duration of menstrual bleeding.

POSTCOITAL HORMONAL CONTRACEPTION

This represents an emergency form of contraception to be used after sexual assaults, condom breakage, or on any occasion a woman is exposed to a high risk of pregnancy. Postcoital contraception cannot be used routinely because very high doses of steroids are used, side effects are consistent, and protection is not complete. Therapeutic abortion is advised if the method fails because of possible harmful effects of high doses of steroids on the fetus. The following treatments have proved effective: (1) conjugated estrogens 15 mg bid for 5 days po or 50 mg iv for 2 consecutive days, (2) estrone 5 mg po tid for 5 days, (3) EE 2.5 mg po for 5 consecutive days, and (4) two combination oral contraceptive pills (each containing norgestrel 0.5 mg + EE 50 µg) taken twice 12 hours apart. Other combination contraceptives are probably equally effective.

Treatment should start as soon as possible after exposure, no later than 72 hours. It is believed that the mechanism of action is an anti-implantation effect of the high dose of steroids. Failure rates are higher with the combined contraceptive method (about 2% versus 1% or less with estrogens alone). Side effects occur frequently and are often severe; they include nausea and vomiting (which occur routinely and often are severe), breast tenderness, headache, dizziness, and leg and abdominal cramps. Contraindications for estrogen-containing contraceptives apply to postcoital contraception.

A promising method of postcoital contraception is the use of an antiprogestin to inhibit implantation. Mifepristone (RU-486), a molecule approved for the induction of medical abortion in the early stages of pregnancy in some countries, has been used successfully in a single oral dose of 600 mg within 72 hours of the unprotected intercourse. In the limited studies available, the success rate and incidence of side effects compare favorably with the combined contraceptive method.

STERILITY TREATMENT: OVULATION INDUCTION

Chronic anovulation, amenorrhea, and infertility may occur for ovarian, pituitary, or hypothalamic failures. These problems occur rather frequently. In fact, it has been reported that anovulation is the leading cause (about 30%) of infertility in couples, and 10 to 15% of couples have infertility problems. Pharmacologic treatments to induce ovulation are aimed in most instances at inducing a few ovulatory cycles, allowing insemination and pregnancy to occur. In these situations, treatment attempts to duplicate the natural cycle, thus limiting the number of follicles selected to one or two. Assisted reproduction techniques, as in vitro fertilization and embryo transfer, gamete intrafallopian transfer, intrauterine insemination, and intracytoplasmatic sperm injection, which are gaining an increasing diffusion, on the contrary need so-called ovarian controlled hyperstimulation, in which multiple follicles simultaneously undergo the maturation process leading to ovulation.

OVULATION INDUCTION WITH ANTIESTROGENS

Clomiphene citrate (CLC) is the drug of first choice in ovulation-induction programs in patients with an intact hypothalamic-pituitary-ovarian axis and adequate estrogen production. Structurally, CLC is not a steroid but a triphenylethylene derivative with the same stilbene nucleus as diethylstilbestrol (DES). The commercially available preparations are racemic mixtures (60-40% *trans-cis*) of two stereoisomers that have different pharmacodynamic and pharmacokinetic properties. Enclomiphene (the *trans* isomer) appears to be responsible for most, if not all, the ovulation-inducing activity of the racemic compound acting mainly as antiestrogen. Zuclomiphene behaves mainly as an estrogen.

The mechanisms and sites of the stimulatory action of CLC are largely unknown. CLC, acting as an antiestrogen, may displace endogenous estrogens from their receptor at the hypothalamic level. According to this view, the compound should block the putative negative feedback exerted by endogenous estrogens, therefore permitting "normalization" of the GnRH pulse frequency. This could represent the triggering event leading to ovulation. As mentioned later, an adequate GnRH pulsatility is the essential minimal requirement to induce the pituitary-ovarian events leading to ovulation. Since the CLC administration is usually limited to the first 5 days of the cycle in which ovulation is expected to be induced, the drug should be better indicated as an ovulation initiator.

The pharmacokinetic profile of CLC is largely incomplete. It is readily absorbed when given orally, and it is mainly excreted in the feces together with its metabolites. A half-life of 2.5 to 11.8 days has been calculated for enclomiphene versus 14.2 to 33.2 days for zuclomiphene. A wide interindividual variability appears to be present.

Clomiphene citrate is indicated in all situations of chronic normogonadotropic, normoprolactinemic oligoovulation with adequate estrogen levels, including luteal-phase dysfunctions, and unexplained infertility.

More than 50% of patients destined to conceive on CLC will do so on the starting dose of 50 mg per day for 5 days. The treatment begins on the third to fifth day after the start of spontaneous or induced (progesterone withdrawal) menstruation. Graded increments of 50 mg per cycle of therapy, up to 200 to 250 mg per day, can be tested. Prolongation of CLC administration for 8 to 10 days is another possible way to overcome drug insensitivity. The mechanisms by which corticosteroids improve CLC efficacy are unknown at the moment. Ovulation is evaluated by monitoring the basal temperature and/or hormonal profile and/or echographic appearance of the ovary. Most of the CLC-initiated conceptions occur within six ovulatory cycles. In the absence of other infertility factors, ovulation rates between 80 and 90% have been reported, with conception rates of over 50%. At variance with other ovulation-induction procedures (see below), the incidence of miscarriage is analogous to that occurring in the normal population. The side effects are hot flashes, probably due to the antiestrogenic effect of CLC. They are rarely severe and occur in about 10% of the patients. Multiple pregnancies, mostly twins, are reported with a frequency several times higher than normal. Contraindications include pregnancy, serious liver disease (since CLC is metabolized at least in part in the liver), and ovarian cysts. The CLC method is relatively simple, cheap, effective, and safe, and it should be used before other ovulation-induction programs that are more expensive and risky.

OVULATION INDUCTION WITH GnRH

The minimal requirement for reproducing the main endocrine events that occur in a normal menstrual cycle and lead to ovulation is the pulsatile secretion of GnRH. The pulsatile administration of GnRH by suitable infusion pumps therefore has become an excellent method to induce ovulation and pregnancy in polycystic ovary syndrome (PCOS) or hypothalamic hypogonadotropic anovulation. The treatment avoids most of the complications associated with exogenous gonadotropin administration. When GnRH is used, ovarian hyperstimulation is absent or occurs very rarely, and multiple pregnancies are present in 5 to 10% of subjects (twins in most cases) because the process of follicular selection is maintained. Also, the incidence of spontaneous miscarriage is rather low (10%).

Both the sc and iv routes have been tested and proved to be effective. However, the sc route appears to be associated with a lower success rate, particularly in PCOS. On the other hand, the theoretical risk of local and septic complications is heavier with the iv route.

The GnRH bolus dose is 20 to 40 µg sc and 2.5 to 20 µg (5 µg in most studies) iv. The pulse frequency is 60 to 90 minutes (spontaneous LH peaks occur every 67-71 minutes in the mid to late luteal phase of the menstrual cycle). The treatment lasts for the whole cycle and is monitored by ultrasound and serum estradiol levels. Ovulation should not be triggered by hCG, which is reserved only for corpus luteum support after documented ovulation.

The GnRH pulsatile regimen produces ovulation in over 85% of treatment cycles and conception in over 25% of patients with hypogonadotropic hypogonadism. The GnRH treatment in PCOS is often started a few days after a cycle of pituitary desensitization with a GnRH agonist analogue (e.g., 4-6 weeks with a short-acting analogue at high doses sc).

Pregnancy rates around 10 to 15% per treatment cycle are achieved in PCOS with pulsatile GnRH treatment alone, whereas figures as high as 21% have been reported in the postdesensitization period. The GnRH agonist pretreatment also seems to reduce the risk of multiple pregnancies. The cost of this therapy is comparable to that with gonadotropins.

OVULATION INDUCTION WITH GONADOTROPINS

Gonadotropins are indicated to induce ovulation in all patients with anovulatory infertility (mainly PCOS and hypogonadotropic hypogonadism) in whom there is resistance or intolerance to antiestrogen treatment or pulsatile GnRH administration has failed. Moreover, they are the treatment of choice to induce superovulations for assisted reproductive techniques.

The available gonadotropin preparations are: (1) human menopausal gonadotropin (hMG), prepared from the urine of postmenopausal women, which has a 1:1 FSH-to-LH content, (2) human chorionic gonadotropin (hCG), prepared from the urine of pregnant women, which has LH-like activity, (3) purified FSH-postmenopausal gonadotropins, in which the LH activity has been largely removed (these include preparations with a 3:1 FSH-to-LH ratio or with a 60:1 FSH-to-LH ratio), and (4) a recombinant human FSH preparation that has an amino acid sequence, structure, and biologic activity analogous to that of the natural hormone.

The conventional dose regimen is represented by 2 to 3 ampules of hMG or purified FSH per day (equivalent to 150-225 IU of FSH) given im for 8 to 12 days. The initial dose can be increased at 5- to 7-day intervals by 75 IU or more, until serum or urinary estrogen concentrations start to increase. Follicular rupture is induced by a single im injection of 5000 IU hCG. If the woman is cycling (e.g., egg donors), the treatment is started on cycle day 2 or 3. Luteal function is supplemented by two additional im injections (2500 IU) of hCG.

In patients with hypogonadotropic amenorrhea or PCOS, the standard procedures lead to pregnancy in about 50% of the cases. Multiple pregnancies (34%), severe hyperstimulation syndrome, in which excessive stimulation of the ovarian follicles may produce ovarian enlargement, possibly progressing to the development of ascites, hypotension, and shock (4.6%), and spontaneous miscarriages (23%) are the complicating factors of therapy.

In controlled studies, which, however, involve a low number of subjects, no clear-cut differences in multiple follicle development have been observed between hMG and purified FSH given in conventional doses. As far as the recombinant preparation is concerned, the few comparison studies with hMG appear to indicate a slightly higher effectiveness of the new preparation in controlled hyperstimulation programs (greater number of oocytes and a better pregnancy rate). On the contrary, in ovulation-induction studies the two preparations behaved similarly, even if the doses of the recombinant FSH were 30% lower than those of hMG.

In the low-dose gonadotropin protocols, the starting dose of hMG or FSH is only 52 IU per day, and follicular growth is monitored primarily by ultrasound with the support of estradiol measurements (at 3- to 4-day intervals). If no dominant follicle appears after 14 days, the dose is increased by 20 to 40 IU per day. When a dominant follicle has reached its optimal size, hCG (5000 IU im) is given. If more than three follicles have a diameter of more than 15 mm, hCG is withheld and the cycle aborted because of the risk of ovarian hyperstimulation and/or multiple pregnancies.

With low-dose protocols, the fecundity rate appears to be about the same, approximately 10% per cycle in PCOS, but the incidence of multiple pregnancies is lower (7%, always twins) in the absence of serious ovarian hyperstimulation.

HORMONAL REPLACEMENT THERAPY IN POSTMENOPAUSAL WOMEN

Menopause represents the permanent cessation of ovarian activity and consequently of the cyclic changes in the endometrium that produce the monthly menstrual bleedings. It occurs in most women between 48 and 53 years of age. Termination of the cyclic ovarian endocrine and gametogenic activity has important biologic conse-

Table 67.5 Estrogen preparations used in HRT and their indicative daily doses

Estrogen preparations	Daily dose
Oral preparations	
Natural estrogens:	
Micronized estradiol	1-2 mg/d
Estradiol valerate	1-2 mg/d
Piperazine estrone sulfate (Estropipate)	1.25-2.5 mg/d
Estriol succinate	2 mg/d
Conjugated estrogens	0.625-1.25 mg/d
Tibolone	1.25-2.5 mg/d
Quinestrol	100 µg/d for 7 d; then 100-200 µg/wk
Chlorotrianisene	10-25 mg/d for 3 wks out of 4
Parenteral preparations	
Transdermal estradiol patches	50-100 µg/d; changed twice weekly
Transdermal estradiol/norethisterone patches	50 µg/d of estradiol + 0.25 mg norethisterone (in 2nd 2 wks of cycle); changed twice weekly
Estradiol implants	50 mg q6mo

quences, the most notable of which is the end of fertility. Moreover, interruption of the steroid secretory activity of the ovary, in particular of estrogens, may lead to the development of pathologic signs and symptoms. The main endocrine alterations related to cessation of ovarian function are represented by the 90 to 95% drop in circulating estradiol. In addition, progesterone almost completely disappears from the circulation, whereas gonadotropins undergo marked elevations following removal of ovarian feedback signals. Even if menopause is a physiologic event, because of the prolongation of life expectancy, a woman today may spend 30 years or longer in a hypoestrogenic state, a situation that may have important negative consequences on her health. Estrogen replacement therapy (i.e., hormone replacement therapy, or HRT) has been developed to provide a safe method to prevent the most serious consequences. Obviously, HRT also can and should be used in all clinical situations in which a hypoestrogenic state is produced by surgical castration or by a pathologic ovarian function.

ESTROGENIC PREPARATIONS

At variance with the use of estrogens for contraceptive purposes, which is limited to a few preparations, several different estrogens and routes of administration are used in HRT (Tab. 67.5).

Oral estrogen preparations

Conjugated equine estrogen (CE). It is the most frequently used preparation. Conjugated equine estrogen contains a combination of the sodium salts of the sulfate ester forms of up to 10 different naturally occurring estrogenic components. These include estrone, estradiol, equilin, equilenin, dihydroequilin, dihydroequilenin, and so on. Sodium estrone sulfate (50-60%) and sodium equilin sulfate (20-30%) are quantitatively the two most important components. CE is still obtained more commonly by extraction from the urine of pregnant mares. The pharmacokinetics of CE is complex and poorly understood because of the intense metabolization, interconversion, and enterohepatic recycling of all the constituents.

The intestinal absorption of CE is rapid and extensive; circulatory estrogens are primarily sulfate conjugates, possibly originating by hepatic reconjugation after intestinal hydrolysis. After absorption, an equilibrium between the predominant sulfated forms, albumin-bound, and the unconjugated estrogens, mainly SHBG-bound, is established. The conjugated forms may represent a large hormonally inert steroid reservoir pool with a substantially longer elimination half-life. After the administration of 0.625 mg per day of CE, the now prevalent HRT dose, estradiol blood levels rise from postmenopausal levels (<20 pg/ml) to those of the early follicular phase (about 40 pg/ml), whereas estrone concentration increases 5 to 10 times.

Indicative estimates of the biologic potency of CE using human biologic endpoints indicate that 3.75 mg of CE corresponds to 0.05 mg of EE. Therefore, the usual effective dose used in HRT, 0.625 mg per day, corresponds to 8.3 µg per day of EE, a dose four times lower than that present in low-dose contraceptives (35 µg).

Estradiol It is the most potent naturally occurring estrogen, but it cannot be given orally as such because of its poor absorption, rapid metabolization, and a large "first pass" effect. To improve absorption, the molecule has been esterified in C-17 position with valeric acid, or the native compound has been micronized in particles of size less than 20 µm. After absorption, the majority of estradiol is metabolized in the gut mucosa and in the liver into estrone (15%) and estrone sulfate (65%). The levels of estrone are therefore three to six times higher than those of estradiol. As with previous oral preparations, the high circulating levels of estrone sulfate are thought to represent a circulating reserve pool. With a 2-mg dose of the micronized preparation, peak levels of estradiol (65-110 pg/ml) are achieved a few hours after ingestion; sustained levels are maintained for about 8 hours, followed by a slow return to baseline in the next 19 hours.

Piperazine estrone sulfate It is the estrone sulfate stabilized with a molecule of piperazine. The sulfate group makes the molecule of estrone water soluble, whereas piperazine, which is pharmacologically inert, has buffering and stabilizing properties. The intestinal absorption of the preparation is good, and peak levels of estrone sulfate and estradiol sulfate are achieved in about 4 hours. The circulating sulfates represent the circulating reserve pool from which sustained levels of the active estrogen estradiol are maintained by hepatic conversion.

Estriol It is a natural metabolite of estradiol and estrone

that cannot be converted back to the former steroids. It exerts its weak estrogenic activity by a short-duration binding to the estrogen receptor. Moreover, the rapid metabolization and excretion in form of glucuronide (only 1-2% of orally administered estriol reaches the systemic circulation) contribute to its weak activity. Estriol has been used in the treatment of vasomotor symptoms of menopause, but it is not clear if it can be used to prevent osteoporosis.

Quinestrol It is the 3-cyclopentyl ether derivative of EE. It does not possess inherent estrogenic activity, but it must be converted in the body into the parent compound. It can be used clinically instead of EE to take advantage of some of its pharmacokinetic properties. The compound is completely absorbed orally, at least in part through lymphatics, and it is partially protected from "first pass" metabolism. Owing to its high lipophilic properties, the drug accumulates in adipose tissue, which acts as a reservoir from which it is thereafter constantly and slowly released. The formation of fat deposit accounts for its long half-life, about 120 hours. This represents an advantage, since the drug may be given once a week, and a disadvantage, because the circulating levels remain high for a long time if the therapy needs to be discontinued.

Tibolone It is a synthetic steroid with mild estrogenic effects and some progestogenic and androgenic actions. It binds to the estrogen receptor directly, whereas its metabolites have some affinity for progesterone and androgen receptors. Because of its inherent androgenic and progestational activity, it has a low stimulating effect on endometrial proliferation; therefore, uterine bleeding occurs less frequently than with conventional unopposed HRT and the incidence of endometrial cancer should thus not be increased, even without the addition of gestagens. Also, the occurrence of breast tenderness appears to be lower than with estrogens. Tibolone seems to have the same bone-sparing effects as conventional HRT, and it is effective in climacteric symptoms. The cardiovascular consequences of long-term therapy are not yet settled. However, its effects on the lipoprotein profile do not appear as favorable as with estrogen therapy, since LDL cholesterol is not decreased and HDL-cholesterol is unchanged or reduced but not increased. In the few studies performed, the overall effect on hemostasis appears to be that of increased fibrinolysis and unchanged coagulation.

Tissue-specific partial estrogen agonist-antagonists presently have become available as an alternative to estrogens in the treatment of osteoporosis. This new, promising form of therapy started when studies in postmenopausal patients treated with *tamoxifen,* widely used as an estrogen antagonist in breast cancer (see Chap. 61), showed a partial bone-protective effect and an estrogen-like effect on lipoproteins. Another molecule of the same class, *raloxifene,* is now available in the United States (see Chap. 46). It has the notable advantage over tamoxifen of acting as an antagonist at the uterine level, therefore producing hypoplasia and not hyperplasia of the endometrium, as does the former compound. It does not, however, antagonize postmenopausal flushes.

Even if the biochemical mechanisms at the base of the selectivity of the agonist-antagonist interactions are not fully understood, it is obvious that the availability of molecules showing estrogen-like activity only on specific targets, such as bone cells, liver, and possibly blood vessels, may represent an advantage.

Transdermal estrogen administration

Trasdermal delivery of drugs is a relatively new administration route with definitive advantages over the classic oral and parenteral routes. Both estrogens and progestins can be absorbed topically, if they are delivered in an appropriate solvent.

Estradiol delivery systems are thin adhesive patches consisting of a drug reservoir containing estradiol in alcoholic solution. Below the reservoir there is a rate-controlling polymeric membrane in immediate contact with the adhesive layer that contacts the skin. Estradiol is delivered to the skin surfaces at a constant rate, 0.21 µg/cm^2 per hour. The 10- and 20-cm^2 patches now available therefore deliver 50 and 100 µg per day of steroid for up to 4 days. The system is applied to the lower abdomen or buttocks and changed twice weekly.

Peak estradiol levels are reached within 4 to 8 hours and are followed by steady-state levels (about 50% of the peak) lasting over 72 hours. In postmenopausal women, mean steady-state estradiol levels are 40 and 75 pg/ml for the 50- and 100-µg patches, respectively, well within the normal range of the early follicular phase. Similar steady-state levels are achieved with 1.25 mg of conjugated estrogen and with 2 mg of micronized estradiol.

However, in contrast to the marked increase in serum estrone levels observed with oral preparations, transdermal estradiol produces only minor increases of circulatory levels of estrone. The ratio of estradiol to estrone is at the normal premenopausal value of 1 or greater.

Finally, transdermal estrogens, because they avoid high levels of steroids in the portal circulation, have a lower effect on liver protein synthesis. However, at the doses used in oral HRT, rarely the impact of estrogen on the liver synthesis of proteins becomes clinically evident.

In addition, HRT by transdermal patches needs to be associated with sequential progesterone supplementation to avoid the risk of inducing endometrial proliferation and carcinoma. Progesterone may be administered orally in a cyclic manner, as in the oral administration schedules, or by patches delivering 50 µg of estradiol and 0.25 mg of norethisterone applied in the second 2 weeks of a 28-day cycle. The levels of progestogen achieved by transdermal administration have been shown to be effective in opposing the proliferative effect of estrogens and in producing the secretory transformation of the endometrium.

Vaginal estrogen preparations

Vaginal administration of estrogens is possible using creams, vaginal tablets, or specifically made silicone devices, such as vaginal rings or cylinders. Steroids placed in the vagina, aside from producing local effects, are absorbed systemically and therefore represent a possible administration route in HRT.

Creams containing CE or estradiol are available but are used rarely because patients find these preparations rather messy to use and difficult to dose. Tablets should give more reproducible estrogen levels, but these preparations are not approved for clinical use everywhere, and studies with these preparations are limited. Administration from polymeric delivery systems is still experimental; however, recent studies appear to indicate that estradiol-releasing (6.5-9.5 µg/d) silicone vaginal rings represent a safe, highly effective, and very well accepted administration form for long-term treatment of urogenital disorders.

WHAT IS THE BEST ESTROGEN REPLACEMENT THERAPY?

At the moment, studies indicating a clear clinical superiority of one preparation over another are not available. A better knowledge of the kinetics of monocomponent estrogen preparations should not conceal the fact that CE has been used safely and successfully for more than 40 years for hundreds of thousands of patient-years. The theoretic advantages of the transdermal preparations have been underlined previously; these must be weighed against the higher economic cost of transdermal therapy (30% or more).

Therapeutic regimens: the association of a progestin

The major risk of HRT appears to be the induction of endometrial hyperplasia, which may progress to adenomatous hyperplasia with atypia, a premalignant condition. In about 1 year of unopposed HRT, a substantial increase in the risk of developing endometrial carcinoma can be documented. The risk increases with increasing duration and dose of HRT and remains elevated for past users for as long as 10 years (odds ratios from 1.7-20 have been reported). Since HRT-induced endometrial cancers are of low stage and grade, the risk of dying from endometrial cancer is increased to a much lesser extent. All types of unopposed estrogen replacement have been incriminated, but most of the data have been obtained in CE users.

Epidemiologic data indicate that the addition of an adequate progestin supplementation reduces the risk of developing endometrial cancer in HRT users to the level observed in nonusers, but it does not show a real protective effect, as occurs in women who use CCs. The duration, doses, and types of progestin used in the different studies are quite different, but it appears that a progestin should be used for at least 10 days per cycle.

A common regimen is a 28-day estrogen cycle with an oral progestin added for the last 10 to 13 days. The dose of progestin should block the effect of estrogens on endometrial cell proliferation but also cause full secretory transformation of the endometrium with subsequent endometrial shedding. Cyclic bleeding is experienced in 80 to 90% of women who use a progestin sequentially; irregular bleeding, expression of a proliferative endometrium, is present in those using only HRT.

Micronized progesterone and a number of progestin derivatives may be used; their recommended daily doses are shown in Table 67.2. No definite difference in the clinical use of one over the other molecule has been reported. In some subjects, progesterone may cause sleepiness because it can be metabolized into 5-α reduced compounds, which interact with the γ- aminobutyric acid (GABA) type A receptors, increasing the activity of endogenous GABA. The safety of treatments in which cyclic progesterone is given at longer time intervals (e.g., 3 months) is under evaluation.

A continuous estrogen and progestin regimen in which both hormones are administered daily also has been used. Lower progestin doses are used in this case. For example, conjugated estrogens (0.625-1.25 mg) are associated with MPA (2.5-5 mg/d) or with norethindrone (0.35-0.7 mg/d). Irregular bleeding is experienced by most patients in the first months of therapy, but in 9 to 12 months, 75 to 95% of the patients become amenorrheic.

The addition of a progestin to HRT is now the standard practice in all women with a uterus. The influence of the progestin does not appear to reduce the therapeutic efficacy or the climacteric symptoms and may even improve the effect on the bone loss.

HRT indications

Climacteric problems Perimenopause or the climacteric is the period when the endocrine, biologic, and clinical signs of decreased ovarian function start to appear. It ends, by convention, after 1 year of amenorrhea, when postmenopause begins. Vasomotor flushes, or "hot flushes," are one of the most frequent and annoying symptoms appearing at climacteric. Psychologic symptoms (e.g., irritability, asthenia, emotional lability, frank depression, reduced libido, etc.), vaginal dryness and atrophy, dispareunia, urinary symptoms (e.g., dysuria, recurrent lower urinary tract infections, and urinary incontinence) have been reported to affect more than 50% of postmenopausal women.

Hot flushes occur in about 75 to 80% of women within 3 months of a surgical, medical, or natural menopause. In most of the women progressing to natural menopause, they are often the reason for starting HRT. Hot flushes may persist for 2 to 5 years in postmenopause. They represent an increased blood flow limited to the skin vessels and lasting from 30 seconds to 5 minutes, from isolated episodes to many a day.

Hot flushes are produced by the acute withdrawal of estrogens, which appears to lower the thermoregulatory set point in the hypothalamic centers, thus activating cutaneous vasodilatation. The action of estrogen is probably mediated by an activation of the noradrenergic system, as indicated by the finding that α_2-agonists reduce hot flushes. Other neurotransmitters or neuromodulators such as dopamine, opioids, and neurosteroids also have been involved in the pathogenesis of hot flushes.

Hormonal repeacement therapy represents the first-choice therapy, with more than 95% efficacy. It requires a minimum of 2 to 4 weeks to be effective. Hot flashes may return after treatment interruption, but HRT is of value because the symptom is self-limiting. Tapering of the doses over several weeks is advised at discontinuation of therapy.

When estrogens are contraindicated, MPA (10-20 mg/per day po or 150 mg per month im) or other progestins, α_2-agonists such as clonidine (0.05-0.10 mg bid), methyldopa (250 mg tid), and lofexidine (0.1-0.6 mg bid), or an antidopaminergic drug such as veralipride (100 mg/per day) have been employed with variable success rates (20-70%).

Postmenopausal problems Osteoporosis (see Chap. 46) is a pathologic condition characterized by reduced bone mass, diminished bone strength, and increased fracture rate. Menopause is a cornerstone in the development of this disease. As a matter of fact, after the achievement of peak bone mass in the third decade, a process influenced by many factors including calcium intake, race, lifestyle, age at menarche, etc., an age-related bone loss begins. Cessation of ovarian function greatly speeds the process. The rate of bone loss varies greatly, ranging from less than 1% to 5% per year. Rapid bone losers rapidly reach the fracture threshold and are therefore vulnerable to fracture for the rest of their lives.

Hormonal replacement therapy stops bone loss independently of the therapeutic regimen, provided that early follicular-phase estrogen levels are achieved; the usual oral doses of 0.625 mg of CE or 1 to 2 mg of estradiol are effective in this regard.

Some recent data indicate the possibility of using even smaller HRT doses, particularly in regimens in which calcium is combined. Also, the incidence of fractures has been shown to be significantly reduced by HRT. Since bone loss is higher in the first 5 to 10 years of menopause, a treatment started early will produce the best benefits in terms of bone mass. HRT appears to stop resorption many years past menopause. The best duration of the hormone replacement is uncertain. A therapy lasting 5 to 10 years, particularly if started early after menopause, should provide enough protection for the rest of life. The ability to monitor easily and safely bone mineral density by new noninvasive methods may help in making the decision to start treatment and makes the monitoring of treatment efficacy easier.

The addition of a progestin to HRT not only does not reduce the efficacy of the therapy but also is possibly associated with an increased effect on bone mass preservation. Progesterone has osteoblast receptors, and when used alone, it has been shown to prevent bone resorption. When used in combination therapy, it also may enhance bone formation.

Other nonestrogen-related treatments for prevention of bone mass loss include calcitonin, bisphosphonates, sodium fluoride, ipriflavone, calcium and vitamin D, anabolic steroids, and parathyroid hormone. Those with alendronate (a bisphosphonate) and with calcium and vitamin D supplementation appear most promising.

Cardiovascular diseases are one of the leading causes of death in postmenopause. In particular, the incidence of coronary heart disease rises with age, due to the combined effect of age and menopause, and the higher prevalence in men greatly decreases. The impact of ovarian function on heart diseases can be appreciated in ovariectomized premenopausal women, a situation in which the risk of nonfatal myocardial infarct rises two to four times. Cerebrovascular diseases possibly show a similar pattern.

The pooled estimate from several studies indicates a substantial protection from cardiovascular risk with HRT: a mean relative risk of 0.49 for current users, who have a higher protection than past users. The duration of estrogen treatment and the doses used (most studies have been performed with conjugated estrogens at 0.625- or 1.25-mg doses) do not seem to affect the size of the benefit.

Several mechanisms may be involved. The most clear is the beneficial impact on the lipid profile. Estrogens lower LDL cholesterol and increase HDL cholesterol. The effect may be reduced by the addition of a progestin in the schedule. In particular, the addition of a progestin blunts the rise in HDL.

Antioxidant properties, preventing LDL oxidation, have been ascribed to estrogens, and the hormones have been shown to prevent paradoxical vasoconstriction in atherosclerotic coronary arteries after acetylcholine and may have calcium channel blocking and α_2 -inhibiting properties. The studies available suggest that the addition of a progestin does not eliminate the effect of HRT on the cardiovascular risks. It should be noted, however, that a prospective, randomized, placebo-controlled study in women with coronary disease, postmenopausal with intact uterus, < 80 years of age, provided negative findings. The HERS study in 2763 women randomized to either 0.625 mg CE/day plus 2.5 mg MPA/day (in one tablet) or a corresponding placebo, failed to show any cardiovascular benefits.

Several reports are now available suggesting that HRT may exert a protective effect on the risk of developing Alzheimer's disease (AD) (see Chap. 12). The risk of AD and related dementia appears to be reduced significantly in estrogen users compared with nonusers (relative risk 0.40) for both oral and nonoral (i.e., injections and/or creams) routes of administration. With CE, the risk decreases significantly with both the doses and the duration of therapy.

Side effects and contraindications

Combined estrogen-progestogen replacement therapy is usually well tolerated. Minor side effects are present in a substantial number of subjects and may lead to discontinuation of therapy in about 20% of cases. As far as the risk of venous thromboembolism is concerned, recent studies, one of which was done on a cohort of 347 252 women without major risk factors for venous thrombosis, indicate that it is two to three times higher among users than among nonusers. This increased risk is limited to the first year of use, and no major differences were found between users of oral and transdermal preparations or between users of unopposed or opposed treatments. Since the risk of idiopathic thromboembolism in postmenopause is 13 per 100 000 women, a risk two to three times higher means having 10 to 20 additional cases per 100 000 women using HRT for 1 year; which is still a very low incidence. When weighted against an almost 50% decrease in cardiovascular diseases, it does not contraindicate HRT but indicates the need to pay attention to a prior history of idiopathic thrombosis.

Systemic side effects include typical estrogen-related effects (e.g., breakthrough bleeding, breast tenderness, and cholestatic jaundice), progesterone-related effects (e.g., gastrointestinal problems, weight gain, headaches, nervousness, depression, and premenstrual-like symptoms), and general complaints (e.g., fatigue, nausea, vomiting, somnolence, insomnia, fluid retention, and changes in libido). The transdermal delivery systems also may induce local tolerability problems, usually mild, due to cutaneous reactions.

Hormonal repacement therapy does not appear to increase the overall risk of breast cancer substantially. However, some evidence of a duration-related increase in breast cancer risk is present across all the studies. An odds ratio of 1.5 after 5 years of HRT use was found in a cooperative case-control Italian study involving over 5000 subjects. The addition of a progestogen to HRT is even more controversial because the few studies available report either a definite protection, no protection, and even an increased risk.

It has been shown that HRT (1.25 mg of conjugated estrogen + cyclic progestogen) does not inhibit ovulation, and therefore, perimenopausal women on HRT should be warned of the possibility of ovulatory cycles and the potential for conception at least for 1 year after cessation of menstruations.

Suggested readings _____

ADASHI EY. Ovulation induction: clomiphene citrate. In: Adashi EY, Rock JA, Rosenwaks Z, eds. Reproductive endocrinology, surgery, and technology. New York: Lippincott-Raven, 1995;1181-1206.

CARR BR, ORY H. Estrogen and progestin components of oral contraceptives: relationship to vascular diseases. Contraception 1997;55:267-72.

FILICORI M. Gonadotropin-releasing hormone and analogues in ovulation induction: Current status and perspectives. J Clin Endocrinol Metab 1996;81:2413-6.

GEURTS TBP, PETERS MJH, VAN BRUGGEN JGC, et al. Puregon (ORG 32489): recombinant human follicle-stimulating hormone. Drugs of Today 1996;32:239-58.

GUTTHANN SP, GARCIA-RODRIGUEZ LA, CASTELLSAGUE J, DUQUE

OLIART A. Hormone replacement therapy and risk of venous thromboembolism: population based control study. Br Med J 1997;314:796-800.

HULLEY S, GRADY D, BUSH T, et al. Randomized trial of estrogen plus progestin for secondary prevention of coronary heart disease in postmenopausal wonen. JAMA 1998;289:605-13.

JACOBS S, HILLARD TC. Hormonal replacement therapy in the aged. A state of the art review. Drugs Aging 1996;8:193-213.

KAUNITZ AM, ROSENFIELD A. Injectable contraception with depot medroxyprogesterone acetate. Drugs 1993;45:857-65.

KUHL H. Comparative pharmacology of newer progestogens. Drugs 1996;51:188-215.

LUUKKAINEN T, TOIVONENT J. Levonorgestrel-releasing IUD as method of contraception with therapeutic properties. Contraception 1995;52:269-6.

PERALTA O, DIAZ S, CROXATTO O. Subdermal contraceptive implants. J Steroid Biochem Mol Biol 1995;53:223-6.

SÖMJEN D, WAISMAN A, KAYE AM. Tissue selective action of tamoxifen methyliodide, raloxifene and tamoxifen on creatine kinase B activity in vitro and in vivo. J Steroid Biochem Mol Biol 1996;59:389-96.

SPEROFF L. Hormonal contraception. In: Adashi EY, Rock JA, Rosenwaks Z, eds. Reproductive endocrinology, surgery, and technology. New York: Lippincott-Raven, 1995;1683-1708.

TRUSSELL J, LEVEQUE JA, KOENIG JD, et al. The economic value of contraception: A comparison of 15 methods. Am J Public Health 1995;85:494-503.

WILLIAMS CL, STANCEL GM. In: Goodman and Gilman's The pharmacological basis of therapeutics, 9th ed. New York: McGraw-Hill, 1996.

68

Treatment of diabetes mellitus

André J. Scheen, Pierre J. Lefèbvre

Diabetes mellitus is a group of metabolic diseases characterized by hyperglycemia resulting from defects in insulin secretion, insulin action, or both. The vast majority of patients with diabetes fall into two broad etiopathogenic categories. In one category (*type 1 diabetes,* previously referred to as *insulin-dependent diabetes mellitus,* or IDDM), the cause is an absolute deficiency of insulin secretion resulting from an autoimmune destruction of the β islet cells of the pancreas. In the other, much more prevalent category (*type 2 diabetes,* previously encompassed by the term *non-insulin-dependent diabetes mellitus,* or NIDDM), the cause is a combination of resistance to insulin action and an inadequate compensatory insulin secretory response. Both forms of diabetes mellitus share numerous common characteristics. Whatever the type, diabetes is a chronic illness that requires continuing med-ical care and education to prevent acute complications and to reduce the risk of long-term complications resulting from chronic hyperglycemia.

Nevertheless, each form has its proper specificities, particularly as far as pharmacologic treatment is concerned (Tab. 68.1). Thus, these two most common forms of diabetes mellitus will be considered separately in this chapter, which will not address other, rarer forms of diabetes (other specific types and gestational diabetes mellitus).

TYPE 1 DIABETES MELLITUS

Disease presentation

Type 1 diabetes mellitus results from a cell-mediated autoimmune destruction of the B cells of the pancreatic Langerhans islets. This phenomenon has multiple genetic predispositions and is also related to environmental factors that are still poorly defined. The disease has strong HLA associations, and various autoantibodies as markers of the immune destruction of the B cells are present in more than 85% of individuals at the diagnosis of hyperglycemia. In some patients, these immunologic markers also may be detected several years before clinical diagnosis of the disease. Immune-mediated diabetes commonly occurs in childhood and adolescence, but it can occur at any age. The rate of B-cell destruction is quite variable, being rapid in some individuals (mainly infants and children) and slow in others (mainly adults). Finally, there is little or no insulin secretion, as manifested by low or undetectable C-peptide plasma levels. Some patients, particularly children and adolescents, may present with ketoacidosis as the first manifestation of the disease, and the risk of ketoacidosis is rather high in most patients, especially in the presence of infection or other stress. Type 1 diabetes is also associated with a high risk of long-term damage, dysfunction, and failure of various organs, especially the eyes, kidneys, nerves, heart, and blood vessels, resulting from both micro- and macroangiopathy.

Table 68.1 Comparison of the most important characteristics of type 1 and type 2 diabetes

Characteristics	Type 1 diabetes	Type 2 diabetes
Prevalence in Europe	0.3-0.5%	2-5 %
Age at diagnosis	Generally < 40 years	Generally > 40 years
Obesity	Rare	Frequent
Pathogenesis	Autoimmune disease	Biochemical (genetic + environmental)
Pathophysiology	Insulin deficiency	Insulin resistance + secretory dysfunction
Associated syndrome X	Rare	Frequent
Main treatment	Insulin	Diet + oral antidiabetic agents
Complications	Micro- > macro-angiopathy	Macro- > micro-angiopathy
Risk of ketoacidosis	High	Low

Treatment

Treatments of general use in the disease

Type 1 diabetes is a chronic disease that requires major modifications in life-style. The role of an integrated team in managing diabetes should not be underestimated. Dietitians and nurse educators can assist patients and physicians in implementing the necessary skills and behaviors needed to achieve desired medical outcomes. Besides antihyperglycemic treatment itself, regular checks of glucose control, combining both self blood glucose monitoring (SBGM) by the patient and laboratory measurement by the physician (glycated hemoglobin or HbA1c, whose level reflects mean glycemia for the last 6-8 weeks), play an essential role in management of the disease. Furthermore, careful detection of incipient complications and early intervention to slow their progression are also highly valuable medical tasks to improve the quality of life of diabetic individuals.

Classic treatment of type 1 diabetes consists of dietary control, exercise, and administration of insulin. It is well known that a proper *diet* is critical in the therapy of diabetes mellitus. Even if it may appear more important in type 2 diabetes, the diet in type 1 diabetes is a dynamic component of the insulin management regimen, and the importance of individualizing the nutrition plan based on desired medical outcomes has been emphasized. Interestingly, recent nutrition recommendations for persons with type 1 diabetes do not advocate sugar restriction for the purpose of blood glucose control, and as high as 55% of the caloric intake as carbohydrates is generally recommended. Although *exercise* has long been considered as an important part of the treatment of diabetes, it often has been difficult to manage by type 1 diabetic patients because of problems with metabolic regulation and/or the presence of diabetic complications. Recommendations about exercise for persons with type 1 diabetes should be made on an individual basis, taking into consideration the patient's personal attitudes and desires about exercise, his/her knowledge and skills in blood glucose management, and the presence or absence of diabetic complications that might pose risks or limitations to exercise.

Insulin administration has been the pivotal treatment of type 1 diabetes since its discovery in 1921. However, as already emphasized by Banting in his Nobel Prize lecture in 1923, insulin is not a cure for diabetes – it is a treatment. Three-quarters of a century afterwards, subcutaneous insulin therapy still remains the key to treatment of type 1 diabetes. The general principles remain the same as those described initially, even if much progress has been made since that time. The most important improvement can be summarized as follows: improvement in the purity of insulin preparations, interference with the duration of action of insulin, improvement of the mode of insulin administration (disposable syringes, pens, pumps), and even more important, the ability to control insulin's efficacy (SBGM) so as to rapidly adjust insulin treatment.

Specific treatments of acute (e.g., ketoacidosis, hypoglycemic coma) or chronic (e.g., retinopathy, neuropathy, nephropathy, foot problems) diabetic complications are beyond the scope of this general review. Similarly, particular situations such as infancy, pregnancy, surgery, or severe acute illnesses will not be further considered

Basic principles

Modern insulin therapy must be integrated into an intensive diabetes treatment plan suited to the needs, goals, and capabilities of each diabetic patient. While the aims of insulin therapy were for several decades restricted to alleviating symptoms (e.g., polyuria, weight loss, fatigue, infections) and to prevent acute complications (e.g., ketoacidosis, severe hypoglycemia), much has changed in the last 20 years. The recent Diabetes Control and Complications Trial (DCCT) definitively confirmed the crucial role of good glycemic control in preventing late degenerative complications. An intensive diabetes treatment program that resulted in a significant improvement in glycemic control (decrease in HbA1c levels from 9 to 7.2%; normal values 3-6%) for up to 8 to 9 years could significantly delay the development and slow down the progression of the microvascular complications of diabetes. However, although most individuals with type 1 diabetes should benefit from an intensive diabetes regimen, not all individuals are candidates for intensive diabetes treatment or are willing to accept the personal commitment inherent in such treatment.

Regimens of insulin therapy

Single insulin dose A single daily dose of insulin is rarely able to achieve normoglycemia. Insulin availability is generally inadequate, with significant hyperglycemia being present at certain times of the day and hypoglycemia occurring at the time of peak insulin action. Therefore, such an insulin regimen should not be recommended anymore for the treatment of type 1 diabetes. However, newly diagnosed diabetic patients occasionally can achieve reasonable glycemic control with one injection of intermediate-acting insulin in the morning, as long as significant residual insulin secretion is present. Older patients or patients with end-stage renal disease also may be candidates for this type of regimen.

Twice-daily insulin dose A twice-daily insulin injection regimen is currently the most frequently used treatment regimen in type 1 diabetes. The regimen generally is given as a twice-daily injection of a combination of regular and intermediate-acting insulin. Although such a regimen provides good insulin availability throughout the day, there are several pitfalls. Hypoglycemia late in the morning or in the early part of night frequently occurs. Furthermore, prebreakfast hyperglycemia results because insulin action has waned. Such side effects are more likely to occur with biosynthetic human insulin, which has a shorter duration of action than animal insulin. Finally, mealtimes must be consistent, because food must be eaten when insulin action peaks, and the ingestion of snacks in addition to meals is usually mandatory to avoid hypoglycemia.

Multiple daily insulin injections Multiple daily insulin injection regimens are a means to improve blood glucose control and reduce wide and erratic excursions in blood glucose levels. Furthermore, they provide additional flexibility in a patient's daily routine and enable the patient to exercise more control over diabetes management. Such a regimen can be achieved in a variety of ways. However, the most common regimen consists of the injection of regular insulin before each main meal (usually three times a day) and the injection of intermediate-acting insulin in the evening (before supper or preferably at bedtime). This regimen minimizes the risk of hypoglycemia. The dosages of regular insulin should be adjusted on the basis of an SBGM, taking into consideration both the amount of carbohydrates ingested and the physical activity to be performed. The use of a cartridge pen type of device for injecting insulin has facilitated successful implementation of multiple daily insulin injections in most well-motivated diabetic patients.

Insulin infusion pumps Continuous subcutaneous insulin infusion (CSII) may be an alternative to multiple daily insulin injections. It permits the greatest degree of life-style flexibility and can facilitate achieving glycemic goals. The reasons for this are that the insulin pump uses only regular insulin, making insulin absorption from subcutaneous tissues more predictable, and that insulin delivery is quite similar to that found in nondiabetic individuals, in that there is a continuous basal insulin delivery supplemented by preprandial boluses to acutely increase plasma insulin levels and compensate for food intake. Although CSII has many advantages, there are several problems unique to insulin pump therapy. Interruption of insulin delivery can result in deterioration of diabetic control in a matter of hours, and ketoacidosis episodes are more frequent with this type of treatment. Another potential problem is infusion-site infections where the needle is inserted. To circumvent these problems and warrant better insulin absorption, implantable programmable insulin pumps with intraperitoneal or intravenous catheters have been tested for the last few years, essentially in France and the United States. Preliminary results showed that long-term implantable pump therapy maintained HbA1c levels in a range similar to that of intensive subcutaneous therapy but with lower indices of glycemic instability and fewer episodes of severe hypoglycemia. Although catheter occlusions remain a limitation, patient satisfaction with implantable pump therapy is high. However, the use of CSII, as well as implantable pumps in particular, requires care by skilled professionals, careful selection of patients, meticulous patient monitoring, and thorough patient education.

Integrated diabetes management

Intensive diabetes treatment is not simply multiple daily injections of insulin or insulin pump therapy. It is a goal-oriented, comprehensive approach to therapy that consists of frequent blood glucose self-monitoring and a systematic approach to quantifying food and physical activity and matching insulin to precise requirements. Thus, the patient is taught to solve problems and make decisions about the treatment plan in response to blood glucose levels and changing circumstances. Because this treatment requires learning and self-management skills that permeate the entire range of life-style behaviors, collaboration among team members, including physicians, nurses, dietitians, and, when necessary, mental health professionals, is essential. An ongoing and comprehensive program of insulin administration, dietary control, self-monitoring, and education directed toward achieving specific health care outcomes is required for diabetes treatment to have the beneficial impact demonstrated by the results of the DCCT.

Risk and benefits

After decades of debate, the beneficial effects of intensified insulin treatment in type 1 diabetes have been demonstrated conclusively in the large DCCT. Overall, the development and progression of microangiopathic complications were reduced by about 50% when the outcomes of the intensive treatment group were compared with those of the conventional treatment group. Fewer macrovascular events also occurred in the intensive treatment group, although the difference did not reach the level of statistical significance.

Body weight gain and severe hypoglycemic episodes are the two most common side effects of intensified insulin therapy. Intensive diabetes treatment was associated with about a 5-kg increase in body weight over the 8- to 9-year duration of the DCCT, and a threefold increment in severe hypoglycemia also was reported. The risk of ketoacidosis also was increased significantly in patients treated with CSII. Thus, while the benefits of intensified insulin treatment in type 1 diabetes are well recognized, the inherent risks cannot be underestimated. However, most of these acute complications should be reduced by appropriate patient education and reasonable glycemic goals tailored to each individual profile.

Drug classes

The introduction of insulin therapy remains the single most important milestone in the history of diabetes. Indeed, over the 75 years since subcutaneous insulin injections were first given, no other therapeutic or ancillary development has displaced insulin therapy as the most important treatment for diabetes. The lack of progress in developing alternatives to insulin therapy does not reflect a lack of commercial and research interest in the hormone, which often has been at the forefront of the application of new biochemical techniques to medicine. Insulin is now available as different preparations and can be administered in different ways.

INSULIN PREPARATIONS

There are four major properties that characterize insulin preparations used for injection: species source, purity, concentration, and type (i.e., certain physicochemical modifications that determine the time course of hypoglycemic action).

Species source

Insulin can be obtained from beef or pork pancreas or is made chemically identical to human insulin by recombinant DNA technology or chemical modification of pork insulin. Human insulin is preferred for use in pregnant women or women considering pregnancy, individuals with allergies or immune resistance to animal-derived insulins (see below), those initiating insulin therapy, and those expected to use insulin only intermittently. Human insulins have a more rapid onset and shorter duration of activity than pork insulins, whereas beef insulins have the slowest onset and longest duration of activity. Thus, changing insulin species may affect blood glucose control and should only be done under the supervision of a health professional with expertise in diabetes. In most countries, especially in Europe, human insulin manufactured using recombinant DNA technology is progressively replacing animal insulin, whose future availability is said to be uncertain.

Purity

In the past, impurities in initial insulin preparations ("dirty insulin") were responsible for many side effects of insulin injection, especially immunologic reactions. The first possible side effect is a local delayed reaction to insulin at the injection site. These reactions are thought to be related to delayed hypersensitivity to impurities in insulin preparations and invariably disappear after several months. The second side effect is true of systemic insulin allergy. This rare complication begins as an immediate reaction (within 30 minutes) at the injection site that can quickly spread over large parts of the body as an urticarial rash. Desensitization is the treatment of choice. The third side effect is immune-mediated insulin resistance, which may require very high daily dosage of insulin. High titers of IgG antibody are present. The fourth side effect is insulin-induced lipoatrophy. This loss of subcutaneous fat at injection sites is enhanced by impurities in insulin preparations and may represent an Arthus reaction between insulin and insulin-binding IgG antibodies. Injection of more pure insulin preparations directly into the atrophic areas is able to reverse this process in most cases. In contrast, insulin-induced lipohypertrophy at the injection site is due to a local lipogenic effect of insulin, and such a side effect may be minimized by the use of varied injection sites. Most of these reactions have become less frequent since the use of purified animal insulins or even rarer with the use of recombinant human insulin. Nevertheless, they occasionally develop in patients starting on purified pork or even human insulins.

Concentration

Insulin is available commercially, depending on the country and the presentation (vials versus cartridges), in concentrations of 40 units/ml (U-40) or 100 units/ml (U-100). A progressive replacement of all U-40 preparations by U-100 preparations is now taking place in all European countries. Before full harmonization, diabetic travelers always should verify that they use appropriate syringes for the insulin preparations in order to avoid hypo- or hyperglycemic accidents. Other concentrations may be used in very special cases, such as insulin resistance (U-500), implantable insulin pump (U-1000), or infancy (dilution to U-10).

Type

Insulin is available in rapid-, short-, intermediate-, and long-acting forms that may be injected separately or mixed in the same syringe. New insulin analogues have been developed by modifying the amino acid sequence of the insulin molecule. From a therapeutic point of view, three characteristics of the time course of action of the different types of insulin preparations are important: onset of action, time of peak activity, and duration of action (Tab. 68.2). These properties depend on the rate of absorption after the subcutaneous injection.

The earliest pharmaceutical preparations of insulin were of insulin dissolved in acidic solution. Such insulin preparations were termed *regular insulin, crystalline insulin,* or *soluble insulin.* They are still recognized as a short-acting insulin. Initial acidic solutions have been replaced with neutral solutions, which are better tolerated and less antigenic. This unmodified insulin was the only insulin that could be administered intravenously.

Intermediate-acting insulins include lente (insulin-zinc suspensions) and NPH (neutral protamine Hagedorn). In the lente series, the size of the crystal determines the rate of absorption. Careful attention to crystal seeding and size is needed to obtain consistent preparations. The protamine in the NPH preparation delays the absorption of insulin; however, its amount is small enough that regular insulin added to the same syringe is still absorbed rapidly (which is not the case after mixing regular insulin with zinc insulin). Insulin

Table 68.2 Profile of action of the various insulin preparations

Type of insulin	Onset of action (h)	Time of peak activity (h)	Duration of action (h)
Rapid lispro insulin	0.2	0.5-2.0	3-4
Soluble or regular insulin	0.25-1.0	1.5-4.0	5-9
Intermediate insulin	0.5-2.0	3.0-6.0	8-14
Long insulin	2.0-4.0	4.0-8.0	12-24

preparations with a predetermined proportion of NPH mixed with regular insulin are also considered intermediate-acting.

The only long-acting insulin is ultralente, which is composed of large crystals. Ultralente insulin is absorbed slowly from subcutaneous tissue, but the rate of absorption is highly dependent on the species of insulin used (beef insulin being the least rapidly absorbed, followed by pork insulin and, lastly, by human insulin).

Lispro is a rapid-acting insulin analogue that has been obtained by switching Pro (B28) and Lys (B29), to Lys (B28) and Pro (B29) amino acids. Lispro insulin is absorbed more rapidly from the subcutaneous tissue than regular human insulin because of a reduced tendency to self-associate. As a consequence, peak serum insulin levels are higher, and they are achieved within less than half the time as regular insulin. In addition, lispro insulin has a shorter duration of action than native insulin. These pharmacokinetic properties allow the injection of lispro insulin immediately before meals (rather than 15-45 minutes before, as for regular insulin) and result in a better control of early postprandial glycemic excursions and a reduced risk of hypoglycemia several hours after injection. However, a late postprandial glucose rise has been reported that can be prevented by combining lispro with a more appropriate basal insulin replacement regimen.

Insulin administration

Subcutaneous injection

The injection of insulin in the subcutaneous adipose tissue is essential for management of patients with type 1 diabetes. Whenever possible, insulin should be self-administered by the patient, and the patient's injection technique should be reviewed periodically with the diabetes care team. Beyond the choices of type and dose of insulin, all steps of insulin administration are important. They include appropriate storage of insulin preparations, correct use of materials of injection, and adequate injection technique itself (i.e., dose preparation, injection site, injection procedure). Conventional insulin administration involves subcutaneous injection with syringes marked in insulin units. Mixing of different insulins in the same syringe is possible but should follow several guidelines to achieve both efficacy and safety. Several penlike devices and insulin-containing cartridges are available that also deliver insulin subcutaneously through a needle. These devices may improve accuracy of insulin administration (e.g., in patients who are visually or neurologically impaired) and/or be more convenient (e.g., in patients using multiple daily injection regimens). Jet injectors that inject insulin as a fine stream into the skin should not be viewed as a routine option for use in patients with type 1 diabetes.

Finally, CSII with an infusion pump is an alternative to multiple-daily-injection therapy for achieving near-normal levels of blood glucose and improved flexibility of life-style and may be proposed in well-selected patients.

Alternative routes of insulin delivery

The classic subcutaneous route for insulin delivery has proved its efficacy and practicability for self-management by diabetic patients over a long period of time. Some disadvantages exist, however, that make it not entirely satisfactory to both doctors and patients. Alternative routes for insulin delivery, such as nasal, gastrointestinal, or transdermal administrations, have been tested without great success. Intranasal insulin administration has the advantage of inducing a rapid and short-lasting hypoglycemic action but has the disadvantage of a poor and highly variable bioavailability. Intraperitoneal and intravenous routes will be in the forefront with the arrival of implanted insulin pumps and probably offer some advantages over the classic subcutaneous injection.

New areas of drug development

NEW ANTIHYPERGLYCEMIC DRUGS

New insulin analogues

Besides the recent development of rapid insulin analogues such as lispro, pharmaceutical companies also attempt to develop long-lasting rather than short-acting insulin analogues. The main objective is the benefit of a more stable and reproducible subcutaneous absorption of the hormone to ensure a better basal insulin delivery rate than with the classic intermediate-acting or lente insulin preparations. This should contribute to improved stability of the glycemic profile, especially during the night.

Other antihyperglycemic agents

Type 1 diabetes is not characterized by a pure insulin deficiency, but it is also associated with defects in other hormonal systems, particularly insulin-like growth factor (IGF-1) and amylin. During recent years, trials have been performed with these two compounds in addition to insulin in an attempt to improve blood glucose control in type 1 diabetic patients.

Recombinant IGF-1 in combination with conventional insulin treatment has been shown to ameliorate the low plasma total and free IGF-1 levels and to be well tolerated in patients with type 1 diabetes. Furthermore, there was a trend toward improved glycemic control, while the regular insulin dose was decreased significantly.

Amylin is a 37-amino-acid polypeptide that is synthesized in and secreted from pancreatic B cells, together with insulin, and has several metabolic effects. A synthetic human amylin analogue (25,28,29-tripro-amylin, or pramlintide) is now in clinical study. Its main action is to slow gastric emptying and therefore slow gastrointestinal absorption of nutrients. An additional antihyperglycemic effect may result from a reduction of meal-induced glucagon release.

INSULIN REPLACEMENT

Islet cell transplantation

Islet cell transplantation has held the promise of a cure for insulinopenic diabetic patients for over three decades, and the failure to reach this goal has been an enormous disappointment to clinicians and patients alike. Nevertheless, the field has witnessed significant progress. Enough islets can now be obtained from a single donor to reverse diabetes after intraportal infusion. Functional and histologic evidence of transplanted islet tissue has been demonstrated 5 years after the islet allotransplantation. The continuous requirement for immunosuppressive drugs still limits the applicability of islet cell transplantation, but the possibility that recipients can be induced to accept islet allografts even in the absence of continuous immunosuppressive therapy (tolerance induction) is currently generating great enthusiasm. Tremendous experimental efforts are under way to create xenogenic porcine/bovine islets and, perhaps over a longer period of time, human/nonhuman engineered insulin-producing cells suitable for graft within special immunoisolation barrier membranes.

Gene therapy

Somatic gene therapy carries great promise for the treatment of a variety of metabolic diseases, including not only rare monogenic disorders but also more common polygenic and multifactorial diseases. The demonstration that liver-directed gene transfer in humans can lead to stable genetic reconstitution is critical to the potential application of somatic gene therapy to diabetes mellitus. Although one potential target for gene therapy for diabetes is the pancreatic B cell, preliminary studies suggested that gene transfer of a regulated insulin gene to extrapancreatic cells, such as hepatocytes, could better be used as therapy for type 1 diabetes.

Implantable artificial pancreas

Finally, insulin also can be replaced through an artificial endocrine pancreas that exerts a closed-loop glycemic control. Unfortunately, until now, none of these closed-loop systems has been used for more than several days in humans because of their large size, volumes of blood needed to measure glucose levels, and the unreliability of glucose sensors and blood access devices. Numerous attempts have been made over the last 10 years to develop a miniaturized implantable artificial or bioartificial pancreas, but a reliable glucose sensor, compatible with human tissues and stable in the long run, still remains a missing link.

Prevention _____

Type 1 diabetes is an autoimmune disease. Several genetic risk factors and immune-related markers are known that accurately identify many first-degree relatives of patients with type 1 diabetes who will develop the disease. Immunologic markers are highly specific and include not only islet cell antibodies (ICA) and anti-insulin antibodies but also new markers such as GAD65 autoantibodies and IA-2 autoantibodies. These autoantibodies have been shown to be detectable in the serum several months or even years before the clinical diagnosis of diabetes. Genetic markers are of more limited use because they probably account for less than 50% of disease susceptibility. It should be pointed out that 90% of cases of type 1 diabetes occur outside affected families. Investigators have begun to explore the use of intervention therapy to halt or even prevent B-cell destruction in such at-risk individuals. It is generally well accepted that interventions for the prevention of type 1 diabetes should be attempted only in the context of defined randomized, controlled clinical studies, even if the latter have their own limitations.

In theory, interventions to prevent the onset or progression of type 1 diabetes could be instituted at various stages of the disease. *Primary prevention*, either in the general population or targeted specifically at high-risk groups, would prevent the earliest stages of type 1 diabetes. Effective primary prevention depends critically on identifying the environmental agents that trigger autoimmune diabetes. Options include vaccinations against diabetogenic viruses (e.g., Coxsackie, retroviruses) and possibly avoidance of cow's milk in neonates (since bovine serum albumin may generate antibodies that crossreact with B-cell antigens). *Secondary prevention* acts at the preclinical stage of the autoimmune B-cell damage and prevents this from progressing to overt diabetes. Secondary interventions currently tested in large randomized clinical trials include nicotinamide and prophylactic insulin. Nicotinamide may preserve B-cell function by preventing excessive consumption of nicotinamide adenine dinucleotide (NAD^+). Low-dose subcutaneous or oral insulin may decrease the expression of potential autoantigens (immunotolerance) and limit the autoimmune process. *Tertiary prevention* applies to people with recent-onset type 1 diabetes and aims to achieve prolonged remission and amelioration of long-term disease. Trials of tertiary prevention have included nonspecific immunosuppression with azathioprine, glucocorticoids or cyclosporine, and nicotinamide, intensified insulin treatment, or bacille Calmette-Guérin (BCG) vaccine. Limited efficacy and/or unacceptable side effects have been reported. Nevertheless, an optimistic view of these exciting developments can be defended, and recent observations justify the hope that acceptably safe, efficacious, and practical interventions will become a reality in a near future.

TYPE 2 DIABETES MELLITUS

Disease presentation_____

Type 2 diabetes mellitus is a heterogeneous condition caused by both genetic and environmental factors in which hyperglycemia results from a dynamic interaction between defects in insulin secretion and insulin action.

Although the specific etiologies of this form of diabetes are not completely known, autoimmune destruction of islet B cells does not occur (in contrast to what is observed in type 1 diabetes), and patients do not have any of other causes of diabetes that have been listed recently. Ketoacidosis seldom occurs spontaneously in this type of diabetes. Most patients are obese or have an increased percentage of body fat distributed predominantly in the intraabdominal region (Tab. 68.1). Diagnosis is usually made after the third decade (*adult-onset diabetes*), but this form of diabetes frequently goes undiagnosed for many years because the hyperglycemia develops gradually and at earlier stages is often not severe enough to be accompanied by clinical symptoms. Nevertheless, such patients are at increased risk of developing microvascular and, especially, macrovascular complications. Indeed, besides hyperglycemia, other abnormalities are frequently present and most probably related to visceral adiposity: dyslipidemias (e.g., hypertriglyceridemia, low HDL-cholesterol, increased small dense LDL particles, postprandial hyperlipemia), arterial hypertension (in about half of overweight patients with type 2 diabetes), and fibrinolytic disturbances (e.g., increased plasminogen-activator inhibitor-1, or PAI-1, levels). All these abnormalities are well-documented cardiovascular risk factors. They are related to insulin resistance (syndrome X or metabolic syndrome) and may be present even in the absence of overt hyperglycemia (e.g., in individuals with so-called impaired fasting glucose, i.e., fasting glucose levels of 110 and <126 mg/dl).

The diagnostic criteria for diabetes mellitus have been modified recently. Three ways to diagnose diabetes are possible, and each must be confirmed, on a subsequent day, by any one of the three following methods: (1) fasting plasma glucose level of 126 mg/dl (instead of 140 mg/dl, as previously considered), (2) a 75-g oral glucose tolerance test (OGTT) with a 2-hour postload plasma glucose value of 200 mg/dl, or (3) symptoms with a casual plasma glucose level of 200 mg/dl. Changing the diagnostic cutoff point for the fasting plasma glucose concentration from 140 to 126 mg/dl was based on the belief that the cutoff points for the fasting and 2-hour OGTT measurements should diagnose similar conditions, given the equivalence in their associations with vascular complications. The use of these new fasting criteria will markedly increase the number of diagnosed diabetic patients (mostly type 2) and raise the crucial question of when to introduce a pharmacologic treatment in such a population with only mild hyperglycemia. The new criteria also should facilitate the diagnosis of numerous adults with diabetes who still are undiagnosed (recent estimates indicate that about half remain undiagnosed in the United States and in most European countries) but are still at significant risk of vascular complications.

Since type 2 diabetes mellitus is characterized by defects in both insulin secretion and insulin action, it may be important to quantify the severity of such defects in a given individual. This may be particularly relevant in clinical research, especially in order to select appropriate patients for pharmacologic trials and to more precisely assess the effect of an antidiabetic drug on the two com-

ponents of the disease. The most widely used tests for evaluating insulin secretion and insulin action are listed in Table 68.3. Assessments based on the simple determination of fasting plasma levels of glucose, insulin, and/or C-peptide are easy to perform but generally less reliable. In contrast, assessments based on dynamic tests are more complicated and time-consuming for both the patient and the medical staff, but they are also more informative. This is particularly the case of the euglycemic hyperinsulinemic clamp, which is now considered the "gold standard" for evaluating insulin sensitivity in vivo. Because of its complexity, however, various alternative methods have been proposed that all have their advantages and limitations. Thus, the most appropriate test should be selected according to the primary objectives and available facilities for each study.

Treatment

Treatments of general use in the disease

In contrast to type 1 diabetes, in which the metabolic abnormality is generally restricted to insulin deficiency and secondary hyperglycemia, type 2 diabetes appears to be a much more complex metabolic disease. Consequently, therapeutic guidelines for type 2 diabetes should focus not only on correction of hyperglycemia but also should encourage consideration of the patient globally and treatment of all risk factors found in each individual, most particularly weight excess and abdominal adiposity, arterial hypertension, and dyslipidemias.

Table 68.3 Classic tests to assess insulin secretion and insulin action in type 2 diabetes

Insulin secretion
Fasting plasma insulin levels (HOMA: homeostatic model assessment)
Fasting plasma C-peptide levels (compared with fasting glycemia)
Stimulated plasma C-peptide levels (postmeal or post-glucagon 1 mg)
Stimulated plasma insulin levels
  Intravenous glucose tolerance test (IVGTT) (acute insulin response, AIR)
  Continuous infusion of glucose with model assessment (CIGMA)
  Stepped intravenous glucose infusion (dose-response curve)

Insulin action
Fasting plasma insulin levels (HOMA)
Euglycemic hyperinsulinemic clamp (CLAMP: gold standard)
Intravenous glucose tolerance test with minimal model analysis (IVGTT)
Varia: insulin tolerance test (ITT)
  Continuous infusion of glucose with model assessment (CIGMA)
  Low-dose insulin-glucose infusion test (LDIGIT)

Type 2 diabetes is a common disease whose prevalence markedly increases with age (>10% of patients are 65 years of age or older). The objectives of therapy should be clearly defined in each patient in order to adapt both treatments and glycemic targets individually. The key recommendation is based on the premise that the benefits of treatment outweigh the risks. As an example, treating a modest hyperglycemia with sulfonylureas or insulin may expose the older patient to severe hypoglycemia, which could be more harmful than the initial metabolic disturbance. However, even if *primum non nocere* should be the rule, the antihyperglycemic treatment of patients with type 2 diabetes should not be neglected, especially in younger individuals (40-60 years), because of the high risk of microangiopathy and macroangiopathy, especially coronary pathology, associated with this complex metabolic disorder and the positive effects of improved glycemic control on the incidence and severity of such complications.

Nonpharmacologic treatment

The initial treatment of choice in patients with type 2 diabetes is optimization of the meal plan and enhancement of physical activity. Reduction of excessive body weight should be a main target in most patients. Unfortunately, traditional dietary strategies, and even very low calorie diets, usually have not been effective in achieving long-term weight loss. Therefore, several additional strategies can be implemented to favor and/or maintain weight loss, such as antiobesity drugs and even, in well-selected extreme cases, bariatric surgery, especially gastroplasty. The emphasis for medical nutrition therapy in type 2 diabetes also should be placed on achieving glucose (55% of

---

Table 68.4 Commercially available oral antidiabetic drugs

Sulfonylureas
First generation:
carbutamide, tolazamide, tolbutamide, chlorpropamide,
Second generation:
glyburide or glibenclamide, glipizide, gliclazide,
gliquidone

Once-daily preparations:
glimepiride, glipizide

Biguanides
Metformin

α-Glucosidase inhibitors
Acarbose

Thiazolidinediones
Troglitazone[1]
Rosiglitazone

---

[1]Not available in most countries; restricted use because of recently described severe hepatotoxicity.

---

energy intake as carbohydrates, with limitation of sucrose and advice to consume more fibers), lipid (reduction in saturated fat and cholesterol consumption), and blood pressure (no more than 3000 mg/day of sodium) goals.

An appropriate exercise program should be an adjunct to diet and/or drug therapy to improve glycemic control, reduce certain cardiovascular risk factors, and increase psychologic well-being in individuals with type 2 diabetes mellitus. However, attention must be paid to minimizing potential exercise complications, and a careful preexercise evaluation should be recommended in all individuals with type 2 diabetes.

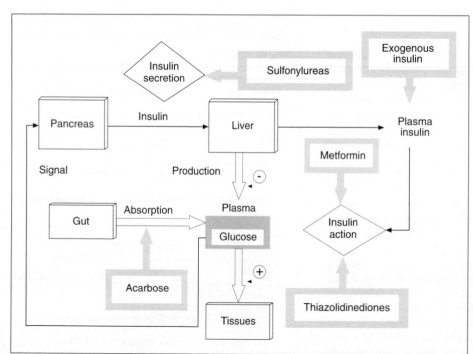

Figure 68.1 Current status of drug treatment of type 2 diabetes: sites of action of sulfonylureas, metformin, acarbose, thiazolidinediones, and exogenous insulin.

Drug therapy

If progress toward glycemic goals is not apparent within a 3-month period after initiation of diet and exercise therapy, then the use of a pharmacologic agent is appropriate. Various oral antihyperglycemic agents have been developed during the last 40 years: first, sulfonylureas and biguanides (metformin is the only one still available in most countries) and, more recently, α-glucosidase inhibitors (acarbose) and thiazolidinediones or glitazones (troglitazone and rosiglitazone) (Tab. 68.4). Insulin also can be used in type 2 diabetes, as initial therapy or most often after secondary failure of oral drug treatment. Criteria for drug selection in daily practice should include not only the patient's clinical characteristics (i.e., body weight, degree of hyperglycemia, age, renal function) but also the pharmacologic properties of the various compounds available (i.e., mode of action, side effects, safety profile) (see below). Updated

recommendations for the management of type 2 diabetes have been published by the European NIDDM Policy Group and by the American Diabetes Association.

First choice: oral monotherapy After diet failure, patients with type 2 diabetes can be treated with one of the four available oral antidiabetic drugs before considering the use of combined therapy or even insulin (Figs. 68.1 and 68.2). It is classically recognized that metformin should be preferred in insulin-resistant, hyperinsulinemic, obese patients, whereas sulfonylureas should be prescribed first in nonobese or only modestly overweight, insulin-deficient patients. However, recent studies have suggested that metformin may be as effective in nonobese as in obese diabetic patients. Acarbose appears to be preferable as monotherapy in diabetic patients with only

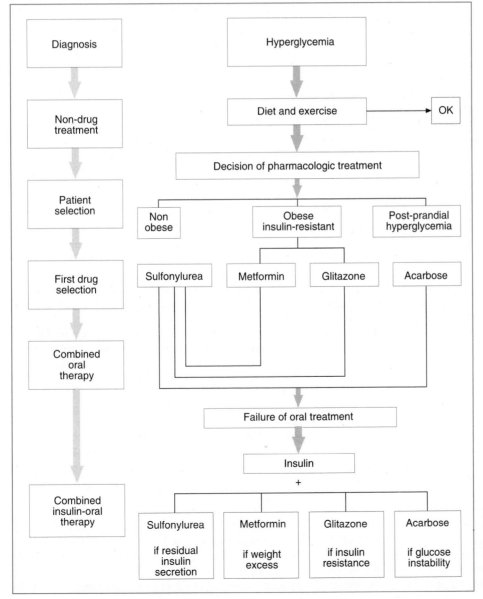

Figure 68.2 Stepwise treatment of type 2 diabetes: a guide to selection of oral antidiabetic agents. Please note that the use of troglitazone has been limited recently because of possible hepatotoxicity.

modest fasting hyperglycemia but rather high postprandial glucose excursions. In such patients, acarbose can improve glycemic control without inducing hypoglycemia. The place of the recently developed glitazones in the general treatment strategy of type 2 diabetes still remains to be more precisely specified. Owing to their mode of action, glitazones should be preferred in insulin-resistant patients, as is the case for metformin. Recent observations have questioned the safety of troglitazone in that a postmarketing survey has reported several cases of severe hepatotoxicity, resulting is its withdrawal from most markets.

Short-term studies on small groups of patients have suggested that the different oral hypoglycemic agents are almost equally effective in glucose control. Unfortunately, long-term studies are very scarce. In this respect, the results of the UKPDS are interesting. They showed that both sulfonylureas (e.g., chlorpropamide and glibenclamide) and metformin are as effective as insulin in controlling fasting plasma glucose concentrations and HbA1c levels, and significantly superior to diet therapy alone. One advantage of metformin in the obese group with type 2 diabetes was the absence of weight gain, which contrasted with a significant weight gain in the group treated with sulfonylureas or insulin. Metformin, in the selected overweight patients appeared to exert a clear reduction of cardiovascular endpoints, whereas glibenclamide and insulin only affected microvascular complications.

Second choice: combined oral therapy Since the four classes of antidiabetic drugs currently available (i.e., sulfonylureas, biguanides, α-glucosidase inhibitors, and glitazones) have different modes and sites of action (see below and Fig. 68.1), they may be combined in a stepwise fashion to provide more ideal glycemic control for most patients. The most common combined therapy associates a sulfonylurea compound and metformin. Numerous studies have demonstrated that both compounds have an at least additive antihyperglycemic effect, without increasing the side effects of either pharmacologic class. Other combinations of oral drugs also may be used, such as acarbose plus sulfonylurea and even acarbose plus metformin. Interesting effects of combining troglitazone and sulfonylureas also have been reported in various clinical trials, at a time when the hepatotoxicity of the drug was still unknown.

Third choice: insulin therapy Seventy-five years after the discovery of insulin, insulin therapy is still controversial in the management of patients with type 2 diabetes, so the questions why, when, and how to prescribe insulin in such individuals remain without definite answers. The minimum goal of insulin therapy is to suppress clinical symptoms of diabetes, and the ultimate goal is to prevent complications. Insulin therapy may be used as an alternative to oral drugs after diet failure, following secondary failure of maximal oral treatment, and when oral agents are contraindicated or become temporarily ineffective. In

most cases, however, insulin is prescribed in patients with type 2 diabetes not as initial therapy after diet failure, as in the UKPDS, but only after secondary failure of oral therapy.

In contrast to the use of insulin as the only treatment in type 1 diabetes, insulin can be combined with various oral antidiabetic drugs in type 2 diabetes. Insulin and sulfonylurea is the combination that has been studied most extensively. Intermediate-acting insulin at bedtime combined with premeal sulfonylurea has been shown to be effective in most studies but requires the persistence of significant residual endogenous insulin secretion. Metformin may be used in combination with insulin to reduce insulin requirements in obese patients, to improve glycemic control, and/or to correct associated metabolic abnormalities. Similar effects of sparing insulin dosage and improving metabolic disturbances are expected from the association of insulin sensitizers such as glitazones with insulin therapy, but these effects remain to be proven in extended studies. Finally, acarbose may be added to insulin to reduce blood glucose variations, especially postprandial early hyperglycemia and late hypoglycemia. In some cases, a combination of three drugs may be used, e.g., insulin, sulfonylurea, and metformin.

Risk and benefits of therapy

Since the prevalence of type 2 diabetes and the risk of severe side effects of oral antidiabetic agents are markedly increased with aging, special attention should be paid to the specific group of elderly diabetic patients. In general, the same measures of management are appropriate in the older as in the younger patient with diabetes but may need to be modified in the presence of comorbidities, polymedication, or social isolation. In particular, the risk of severe sulfonylurea-induced hypoglycemia or biguanide-associated lactic acidosis is higher in the elderly, so these drugs must be prescribed with caution in the older population.

Attempts to compare the risks of the two most prescribed classes of oral antidiabetic agents, sulfonylureas and biguanides, concluded that the risk of developing lactic acidosis on metformin is less important than that of developing severe hypoglycemia on sulfonylurea therapy. However, it is difficult to draw any definite conclusion from such population surveys because the individual risk essentially depends on the type of patient, the dose of the medication, and the recommendations for proper use. As far as acarbose is concerned, no severe side effects have been reported as yet. In contrast, the hepatotoxicity of glitazones may be a major problem, so the safety of this new class of pharmacologic compounds for treating type 2 diabetic patients still requires intensive research.

As for hypertension, the increase in the different available drugs probably will favor the use of combined therapy, although it remains to be established which combination will provide the best results in a given patient. In addition, the cost/benefit ratio of combined therapy remains to be assessed in large randomized trials. In addition, it remains to be answered whether better metabolic control can be maintained in the long term with combined therapy as compared with monotherapy. Finally, it is noteworthy that until now, no long-term studies in type 2 diabetic patients have shown the superiority of any kind of antihyperglycemic oral agent for postponing or preventing micro- or macroangiopathic complications except for metformin in overweight patients. The UKPDS has shown therapy with ultralente to be an acceptable therapy. This study, in addition showed that insulin clearly resulted in reduced microvascular complications, at the expense, however, of an increased risk of hypoglycemia.

Drug classes

Currently available oral antidiabetic agents include sulfonylureas, biguanides, α-glucosidase inhibitors, and in some countries, thiazolidinediones (see Tab. 68.4).

SULFONYLUREAS

Sulfonylureas remain the most popular drug treatment of type 2 diabetes, and numerous compounds are available in most countries. They are classically divided in sulfonylureas of the first and second generation (see Tab. 68.4). Several pharmacokinetic properties may differentiate the various compounds, especially elimination half-life or presence of active metabolites (Tab. 68.5). It remains unclear whether such differences have important clinical implications in daily practice, at least in the vast majority of diabetic patients. Nevertheless, the risk of severe and prolonged hypoglycemia appears to be higher for compounds with longer elimination half-lives and/or those which generate active metabolites. New compounds such as glimepiride or glipizide are presented as

once-daily formulations. Sulfonylureas essentially stimulate insulin secretion, even if some extrapancreatic effects also have been described. Sulfonylureas appear to be a rational choice to begin pharmacologic intervention, especially in the absence of massive obesity, because almost all patients are relatively insulin deficient. If such treatment with a sulfonylurea compound undoubtedly can ameliorate glycemic control in most patients, it remains unclear, however, whether it can influence the natural history of the disease.

Hypoglycemia is the main side effect of sulfonylurea derivatives, especially in elderly people. Hypoglycemic episodes appear to be more often associated with chlorpropamide and glibenclamide, although all sulfonylureas can have such a side effect. Drug interactions have been reported between sulfonylureas and various other pharmacologic compounds that can increase the hypoglycemic risk of the antidiabetic drug (see Chap. 6). Weight gain, sometimes of several kilograms, usually occurs with sulfonylureas and is undesirable in already overweight patients. Sulfonylureas should not be used in pregnant or lactating women.

BIGUANIDES

The glucose-lowering effect of the biguanide compound metformin does not depend on stimulation of insulin secretion but is rather attributed to enhanced non-insulin-mediated and insulin-mediated glucose metabolism. The underlying mechanisms are still unclear, but metformin has been shown to decrease hepatic glucose output, stimulate peripheral glucose uptake, and increase intestinal use of glucose. Since insulin resistance is a key feature of type 2 diabetes, especially when obesity is present, met-

Table 68.5 Main pharmacokinetic properties of most commonly used antihyperglycemic compounds in humans

Drug	Bioavailability (%)	Distribution volume (l/kg)	$t_{1/2}$ (h)	Systemic clearance (ml/min)	Active metabolites
Sulfonylureas					
Carbutamide	95-98	0.26	40	8	No
Chlorpropamide	100	0.11-0.18	33-50	1.8-3.3	Yes
Glibenclamide/glyburide	100	0.13-0.20	13-15	50-170	Yes
Gliclazide	80	0.19-0.26	8-17	13-26	No
Glimepiride	100	0.18	1.3-3.4	48	Yes
Gliquidone	80-100	0.16	1.4	90	Weak activity
Glipizide	100	0.12-0.26	2-9	33-52	No?
Tolbutamide	85-100	0.10-0.15	7-9	12-17	Weak activity
Tolazamide	85	0.16	3-7	?	Yes
Biguanide					
Metformin (850 mg)	40-55	5-6	2-4	450	No

Note: Protein binding is greater than 95% for all sulfonylurea compounds except for carbutamide (50-60%). Binding to plasma proteins does not occur with metformin.

formin would be more appropriate as a first-line antidiabetic drug in obese diabetic patients. Another interesting effect of metformin is its favorable action on various disorders associated with insulin resistance, such as high triglyceride levels, low HDL-cholesterol concentrations, and high plasminogen activator inhibitor-1 (PAI-1) levels, frequently seen in android obese subjects with type 2 diabetes. The usual dosage is 500 mg three to four times per day or 850 mg two to three times per day. The main pharmacokinetic parameters of metformin (850-mg tablet) are summarized in Table 68.5.

Gastrointestinal side effects, despite progressive increases in dosage, may hinder the use of metformin in some patients. In contrast to sulfonylureas, metformin does not cause weight gain, reduces rather than increases plasma insulin levels, and only rarely causes overt hypoglycemia. Lactic acidosis remains the major potential side effect of biguanide therapy. Two compounds, buformin and phenformin, are not more commercialized (or strictly limited) because of this serious complication. In contrast, lactic acidosis is rare with metformin. Since metformin is excreted by kidney, renal insufficiency represents an absolute contraindication to use of this drug, and metformin overdose or lactic acidosis can be treated with hemodialysis. In fact, metformin is safe if its use is avoided in patients with contraindications to its use, i.e., any person with decreased renal function, severe liver disease, or cardiac or respiratory insufficiency. Its use in elderly patients remains controversial and is a matter of individual clinical judgment. Metformin should not be used in pregnant or lactating women. No major drug interactions have been described with metformin, with the exception of nephrotoxic compounds, which may increase drug levels and favor lactic acidosis.

GLUCOSIDASE INHIBITORS

α-Glucosidase inhibitors exert a competitive, dose-dependent inhibition of small intestinal α-glucosidase enzymes that break down nonabsorbable complex carbohydrates into absorbable monosaccharides. Such an action leads to a delayed and reduced rise in postprandial blood glucose levels and consequently plasma insulin concentrations. Several studies have shown that acarbose improves indices of blood glucose stability in type 2 diabetic patients treated with diet, oral hypoglycemic agents, or insulin. Improvement in glycated hemoglobin (HbA1C) levels by about 0.6 to 0.7 % was obtained without increasing, or even reducing, body weight and the incidence of hypoglycemic episodes.

Since acarbose is not absorbed, no systemic adverse effects are expected. The major side effect of α-glucosidase inhibitors is gastrointestinal intolerance (flatulence, soft stools or diarrhea, mild abdominal pain) due to both osmotic effects and bacterial fermentation of undigested carbohydrates in the distal bowel. Many of these symptoms are dose-related and transient. Thus, the dosage should be increased very slowly (starting with 50 mg per day) and adjusted for each patient (up to 100 mg up to three times per day) in order to limit gastrointestinal symptoms and improve compliance. Acarbose may represent a good alternative in elderly people at higher risk of sulfonylurea-induced hypoglycemia and metformin-induced lactic acidosis.

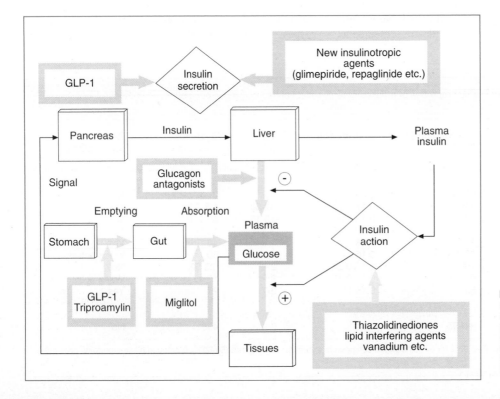

Figure 68.3 Future developments in drug treatment of type 2 diabetes: new pharmacologic strategies designed to improve insulin secretion, ameliorate insulin action, or delay carbohydrate absorption.

THIAZOLIDINEDIONES

Thiazolidinediones are a new class of compounds that work by enhancing insulin action and thus promoting glucose utilization in peripheral tissues, possibly by stimulating nonoxidative glucose metabolism in muscle and suppressing gluconeogenesis in the liver. They have no effect on insulin secretion and are known as *insulin sensitizers*. This action is attributed to the stimulation of a new class of nuclear receptors (PPAR-γ).

Troglitazone (as well as other thiazolidinediones in clinical development) has been shown to improve insulin resistance and glucose tolerance in obese subjects with impaired glucose tolerance and in patients with type 2 diabetes without inducing weight gain or drug-related hypoglycemia. However, the antihyperglycemic activity of the drug does not appear to be constant, and nonresponders to troglitazone have been reported in several reports. Interestingly enough, several components of the insulin resistance syndrome, e.g., lipid abnormalities and arterial hypertension, appear also to be improved by troglitazone. Whereas troglitazone seemed to be devoid of severe side effects in clinical trials, several cases of fatal hepatotoxicity have been reported after commercial drug availability in Japan and United States. At the present time, troglitazone has been withdrawn from the market in the United Kingdom and US and its use submitted to very strict liver enzymes monitoring in Japan.

INSULIN

Exogenous insulin may become necessary to compensate for the secretory failure of the B cell in the presence of marked insulin resistance in type 2 diabetes. Despite the absence of consensus, the dominance of a single morning injection of intermediate-acting insulin as a standard initial approach is being challenged by innovations such as bedtime insulin, alone or in combination with sulfonylureas. Sometimes, twice-daily (more particularly premixed NPH-regular insulins) and, more rarely, multiple insulin injections may be required. The feasibility of intensive insulin management in type 2 diabetes mellitus has been demonstrated recently, but the benefits of such an approach remain to be demonstrated in this population. The general principles of insulin therapy in type 2 diabetes are similar to those described in patients with type 1 diabetes (see above).

The most important side effect of insulin therapy is weight gain. However, such weight increase may remain rather modest when appropriate dietary advice is provided. The risk of hypoglycemia is far less in type 2 than in type 1 diabetic patients. Hyperinsulinemia associated with insulin resistance has been suspected to promote atherosclerosis in diabetic patients. However, no data have been published yet demonstrating deleterious effects of exogenous insulin therapy in type 2 diabetic patients as far as atherosclerotic cardiovascular complications are concerned, and in fact, some prelimi-

nary data rather suggest that insulin therapy may be beneficial.

New areas of drug development

Although a number of pharmacologic approaches to the treatment of type 2 diabetes are currently available (see Fig. 68.1), it is clear that none is ideal for the treatment of most patients who cannot be controlled adequately by monotherapy and even combined drug therapy. The quite frequent progression toward secondary failure to oral treatment and insulin requirement explains the intensive pharmaceutical research to find new drugs able to stimulate insulin secretion, improve insulin action, or delay carbohydrate absorption (Fig. 68.3).

Enhancers of insulin release

New agents that stimulate insulin secretion include nonsulfonylurea insulin secretagogues such as repaglinide and, of most interest, glucagon-like peptide-1 (GLP-1). This latter amide is a hormone from the lower intestine that functions as a so-called incretin hormone; i.e., it is released after meals and potentiates insulin secretion during the postprandial phase. It also inhibits gastric emptying rate. GLP-1 may promote insulin secretion in type 2 diabetic patients, as well as in those failing on maximal oral hypoglycemic agents. It has the major and unique advantage not to further lower blood glucose level at normal blood glucose concentrations, and so, unlike sulfonylureas, it does not potentiate the risk of hypoglycemia.

Enhancers of insulin action

The crucial role attributed to insulin resistance has promoted the development of strategies to improve insulin action. Agents that reduce insulin resistance may include compounds that interfere with lipid metabolism, especially nonesterified fatty acid production and/or oxidation; glucagon antagonists; vanadium compounds that have insulinomimetic properties; anti-tumor necrosis factor α agents; and agonists of the PPAR or RXR nuclear receptors.

Subclinical magnesium deficiency is a common finding in diabetic patients (due to low intake and excessive urinary loss associated with chronic glycosuria) and may contribute to or aggravate insulin resistance. Magnesium supplementation can improve insulin action and glucose control in magnesium-deficient diabetic patients.

Agents acting on gastrointestinal tract

New agents that slow carbohydrate absorption may exert their action either by inhibiting α-glucosidase enzymes (1-deoxynojirimycin derivatives such as miglitol and voglibose) or, even at a more proximal step, by slowing gastric emptying (amylin analogues such as 25,28,29-triproamylin, called pramlintide, or GLP-1).

Suggested readings

ALBERTI KGMM, GRIES FA, JERVELL J, KRANS HMJ for the European NIDDM Policy Group. A desktop guide for the management of non-insulin-dependent diabetes mellitus (NIDDM): an update. Diabetic Med 1994;11:899-909.

ALBERTI KGMM, ZIMMET P, DEFRONZO RA, KEEN H, eds. International textbook of diabetes mellitus, 2nd ed. Chichester, UK: Wiley, 1997.

AMERICAN DIABETES ASSOCIATION. Clinical practice recommendations, 1998. Diabetes Care 1998;21:S1-98.

THE DIABETES CONTROL AND COMPLICATIONS TRIAL RESEARCH GROUP. The effect of intensive treatment of diabetes on the development and progression of long-term complications in insulin-dependent diabetes mellitus. N Engl J Med 1993;329:977-86.

HENRY RR. Thiazolidinediones. Endocrinol Metab Clin North Am 1997;26:553-73.

HOLLEMAN F, HOEKSTRA JBL. Insulin lispro. N Engl J Med 1997; 337:176-83.

KUHLMANN J, PULS W, eds. Oral antidiabetics: handbook of experimental pharmacology. Berlin: Springer-Verlag, 1995.

PICK UP J, WILLIAMS G, eds. Textbook of diabetes, 2nd ed. Oxford, UK: Blackwell Scientific, 1997.

PORTE D JR, SHERWIN RS, eds. Ellenberg & Rifkin's Diabetes mellitus, 5th ed. New York: Appleton & Lange, 1996.

REAVEN GM. Role of insulin resistance in human disease. Diabetes 1988;37:1595-607.

REPORT ON THE EXPERT COMMITTEE ON THE DIAGNOSIS AND CLASSIFICATION OF DIABETES MELLITUS. Diabetes Care 1997; 20:1183-97.

SCHEEN AJ. Non-insulin-dependent diabetes mellitus in the elderly. Baillières Clin Endocrinol Metab 1997;11:388-406.

SCHEEN AJ. Drug treatment of non-insulin-dependent diabetes mellitus in the 1990s: achievements and future developments. Drugs 1997;54:355-68.

SCHEEN AJ, LEFÈBVRE PJ. Oral antidiabetic agents: a guide to selection. Drugs 1998;55:225-36.

UNITED KINGDOM PROSPECTIVE DIABETES STUDY GROUP. Intensive blood glucose control, with sulphonylureas or insulin compared with conventional treatment and risk of complications in patients with type 2 diabetes. Effect of intensive blood glucose control on complications in overweight patients with type 2 diabetes. Br Med J 1998;352:837-65.

UNITED KINGDOM PROSPECTIVE DIABETES STUDY GROUP. Effect of intensive blood glucose control with metformin on complications in overweight patients with type 2 diabetes. Br Med J 1998;352:854-65.

69

Hyperlipidemias

Franco Pazzucconi, Cesare R. Sirtori

The history of cholesterol and lipoprotein profiling is nearly as long as the history of biochemistry. For nearly 200 years, the sterol molecule has held the attention of biochemists and life scientists, probably due to the intriguing complexity of the molecule itself and the double-faced characteristics of its action: cholesterol and other lipids are necessary to life but become life-threatening when they reach elevated levels. The relationship between alterations in lipid metabolism and atherosclerosis has been observed clearly since the beginning of the century.

The first description of a lipoprotein was by Hewson in 1771. He noted that chylomicrons were absent in human plasmas during fast but that some subjects had a longer permanence in plasma after a meal, thus making plasma turbid even in fasting conditions. Later Hewson himself also identified the other triglyceride-rich lipoproteins, now known as the *very low density lipoproteins* (VLDLs).

The first description of cholesterol was by Chevreul in 1816. Christison later discovered the presence of cholesterol-rich lipoproteins in perfectly clear human plasma. A few years later, Vogel, in Lipsia, found that cholesterol was one of the major components of atheromatous lesions. In 1913, Anitschkow showed that feeding rabbits a cholesterol-rich diet induced severe arterial disease. At the same time, again in Russia, Ignatowsky provided epidemiologic evidence that opulent citizens, consumers of fat and animal protein, were more frequent victims of complications of arterial disease than were poor citizens, whose diet was based on vegetables.

Subsequently, starting in the 1950s, a number of "intervention trials" based on a reduction in the dietary intake of saturated fat in particular showed both a reduction in cholesterolemia and a lower incidence of coronary heart disease (CHD) in the treated groups. Classic studies were carried out in New York (Anti-Coronary Club), Los Angeles, and Helsinki (Psychiatric Hospital Study) and provided the basis for the lipid hypothesis, correlating blood lipid levels with increased cardiovascular risk. Definitive proof of the lipid hypothesis in humans was then obtained from a number of randomized, controlled trials (RCTs) with drugs or with a surgical procedure. The two earlier drug studies, the Lipid Research Clinics (LRC) study in the United States and the Helsinki Heart Study (HHS) in Finland, both of primary prevention, used, respectively, an anion-binding resin and the drug gemfibrozil.

In the LRC study, 3806 hypercholesterolemic subjects with a mean total cholesterol level of 290 mg/dl (7.5 mmol/l) with no symptoms of coronary heart disease were followed for an average of 7.4 years, receiving 24 g per day of a bile acid-binding resin (cholestyramine) or a corresponding placebo. The treated group, despite a wide variability in compliance to the drug regimen, achieved a mean *low-density lipoprotein* (LDL)-cholesterol reduction of around 20% (versus 7% in the placebo group), obtaining a 24% decline in death due to myocardial infarction (MI) and a 19% reduction in nonfatal MI (both $p < 0.05$). In addition, other endpoints of arterial disease (i.e., angina pectoris and coronary bypass surgery) were reduced by 20 and 21%, respectively, in the cholestyramine group.

The HHS evaluated employees of the Finnish railways with a non-HDL-cholesterol (VLDL + LDL) level of over 200 mg/dl (5.2 mmol/l). Therefore, Finnish subjects had a lower cholesterolemia [mean 250 mg/dl (6.45 mmol/l)] compared with the LRC participants, whereas hypertriglyceridemia was rather common: 36% had mean plasma triglycerides levels of greater than 175 mg/dl (2.0 mmol/l), showing either type IIb or type IV hyperlipoproteinemia (see below). During the 5 years of the study, 2051 of the subjects received gemfibrozil (600 mg bid) and 2030 a corresponding placebo. In treated subjects, significant reductions were noted in both cholesterol (11% total and 10% LDL) and particularly triglycerides (43%), with a concomitant rise in *high density lipoprotein* (HDL)-cholesterol (+14%). The HHS confirmed a striking reduction in the incidence of coronary heart disease (34% in the gemfibrozil group), evident from the second year of the study onward, while nonfatal MI was reduced by 37 percent. Both the LCR study and the HHS showed a slight, nonsignificant rise in total mortality in the drug-treated groups.

More recent studies have evaluated the preventive potential of novel hydroxymethylglutaryl CoA reductase inhibitors (statins). These studies were both of primary prevention (in normal individuals) and of secondary prevention (in subjects with ascertained CHD).

The Scandinavian Simvastatin Survival Study (4S) was

Table 69.1 Major study characteristics and relative/absolute risk reductions

	LRC	HHS	WOSCOPS	CAPS	POSCH	4S	CARE	LIPID	VA-HIT
Prevention	Primary	Primary	Primary	Primary	Secondary	Secondary	Secondary	Secondary	Secondary
Number of enrolled patients	3806	4081	6595	6605	838	4444	4159	9014	2531
Average cholesterol levels (mg/dl)	292	289	272	221	237	262	209	218	175
Cholesterol reduction	-8%	-11%	-20%	-18%	-23%	-28%	-20%	-18%	-4%
Absolute risk (CHD death, MI)	8.6	4.1	7.9	5.5	18.0	22.6	13.2	15.9	21.7
Relative risk reduction (%)	19	34	31	37	35	34	24	24	22
Absolute risk reduction (ΔAR) (%)	1.63	1.31	2.45	2.03	6.10	7.68	3.17	3.54	4.40
NNT[1] (100/ΔAR)	61	76	41	50	10	13	32	28	23

[1]Number needed to treat: see text.
(POSCH = Program on the Surgical Control of the Hyperlipidemias.)

a 5.4-year secondary prevention study on 4444 men with mean total cholesterol levels around 260 mg/dl, range of 212 to 309 mg/dl (mean 6.7 mmol/liter, range of 5.46-7.97 mmol/l). Treatment with simvastatin (an HMG-CoA reductase inhibitor) led to a mean total cholesterol and LDL-cholesterol reduction of 25 and 35%, respectively, with a 34% fall in major coronary events, a 42% reduction in coronary deaths, and a 30% fall in all-cause mortality (Tab. 69.1).

A very large primary prevention study, the West of Scotland Prevention Study (WOSCOPS), followed 6595 men aged 45 to 64 years with a mean plasma cholesterol level of 272 ± 23 mg/dl (7.0 ± 0.6 mmol/l) for 5 years. This study, designed to verify the efficacy of pravastatin, an HMG-CoA reductase inhibitor, in mildly hypercholesterolemic subjects, obtained an LDL-cholesterol reduction of about 26%, achieving a 32% reduction in deaths from all cardiovascular causes, corresponding to a 22% reduction in all-cause mortality (this latter close to statistical significance).

In the Cholesterol and Recurrent Events (CARE) study, 4159 subjects (3583 men and 576 women) with cholesterol levels below 240 mg/dl (6.2 mmol/l) and LDL-cholesterol levels between 115 and 174 mg/dl (3.0-4.5 mmol/l) with previous MI were randomly allocated to either pravastatin (40 mg/d) or a corresponding placebo. In the 5 years of follow-up, a mean 32% LDL-cholesterol decline was noted, with a reduction in coronary events of 24%. The frequency of stroke also was diminished by 31%, demonstrating that in high-risk patients, lowering cholesterol is appropriate even in presence of "average" lipid levels.

The Long Term Intervention with Pravastatin in Ischaemic Disease (LIPID) study evaluated a general population of MI patients, also with the objective of monitoring total mortality changes. A population of 9014 patients 31 to 75 years of age with total cholesterol levels between 155 and 271 mg/dl (4.0-6.9 mmol/l) was randomly allo-

cated either to pravastatin (40 mg/per day) or placebo and followed for a period of 6.1 years. The LIPID study, specifically designed with the aim of testing pravastatin effects on total mortality, proved that treating subjects with previous CHD events, even in presence of low LDL-cholesterol levels, may improve risk. Overall mortality was 11.0% in the treated group versus 14.1% in the placebo group.

Another primary prevention study, the Air Force/Texas Coronary Atherosclerosis Prevention Study (AFCAPS/TexCAPS), followed a design similar to the HHS by examining a total of 5608 men (45-73 years old) and 997 postmenopausal women (55-73 years old) without any sign of vascular pathology with average mean total and LDL-cholesterol levels of 221 and 150 mg/dl (5.71 and 3.89 mmol/l), respectively, the only lipid abnormality being low HDL-cholesterol levels below 50 mg/dl (mean of 36 mg/dl, 0.94 mmol/l). Participants were randomly allocated to either lovastatin 20 mg per day or placebo. Patients on lovastatin were titrated to 40 mg per day if their LDL-cholesterol levels exceeded 110 mg/dl (2.84 mmol/l). Reducing total and LDL-cholesterol levels by 25 and 18%, respectively, and increasing HDL-cholesterol levels by 6%, patients on lovastatin experienced 37% fewer first acute coronary events versus those on placebo, with no change or a slight decrease in total mortality in the treated group.

More recently the Department of Veterans Affairs High-Density Lipoprotein Cholesterol Intervention Trial (VA-HIT study) was designed to assess whether lipid-lowering therapy could reduce the combined incidence of CAD deaths and nonfatal MI in men with established CAD with low levels of HDL-cholesterol and "desirable" levels of LDL-cholesterol. Twenty-five hundred men with CAD and HDL-cholesterol levels of 40 mg/dl or less, LDL-cholesterol levels of 140 mg/dl or less, and TG levels of 300 mg/dl or less were randomized to either gemfibrozil, 600 mg bid, or placebo and followed in a double-blind manner for an average of 6 years. Patients on gemfibrozil had a 22% lower incidence of heart attack and coronary deaths, a 25% reduction in risk of stroke, and a 60% reduction in minor strokes (Tab. 69.1).

Together the LRC study and the HHS, WOSCOPS, and AFCAPS/TexCAPS indicate that a reduction in plasma lipids, both cholesterol and triglycerides, and possibly a rise in HDL-cholesterol levels are major goals in the prevention of cardiovascular disease. The benefit of these therapeutic measures in patients with previous coronary disease appears to be even more significant than that resulting from lowering elevated blood pressure, as demonstrated by 4S, CARE, LIPID and VA-HIT studies.

Emphasis thus has been placed recently on the role of lipid lowering in the therapy of established cardiovascular conditions as well as in their prevention. Such studies, both in animals and in humans, have described the potential for "regression" of atherosclerotic lesions. Studies in both monkeys and pigs, clearly indicate that high-fat diets can induce the formation of atherosclerotic lesions and that by replacing such diets with low-fat regimens, lesions can to some extent "regress." Regression may be further accelerated by the addition of different lipid-lowering drugs. In humans, angiographically documented lesions are less prone to progress when patients are placed on low-fat regimens with drugs. Also, the possibility of regression in humans recently has been firmly established, although highly aggressive drug regimens, including inhibitors of HMG-CoA reductase or high-dose nicotinic acid combined with anion-binding resins, a surgical procedure (partial ileal bypass, as shown in the POSCH study), or the application of an extracorporeal apheretic treatment for LDL, are required to induce the regression of some lesions. In the last 50 years, the so-called lipid hypothesis has been investigated thoroughly and has provided indisputable evidence. Only in the last decade has it been widely accepted by the medical community, and only in very recent years has it become general knowledge.

The wide interest in managing atherosclerosis-related risk is obviously due to the fact that this is the major cause of death and morbidity in western countries. Over 50% of all deaths in the United States and Europe have atherosclerosis as an underlying cause. No possible doubt remains that decreasing total cholesterol plasma levels

induces a parallel lowering in MI both in primary prevention (WOSCOPS, LRC, HHS, and AFCAPS- TexCAPS) and more so in secondary prevention (4S, CARE, LIPID and VA-HIT studies). Decline in cardiovascular morbidity and mortality has been proven to be independent of all other risk factors or therapies such as antiplatelets, ACE inhibitors, etc.

Treatment with lipid-lowering drugs is therefore of growing significance in preventive medicine. Prescription of such agents is necessary both for patients poorly responsive to dietary management and for those whose plasma lipid/lipoprotein abnormalities coexist with an increased genetic risk of atherosclerosis. Alterations in the lipoprotein spectrum, particularly a reduction in the protective HDLs, and/or increased levels of specific apolipoproteins (B and E) also carry a significant risk.

Disease presentation

MAJOR ASPECTS OF LIPID METABOLISM IN THE CLINIC

Cholesterol and triglycerides (TGs) are hydrophobic substances. To ensure their circulation in an aqueous milieu such as plasma, lipids are complexed with phospholipids and proteins in spherical structures called *lipoproteins.* Lipoproteins are a very heterogeneous family of large particles composed of a hydrophobic core of triglycerides and cholesterol esters and a hydrophilic surface of phospholipids and proteins (Tab. 69.2). The protein components of these macrocomplexes are referred to as *apolipoproteins,* and they have two primary functions: together with phospholipids, they ensure an optimal fat solubility in the aqueous environment of plasma, and moreover, they regulate lipoprotein interactions with cells and their catabolism. Both cholesterol and TGs are indispensable to life, cholesterol as a structural component of cell membranes and as a precursor of steroid hormones and bile acids and TGs as major energy supplies.

Metabolism of lipids and lipoproteins can be divided into two major pathways: an exogenous pathway, respon-

---

Table 69.2 Lipoprotein classes and composition

Lipoprotein	Density (water = 1 000)	Composition (weight %) C	TG	Protein	Major apolipoprotein
Chylomicrons	0.940	5	85-90	1-2	B-48, E, CII
VLDL	0.940-1.006	20	60-70	5-10	B-100, E, CII
Chylomicron remnants	1.006-1.019	30	30	15-20	B-48, E
VLDL remnants (IDL)	1.006-1.019	30	30	15-20	B-100, E
LDL	1.019-1.063	50-60	4-8	20	B-100
HDL	1.063-1.210	15-20	2-7	45-55	AI, AII

(C = cholesterol; TG = triglyceride; VLDL = very-low-density lipoprotein; IDL = intermediate-density lipoprotein; LDL = low-density lipoprotein; HDL = high-density lipoprotein.)

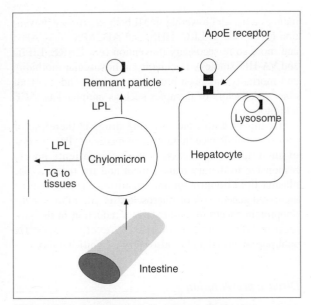

Figure 69.1 Exogenous lipid pathway. Chylomicrons, once formed from the dietary intake of fat, are secreted into the lymphatic system and enter the systemic circulation. In the capillaries of adipose tissue and muscles, apoCII activates lipoprotein lipase (LPL), the enzyme hydrolyzing triglycerides (TGs), making them available to surrounding tissues, either for providing energy or for storage. The reduction in core mass due to TG hydrolysis results in the permanence of chylomicron remnants, which are then taken up by the liver through specific receptors for apolipoprotein E (apoE) and digested in lysosomes.

sible for lipid absorption and distribution, and an endogenous pathway that directly supplies body requirements during fasting.

Exogenous pathway

The dietary intake of fats is rather conspicuous. Humans in western societies have an approximate daily intake of 80 to 100 g of TGs, 4 to 6 g of phospholipids, and 0.5 g of cholesterol. After absorption in the intestinal microvilli, dietary cholesterol is esterified to cholesterol esters (via the microsomal enzyme acylCoA cholesterol acyltransferase, ACAT). Chylomicrons, very large particles (diameters up to 500 nm) mainly containing TGs and cholesterol esters (CEs), are characterized by the presence of apolipoprotein B-48 (apoB-48), apolipoprotein E (apoE), and apolipoprotein CII (apoCII). Once formed, they are secreted into the lymph and enter systemic circulation. In the capillaries of adipose tissue and muscles, apoCII activates lipoprotein lipase (LPL), the enzyme hydrolyzing TGs into diglycerides, monoglycerides, and free fatty acids, making them available to surrounding tissues as an energy source or for reesterification to storage TGs.

The reduction in core mass due to TG hydrolysis results in an excess of surface components transferred to high-density lipoproteins (HDLs). The remainder of chylomicron particles, so-called chylomicron remnants, are then taken up by the liver through specific receptors for

apolipoproteins E and B-48 and digested in the lysosomes (Fig. 69.1). This process allows the liver to obtain free cholesterol and TGs from chylomicrons. Exogenous cholesterol is then eliminated through the bile or, most frequently, used for either membrane synthesis or synthesis of lipoproteins of the endogenous pathway; TGs are mostly stored for endogenous lipoprotein synthesis.

Endogenous pathway

The endogenous pathway begins in the liver with the synthesis of very-low-density lipoproteins (VLDLs) (diameter 200 nm), similar in composition to chylomicrons, except for the presence of apoB-100 instead of apoB-48. VLDLs, like chylomicrons, are processed by lipoprotein lipase (LPL), thereby providing peripheral tissues with TGs as a source of energy (Fig. 69.1). VLDL catabolism results in VLDL remnants, also known as *intermediate-density lipoproteins* (IDLs). About 50% of IDLs are removed by the liver by a receptor-mediated process. LDL receptors recognize apoE on the IDL surface. The remainder of IDLs are transformed into low-density lipoproteins (LDLs), highly atherogenic particles containing minimal amounts of TGs but a large amount of cholesterol ester (CE) and apoB-100 as the sole apolipoprotein. LDLs have a far smaller diameter (around 20-50 nm) than chylomicrons or VLDLs, have a relatively long circulation in the periphery (half-life of 1.5-2 days), and constitute the major source of cholesterol for body tissues, delivering cholesterol to cholesterol-requiring tissues such as the gonads, adrenals, and rapidly dividing cells.

LDLs are normally removed from plasma by the liver via the LDL receptor that also recognizes apoB-100, providing a cholesterol source for bile acids and lipoprotein synthesis (Fig. 69.2). In both the liver and extrahepatic tissues, LDL uptake is regulated by high-affinity specific receptors, whose presence is genetically determined and whose number may increase or decrease based on metabolic demands. In normal subjects, receptor biosynthesis is increased in all

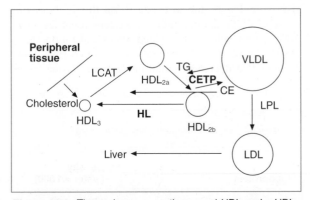

Figure 69.2 The endogenous pathway and HDL cycle. HDLs promote free cholesterol efflux from peripheral cells, then absorbing and storing it in their core as a consequence of its esterification by the enzyme lecithin: cholesterol-acyltransferase (LCAT). HDLs are not only cleared directly from plasma by the liver, but in addition, they interact with VLDLs and LDLs in plasma, transferring back their cholesteryl esters to the lower-density lipoproteins by way of the cholesteryl ester transfer protein (CETP). Excess cholesteryl esters in LDLs are then disposed of by the high-affinity LDL receptor pathway.

Table 69.3 Genetic classification of hyperlipoproteinemias and dyslipoproteinemias and major changes in lipoprotein levels

Pathology/Phenotype	Chylomicrons	VLDL	LDL	HDL	IDL	Phenotype
I	↑	–	↓	– or ↓	–	
IIa	–	–	↑	–	–	
IIb	–	↑	↑	– or ↓	–	
III	–	–	–	– or ↓	↑	
IV	↑	–	–	– or ↓	–	
V	↑	↑	↓	– or ↓	–	
LPL deficiency	↑	↑	↑	–	↑	I
ApoCII deficiency	↑	↑	↑	–	↑	I
Familial hypertriglyceridemia	– or ↑	↑	–	– or ↓	↑	IV, rarely V
Familial combined hyperlipoproteinemia	–	↑	↑	– or ↓	–↑	IIa, IIb, IV
Dysbetalipoproteinemia	–	–	–	– or ↓	↑	III
Familial hypercholesterolemia	–	–	↑	– or ↓	–	IIa
Polygenic hypercholesterolemia	–	–	↑	– or ↓	–	IIa

conditions where the tissues need cholesterol. For conditions where the influx of both VLDLs and LDLs is steadily raised, these lipoproteins, and particularly their metabolic derivatives in the circulation (oxidized products, acetyl or malondialdehyde conjugates), may not be cleared by the receptor pathway but are instead removed from plasma in a non-LDL-receptor-mediated pathway active in Kupffer's cells, smooth muscle cells, and macrophages. This secondary or "scavenger" pathway of lipoprotein metabolism allows lipid deposition in different sites, particularly the arterial walls (thus inducing atheromas), tendons, and skin (with resulting xanthomas and xanthelasmas). This appears to be the major mechanism in the development of foam cells and atheromas.

Accumulation of cholesterol in peripheral cells is prevented by continuous removal via HDLs synthesized in both the liver and the intestine (Fig. 69.2). These very small particles (diameter around 10 nm) have apolipoproteins AI and AII as their major protein components. HDLs can efficiently absorb free cholesterol from peripheral cells, with consequent esterification by the enzyme lecithin:cholesterol-acyltransferase (LCAT). HDLs have a constant mobility from tissues to liver, where possibly part of the lipoprotein-free cholesterol may be used as the precursor of bile acids. In addition, HDLs interact with VLDLs and LDLs in plasma, transferring back their cholesteryl esters to the lower-density lipoproteins by way of the cholesteryl ester transfer protein (CETP) (Fig. 69.2). Excess CEs in LDLs are then disposed of by the high-affinity receptor pathway. In this way, HDLs may act as an important defensive mechanism against excess deposition of cholesterol in body tissues, particularly in arterial walls. HDL metabolism has been the subject of a large number of studies, with the aim of providing tools to further reduce the risk of CHD through the development of agents raising HDL levels and improving their ability to remove cholesterol.

HYPERLIPOPROTEINEMIAS AND DYSLIPOPROTEINEMIAS

In the fasting state, the predominant circulating lipoproteins are LDLs and HDLs (accounting for most of the cholesterol in plasma) and VLDLs (carrying most TGs and a smaller percentage of cholesterol). Abnormalities in the physiologic mechanisms regulating plasma lipid/lipoprotein levels may result in significant impairment in the removal or increased production of these lipoproteins, leading to elevation of cholesterol, TGs, or both. If LDLs accumulate, the patient will present with hypercholesterolemia. An increase in chylomicrons or VLDLs will result primarily in hypertriglyceridemia, but since LDLs derive from VLDLs, high levels of VLDLs also may determine hypertriglyceridemia associated with hypercholesterolemia. This double condition also will be present in states of elevated remnant particle levels.

A commonly used term for these disorders is *hyperlipoproteinemia*. However, recently, different syndromes have been described where the abnormality may be either lower levels of a protective lipoprotein such as HDL or qualitative changes, reflecting an altered distribution of either the lipids or the protein (apolipoprotein) components. Thus, the terms *dyslipidemia* and *dyslipoproteinemia* are being applied more frequently. The causes of dyslipidemia can be either acquired or genetic, although an acquired defect can coexist with a genetic one.

Primary hyperlipoproteinemias

Individuals with hyperlipoproteinemias are frequently classified according to Frederickson phenotypes I to V or in terms of familial (monogenic) versus polygenic disease. Frederickson phenotypes are determined by electrophoretic or lipoprotein analysis. Phenotype I shows severe chylomicronemia. Type IIa disease is characterized by elevated LDL levels, whereas patients with type IIb disease have raised levels of both LDL and VLDL. Type III patients show increased prebeta or IDLs due to structural abnormalities of apolipoprotein E, type IV patients have raised VLDLs, and finally, type V patients exhibit both VLDL and chylomicron elevations (Tab. 69.3).

From an epidemiologic point of view, types IIa, IIb, and IV are the most common phenotypes, whereas types I and V are very rare. The consequences of these metabolic situations are increased cardiovascular risk for phenotypes II (both IIa and IIb) III, and IV and increased TG-related complications such as pancreatitis for phenotypes I and V.

The genotype-based classification of hyperlipoproteinemias is summarized in Table 69.3. Very rare conditions of LPL or apoCII deficiency cause a marked impairment in chylomicron catabolism and, in the case of apoCII deficiency, also of VLDL catabolism, which leads to very high TGs levels (1500-10,000 mg/dl, or 20-120 mmol/liter). Patients corresponding to Frederickson phenotypes I and V may present with early pancreatitis. They seldom have an accelerated vascular pathology, underlying the nonatherogenic nature of chylomicrons.

A more common cause of hypertriglyceridemia is familial hypertriglyceridemia, corresponding to Frederickson phenotype IV. Here, increased biosynthesis and decreased removal of TG-rich lipoproteins (primarily VLDLs) induce a moderate TG rise (400-800 mg/dl, or 4.50-9.0 mmol/l). This is correlated with increased atherosclerosis risk particularly when it is associated with other risk factors, e.g., frequently with reduced HDL levels. Hypertriglyceridemia may then amplify the risk of disease exponentially.

Another common cause of hypertriglyceridemia is familial combined hyperlipoproteinemia (FCHL). In this disease, patients have increased apoB containing lipoproteins (mostly VLDLs) that results in moderately elevated cholesterol and/or TG levels. A distinctive characteristic of FCHL is that its presentation varies in the different affected relatives, showing, in the same family, different phenotypes, such as IIa, IIb, IV, and rarely V, and a strong family history of premature CHD.

A less common hyperlipidemia is dysbetalipoproteinemia (type III), also called *broad beta disease* because the beta band in electrophoresis typically is widened. Affected patients are homozygous for a particular allele of apolipoprotein E, apoE2. ApoE2 has a reduced affinity for the specific hepatic receptor compared to apoE3, resulting in an accumulation of IDL remnants. These particles contain both cholesterol and TGs in nearly equal amounts,

resulting in moderately elevated cholesterol and TG levels; typically, the two levels are very similar in magnitude, ranging from 270 to 500 mg/dl. Interestingly, the E2/E2 genotype is present in 1 in 100 persons in the population, but the phenotypic expression of the disease can be found in only 1 in 10 000 persons. Most individuals therefore can compensate for the defect, and its expression is thought to require the presence of other inherited or acquired lipid defects.

The type IIa hyperlipoproteinemia phenotype underlies two metabolic disorders: familial hypercholesterolemia (FH) and polygenic hypercholesterolemia. In the first, the defect is well established, resulting in various degrees of LDL receptor deficiency (or mutation) and causing a reduced tissue (mainly liver) uptake of cholesterol. The disease is transmitted in an autosomal dominant pattern with incomplete penetrance. Heterozygous subjects have an incidence of 1 in 500 persons in the population, representing some 4% of all hypercholesterolemic patients; they have cholesterol levels in the range of 300 to 500 mg/dl (7.7-12.9 mmol/l). Homozygotes are extremely uncommon, with an incidence of 1 in 2-3 million persons as opposed to the expected frequency of 1 in 1 million, probably due to a high unrecognized incidence of prenatal lethality. These subjects have cholesterol levels ranging from 600 to 1000 mg/dl (25.8 mmol/l), tendon xanthomas, and CHD in early life and frequently are unresponsive to treatment. Many homozygotes are double heterozygous with two defective LDL receptor alleles. There are over 300 known mutations at the LDL receptor locus that can determine FH, divided in four classes.

Recently, a new genetic abnormality has been recognized: familial defective apoB (FDB), consisting of apolipoprotein B with an altered sequence that leads to defective binding to a normal LDL receptor. These conditions (three are known at present) have an estimated frequency of 1 in 500 persons, resulting in a moderate hypercholesterolemia with raised LDL levels.

The most common and yet least understood type of hypercholesterolemia is the so-called polygenic hypercholesterolemia. These subjects have an increased production of LDL or, at times, a decreased removal. The genetic cause is not a single mutation in a specific gene but rather a collective gene pattern inducing a moderate incapacity in LDL hepatic clearance together with an increased VLDL production.

Secondary hyperlipoproteinemias

They are relatively infrequent and may be associated with any endocrine or parenchymal disease affecting lipid/lipoprotein metabolism. In some cases, iatrogenic dyslipidemia can be observed.

A typical cause of secondary hyperlipoproteinemia is diabetes mellitus, both insulin-dependent (IDDM) and non-insulin-dependent (NIDDM), generally with increased TG and VLDL levels (see Chap. 68). In IDDM, lack of insulin, a potent stimulator of LPL, causes a reduced VLDL catabolism and in some cases also hyperchylomicronemia. Moreover, lack of insulin induces an enhanced lipolysis with increased free fatty acid concentrations and raised VLDL biosynthesis. The situation in NIDDM is somewhat more complex; these patients often having preexisting alterations in lipid metabolism and frequently being obese. Such deranged metabolic situations are additive to the lack of insulin. Indeed, whereas in patients with IDDM, good glycemic control can reverse lipoprotein abnormalities, the same may not be true for NIDDM patients.

Hypothyroidism (see Chap. 65) is associated with increased LDL levels due to a reduced receptor-regulated catabolism, together with reduced VLDL biosynthesis, but the first mechanism is quantitatively more important. Another endocrine disorder associated with hypercholesterolemia/hypertriglyceridemia is Cushing's disease. The abnormalities in corticosteroid hormones in this syndrome reduce LPL activity.

In the nephrotic syndrome, when plasma albumin concentrations decrease under 3 g/dl, a hyperlipemia often can be seen with increased secretion of both VLDLs and LDLs, probably related to inhibition of both LPL and LCAT. Similarly, in uremia, increased VLDL levels are part of the clinical picture, due to reduced catabolism.

As mentioned previously, the liver is the key organ in lipid metabolism. Every pathologic condition of the liver will induce abnormalities in lipoprotein metabolism. Extensive organ damage will result in reduced VLDL and LDL levels. In biliary cirrhosis and cholestasis, instead, an increase in the formation of an abnormal lipoprotein, lipoprotein X (LpX), results from the interaction of bile acids with LDLs in the circulation. LpX is not able to activate the feedback mechanism of inhibition of cholesterol synthesis, resulting in an enhanced cholesterol biosynthesis.

Other dyslipoproteinemias are iatrogenic. Use of oral contraceptives occasionally may result in increased triglyceridemia, stimulated by the estrogen content of the pill (see Chap. 67). Similarly, β-blockers may be associated with hypertriglyceridemia and at times also with reduced HDL-cholesterol. A particular cause of secondary iatrogenic hyperlipoproteinemias is alcohol, due to the potent stimulatory activity of ethanol on VLDL secretion. Finally, protease inhibitors, which are used in the treatment of AIDS (see Chap. 40), may lead to severe hypertrygliceridemia with elevated cholesterol and reduced HDL levels; this may be associated with abdominal or truncal fat deposition and early coronary disease.

Dyslipoproteinemias

More recently described lipid-associated mechanisms for the development of arterial disease are abnormalities in the distribution/composition of lipoproteins. Dyslipoproteinemias are clinical conditions not strictly associated with quantitative abnormalities in lipid levels but rather with increases/decreases of specific lipoproteins or even of apolipoproteins.

The most common is hypo-α-lipoproteinemia, characterized by low HDL-cholesterol levels. This abnormality may be present in as many as 10% of atherosclerotic patients and is considered to be an independent risk factor for arterial disease. Low HDL-cholesterol is frequently associated with hypertriglyceridemia and may be the consequence of different biochemical abnormalities and of some acquired disorders (physical inactivity, intake of some α-blockers).

There are three known syndromes associated to hypo-α-lipoproteinemia: Tangier disease, familial hypo-α-lipoproteinemia, and lecithin:cholesterol-acyltransferase (LCAT) deficiency. Tangier disease is an autosomal recessive syndrome characterized by a low plasma cholesterol level (<100 mg/dl, 2.58 mmol/l), normal or elevated triglycerides, and reduced HDL-cholesterol (heterozygotes) or completely absent HDL-cholesterol (homozygous subjects). The composition of every class of lipoproteins is altered, and there is cholesterol ester (CE) deposition in macrophages, liver, spleen, intestinal mucosae, skin, and lymphatic organs. Although deposition in the cells of the arterial walls is not the rule, these subjects frequently present with atherosclerotic lesions.

Familial hypo-α-lipoproteinemia is an autosomal dominant genetic defect associated with a decrease in HDL-cholesterol concentrations with normal lipase and LCAT activity and early onset of atherosclerotic disease. Diagnostic criteria are HDL-cholesterol level < 25 mg/dl (0.64 mmol/l) with the exclusion of secondary forms, such as obesity, hypertriglyceridemia, diabetes mellitus, and presence in other family members of hypo-α-lipoproteinemia. Among the causes of HDL-cholesterol reduction, often an apoAI mutation may be shown. Many different apoAI mutations have been reported, some of which (apoAI$_{Milano}$, apoAI$_{Paris}$) are apparently associated with protection from atherosclerotic disease. LCAT deficiency finally is a very uncommon autosomal recessive disorder characterized by corneal opacity, anemia, proteinuria, and renal insufficiency.

Hyper-apoB-lipoproteinemia has been described in numerous cohorts of CHD patients. It is characterized by an enrichment of apoB in LDL, which otherwise is of relatively normal composition, except for a slight triglyceride (TG) excess; mild hypertriglyceridemia also may occur. LDL particles of these patients are also smaller than those of normal subjects (so-called pattern B).

The accumulation in plasma of a newly described form of lipoprotein, lipoprotein (a) [Lp(a), previously called sinking pre-β-lipoprotein, slow migrating pre-β-lipoprotein recently has stimulated considerable interest. Lp(a) is detected in the density range of LDL and is composed of apoB and an apoprotein [apo(a)] of variable molecular weight (from 400-700 kDa) with considerable homology with plasminogen. About 30% of adults have elevated levels of Lp(a) (>35 mg/dl) and an enhanced risk of cardiovascular disease, possibly due to an interaction of the Lp(a) particles with arterial plasminogen binding sites, followed by local deposition of cholesteryl esters. Drug treatment of elevated Lp(a) levels thus far has had discouraging results except for the case of postmenopausal hormone replacement therapy, which is of moderate effectiveness but with restricted indications.

Hyperlipoproteinemias also may be linked to mutations in the major apolipoproteins (apoAI, apoB, apoE). These mutants show amino acid changes in the sequence of the

Table 69.4 National cholesterol education panel (NCEP) guidelines for lipid management

Concomitant risk factors[1]	Definite atherosclerotic disease[2]	LDL-Cholesterol (mg/dl)	
		Mandatory to therapy	Goal
1 or less	No	>190	<160
2 or more	No	>160	<130
No[3]	Yes	>130	<100[4]

[1]Concomitant risk factors for coronary heart disease (CHD) include age (males > 45 years and females > 55 years or with premature menopause without estrogen replacement therapy), familiar history of premature CHD, current cigarette smoking, hypertension, confirmed HDL-cholesterol < 35 mg/dl, and diabetes mellitus. Subtract 1 risk factor if HDL-cholesterol > 60 mg/dl.
[2]Presence of CHD, cerebrovascular disease, or peripheral vascular disease.
[3]Definite atherosclerotic disease totally blunts the presence of other concomitant risk factors.
[4]In CHD patients with LDL-cholesterol levels 100 to 129 mg/dl, the physician should exercise clinical judgment in deciding whether to initiate drug treatment.

apoprotein, which may lead to an increase in some lipoprotein fractions. The list of mutants is now large and still growing and includes apoB abnormalities linked to arterial disease.

Treatment

Therapeutic strategy

The treatment of dyslipidemias/dyslipoproteinemias is based on the concept of *individual absolute risk assessment*. This is dictated by age, sex, and family history of CHD, hypertension, diabetes mellitus, etc. The higher the absolute risk, the more effective is the selected intervention strategy. In clinical studies of lipid-lowering agents, a *relative risk* reduction was evaluated, which is a statistical comparison of treated versus control groups. The absolute cardiovascular risk of a single patient can now be calculated easily through the use of computer programs (e.g., CERCA, Internet: *http//www.chd-taskforce.de/calculator*), providing a reliable assessment of the individual risk and the impact of correction. Absolute risk evaluation takes into account the presence of other risks in addition to lipids. Risk factors can be grouped into major and contributing risk factors. *Major risk factors* are those definitely associated with a significant increase in the risk of atherosclerosis development. *Contributing risk factors* are those associated with increased risk of cardiovascular disease, but their significance and prevalence have not yet been established. Some of them can be treated or modified, and some cannot.

Smoking, high blood pressure, physical inactivity, obesity, and diabetes are with dyslipoproteinemias the six major, independent, treatable risk factors for CHD.

Cigarettes and tobacco smoke A smoker's risk of heart attack is more than twice that of a nonsmoker. Cigarette smoking is the biggest risk factor for sudden cardiac death. Smokers have two to four times the risk of nonsmokers; moreover, smokers who have a heart attack are more likely to die and die suddenly versus nonsmokers. Cigarette produces a greater risk in persons under 50 years of age than in those over age 50. Interestingly, the ratio of HDL to LDL is lower in smokers than in nonsmokers.

High blood pressure High blood pressure raises the risk of stroke, heart attack, kidney failure, and congestive heart failure. When high blood pressure coexists with obesity, smoking, a high cholesterol level, or diabetes, the risk of heart attack or stroke increases several times.

Physical inactivity Lack of physical activity is a risk factor for coronary heart disease. Regular exercise plays a significant role in preventing heart and blood vessel disease. Even modest levels of regular low-intensity physical activity are beneficial.

Obesity and overweight People who have excess body fat (particularly at the abdominal level) are more likely to develop heart disease and stroke even if they have no other risk factors. Obesity directly influences blood pressure, blood cholesterol level, TG level and negatively influences HDL-cholesterol levels and leads to an enhanced diabetes risk.

Diabetes mellitus Diabetes severely increases the risk of developing cardiovascular disease. Even when glucose levels are under control, diabetes increases the risk of heart disease and stroke approximately twofold.

Increasing age, gender, family history of heart disease, and previous CHD are nonmodifiable major risk factors.

Increasing age About four of five people who die of CHD are 65 years of age or older. At older ages, women with heart attacks are twice as likely as men are to die from these events.

Gender Men have a greater risk of heart attack than women, and they have attacks earlier in life. Even after menopause, when women's death rate from heart disease doubles, it is lower than that of men.

Family history Children of parents with heart disease are more likely to develop it.

Previous CHD A subject who already has CHD has an absolute risk four times higher than a healthy subject.

Finally, individual response to stress may be a contributing factor. A relationship between CHD risk and a person's life stress, behavior, habits, and socioeconomic status has been noted, even if not proven. These factors may affect established risk factors. For example, stressed people overeat and start smoking or smoke more than they would otherwise. Low social class and economic problems in general are significant risk factors for CHD.

On the basis of absolute risk assessment, the US National Cholesterol Education Panel recently has classified different LDL-cholesterol levels as desirable to mandatory for pharmacologic treatment (Tab. 69.4). The general therapeutic strategy of intervention in the United States and Europe begins with a life-style intervention involving modifications in dietary habits (excess consumption of saturated fat, total calories, animal proteins, etc.), smoking cessation, introduction of physical activity, etc. The major dietary changes are aimed at reduction of excess body weight and the controlled intake of nutrients generally linked to plasma lipids. Reduction of body weight may lead to an improved control of several forms of hypertriglyceridemia; the same goal can be achieved by a reduction of ethanol intake. In the case of hypercholesterolemia, the total amount of dietary fat is correlated with raised cholesterol; saturated fats (of animal origin) are among the most potent causative factors in hypercholesterolemia. In addition to these, animal protein intake may be a significant factor in many hypercholesterolemic patients; the change from animal to vegetable proteins (e.g., soy proteins) as the major dietary protein frequently leads to correction of the hypercholesterolemia. Physical activity always should be encouraged as it may increase HDL-cholesterol levels.

When the first intervention (lasting at least 3 months) has not achieved the desired change in the abnormal lipid pattern and has not improved the individual absolute risk assessment enough, bile acid sequestrants, nicotinic acid, probucol, fibrates, or HMG-CoA reductase inhibitors may be indicated.

Drug therapy

The therapeutic approach to high-risk patients with elevated lipids is obviously a combination of different strategies, i.e., the already mentioned life-style changes and elimination of other risk factors, in addition to a pharmacologic intervention specific to the lipid/lipoprotein alteration of the subject. The individual absolute cardiovascular risk generally indicated by most guidelines for drug intervention is approximately 1.5 to 2% per year. Clinical studies have shown that even patients with a lower cardiovascular risk may benefit from drug treatment. However, this may prove very costly. A widely used major index of benefit, ie, the *number needed to treat* (NNT)

$$NNT = 100/\text{absolute risk reduction}$$

which expresses the number of subjects needing treatment to have one less instance of the disease, may prove very high. *NNT* in previously reported prevention studies ranged from as low as 13 (4S) to well over 60 (HHS and AFCAPS) (Tab. 69.1).

Drug classes

Plasma lipid-modifying agents are pharmacologic compounds that affect the levels of major circulating lipids, i.e., cholesterol and TGs. This effect is generally exerted through changes in absorption, synthesis, or catabolism of the lipid vectors in plasma, the lipoproteins.

Lipid-lowering drugs can be divided into nonsystemic (nonabsorbable) and systemic drugs, the former including only hypocholesterolemic compounds. Nonsystemic compounds generally act at the intestinal level by affecting the absorption/excretion of neutral and acidic steroids; the latter act by a variety of mechanisms, from activation of lipoprotein catabolism (e.g., fibric acid derivatives) to antagonism of cholesterol biosynthesis (hydroxymethylglutaryl-CoA reductase inhibitors). The different drug groups may share, to a large extent, their major indications, but specific targets of activity differ for each drug class. Moreover, the pattern of side effects and/or contraindications may favor the selection of one or the other agent in specific clinical syndromes.

NONSYSTEMIC LIPID-LOWERING DRUGS

The major nonabsorbable agents are the anion-exchange resins, which bind bile acids in the intestine, and the antibiotic neomycin, which precipitates micelles in the intestinal lumen that contain both bile acids and neutral sterols.

Anion-exchange resins

The bile acid-binding resins include cholestyramine, colestipol and colesevelam. Cholestyramine was developed and used originally for the treatment of itching secondary to elevated concentration of bile acids in cholestasis. Very soon thereafter, however, attention focused on its ability to lower plasma total and LDL-cholesterol levels. Both cholestyramine and colestipol are not absorbed in the gastrointestinal (GI) tract (less than 5% of the dose of a radioactively labeled drug may appear in urine), and they have a very limited range of systemic side effects. For this reason, they are particularly useful in the treatment of hypercholesterolemia in pregnant women and children. The major problem with ion-exchange resins is their unpleasant taste and the frequent GI side effects.

Cholestyramine is the chloride salt of a basic anion-exchange resin formed by a polymer of styrene and divinylbenzene. Colestipol is the chloride form of a basic anion-exchange resin made up of a copolymer of diethylenetriamine and 1-chloro-2,3-epoxypropane.

Both compounds are hydrophilic and yet insoluble in water, so they are given orally after being suspended in water or juice. In some European countries, DEAE-Sephadex is used with similar indications; the product is as active as cholestyramine. A novel, lower dose resin, colesevelam, has been recently approved in the US.

Mechanism of action

Bile acids are synthesized in the liver from cholesterol as their sole precursor. Secreted in the GI tract during digestion, bile acids form micellar structures with dietary lipids, allowing absorption, following which they can thus be resecreted. Resins bind bile acids and prevent their reabsorption, thus resulting in fecal loss. Normally, daily intestinal loss of bile acids is seldom above 1 g; following treatment with cholestyramine, the loss goes up to 2 to 3 g per day. In addition to impairing dietary sterol absorption, the marked bile acids loss leads to activation of cholesterol 7α-hydroxylase, the rate-limiting enzyme in bile acid biosynthesis. This induces an increase in cholesterol consumption to which hepatocytes respond both with an increase in the activity of 3-hydroxy-3-methyl glutaryl-coenzyme A reductase and an upregulation of LDL receptors expressed on the cell surface, thus resulting in a decrease in LDL plasma concentrations.

Pharmaceutical forms

Cholestyramine is available in most countries in packets containing 4 g of resin, and colestipol is available in packets containing 5 g of resin. Daily doses for both resins range from 8 to 24 g (cholestyramine) or from 10 to 30 g (colestipol), divided into two to three portions. Some patients find it beneficial to take resins in a single administration in the morning. Colesevelam is available in 3 g doses (max 9 g/day).

Pharmacokinetics and pharmacodynamics

Anion-exchange resins do not undergo any metabolic conversion. Resins significantly reduce the concentration of total and LDL-cholesterol, particularly in hypercholesterolemic patients. These effects are rapid in onset (within 1 week of treatment) and usually in the range of 20 to 30% versus starting levels. In some patients, a transient increase in VLDLs and TGs may be seen early in treatment. During the LRC study (see above), significant rises in HDL-cholesterol levels also were noted. This last finding may be linked to the increased cholesterol mobilization from tissues during therapy. Resins are contraindicated in patients with significant hypertriglyceridemia, in whom a further rise in plasma TGs and VLDLs is not desirable.

Clinical indications

Numerous studies have shown that resins are quite effective on total and LDL-cholesterolemia. Moreover, other studies have shown that the LDL reduction obtained is correlated with a slowing of progression of coronary atherosclerosis and a lowered incidence of coronary events. The LRC study (mentioned earlier) is the most extensive study on the therapeutic potential of cholestyramine, but many others have been performed. Studies in hypercholesterolemic children have shown satisfactory activity but a difficult compliance. No reduction in growth and no evidence of major side effects were reported.

The effect of ion-exchange resins also is maintained when such agents are given in combination therapy. The combination of cholestyramine and nicotinic acid (CLAS study) has been shown to markedly improve long-term prognosis. Colestipol gave excellent results when combined with either nicotinic acid or lovastatin in the FATS study that evaluated coronary progression in mildly hypercholesterolemic patients with angina or previous MI.

Adverse effects and interactions

Since resins are not absorbed, the range of systemic side effects is limited. Aside from this very favorable property, therapy with these drugs is subject to problems with patient compliance. The unpleasant taste and sandy consistency of these preparations has always restrained their use. Resin use frequently is associated with constipation (10-30% of treated subjects), most often in the elderly. Although most cases of constipation are mild and self-limited, progression to fecal impaction can occur. Not uncommon also are flatulence, belching, vomiting, abdominal distress, and nausea. Such unpleasant feelings are difficult to control. One method to avoid such difficulties is to administer cholestyramine once daily after mixing with fruit juices and crushed ice in a shaker, thus masking the sandy consistency. Less than 1% of patients experience modest and transient biochemical alterations such as increases in the levels of transaminase or alkaline phosphatase. Rarely, absorption of the chloride ion of the molecule may lead to hyperchloremic acidosis.

Interactions with different drugs and vitamins may be common; in the case of vitamins, such interactions generally are modest. Drugs commonly bound by resins include ferrous sulfate, acidic anti-inflammatory drugs, phenobarbital, thyroxine, and the various digitalis molecules. Aside from chemical interactions, anion-exchange resins also may delay absorption of certain medications simply because of their bulk-forming properties. For this reason, it is advisable to administer cholestyramine or other resins at least 4 hours before or 2 hours after the intake of other drugs.

Neomycin

Neomycin is an aminoglycoside antibiotic that generally is used for the prevention of hepatic coma. A significant cholesterol reduction was noted as a side effect in treated patients. Such activity can be of therapeutic interest in hypercholesterolemic patients with normal liver function. It appears that the cholesterol reduction is independent of the antimicrobial activity. Neomycin seems to perturb the formation of micelles of bile acids and neutral sterols, thus leading to a significant loss, particularly of neutral sterols, in the feces. An interesting effect emerging in patients with elevated Lp(a) levels is their decline after neomycin treatment.

Administration of neomycin is not always well tolerated. Absorption of the compound may lead to possible impairment of kidney function. Subjective side effects also are often reported (e.g., itching and abnormalities in intestinal function).

Neomycin is usually given in divided doses, ranging from 0.5 to 2 g per day. Cholesterol and LDL reductions of up to 20% or more may be observed in responsive patients. Neomycin may be the best available agent for reducing

Lp(a) levels, particularly in association with nicotinic acid.

SYSTEMIC LIPID-LOWERING DRUGS

Systemic lipid-lowering agents include a variety of chemical structures with widely different mechanisms of action. Some of these agents, e.g., fibric acids, have been in use for many years and are still the mainstay of therapy in some countries; others, e.g., the HMG-CoA reductase inhibitors, are relatively new, but they have gathered growing importance and are actually the most used drugs in the field and among the most widely used drugs in general.

Fibrates

Fibric acid derivatives, or fibrates, constitute a rather large series of compounds characterized by the presence of an aryloxy acid moiety. The first available drug of this class, clofibrate, was tested initially more than 35 years ago and found to be effective in reducing plasma triglyceride levels and in increasing HDL-cholesterol. Unfortunately, although a decline in the rate of nonfatal MI could be observed in a WHO-sponsored study, an increase in noncardiac deaths and overall mortality, yet unexplained, also was noted.

During the 1960s and 1970s, several other fibrates were developed, most notably bezafibrate, fenofibrate, gemfibrozil, and ciprofibrate. Clofibrate is the ethyl ester of *p*-chlorophenoxyisobutyric acid (CPIB). The other major fibrates show a similar basic structure, except for gemfibrozil, possibly the most peculiar molecule among fibrates because it does not have a chloride atom in the *para* position.

Mechanism of action

Fibrates activate a catabolic system for fatty acids in liver cells by interacting with a nuclear receptor (peroxisome proliferator-activated receptor, or PPAR). There are three types of PPARs, termed α, σ (or β) and γ. These nuclear receptors, once activated, dimerize with the retinoic X receptor (RXR) and then bind the response element of the DNA-binding domains of PPARs (PPREs). Several substances are known to be PPAR ligands/activators or "fraudulent fatty acids"; among these, fibrates, ω-3 fatty acids from fish oil, thiazolidinedione antidiabetics (see Chap. 68), and natural fatty acids, particularly the long-chain unsaturates believed to be the endogenous ligands for these nuclear receptors.

Fibrates, through PPARs, increase fatty acid catabolism by enhancing different enzymes. Acyl-CoA synthetase prevents their efflux from the cell and activates them for further catabolism. Both peroxisomal and mitochondrial β and ω-oxidation-related enzymes are increased. Conversely, fibrates induce a net decrease in acetyl-CoA carboxylase and fatty acid synthase, thus reducing de novo TG synthesis.

Extracellularly, as a consequence of the intracellular mechanism, fibrates increase lipoprotein lipase (LPL) gene expression, thus enhancing VLDL-TG removal, while decreasing apoCIII gene expression and therefore increasing LPL-mediated catabolism. Although depressive effects on fatty acid hepatic synthesis and release have been shown in experimental animals, similar conclusions have not been reached consistently in humans.

By activating these different mechanisms, fibrates can reduce VLDLs and TGs in about 80% of patients with elevated TGs, reducing triglyceridemia to normal values in the large majority. Consequences of increased VLDL catabolism are a rise of HDL-cholesterol, occurring in most patients, and a paradoxical rise of LDL-cholesterol in some hypertriglyceridemic patients due to the enhanced formation of LDLs from VLDLs. Normally, however, these compounds significantly reduce cholesterolemia, particularly in patients with relatively marked elevations and normal triglyceridemia (familial type IIa), this effect probably being linked to the improved delipidization of LDL because of the increased lipase, leading to a better interaction with LDL receptors.

From a general point of view, fibrates can markedly reduce both cholesterol and TGs, frequently elevating HDL-cholesterol and leading to a decrease in the body cholesterol pool and cholesterol deposits in tissues, occasionally resulting in xanthoma regression. These clinical observations are particularly dramatic in patients with familial dysbetalipoproteinemia (Fredrickson's type III). In these patients, the reduction in cholesterol and TGs is accompanied by clear-cut improvements in vascular disease.

New aspects of the activity of fibrates are related to nonlipid parameters. Some (in particular, bezafibrate but not gemfibrozil) display a potent plasma fibrinogen-reducing activity. In addition, an activity on platelet aggregation, reducing sensitivity to different aggregants in treated patients, also has been demonstrated. Fenofibrate has been shown to decrease platelet-derived growth factor, a stimulus for smooth muscle cell proliferation.

Pharmaceutical forms

Fibrates are available in a wide range of doses, with different therapeutic schedules. Bezafibrate is usually given in two daily doses of 300 mg; a slow-release formulation of 400 mg is also available in most countries. Fenofibrate can be given in three divided doses of 100 mg or, because of the long half-life, as a single daily administration of 250 to 300 mg; it is also available in a single daily dose of 200 mg in a comicronized formulation (maximum dosage 400 mg per day). Gemfibrozil generally is given as 600 mg bid; in some countries, a 900-mg tablet or sachet form is available for daily administration. Less widely available are ciprofibrate, clinofibrate, and others.

Clinical activity

Fibrates were widely used initially to lower LDL-cholesterol. After the introduction of statins, their role shifted more to the reduction of VLDL and plasma TG levels

Table 69.5 Fibric acid derivatives: pharmacokinetic properties

	Oral bioavailability (%)	Volume of distribution (l)	$t_{1/2}$ (h)
Bezafibrate	100	17	1.5-30
Ciprofibrate	80	12	40-80
Clofibrate	100	14.5	15
Fenofibrate	60 (100[1])	62.5	20-25 (15-30[1])
Gemfibrozil	100	9-10	1.3

[1]Comicronized fenofibrate.

and/or to raising HDL. It has been suggested that the rise in HDL is responsible for the reduction in CHD observed in the Helsinki Heart Study as well as in the VA-HIT trial.

The highest efficacy of fibrates is achieved in type IV hyperlipoproteinemia, with a reduction in TGs up to 60% or more and a concomitant increase of HDL-cholesterol levels. Hypercholesterolemias (types IIa and IIb) show a less clear-cut response. In general, plasma cholesterol response is more marked in severe hypercholesterolemia (familial type II), with a 15 to 30% reduction, possibly because of a more prolonged elimination half-life and higher blood levels in these patients. For the same reason, fibrates with a longer elimination half-life (e.g., fenofibrate, ciprofibrate) may be more effective in severe type II hyperlipidemia. In type IIb hyperlipoproteinemia, fibrates can reduce TG levels by about 35 to 40% and LDL-cholesterol levels by 15 to 30% and raise HDL-cholesterol levels by approximately 20%. The most responsive hyperlipoproteinemia is type III, because of the potent stimulation of lipoprotein clearance induced by fibrates, both LDL-cholesterol and TGs being decreased by 30 to 50%. Finally, fibrates, in particular gemfibrozil, can be usefully prescribed in patients at risk for acute pancreatitis with type V hyperlipoproteinemia with TG levels between 1000 and 2000 mg/dl (11.5-23 mmol/l).

Although it is difficult to clearly identify specific differences among fibrates, long-acting fibrates generally are more effective in hypercholesterolemia, whereas compounds with a shorter half-life are more effective in type IV hyperlipoproteinemia. Gemfibrozil seems to be most effective in raising HDL and apoAI levels and fenofibrate in reducing apoB concentrations. Clinical experience suggests, however, that resistance to treatment with one fibrate does not exclude sensitivity to another.

The efficacy of fibrates in the primary and secondary prevention of CHD is supported by the results from Helsinki Heart Study and the VA-HIT study (see above), strongly suggesting that hypertriglyceridemic subjects with low HDL levels can obtain a protective effect. Fibrates have demonstrated a favorable activity in coronary lesions. The BECAIT study with bezafibrate and the LOCAT study with gemfibrozil both showed a reduced progression of lesions and even regression in a significant percentage of young coronary patients mainly with hypertriglyceridemia and low HDL levels.

Absorption, fate, and excretion

The pharmacodynamic activity of fibrates is only partially linked to their kinetics, since PPAR activation seems to be independent of a continued presence of the drug in plasma. On the other hand, fibrates with a long elimination half-life have the advantage of single daily administrations (in some cases, patients may skip one or both weekend treatments without changes in the effects on plasma lipids). The major kinetic characteristics of the most widely available fibrates are summarized in Table 69.5. With the exception of gemfibrozil, fibrates are prodrugs, being deesterified to the active acid.

Metabolite formation differs with the different agents, major metabolites including hydroxylated products, phenol metabolites, etc. In general, most of the transformation products are excreted in the urine in the form of glucuronide conjugates. Fibrates are extensively bound to plasma proteins, particularly albumin. A portion is also bound to lipoproteins, and it has been suggested that this latter binding may partly influence the pharmacodynamic properties. Most fibrates, with the exception of gemfibrozil, also display interactions of some clinical usefulness by reducing uric acid and competing for reabsorption (see Chap. 71).

Adverse effects and interactions

Fibrates generally are well tolerated. Subjective side effects, e.g., GI or skin manifestations, are quite uncommon (2% or less in large series). Impotence and/or loss of libido have been reported occasionally, particularly with gemfibrozil and fenofibrate. Some of the newer agents, particularly those with the longest half-lives (e.g., fenofibrate), have been associated with increased transaminase levels in plasma. Clinical myositis was described in an early patient series with clofibrate, associated with a flu-like syndrome and marked increases of plasma creatine phosphokinase (CPK); such findings are rarely encountered with the newer agents.

Fibrates may increase bile cholesterol elimination, thus leading to an increased risk of lithogenicity. This risk has been well established only for clofibrate; reports on other agents are contradictory and do not seem to support a similar risk.

A species-specific increased incidence of liver tumors in rodents due to peroxisomal proliferation was reported previously. In the WHO study with clofibrate, a significant rise in assorted malignancies was found. However, there is no convincing evidence of an increased risk of tumors of any kind in humans receiving currently available fibrates. It may be concluded generally that the profile of risk attributed to fibric acid derivatives after the WHO study with clofibrate (i.e., gallstone disease, increased incidence of tumors, liver toxicity, etc.) does not appear to be shared to any significant extent by any of the newer derivatives.

The most clinically significant drug interaction is the

potentiation of coumarin anticoagulants. Both clofibrate and gemfibrozil have been reported to displace warfarin from albumin binding, but this mechanism is certainly not responsible for the observed effect. Some authors have suggested a sensitization of the binding sites for vitamin K antagonists. Whatever the mechanism, this interaction usually requires a lowering of the dose of concomitantly given coumarins with careful monitoring of the prothrombin time.

Clinical interactions have been reported between fibrates and statins. The association of fibrates with statins can provoke with CPK elevations, myopathy, myoglobinuria, and/or acute renal failure. This potential interaction advises caution in the concomitant administration of fibrate and statin that may be prescribed to patients with severe cases of hypercholesterolemia/hypertriglyceridemia. Large studies have indicated that, with proper care, this association may be administered safely.

Nicotinic acid

Nicotinic acid (NA) or niacin (pyridine-3-carboxylic acid) is a water soluble B vitamin used in the prophylaxis and treatment of pellagra. Activity is exerted in the body after conversion to either nicotinamide adenine dinucleotide (NAD) or nicotinamide adenine dinucleotide phosphate (NADP).

NA activity on plasma cholesterol concentrations at very high doses (in excess of 2 g/d) was demonstrated more than 40 years ago. This action is typical of NA and not shared by nicotinamide and is completely separated from its role as a vitamin. Subsequently, NA was found to reduce plasma TG levels and to exert other favorable effects on the lipid and lipoprotein pattern. Specifically, it decreases TGs in VLDLs (20-80%) and cholesterol content in LDLs (10-15%); moreover, it raises HDL level, mainly the HDL_2 subfraction.

There are several mechanisms by which NA alters serum lipoprotein levels. Earlier studies found that NA was able to inhibit lipolysis in adipose tissue with a subsequent fall in plasma free fatty acids starting from 1 hour after dosing, with the effect lasting up to 3 hours. Free fatty acids are taken up by the liver to act as VLDL precursors; consequently, the synthesis of TG-rich lipoproteins was found to be reduced. A reduction in LDL synthesis can be less clearly demonstrated, and the observed decline in total and LDL-cholesterol levels may be linked to the reduction in VLDLs as LDL precursors or to an enhanced hepatic clearance of IDLs, which, with their reduced content in TGs, appear to have an improved affinity for the liver LDL receptors. Finally, NA inhibits hepatic lipase, preventing the transformation of the more efficient HDL_2 subfraction to the less efficient HDL_3.

Nicotinic acid, when available, is usually prepared in tablets of 100 to 500 mg. Treatment should be started with low doses (100 mg qd or bid), gradually reaching the effective dose. If NA is given concomitantly with a bile acid-binding resin, daily doses of 3 g are generally adequate. Niceritrol, acipimox, nicotinyl alcohol, and others are given in different doses (tablets of 250-500 mg) and usually do not require gradual dose adjustments.

The primary indications for NA are combined hyperlipidemias and isolated hypercholesterolemia. At a dose of 2 to 8 g per day, NA can achieve reductions in plasma TG and cholesterol levels of 30 to 40% and 15 to 20%, respectively. LDL-cholesterol levels may be reduced by 20% or more. Increased levels of HDL-cholesterol, 30% or more, may be the highest response among lipid-lowering agents. Unlike most other lipid-lowering agents, high-dose NA can reduce plasma levels of Lp(a). For this reason, NA potentially has the widest range of therapeutic activity.

Unfortunately, these beneficial effects are counteracted by serious side effects, ranging from impaired glucose tolerance to hyperuricemia and GI intolerance, gastritis, abnormal liver function tests, and the occasional development of toxic hepatitis. Subjectively, the administration of NA is accompanied by severe skin flushing, headache, itching, tingling, warmth, and occasionally, nausea. All subjective side effects are possibly related to an enhanced vascular release of prostacyclin and are blunted by the previous administration of aspirin or, to a lesser extent, by the use of sustained-release formulations of NA.

These side-effects have curtailed the use of NA in warmer countries. In these locations, some NA derivatives, such as nicotinyl alcohol, niceritrol, and acipimox, have been marketed with some success. Apparently, however, the newer agents do not share the remarkable activity of the parent compound in all forms of hyperlipidemia. Some of these drugs, e.g., acipimox, have a better and longer-lasting antilipolytic activity versus plain NA despite the less marked hypolipidemic activity, thus casting doubt on the identity of the postulated mechanism of action.

Interest in NA has been maintained because of the positive results obtained in the Coronary Drug Project, a trial that examined hypolipidemic drugs in the secondary prevention of CHD. In this study, NA was the only drug that reduced the recurrence of nonfatal MI when examined 9 years after discontinuing treatment. In the FATS study, the best results in terms of coronary regression/inhibited progression were achieved with a combination of NA and colestipol.

Probucol

Probucol (4-4'-[(1-methylethyldene)bis(thio)]bis[2,6-bis(1,1-dimethylethyl) phenol), chemically related to the potent antioxidant-hydroxytoluene (BHT), was first developed as an antioxidant for industrial use about 40 years ago. Because of a potent hypolipidemic activity detected in animals, it was introduced in the early 1970s into therapy. Probucol has a rather unusual property, in that, in patients, it tends to lower HDL-cholesterol levels more than LDL-cholesterol levels. This mechanism may prove crucial for an understanding of the drug's therapeutic activity, but since it is believed that lowering of HDL-cholesterol may not counterbalance the atherogenic effect of elevated LDL-cholesterol, physicians generally have not favored the use of probucol, except in nations such as Japan. In other countries, use has been limited, for many years, to hypercholesterolemic patients unable to tolerate the side effects of other lipid-lowering drugs. Recently, probucol has regained popularity for its antioxidant properties, and several studies have been conducted to characterize this significant peculiarity.

Noteworthy are studies indicating a powerful protective effect against arterial restenosis after angioplasty. Among these, in the large Multivitamins and Probucol Study, probucol markedly reduced the incidence and severity of restenosis when administered 1 month prior to the procedure and for 6 months after versus no effect of antioxidant vitamins. Nonetheless, probucol was voluntarily removed from the US market in 1995 and later from other countries primarily because of concern about safety, in particular proarrhythmic properties. Unfortunately, this has resulted in the dismissal of a drug with very peculiar features that can be used very effectively in the therapy of dyslipidemias. Generic formulations of probucol have now become available in a number of western countries.

Mechanism of action

Initial studies on probucol indicated that this compound may affect cholesterol absorption and, by unknown mechanisms, increase the catabolism of LDL and decrease the synthesis of HDL apolipoproteins. Other studies have shown that probucol, being incorporated into LDL, may affect their metabolic properties, improving receptor and nonreceptor clearance. For this reason, probucol also may be effective in patients with no available LDL receptors, such as homozygous type II patients.

The most interesting property of probucol is the remarkable reduction in HDL-cholesterol it produces. This reduction, paradoxically, occurs in the face of very evident decreases in the size of tendon xanthomas and xanthelasmas in treated patients. This apparent discrepancy is probably due to the ability of probucol to improve the function of the cholesteryl ester transport protein (CETP) system, delivering cholesteryl esters from HDL to lower-density lipoproteins, thus increasing reverse cholesterol transport (see Fig. 69.2). The reduction of HDL is, in fact, accompanied by a similar increase in the transfer reaction, suggesting that this may be a major mode of action. Moreover, the stimulated CETP system leads to the formation of smaller HDL particles, known to be more effective in the removal of tissue cholesterol than larger HDL particles. In fact, HDLs obtained from probucol-treated patients demonstrate an enhanced capacity to remove CEs from macrophages versus control HDLs.

Finally, probucol has a potent antioxidant action, particularly significant because oxidized LDLs are directly atherogenic and have a decreased affinity for the LDL receptors. Moreover, probucol can reduce the expression of specific adhesion molecules on vascular endothelial cells, inhibiting monocyte adhesion.

Pharmaceutical forms

Probucol is available in 250- and 500-mg tablets. The recommended dose is 500 mg bid, taken with meals.

Pharmacokinetics

Only 2 to 8% of the drug is absorbed in the GI tract; it is then transported to the systemic circulation in chylomicrons. This may have to do with the demonstrated activity on intestinal apolipoprotein biosynthesis. When, however, the drug is taken with food, peak plasma concentrations are definitely higher. Probucol accumulates in the adipose tissue, where it persists for several months (up to 6 months), and the circulating drug is almost totally contained in VLDL, LDL, and HDL particles. This phenomenon is probably responsible for the long period (3 months) necessary to achieve a steady-state kinetic during oral administration of a dose of 500 mg bid. Probucol is mostly excreted through bile and feces, only a small amount being eliminated in urine. The persistence of the drug in body tissues does not lead to permanence of the hypocholesterolemic activity, which generally fades away within a month or so. The high lipophilicity of this compound allows its passage through the placenta and in milk, and therefore, use should be avoided in nursing or pregnant women.

Clinical activity

Probucol lowers LDL-cholesterol levels by 10 to 15% and HDL-cholesterol levels by 25% or more, this being secondary to the 30% increase in plasma CETP activity. The maximal effect on plasma cholesterol (LDL plus HDL) occurs after 1 to 3 months of treatment. Other effects (on TGs or VLDLs) are minimal.

Adverse effects and interactions

Subjectively, probucol can induce abdominal side effects such as diarrhea, flatulence, and nausea in 10% of patients, these problems usually being transient. The safety of probucol has not been established for children or during pregnancy. Since probucol tends to remain in the body for prolonged periods, it is prudent to discontinue the drug at least 6 months before attempting pregnancy.

The major side effect of probucol occurs in the cardiac conduction system, with prolongation of the QT interval on ECG that may lead to tachyarrhythmias, particularly torsades de pointes. Interestingly, however, published articles and adverse reaction reports from the Food and Drug Administration indicate that 94% of tachyarrhythmias and QTc prolongations associated with probucol therapy occur in women. Specifically, torsades de pointes were seen only in women, and probucol-associated QTc prolongation responses at doses of 500 to 1000 mg per day were observed three to four times more frequently in women.

HMG-CoA REDUCTASE INHIBITORS (STATINS)

Development of drugs affecting cholesterol synthesis was suggested by the well-known metabolic fate of this chemical: only 300 to 500 mg of cholesterol is absorbed daily from the diet, whereas an additional 700 to 900 mg is synthetized de novo by various organs in the body, mainly by the liver. Biosynthesis follows a series of 25 separate reactions, starting with three successive condensations of acetyl-coenzyme A units to form 3-hydroxy-3-methylgutaryl-coenzyme A (HMG-CoA). HMG-CoA is then reduced to mevalonate via the action of the microsomal enzyme 3-hydroxy-3-methylgutaryl-coenzyme A reductase (HMG-CoA reductase). This first committed step in cholesterol synthesis is also a rate-limiting reaction. HMG-CoA is a water-soluble intermediate that is easily catabolized, and accumulation would not lead to any toxicity problems. Thus, HMG-CoA reductase was a natural target for a possible pharmacologic intervention.

A specific HMG-CoA reductase inhibitor, mevastatin (or compactin), a fungal metabolite from *Penicillum citrinum,* was described in 1976. Soon after, lovastatin (mevinolin) was isolated from *Aspergillus terreus* cultures. After specific structure/activity studies, two semisynthetic derivatives become available some years later: simvastatin (the 2,2-dimethyl-butyrate analogue of lovastatin) and pravastatin (the 6-hydroxy open acid analogue of mevastatin). More recently, three totally synthetic statins have been marketed: fluvastatin, atorvastatin, and cerivastatin.

All HMG-CoA reductase inhibitors have a chemical structure with a moiety resembling hydroxymethylglutaric acid. The HMG-resembling moiety may be present in a closed (lactone) or an open (hydroxyacid) form. The lactone ring is present in lovastatin, simvastatin, fluvastatin, atorvastatin, and cerivastatin; the open acid in pravastatin. Lactones are prodrugs, the open ring hydroxyacids being the active compounds. Ring opening occurs at an alkaline pH or in the liver.

Mechanism of action

Statins are reversible inhibitors of microsomal HMG-CoA reductase. Inhibition of HMG-CoA reductase decreases intracellular cholesterol biosynthesis, which then leads to transcriptionally upregulated production of microsomal HMG-CoA reductase and cell surface LDL receptors. No inhibition of other metabolic pathways, including synthesis of fatty acids, proteins, or nucleic acids, is observed.

The upregulation of LDL receptors in hepatocytes causes a dramatic fall in plasma LDL-cholesterol. This occurs with minimal daily dosages, generally from a minimum of 5 to a maximum of 80 mg per day (0.1-0.4 mg in the case of cerivastatin). Unfortunately, in addition to the positive effect on LDL receptor expression and upregulation, statins also cause a compensatory overexpression of HMG-CoA reductase, attributed to an increased transcription of the enzyme gene and decreased protein degradation. Through these mechanisms, cultured fibroblasts can restore a normal cholesterol synthesis even in the presence of high concentrations of the inhibitor. The raised production of HMG-CoA reductase therefore allows a significant plasma cholesterol reduction in the face of unchanged total-body cholesterol in treated patients. These data suggest an explanation for some cases of poor responses or loss of response to statin therapy. Loss of response and resistance to statins are indeed not so infrequent in the clinic (9-10% and 7-8%, respectively) and, in our experience, are the major problem of statin therapy.

More recent studies suggest that, in addition to reducing cholesterol biosynthesis, statins also may slightly reduce cholesterol absorption.

All statins have similar qualitative effects on plasma lipid/lipoprotein changes (Tab. 69.6), with the possible exception of atorvastatin, which has been found also to significantly reduce TG levels. All statins act in an additive fashion with bile acid-binding resins.

The selectivity in the mode of action is confirmed by lipoprotein data in humans that indicate that aside from a small increase in HDL-cholesterol level, lipoprotein structure and composition are only moderately affected. These findings allow one to conclude that the mode of action of HMG-CoA reductase inhibitors in lowering cholesterol is by reducing biosynthesis and, as a consequence, raising LDL receptors, thus decreasing the number of circulating LDL particles.

Pharmaceutical forms

Lovastatin is available commercially in the US, Canada, and some European countries (20- and 40-mg tablets); the daily dose should not exceed 80 mg. All other statins are essentially available worldwide. Simvastatin is available in tablets of 10, 20, and 40 mg (maximal daily dose 40 mg), whereas pravastatin is available in 10-, 20-, and 40-mg tablets (maximal dose 80 mg). Fluvastatin is available in 20- and 40-mg capsules, doses ranging from 20 to 80 mg per day. Atorvastatin (maximal dose of 80 mg per day) is available in 10-, 20-, and 40-mg tablets. Cerivastatin is available in 0.2- and 0.4-mg tablets, the dose ranging from 0.1 to 0.4 mg per day.

Pharmacokinetics

Generally, 30 to 50% of HMG-CoA reductase inhibitors are absorbed. All of them, except cerivastatin, undergo a

---

Table 69.6 Effects on lipid/lipoprotein of different statins

	TC	TG	LDL-C	apoB	HDL-C
Atorvastatin (10 mg/d)	28	15	38	32	+7
Cerivastatin (0,2 mg/d)	20	10	27	20	+5
Fluvastatin (40 mg/d)	18	10	26	18	+5
Lovastatin (20 mg/d)	19	6	27	20	+7
Pravastatin (20 mg/d)	17	9	23	16	+6
Simvastatin (10 mg/d)	24	10	30	30	+7

Note: Data are expressed as mean % changes versus baseline and reflect the experience of the authors.

conspicuous "first pass" effect so that after a short time (1-4 hours), no drug is detectable in plasma. Atorvastatin differs from the other statins in that it has a prolonged plasma half-life (14-16 h). This peculiar characteristic of this newer statin probably accounts in part for its higher effectiveness. All statins are highly bound to plasma proteins, and the major elimination route is fecal.

Probably because of the structural similarity between these molecules and HMG, they have a unique profile of competitive, specific, and reversible inhibition of the HMG-CoA reductase enzyme. Interestingly, their affinity for the enzyme (Ki = 10 nM) is more than 1000-fold higher than the affinity of the natural substrate HMG CoA (Km = 10 μM). For this reason, even the apparently inactive metabolites of the three drugs (activities 10- to 100-fold lower) may contribute significantly to the pharmacodynamic activity.

There was a question on the "selectivity" of action of these agents in different tissues. Apparently, pravastatin's chemical and physical characteristics do result in a higher affinity for liver cells, and this may be associated with a reduced incidence of side effects. After many years of extensive use, however, statins have demonstrated a very favorable side effects profile, and this issue of selectivity has lost some interest.

Clinical activity

HMG-CoA reductase inhibitors presently provide the most potent drug treatment for hypercholesterolemia. In large clinical series of patients with type II hyperlipoproteinemia (both IIa and IIb), total and LDL-cholesterol reductions were generally on the order of 25 to 40%, and even beyond for atorvastatin (60% at the higher dose of 80 mg/d). These results, at low daily doses, are generally encouraging for patients and are followed by excellent compliance.

Other lipoprotein changes are minimal: TG reduction seldom exceeds 20% and is mostly related to a decrease in TGs in the LDL fraction, with the above-reported exception of atorvastatin, which lowers not only LDL levels but also to a lesser extent VLDL levels, thus achieving a net TG reduction of around 30%. Changes in HDL-cholesterol, although statistically significant in large series, are often unpredictable and not dose-related. Although it can be excluded that the mild microsomal enzyme-inducing properties of these compounds are in play, the mechanism and clinical significance of HDL rises are difficult to evaluate. Possibly, the rise in HDLs may be only the consequence of improved removal of cholesterol from tissues.

Clinical and animal experience has suggested that the association of reductase inhibitors with other drugs may prove extremely effective in patients with severe hypercholesterolemia (e.g., familial heterozygous cases). The association with anion-binding resins is among the most widely tested and achieves maximal effectiveness. Plasma cholesterol and LDL reductions with this association may be as high as 40 to 50% or more. Statin treatment does not affect serum Lp(a) levels, however.

A good activity also has been shown by combining probucol and also fibrates in type IIb hyperlipoproteinemia. This combination, however, may carry some risk in terms of an increased incidence of myalgia (see Fibrates, above).

The reduction in cardiovascular events with statin therapy observed in the recent major lipid-lowering trials is better in terms of absolute risk reduction than that seen in earlier studies, possibly because of the choice of patients with higher absolute risk (see above).

Aside from the lipid effects, statins have demonstrated a number of interesting activities. Statin therapy has been shown to reduce platelet aggregation via a dual mechanism involving reduced thromboxane B_2 formation and also, at least for fluvastatin and lovastatin, a direct binding to platelets. Moreover, hypercholesterolemia has a detrimental effect on endothelial function in both the epicardial coronary arteries and resistance vessels. Exercise induces a metabolic vasodilatation in the resistance vessels and a flow-mediated endothelium-dependent dilatation of the epicardial vessels. Endothelial dysfunction leads to paradoxical vasoconstriction with impairment of myocardial perfusion and contributes to the pathogenesis of myocardial ischemia. Cholesterol lowering with statins has been shown to restore to some extent a normal endothelial function.

Finally, all statins, with the exception of pravastatin, can inhibit the proliferation, migration, and signaling of vascular smooth muscle cells. Inhibition of farnesol and of geranylgeraniol synthesis by HMG-CoA reductase blockade and the resulting reduction in prenylation of key cellular proteins, activating cell proliferation and protein synthesis, may underlie this effect.

Adverse effects and interactions

Experience with statins involving several thousands of patients treated for 15 years or longer does not show an increased incidence of severe side effects. Atorvastatin, fluvastatin, and cerivastatin studies provide similar findings but have a shorter follow-up. Previously claimed effects on the refractory system of the eye, found in dogs treated with very high doses of both lovastatin and simvastatin, were never demonstrated in humans. In treated patients, a small incidence of liver (ALT, AST rises) and muscular (CPK rises) toxicities has been described with all inhibitors. Clinical myalgia occurs with a higher frequency (5% or more) in patients concomitantly treated with a statin and a fibrate derivative (see Fibrates, above). Such side effects definitely occur more rarely with pravastatin, and the association of fluvastatin with fibrates, in particular bezafibrate, seems to avoid this problem completely.

Statins, like fibrates, may potentiate coumarin anticoagulants by an unclear mechanism. Increased steady-state digoxin levels have been reported in volunteer studies with simvastatin. Most statins may interact with several drugs catabolyzed by the CYP3A4 system. Among them are erythromycin, dihydropyridine calcium antagonists, azole antifungals, midazolam, and grapefruit juice (see

Chap. 6). These last interactions are not present with flu-vastatin, since this drug is metabolized by a different P450 isoform (namely, CYP2C9) that is responsible for diclofenac and tolbutamide metabolism, as well as with cerivastatin, which undergoes a dual metabolic handling (CYP3A4 and CYP2C8).

Because of the critical role of HMG-CoA reductase in embryogenesis, these compounds should not be given to pregnant women and should be withheld for several months before a planned pregnancy.

OTHER DRUGS

Numerous other agents are available, in different countries, for the management of hyperlipoproteinemias. Most of these are absorbable, and a few are of natural origin. Among the most widely used, the following may be listed:

- β-Sitosterol is a plant sterol that is available in some countries for the treatment of hypercholesterolemia. It exerts a selective lowering of LDL-cholesterol at daily doses of 6 g or higher. Occasionally it may induce nausea with mild laxative effects. β-Sitosterol generally has been superseded by the newer anion-exchange resins.
- Metformin, a biguanide antidiabetic (see Chap. 68), exerts a significant hypotriglyceridemic activity in non-diabetic patients. The mechanism is linked to a reduced liver intestinal biosynthesis of VLDLs and possibly to stimulated activity of the glucose transporter mechanisms in peripheral cells. Metformin is available in 500- or 850-mg tablets to be taken bid or tid with meals. Metformin generally is used in daily doses of 1000 to 2550 mg. Although the risk of lactic acidosis with this compound in nondiabetic patients is negligible, care should be taken in the management of elderly people.
- Tiadenol is a substituted decane affecting both cholesterol and TG levels in different forms of hyperlipoproteinemia. The mechanism is probably linked to an increased lipoprotein catabolism, as in the case of fibrates, but in addition, the drug apparently reduces liver lipoprotein secretion. Tiadenol is available in 800-mg tablets to be taken tid. Although short-term trials have clearly indicated a potent activity of tiadenol in numerous patient series, long-term results are less satisfactory. Recent animal data indicate that chronic administration may lead to activation of the liver microsomal enzyme system, thus lowering activity. Tiadenol is otherwise generally well tolerated, and cautionary notes are similar to those of fibric acids.
- Pantethine is the disulfide dimer of pantetheine, the amide conjugate of pantothenic acid with cysteamine. It is available in 250- or 500-mg tablets, for total daily doses of 750 to 1000 mg. Pantethine has been shown in numerous clinical trials to reduce significantly, although not markedly, serum total (10-12%) and LDL-cholesterol (12-15%) levels; some activity is also exerted in hypertriglyceridemias. The mechanism of pantethine is rather unique, being linked to a reduced activation of HMG-CoA reductase in the presence of high concentrations of cholesterol precursors. Pantethine is well tolerated, and reported side effects are minimal.

n-3 free fatty acids

The potentially beneficial effects of dietary ω-3 or n-3 polyunsaturated fatty acids (PUFAs) on vascular disease continue to generate intense clinical and investigative interest throughout the world. The very low incidence of MI in the Greenland Eskimos suggested that a high dietary n-3 PUFA intake with marine food might protect against coronary heart disease.

The two major n-3 fatty acids are eicosapentaenoic acid (EPA, 20:5, n-3), with five double bonds, and docosahexaenoic acid (DHA, 22:6, n-3), with six double bonds. Unlike many of the pharmaceutical agents used in patients with coronary artery disease that have just a single mechanism of action, the EPA and DHA from fish oil have multifaceted actions. They reduce fasting and postprandial TG levels (by 20-30%) and decrease platelet reactivity, particularly by inhibiting the synthesis of thromboxane A_2, the prostaglandin that causes platelet aggregation and vasoconstriction. Both n-3 PUFAs improve fibrinolysis, delay the growth of the atherosclerotic plaque by inhibiting both cellular growth factors and the migration of monocytes, promote the synthesis of beneficial NO in the endothelium, and may slightly decrease blood pressure. Furthermore n-3 PUFAs also may beneficially influence vessel wall characteristics and blood rheology. Finally, they have been shown to inhibit ventricular tachyarrhythmias in animals. A recent controlled study (GISSI-Prevenzione) showed a significant 15% reduction of sudden death in coronary patients. Commercially available n-3 PUFA formulation, mostly gel capsules, are innumerable, containing from 400 to 1000 mg of EPA + DHA in variable proportions. Doses are from 1000 to 6000 mg per day.

Suggested readings

BLOOMFIELD RUBINS H, ROBINS SJ, COLLINS D, et al. Gemfibrozil for the secondary prevention of coronary heart disease in men with low levels of high-density lipoprotein cholesterol. N Engl J Med 1999;341:410-8

DOWNS JR, CLEARFIELD M, WEIS S, et al. Primary prevention of acute coronary events with lovastatin in men and women with average cholesterol levels. J Am Med Ass 1998;279:1615-22.

FRANCESCHINI G, SIRTORI M. VACCARINO V, et al. Mechanisms of HDL reduction after probucol - Changes in HDL subfractions and Increased reverse cholesteryl ester transfer. Arteriosclerosis 1989;9:462-9.

FRIK MH, ELO O, HAAPA K, et al. Helsinki Heart Study: primary-prevention trial with gemfibrozil in middle-aged men with dyslipidemia. N. Engl J Med 1987;317:1237-45.

FRUCHART JC, BREWER HB, et al. Consensus for the use of fibrates in the treatment of dyslipoproteinemia and coronary heart disease. Am J Cardiol 1998;81:912-16.

GISSI - Prevenzione Investigators. Dietary supplementation with n-3 polyunsaturated fatty acids and vitamin E after myocardial infarction: results of the GISSI-Prevenzione trial. Lancet 1999;447-55.

Lipid Research Clinics Program. The Lipid Research Clinics Coronary Primary Prevention Trial results I: Reduction in incidence of coronary heart disease, J Am Med Ass 1984;251:351-64.

Miller Bass K, Newschaffer CJ, Klag MJ, Bush TL. Plasma lipoprotein levels as predictors of cardiovascular death in women. Arch Intern Med 1993;153:2209-16.

Neuvonen PJ, Kantola T, Kivistö KT. Simvastatin but not pravastatin is very susceptible to interaction with the CYP3A4 inhibitor itraconazole. Clin Pharmacol Ther 1998;63:332-41.

Pazzucconi F, Dorigotti F, Gianfranceschi G. Therapy with HMG CoA reductase inhibitors: characteristics of the long-term permanence of the hypocholesterolemic activity. Atherosclerosis 1995;117:189-98.

Scandinavian Simvastatin Survival Study Group. Randomized trial of cholesterol lowering in 4444 participants with coronary heart disease: the Scandinavian Simvastatin Survival Study (4S). Lancet 1994;344:1383-9.

Sacks FM, Pfeffer MA, Moye LA, et al. The effect of pravastatin on coronary events after myocardial infarction in patients with average cholesterol levels. N Engl J Med 1996;335:1001-9.

Shepherd J. Cobbe SM, Ford I, et al for the West of Scotland Coronary Prevention Study Group. Prevention of coronary heart disease with pravastatin in men with hypercholesterolemia. N Engl J Med 1995;333:1301-7.

Sirtori CR. Tissue selectivity of hydroxymethylglutaryl coenzyme A (HMG CoA) reductase inhibitors. Pharmacol Ther 1993;60:431-59.

Staels B. Vu-Dac N, Kosykh VA, et al. Fibrates downregulate apolipoprotein C-III expression independent of induction of peroxisomal acyl coenzyme A oxidase. J Clin Invest 1995;95:705-12.

Obesity

Anne-Marie Glenny, Susan O'Meara

Obesity and overweight are serious public health problems for the western world, where energy-rich diets and sedentary lifestyles are becoming more common. Existing evidence shows that avoiding obesity and achieving weight loss are beneficial to health. Health care professionals and purchasers are under increasing pressure to intervene to reduce the prevalence of obesity.

The prevalence of obesity and overweight continues to increase in developed countries. Data from the 38 European centers included in the World Health Organization's MONICA project show the average European age-standardized 90th percentiles of body mass index (BMI) to be 31 kg/m^2 in men and 33 kg/m^2 in women. The prevalence of obesity, defined as a BMI of greater than 30 kg/m^2, is shown to be greater than 10% across Europe, with much geographic variation. Estimates of the prevalence of male obesity (40-60 years) range from 10% in northern Europe to 18% in eastern Europe. There is greater variation for women of the same age, with estimates of 15% in northern Europe and 30% in Mediterranean and eastern Europe.

Certain high-risk groups have been identified. In families where one or both parents are overweight or obese, children are at greater risk of developing the condition. The risk of obesity varies during the life cycle, with men being at greater risk during their late 30s. Women face an increased risk at several stages, e.g., when newly married, during pregnancy, during menopause, and at retirement.

Risk of obesity is also associated with social class and education. In England, the age-standardized prevalence of obesity in women is around 21% for manual workers, compared with approximately 13% for those in professional or managerial occupations. A similar trend exists for men, but within a narrower range. Women with no qualifications show a mean BMI of 26.7 kg/m^2 as opposed to 24.6 kg/m^2 in those educated to C level or above; this trend is repeated for men.

The risk of obesity varies among different ethnic groups. It has been suggested that Asian people are at greater risk of developing obesity when compared with Afro-Caribbean and Caucasian people. Asians are particularly at risk of developing abdominal obesity, and there is also an increased prevalence of insulin resistance in this group. Such racial differences in the risk of developing obesity appear to be more pronounced in women than in men.

People who are overweight or obese are more likely to suffer from coronary heart disease, hypercholesterolemia, hypertension, diabetes, cholelithiasis, degenerative joint disease, and obstructive sleep apnea. Obese men and women may experience a reduction in daily functioning and quality of life and suffer from social and psychologic problems. In addition to these, life expectancy is also reduced by obesity. Health benefits are associated with even modest reductions in weight, with reductions in blood pressure, cholesterol, and triglycerides achievable with just a 5 to 10% reduction in initial weight. In order to obtain long-term health benefits, however, weight loss must be maintained. There is concern that "weight cycling" or "yo-yo dieting," whereby individuals fluctuate between periods of weight loss and weight regain, may be associated with an increased risk of mortality, especially cardiovascular mortality. A recent literature review, however, highlighted methodologic problems and suggested that such results should be treated with caution.

Measurements of obesity

The BMI is frequently used as a measure of overweight and obesity. However, health professionals need to be aware that BMI does not take into account factors such as size of body frame, proportion of lean mass, gender, and age. A better predictor of cardiovascular risk is the girth-to-height ratio (waist circumference divided by height), because it is a good measure of central (abdominal) fat distribution. This is associated with an increased risk of cardiovascular mortality, hypertension, and non-insulin-dependent diabetes. Other measurements of obesity include body weight, percentage over ideal body weight, skinfold thickness, and body composition.

Prevention of obesity

Despite the fact that obesity is generally considered to be a preventable condition, there are few good-quality evaluations of primary prevention programs. Community education programs, either with or without a financial incentive to maintain a healthy weight, may be of value in adults. However, long-term follow-up data (6-10 years) indicate that the benefits of such programs diminish over time, and health outcomes are no better than for those receiving no intervention.

Options for the management of obesity

It is generally accepted that pharmacologic and surgical interventions for the management of obesity should not be considered as a first-line strategy. Dietary, exercise, and behavioral interventions should be the first options for both weight reduction and weight maintenance.

Dietary interventions

Dietary restriction, accompanied by adequate support and encouragement, remains one of the most important elements of a weight-reduction program. Despite the multitude of available prescribed diets, including low-calorie diets, very-low-calorie diets, fat restriction, high-fiber regimens, protein-sparing modified fasts, and liquid (formula) diets, no single regimen has emerged as being more effective than any other.

Behavioral interventions

Behavioral techniques such as conditioning and managed reinforcement, based on the idea that much behavior is learned and reinforced by social circumstances, are used commonly for the management of obesity. Research evidence suggests that behavioral modification is most effective when carried out in conjunction with other weight-reduction programs. There is some evidence to suggest that cue avoidance (i.e., avoidance of situations that provide the temptation to overeat) may be more effective than cognitive approaches involving role play to rehearse resisting overeating or social pressure. Daily weight charting has been shown to increase the effectiveness of a behavioral program. Other promising approaches that require further evaluation include behavioral therapy by correspondence and the extension of the behavioral intervention period.

Exercise Weight gain occurs when energy intake exceeds energy expenditure. Modernization has, in general, led to sedentary life-styles for both children and adults in the western world. One way of resolving the positive energy balance that results from today's life-style is to increase physical activity. A recent systematic review in this area identified only four randomized, controlled trials evaluating the role of exercise alone in obese patients who were monitored for 12 months or longer. Although different types of activity were evaluated, including varying levels of aerobic exercise as well as less strenuous stretching sessions, the optimal type and frequency of activity remain unclear.

Pharmacologic interventions

Much controversy exists over the role of "slimming drugs." It is generally agreed that they are unsuitable for use as a sole treatment but rather should be employed as an adjunct to other weight-loss interventions such as prescribed diet, exercise, or behavioral therapy. At present, drugs are not used for childhood obesity because of the risks of growth suppression. The research literature reflects their use in adults aged up to 75 years.

Surgical interventions

Surgical treatment is usually considered only for those suffering from morbid obesity (BMI greater than 40 kg/m^2), for whom less invasive methods of weight loss have failed. In general, the weight loss associated with surgical interventions is greater and more sustained than that achieved by nonsurgical methods, with gastric bypass surgery and vertical banded gastroplasty showing typical weight losses of 45 to 65 kg and 30 to 35 kg, respectively, 1 year postoperatively. Surgery is, however, linked with complications, such as revision of the initial procedure, dumping syndrome, vitamin and mineral deficiencies, and associated mortality.

Maintenance of weight loss

Many people lose weight successfully but regain it later, negating any improvement in health and causing yet further anxiety for the patient. It is imperative that weight management is viewed as a long-term intervention, incorporating strategies for both weight reduction and the maintenance of weight loss. Continued contact with either a health professional or a self-help group has been shown to be beneficial as a maintenance program.

Drug classes

Slimming drugs date back to the nineteenth century when ephedrine, a sympathomimetic amine, was extracted from the Chinese plant *Ephedra sinica* and used as a stimulant. The development of amphetamines arose from experimentation with ephedrine-like compounds, their appetite-suppressant effects first being reported in the late 1930s. During the 1950s and 1960s, amphetamines made up the bulk of the medications used for the treatment of obesity. As improvements were made in behavioral and dietary interventions, the use of pharmacologic interventions for the promotion of weight loss declined. Due to the severe adverse effects associated with amphetamines, such as anxiety, insomnia, irritability, and possible dependency, it was soon felt that their disadvantages outweighed their benefits. Amphetamines are no longer recommended for the management of obesity. However, the development of drugs for the management of obesity continued, and with the introduction in the early 1980s of fenfluramine, a drug chemically but not pharmacologically resembling the amphetamines, interest in the pharmacologic treatment of obesity was renewed.

There are three principal mechanisms by which pharmacologic interventions act to promote and maintain weight loss: reduction of energy intake, reduction of energy absorption, and increase in energy expenditure (Tab. 70.1).

Table 70.1 Pharmacologic interventions for the management of obesity

Drug	Daily dosage range (mg)	Peak blood levels (h)	Plasma half-life (h)	Main side effects	Contraindications
Mazindol	1-3	–	10	Overstimulation of the central nervous system (e.g., insomnia, nervousness, restlessness, irritability)	Cardiovascular disease, hyperthyroidism, glaucoma, extrapyramidal disorders, hyperexcitability, extrapyramidal states; should be avoided for pregnant and breast-feeding mothers; should not be given to those with a history of drug abuse
Phentermine	15-37.5	–	12-24	Dry mouth, headache, rashes, euphoria, and dependence; risk of pulmonary hypertension (rare)	Cardiovascular disease, glaucoma, hyperthyroidism, epilepsy, unstable personality, history of drug or alcohol abuse, pregnancy and breast-feeding
Dexfenfluramine hydrochloride[1]	30	4	18 (range 11-30)	As for fenfluramine, but may be better tolerated	As for fenfluramine
Fenfluramine hydrochloride[1]	60-120	2-6	20 (range 11-30)	Diarrhea, drowsiness, dizziness, and lethargy	Pulmonary hypertension, cardiovascular or cerebrovascular disease, and current or past medical history of psychiatric disorder; not to be given to children under 12 years of age; not to be given to those on monoamine oxidase inhibitors or within 2 weeks of discontinuation of such treatment
Fluoxetine hydrochloride	60	6-8	24-72	Gastrointestinal and nervous system symptoms (e.g., nausea, vomiting, dyspepsia, diarrhea, anxiety, insomnia, nervousness, and drowsiness)	Not recommended for nursing mothers; not to be given to those on monoamine oxidase inhibitors; the long half-life of fluoxetine should be taken into account following treatment with monoamine oxidase inhibitors
Sertraline hydrochloride	50-200	4.5-8.4	26 (mean half-life for young and elderly adults ranges from 22-36 h)	As for fluoxetine hydrochloride	Avoid abrupt withdrawal; as for fluoxetine hydrochloride
Sibutramine	10-15	–	14-16	Dry mouth, constipation, insomnia, dizziness, and nausea	Unclear as yet; should be similar to mazindol
Orlistat	120-360	–	7	Gastrointestinal disturbances including increased defecation and oily spotting	Chronic malabsorption syndrome, cholestasis, breast-feeding; not recommended for use during pregnancy

[1]Fenfluramine hydrochloride and dexfenfluramine hydrochloride have both been withdrawn from the market due to associated increased risk of pulmonary hypertension.

Reduction of energy intake

The reduction of energy intake can be achieved through the use of appetite suppressants, known as *anorexiant* or *anorectic drugs*. Such drugs can be divided into the bulk-forming drugs (e.g., methylcellulose) and the centrally acting appetite suppressants. There is no published research evidence to support the use of bulk-forming agents, which claim to reduce intake by producing feelings of satiety. However, there is continuing interest in the role of centrally acting appetite suppressants. These drugs can be subdivided into two categories.

Drugs acting via catecholaminergic (noradrenergic) pathways

Drugs affecting the catecholaminergic system include the amphetamines, benzphetamine hydrochloride, phendimetrazine tartrate, phentermine, mazindol, diethylpropion hydrochloride (amfepramone hydrochloride), and phenylpropanolamine. As discussed previously, amphetamines and their closely related derivatives are not recommended for the treatment of obesity. Of the remaining catecholaminergic drugs, only mazindol and phentermine have been evaluated in good-quality randomized, controlled trials monitoring patients for a period of 12 months or more.

Mazindol is readily absorbed from the gastrointestinal tract and excreted, partly as metabolites and partly unchanged, in the urine. The dosage of mazindol is 1 mg up to a maximum of three times a day. Adverse effects of mazindol are commonly overstimulation of the central nervous system, gastrointestinal disturbances, headache, tremor, sweating, tachycardia, palpitations, dizziness, and altered libido. The possibility of dependence also should be considered. The effectiveness of mazindol has been compared with that of a standard anorexiant (D-amphetamine) and a placebo. Both drugs showed significantly greater weight loss than the placebo during the 12 weeks of treatment. However, weight regain commenced postintervention. No statistically significant difference was demonstrated between the three groups at 1-year follow-up.

Phentermine (at present the only centrally acting appetite suppressant licensed for use in the United Kingdom) is administered orally either as base or hydrochloride. Phentermine has minor sympathomimetic and stimulant properties. It is well absorbed from the small intestine when given as an oral sustained-release complex (15-30 mg daily before breakfast). Phentermine has been associated with the rare yet serious risk of pulmonary hypertension. Patients reporting dyspnea or reduction in exercise tolerance should be taken off the drug immediately. A common side effect associated with the use of phentermine is dry mouth. Other adverse effects include headaches, rashes, euphoria, agitation, dependence, nausea and vomiting, dizziness, hallucinations, depression, psychosis, palpitations, tachycardia, hypertension, constipation, urinary frequency, and facial edema. Phentermine is not recommended for use in the elderly, childhood obesity, or during pregnancy/breast-feeding. It is also contraindicated for those with ischemic cardiovascular disease, epilepsy, glaucoma, hyperthyroidism, or a history of psychiatric illness or alcohol/drug abuse.

Drugs acting via the serotoninergic pathways

The principal aim of drugs in this group is to increase serotonin (5-hydroxytryptamine, 5-HT) levels in the neuronal cleft, which is believed to reduce food intake. The mechanisms by which this is achieved vary. Certain drugs inhibit serotonin reuptake into the nerve terminals, some affect both serotonin release and reuptake, and others act directly on serotonin receptors. Drugs affecting the serotonergic system include fenfluramine hydrochloride, dexfenfluramine hydrochloride (the dextrorotatory isomer of fenfluramine), fluoxetine hydrochloride, sertraline hydrochloride, and other antidepressant selective serotonin reuptake inhibitors (SSRIs). Of these, dexfenfluramine hydrochloride has undergone the most thorough evaluation in published randomized controlled trials (RCTs), the largest being the multicenter INDEX study.

Dexfenfluramine hydrochloride works by both stimulating the release of serotonin and inhibiting its reuptake. Research evidence has demonstrated statistically significant weight loss in favor of dexfenfluramine hydrochloride (15 mg twice daily for periods of up to 12 months) when compared with placebo. However, there is a tendency for weight regain to commence around 6 to 9 months after the start of therapy, independent of whether treatment is continued or not.

Recent developments, however, have led to the withdrawal of both fenfluramine hydrochloride and dexfenfluramine hydrochloride. Like phentermine, fenfluramine hydrochloride and dexfenfluramine hydrochloride have been associated with an increased risk of pulmonary hypertension. In addition, a series of case reports on women suggests that there also may be an association between valvular heart disease and use of the combination therapy fenfluramine-phentermine, as used in the United States. Further reports of valvular heart disease have been received by the Food and Drug Administration (FDA), mainly in association with fenfluramine-phentermine treatment but also where fenfluramine hydrochloride and dexfenfluramine hydrochloride have been used as single agents. The manufacturers of these drugs (Wyeth-Ayerst in the United States and Servier Laboratories in Europe) voluntarily removed them from the market in 1997. It is anticipated that further research will be carried out to explore the possible associations more rigorously.

The SSRIs fluoxetine hydrochloride and sertraline hydrochloride (see Chap. 13) have both been evaluated for their effectiveness in the promotion of weight loss, although both drugs are classed primarily as antidepressants. Fluoxetine hydrochloride (maximum dose 60 mg/d) is readily absorbed from the gastrointestinal tract. It has a long half-life, and peak plasma concentrations occur around 6 to 8 hours after administration. Metabolism occurs in the liver, producing the primary active metabolite norfluoxetine through demethylation. SSRIs are associated with many adverse effects, the most common of which are gastrointestinal disturbances and neurologic problems (including anxiety, nervousness, insomnia, and drowsiness). Fluoxetine hydrochloride also has been associated with headaches, dizziness, convulsions, and sexual dysfunction. SSRIs are not recommended for the use in children or nursing mothers, and caution should be taken in epilepsy.

A 1-year multicenter RCT of fluoxetine hydrochloride (60 mg/d) versus placebo was undertaken in 458 obese patients. Both groups received dietary advice and behavioral counselling. Fluoxetine hydrochloride produced a statistically significant greater mean weight loss from weeks 2 to 28 compared with placebo. After this period, the difference in weight loss between the two groups was no longer statistically significant, with weight regain commencing even though treatment continued. Similar results were obtained in a smaller placebo-controlled trial of fluoxetine hydrochloride, in which non-insulin-dependent obese diabetics were recruited.

Sertraline hydrochloride is slowly absorbed from the gastrointestinal tract, undergoing extensive metabolism in the liver. It is excreted in both urine and feces, in approximately equal quantities. Sertraline hydrochloride is associated with similar adverse effects to fluoxetine. In addition, hyponatremia, mainly in elderly patients, has been reported.

Sertraline hydrochloride was evaluated as part of a weight-maintenance program following successful weight reduction. Participants were required to have lost at least 10% of their initial weight, through a very-low-calorie diet and behavioral therapy, before being randomized to either sertraline hydrochloride (50-200 mg/d) or placebo. Six weeks following randomization, a small mean weight loss was observed in the sertraline group compared with a slight weight gain in the placebo group. However, weight regain then occurred in both groups, and by the end of the 26-week maintenance program, there were no statistically significant differences.

A newer agent, sibutramine hydrochloride is both a catecholaminergic and serotonergic reuptake inhibitor. It also stimulates thermogenesis, thus increasing energy expenditure. A review of clinical trials of this drug has demonstrated a dose-related weight loss, with optimal doses of 10 and 15 mg per day. A multicenter, double-blind, placebo-controlled trial of sibutramine hydrochloride (10 and 15 mg once daily for 52 weeks) showed weight loss during the first 6 months, with weight remaining stable for the following 6 months. At 12 months, average weight loss was 1.6 kg for the placebo group and 3.3 and 4.4 kg for the 10- and 15-mg sibutramine hydrochloride groups, respectively. Adverse events in the sibutramine hydrochloride groups commonly were headache, constipation, dry mouth, and pharyngitis.

Reduction of energy absorption

Pharmacologic interventions can be used to decrease energy absorption in the gastrointestinal tract. A new drug in this field is orlistat, an inhibitor of the gastric and pan-

creatic lipases. A derivative of lipstatin, orlistat works by forming covalent bonds to the serine residue of the active site of the gastrointestinal lipases. In doing this, orlistat inhibits the hydrolysis of dietary triglycerides, consequently limiting the absorption of monoglycerides and free fatty acids. Orlistat's activity appears to be dose-dependent. At doses of 120 mg tid with main meals, orlistat reduces dietary fat absorption by approximately one-third. The reduction in fat absorption tends to plateau at doses greater than 120 mg. An adverse effect associated with orlistat is anal leakage.

A 2-year randomized, controlled trial of orlistat has been conducted across 15 European centers. Patients underwent a 4-week, single-blind placebo lead-in period, after which they were randomized to receive either 52 weeks of treatment with orlistat (120 mg tid) or placebo in conjunction with a hypocaloric diet. Patients were then reassigned to orlistat or placebo, in conjunction with a weight-maintenance diet for a second 52-week period. At the end of the first year, those receiving orlistat had lost 10.3 kg, in comparison with 6.1 kg for patients receiving placebo. During the second year, patients continuing with orlistat treatment regained approximately half the amount of weight regained by those who switched to placebo. The trial concluded that orlistat, when taken in conjunction with an appropriate diet, promotes clinically significant weight loss and limits weight regain over a 2-year period. Further clinical trials assessing the safety of orlistat and other drugs that inhibit the action of the digestive enzymes are ongoing.

Increase in energy expenditure

If obesity is seen as a positive energy balance, then one way to correct this imbalance is to increase the amount of energy an individual expends. This can be done through increased amounts of physical exercise, as discussed earlier in this section, or through the use of drugs that mimic some of the effects of moderate exercise, increasing metabolic rate. Thermogenic adrenergic agonists, such as ephedrine, have been used in the past for the treatment of obesity, although none are recommended at present for weight control. Second-generation thermogenic drugs are currently under study.

COST CONSIDERATIONS AND FUTURE DEVELOPMENTS

Very little data exist on the cost-effectiveness of obesity-related interventions and nothing specifically relating to drug treatment. There is an urgent need to collect good-quality cost-effectiveness data for antiobesity drugs. This should be done in parallel with rigorous evaluations of clinical effectiveness. Since many patients tend to regain weight either during or after treatment, both short- and long-term data are required reflecting the longer-term patterns of weight loss and regain.

The principal aims of obesity treatment are a reduction in both body fat and incidence of associated morbidity. Due to the chronic nature of the condition, successful treatment is often elusive, causing frustration for both patient and health professional. Given that obesity is a heterogeneous condition, treatment choices should take account of psychologic and sociodemographic characteristics of patients, since such factors may influence weight-loss patterns or even constitute barriers to successful treatment outcomes. Programs tailored to individuals' requirements, using a combination of intervention types, may be the most favorable approach. Dietary, exercise, and behavioral interventions should continue to be the first line of treatment, but such approaches are most likely to be effective when at least two are used in combination (e.g., diet combined with exercise). Patients also should be educated as to the health benefits of even modest weight loss (around 5-10% of initial body weight) and encouraged to aim toward realistic weight-loss goals, not necessarily an ideal body weight.

Drug therapy may have a role in the treatment of carefully selected patients who have failed to lose weight after a genuine attempt using the preceding methods. Currently, prescriptions are of limited duration. Drug treatment should be combined with other weight-loss strategies, and the relevant life-style issues should be addressed. Patients should be supported and carefully monitored throughout therapy. The issue of weight regain has emerged as an important problem that needs to be addressed. The methodologic standard of obesity-related research is generally poor, and further evaluation is required to establish more clearly the role of all weight-control interventions.

Suggested readings

BRAY G. Use and abuse of appetite-suppressant drugs in the treatment of obesity. Ann Intern Med 1993;119:707-13.

CONNOLLY HM, CRARY JL, MC GOON MD, et al. Valvular heart disease associated with fenfluramine-phentermine. N Eng J Med 1997;337:581/87.

GLENNY A, O'MEARA S, MELVILLE A, et al. The prevention and treatment of obesity: A systematic review of the literature. Int J Obes Relat Metab Disord 1997;21:715-37.

GUERCIOLINI R. Mode of action of orlistat. Int J Obes 1997;21:S12-S23.

JAMES W, AVENELL A, BROOM J, WHITEHEAD J. A one-year trial to assess the value of orlistat in the management of obesity. Int J Obes 1997;21:S24-S30.

LEAN M. Sibutramine: a review of clinical efficacy. Int J Obes 1997;21:S30-S36.

NATIONAL TASK FORCE ON THE PREVENTION AND TREATMENT OF OBESITY. Long-term pharmacotherapy in the management of obesity. JAMA 1996;276:1907-15.

SEIDELL J. Obesity in Europe: prevalence and consequences for use of medical care. Pharmacoeconomics 1994;5:38-44.

SEIDELL J. Obesity in Europe. Obes Res 1995;3(suppl. 2):89S-93S.

SEIDELL J. The impact of obesity on health status: some implications for health care costs. Int J Obes 1995;19:S13-S16.

SJOSTROM L, RISSANEN A, ANDERSEN T, et al. Randomised placebo-controlled trial of orlistat for weight loss and prevention of weight regain in obese patients. European Multicentre Orlistat Study Group. Lancet 1998;352:167-73.

Gout

Cesare R. Sirtori

Gout is the end result of a group of disorders characterized by *hyperuricemia,* defined as plasma urate levels greater than 420 μM (7.0 mg/dl), indicative of an increased total-body urate. The major clinical consequence of hyperuricemia is gouty arthritis. Typically, a monarthric disease, gout has been known since the beginning of mankind and has been the object of an extensive number of earlier reports. Among the gouty patients can be listed King Louis XIV (Le Roi Soleil), Galileo, Ben Franklin, and many others. Acute gout is characterized by swelling of joints, mainly the toes, acccompanied by local warmth, tenderness, and occasionally low-grade fever. If untreated, the gouty attack usually peaks 24 to 48 hours after the first symptoms and subsides within 7 to 10 days.

Disease presentation

Hyperuricemia, i.e., a plasma (or serum) urate level above 420 μM (7.0 mg/dl), defines the concentration of urates in blood exceeding the solubility limit of monosodium urate (415 μM, or 6.8 mg/dl). It also corresponds to the mean + 2 standard deviations (SDs) of values determined in randomly selected populations. The risk of developing gouty arthritis or urolithiasis increases with urate levels above 7.0 mg/dl. The total-body urate pool is the result of, in selected patients, increased urate production and, in the majority of hyperuricemic patients, decreased excretion.

Increased urate production

Increased urate production is partly derived from the diet, particularly as a consequence of high purine intake. On the other hand, restriction of dietary purines (food items rich in nucleic acids, e.g., liver, kidney, and anchovies) may reduce urate levels by no more than 60 μM (1.0 mg/dl). Endogenous purine synthesis also influences the serum urate level to a significant extent. Purine biosynthesis starts by conjugating phosphoribosyl pyrophosphate (PRPP) and glutamine, a reaction catalyzed by amidophosphoribosyl transferase (amido PRP). The availability of PRPP drives the reaction forward, whereas the end products of biosynthesis, mainly inosine monophosphate and other ribonucleotides, provide feedback inhibition. A

second regulatory pathway is the salvage of purine bases, catalyzed by hypoxanthine phosphoribosyl transferase (HPRT), combining the purine bases hypoxanthine and guanine with PRPP to form the respective ribonucleotides. Increased salvage thus may reduce de novo synthesis by reducing PRPP levels and increasing the concentrations of inhibitory ribonucleotides. Congenital hyperuricemia may derive from an increased activity of PRPP synthetase, resulting in overproduction of purines, hyperuricemia, uric acid stones, and gout before age 20. Conversely, deficiency of HPRT results in hyperuricemia, uric acid calculi, and gout because of urate overproduction. Complete lack of HPRT finally causes the Lesch-Nyhan syndrome, associated with self-mutilation, choreoathetosis, and other neurologic disorders.

Decreased uric acid excretion

Decreased uric acid excretion characterizes as many as 98% of individuals with primary hyperuricemia and gout. Urinary excretion of uric acid is, in fact, about 40% lower in gouty individuals versus normal subjects. The mechanism appears to be consequent to a lower sensitivity of the excretory mechanisms to increased urate concentrations. It results from a decreased proximal tubular secretion of urate rather than from reduced glomerular filtration. In some cases, decreased uric acid excretion might be consequent to metabolic acidosis, e.g., as in diabetic ketoacidosis, starvation, or intoxication by ethanol or by some acidic drugs (salicylates). This situation leads to the accumulation of organic acids competing with urates for secretion. Alcohol intoxication, in addition, leads to an accelerated breakdown of ATP, increased urate production, and hyperlactacidemia, reducing urate secretion. A scheme of uric acid production/excretion and possible pharmacologic control is provided in Figure 71.1.

Treatment

Nonpharmacologic treatment

Hyperuricemia is, in the vast majority of patients, related to a generalized metabolic disorder described as the *polymetabolic syndrome (syndrome X)* and characterized by

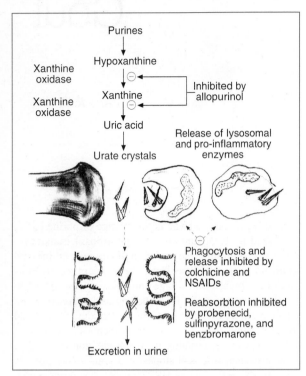

Figure 71.1 Biochemical pathway of uric acid biosynthesis, development of gout, and drug interactions at the different levels.

hyperinsulinemia, insulin resistance, glucose intolerance, hypertriglyceridemia with low high-density lipoprotein (HDL)-cholesterol levels, and excess abdominal fat (see Chap. 68). Dietary treatment of this disorder (e.g., low-calorie diet, reduction of body weight, etc.) can by itself reduce hyperuricemia. Hyperuricemia also can be reduced by some drug treatments for other indications; e.g., some fibric acid derivatives such as fenofibrate increase urate excretion to a similar extent as classic uricosuric agents (see Chap. 70).

In a significant number of patients, uric acid levels thus can be reduced to below 7.0 mg/dl only by improving general metabolic conditions, particularly reducing body weight and improving glycemic control. It, therefore, can be concluded safely that prescription of urate-lowering agents for asymptomatic hyperuricemia is, in most cases, neither cost-effective nor beneficial. While the risk of developing gouty arthritis is, in fact, significant in patients with high serum urate levels, the treatment of asymptomatic hyperuricemia to prevent the first attack of gouty arthritis is not appropriate because most such patients never develop gout. Target-organ disease, particularly kidney damage or tophi, may never be identified before a first gouty attack, and a reduction in renal function may not necessarily depend on asymptomatic hyperuricemia. The risk of stone formation in people with asymptomatic hyperuricemia is not established. The possibility that hyperuricemia may be an independent risk factor for atherosclerotic cardiovascular disease has been proposed by a number of authors; however, as noted previously, isolated hyperuricemia seldom occurs, and its

association with other major risk factors (e.g., insulin resistance, reduced HDL-cholesterol, hypertriglyceridemia) does not indicate asymptomatic hyperuricemia as a specific target for treatment. On the other hand, epidemiologic data do suggest that patients with serum urate concentrations above 10 mg/dl have a greater than 50% chance of developing gouty arthritis if this abnormality persists. The risk may be higher in elderly patients. Data on patients with kidney stones suggest that the risk of developing nephrolithiasis is above 20% when daily urate excretion is less than 700 mg but is 50% when this value exceeds 1100 mg.

Drug therapy

Hyperuricemia and gout Drug treatment of hyperuricemia, once the appropriate dietary steps have been taken, is addressed to patients with a high risk of gouty attacks because of previous symptomatic episodes of gout, significant family history, or disorders such as blood dyscrasias and cancer treated with chemotherapeutic agents that increase serum urate levels. In these patients, the start of treatment should be preceded by prophylaxis with colchicine (see below) or with a potent nonsteroidal anti-inflammatory drug (NSAID) in doses adequate to prevent a possible gouty attack. This may occur because of the rapid mobilization of tissue/serum urates after the start of allopurinol or uricosuric therapy (including drugs with a uricosuric mechanism, e.g., fenofibrate or high-dose aspirin). Colchicine therapy at a dose of 0.6 mg po qd to tid is about 90% effective in preventing gouty attacks induced by the initiation of hypouricemic therapy.

Antihyperuricemic therapy should aim toward a reduction of serum urate at or below 300 μM (5.0 mg/dl). This will, in fact, not allow tissue deposition of urate crystals, which would continue if the serum urate level were kept at 415 μM (6.8 mg/dl) or higher. Keeping urate concentrations at the indicated levels will allow dissolution of urate crystals and the consequent reduction of the urate pool.

Gouty attacks The gouty attack is a dramatic phenomenon resulting from the inflammatory reaction of articular tissue to urate crystals. Leukocytes, accompanying the inflammatory process, have an elevated lactate production, resulting in a local decrease in pH, favouring urate deposition, particularly in patients with increased urate production and/or decreased excretion. In order to treat gouty attacks or to prevent their occurrence, when tissue urates are rapidly mobilized by allopurinol/uricosuric agents, two types of drugs are available. Colchicine is an anti-inflammatory agent active only against gouty arthritis. As an alternative, most NSAIDs can favorably affect the symptoms of gout or prevent their occurrence.

Drug classes

ALLOPURINOL

Allopurinol is the prototype of substrate-competitive inhibitors of xanthine oxidase. Oxipurinol, the major metabolite of allopurinol is also an effective, long-acting inhibitor of the enzyme. Allopurinol is well absorbed from the gastrointestinal tract and has a half-life of about 3 hours (Tab. 71.1).

Allopurinol is the most widely used and most effective preventive treatment for the major complications of gout. It acts on essentially all types of hyperuricemia but mainly so in patients with gout and urate overproduction (24-hour urinary urate > 800 mg on a general diet or > 600 mg on purine-restricted diet). Patients with nephrolithiasis, renal insufficiency, and a general inability to take uricosuric agents because of ineffectiveness or intolerance have a primary indication for allopurinol treatment. Allopurinol is also the drug of choice for patients at risk of developing acute urate nephropathy, i.e., with hyperuricemia secondary to polycytemia vera, myeloid metaplasia, or other blood disorders.

Allopurinol administration decreases serum urate concentrations and urinary excretion in the first 24 hours of treatment, with maximal reduction occurring in about 2 weeks. The effective dose, 300 mg qd, may be reduced in very sensitive patients or in the presence of renal dysfunction. Daily doses should not exceed 400 mg; if such a dosage is ineffective, lack of compliance should be suspected. Because of the long half-life of the active metabolite oxipurinol, allopurinol may be given once daily. Side effects are relatively unusual and include skin rashes, gastrointestinal distress, diarrhea, and headache. More serious side effects may include eosinophilia, alopecia, bone marrow suppression, liver toxicity, and hypersensitivity vasculitis. Sensitivity in patients with renal insufficiency or in those taking thiazide diuretics is enhanced.

Allopurinol, a potent enzyme inhibitor, may potentiate drugs metabolized by a similar or different routes. The major problem is that of purine drugs used in cancer therapy, mainly mercaptopurine and its derivative, azathioprine; doses of both should be reduced when given together with allopurinol. The drug also may interfere with the liver inactivation of other drugs, including oral anticoagulants, that should be monitored more carefully. Similarly, allopurinol increases the accumulation of the active metabolite of theophylline, 1-methylxanthine, thus potentially increasing theophylline levels in plasma.

Allopurinol increases the half-life of probenecid and its uricosuric effect, whereas probenecid may increase elimination of the metabolite alloxanthine and therefore increase the necessary daily doses of allopurinol. Finally, a repeatedly described increased incidence of skin rashes in patients treated with allopurinol and ampicillin is as yet unexplained.

URATE OXIDASE

Urate oxidase, a bacterial enzyme (generally from *Arthrobacter protoformiae*), can be used for a short period of time in gouty patients with strong contraindications to both allopurinol and uricosuric agents, e.g., heart transplant recipients. Parenteral administration in a dose of 1000 units per day, 7 days per month, reportedly leads to shrinking of the tophi and improved motility of fingers. This first-phase treatment of gout should be followed by administration of another agent.

URICOSURIC AGENTS

Induction of increased uricosuria by *uricosuric agents* appears to be a plausible approach to the management of an elevated plasma urate level. On the other hand, this approach enjoys less and less popularity because of the potential risk of inducing an increased urate load on the kidney, resulting in possible damage.

In humans, unlike other species, urates are transported to the kidney by a bidirectional mechanism with a prevalent reabsorption; excretion of urates is about 10% of the filtered amount. In the tubular system, urate reabsorption is facilitated by a transporter, acting as an anion exchanger (see Chap. 21). Tubular urates may be exchanged for an organic/inorganic anion moving in the opposite direction. It is therefore possible that a drug may cause retention of urates or uricosuria according to the given dose

Table 71.1 Drugs for hyperuricemia/gout. Major kinetic parameters

	Bioavailability (%)	Volume of distribution (l/kg)	t_{max} (h)	$t_{1/2}$ (h)	Total clearance (ml/min)
Allopurinol	90	1.5	1.5	1.5	993
(Oxipurinol)	-	-	4.5	40	25
Probenecid	100	0.2	3-4	2-4	28
Sulfinpyrazone	100	2.4	3	5	47
Benzbromarone	50	0.7	1.5	3	91
(Slow eliminators)	-	3.1	1.5	13	11.5
Colchicine	47	1-2	1.1	58	8.5

(Mean values or ranges thereof).

and, furthermore, that uricosuric agents may potentiate or antagonize each other.

Uricosuric drugs, when present in the tubular lumen, compete with urates for the membrane transporter, inhibiting reabsorption by the urate-anion exchanger. They may display a paradoxic effect, i.e., reducing excretion of uric acid at low doses and increasing it at high doses. This "low dose" phenomenon may depend either on the inhibition of a small physiologic secretory mechanism of urates or on a promoted reabsorption if the product is not delivered to the lumen but is kept in tubular cells, thus needing to exchange with urates. A clinically significant interaction is that between two uricosuric agents given at the same time. In this case, the lack of tubular secretion of one agent induced by the other will lead to urate reabsorption. Such also may be the case with specific uricosuric agents given concomitantly with high-dose aspirin or fenofibrate.

Probenecid Probenecid, initially developed for reducing tubular secretion of penicillin is an organic, lipid-soluble derivative of benzoic acid (pK_a 3.4). Probenecid reduces the tubular secretion of a number of acidic drugs, including methotrexate, clofibrate, and numerous NSAIDs, as well as the transport of monoamines into the cerebrospinal fluid. By a similar mechanism, probenecid, secreted into the tubular lumen, reduces reabsorption of uric acid, thus increasing excretion. This effect is antagonized by salicylates. Probenecid, given orally in doses of 250 mg bid, gradually increased up to 2 g per day in four doses, is used now for the rapid induction of urate excretion, although a number of fixed-dose associations with oral or parenteral penicillins are available in the US. Probenecid needs to be associated initially with colchicine or an NSAID and followed by continuation of treatment with allopurinol. The drug is generally well tolerated, except for some gastrointestinal intolerance and potential skin rashes. Major kinetic parameters are reported in Table 71.1.

Sulfinpyrazone Sulfinpyrazone is a synthetic anti-inflammatory agent with a potent platelet antiaggregating activity. At low doses, it can inhibit tubular reabsorption of uric acid. It is a strong organic acid (pK_a 2.8), giving rise to soluble salts. Sulfinpyrazone is well absorbed after oral administration, and it has a half-life of approximately 3 hours (Tab. 71.1). Generally it is given at initial doses of 100 to 200 mg bid, eventually to be increased to 200 to 800 mg per day in two to four doses. It is generally well tolerated, except for gastrointestinal intolerance in 10 to 15% of patients, i.e., similar to major NSAIDs. It may potentiate the anticoagulant effect of warfarin by inhibiting the P450-2C9-mediated metabolism to (*S*)7-hydroxywarfarin (see Chap. 6).

Benzbromarone Benzbromarone is used in some European countries. An iodinated derivative, benziodarone, is available in Spain and Italy. Benzbromarone is a potent and reversible inhibitor of the urate-anion exchanger in proximal tubules. It is more potent than other uricosuric agents, being highly effective in single daily doses of 40 to 80 mg. In some countries it is provided in a fixed-dose combination with allopurinol (generally 100 mg allopurinol plus 50 mg benzbromarone). The major kinetic characteristics reported in Table 71.1 indicate the existence of a small number of subjects with a considerably reduced elimination, most likely due to genetically impaired renal handling. Benzbromarone has been associated with a small number of cases of severe idiosyncratic liver toxicity (occasionally leading to liver failure); a relationship with altered drug elimination has not been established. Benzbromarone can potentiate the anticoagulant effect of warfarin by inhibiting its metabolism.

COLCHICINE

Colchicine, an alkaloid of *Colchicum autumnale*, has been known since the time of Dioscorides and was introduced to the United States by Benjamin Franklin, himself a gouty patient. The anti-inflammatory effect of colchicine in acute gouty arthritis is selective. The drug is only occasionally effective in other types of arthritis, is not analgesic, and does not alleviate other types of pain. Colchicine acts as an antimitotic, affecting cell division in plants and animals by interacting with cell spindle formation in a manners similar to the action of *Vinca* alkaloids and the podophyllotoxins (see Chap. 49). By selectively binding tubulin in proliferating leukocytes, colchicine causes depolymerization and disappearance of fibrillar microtubules, and this seems to be the basis of its beneficial effects. Colchicine exerts other interesting effects; e.g., it inhibits secretion of histamine-containing granules from mast cells, reduces insulin secretion from pancreatic beta cells, and reduces body temperature. The major indication is the prevention/treatment of gouty attacks; in the Mediterranean region it also has been used with some success in the treatment of the Mediterranean fever.

After oral administration, it is well absorbed and reaches maximal concentration in 0.5 to 2 hours (Tab. 71.1). Because of its long half-life, it can be detected in leukocytes and in the urine for at least 9 days after a single administration. Major toxic effects occur at the gastrointestinal level, including nausea, vomiting, diarrhea, and abdominal pain. Colchicine may cause leukopenia and has a definite risk, on long-term treatment, of bone marrow suppression with aplastic anemia, myopathy, alopecia, and azospermia. Administration of a single dose of 2 mg colchicine, generally diluted in saline (never to exceed 4 mg), is adequate to control the acute gouty attack. Prophylactic doses, as small as 0.5 mg two to four times per week (highest doses may be up to 1 mg per day) can be given safely to prevent recurrent gout in patients initiating chronic treatment with allopurinol or uricosuric agents. Before and after surgery in gouty patients, colchicine should be given for 3 days (0.5-0.6 mg tid) to reduce the high incidence of attacks after the procedure.

NONSTEROIDAL ANTI-INFLAMMATORY DRUGS (NSAIDs)

NSAIDs, discussed in other parts of this book (see Chaps. 44 and 45) are effective for the treatment of acute gouty attacks and can be used safely for their prevention. Anti-inflammatories also can compete for uric acid reabsorption, i.e., exerting a uricosuric activity. Their side effects are well-known and do not need to be repeated here. Essentially all NSAIDs can be used safely; possibly a larger experience has been gained with indomethacin and its derivatives. Indomethacin, because of its very potent anti-inflammatory activity, can effectively reduce leukocyte proliferation/degranulation, thus alleviating gouty symptoms. It also can be used for the prevention of gouty attacks. Although with a lesser experience, other NSAIDs, such as propionic acid derivatives (e.g., naproxen, ibuprofen, and piroxicam, this latter with the advantage of the long half-life), have been used with success, particularly in the therapy of painful acute attacks.

Suggested readings

BECKER MA, et al. Purines and pyrimidines. In: Scriver CR et al, eds: The molecular and metabolic bases of inherited disease, 7th ed. New York: McGraw-Hill, 1995:1655-841.

DAN T, KOGA H. Uricosurics inhibit urate transporter in rat renal brush border membrane new vescicles. Eur J Pharmacol 1990;187:303-2.

EMANUELSSON BM, BEERMANN B, PAALZOW LK. Non-linear elimination and protein binding of probenecid. Eur J Clin Pharmacol 1987;32:395-401.

FERRON GM, ROCHDI M, JUSKO WJ, SCHERRMANN JM. Oral absorption characteristics and pharmacokinetics of colchicine in healthy volunteers after single and multiple doses. J Clin Pharmacol 1996;36:874-83.

MAHONY C, WOLFRAM KM, NASH PV, BJORNSSON TD. Kinetics and metbolism of sulfinpyrazone. Clin Pharmacol Ther 1983;33:491-7.

McCARTHY GM, BARTHELEMY CR, VEUM JA, WORTMANN RL. Influence of antihyperuricemic therapy on the clinical and radiographic progression of gout. Arthritis Rheum 1991;34:1489-94.

ROZENBERG S, ROCHE B, DORENT R, et al. Urate-oxidase for the treatment of tophaceous gout in heart transplant recipients. A report of three cases. Rev Rheum Engl Ed 1995;62:392-4.

RUNDLES RW. The development of allopurinol. Arch Intern Med 1985;145:1492-503.

SACK W, DE VRIES JX, KUTSCHKER C. Disposition and uric acid lowering effect of oxipurinol: comparison of different oxipurinol formulations and allopurinol in healthy individuals. Eur J Clin Pharmacol 1995;49: 215-20

SACK WI, DE VRIES JX, ITTENSOHN A, WEBER E. Rapid and slow benzbromarone elimination phenotypes in man: benzbromarone and metabolite profiles. Eur J Clin Pharmacol 1990;39:577-81, .

WALLACE SL. COLCHICINE. Clinical pharmacology in acute gouty arthritis. Am J Med 1961;30:439-48.

WORTMANN RL. Gout and other disorders of purine metabolism, In: Fauci AS et al, eds. Harrison's Principles of internal medicine, 14th ed. New York:McGraw-Hill, 1998, chap. 34:2158-66.

Nutrition: deficiencies and effects of drug therapy

Vitamins, oligoelements, and functional foods

Claudio Galli, Francesco Visioli

Vitamins and mineral salts represent the fraction of the diet that does not provide energy out of the 40 or more components of the diet. *Vitamins,* which have very diversified chemical structures, are organic substances that must be provided to the organism in small quantities because they are not synthesized de novo or the rate of synthesis is inadequate for the maintenance of health [e.g., the production of nicotinic acid (niacin) from tryptophan]. The primary environmental source of vitamins is diet, but

an obvious exception is represented by the endogenous synthesis of vitamin D in the skin under the influence of ultraviolet (UV) light.

Substances required exclusively by microorganisms and by cultured cells are defined as *growth factors* in order to avoid claims of potential therapeutic applications not based on scientific evidence in humans. When vitamins are present in more than one chemical form (e.g., pyridoxine, pyridoxal, pyridoxamine), they may be called

Table 72.1 Recommended dietary allowances (RDAs) for vitamins

Category	Age (years)	Liposoluble vitamins				Hydrosoluble vitamins						
		A (µg RE)[1]	D (µg)[2]	E (mg α-TE)[3]	K (µg)	C (mg)	Thiamine (mg)	Riboflavine (mg)	Niacine (mg)[4]	B₆ (mg)	Folate (µg)	B₁₂ (µg)
Newborns	0.0-0.5	375	7.5	3	5	30	0.3	0.4	5	0.3	25	0.3
	0.5-1.0	375	10	4	10	35	0.4	0.5	6	0.6	35	0.5
Children	1-3	400	10	6	15	40	0.7	0.8	9	1.0	50	0.7
	4-6	500	10	7	20	45	0.9	1.1	12	1.1	75	1.0
	7-10	700	10	7	30	45	1.0	1.2	13	1.4	100	1.4
Males	11-14	1000	10	10	45	50	1.3	1.5	17	1.7	150	2.0
	15-18	1000	10	10	65	60	1.5	1.8	20	2.0	200	2.0
	19-24	1000	10	10	70	60	1.5	1.7	19	2.0	200	2.0
	25-50	1000	5	10	80	60	1.5	1.7	19	2.0	200	2.0
	51+	1000	5	10	80	60	1.2	1.4	15	2.0	200	2.0
Females	11-14	800	10	8	45	50	1.1	1.3	15	1.4	150	2.0
	15-18	800	10	8	55	60	1.1	1.3	15	1.5	180	2.0
	19-24	800	10	8	60	60	1.1	1.3	15	1.6	180	2.0
	25-50	800	5	8	65	60	1.1	1.3	15	1.6	180	2.0
	51+	800	5	8	65	60	1.1	1.2	13	1.6	180	2.0
Pregnancy		800	10	10	65	70	1.5	1.6	17	2.2	400	2.2
Breast-feeding	1st sem.	1300	10	12	65	95	1.6	1.8	20	2.1	280	2.6
	2nd sem.	1200	10	11	65	90	1.6	1.7	20	2.1	260	2.6

Values are expressed as the average, prolonged daily intake and take into consideration the singular variations among normal individuals.
[1]Retinol equivalents. 1 retinol equivalent = 1 µg of retinol or 6 µg of beta carotene.
[2]As cholecalciferol. 10 µg of cholecalciferol = 400 IU of vitamin D.
[3]Equivalents in α tocopherol. 1 mg d-α tocopherol = 1 α-TE.
[4]1 NE (niacin equivalent) corresponds to 1 mg of niacin or 60 mg of tryptophan in the diet.

vitamers. Vitamins conventionally are classified as lipid soluble (or liposoluble) and hydrosoluble (or water soluble). The former can be stored in appreciable quantities in the body, and this property confers a greater potential toxicity. Hydrosoluble vitamins are stored to a limited extent and therefore must be consumed frequently to maintain saturation levels in tissues.

Several vitamins are not biologically active in the form in which they are ingested and must be converted to an active form in vivo. In the case of hydrosoluble vitamins, the activation includes phosphorylation processes (e.g., thiamine, riboflavine, nicotinic acid, and pyridoxine), and it may require the coupling with purine and pyrimidine nucleotides (e.g., riboflavin, nicotinic acid). In their main actions, hydrosoluble vitamins participate as cofactors of specific enzymes, whereas the lipid-soluble vitamins A and D behave as hormones by interacting with specific nuclear receptors in target tissues.

The evidence concerning the requirements and recommendations for individual nutrients and the Recommended Dietary Allowances (RDAs) that will serve as guidelines for healthy nutrition are regularly reevaluated in several countries. The RDAs for vitamins and minerals proposed by the Food and Nutrition Board in the United States since 1941, and revised regularly, are summarized in Tables 72.1 and 72.2, respectively. These values are sufficient to cover the requirements of a large proportion (95%) of the healthy population in a given age interval of both genders.

Recommendations also have been prepared, in the form of ranges, for those nutrients whose requirements have not been completely defined. These provisional RDAs apply to two water-soluble vitamins (i.e., biotin and pantothenic acid), as well as to several trace elements (e.g., copper, manganese, fluorine, chrome, and molybdenum). All levels of intake within these ranges are safe and effective, but consumption of higher or lower quantities for prolonged periods may enhance the risk of marginal toxicity or of marginal deficiency, respectively. The Food and Nutrition Board of United States also has prepared recommendations for other food components that occasionally have been proposed to be nutritionally essential. These are divided into (1) substances known to be essential for certain animal species but not for humans (e.g., nickel, vanadium, and silicone), (2) substances that act as growth factors only for lower forms of life (e.g., *para*-aminobenzoic acid, carnitine, and pimelic acid), (3) substances present in foods that have been proposed as vitamins but which in reality show only a pharmacologic activity or do not possess any biologic activity (e.g., rutin, with possible antihemorrhagic activity), and (4) substances for which no scientific evidence of a nutritional role is available (e.g., pangamic acid, erroneously defined as vitamin B_{15}, and laetrile, also called vitamin B_{17}).

Millions of individuals regularly consume quantities of vitamins in large excess with respect to the RDAs in the belief that vitamin preparations provide additional energy and may help them to "feel better". The use of vitamin supplements is advisable when there is the possibility that deficiencies may develop (e.g., inadequate intake, malabsorption, enhanced tissue requirements, or genetically derived metabolic alterations with structural anomalies of the enzymes for which vitamins are cofactors). Deficiencies may occur in population groups living below the poverty level, especially in the elderly and with respect of vitamins

Table 72.2 Recommended dietary allowances (RDAs) for minerals

Category	Age (years)	Calcium (mg)	Phosphorus (mg)	Magnesium (mg)	Iron (mg)	Zinc (mg)	Iodine (µg)	Selenium (µg)
Newborns	0.0-0.5	400	300	40	6	5	40	10
	0.5-1.0	600	500	60	10	5	50	15
Children	1-3	800	800	80	10	10	70	20
	4-6	800	800	120	10	10	90	20
	7-10	800	800	170	10	10	120	30
Male	11-14	1.200	1.200	270	12	15	150	40
	15-18	1.200	1.200	400	12	15	150	50
	19-24	1.200	1.200	350	10	15	150	70
	25-50	800	800	350	10	15	150	70
	51+	800	800	350	10	15	150	70
Female	11-14	1.200	1.200	280	15	12	150	45
	15-18	1.200	1.200	300	15	12	150	50
	19-24	1.200	1.200	280	15	12	150	55
	25-50	800	800	280	15	12	150	55
	51+	800	800	280	10	12	150	55
Pregnancy		1.200	1.200	320	30	15	175	65
Weaning	1st sem.	1.200	1.200	355	15	19	200	75
	2nd sem.	1.200	1.200	340	15	16	200	75

(Values represent the average daily intake as maintained in time and include variations among normal individuals.)

A and C. Furthermore, peculiar dietary habits or conditions, such as diets for losing weight or refusal of food (anorexia), may expose certain individuals to deficiencies. Additional causes of vitamin deficiencies are hepatobiliary and pancreatic diseases, prolonged diarrhea, hyperthyroidism, pernicious anemia, sprue, and intestinal bypass interventions. Antibiotic treatments also may alter the intestinal flora and may reduce the bioavailability of vitamins that are locally synthesized (e.g., vitamin K and biotin).

Oral supplementation of vitamins is indicated when there is an increased risk of deficiency. Although the position of the American Dietetic Association is to strictly follow the RDAs, on the assumption that supplementations above these levels have not been proved to be beneficial, a large number of people do take vitamin supplements in excess of the RDAs. In many cases vitamins are used in the prevention or treatment of various diseases. In fact, there is evidence that consuming certain vitamins greatly in excess of the RDA appears to exert preventive or possibly even therapeutic effects with respect to such diseases as those affecting the cardiovascular system and, possibly, certain cancers.

This chapter considers the biologic roles and possible therapeutic applications of the lipid-soluble vitamins. Only a schematic presentation is made of the metabolic actions and possible clinical applications of the water-soluble vitamins.

LIPID-SOLUBLE VITAMINS

VITAMIN A

Although vitamin A must be supplied to the organism, the majority of its actions, as is the case with vitamin D, involve receptors of a hormonal nature and have to do with the modulation of functions and differentiation at the cellular level, i.e., types of actions that are beyond the classic functions of vitamins.

Structure and biologic activity

The term *vitamin A* refers to defined chemical entities such as retinol and its esters, but it is also used to describe all the compounds that exert the biologic activities of retinol. *Retinol* (vitamin A_1) is a primary alcohol present in esterified form in tissues of terrestrial animals and of salwater fish (liver). Other compounds related to retinol are *3-dehydroretinol* (vitamin A_2) and a series of isomers. Interconversions between isomers take place in the whole organism and in the visual cycle. However, the reaction between *retinal* (the aldehyde of vitamin A) and opsin to form rhodopsin takes place only with the 11-*cis* isomer. *Retinoic acid* (vitamin A acid) has some of the activities of retinol (e.g., promotion of cell growth, control of differentiation, and maintenance of epithelial tissues) but not others (e.g., involvement in visual and reproductive functions).

In essence, all-*trans* retinoic acid (tretinoin, ATRA) is the active form of vitamin A in all tissues except for the retina and is much more potent than retinol. Synthetic compounds,

including the prodrug *etretinate,* a prototype of second-generation retinoids, are more potent than tretinoin in several systems in vitro. Third-generation synthetic retinoids also exist in the form of very potent aromatic retinoids called *carotenoids.*

The richest source of vitamin A and carotenoids is the liver, in association with other animal sources both terrestrial and fish, which provide appreciable amounts of preformed vitamin. After being absorbed, retinol is transported by chylomicrons to the liver, were it is stored as retinyl ester or exported to the plasma compartment as free alcohol bound to retinol-binding protein (RBP). This carrier is responsible for delivery to the critical sites in tissues. Two important active metabolites are *retinal* (or retinaldehyde), the active component of the visual pigment, and *retinoic acid,* an intracellular messenger that modulates cellular differentiation.

There are also several types of carotenoids in plants, such as β-carotene and β-cryptoxanthine, which can be converted to vitamin A in the intestine and in other sites. Rich sources of provitamin carotenoids include green leaves and several types of fruits and vegetables with yellow or orange colors, and it is currently assumed that between a tenth and a half, by weight, of these carotenoids may be converted to vitamin A (the efficiency of this conversion process is variable and depends on several factors, such as the fat content of the diet, the accessibility of dietary carotenoids to the biologic surfaces where absorption takes place and to the metabolic enzymes, and the concentrations of biliary salts). Some carotenoids cannot be converted to vitamin A, but even those which are not (e.g., lutein) may exert antioxidant activities, thus becoming potentially relevant nutrients. Carotenoids are absorbed in the ileum and are detectable in several tissues, but as opposed to vitamin A, they do not bind to specific carrier proteins and are transported mainly as nonpolar lipids.

The functions of vitamin A in the organism are quite diverse. In addition to visual function, vitamin A is essential for growth and differentiation of epithelial tissues and is required for the growth of bones and for reproduction and embryonal development.

Metabolism

Together with some carotenoids, vitamin A enhances immune functions, thus reducing the consequences of infectious diseases, and it may exert a protective action against certain types of tumors. There is therefore marked interest in the pharmacologic applications of retinoids in the prophylaxis of tumors and in the treatment of preneoplastic conditions. Retinoids are also employed in the treatment of skin pathologies, including those related to aging and prolonged exposure to sunlight.

Visual cycle Vitamin A deficiency is responsible for a condition known as *nyctalopia* (night blindness) consequent to dysfunction of the retinal rods, normally sensitive to low-intensity light. 11-*cis*-Retinal, metabolically derived from

11-*cis*-retinol, combines with opsin to form rhodopsin, which, in turn, is localized in the membranes of rod-containing disks and is characterized by a structure typical of receptors, whose function is transduced by G-proteins. The absorption of a photon activates a series of reactions at the end of which 11-*cis*-retinal isomerizes to the all-*trans* form, while opsin dissociates. Activated rhodopsin interacts with trasducin, a G-protein, that in turn triggers a cyclic-GMP-specific phosphodiesterase. The subsequent reduction of cGMP results in reduced conductance of the Na^+ channels in the plasma membrane with a consequent increment of trans-membrane potential. This potential, after subsequent processes, finally results in the action potential, which reaches the central nervous system (CNS) through the optic nerve.

Vitamin A and epithelia Vitamin A activates and controls the differentiation of epithelial cells in mucus-secreting tissues or in keratinized tissues. In the presence of retinol or retinoic acid, basal epithelial cells are stimulated to produce mucus, with a thick layer of mucin, in association with inhibition of keratinization and the appearance of goblet cells when retinoid concentration is in excess. Retinoid action takes place through enhanced synthesis of certain proteins (e.g., fibronectin) together with reduced synthesis of others (e.g., collagenase, keratin). These effects are mediated by changes in nuclear transcription. Retinoic acid in fact modulates gene expression by interacting with nuclear receptors. Three of these (α, β, and γ) are located on human chromosomes 17, 3, and 12 and belong to a superfamily of receptors that includes receptors for steroids, thyroid hormones, and calcitriol. An additional group of receptors, called *retinoid X receptors* (RXRs), has been added recently to this superfamily. Genic activation by these hormones involves binding with the hormone-receptor complex followed by dimerization with an RXR-ligand complex. The endogenous ligand for RXR is 9-*cis*-retinoic acid, whereas an analogous receptor for retinol has not yet been discovered.

Vitamin A and carcinogenesis Since vitamin A regulates cell differentiation and proliferation, there is great interest in its possible interference with carcinogenesis. Vitamin deficiency enhances the susceptibility to cancer induction in experimental animals, and this effect is reduced by retinoid administration, even long after exposure to carcinogens. The antitumor effect is observed in several models of experimental tumors. The mechanisms underlying these effects have not been clarified, but they may be mediated by regulation of the synthesis of glycoproteins and glycolipids involved in cellular adhesion and in intercellular communication. Several epidemiologic studies have shown an inverse correlation between intake of vitamin A and tumor morbidity and mortality, but correlations with the intake of retinol are inconsistent.

Vitamin A and immune functions A correlation between vitamin deficiency and enhanced susceptibility to infec-

tions in several animal models has long been known. These effects are mediated by lymphatic tissue changes, especially reductions in cytotoxic and killer cell functions, as well as by altered antibody response. However, differences also have been observed between various animal models. The relationship between vitamin A intake and measles has been investigated thoroughly, and clinical studies have shown that vitamin administration reduces morbidity and mortality in children. The World Health Organization (WHO) and UNICEF therefore recommend administration of 30 to 60 mg per day (100.000-200.000 units/d) of vitamin A to all children affected by measles in countries where the mortality from this disease exceeds 1%.

Requirements and tolerability

Retinoid stores in healthy adults are sufficient to guarantee adequate levels in tissues for prolonged periods of time. Deficiencies occur more commonly during chronic diseases affecting lipid absorption. Vitamin A deficiency is one of the most severe forms of nutritional deprivation seen in several countries in Africa, Southeast Asia, and Central and South America, and if it is associated with severe malnutrition, it may be fatal. Over 250000 children suffer from irreversible blindness every year globally as a result of vitamin A deficiency. Deficiency symptoms are frequently overlooked and consist of cutaneous alterations (e.g., hyperkeratosis and infections) and night blindness (in the case of more severe deficiencies). Alterations can be observed in various systems and organs: eyes (e.g., emeralopia, keratomalacia, and xerosis of the cornea and conjunctiva), respiratory tract (e.g., keratinization and infections), skin (e.g., keratinization and dryness), genitourinary system (e.g., urinary stones, altered spermatogenesis, testicular degeneration, etc.), gastrointestinal tract (e.g., reduction of goblet cells without keratinization), sweat glands (e.g., atrophy and keratinization), and bones (e.g., defects in bone deposition).

Therapeutic applications

Interest in the clinical use of vitamin A has centered mainly on the prevention of xerophthalmia and blindness in less developed countries, and research has been devoted mainly to the development of synthetic retinoids that are less toxic than vitamin A in the treatment of skin diseases. The growing concern that substances present in the diet and in the environment may induce long-term damage in tissues at the gene level, with a subsequent greater risk of tumors and other degenerative diseases, recently has stimulated interest in the possible protective effects of such nutrients as carotenoids in these pathologies. This potential protective role is distinct from the well-known role of certain carotenoids as vitamin A precursors and may involve antioxidant activities and protection from free radicals. Finally, the use of all-*trans* retinoic acid (ATRA), in combination with anthracycline, in the treatment of acute promyelocytic leukemia produces an approximately 90% complete remission rate through a cytodifferentiating mechanism involving the leukemic clone (see Chap. 63).

Vitamin A in infant malnutrition In the past 20 to 30 years, vitamin A has been given in high doses to school-aged children in several communities in which vitamin A deficiency is a cause of xerophthalmia and blindness. Evaluation of the effects of treatment has been restricted to the reduction in mortality, a parameter that can be measured much more easily in places where clinical competence is limited. In addition, there is a strong correlation between mortality and xerophthalmia, and vitamin A deficiency is a more common cause of death than of blindness. Controlled double-blind studies carried out in several countries, such as Indonesia, India, and Ghana, using doses on the order of 200 000 IU [1 International Unit (IU) = 0.3 µg retinol = 1.05 nmol retinol] have shown in six of eight studies a reduction in mortality in the range of 26 to 54%. These data, reevaluated in a series of metaanalyses, have led to the general conclusion, presented in a United Nations publication, that the net benefit of vitamin supplementation in reducing childhood mortality is highly significant. Additional investigations of the effects of vitamin A supplementation have shown that certain infections, such as chicken pox, undergo a milder course, resulting in higher survival rates, with the use of high vitamin doses (e.g., 120 mg), whereas gastrointestinal and respiratory infections are not appreciably affected, although progression toward more severe forms is somewhat reduced.

On the other hand, several infectious diseases cause an initial reaction that reduces the synthesis of retinol-binding protein (RBP) in the liver, resulting in a fall in circulating retinol, despite the lack of reduction of vitamin stores. In addition to its role in basic physiologic processes, vitamin A interacts with various nutrients, such as protein and iron, and with the homeostasis of these compounds.

Hypervitaminosis A Intakes greatly exceeding the RDA result in the toxic hypervitaminosis syndrome. These major toxic effects may occur in the treatment of skin disorders with natural and synthetic retinoids. Toxicity in children generally is the result of excessive prophylactic treatment on the part of the parents, whereas in adults it may result from extended self-medication for acne or other skin lesions. The age of the patient, dose, and duration of treatment are the major factors in retinol toxicity. Mild symptoms of intoxication are observed rarely in adults who consume less that 30 mg retinol per day, but daily consumption of 7.5 to 15 mg for 30 days has induced toxicity in infants. Poisoning is observed frequently with acute doses in excess of 500 mg in adults, 100 mg in children, and 30 mg in infants. Despite the fact that the Food and Nutrition Board of the National Research Council (1980) has warned that the ingestion of more than 7.5 mg of retinol daily is ill advised, an appreciable proportion of vitamin A users, at least in the United States, exceed this amount. Chronic retinoid intoxication is characterized by skin dryness, hepatosplenomegaly, increased intracranial pressure and hyperlipidemia.

VITAMIN E

Structure and biologic activity

The term *vitamin E* encompasses eight compounds, four tocols and four tocotrienols, that share vitamin E activity. Mono-, di-, and trimethyltocols are identified as *tocopherols*. They all have a basic structure with a 6-chromanol ring and several methyl groups in positions 5, 6, and 7 and a saturated or unsaturated side chain. The four isomers, α, β, δ, and γ, contain saturated side chains with 16 carbon atoms (tocotrienols).

Metabolism

Due to its lipid soluble nature, vitamin E is absorbed at the intestinal level, with mechanisms depending on bile secretion, micelle formation, and transport across intestinal membranes. Tocopherols are transported in the circulation in association with lipoproteins; there is a strong correlation between plasma vitamin levels and total lipid concentrations. Vitamin E supplementation results in rapid and parallel increments in tocopherol levels both in plasma and in erythrocytes. Vitamin E deposition in peripheral tissues takes place through the low-density lipoprotein (LDL) receptor system (apoB/E). Studies with the use of radioactive α-tocopherol suggest that vitamin E is removed mainly in association with chylomicron remnants. The biologic metabolism of vitamin E is quantitatively limited, with the exception of the oxidoreductase reactions in which tocopherols play an important role, as will be described below.

Requirements and tolerability

Because it is lipid-soluble, vitamin E accumulates in adipose tissue. Deficiency syndromes therefore are more rare in adults than in children. Vitamin E requirements depend essentially on three factors: basal requirement of *RRR*-tocopherol, factors in the diet that are correlated with vitamin E such as dietary fatty acids, and finally, exposure to environmental factors such as smog and cigarette smoking that initiate oxidative processes and enhance vitamin E requirements. The RDA of 10 mg should be increased in parallel with an enhanced dietary intake of polyunsaturated fatty acids (more susceptible to nonenzymatic oxidation), such as the fatty acids of the n-3 series, typically present in fish and fish oils (see Chap. 6). Exposure to certain environmental oxidative stresses (e.g., cigarette smoking, smog, chemical factors, prolonged exposure to UV radiation, etc.) further enhances vitamin E requirements.

Inadequate intake of tocopherols leads to anemia, reduced fertility, muscular dystrophy, and neurologic disorders. Generally, vitamin E deficiency syndromes are correlated with dysfunctions in the absorption of lipids or with genetic abnormalities involving a tocopherol transport. Among the former are apolipoproteinemia and cholestatic liver, whereas the latter include a lack of a tocopherol-binding protein that, in the liver, is responsible for the incorporation of vitamin E into lipoproteins. In these patients, supplements containing high doses of vitamin E restore the normal plasma levels of α-tocopherol and stop the progression of neurologic damage.

The reported side effects of high doses vitamin E are very modest: Doses up to 600 mg per day did not cause any negative effects in healthy volunteers, suggesting that vitamin E has a tolerability that is much higher than that of the other lipid-soluble vitamins.

Therapeutic applications

Growing scientific evidence indicates that vitamin E can play a protective role with respect to the development of atherosclerosis and coronary heart disease (CHD). However, whereas most epidemiologic studies have thus far indicated an inverse correlation between plasma vitamin E levels or between vitamin E consumption, as evaluated through questionnaires, and mortality from CHD, other intervention studies have so far failed to clearly demonstrate a protective effect of tocopherols on the progression of atherosclerotic lesions. Thus, further studies are needed to clarify this important issue and to establish any eventual recommendations.

VITAMIN D

Structure and biologic activity

Vitamin D (cholecalciferol) is formed in the skin following the photochemical conversion of its precursor, 7-dihydrocholesterol. The term *vitamin D₃* refers to cholecalciferol and distinguishes it from ergocalciferol (vitamin D₂), found in mushrooms and rare in nature, since mushrooms do not flourish in sunlight. The term *vitamin D₁*, not in use any more, formerly identified a mixture of ergocalciferol and other sterols. The common dietary sources are quite low in vitamin D, whose level in the body is maintained through photoirradiation. Thus, vitamin D functions as a hormone, which together with parathormone plays a fundamental role in calcium homeostasis. The hormonal characteristics of vitamin D are supported by the following properties: it is synthesized in the skin and, under normal conditions, is not required in the diet; it is transported in blood far from the sites of synthesis to be activated by a well-tuned enzymatic system; its active form binds specific receptors in target tissues yielding an increase in plasma Ca^{2+} concentrations. These receptors are also expressed in several tissues and cells, such as hematopoietic cells, lymphocytes, skin and pancreas cells, muscle cells, and neurons, mediating several events not related to calcium homeostasis. Vitamin D, both of dietary sources and endogenous synthesis, in order to be biologically active,

has to be converted to its trihydroxylated metabolite, $1,25(OH)_2D$, through two metabolic steps. The first step (hepatic) leads to the formation of 25-hydroxycholecalciferol (25-OHD, or calcifediol) that enters the bloodstream and is transported by a globulin that binds vitamin D. The final activation to calcitriol, $1,25(OH)_2D$, takes place mostly in the kidney, the primary source of circulating calcitriol.

Metabolism

The primary biologic functions of $1,25(OH)_2D$ include maintenance of serum calcium and phosphate levels within normal ranges to maintain essential cellular functions and promote bone mineralization. The primary effect is to promote the absorption of calcium and phosphate in the small bowel, to interact with parathormone in increasing their mobilization from bone, and to reduce their renal excretion. Calcitriol binds to a cytoplasmic receptor in the target cells, and the receptor-hormone complex interacts with DNA, increasing or inhibiting genic transcription.

Requirements and tolerability

Vitamin D deficiency leads to a reduced capacity of the small bowel to absorb calcium. There appear to be modest direct effects on bone mineralization, whereas, together with parathormone, calcitriol promotes the mobilization of calcium from bone. The amount of vitamin D necessary to the body is very small: 10 µg per day with the diet maintains constant levels of vitamin D in adults.

Vitamin D deficiency, which is now rare, is due to a concomitant lack of biosynthesis (insufficient exposure to sunlight), to a reduced dietary intake, or to a malabsorption of calcium. As a consequence, rickets and osteomalacia, due to the alteration of calcium homeostasis, are observed.

Some pathologic conditions, such as hyperparathyroidism, accelerate removal of the dihydroxylated metabolite of vitamin D by the liver, with a consequent lower biologic activity of cholecalciferol. Both osteomalacia (a defect in bone mineralization) and osteoporosis (in which a reduction in bone mass is observed) consequent to the vitamin D deficiency can be prevented rapidly and effectively, especially in the elderly, by treatment with vitamin D at 10 µg per day orally.

Excessive exposure to sunlight does not stimulate the production of toxic quantities of vitamin D. The only way in which vitamin D can accumulate in toxic amounts is through the uncontrolled supplementation of several milligrams per day for weeks. The mechanisms responsible for the toxic, often lethal, effects of vitamin D are still unknown. In laboratory animals, death occurs before an altered calcium homeostasis (hypercalcemia) can be recorded, as opposed to what is observed in individuals affected by hypervitaminosis D.

Recent theories suggest that the accumulation of $1,25(OH)_2D$ after saturation of the 25(OH)D-binding circulating proteins is responsible for the toxic effects of vitamin D. Such effects are so potent that ergocalciferol is employed as a rat poison.

Treatment with vitamin D_3 (800 IU/ day) and calcium (1.2 g/ day) was carried out in a controlled study that lasted 3 years on 3270 menopausal women, and it effectively prevented a reduction of bone mass, increased plasma levels of 25(OH)D, and reduced the compensatory hyperparathyroidism and femoral fractures. Supplementation with vitamin D and calcium therefore represents an important approach to the prevention of senile osteoporosis, when a deficiency of calcium and vitamin D are common, and the consequent loss of bone mass Osteoporosis and an increased frequency of falls represent the two most frequent causes of fractures.

VITAMIN K

Structure and biologic activity

The term *vitamin K* includes several molecular species sharing a 2-methyl-1,4-naphthoquinonic structure. The length of the prenylic chain in the 3 position is not fixed and originates the menaquinone class (MK-*n*, in which *n* designates the number of prenylic units). Phylloquinone in particular (*n* = 3) is the form of vitamin K usually found in vegetables.

Vitamin K is widespread in foods and tissues. Green leaves, legumes, vegetable oils, fish, and cereals are particularly rich in phylloquinone, whose bioavailability is still under investigation. The distribution of menaquinones in foodstuffs is more limited and probably restricted to aged cheese and liver. The main source of menaquinones in the human body is the intestinal flora, which synthesizes in particular MK-7-13. In the bloodstream, vitamin K is mainly associated with lipoproteins, especially with the triglyceride-rich ones. Bones and liver are the body stores of vitamin K, whose levels are actually hard to determine with precision due to the extremely low values.

Metabolism

Vitamin K catalyses the reactions of carboxylation that lead to the formation of clotting factors II (prothrombin and factors VII, IX, and X). Deficiency of vitamin K in adults leads to bleeding. In the newborn, oral or im prophylaxis is still a subject of debate. On the one hand, neonatal bleeding may lead to very serious complications, especially when it involves the central nervous system. On the other hand, there is epidemiologic evidence of an increased incidence of cancer correlated with vitamin K prophylaxis, possibly due to the presence of potentially carcinogenic excipients.

The discovery of three vitamin K-dependent proteins, osteocalcin, protein S, and protein Gla, that play an important role in bone formation led to the suggestion of an involvement of vitamin K in the development and maintenance of bone. In particular, the use of vitamin K antagonists such as warfarin produced an irregular development of the skeleton in laboratory animals. In human volunteers, including postmenopausal women, doses of 1 mg per day of vitamin K for 14 days induced a significant reduction in the urinary excretion of calcium. These data suggest a so far unexpected role for vitamin K in the maintenance of bone integrity.

Requirements and tolerability

The RDA for vitamin K has not yet been determined precisely, owing to the limited number of studies concerning the metabolism and biologic role of menaquinones. The role played by vitamin K in clotting suggests that a daily dose of 1 mg/kg of body weight might satisfy the metabolic needs of the body, even if recent studies on the interaction between menaquinones and bone proteins indicate that the latter may be more affected by vitamin K deficiency.

Therapeutic applications

Vitamin K is administered to a large number of children at high risk of bleeding, but there are no clear-cut data to determine if such prophylactic treatments are devoid of risks. Patients with cystic fibrosis also have been treated in various clinical trials, evaluated by a metaanalysis, that nonetheless have not identified specific conditions for the administration of vitamin K under such circumstances.

WATER-SOLUBLE VITAMINS

Vitamins of the B complex play physiologic roles in intermediate metabolism. Symptoms of vitamin B deficiency and therapeutic applications are listed in Table 72.3.

Some interesting observations about the potentially protective role of vitamin C in atherosclerosis appeared recently in the literature. Such interest centers around the putative protective effects of natural antioxidants, such as vitamins C and E, on these processes. A literature analysis suggests that there is an association between vitamin C and plasma lipid concentrations. A critical review of in vitro and in vivo studies carried out in animals and humans reveals that vitamin C, although not lipid-soluble, reduces LDL susceptibility to oxidation. On the other hand, plasma vitamin C concentrations are reduced in diabetic patients, in whom a strong increase in LDL oxidizability is observed. Conversely, supplementation of smokers with high doses of ascorbic acid reduces LDL susceptibility to oxidation, and vitamin C administration also can reverse the endothelial vasomotor dysfunction in patients with coronary artery disease. The antioxidant effects of vitamin C on LDLs initially observed in vitro is also mediated by a sparing effect on vitamin E oxidation.

A potentiation by vitamin C of the preventive effect of vitamin E on LDL peroxidation and vessels protection also has been observed in laboratory animals, suggesting that a combined intake of the two vitamins represents the best approach to affording protection.

The RDA of vitamin C, so far estimated to be on the order of 60 mg per day, recently has been recently increased to the 250-mg range, based on determinations

Table 72.3. Hydrosoluble vitamins: symptoms of deficiency and therapeutic uses

Vitamins	Symptoms of deficiency	Therapeutic utilizations
B$_1$ or thiamine	Beriberi (with cardiovascular and neurologic symptoms) in alcoholics and in patients with renal failure	Treatment of deficiency, neuropathic alcoholics, subacute necrotic encephalomyelopathies, pregnancy neuritis
B$_2$ or riboflavine	Stomatitis, glossitis, seborrhea, dermatitis, anemia and neuropathia	Treatment of deficiency
Nicotinic acid (converted to NAD or NADP)	Dermatitis (pellagra), diarrhea, nervous disorders	Prevention and treatment of pellagra (symptomatic in Hartnup disease and in carcinoid tumors)
B$_6$ or piridoxine (piridoxine, piridoxal, piridoxamine)	Skin lesions, nervous disorders, anemia	Incorporated in several multivitamin preparations
Panthotenic acid	Neuromuscular degeneration and adrenal gland failure	Incorporated in several multivitamin preparations
Biotin	Consequent to treatments with antibiotics or to prolonged biotin-free parenteral nutrition; dermatitis	Childhood seborrhea, genetic alterations of biotin dependent enzymes
Choline (included as hydrosoluble vitamin, but the real need is yet to be established)	Symptoms in animals only	Treatment of hepatic diseases and cirrosis and neurologic disorders linked to a reduced acetylcholine synthesis; efficacy not proven
Carnitine	Rare genetic diseases with functional cardiac and muscular alterations	Treatment of primary deficiency, variable results; kidney dysfunctions in dialysis patients with miocardial disorders
	Secondary deficiency in renal dysfunction or in genetic metabolic diseases	Cardiomyopathy and ischemic cardiovascular disease

that examined not just the renal excretion threshold but also the active uptake by circulating cells (leukocytes) in relation to consumption.

MINERALS

The daily requirements for minerals are listed in Table 72.2; as far as calcium metabolism is concerned (see also Chap. 46). This section will consider other minerals that play an important role in human nutrition and their links to human pathology.

ZINC

Biochemical and physiologic functions

The human body contains about 1 to 2 g of zinc, distributed uniformly throughout all tissues. There are more than 70 zinc-containing enzymes, through which zinc plays

catalytic, regulatory, or structural roles. For example, carbonic anhydrase, Cu-Zn superoxide dismutase, and fructose bisphosphatase activities are regulated by zinc.

One of the fundamental activities of zinc involves the regulation of membrane function. In addition, the association of zinc with metalloproteins is considered to be involved in the chain breaking of free-radical reactions, leading to lipid peroxidation. Finally, a structural and stabilizing role of zinc on receptors also has been proposed following the identification of the "zinc finger" DNA-binding proteins.

The absorption of zinc depends on the presence in the diet of other nutrients capable of altering zinc solubility and absorption. For instance, meat, eggs, and fish are considered to be good sources of zinc because they do not contain other compounds that inhibit its absorption but do contain amino acids such as cysteine and histidine that facilitate solubility. On the other hand, the bioavailability of vegetable-derived zinc is much lower because of the presence in these foods of zinc-binding substances such as phytates.

The net absorption of zinc is also affected by competition with other metals such as cadmium and copper. Overall, the absorption of zinc from food, which takes place in the small bowel, can be estimated to be between 25 and 40% of the ingested amount. There seem to be two distinct mechanisms that regulate the uptake of zinc by the intestinal mucosa, the first mediated by a carrier and the other by simple diffusion.

The intestinal absorption of zinc plays an important role in the regulation of its homeostasis. A linear increase in the total amount of zinc absorbed by the gut has been observed following an increased intake. Thus, there seems to be no adaptation process of the intestinal mucosa to increased amounts of zinc that transit the gut. Other factors that may influence the absorption of zinc include age (absorption decreases with age) and pregnancy, which usually increases zinc bioavailability. There is no specific deposit of zinc in the body, and thus any dietary shortage of zinc rapidly translates into deficiency.

Requirements and tolerability

One of the earliest signs of zinc deficiency is a slower rate of growth and development of living organisms. Other clinical manifestations include alopecia, skin damage, photophobia, and deficiencies of the immune system. There appears to be no "gradual" deficiency, in terms of limited effects. It is possible that the need of zinc for nucleic acid metabolism could explain the observed effects of zinc deficiency on growth. In any event, zinc deficiency among adults is extremely rare and can be connected to the concomitant intake of chelators such as phytates.

The recommended levels of zinc intake can be estimated by measuring the amount of cation necessary to replenish its physiologic levels (through the use of isotopes) and the amount necessary to maintain a correct balance. Assuming that the amount of dietary zinc that is absorbed is 35%, the U.S. RDA suggests a daily intake of 15 mg for men and 1 mg for women. Intake should be increased during pregnancy. The lack of zinc during pregnancy, in fact, has teratogenic effects. Other conditions that require higher levels of zinc consumption include alcohol dependency, possibly AIDS, and advanced age.

High amounts of zinc, often following consumption of food that have been kept in zinc-rich containers, lead to gastrointestinal episodes including nausea, vomiting, and abdominal pain. Doses higher than 200 mg are emetic.

IRON

Aerobic metabolism depends on iron. The respiratory chain and other redox systems require a heme-bound Fe^{2+} ion. Iron plays several important roles in redox reactions because of its ability to (1) easily change its redox status and (2) form coordination complexes with electron-donating atoms.

Biochemical and physiologic functions

Despite the abundance of iron in the earth's crust, the exchanges between the human body and the environment are very limited. In fact, without massive bleeding, loss of iron from the body is very small, and the overall levels in the body mostly depend on iron absorption. Only 10% of the total is lost each year by healthy men, usually excreted from the gastrointestinal tract. Most of the iron ingested with the diet is chelated by appropriate agents in the stomach and is absorbed by the small bowel. This explains why chelating substances such as ascorbate, sugars, and amino acids facilitate the absorption of iron. Healthy subjects absorb 5 to 15% of dietary iron, although these levels can increase in iron-deficient individuals. Because of this fine regulation of iron absorption, iron overloads following oral administrations are quite rare; conversely, iv administration can lead to iron intoxication.

In the body, iron circulates bound to transferrin, which can bind two Fe(III) atoms. The half-life of transferrin is 8 to 19 days, whereas iron turnover is faster: 25 to 30 mg per day. Between 70 and 90% of the plasma iron is taken up by red blood cells, whereas lower quantities are taken up by muscle cells to form myoglobin and by other cells to form cytochromes, peroxidases, etc. The normal levels of sideremia fluctuate between 40 and 160 µg/dl.

Most excess iron is stored, bound to ferritin, in the liver, spleen, bone marrow, and other tissues. Plasma transferrin accomplishes the internal iron exchanges by binding to specific receptors in membranes. The levels of human transferrin receptors, as well as those of ferritin, are self-regulated according to iron supply.

Requirements and tolerability

In the adult male, the normal requirement for iron is 13 mg/kg per day, whereas menstruating women need about 21 mg/kg per day, and this increases to up to 80 mg/kg per day during the last two trimesters of pregnancy. Under normal dietary conditions, the supply of iron compensates for the low excretion.

Iron deficiency anemia (see Chap. 73) is extensive in developing countries, where 20 to 40% of pregnant women and infants may be affected. The use of fortified foods compensates for the limited availability of iron-rich foods in some countries or for impaired absorption resulting from gastrectomy or malabsorption in the small intestine.

The treatment of choice for iron deficiency is ferrous sulfate, which is absorbed about three times more than ferric salts. Other iron compounds are employed in food fortification, mostly in the form of ferric edetate. The average dose for the treatment of anemia is 200 mg iron per day (2-3 mg/kg). It is best to administer iron salts in the fasting state, despite potential untoward gastrointestinal effects. Side effects include heartburn, nausea, constipation, and diarrhea. Iron overload (hemochromatosis) induces oxidative damage to the liver and results in hemorrhagic gastroenteritis and hepatic damage. Parenteral administration of iron, as an alternative to oral preparations, rapidly replenishes iron stores and is indicated in patients with gastrointestonal complications such as inflammatory bowel disease.

FUNCTIONAL FOODS

The concept of functional foods, i.e., foods containing specific physiologically active components, originated as a means of improving the health status of the population and thus reducing the drain on economy caused by escalating health costs. This area is attracting mainly food manufacturers in Europe and the United States, and a number of functional food products are appearing on the market. It is likely that there will be competition between the food industry and the pharmaceutical industry in areas of overlapping interest. The regulatory aspects of functional foods have yet to be resolved satisfactorily in Europe and the United States, but incorporation of the concept of functional foods into food regulations will be accelerated under pressure from consumers. The consumer perception of the benefits of functional foods compared with normal foods, however, will not be very uni-

form because some consumer groups question the need for such foods from a health point of view and see the concept rather as a marketing strategy. A number of foods for which anticarcinogenic and other well-defined properties are likely to be claimed will appear on the market, the active components being present in the raw materials or produced or enhanced by the manufacturing process. For instance, there is increasing demand for soy protein products in human food applications; the favorable effects of such proteins on plasma cholesterol levels may hold important implications in CHD prevention. The anti-CHD claim for soy protein very recently has been approved by the US FDA.

From the point of view of a science-based approach to this area, necessary steps are to critically assess the scientific evidence that specific nutrients positively affect bodily functions, to examine the available science from the point of view of function rather than form of the product, and to reach a consensus on targeted modifications of food and food constituents and options for their application. This approach will provide key actors from the food and agricultural industry, governmental and intergovernmental bodies, and the scientific community, with an opportunity to exchange ideas and interact on a neutral platform.

Suggested readings

ABRAMS SA, SILBER TJ, ESTEBAN NV, et al. Mineral balance and bone turnover in adolescents with anorexia nervosa. J Pediatr 1993;123:326-31.

CHAN GM, HOFFMAN K, McMURRY M. Effects of dairy products on bone and body composition of pubertal girls. J Pediatr 1995;126:551-6.

DURIE PR. Vitamin K and the management of patients with cystic fibrosis. Can Med Assoc J 1994;151:933-6.

FULLER CJ, GRUNDY SM, NORKUS EP, JIALAL I. Effect of ascorbate supplementation on low-density lipoprotein oxidation in smokers. Atherosclerosis 1996;119:139-50.

HOWARD PA, MEYERS DG. Effect of vitamin C on plasma lipids. Ann Pharmacother 1995;29:1129-36.

LEVINE GN, FREI B, KOULORIS SN, et al. Ascorbic acid reverses endothelial vasomotor dysfunction in patients with coronary artery disease. Circulation 1996;93:1107-13.

MANDELLI F. New strategies for the treatment of acute promyelocytic leukemia. J Int Med 1997;740:23-7.

MOYER-MILEUR L, LUETKEMEIER M, BOOMER L, CHAN GM. Effect of physical activity on bone mineralization in premature infants. J Pediatr 1995;127:620-5.

RETSKY KL, FREI B. Vitamin C prevents metal ion-dependent initiation and propagation of lipid peroxidation in human low-density lipoprotein. Biochim Biophys Acta 1995;1257:279-87.

SIRTORI CR, LOVATI, MR GIANOSSE et al. Reduction of serum cholesterol by soy proteins: clinical esperience and potential molecular mechanisms. NMCD 1999;8:334-40.

SLATTERY JM. Why we need a clinical trial for vitamin K. Br Med J 1994;308:908-10.

WELSBY D. Isolated soy protein and its use in beverages. Inform 1998;9:250-3.

Blood and the immune system

Anemia

Timothy A. Denton

Anemia is one of the most common maladies encountered by practitioners throughout the world. Accurate, efficient diagnosis is imperative because anemia is not itself a disease; rather, it is a companion of other, often serious conditions. Its presentation therefore must be distinguished from primary disease, and the unequivocal cause should be determined before therapy is prescribed.

Disease presentation

Anemia's clinical manifestations are derived primarily from lowered blood oxygen content by way of a reduced total red cell mass. The equation for oxygen content, that is,

$$O_2 \text{ content} = (1.34 \times [\text{Hb}] \times SaO_2) + (0.003 \times PO_2)$$

demonstrates that the concentration of hemoglobin, (Hb), is the major determinant of oxygen transport, given normal pulmonary and cardiac physiology. Lowered hemoglobin (acutely or chronically) leads to low oxygen delivery (SaO_2) and the manifestations of peripheral hypoxia.

Depending on the severity of the anemia and how quickly oxygen delivery falls, there are a number of normal physiologic responses. One of the first is an increase in erythrocyte-2,3-diphosphoglycerate concentration, resulting in a right shift of the oxyhemoglobin dissociation curve. This shift decreases the affinity of hemoglobin for oxygen and provides easier unloading at the tissue level. Further, the shift to anaerobic metabolism causes a mild acidosis, which, in turn, induces vasodilatation. This peripheral dilatation increases cardiac output, improving oxygen delivery (O_2 delivery = O_2 content cardiac output) at any level of oxygen content. These physiologic changes are not usually significant until the hematocrit is lowered to the 20 to 24% range.

Each of the above-described physiologic alterations causes specific symptoms and signs. Small decrements in hemoglobin concentration (down to 9 g/dl or a hematocrit of 27%) usually result in few, if any, symptoms or signs. Below this level, and as a function of the rate of fall of hemoglobin concentration, initial symptoms and signs may become apparent. In acute anemias (i.e., severe blood loss or hemolysis), there are few compensatory mechanisms; thus, symptoms and signs tend to be more severe. The presence of other diseases also can worsen the symptoms of anemia. A patient with either a carotid or coronary artery obstructive lesion may be asymptomatic. In the presence of an acute gastrointestinal bleed, however, a significant fall in oxygen delivery may result in a stroke or cardiac ischemia. Hemoglobin levels that fall to less than 7.5 g/dl (hematocrit of ~23%) with an increase in cardiac output may result in heart failure if there is poor cardiac reserve.

The symptoms of anemia may be manifest in many organ systems. Systemic symptoms usually include extreme fatigue and mild to moderate shortness of breath. Central nervous system (CNS) oxygen deprivation can cause subtle alterations in mental status, inability to concentrate, loss of memory, dizziness, headache, and inability to sleep. Additional CNS complaints can include tinnitus, vertigo, and syncope. Various types of anemia may present with strength and coordination abnormalities, as in vitamin B_{12} deficiency, where demyelination can cause abnormalities in long motor tracts of the spinal cord. Cardiac symptoms, such as palpitations, also may be noted if the anemia is severe enough to cause peripheral vasodilatation and compensatory tachycardia. Shunting of blood to critical organ systems can cause the gastrointestinal symptoms of nausea and anorexia, while there will be excessive cold sensitivity due to poor skin perfusion.

The diagnosis of anemia is confirmed by the demonstration of a low circulating red blood cell mass, a reasonable surrogate being a hematocrit of less than 41% in males and 37% in females (approximately 10% below the normal range). A low hematocrit does not necessarily mean a low red cell mass, since hemodilution decreases hemtocrit without changing the total number of red cells. Thus, anemia may be misdiagnosed in cases of intravenous volume infusions or volume shifts. Other abnormal laboratory findings are a function of the type of anemia (see below).

Etiology

The evaluation of anemia is a search for the underlying cause. In some cases, the diagnosis is quite easy to make, as in massive gastrointestinal bleeding or a myelophthisic anemia, but in other situations the diagnosis may be more difficult. Presented here is the classic approach to the etiologies of anemia, with a division into three types: poor erythrocyte production, extravascular erythrocyte loss, and increased erythrocyte destruction. A simplified classification according to this scheme is presented in Table 73.1.

Underproduction The vast majority of anemias associated with depressed production of erythrocytes are related to the inability to produce one of the components of hemoglobin – iron, heme, or globin. Each of these deficiencies is represented by one or more types of anemia. Low iron levels do not allow the complete production of heme; thus, the red cells that are made tend to be small and hypochromic. Deficient or abnormal production of the globin protein is seen in many anemias, such as thallassemia, B_{12} deficiency, folate deficiency, chemotherapy, and various metabolic disorders. Poor production is also associated with conditions that destroy functioning bone marrow.

Increased destruction Red cells are easily destroyed in situations of high shear stress, turbulence, or mechanical obstruction. This type of hemolysis is possible with endovascular prostheses such as mechanical heart valves. In the presence of nonbiologic surfaces and high pressure gradients, red cells are subjected to high shear rates, which can damage membranes. Abnormal red cells (in cases of spherocytosis or eliptocytosis) are even more susceptible to this type of lysis. This is also the case with enzyme deficiencies (e.g., glucose-6-phosphodehydroge-

nase), in which the metabolic demands of the membrane cannot be met by cytosol enzymes. Hemoglobinopathies also predispose to increased lysis. The final mechanism for red cell lysis is immune-mediated. Antibodies directed against surface proteins can stimulate the activation of complement and lead to lysis.

Extravascular loss The term *extravascular loss* is chosen carefully to include all potential etiologies of blood-loss anemia. The most common and intuitive is gastrointestinal loss, from acute or chronic gastrointestinal bleeding. However, it is possible to lose a significant amount of blood in various other body compartments. For example, bleeding into the thorax after trauma or a surgical procedure can cause significant blood loss, as can a retroperitoneal bleed after a catheter procedure performed from the groin.

Clinical findings

Anemia typically is diagnosed by comparing a patient's hemoglobin or hematocrit with published tables based on age and sex. As stated earlier, a reasonable level for the diagnosis of anemia is a hematocrit of less than 41% in males and 37% in females (10% below the normal range). This, of course, assumes that there has been no significant dilutional effect. After the diagnosis of anemia, a reasonable first step is the assessment of red cell indices and reticulocyte count. Table 73.2 presents a scheme in which most anemias can be classified by these two variables. The mean corpuscular volume (MCV) is probably the most important index, since anemias can be classified as microcytic (<80 fl), normocytic (80 fl < MCV < 100 fl), or macrocytic (>100 fl) according to the size of the erythrocyte. A reticulocyte count can distinguish between anemias in which the marrow response is normal (e.g., high reticulocyte count in extravascular loss, hemolysis) and in which it is low (e.g., bone marrow failure anemias).

Treatment

Once the etiology of an anemia is determined, the primary disease must be treated. An iron-deficiency anemia from diverticular blood loss would be treated by coagulation of the bleeding site or partial colectomy. A second decision involves the treatment of anemia itself. The goal of anemia treatment is to return the hemoglobin concentration to a level that relieves a patient's symptoms.

Emergency anemia treatment is usually limited to the use of red cell products. The primary concern in these situations is to maintain adequate hemodynamics (i.e., blood pressure and cardiac output) through rapid volume infusions of either crystalloid (e.g., saline, Ringer's lactate solution) or colloid (e.g., albumin, dextran, hetastarch). In the course of volume resuscitation, blood may be needed not only for hemodynamic purposes but also for replacement of lost oxygen-carrying capacity.

During therapy, serial determinations of hematocrit can

Table 73.1 Etiologic classification of anemias

Underproduction
 Inadequate biochemical synthesis:
  Globin (thalassemias, B_{12}, folate, chemotherapy, metabolic disorders)
  Heme (sideroblastic)
  Iron (iron deficiency)
 Bone marrow replacement
  Myelophthisic anemia
 Aplastic
  Stem cell failure (drugs, thymoma, antibodies, infection, idiopathic)

Destruction
 Mechanical
  Intravascular prostheses
  Microangiopathic hemolytic anemia (MAHA)
 Red blood cell anomalies
  Membrane – spherocytosis, elliptocytosis
  Hemoglobinopathies – Hb SS, Hb SC
  Enzyme deficiency
 Immune lysis

Extravascular loss
 External (gastrointestinal, genitourinary)
 Internal (retroperitoneal, thoracic, proximal thigh)

Table 73.2 Clinical classification of the anemias

	Microcytic MCV <80 fl	Normocytic 80 fl < MCV < 100 fl	Macrocytic >100 fl
Reticulocyte count low or normal	Iron deficiency Hemoglobinopathy Chronic disease Sideroblastic Bone marrow failure	Iron deficiency (early) Renal failure Liver failure Chronic disease Endocrine Bone marrow failure	B_{12} deficiency Folate deficiency Liver failure Endocrine Drugs Bone marrow failure
Reticulocyte count high	RBC loss Hemolysis	RBC loss Hemolysis Hypersplenism	RBC loss Hemolysis Hypersplenism Treated disease

(fl = femptoliters; MCV = mean corpuscular volume.)

aid in the transfusion decisions. In the acute emergency, there are no clear guidelines regarding the use of blood products, and arbitrary cutpoints for transfusion may be needed.

The therapy of chronic anemia is a function of its etiology. Once the etiology is determined, the underlying condition must be treated. If the primary cause is treatable, such as myxedema, iron, B_{12}, or folate deficiency, the anemia may be cured. In many situations, however, such as renal failure, liver failure, or chronic hemolysis, ongoing decisions must be made regarding the use of blood products, erythropoietin, vitamins, minerals, and bone marrow stimulants. The use of red cell transfusions is usually limited to patients who have become symptomatic from low oxygen delivery and the cause of the anemia has not yet responded to pharmacologic therapy.

Nonpharmacologic treatment

Red blood cell transfusions

Although the first blood transfusion was performed in 1667, it was not until the discovery of the ABO blood grouping system in the early 1900s that transfusion became generally accepted. Since then, continuous improvements in testing for potential donor/recipient interactions (e.g., ABO, Rh, and other antigenic systems), infections (e.g., hepatitis A, B, and C and HIV), and alternatives to homologous transfusions (e.g., autologous blood) have made the blood pool quite safe. However, blood products are not perfectly safe, and the clinician needs to weigh the benefits and risks of each transfusion decision.

In nonemergency anemia there are conflicting data regarding the impact of transfusions on survival. Some investigators have demonstrated that postoperative survival is inversely related to the preoperative hemoglobin level, but studies in Jehovah's witnesses and other populations demonstrate that extremely low hematocrit levels had little or no survival impact and that transfusions may be overused. The presence of symptoms, not an

arbitrary cutpoint for hemoglobin, is the recommended therapeutic trigger for transfusions. Most published data indicate that transfusion is rarely indicated for hematocrits greater than 24% unless there are mitigating circumstances.

Autologous blood transfusion has been developed as an alternative strategy to reduce the use of allogeneic blood products. Patients who are candidates for transfusion because of a planned procedure may donate units of blood for storage and retransfusion. Some patients request directed-donor blood-blood from friends or family members who are donation candidates. There are no data to indicate that directed-donor blood is any safer than random-donor blood.

Cost is another issue to be considered carefully. Although the cost of a single unit of packed red cells varies from $ 160 to $ 350, population-based costs for infections and transfusion reactions can raise total cost to very near $ 500 in the United States. Collection and storage of autologous units of blood add incrementally. The effectiveness, complications, and costs associated with blood products must be weighed carefully against the effectiveness, complications, and costs of pharmacologic therapy. Although not yet used routinely, artificial blood substitutes would allow a pharmacologic method to increase oxygen delivery without the associated complications. As of this writing, perfluorocarbons (i.e., specific compounds that avidly bind oxygen) and modified hemoglobins (i.e., chemical congeners or genetically engineered variants) offer the most promise, although none has proved successful in general practice.

Drug therapy

Iron therapy

Iron therapy is used to treat primary iron store deficiency and serves to augment iron stores during therapy for other types of anemia. It is one of the most common therapies prescribed. Yet, like any other medication, it

Table 73.3 Pharmacologic regimens for anemia therapy

Therapeutic regimen	Dose range	Typical dose	Comments
Iron			
Ferrous sulfate	325-975 mg qd	325 mg po tid	Gastrointestinal symptoms less if taken with meals
Carbonyl iron	50-150 mg qd	50 mg po tid	Fewer gastrointestinal side effects
Ferrous fumarate	1-3 tablets qd	3 tablets qd	Fewer gastrointestinal side effects
Ferrous gluconate	1-3 tablets qd	3 tablets qd	Fewer gastrointestinal side effects
Polysaccharide iron	1-3 tablets qd	3 tablets qd	Fewer gastrointestinal side effects
Iron dextran	0.5-2 ml qd (50 mg/ml)	Total dose must be calculated, 1 ml im or slow iv infusion over 6 h qd	Indicated only if cannot take orally. Always administer test dose of 0.5 ml, iv infusion preferred
Iron ovotransferrin	200-400 mg qd	200 mg qd	Reduced interaction with quinolones
Cyanocobalamin (Vitamin B$_{12}$)			
B$_{12}$ injection	1-1000 µg every month	100 µg every month im or sc	100 µg qd x 7 days, alternate day x 2 weeks, q3 x 3 weeks, then monthly for life
B$_{12}$ oral	300-1000 µg qd	100 µg every week	Vegetarians, normal gastrointestinal tract
B$_{12}$ nasal	500 µg weekly	500 µg every week	Use only as maintenance therapy, intradermal test dose recommended
Folic acid			
Folic acid (po)	1-5 mg/d	1 mg/d	May mask B$_{12}$ deficiency
Folic acid (iv, im)	5 mg/ml	1 mg/d	May mask B$_{12}$ deficiency
Pyridoxine	50-500 mg/d	200 mg qd	Rarely effective in sideroblastic anemia
Androgens			
Oxymetholone	50-150 mg/d	50 mg bid	Rarely effective, replaced by epoetin
Danazol	50-800 mg/d	200 mg po bid	Rarely effective, replaced by epoetin
Erythropoietin, Epoetin, EPO	50-300 units/kg/tiw Starting 15-300 units/kg/tiw Maintenance	100 units/kg/tiw Starting 75 units/kg/tiw Maintenance	Adjust dose monthly as a function of hematocrit response, watch blood pressure three times per week and hematocrit weekly.

should be used only when appropriate. Table 73.3 presents a compilation of the forms of iron and other commonly used drugs in anemia therapy, their typical dosing, and special considerations in treatment.

Pharmacokinetics/metabolism Oral ferrous iron, in the presence of gastric acid, is absorbed rapidly from the duodenum and proximal ileum. It is converted to the ferric form, bound to the serum protein transferrin (existing in multiple forms), and taken up by the reticuloendothelial system. From there it can be transferred to the erythrocytic cell line. A typical diet provides approximately 1 mg of iron per day, which is the rate of loss of iron from the gastrointestinal tract, skin, nails, hair, and urine. Iron absorption is reduced when taken with calcium supplements. Intramuscular injections of parenteral iron are absorbed by the lymphatic system and presented to the reticuloendothelial system or deposited in macrophages. Within 3 days of the im injection, approximately two-thirds of the iron is metabolized, and up to 90% is gone by 1 to 3 weeks.

Indications Iron therapy is clearly indicated in documented cases of iron-deficiency anemia (i.e., normocytic or microcytic anemia with either low ferritin, low serum iron with high total iron-binding capacity, or low bone marrow iron stores). It also may be used as a diagnostic trial in patients with mild anemia that is thought to be iron deficient. Therapeutic iron is also indicated in patients in whom depletion of iron stores is common and predictable. For example, pregnancy predisposes to iron loss; thus supplemental iron is prescribed not only during pregnancy but also during lactation. Women who have moderate losses of blood during menstruation also may benefit from routine iron supplementation. Patients treated with epoetin need iron supplementation because the drug initiates a rapid depletion of total-body iron stores.

Side effects The side effects of oral iron usually are limited to the gastrointestinal tract. Nausea, diarrhea, abdominal pain, constipation, and dark stools are not uncommon. With parenteral iron, severe allergic reactions can occur in 0.2 to 0.3% of patients. Test doses of

0.5 cc iv over 30 seconds can identify these patients. If there is no reaction after 1 hour, the usual dose may be given, but anaphylaxis is still possible after a seemingly benign response to a test dose. Delayed reactions are also possible (1-2 days after the dose) and may last 3 to 4 days. Hemosiderosis may occur with long-term administration of iron compounds. With the exception of chronic blood loss, iron therapy should be limited to 6 months.

Contraindications   Oral iron should not be used in patients with a known sensitivity to the product or in those who have known elevated iron stores. Parenteral iron should not be used in patients with a prior reaction to the drug, hepatic dysfunction, hemochromatosis, or repeated blood transfusions (they may be iron overloaded). Iron-overload states (e.g., hemochromatosis and hemosiderosis) are contraindications to any form of iron.

Drug forms, dosage   There are hundreds of forms of oral iron, both prescription and over-the-counter, with iron alone or in combination with other vitamins and minerals. The following discussion identifies the major forms of iron and their typical doses. The goals of iron therapy are the delivery of approximately 50 to 100 mg of elemental iron three times daily.

Ferrous sulfate   This common form of oral iron is absorbed rapidly from the gastrointestinal tract and contains 200 mg of elemental iron per gram of compound. The elixir should be mixed with fruit juice or water, not milk or wine. There are over 45 commercial forms of ferrous sulfate and an even greater number in combination with other vitamins and minerals.

Carbonyl iron   This form of iron is highly purified elemental iron – $Fe(CO)_5$. It has equal efficacy to ferrous sulfate but fewer side effects and lower toxicity. The 50-mg tablet has the same amount of iron as the 250 mg of the sulfate.

Ferrous fumarate   This has a greater gastrointestinal tolerability than the preceding two. It provides a greater amount of elemental iron per gram than the sulfate (330 mg/g).

Ferrous gluconate   This also has excellent kinetics but a lower elemental iron availability (120 mg of elemental iron per gram of compound).

Polysaccharide-iron complex   This compound is hydrolyzed starch in combination with iron, and it has similar kinetics as the sulfate form and contains 150 mg of elemental iron per gram. The cost is as high as that for ferrous sulfate.

Iron-ovotransferrin complex   An oral iron complex with a reduced potential to affect quinolone absorption (see Chap. 6).

Iron dextran   Parenteral iron is indicated under very limited circumstances. The dosage is calculated based on published formulas that are a function of the required increment in hemoglobin and the patient's lean body weight. Dosing typically is done at a rate of 1-2 ml per day (given slowly by intravenous drip over 6 hours), but only after an initial test dose of 0.5 ml intravenously over 30 seconds. Parenteral and oral iron should not be given concurrently. There has been a report of an increased incidence of cancer in animals at the intramuscular injection site.

Therapeutic strategy/expected response   Oral therapy is the preferred route in iron-deficiency anemia, and ferrous sulfate is used commonly and is given at 325 mg orally tid. For optimal absorption, the drug should be taken on an empty stomach, but this can lead to gastrointestinal symptoms; thus, many patients must take the drug with meals. With this dosing strategy, from 10 to 20 mg of iron is absorbed per day, allowing for rapid replenishment of iron stores. The reticulocyte count should peak in 2 weeks; there should be a significant increase in hematocrit in 3 to 4 weeks, and the red cell mass should return to normal in 3 to 4 months. When patients are intolerant of oral iron, do not respond to oral therapy, or have blood losses exceeding the ability to replace iron stores with oral forms, parenteral iron may be indicated.

Overdose   Overdose from oral iron occurs in thousands of children each year, multivitamins being the most common form. The effects are variable and include a direct corrosive effect on the gastrointestinal mucosa, hypotension, low cardiac output, altered mental status, renal failure, multiorgan failure, and coagulopathy. The initial therapy includes complete bowel irrigation and, if necessary, iv fluids for hemodynamic support. In the presence of severe toxicity, desferrioxamine 15 mg/kg per hour by iv infusion should be initiated. The treatment of allergic reactions to parenteral iron may include epinephrine (sc or iv), antihistamines, and steroids.

Vitamin B_{12}

Vitamin B_{12}, or cobalamin, plays an important role in cellular metabolism, serving as a coenzyme in one-carbon transfers and is absolutely essential for cell growth. Megaloblastic anemias were identified in the early 1800s, and in the 1920s, intrinsic and extrinsic (vitamin B_{12}) factors were found to reverse pernicious anemia. B_{12} is absorbed in the distal ileum and bound to a small gastric-derived glycoprotein called *intrinsic factor,* and the combination escapes digestion by the upper gastrointestinal tract. The method of treatment with B_{12} depends on the etiology. In cases of intrinsic factor deficiency, it is possible to give B_{12} parenterally or orally along with intrinsic factor, but in a large number of cases, patients will develop antibodies to intrinsic factor that limit its activity. Strict vegetarians may need only supplementation with oral B_{12}. In cases of malabsorption, parenteral therapy may be necessary, and if the malabsorption is from intestinal overgrowth syndrome, antibiotics are needed.

Great care must be taken to ensure that an accurate diagnosis of megaloblastic anemia is made because treatment with folate alone can improve the anemia of B_{12} deficiency but will not improve the neuropathy. Indications for the use of B_{12} are the existence of any pathology that leads to inadequate uptake of the vitamin. A clear documentation of B_{12} deficiency (low serum B_{12} level, although it has limitations) and the etiology of the deficiency is necessary before determining therapy. In patients in whom there is inadequate oral intake, oral forms may be all that is needed. However, in patients with intrinsic factor deficiency, parenteral forms are necessary. After initiation of therapy, the bone marrow usually responds in 48 hours, and an increased reticulocyte count is seen in 2 to 4 days.

All types of B_{12} can be classified into three groups: parenteral, oral (with or without intrinsic factor and/or other vitamins and minerals), and intranasal. With severe anemia, 100 µg should be given daily (im, deep sc, but never iv, since it will all be excreted in the urine) for 7 days, every other day for 2 weeks, every 3 days for 3 weeks, and every month for life if there is a total lack of B_{12} absorption.

B_{12} also may be used in the Schilling test, where a dose of up to 1000 µg of B_{12} is administered parenterally, and then a radioactively labeled B_{12} is given orally. A 24-hour urine collection will show less than 3% excretion of radioactive B_{12} in the absence of intrinsic factor, whereas a normal response is to excrete more than 7% of radioactive B_{12}.

There are over 55 types of injectable B_{12}. The oral B_{12} form should be limited to patients who have adequate gastrointestinal function but who also may have diets deficient in B_{12} (vegans) or those who need supplements (pregnancy). Oral forms can be used rarely in malabsorption, and very large doses are needed, usually 300 to 1000 µg weekly for 3 weeks and then 250 µg monthly. Intranasal B_{12} is applied to the nasal mucosa for rapid uptake. The bioavailabilty of intranasal B_{12} is approximately 9% compared with an im dose. An intradermal test dose is recommended before initiating therapy. The dose is usually 500 µg weekly, delivered by a metered-dose device.

Folic acid

Folic acid is a precursor of tetrahydrofolate that is required for 1-carbon transfers and, ultimately, nucleoprotein synthesis. The effects of folate depletion are similar to those of B_{12} depletion, since the two compounds are used in the same pathway.

Folic acid is indicated for the treatment of megaloblastic anemia in which low folic acid levels have been demonstrated. Because folate may improve the anemia of

B_{12} deficiency but will not reverse the neurologic pathology, it should not be used alone unless the diagnosis of isolated folate-deficiency megaloblastic anemia is clearly made. In patients with a high turnover of erythrocytes, such as those with uncontrolled hemolytic anemias, folate may be needed as a supplement. The nonanemic indications for the use of folate include pregnancy (to decrease neural tube defects), liver disease, and malabsorption. Folate is also dialyzed; thus supplementation is needed in patients on hemodialysis. Folate is usually well tolerated. As mentioned earlier, it should be used cautiously in patients with undiagnosed anemia because it can improve the anemia of B_{12} deficiency but will have no effect on neurologic sequelae. Reactions to folic acid are rare and may include pruritus and a rash. Folate can be given orally, by sc injection, by im injection, and iv. The decision as to which form to give depends on the severity of the anemia and the patient's clinical state (i.e., able to take oral nutrition or on total parenteral nutrition). There is a rapid onset of action, with a bone marrow response in approximately 2 days and a 5-day response for an increase in reticulocyte count. Typical doses range from 0.05 to 1 mg per day to treat anemia and replenish stores. The prophylactic dose of folate is approximately 0.4 mg per day (3 months before pregnancy), 0.8 mg per day for pregnant women, and higher doses required in malabsorption. If a woman has previously given birth to a child with a neural tube defect, 4 mg per day is indicated.

Pyridoxine (vitamin B_6)

Pyridoxine is an important coenzyme in amino acid metabolism and has a very limited use in the therapy of idiopathic sideroblastic anemia. If used, successful responses do not exceed 50%, but there is little risk in treatment. Oral pyridoxine is absorbed rapidly from the intestinal mucosa and stored in the liver. The use of pyridoxine in sideroblastic anemia should be undertaken only by those expert in the disease and its therapy. The response rates are less than 50%, and the typical dose is 200 mg per day (ranging from 50-600 mg/d) given over at least 2 months. If there is no response, the patient should be switched to a different agent. Pyridoxine can be given orally, by sc injection, by im injection, or iv. The decision as to which form to give depends on the severity of the anemia and the patient's clinical state (i.e., able to take oral nutrition or on total parenteral nutrition). At least 28 forms are available commercially.

Androgens

Androgens are direct stimulants of bone marrow (via erythropoietin) and account for the differences in hemoglobin levels between normal males and females. Historically, they have been used as bone marrow stimulants, but they have been replaced in part by the use of epoetin-alpha. They should be used only by those knowledgeable and experienced in the treatment of complicated anemias. There is little risk in their use but very low benefit. Occasionally, they may increase red cell mass in immune hemolysis, lymphomas, and other primary bone marrow anomalies. Androgens have been used in angiogenic myeloid metaplasia, aplastic anemia, myelodysplastic syndrome, and idiopathic thrombocytopenia after the initiation of standard therapy. Prior to the use of androgens, men must be screened for prostate cancer. Porphyria, renal failure, liver failure, and heart failure are contraindications to the use of androgens. A worsening of anemia has been reported in some forms of myelodysplastic syndrome. Allergic reactions are rare. Typical androgenic effects include menstrual disturbances, hirsutism, change in voice, acne, cholestatic jaundice, headaches, and hair loss. Androgens also can raise the serum low-density lipoprotein (LDL) level and lower the high-density lipoprotein (HDL) level. There do not appear to be any immediate effects from large overdoses. Androgens are often used to stimulate bone marrow when other measures have failed. The response to androgens is variable and should not be expected to occur for a few weeks. There are many commercialy available androgens. Danazol (200 mg orally bid) and oxymetholone (50 mg 1-3 times per day) and testosterone forms have all been used in this context.

Epoetin-alpha

Erythropoietin is a protein growth factor synthesized in the kidney (renal peritubular cells, 90%) and liver (10%) that stimulates the production of erythroid precursors (see Chap. 51). Production of the protein is increased with tissue hypoxia (hypoxemia or anemia) and decreased in chronic renal failure. The recombinant form (rHuEPO) was designated an orphan drug in 1986 and approved for use in chronic renal failure in 1989. Since then, its use has expanded to the anemia associated with human immunodeficiency virus (HIV) infection and zidovudine therapy (1990), and in 1993 it was approved for anemia therapy in patients with cancer undergoing chemotherapy. There are three forms of recombinant erythropoietin, epoetin-alpha, epoetin-beta, and epoetin-gamma, each having the same amino acid sequence but differing in their manner of glycosylation.

Epoetin-alpha has had a tremendous impact on patients with chronic renal failure. Prior to its introduction, patients on hemodialysis had hematocrits in the 18 to 25% range and required serial transfusions. After its introduction, most patients were able to maintain a near-normal hematocrit with three times per week therapy. There has not been a demonstrated impact on survival, but a reduction in transfusions and their infectious complications should translate into lower numbers of chronic viral infections. To a much greater extent, epoetin has had a large impact on improving the quality of life. The specific indications for epoetin are anemia associated with chronic renal failure, anemia of HIV with zidovudine, and the anemia of patients undergoing chemotherapy for cancer. It also has been used as a bone marrow stimulant to increase autologous blood collection and to decrease the rate of allogeneic transfusion after procedures with significant potential for blood loss.

Only physicians experienced in the treatment of anemia with bone marrow stimulants should use this med-

ication routinely. Potassium must be watched carefully during the initiation of therapy. Oral iron should be given because the drug can rapidly deplete iron stores. Patients with hypertension should be monitored carefully because a rapid rise in hematocrit can exacerbate this condition. Absolute contraindications include uncontrolled hypertension, any known sensitivity to the drug, and sensitivity to human albumin. Some highly competitive athletes have used epoetin to augment their oxygen-carrying capacity – one form of "blood doping."

Side effects can include nausea, vomiting, abdominal pain, fever, hypertension, thrombosis (especially of dialysis shunts), seizures (thought to be related to uncontrolled hypertension), and alterations in serum potassium concentration.

Because of the drug's expense, the decision-making process for the use of epoetin is similar to the transfusion decision-making process. The typical starting dose for the anemia of chronic renal failure is 50 to 150 units/kg three times per week (generally no more than 600 IU/kg per week should be given). An elevation in the reticulocyte count should be seen in approximately 10 days, and hematocrit will rise significantly in 1 to 6 weeks. During initiation of therapy, hematocrit should be measured weekly along with the potassium level, and blood pressure should be checked at least three times per week. An increase in hematocrit greater than 4% should initiate a reduction in dose. Dosages should be adjusted every 4 weeks. Many patients require oral iron (40-200 mg of elemental iron orally per day) to ensure that their stores are maintained during the rapid induction of red cell production. Once the target hematocrit is reached (~36%, the goal not being a normal hematocrit), drug usage is adjusted to an individualized maintenance dose. For chronic renal failure, a typical maintenance dose is 75 to 100 IU/kg three times a week. The drug may be given sc or im, but for patients on hemodialysis, it can be given iv, since they are usually dialyzed three times per week.

Patients with the anemia of cancer chemotherapy present special problems. They may have normal or high levels of intrinsic erythropoietin, in which case they probably will not respond to exogenous epoetin-alpha. A reasonable starting dose in these patients is 150 to 300 IU/kg three times per week for 8 weeks. Beyond 300 IU/kg, patients generally do not respond because of high endogenous erythropoietin. Patients with HIV infection on zidovudine may need a starting dose of 100 to 300 units/kg three times per week, with a maintenance dose of 100 units/kg three times per week. To stimulate red cell production prior to a surgical procedure, some clinicians use 300 units/kg per day for 10 days and continue that therapy for 4 days after surgery. To augment red cell production for autologous donation, 600 units/kg two to three times per week can be used. The drug may be given by the intramuscular or subcutaneous route.

Cost is an important consideration in the use of epoetin-alpha, with a typical price of $12 per 1000 units. For patients on hemodialysis, the annual cost of the drug is over $ 6000 per year in the United States. The deci-

sion to treat must be made carefully based on the individual patient's physiology, comorbidity, quality of life, and the potential need for blood transfusions and their complications.

Suggested readings

AMERICAN COLLEGE OF PHYSICIANS. Practice strategies for elective red blood cell transfusion. Ann Intern Med 1992;116:403-6.

BENNETT JC, PLUM F. Cecil's Textbook of medicine, 20th ed. Philadelphia: WB Saunders, 1996.

BEUTLER E, LICHMAN MA, COLLER BS, KIPPS TJ. William's Hematology, 5th ed. New York: McGraw-Hill, 1995.

CARSON JL, DUFF AM, BERLIN JA, et al. Perioperative blood transfusion and postoperative mortality. JAMA 1998;279:199-205.

DENTON TA, DIAMOND GA, MATLOFF JM, GRAY RJ. Anemia therapy: Individual benefit and societal cost. Semin Oncol 1994;21:29-35.

DEVITA VT, HELLMAN S, ROSENBERG SA. Cancer: principles and practice of oncology, 5th ed. New York: Lippincott-Raven, 1997.

ELLENHORN MJ. Ellenhorn's Medical toxicology: diagnosis and treatment of human poisoning, 2nd ed. Baltimore: Williams & Wilkins, 1997.

HARDMAN JG, LIMBIRD LE. eds. Goodman & Gilman's The pharmacological basis of therapeutics, 9th ed. New York: McGraw-Hill, 1996.

HOLLAND JF, FREI E, BAST RC, et al, eds. Cancer medicine. Baltimore: Williams & Wilkins, 1997.

KITCHENS CS. Are transfusions overrated? Surgical outcome of Jehovah's Witnesses. Am J Med 1993;94:117-9.

LEE R, BITHELL TC, FOERSTER J, et al, eds. Wintrobe's Clinical hematology, 9th ed. Philadelphia: Lea & Febiger, 1993.

MCEVOY GK, ed. American Hospital Formulary Service, Drug Information. Bethesda, Md: AHFS, 1997

OTT DA, COOLEY DA. Cardiovascular surgery in Jehovah's Witnesses: report of 542 operations without blood transfusion. JAMA 1977;238:1256-8.

PHYSICIAN'S DESK REFERENCE, 1998. Oradel, NJ: Medical Economics Company, 1998.

WILSON JD, BRAUNWALD E, ISSELBACHER KJ, et al, eds. Harrison's Principles of internal medicine, 12th ed., New York: McGraw-Hill, 1991.

WINSLOW RM, VANDEGRIFF KD, INTAGLIETTA M. Blood substitutes: new challenges. Birkhauser, 1996.

74

Atherothrombosis

Raffaele De Caterina, Carlo Patrono

Despite a decline started about 30 years ago in the United States (53% decline in the age-corrected death rate between 1964 and 1994) and more recently observed throughout Europe, cardiovascular diseases are the leading cause of morbidity and mortality in western populations. According to recent estimates, deaths from cardiovascular disease amount to 42% of total deaths, the vast majority of these being due to coronary artery disease (CAD), with its clinical manifestations of acute myocardial infarction (MI), angina, sudden ischemic cardiac death, and ischemic cardiomyopathy. Stroke, mostly ischemic and on the background of hypertension, is presently ranked as the second single cause of mortality and morbidity among cardiovascular diseases and the third leading cause of death and has dramatic consequences in terms of disability and social burden for afflicted people.

Atherosclerosis is the common substrate to these diseases, and thrombosis is the leading cause of the clinical manifestations of atherosclerosis. Because of its generalized nature, it comes as no surprise that the first manifestations of atherosclerosis in one area – the heart, the brain, the abdominal aorta, or the iliac arteries – is quite often the hallmark of an increased risk of ominous consequences in any of the other areas. Because atherosclerosis is the common background and thrombosis the ultimate mechanism leading to clinical complications, and because of the intimate interrelationships between the two, the concept of *atherothrombosis* recently has gained acceptance to designate a common pathogenesis for a number of district-specific diseases. Of the long-respected Virchow's triad of mechanisms of thrombosis – the vessel wall, the blood, and blood flow – the first plays a prominent role in atherothrombosis and a minor one in venous thrombosis. Arterial thrombosis typically is precipitated by a rapid change in the usually non-thrombogenic properties of the vessel wall. Rupture of an atherosclerotic plaque, suddenly exposing thrombogenic material of the atherosclerotic intima, is considered as the most common trigger, with an accessory role played by superficial erosion. Plaque fissuring or erosion, although most likely necessary to the triggering of acute thrombosis, is probably not sufficient to explain the occurrence of a clinically relevant thrombotic event.

In most cases, the formation of a mural thrombus is likely to provide a mechanism of repair of this acute vascular lesion. Depending on the contribution of other factors, such as the reaction of the hemostatic system and adequacy of blood flow, thrombosis is more or less likely to be occlusive. Even then, its occurrence does not necessarily imply the development of a clinical syndrome, because of accessory variables such as the state of the dependent circulatory bed (e.g., the presence of collaterals), the metabolism of the dependent tissue, and its susceptibility to ensuing ischemia.

Disease presentation

Myocardial infarction and unstable angina

These are described in detail in Chapter 25.

Ischemic stroke

The term *stroke* is used to describe a number of cerebrovascular disorders. Stroke is usually categorized as *ischemic* or *hemorrhagic* on the basis of the involved vascular territory, temporal evolution, and etiology. About 15% of strokes are hemorrhagic, usually due to a lesion in a cerebral vessel, usually an arterial aneurysm, with subarachnoid or intraparenchymal hemorrhage. Most strokes (about 85%) are caused by an arterial occlusion, with subsequent cerebral ischemia and infarction. The objective of restoring flow into an ischemic area is complicated by the reperfusion damage that occurs in the ischemic tissue after a few hours of ischemia, likely causing hemorrhagic evolution of an initially purely ischemic stroke. It is important to distinguish between primitive cerebral hemorrhage, in which the primary event is the rupture of a cerebral artery, and strokes with secondary hemorrhagic complications. Primitively hemorrhagic strokes have a worse prognosis (40% mortality rate as compared with 15-20% mortality of ischemic strokes). Computed tomography (CT scan) and magnetic resonance imaging (MRI) now allow clinicians to distinguish between the two types of stroke in most cases, with practical implications for their management.

Peripheral arterial disease

Atherosclerotic narrowing of the abdominal aorta, the ilial arteries, or the arteries of the lower limbs reduces blood flow to lower limbs during exercise or at rest. The resulting symptoms depend on the severity of arterial narrowing and on the extent of development of collateral circulation. Symptoms range from intermittent claudication to pain at rest. Ulcerations and gangrene are late consequences of trophic abnormalities in the affected tissues. The term *critical limb ischemia* refers to symptomatic lower extremity arterial disease in which the ischemic process endangers all or part of the involved territory. *Intermittent claudication* denotes pain developing in the affected limb with exercise and relieved by rest. Most often pain is localized in the calf and depends on narrowing in the superficial femoral and popliteal arteries. Intermittent claudication is present in up to 5% of men and 2.5% of women older than 60 years of age. When more sensitive techniques are used to detect atherosclerotic narrowings in asymptomatic individuals, prevalence may be up to three times higher.

With increasing degrees of arterial narrowing there is a progressive fall in systolic blood pressure distal to the obstruction. Thus, by measuring the systolic blood pressure at different levels of the limbs, combining cuff inflation with the use of sensors to detect blood flow, one can localize the site of the obstruction. In normal individuals, the systolic blood pressure at the ankle is greater than at the arm, so the ankle/arm pressure index is usually greater than 1.0. To account for variability of the method, a lower limit of normality is set at greater than 0.95. Values lower than this denote the existence of significant peripheral arterial disease. Assessment of this index can help in the diagnosis and serves as a baseline measure for follow-up purposes.

Drug classes

ANTIPLATELET DRUGS (Tab. 74.1)

Aspirin

Mechanism of action

Aspirin acetylates prostaglandin (PG)H-synthase and irreversibly inhibits its cyclooxygenase (COX) activity. This enzyme catalyzes the first committed step in prostanoid biosynthesis, i.e., the conversion of arachidonic acid to PGH_2. There are two isoforms of PGH-synthase (PGHS) referred to as PGHS-1 and PGHS-2 or COX-1 and COX-2.

COX-1 is constitutively expressed in most cell types, including platelets. COX-2 is undetectable in most mammalian tissues, but its expression can be induced rapidly in response to inflammatory and mitogenic stimuli (see Chap. 48). Aspirin is a more potent inhibitor of platelet COX-1 than monocyte COX-2. Thus, the existence of two isozymes with different aspirin sensitivities, coupled with extremely different rates of recovery of their cyclooxygenase activity following inactivation by aspirin, at least in part explains the different dose requirements and durations of aspirin effects on platelet function versus its analgesic and anti-inflammatory actions. Human platelets and vascular endothelial cells process PGH_2 to produce thromboxane A_2 (TXA_2) and prostacyclin (PGI_2), respectively. TXA_2 induces platelet aggregation and vasoconstriction, whereas PGI_2 inhibits platelet aggregation and induces vasodilation. Vascular PGI_2 production appears to be largely dependent on COX-2 activity of endothelial cells, a finding that may explain the relative biochemical selectivity of aspirin in inhibiting TXA_2 but not PGI_2 at very low doses.

Pharmacokinetics

Aspirin is absorbed rapidly in the stomach and upper intestine. Peak plasma levels occur 30 to 40 minutes after aspirin ingestion, and inhibition of platelet function is evident by 1 hour. In contrast, it can take up to 3 to 4 hours to reach peak plasma levels after administration of enteric-coated aspirin. If only enteric-coated tablets are available and a rapid effect is required, the tablets should be chewed. The oral bioavailability of regular aspirin tablets is approximately 40 to 50% over a wide range of doses. A considerably lower bioavailability has been reported for enteric-coated tablets and sustained-release, microencapsulated preparations. Because platelet COX-1 is acetylated in the presystemic circulation, the antiplatelet effect of aspirin is largely independent of systemic bioavailability.

Recent studies have raised the possibility that about 10 to 15% of patients have a poor response to aspirin therapy and that some patients develop progressive "resistance" to its antiplatelet effect over time. It is unclear if these observations reflect noncompliance, poor absorption, or altered pharmacodynamics. Drug interactions with reversible COX inhibitors potentially preventing acetylation of platelet COX-1 by aspirin also should be considered in elderly patients who are often on nonsteroidal anti-inflammatory drugs (NSAIDs) because of arthritic problems.

The plasma concentration of aspirin decays with a half-life of 15 to 20 minutes. Despite the rapid clearance of aspirin from the circulation, the platelet-inhibitory

---

Table 74.1 Currently available antiplatelet drugs

Inhibitors of platelet cyclooxygenase activity
  Aspirin
  Reversible inhibitors (sulfinpyrazone, indobufen, triflusal)
Inhibitors of platelet phosphodiesterase
  Dipyridamole
ADP-receptor inhibitors
  Ticlopidine, clopidogrel
GPIIb/IIIa antagonists
  Abciximab
  Tirofiban
  Eptifibatide

effect lasts for the life span of the platelet because aspirin irreversibly inactivates platelet COX-1. The mean life span of human platelets is approximately 10 days. Therefore, approximately 10% of circulating platelets is replaced every 24 hours, and 5 to 6 days following aspirin ingestion, approximately 50% of the platelets function normally.

Pharmacodynamics

Acetylation of platelet COX-1 by aspirin results in blockade of TXA_2 production, as reflected by lower serum TXB_2 levels measured ex vivo. When given orally to healthy subjects, aspirin inhibits TXA_2 production in a dose-dependent fashion. A log-linear inhibition of platelet TXB_2 production is found after single doses in the range of 10 to 100 mg (Fig. 74.1). Because of irreversible enzyme inactivation and lack of de novo enzyme synthesis in platelets, acetylation of platelet COX-1 and the consequent inhibition of TXA_2 production by low doses of aspirin (20-50 mg daily) are cumulative on repeated daily dosing. A log-linear relationship also exists between the oral dose of aspirin and the inhibition of platelet TXB_2 production, measured at steady state on repeated daily dosing (Fig. 74.2). When comparing this dose-response relationship with that based on measurements performed after single dosing, an 8-fold shift to the left is apparent, with the ID_{50} values (the dose required to inhibit enzyme activity by 50%) approximating 3 and 26 mg, respectively. Such a dose-response relationship predicts saturability of the antithrombotic effect of aspirin at low doses (i.e., <100 mg daily).

Although there is some evidence from in vitro experiments and in vivo studies that aspirin may inhibit platelet function by a mechanism that is unrelated to inhibition of TXA_2 synthesis, the results of clinical trials, in which different doses of aspirin ranging from 30 to 1500 mg per day have been used, are consistent with the hypothesis that the antithrombotic effect of aspirin is caused by inhibition of platelet TXA_2 synthesis. Thus the reduction in risk of both MI or death in unstable angina and stroke or death in transient cerebral ischemia has been reported with daily doses of aspirin as low as

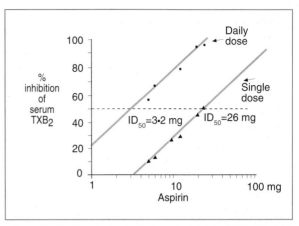

Figure 74.2 Cumulative inhibition of platelet PGHS-1 by low doses of aspirin, on repeated daily dosing, shifts the dose-response curve to the left by a factor equivalent to the fractional daily platelet turnover. Serum TXB_2 was measured before and after single or daily dosing with aspirin in four healthy subjects. Individual data are expressed as percent inhibition, with each subject serving as his/her own control. Daily dosing values represent measurements obtained at steady-state inhibition. Such a dose-response relationship predicts saturability of the antithrombotic effect of aspirin at doses as low as 30 to 50 mg daily. ID_{50} = dose required to inhibit TXB_2 production by 50%. (Reproduced from Patrono C, et al: Circulation 1985;72:1177 with permission.)

50 to 75 mg, and no greater benefit was obtained with 20- to 30-fold higher doses.

There are both practical and theoretical reasons to choose the lowest effective dose of aspirin (Tab. 74.2). The gastrointestinal (GI) side effects of aspirin appear to be dose-dependent (see below). There are also theoretical reasons to select a dose of aspirin that inhibits TXA_2 synthesis without inhibiting PGI_2 synthesis. Thus, a low dose may be more antithrombotic because it inhibits PGI_2 less than a high dose. This hypothesis is supported by indirect comparisons of the results of placebo-controlled trials using different daily doses of aspirin in the same clinical setting, as well as by a recently completed trial directly comparing four aspirin regimens (81, 325, 650, and 1300

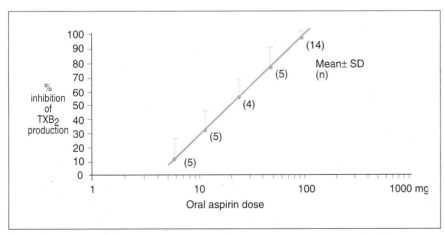

Figure 74.1 Single oral doses of aspirin produce log-linear inhibition of platelet TXB_2 production measured ex vivo in healthy subjects. TXB_2 production during whole blood clotting was measured before and 24 h after aspirin ingestion. The results are expressed as percent inhibition, each subject serving as his or her own control. (Reproduced from Patrignani P, Filabozzi P, Patrono C: J Clin Invest 1982; 69:1366 with permission.)

Table 74.2 Minimum effective dose of aspirin in vascular disorders

Disorder	Daily dose (mg)
Hypertension	75
Stable angina	75
Unstable angina	75
Acute myocardial infarction	160
Transient ischemic attack and ischemic stroke	50
Acute ischemic stroke	160

mg daily) in patients undergoing carotid endarterectomy.

Clinical activity

The efficacy and safety of aspirin are documented from analysis of over 50 randomized clinical trials that included approximately 100 000 patients at variable risk of thrombotic complications of atherosclerosis. Aspirin has been tested in patients demonstrating the whole spectrum of atherosclerosis, from apparently healthy low-risk individuals to patients presenting with an acute MI or an acute ischemic stroke; similarly, trials have extended for as short as a few weeks duration or as long as many years. Although aspirin has been shown consistently to be effective in preventing fatal and/or nonfatal vascular events in these trials, both the size of the proportional effects and the absolute benefits of antiplatelet therapy are somewhat heterogeneous in different clinical settings.

In the Second International Study of Infarct Survival (ISIS-2), a single 162.5-mg tablet of aspirin started within 24 hours of the onset of symptoms of a suspected MI and continued daily for 5 weeks produced highly significant reductions in the risk of vascular mortality (by 23%), nonfatal reinfarction (by 49%), and nonfatal stroke (by 46%). It should be emphasized that this is the only trial of any antiplatelet drug having vascular mortality as the primary endpoint. There was no increase in hemorrhagic stroke or GI bleeding in the aspirin-treated patients and only a small increase in minor bleeding. Thus, aspirin confers

conclusive net benefits in the acute phase of evolving MI and should be administered routinely to virtually all patients with suspected acute MI. Treatment of 1 000 such patients with aspirin for 5 weeks will result in approximately 40 patients in whom a vascular event is prevented.

Two separate trials with a similar protocol, the International Stroke Trial (IST) and the Chinese Acute Stroke Trial (CAST), tested the efficacy and safety of early aspirin use in acute ischemic stroke. Approximately 40 000 patients were randomized within 48 hours of the onset of symptoms to 2 to 4 weeks of daily aspirin therapy (300 and 160 mg, respectively) or placebo. An overview of the results of both trials suggests an absolute benefit of about 10 fewer deaths or nonfatal strokes per 1000 patients in the first month of aspirin therapy plus an extra 10 patients per 1000 with complete recovery. The proportional odds reduction in fatal or nonfatal vascular events is only 10% in this setting. Although the background risk of hemorrhagic stroke was threefold higher in CAST than in IST, the small absolute increase in this risk associated with early use of aspirin was similar in the two studies (excess 2 per 1000 patients). These results are consistent with biochemical evidence of episodic platelet activation during the first 48 hours after the onset of symptoms of an acute ischemic stroke and with suppression of in vivo TXA_2 biosynthesis in patients receiving low-dose aspirin in this setting. However, when contrasting the effects of aspirin in acute MI with those in acute stroke, it seems reasonable to assume that thromboxane-driven amplification of the platelet response to acute vascular injury plays a more important role in the coronary than in the cerebrovascular territory.

Long-term aspirin therapy confers conclusive net benefit on risk of subsequent MI, stroke, and vascular death among subjects with intermediate- to high-risk of vascular complications. These include patients with chronic stable angina, patients with prior MI, patients with unstable angina, as well as patients in other high-risk categories. The proportional effects of aspirin therapy on vascular events in these different clinical settings are rather homogeneous, ranging between 20 and 25% odds reduction based on an overview of all randomized trials. However, individual trial data show substantial heterogeneity, ranging from no statistically significant benefits in patients with peripheral vascular disease to greater than

Table 74.3 Reduction in the risk of death or acute myocardial infarction associated with different regimens of aspirin therapy in patients with unstable angina[1]

Trial	Daily aspirin dose (mg)	Risk reduction (%)	
		at 3 mos	at 1 yr
Cairns et al., 1985	1300	NA	30
Lewis et al., 1983	324	41	NA
Wallentin and the RISC Groups, 1990	75	64	48

[1]All analyses were conducted according to the intention-to-treat principle.
(NA = not available.)

50% relative risk reduction in patients with unstable angina. These findings can be interpreted as reflecting the variable importance of TXA$_2$ as a mechanism amplifying the hemostatic response to plaque destabilization in different clinical settings. In terms of absolute benefit, these protective effects of aspirin translate into avoidance of a major vascular event in 50 patients per 1000 patients with unstable angina treated for 6 months and in approximately 35 patients per 1 000 patients with prior MI treated for 30 months.

For patients with different manifestations of ischemic heart disease, a vast consensus exists in defining a rather narrow range of recommended daily doses (i.e., 75 to 160 mg) for secondary prevention. This is supported by separate trial data in over 20 000 patients randomized to low-dose aspirin or placebo as well as by an overview of all antiplatelet trials showing no obvious dose dependence for the protective effects of aspirin.

Table 74.3 demonstrates saturation of the antithrombotic effect of aspirin at low dose by comparing the relative risk reductions obtained with daily doses of 75, 324, and 1300 mg in the Swedish, American, and Canadian trials, respectively, carried out in patients with unstable angina. There is no obvious dose dependence of the antithrombotic effect of aspirin in this setting. If anything, an inverse relationship is apparent between the aspirin dose and the reported risk reductions at 3 and 12 months.

In contrast, for patients with cerebrovascular disease, a much larger degree of uncertainty still exists about the optimal aspirin dose, with recommendations ranging from 30 to 1300 mg per day. In the absence of definitive evidence from direct randomized comparisons of low-dose versus high-dose aspirin in trials of adequate size to detect a moderate difference (one way or the other) between the two, good clinical practice should recommend the use of the lowest dose of aspirin shown to be effective in patients with transient cerebral ischemia because of safety considerations.

Adverse effects

Aspirin does not cause a generalized bleeding abnormality unless it is given to patients with an underlying hemostatic defect, such as hemophilia, uremia, or that induced by anticoagulant therapy. The balance between preventing vascular occlusion and causing excess bleeding with aspirin depends critically on the absolute thrombotic versus hemorrhagic risk of the patient. Thus in individuals at very low risk for vascular occlusion (e.g., 1% per year), a very small absolute benefit is offset by exposure of a large number of healthy subjects to undue bleeding complications. In contrast, in patients at high risk of cardiovascular or cerebrovascular complications (i.e., >5% per year), the substantial absolute benefit of aspirin prophylaxis clearly outweighs the risk. For example, the absolute excess of major bleeds (i.e., those requiring transfusion) in acute MI is approximately 100 times smaller than the absolute number of major vascular events avoided by aspirin therapy.

Hypertension often has been considered a contraindication to aspirin because of the concern that possible benefits in the prevention of cardiovascular events may be counterbalanced by an increased risk of cerebral bleeding. The results of the aspirin component of the Hypertension Optimal Treatment study (see Chap. 23) are somewhat reassuring in this regard, by showing that hypertensive patients whose blood pressure was well controlled were protected from MI without an increase in cerebral bleeds or strokes associated with aspirin therapy.

Aspirin-induced GI toxicity, as detected in randomized clinical trials, appears to be dose-related in the range of 30 to 1300 mg daily. This is based largely on indirect comparisons of different trials and on a limited number of randomized, direct comparisons of different aspirin doses. Such a dose-response relationship is thought to reflect at least two COX-1-dependent components, i.e., dose-dependent inhibition of COX-1 in the GI mucosa and dose-independent (within the range of examined doses) inhibition of COX-1 in platelets. The cyclooxygenase activity of gastric mucosa lining cells is hardly affected after single oral dosing with 100 mg of aspirin, whereas COX-1 activity in platelets is completely abolished. Thus, it is not surprising that the antithrombotic effect of aspirin can be dissociated, at least in part, from its most common side effect. However, even when administered at low doses, aspirin can cause serious GI bleeding, as reported in studies using 30 to 50 mg daily. The relative risk of hospitalization due to upper GI bleeding and/or perforation associated with low-dose aspirin (mostly 100 to 300 mg daily) is approximately 2.0 and comparable with that of other antiplatelet agents and anticoagulants in a large population-based observational study. When the estimated overall relative risks of GI complications with the use of NSAIDs (including aspirin at analgesic/anti-inflammatory

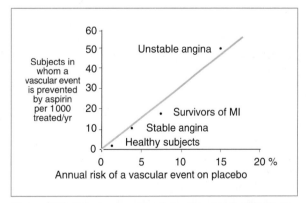

Figure 74.3 The absolute risk of vascular complications is the major determinant of the absolute benefit of antiplatelet prophylaxis. Data are plotted from placebo-controlled aspirin trials in different clinical settings. For each category of patients, the abscissa denotes the absolute risk of experiencing a major vascular event as recorded in the placebo arm of the trial(s). The absolute benefit of antiplatelet treatment is reported on the ordinate as the number of subjects in whom an important vascular event (nonfatal MI, nonfatal stroke, or vascular death) is actually prevented by treating 1000 subjects with aspirin for 1 year. (Reproduced from Patrono C, et al: The relationship among dose, effectiveness, and side effects. Chest 1998;114:470S with permission.)

doses) were calculated, they lay mainly in the interval 3.0 to 5.0 as compared with nonusers.

Thus, in summary, inhibition of TXA_2-dependent platelet function by aspirin may lead to prevention of thrombosis as well as to excess bleeding. The balance between the two depends critically on the absolute thrombotic versus hemorrhagic risk of the patient. In individuals at very low risk for vascular occlusion, a very small absolute benefit may be offset by exposure of very large numbers of healthy subjects to undue bleeding complications. As the risk of experiencing a major vascular event increases, so does the absolute benefit of antiplatelet prophylaxis with aspirin, as shown in Figure 74.3, for a number of clinical settings where the efficacy of the drug has been tested in randomized clinical trials. Based on the results of such trials, the antithrombotic effect of aspirin does not appear to be dose-related over a wide range of daily doses (30-1300 mg), an observation consistent with saturability of platelet cyclooxygenase inhibition by aspirin at very low doses. In contrast, GI toxicity of the drug does appear to be dose-related, consistent with dose- and dosing interval-dependent inhibition of cyclooxygenase activity in the nucleated lining cells of the GI mucosa. Thus aspirin once daily is recommended in all clinical conditions where antiplatelet therapy is effective. Because of safety considerations, physicians are encouraged to use the lowest dose of aspirin shown to be effective in each clinical setting.

Reversible cyclooxygenase inhibitors

A number of NSAIDs can inhibit TXA_2-dependent platelet function through competitive, reversible inhibition of platelet COX-1. In general, these drugs, when used at conventional anti-inflammatory dosages, inhibit platelet cyclooxygenase activity by only 70 to 85%. This level of inhibition may be insufficient to block adequately platelet aggregation in vivo because of the very substantial biosynthetic capacity of human platelets to produce TXA_2.

The only reversible cyclooxygenase inhibitors that have been tested in randomized clinical trials for their antithrombotic efficacy are sulfinpyrazone, indobufen, and triflusal. Sulfinpyrazone is a uricosuric agent (see Chap. 71) that is structurally related to the anti-inflammatory agent phenylbutazone. When used at the highest approved dosage of 200 mg four times daily, the drug inhibits platelet cyclooxygenase activity by approximately 60%, after conversion from an inactive sulfoxide to an active sulfide metabolite. The conflicting or negative results obtained in randomized clinical trials of sulfinpyrazone in patients with MI or unstable angina are not surprising in light of the fact that the drug is a weak cyclooxygenase inhibitor with no other established antiplatelet mechanism of action.

In contrast, indobufen is a very potent inhibitor of platelet cyclooxygenase activity and has comparable biochemical, functional, and clinical effects to those of a standard dose of aspirin. Thus, at therapeutic plasma levels achieved after oral dosing of 200 mg bid, indobufen inhibits serum TXB_2 by greater than 95% throughout the dosing interval and reduces urinary thromboxane metabolite excretion to an extent quite comparable with that of aspirin. Indobufen also has been investigated in a placebo-controlled study of patients with heart disease at increased embolic risk and compared with warfarin and ticlopidine in patients with nonrheumatic atrial fibrillation and patients with recent reversible cerebral ischemia, respectively. However, none of these studies in over 4000 patients clearly established an advantage of indobufen versus standard treatments, although the confidence intervals for these comparisons are wide. Indobufen has been reported to suppress in vivo TXA_2 biosynthesis more effectively than low-dose aspirin in patients with unstable angina, an effect possibly related to inhibition of monocyte COX-2 by therapeutic plasma levels of indobufen. The clinical relevance of these findings remains to be established.

Another platelet antiaggregant, structurally related to the salicylate groups of compounds, is triflusal, available in some European countries. Triflusal and its major metabolite act on the arachidonate pathway similar to acetylsalicylic acid, with better tolerability. Positive studies have been reported in unstable angina and in peripheral arterial disease.

Dipyridamole

Dipyridamole is a pyrimidopyrimidine derivative with vasodilator and antiplatelet properties. The mechanism of action of dipyridamole as an antiplatelet agent has been the subject of controversy. Both inhibition of cyclic nucleotide phosphodiesterase (the enzyme that degrades cAMP to 5'-AMP) and blockade of the uptake of adenosine (which acts at A_2 receptors for adenosine to stimulate platelet adenylyl cyclase) have been suggested. Moreover, direct stimulation of PGI_2 synthesis and protection against its degradation have been reported, although the dipyridamole concentrations required to produce these effects far exceed the low micromolar plasma levels achieved after oral administration of conventional doses (100-400 mg/day).

The absorption of dipyridamole from conventional formulations is quite variable and may result in low systemic bioavailability of the drug. A modified-release formulation of dipyridamole with improved bioavailability has been developed in association with low-dose aspirin. Dipyridamole is eliminated primarily by biliary excretion as a glucuronide conjugate and is subject to enterohepatic recirculation. A terminal half-life of 10 hours has been reported. This is consistent with the twice-daily regimen used in recent clinical studies.

Although the clinical efficacy of dipyridamole, alone or in combination with aspirin, has been questioned on the basis of earlier randomized trials, the whole issue has been reopened by the results of the recently published European Stroke Prevention Study 2 (ESPS-2). In this study of 6602 patients with prior stroke or transient ischemic attack (TIA), stroke risk in comparison with placebo was reduced by 18% with low-dose aspirin ($p = 0.013$), by 16% with dipyridamole alone ($p = 0.039$), and by 37% with aspirin plus dipyridamole ($p < 0.001$). The corresponding relative risk reductions for the outcome of stroke or death were 13% ($p = 0.016$), 15% ($p = 0.015$), and 24% ($p < 0.001$), respectively. Headache was the most common adverse effect of dipyridamole. Bleeding at any site was almost doubled in the two aspirin arms but was indistinguishable from placebo in the dipyridamole-treated patients. This study has been criticized for the continued inclusion of a placebo arm after the place of aspirin in the secondary prevention of stroke had been established.

ADP-RECEPTOR INHIBITORS

A different class of antiplatelet agents is represented by the thienopyridines ticlopidine and clopidogrel. The two are structurally related, and clopidogrel was developed with the aim of separating the desired antiplatelet effect from the potential myelotoxicity associated with the use of ticlopidine. Both drugs selectively inhibit ADP-induced platelet aggregation with no direct effects on arachidonic acid metabolism. Although ticlopidine and clopidogrel also can inhibit platelet aggregation induced by collagen and thrombin, these inhibitory effects are abolished by increasing the agonist concentration and therefore are likely to reflect blockade of ADP-mediated amplification of the platelet response to other agonists.

Clopidogrel, and most likely also ticlopidine, induces irreversible alterations in the platelet receptor mediating the inhibition of stimulated adenylyl cyclase activity by ADP. The inhibition of platelet function by clopidogrel is associated with a selective reduction in the number of ADP binding sites, with no consistent change in the binding affinity. The hypothesis of permanent modification of a putative ADP receptor by thienopyridines is consistent with time-dependent cumulative inhibition of ADP-induced platelet aggregation on repeated daily dosing with ticlopidine or clopidogrel and with slow recovery of platelet function on drug withdrawal.

Up to 90% of a single oral dose of ticlopidine is rapidly absorbed in humans. Peak plasma concentrations occur 1 to 3 hours after a single oral dose of 250 mg. Plasma levels of ticlopidine increase by approximately threefold on repeated twice-daily dosing over 2 to 3 weeks because of drug accumulation. Greater than 98% of ticlopidine is reversibly bound to plasma proteins, primarily albumin. Ticlopidine is metabolized rapidly and extensively. A total of 13 metabolites have been identified in humans. Of these, only the 2-keto derivative is more potent than ticlopidine in inhibiting ADP-induced platelet aggregation.

The apparent elimination half-life of ticlopidine is 24 to 36 hours after a single oral dose and up to 96 hours after 14 days of repeated dosing. The recommended regimen of ticlopidine is 250 mg bid, although it is unclear how a bid regimen is justified by the pharmacokinetic and pharmacodynamic features noted earlier.

Ticlopidine has been shown to be effective in patients with stroke, transient cerebral ischemia, unstable angina, and intermittent claudication and those having aortocoronary bypass surgery. Ticlopidine was shown to be more effective than conventional antianginal therapy in reduc-

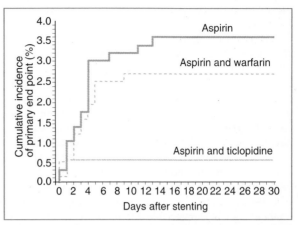

Figure 74.4 Cumulative incidence of the primary endpoint (death from any cause, revascularization of the target lesion without death, evidence of thrombosis of the target vessel on repeated angiography without revascularization, or nonfatal MI in patients who did not undergo repeated angiography) among 1653 patients who underwent coronary stenting and were randomly assigned to one of three antithrombotic regimens: aspirin alone, aspirin and warfarin, or aspirin and ticlopidine. (Reproduced from Leon MB, et al: N Engl J Med 1998; 339:1665 with permission.)

ing vascular death or MI in patients with unstable angina, and the 50% relative risk reduction at 6 months of follow-up is quite comparable with the effects of low-dose aspirin in this setting. However, a delayed antithrombotic effect of ticlopidine was noted in this trial, with no apparent protection during the first 2 weeks of drug administration. This clinical finding is consistent with pharmacokinetic evidence of ticlopidine accumulation over 2 weeks of daily dosing with 250 mg bid as well as with pharmacodynamic evidence of a delayed antiplatelet effect of the drug. On the other hand, the additive antithrombotic effect of ticlopidine and aspirin versus aspirin alone becomes apparent during the first few days after coronary stenting (Fig. 74.4). These results also illustrate the potential advantage of combining two different drugs blocking two distinct mechanisms of amplification of the platelet response to vascular injury, i.e., TXA_2 and ADP, in a high-risk setting.

The association of ticlopidine therapy with hypercholesterolemia and neutropenia (for which the reported rate of occurrence is 2.4% for neutrophils $< 1.2 \times 10^9/l$ and 0.8% for neutrophils $< 0.45 \times 10^9/l$) and its cost have reduced enthusiasm for this drug as an alternative to aspirin in most situations.

The pharmacokinetics of clopidogrel are somewhat different from those of ticlopidine. Thus, after administration of single oral doses (up to 200 mg) or repeated doses (up to 100 mg daily), unchanged clopidogrel was not detectable in peripheral venous plasma. Concentrations of 1 to 2 ng/ml were measured in the plasma of patients who received clopidogrel 150 mg per day (twice as much as the dose used in the CAPRIE study and recently approved for clinical use) for 16 days. The main systemic metabolite of clopidogrel is the carboxylic acid derivative SR26334.

ADP-induced platelet aggregation was inhibited in a dose-dependent fashion, with an apparent ceiling effect (40% inhibition) at 400 mg, after single oral doses of clopidogrel administered to healthy volunteers. Inhibition of platelet aggregation was detectable at 2 hours after oral dosing of 400 mg and remained relatively stable up to 48 hours. On repeated daily dosing of 50 to 100 mg of clopidogrel to healthy volunteers, ADP-induced platelet aggregation was inhibited from the second day of treatment (25-30% inhibition) and reached a steady state (50-60% inhibition) after 4 to 7 days. This level of maximal inhibition was comparable with that achieved with ticlopidine (500 mg/day). No appreciable differences in the inhibitory effects of 50, 75, and 100 mg of clopidogrel were noted in this study, suggesting that 50 mg daily may be at or close to the top of the dose-response curve.

These findings suggest that the active metabolite(s) of clopidogrel has a pharmacodynamic pattern quite similar to that of aspirin in causing cumulative inhibition of platelet function on repeated daily administration of low doses. As in the case of aspirin, platelet function returned to normal 7 days after the last dose of clopidogrel. Both the cumulative nature of the inhibitory effects and the slow rate of recovery of platelet function are consistent with the active moieties of aspirin (acetylsalicylic acid) and clopidogrel active metabolite causing a permanent defect in a platelet protein that cannot be repaired during the 24-hour dosing interval and can only be replaced as a function of platelet turnover. This also justifies the once-daily regimen of both drugs despite their short half-life in the human circulation.

Bleeding time measurements performed in the same multiple-dose study showed a comparable prolongation (by 1.5- to 2.0-fold over control) at 50 to 100 mg daily of clopidogrel or ticlopidine 500 mg daily.

Clopidogrel has undergone a quite unusual clinical development, with very limited phase II studies and a single, very large phase III trial, i.e., CAPRIE, to test its efficacy and safety at 75 mg daily versus aspirin 325 mg daily. CAPRIE is unique among the studies that have directly compared antiplatelet agents against aspirin in that it incorporated three groups of patients, all of whom are recognized to be at an increased risk of recurrent ischemic events: those who have experienced a recent stroke or recent MI and those presenting with symptomatic peripheral arterial disease.

Overall, CAPRIE showed a modest difference in effectiveness; the annual event rate calculated for aspirin was 5.83% compared with 5.32% for clopidogrel, a relative risk reduction of 8.7% (95% CI, 0.3-16.5%; $p = 0.043$). What is particularly interesting, however, are the results obtained when the effects of aspirin and clopidogrel in the three separate groups of patients are compared (Fig. 74.5). This analysis shows that the majority of the difference in effectiveness occurred in patients who entered the trial because of symptomatic peripheral arterial disease. A

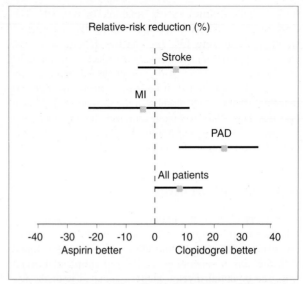

Figure 74.5 Relative risk reduction and 95% confidence interval by disease subgroup in the CAPRIE study. MI = myocardial infarction; PAD = peripheral arterial disease. (Reproduced from CAPRIE Steering Committee Lancet 1996;348:1329 with permission.)

highly significant 24% reduction in relative risk over aspirin was seen in the clopidogrel-treated patients with peripheral arterial disease, whereas a nonsignificant 7.3% reduction in relative risk and a nonsignificant 3.7% increase in risk were calculated in the clopidogrel-treated groups of stroke and MI patients, respectively. Although it is possible that such a differential effect of clopidogrel versus aspirin may reflect the play of chance, the possibility also exists that ADP and TXA_2 may be equally important in amplifying the platelet response to plaque destabilization when this occurs in the absence of peripheral arterial disease, whereas ADP may be the key player of platelet activation when this occurs in the presence of peripheral arterial disease.

Both clopidogrel and medium-dose aspirin were well tolerated in the CAPRIE study. The frequency of severe rash and severe diarrhea was higher with clopidogrel than with aspirin, whereas GI discomfort and hemorrhage were more frequent with aspirin than with clopidogrel. No excess neutropenia was found in the clopidogrel group, thus demonstrating the validity of the structural modifications vis-à-vis ticlopidine. Based on these findings, clopidogrel was approved recently for the reduction of atherothrombotic events in patients with recent stroke, recent MI, or established peripheral arterial disease.

Studies are ongoing to test the efficacy and safety of combining clopidogrel with low dose aspirin in high-risk settings (e.g., acute coronary syndromes).

INTEGRIN $\alpha_{IIb}\beta_3$ (GPIIb/IIIa) ANTAGONISTS (see also Tab. 25.7)

Following recognition that the expression of functionally active integrin $\alpha_{IIb}\beta_3$ (GPIIb/IIIa) on the platelet surface is the final common pathway of platelet aggregation,

Table 74.4 Clinical trials of GP IIb/IIIa antagonists in coronary syndromes

Trial	Number of patients	Compound	Placebo (%)	GPIIb/IIIa antagonist (%)	Relative risk reduction (%)
Percutaneous coronary interventions					
EPIC	2099	Abciximab	10.3	6.9	30.0
EPILOG	2792	Abciximab	9.1	3.8[1]	58.2
CAPTURE	1265	Abciximab	9.0	4.8	46.7
IMPACT-II	4010	Eptifibatide	8.4	6.9	17.9
RESTORE	2139	Tirofiban	6.4	5.0	21.9
Unstable angina and non-Q-wave myocardial infarction					
PRISM	3232	Tirofiban	7.1	5.8	18.3
PRISM-Plus	1570	Tirofiban	11.9	8.7	26.9
PURSUIT	10948	Eptifibatide	15.7	14.2	9.6

Note: Rates of death or myocardial infarction at 30 days are shown for each trial.
[1]Abciximab + low-dose heparin.

regardless of the initiating stimulus, this glycoprotein has become the target of novel antiplatelet drugs. The inhibitors of GPIIb/IIIa include monoclonal antibodies against the receptor, naturally occurring Arg-Gly-Asp sequence (RGD)-containing peptides isolated from snake venoms, synthetic RGD- or Lys-Gly-Asp sequence (KGD)-containing peptides, as well as peptidomimetic and nonpeptide RGD mimetics that compete with fibrinogen, von Willebrand factor, and/or perhaps other ligands, for occupancy of the platelet receptor.

Abciximab

Blockade of GPIIb/IIIa receptors by murine monoclonal antibodies such as 7E3 essentially induces a functional thrombasthenic phenotype. Platelet aggregation is significantly inhibited at antibody doses that decrease the number of available receptors to less than 50% of normal. Platelet aggregation is nearly completely abolished at approximately 80% receptor blockade, but the bleeding time is only mildly affected at this level of receptor blockade. It is only with more than 90% receptor blockade that the bleeding time becomes extremely prolonged. Because of concerns about immunogenicity of the original 7E3 antibody, a mouse/human chimeric 7E3 Fab (abciximab) was created for clinical development.

Pharmacokinetic data on abciximab indicate that following intravenous bolus administration, free plasma concentrations decrease rapidly (initial half-life of about 30 minutes) as a result of rapid binding to platelet GPIIb/IIIa receptors, with approximately 65% of the injected antibody becoming attached to platelets in the circulation and spleen. After bolus injection of abciximab, a dose-dependent inhibition of ADP-induced platelet aggregation was recorded in patients judged to be at moderate to high risk

of percutaneous transluminal coronary angioplasty (PTCA)-associated ischemic complications. A bolus dose of 0.25 mg/kg was found to result in blockade of more than 80% of platelet receptors and reduce platelet aggregation in response to 20 μM ADP to less than 20% of baseline. A steep dose-response curve was apparent in this study. Peak effects on receptor blockade, platelet aggregation, and bleeding time were observed at the first sampling time of 2 hours after bolus administration of 0.25 mg/kg. Gradual recovery of platelet function then occurred over time, with bleeding times returning to near-normal values by 12 hours. Platelet aggregation in response to 20 μM ADP returns to more than 50% of baseline within 24 hours in most patients and within 48 hours in nearly all patients.

The receptor blockade, inhibition of platelet aggregation, and prolongation of bleeding time produced by administering a 0.25 mg/kg bolus dose of abciximab could be maintained for 12 hours by administering a 10 μg per minute infusion during that time period. This regimen was chosen for the pivotal phase III trial (EPIC) that demonstrated the clinical efficacy of abciximab, added to conventional antithrombotic therapy, in reducing the incidence of ischemic events in patients undergoing PTCA (see also Chap. 25).

Major bleeding increased significantly in abciximab-treated patients in the EPIC trial. Subsequently, however, it was found that a reduction in the dosage of concomitant heparin and more rapid sheath removal can greatly reduce the bleeding complications attendant to abciximab administration. Besides hemorrhage, thrombocytopenia represents an important side effect of abciximab treatment. Approximately 1 to 2% of patients treated with abciximab develop platelet counts of less than 50 000/μl, of which approximately 0.5 to 1% reflect very rapid decreases (beginning within 2 hours of administration) due to abciximab. Thus far, all reports indicate that the thrombocytopenia can be treated effectively with platelet transfusions and is reversible, with recovery occurring over several days. In the EPIC trial, approximately 6% of patients treated with abciximab developed antibodies to the variable region(s) of abciximab (human antichimeric antibody). Few data are currently available to assess the potential risks of reinjecting abciximab.

Tirofiban

Tirofiban (MK-383, Aggrastat) is a nonpeptide derivative of tyrosine that selectively inhibits the GPIIb/IIIa receptor, with minimal effects on the $\alpha_v \beta_3$ vitronectin receptor. When administered to humans at 0.15 µg/kg per minute for 4 hours, tirofiban produced a 2.5-fold increase in bleeding time and a 97% inhibition of ADP-induced platelet aggregation. The mean plasma clearance was 329 ml per minute, and the half-life in plasma was 1.6 hours. After stopping tirofiban, within 4 hours, bleeding times returned to normal and inhibition of platelet aggregation declined to approximately 20%. When tirofiban was administered with aspirin, the bleeding time increased 4.1 ± 1.5-fold, even though tirofiban plasma levels were unaffected. The plasma concentration of tirofiban needed to inhibit platelet aggregation by 50% decreased, however, from approximately 12 to approximately 9 ng/ml when aspirin was coadministered.

In a pilot study, 73 patients undergoing PTCA were treated with aspirin, heparin, and bolus doses of tirofiban of 5, 10, or 15 µg/kg followed by tirofiban infusions of 0.05, 0.10, and 0.15 µg/kg per minute, respectively. The onset of platelet inhibition was rapid, with platelet aggregation in response to 5 µM ADP inhibited by 93% and 96%, respectively, within 5 minutes of administering the two higher-dose regimens. Bleeding times at 2 hours after starting the infusion were 19.5, more than 30, and more than 30 minutes. At the end of the infusion (16-24 h), platelet aggregation was inhibited by 57%, 87%, and 95% in response to the escalating tirofiban regimens, respectively. Platelet aggregation began to return toward normal within 1.5 hours after discontinuing the infusion in all groups; 4 hours after discontinuing therapy, platelet aggregation inhibition decreased to less than 50%, even in the group receiving the highest dose.

Severe but reversible thrombocytopenia has been reported in a small percentage of patients treated with tirofiban; an immunologic mechanism has been proposed, mediated by preformed antibodies to a conformation of the GPIIb/IIIa receptor induced by the binding of tirofiban to the receptor. No data are available on the safety of reinfusing tirofiban.

Eptifibatide

Eptifibatide (Integrilin) is a synthetic disulfide-linked cyclic heptapeptide with high specificity for inhibition of GPIIb/IIIa compared with inhibition of the $\alpha_v \beta_3$ vitronectin receptor. Four eptifibatide regimens were tested in 54 patients undergoing coronary interventions who also were treated with aspirin and heparin: (1) 180 µg/kg bolus + 1 µg/kg per minute infusion for 18 to 24 hours, (2) 135 µg/kg bolus + 0.5 µg/kg per minute infusion for 18 to 24 hours, (3) 90 µg/kg bolus + 0.75 µg/kg per minute infusion for 18 to 24 hours, and (4) 135 µg/kg bolus + 0.75 µg/kg per minute for 18 to 24 hours. Fifteen minutes after the 180 µg/kg bolus dose, platelet aggregation was inhibited by more than 95% in response to 20 µM ADP, with virtually no interindividual variation, whereas the 135 µg/kg bolus dose resulted in 80 to 90% inhibition in 75% of the patients, and the 90 µg/kg bolus produced only slightly less inhibition than the 135 µg/kg dose. The inhibition of platelet aggregation achieved with the 180 µg/kg bolus dose was sustained throughout the infusion by the 1 µg/kg per minute dose, but there was a tendency for the platelet aggregation response to return toward normal during the infusion in some patients given the 0.75 µg/kg per minute dose, and the return of the platelet aggregation response toward normal was more marked in those given the 0.5 µg/kg per minute infusion dose. Two hours after discontinuing the eptifibatide infusion, there was substantial return of platelet function in all groups, and return of more than half the baseline aggregation response was seen in all groups after 4 hours. Median bleeding times were prolonged in all groups at the time the infusion was terminated (22, 12, 12, and 17 minutes, respectively, compared with control values of 7-8 minutes), and they returned toward normal after 1 hour (9, 10, 9, and 11 minutes, respectively). As in the previous study, activated clotting times were longer in patients treated with eptifibatide + heparin than in those treated with placebo + heparin. A modest increase in hemorrhagic complications has been reported in patients treated with eptifibatide in the PURSUIT trial. Eptifibatide treatment has not been associated with an increased frequency of overall thrombocytopenia, but it may be associated with a small increase in profound thrombocytopenia. No data are available concerning the safety of reinfusing eptifibatide.

Clinical activity (see also Chap. 25)

The efficacy and safety of GPIIb/IIIa antagonists was evaluated initially in patients undergoing PTCAs. Over 12 000 patients have been enrolled in five studies of abciximab, eptifibatide, and tirofiban (Tab. 74.4). The first of these phase III trials, the EPIC trial, resulted in approval in many countries of abciximab (ReoPro) in 1994 for PTCA patients at high risk of developing ischemic complication. Eptifibatide and tirofiban have been studied in the IMPACT-II and RESTORE trials, respectively. Although neither of these trials achieved their predefined efficacy endpoints, there was a positive trend in each case (see Tab. 74.4). Eptifibatide received approval from the Food and Drug Administration (FDA) for PTCA in 1998 based on data from the IMPACT-II and PURSUIT trials. The CAPTURE trial demonstrated the efficacy of an 18- to 24-hour abciximab treatment prior to PTCA in patients with unstable angina refractory to conventional antithrombotic and antianginal therapy. The EPILOG trial demonstrated the efficacy of abciximab in a broad patient population undergoing PTCA, not just high-risk patients as enrolled in the EPIC and CAPTURE trials. The EPISTENT trial demonstrated that abciximab decreases the frequency of ischemic complications of PTCA associated with stent insertion during the first 30 days and that there are fewer ischemic complications during this time period in patients treated with PTCA and abciximab alone without stent insertion versus those treated with stent alone.

Three completed trials have examined the efficacy and safety of tirofiban, and eptifibatide in approximately 16 000 patients with unstable angina or non-Q-wave MI randomized to receive a GPIIb/IIIa antagonist or placebo in addition to conventional antithrombotic therapy (Tab. 74.4). These studies demonstrated a 10 to 27% relative risk reduction in MI or death at 30 days. Although the results of short-term, high-grade blockade of GPIIb/IIIa with intravenous antagonists in unstable coronary syndromes are encouraging, as exemplified by the effects of eptifibatide in the PURSUIT trial, it is obvious from the time course of major vascular events over 30 days that a substantial proportion of these events continues to occur despite a very aggressive antithrombotic strategy (Fig. 74.6). This most likely reflects the presence of a persistently thrombogenic surface weeks after the acute clinical presentation and/or persistent platelet and coagulation activation in response to other stimuli (e.g., inflammation, dyslipidemia).

Oral agents

Orally active nonpeptide GPIIb/IIIa inhibitors have been developed, and they have the potential to be given long term. However, a number of issues remain unsolved. These include the uncertainty as to the optimal degree of GPIIb/IIIa receptor blockade compatible with superior efficacy vis-à-vis aspirin (and/or clopidogrel) and acceptable bleeding risk during long-term administration, the inadequacy of currently available surrogate markers for efficacy (ADP-induced platelet aggregation) and safety (skin bleeding time) on which dose-finding studies are based, and the steep dose-response curve displayed by many of these agents, requiring dose titration and monitoring. The disappointing results of recently reported phase III trials of oral GPIIb/IIIa antagonists (e.g., OPUS-TIMI 16) underscore the importance of the preceding limitations.

ANTICOAGULANTS

Unfractionated heparin

Heparin is the most time-honored anticoagulant medication, having been introduced into clinical practice in 1937. Since then, considerable progress has been made in purification of the molecule and in understanding its mechanism of action. Heparin still remains the drug of choice for achieving rapid anticoagulation because of the immediate onset of its effect when it is administered intravenously. Heparin consists of a polysaccharide chain composed of repeated units containing glucosamine and glucuronic or iduronic acid. One to three sulfate groups are present every two monosaccharide units and confer a characteristic acidity to the molecule. Interaction of heparin with antithrombin III is mediated by a unique pentasaccharide sequence. Macromolecular heparin consists of a core protein of unknown dimensions and a variable number of mucopolysaccharide units, with molecular weights ranging between 30 000 and 100 000 Da. Pharmaceutical preparations contain only the polysaccharide chain, with mean molecular weights between 12 000 and 15 000 Da.

Mechanism of action

Heparin molecules possess a number of properties of potential clinical usefulness, including the ability to inhibit smooth muscle cell proliferation, to activate lipoprotein lipase, and to suppress aldosterone synthesis. The anticoagulant activity of heparin is mostly due to its property of accelerating (by a factor of approximately 1000) the formation of complexes between a liver-produced plasma protein, i.e., antithrombin III (AT III), and several serine proteases of the coagulation cascade, including activated factors XII, XI, IX, X and thrombin. The inhibitory activity on factor Xa and thrombin are particularly relevant clinically. For the acceleration of thrombin degradation, the formation of a ternary complex between heparin, AT III, and thrombin is thought to be necessary, with heparin molecules embracing both AT III and thrombin molecules, whereas for acceleration of the formation of factor Xa-thrombin complexes, heparin only needs to bind AT III. For this reason, small heparin molecules can still inactivate factor Xa, provided they have the AT III-binding domain, even if they are virtually devoid of the ability to inactivate thrombin. This is the basis for the relative selectivity for factor Xa inactivation of heparin molecules of low molecular weight (low-molecular-weight heparins, LMWHs) produced by a variety of techniques and recent-

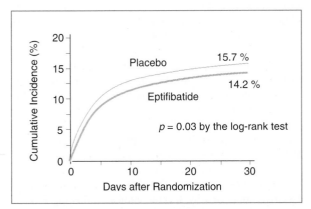

Figure 74.6 Kaplan-Meier curves showing the incidence of death or nonfatal MI at 30 days among 9461 patients with acute coronary syndromes randomized to eptifibatide or placebo. (Reproduced from The PURSUIT Trial Investigators: N Engl J Med 1998;339:436 with permission.)

ly introduced into clinical practice (see below). At concentrations higher than therapeutically effective, heparin and heparin-like mucopolysaccharides also catalyze the inhibition of thrombin by another plasma protein, heparin-cofactor II. At least partially in response to negative surface charges, heparin also binds to platelets and induces a stimulation of some thrombin-independent pathways of platelet activation.

Pharmacokinetics

Heparin is not absorbed though the GI mucosa and therefore must be given parenterally. The disappearance of anticoagulant activity after heparin iv injection (half-life values reported between 23 and 360 minutes) is thought to be best explained by a model based on the combination of a saturable nonlinear mechanism (most likely endothelial uptake and reticuloendothelial desulfatation) and a linear nonsaturable mechanism (most likely renal clearance). This accounts for the clear increase in heparin half-life values when switching from a first low-dose administration (practically, up to around 5000 units) when the first mechanism predominates to higher dosing. In addition, the more rapid elimination of higher-molecular-weight fractions is suggested by the more rapid disappearance of antithrombin versus anti-factor Xa activity. Conventional heparins (in the form of either sodium or calcium salts) can be administered sc, with therapeutic levels achieved with twice- or thrice-daily dosing. Bioavailability of these formulations is low (typically around 30%) and individually variable, being one of the major limitations in the administration of fully anticoagulant doses by this route.

Pharmacodynamics

The need for monitoring heparin therapy is due to the large patient variability in the anticoagulant response, in part related to variability of plasma proteins binding heparin and competing with AT III, variability in the concentration of coagulation factors, and variability in the clearance mechanisms. The coagulation time and its derivative activated partial thromboplastin time (aPTT) are both suitable for monitoring heparin therapy in that they are sensitive to the antithrombin action of heparin and, less, to inhibition of serine proteases upstream in the coagulation cascade. The aPTT, which is performed on citrate-anticoagulated plasma, is thought to be more standardized than conventional measurement of the coagulation time, either in whole blood or in plasma. For most practical indications when iv heparin administration is deemed necessary, adequate anticoagulation is thought to be reached when the aPTT reaches 1.5 to 2.5 times the baseline value before the onset of therapy. Because of individual variations in the aPTT, this recommendation appears preferable to that of indicating a range of optimal aPTT values. In situations where higher levels of anticoagulation are felt to be necessary, the aPTT has limitations in providing nondiscriminative values on most automated coagulometers, and the performance of a stan-

dardized "activated" coagulation time (aCT) has become popular. This technique has the advantage of being directly performable at the bedside or in the catheterization laboratory. However, attention has to be paid to the fact that the results with the Hemocron device are approximately 50 seconds higher than with the HemoTec device in the 300-second range. For standard PTCA procedures, a priming dose on the order of 10 000 units for a 70-kg patient (or a weight-adjusted 100 unit/kg dose) is usually given, and subsequent doses are given in order to keep the aPTT above 300 seconds (HemoTec) or above 350 seconds (Hemocron).

Clinical activity

The efficacy of heparin without thrombolysis in acute MI has been evaluated in two open randomized trials as compared with an untreated control group, but in neither of these trials has there been an assessment of the potential benefit of adding heparin on top of aspirin. Therefore, these results may not be practically relevant. The use of heparin as an adjunct to thrombolysis in acute MI is presently debated. A meta-analysis summarizing data from 26 randomized studies indicated that in the presence of aspirin and with thrombolysis, heparin prevents only 5 deaths per 1000 patients treated ($p = 0.03$), at a cost of 3 additional major bleeding episodes per 1000 patients ($p = 0.0001$). The use of heparin as an adjunct to tissue-type plasminogen activator (tPA), as used in the GUSTO trial, had been based on relatively limited previous experience and is considered questionable, despite being routine at the moment. A subgroup analysis of the GUSTO I study demonstrated that the risk of major bleeding, including intracranial bleeding, increases progressively with an aPTT of greater than 75 seconds without a concomitant decrease in the risk of death and acute MI. Accordingly, and consistent with ACC/AHA practice guidelines, it seems prudent not to exceed this when heparin is used with thrombolytics (see Chap. 25).

The use of sc heparin (12 500 units every 12 h) in the presence of mural thrombosis alone or as a bridge to longer-term anticoagulation with warfarin is more adequately supported by clinical data, resulting in a reduction in the incidence of mural thrombosis, as detected by two-dimensional (2D) echocardiography, by 72% and 58% as compared with untreated control and low-dose heparin (5 000 units every 12 h), respectively. Such a treatment schedule is also generally used in the prophylaxis of thrombotic complications, e.g. after major orthopedic surgery. Intravenous heparin is presently considered a mainstay in the therapy of acute unstable angina because it is quite effective in relieving symptoms of myocardial ischemia as well as in reducing progression to acute MI. However, in studies with longer follow-up, there is only a trend toward fewer deaths and MIs.

The use of heparin at the above-noted doses during PTCA is supported by several studies. Following PTCA, heparin administration should not be prolonged, and there is an additional advantage in allowing a significant reduction of bleeding by early sheath removal. As a result of higher rates of bleeding concomitant with the use of abciximab in high-risk PTCA procedures, the EPILOG trial has documented the safety and advantage of reducing the optimal aCT to 200 to 300 seconds after heparin boluses of 70 units/kg concomitant with bolus plus infusion administration of abciximab. This infusion rate was later used in the CAPTURE trial in patients with unstable angina, demonstrating efficacy compared with "conventional" heparin infusion rates without abciximab, and is likely to become the reference treatment as an adjunct to abciximab.

Safety

A major drawback of heparin use is bleeding connected to its antithrombin properties, as discussed earlier. In addition, heparin can cause other less common complications, including thrombocytopenia, osteoporosis, skin necrosis, urticarial lesions, erythematous papules and plaques, lipoprotein-lipase induction, and suppressive effects on aldosterone synthesis. Thrombocytopenia can appear as an early, benign, reversible, nonimmune form, possibly caused by platelet activation, and a late, more serious, IgG-mediated immune form. The latter is much more serious because of its risk of thrombotic complication and demands heparin discontinuation. It occurs in about 5 to 6% of patients receiving heparin for more than 5 days (e.g., after orthopedic surgery in the prevention of complications of thrombophlebitis), is followed by thrombosis (more frequently venous than arterial) in about 1% of those patients, and is influenced by previous exposure to heparin. It requires prompt recognition and sometimes specific treatment (e.g., danaparoid, argatroban, hirudin) besides heparin discontinuation.

Reports from recent studies suggest that 2 to 3% of patients receiving heparin for more than 3 months develop symptomatic bone fractures and that approximately one-third of patients show an asymptomatic reduction in bone density, as determined by dual photon absorptiometry.

Low-molecular weight heparins (LMWHs)

LMWHs are produced by a variety of depolymerization methods starting from unfractionated heparin. Like classic "unfractionated" heparin, LMWHs produce most of their anticoagulant effects through the binding of AT III, an effect mediated by a unique pentasaccharide sequence found in less than one-third of LMWH molecules. This sequence is sufficient for the inactivation of factor Xa. A longer 18-saccharide sequence that includes the pentasaccharide is required for the formation of the ternary complex with AT III and thrombin. This sequence is much less frequent in LMWHs compared with classic heparin, in which virtually all molecules have 18 or more saccharide units. Consequently, while classic heparin has an anti-factor Xa to anti-thrombin ratio of 1:1, LMWHs have a ratio varying between 4:1 and 2:1 depending on their molecular size distribution.

Mechanism of action

Depolymerization of standard heparin into LMWH results in five main changes in its properties, all due to reduced

Table 74.5 Differential characteristics of standard heparin, low-molecular weight heparins (LMWHs) and hirudin

Standard heparin	LMWHs	Hirudin
Inhibits to the same extent thrombin and factor Xa generation, less factors IXa and XIa	Mostly inhibit Xa, inhibits thrombin less effectively	Specific and potent thrombin inhibitor
Dependent on antithrombin III	Dependent on antithrombin III	Independent on antithrombin III
Neutralized by heparinase, many plasma proteins, platelet factor 4, fibrin monomers, avid binding to endothelium and macrophages	Neutralized by heparinase, weak binding to endothelium	Not neutralized by heparinase, endothelium, macrophages, plasma proteins, fibrin monomers
Does not inactivate thrombin and factor Xa bound to clot	Does not inactivate thrombin and factor Xa bound to clot	Inactivates thrombin bound to clot
Inhibits thrombin-induced platelet function, may activate platelets	Inhibits thrombin-induced platelet function, may activate platelets	Inhibits thrombin-induced platelet function, does not otherwise activate platelets
Thrombocytopenia not rare	May induce thrombocytopenia	Does not induce thrombocytopenia
Bioavailability after subcutaneous injection around 30%	Bioavailability after sc injection >90%	Bioavailability after sc injection around 85%
Nonlinear dose-effect relationship	Linear dose-effect relationship	Linear dose-effect relationship
Not immunogenic	Not immunogenic	Weakly immunogenic
Constantly induces some transient elevation of hepatic enzymes	May induce some transient elevation of hepatic enzymes	No hepatic toxicity
Increases vascular permeability	No increase in vascular permeability	No increase in vascular permeability

binding of LMWHs to proteins or cells: (1) reduced ability to catalyze AT III–mediated thrombin inactivation, (2) reduced nonspecific binding to plasma proteins, resulting in an increase in the predictability of the dose-response relationship, (3) reduced binding to endothelial cells and macrophages, with a marked reduction in the fast saturable component of the heparin plasma disappearance curve and consequent increase in plasma half-life, (4) reduced binding to platelets and platelet factor IV, accounting for a lower incidence of heparin-induced thrombocytopenia, and (5) reduced binding to osteoblasts and reduced osteoclast activation, resulting in less bone loss. Although the original hypothesis on the anticoagulant action of LMWHs held that this was mainly due to upstream inhibition of the coagulation cascade through factor Xa inhibition, more recent studies have shown that thrombin inactivation is still likely to be the main mechanism of action.

Pharmacokinetics

LMWHs are characterized by excellent bioavailability by the sc route and a very predictable anticoagulant response when administered in fixed doses. Lesser binding to von Willebrand factor may explain the fewer bleeding complications for equivalent anticoagulant effects. Lesser binding to endothelial cells can explain the longer plasma half-life (2-4 times longer than heparin). LMWHs are mainly excreted by the renal route.

Pharmacodynamics, efficacy, and safety

Since the use of heparin in conjunction with aspirin is the antithrombotic treatment of choice for unstable angina and non-Q-wave MI, and since LMWHs have proved successful in substituting for heparin in the treatment of venous thromboembolism, a number of recent studies have investigated the use of LMWHs instead of standard heparin in unstable coronary syndromes. Four randomized trials comparing LMWH with standard heparin in acute coronary syndromes have been reported. The first was a small open-label trial comparing nadroparine versus standard heparin as an adjunct to aspirin in unstable angina and suggested a reduction by LMWH of the subsequent risk of acute MI. This prompted further investigation. In the FRISC study, another LMWH, dalteparin, was administered at 120 anti-factor Xa units/kg bid for 6 days in 1506 patients with unstable angina and non-Q-wave MI, followed by 7500 units qd for 35 to 45 days. The control group received placebo injections. The study showed the efficacy of dalteparin in decreasing the short-term risk of acute MI, but there was some rebound after cessation of the high-dose treatment, and the trial was not controlled with standard heparin. In the FRIC study, dalteparin at the same dosage used in the first phase of the FRISC study (120 units/kg bid) was compared with standard heparin infusion for 6 days in an open randomized design. In the second phase, a double-blind comparison of LMWH con-

tinuation (7500 units qd) or placebo (instead of standard heparin) was performed. The two treatments were equivalent in terms of efficacy and safety. However, after 6 days, dalteparin was no more effective than placebo, a finding consistent with the results of the FRISC study. The fourth study, the ESSENCE trial, randomized 3171 patients with unstable angina or non-Q-wave MI to another LMWH, enoxaparin, at 100 units/kg bid or standard heparin infusion. Mean duration of treatment was 2.6 days. Death, MI, and recurrent angina were less common in the LMWH group at 14 and 30 days. Most of the difference was accounted for by a lower incidence of recurrent angina. There were no differences in the incidence of major bleeding at 30 days. Thus, in this study, LMWH proved superior to standard heparin in the management of unstable coronary syndromes. A recent comparison between LWMH and heparin in the treatment of stroke in patients with atrial fibrillation did not provide evidence for LMWH superiority.

Besides data on bleeding, safety data on LMWHs suggest that they do not cross the placenta, like standard heparin, and that they are safe and effective in pregnancy. There is a suggestion that their long-term use may be associated with less incidence of osteoporosis. Immune thrombocytopenia and consequent thrombosis also may be less than with standard heparin, although there is a clear cross-reaction with standard heparin. Because of this cross-reactivity, LMWHs are contraindicated in the treatment of acute heparin-induced thrombocytopenia.

Direct thrombin inhibitors

Mechanism of action

Unlike standard heparin and LMWHs, direct thrombin inhibitors act independently of AT IIII and inactivate both free thrombin and thrombin bound to fibrin. Direct thrombin inhibitors include hirudin, synthetic hirudin fragments (hirugen and hirulog), low-molecular-weight inhibitors that act directly on the thrombin active site [D-Phe-Pro-ArgCH$_2$Cl (PPACK) and its derivative, argatroban], and the newly described thrombin-binding DNA aptamer. A comparison of the general properties of this class of compounds with those of standard heparin and LMWHs is given in Table 74.5. Clinical trials in atherothrombotic syndromes have been performed with hirudin and hirulog.

Pharmacokinetics

The best known thrombin inhibitors, i.e., hirudin, hirulog, and argatroban, have a pattern of linear disappearance from the circulation when administered intravenously. Their pharmacokinetic properties, in addition to the lack of cofactor requirement, result in stable and reproducible anticoagulation.

Efficacy and safety

The GUSTO-II trials evaluated the efficacy and safety of recombinant hirudin in patients with acute chest pain with or without ST-segment elevation. The first phase of the trial, GUSTO-IIA, was stopped prematurely after enrollment of more than 2 500 patients because of excess bleeding in patients receiving hirudin. The dose subsequently was reduced to a 0.10 mg/kg bolus and a 0.1 mg/kg per hour infusion for the second phase. In GUSTO II-B, the primary endpoint — death or nonfatal MI at 30 days — occurred in 8.9% of patients with hirudin and 9.8% with heparin ($p = 0.06$). The benefit was much more striking during the first 24 hours (1.3 versus 2.1%, risk reduction 25%, $p = 0.001$). The Organization to Assess Strategies for Ischemic Syndromes (OASIS) pilot study used an intermediate dose of hirudin, a 0.4 mg/kg bolus and 0.15 mg/kg per hour infusion, with dose titration to achieve an aPTT value of 60 to 100 seconds. The rate of death, MI, and refractory angina at 7 days was reduced from 7.1% with heparin to 3.7% with hirudin ($p = 0.15$). When severe angina also was included, the difference was statistically significant ($p = 0.05$). Based on this study, a larger study enrolling more than 10 000 patients has been performed. A preliminary report confirms the significant benefit over standard heparin in acute coronary syndromes. The other direct thrombin inhibitor that has undergone phase III evaluation, hirulog, has been tested in the TIMI 7 trial, a randomized, double-blind study of hirulog, given with 325 mg per day of aspirin to 410 patients with unstable angina. Patients received a constant infusion of hirulog for 72 hours at one of four doses: 0.02 ($n = 160$), 0.25 ($n = 81$), 0.5 ($n = 88$), and 1.0 ($n = 81$) mg/kg per hour. The primary efficacy endpoint was "unsatisfactory outcome," defined as death, nonfatal MI, rapid clinical deterioration, or recurrent ischemic pain at rest with ECG changes by 72 hours. Unsatisfactory outcome was not different among the four dose groups: 8.1, 6.2, 11.4, and 6.2% ($p = NS$). However, the secondary endpoint of death or nonfatal MI through hospital discharge occurred in 10.0% of patients treated with 0.02 mg/kg per hour compared with 3.2% of patients treated with the three higher doses of hirulog (0.25, 0.5, and 1.0 mg/kg per hour, $p = 0.008$). Results of recent angiographic studies also support some superiority of hirulog as well as hirudin over standard heparin in increasing patency associated with thrombolysis.

ORAL ANTICOAGULANTS

Oral anticoagulants are the mainstay of long-term anticoagulation. They include a number of substances antagonizing the effects of vitamin K and belonging to either coumarin (dicumarol, warfarin, acenocoumarol, phenprocoumon) and indanedionic derivatives (phenindione). The largest experience has been obtained with warfarin, which therefore will be discussed as the prototypical drug of this family.

Mechanism of action

The anticoagulant effect of coumarin derivatives occurs by interference with the carboxylation of glutamic acid residues on a number of coagulation factors synthesized by the liver, namely, prothrombin and factors VII, IX, and X. Two natural anticoagulants, protein C and protein S, also require analogous carboxylation to be active. Glutamic acid gamma-carboxylation is required by these coagulation factors to allow their binding to Ca^{2+} and, indirectly, to a negatively charged phospholipid surface and occurs in the presence of the reduced form of vitamin K, to which oral anticoagulants have a close structural resemblance, competing for one or two enzymes implicated in vitamin K reduction.

Pharmacokinetics

Warfarin is a racemic mixture of two enantiomers, the *R* and *S* forms, the latter being about 5 times more potent than the former. It has an excellent bioavailability after oral administration, is rapidly absorbed from the GI tract, reaches a peak plasma concentration in about 2 to 8 hours, and has a plasma half-life of 25 to 60 hours. Warfarin circulates bound to plasma proteins and rapidly accumulates in the liver. Variability in drug metabolism as well as numerous dietary and environmental factors affect the kinetics and anticoagulant effects of warfarin. In particular genetically regulated CYP2C9 metabolic handling recently has been shown to dramatically affect warfarin metabolism. Patients with a variant allele may be at higher risk of bleeding complications. A large number of drugs can affect warfarin pharmacokinetics by interfering with absorption (e.g., cholestyramine) or by inhibiting the metabolic clearance of one or both enantiomers. Food can affect warfarin effects by altering its absorption or metabolic clearance or by supplying large amounts of antagonizing vitamin K. Phylloquinone in plant material and in vegetarian diets is the main source of vitamin K and is possibly associated with seasonal fluctuations in warfarin sensitivity in subjects receiving long-term therapy. Drugs affecting hemostasis independent of warfarin's mode of action can potentiate warfarin-associated bleeding; this is the case for aspirin, other NSAIDs, and high-dose β-lactam antibiotics. A combination of aspirin 100 mg per day and high-intensity warfarin (INR 3.0-4.5) has been used in patients at high risk of thromboembolic events, such as those with prosthetic heart valves. In this setting, this combination increases the risk of minor hemorrhage with a trend for increased risk of major bleeding. Hereditary resistance to warfarin has been described, with some patients requiring 10 times higher doses than average.

Pharmacodynamics

Traditionally, the prothrombin time (PT) has been used to monitor oral anticoagulant therapy. This test is sensitive to decreases in the activity of factors II, VII, and X in both pathways of blood coagulation. At the beginning of warfarin therapy, these factors are reduced in their plasma activity at a rate proportional to their half-life, which is minimum (6 h) for factor VII and maximum (60 h) for prothrombin. Since there is some evidence that most of the antithrombotic effect of warfarin is related to the decrease in prothrombin activity, it is likely that the initial PT values do not closely reflect the antithrombotic activity of the drug. Also, depression in the activity of the anticoagulant proteins C and S, having half-lives shorter than prothrombin, possibly can cause a transient prothrombotic state at the beginning of warfarin therapy when started with loading doses that may cause skin necrosis. This supports the use of a lower dose of warfarin (around 5 mg) from the beginning of warfarin therapy; this would be associated with a similar rate of lowering of prothrombin levels but a slower decline in protein C as compared with higher doses.

Thromboplastins used in the PT test vary widely in their responsiveness to the anticoagulant effect of warfarin depending on their origin, phospholipid content, and method of preparation. When the PT was expressed in seconds or as a ratio of the patient's plasma to a normal pool of plasmas, there was no generalization of indications for an appropriate therapeutic range. This problem is overcome by expressing the PT as the *International Normalized Ratio* (INR), which is given by the formula INR = (patient PT/plasma pool control PT) elevated to ISI, where ISI (International Sensitivity Index) is a measure of the responsiveness of a given thromboplastin to the reduction of the vitamin K-dependent factors compared with the World Health Organization (WHO) International Reference Thromboplastin, which is given the value of 1.0. Therefore, the INR corrects and normalizes the PT ratio as a function of the sensitivity of the reagent, thus allowing comparability of values among laboratories using different reagents.

Efficacy

Both the efficacy and safety of warfarin depend on maintaining the INR in the therapeutic range. This requires balancing the thrombotic and hemorrhagic risks of the individual patient in consideration of the underlying disease. The optimal therapeutic range has been reviewed repeatedly by the Consensus Conference on Antithrombotic Therapy of the American College of Chest Physicians (ACCP) and the National Heart, Lung and Blood Institute (NHLBI), most recently in 1998. At present, a recommendation of a target INR of 2.5 (range 2.0-3.0) is made for most indications. Exceptions are patients with mechanical heart valves and some patients with venous thrombosis and the antiphospholipid antibody syndrome, for whom a target INR of 3.0 (range 2.5-3.5) is recommended. Results of a number of studies have indicated that the effectiveness of warfarin is reduced for INR values of less than 2.0 and is practically lost for values of less than 1.5, with the exception of the recently reported Thrombosis Prevention Trial, which showed efficacy in the reduction of myocardial ischemic events when the PT was used at a targeted range of 1.3 to 1.8. Results do not support the use of unadjusted, fixed-dose warfarin.

With regard to atherothrombosis, the following conclusions from clinical trials can be drawn:
- primary prevention of MI has been investigated in the Thrombosis Prevention Trial, in which 5499 men at high risk of ischemic heart disease were treated with low-

intensity warfarin (targeted INR 1.3-1.8), low-dose aspirin, both, or neither. The primary outcome was the occurrence of acute ischemic coronary events (coronary death and nonfatal MI). The event rate was 1.4% per year in the placebo group. A nonsignificant reduction in the primary outcome by 22 and 23% was seen in the warfarin and aspirin groups, respectively, whereas the combination produced a highly significant ($p = 0.006$) reduction by 34%. Combined treatment also was associated, however, with an increased risk of hemorrhagic stroke;
- studies performed in the 1960s provided some evidence that moderate-intensity anticoagulation with warfarin (INR 2.0-3.0) is effective in preventing stroke and venous thromboembolism in patients with acute MI. Analysis of pooled data indicated a 20% reduction in mortality and nonfatal reinfarction. More recent studies have reopened interest in this area. In the Sixty-Plus Reinfarction Study, patients over age 60 who had been treated with oral anticoagulants for at least 6 months were assigned to continuation of therapy or to its withdrawal. Patients continuing to receive oral anticoagulants had fewer reinfarctions and stroke than control patients. In the WARIS study, a 50% reduction in the incidence of the combined endpoint of recurrent infarction, stroke, and death was observed. The recently reported ASPECT study also showed a consistent greater than 50% reduction in reinfarction and a 40% reduction in stroke. All three studies used high-intensity regimens (INR 2.7-4.8), and all reported an increased incidence of bleeding in patients treated with anticoagulants. Indirectly supporting evidence for the efficacy of such regimens comes from a recently reported randomized trial in patients with peripheral arterial disease, in which a high-intensity regimen produced a statistically significant 50% reduction in mortality. In contrast, the CARS study showed no greater effectiveness of fixed low-dose warfarin plus aspirin compared with aspirin alone in the long-term management of MI patients. Cumulatively, these results indicate efficacy of high-intensity regimens that has to be balanced with some increase in bleeding.

Safety

Bleeding is the main complication of warfarin therapy. Main factors affecting the bleeding risk are the intensity of anticoagulation, the patient's underlying clinical disorder, and the concomitant use of aspirin. Four randomized trials have shown that the risk of clinically important bleeding can be reduced by lowering the therapeutic range from high (INR 3.0-4.5) to moderate intensity (INR 2.0–3.0). Bleeding risk also increases with age over 65, a history of stroke or GI bleeding, atrial fibrillation, and the presence of renal insufficiency or anemia. The enhanced sensitivity of elderly people to warfarin may be caused by a reduced clearance. The other most important side effect of warfarin is skin necrosis, which occurs usually between days 3 and 8 of therapy and is caused by extensive thrombosis of venules and capillaries in the subcutaneous fat. A role for iatrogenic deficiency of protein C and S has been strongly suspected, although the mechanism(s) for skin localization of the complications is still speculative. Oral anticoagulants are teratogenic, especially during the first trimester of pregnancy, and therefore should be avoided in this setting.

FIBRINOLYTIC AGENTS

All thrombolytics are activators of plasminogen, catalyzing – directly or indirectly – its conversion to the active enzyme plasmin, which in turn degrades fibrin and thereby contributes to the dissolution of a clot. Prourokinase, urokinase, tissue-type plasminogen activator (tPA), and tPA mutants represent natural human products or derivatives. Streptokinase, plasminogen-streptokinase complexes, staphylokinase, and bat tPA are nonhuman products.

Pharmacokinetics

Streptokinase is a single-chain, 414-amino-acid nonenzymatic protein synthesized by various families of hemolytic streptococci with a molecular weight of about 50,000 Da. Streptokinase does not activate plasminogen directly but rather through the initial formation of a 1:1 complex with plasminogen, subsequently becoming activated to plasmin through a conformational change. Most subjects have measurable levels of antibodies to streptokinase, likely as a result of previous streptococcal infections. The levels of these antibodies may influence the outcome of fibrinolysis with streptokinase. Since there is a clear-cut increase in the titer of these antibodies for 4 to 6 months after thrombolysis with streptokinase, the drug may be ineffective during this time.

Anisoylated plasminogen-streptokinase complex (APSAC, anistreplase) is a 1:1 noncovalent complex between human Lys-plasminogen and streptokinase. The reversible acylation (anisoylation) of the catalytic nucleus protects the activity of the complex for some time after injection, ensuring a longer half-life (70 versus 25 minutes for streptokinase) of the fibrinolytic activity. The active complex after deacylation is a direct activator of plasminogen. Antibodies against streptokinase also can interfere with APSAC activity.

Urokinase (twin-chain, urokinase-type plasminogen activator, tcuPA, saruplase) is a serine protease first isolated from human urine and then obtained from cultured renal embryonic cells. Urokinase is a direct plasminogen activator without specific affinity for fibrin, thereby also activating free plasminogen and leading to a consumption of α_2-antiplasmin and subsequent degradation of fibrinogen and other coagulation factors.

Prourokinase (single-chain, urokinase-like plasminogen activator, scuPA) is the single-chain precursor of urokinase now obtained by recombinant DNA technology. Prourokinase becomes a direct plasminogen activator by generating the active form urokinase by proteolytic cleavage of a single peptide bond by plasmin or kallikrein in the proximity of fibrin, and this allows for some greater fibrin specificity as compared with urokinase.

Tissue-type plasminogen activator (tPA, Activase, Actilyse) is a single-chain inactive serine protease cleaved by plasmin to a double-chain active form. For clinical use

it is now produced by recombinant DNA technology (rtPA) in the single-chain form. tPA has specific affinity for fibrin. Fibrin potentiates the efficacy of plasminogen activation by tPA by two to three orders of magnitude, due to the formation of a cyclic ternary complex of fibrin, tPA, and plasminogen. Fibrin acts by increasing the local concentration of plasminogen, thus creating further interaction between tPA and its substrate. In naturally occurring fibrinolysis, this results in specific activation of fibrinolysis only on the surface of the thrombus. This does not necessarily occur at thrombolytic doses of tPA. In vivo, tPA has a short half-life with a rapid and slow component of 4 and 46 minutes, respectively.

A number of recombinant tPA mutants have been produced, allowing slower clearance from the circulation, more selective binding to fibrin, greater rate of activation by fibrin, and resistance to plasma protease inhibitors. Some of these mutants are undergoing phase III and IV trials at the moment. Reteplase (Retavase) is a single-chain nonglycosylated variant of rtPA lacking two domains (the index domain and the epidermal growth factor domain) involved in binding with endothelial cells and monocytes. This results in a considerable prolongation of the half-life, with a clearance 4.3 times slower. This renders reteplase suitable for bolus administration. TNK-tPA is a combination in the same molecule of three rtPA mutants; in one (rtPA-K), some amino acid substitutions allow a prolonged half-life and resistance to PAI-1 inactivation, thereby potentially offering greater effects on platelet-rich arterial thrombi (which are rich in PAI-1); by another amino acid substitution (rtPA-N), another tPA variant characterized by a clearance 8 times slower and 200 times more resistant to PAI-1 is obtained. The resulting molecule has greater thrombolytic efficacy in platelet-rich thrombi, shows higher sparing of fibrinogen, and is effective as a bolus at half the dosage of rtPA. In patients with acute MI, TNK-tPA has a significantly longer half-life and less clearance than native tPA. *Desmodus* plasminogen activator (DSPA) originally was obtained from the saliva of *Desmodus* vampire bats. Two high-molecular-weight forms have specific activity in vitro similar to or greater than tPA, a greater resistance to PAI-1, and a considerably higher fibrin specificity, strictly requiring polymeric fibrin as a cofactor. ZK152387 is a variety of DSPA-α_1 obtained by recombinant DNA technology in mammalian cells and likely suitable for bolus administration. Staphylokinase, produced by some strains of staphylococci, is similar to streptokinase in being an indirect plasminogen activator and by forming 1:1 complexes with plasminogen. At variance with streptokinase, staphylokinase shows some fibrin specificity due to the rapid inhibition of the free plasmin-staphylokinase complex in plasma by α_2-antiplasmin and a reduction by more than 100-fold in the rate of inhibition on the fibrin surface. Recombinant staphylokinase (STAR) appears to be more potent than streptokinase in the lysis of platelet-rich thrombi and also less immunogenic and allergenic in baboons.

Pharmacodynamics, efficacy, and safety

Clinical experience with thrombolytic drugs changed the standards of therapy for acute MI in the 1980s, whereas initial attempts for use in other acute coronary syndromes have later been abandoned (see Chap. 25). This difference in success is likely due to the different nature of coronary thrombi in the two conditions. Thus, in acute Q-wave MI, thrombosis is most often occlusive and with a large fibrin component (prevalently red thrombus). In non-Q-wave MI and unstable angina, coronary occlusion is usually more transient, mostly due to a nonocclusive thrombus that is platelet-rich (white thrombus).

Three main types of clinical studies have been performed to evaluate the clinical efficacy of coronary thrombolysis. Recanalization studies, documenting the reopening of a previously closed infarct-related artery, are those which have yielded the largest amount of comparative information for different thrombolytics, but they are limited by the need to perform a coronary angiogram before starting treatment. A second type of study evaluates the time-related patency of the infarct-related artery. Such studies can only document the angiographic status after the beginning of treatment and are biased by the lack of information before treatment and by the frequent occurrence of spontaneous recanalization. They often do not show a relationship between (late) patency and myocardial salvage. Thus, conclusions about the similarity of different thrombolytics based on the similarity of effects on late reperfusion appear unwarranted. The third type of clinical assessment of thrombolytics is based on indirect markers of patency, such as the persistence of wall motion abnormalities, and global changes in ventricular function, as well as – most important – on mortality. We will consider only major studies with assessment of mortality as the primary endpoint because these can provide information directly useful for translation into clinical practice. The GISSI-1 study, conducted in more than 12 000 patients, showed a global reduction in 21-day mortality from 13 to 10.7% associated with treatment with intravenous streptokiase and an impressive 47% reduction in mortality in patients in whom treatment had been given within 1 hour of the onset of symptoms. A subsequent cumulative analysis of the data from four studies in which a comparison had been performed between streptokinase and tPA showed a total mortality rate of 8% in patients treated with streptokinase and 8% in those treated with tPA. Consequently, for many investigators, the results of the more recently performed GISSI-2 and t-PA/SK International studies were surprising. In these studies, a direct comparison between tPA and streptokinase was performed on 20 891 patients. No significant differences in terms of mortality were detected in these studies, but early mortality (21-30 days) was 8.7%, higher than in a cumulative evaluation of previous studies with tPA. This was interpreted as due to an inadequate anticoagulant treatment in the GISSI-2 and tPA/SK International studies. The GUSTO study more recently addressed the issue of a direct comparison between the two thrombolytics on mortality. Results of the GUSTO study have generated a long-standing debate. Despite confirming in general the open artery hypothesis (i.e., that thrombolytics providing higher early recanalization rates are associated with higher efficacy in mortality reduction), differences are small, albeit statistically significant, and restricted mostly to anterior (as opposed to inferior) MI and to younger age groups.

Two clinical studies with mortality as the primary endpoint have been performed so far with reteplase in patients with acute MI. The INJECT study was aimed at demonstrating at least the equivalence of reteplase as compared with streptokinase. At 6 months, mortality was 11.0 and 12.0%, respectively. The rate of hemorrhagic episodes also was similar (0.7% reteplase, 1.0% streptokinase). The incidence of stroke during admission was 1.23% for reteplase and 1% for streptokinase. In the GUSTO III study, a comparison of reteplase (at the same dosages noted earlier) with front-loaded tPA (100 mg in 90 minutes) was performed in 12 000 patients submitted to thrombolysis within 6 hours after the onset of symptoms. Results were similar in the two groups. These studies do not allow conclusions on the superiority of reteplase over streptokinase or tPA and do not justify using reteplase instead of streptokinase (much less expensive) or tPA (for which a much larger experience has been gathered). However, the possibility of bolus administration of reteplase in the setting of prehospital thrombolysis would open the possibility of reducing the delay between the onset of symptoms and administration of the drug, which is likely to be one of the next frontiers in thrombolysis in the years to come.

Phase III studies with TNK-tPA are being performed to evaluate this drug as compared with accelerated tPA.

The meta-analysis performed by the Fibrinolysis Therapy Trialists' (FTT) Collaborative Group, pooling data from nine large trials evaluating the efficacy of thrombolysis versus placebo in acute MI, has confirmed that this treatment, performed within 12 hours after the onset of symptoms, reduces 5-week mortality by $21 \pm 3\%$. Despite these clearly positive results, several problems are still open in pharmacologic thrombolysis for acute MI, including the following:

1. significant mortality (6.3% in the GUSTO study) still persists;
2. an effective reperfusion (TIMI 3 flow in the infarct-related artery) is presently possible only in 50% of patients;
3. reocclusion after effective reperfusion is not infrequent;
4. the risk of cerebral hemorrhage during the procedure is still elevated, especially in elderly patients.

AITHAL GP, DAY CP, KESTEVEN PJL, DALY AK. Association of polymorphisms in the cytochrome P450 CYP2C9 with warfarin dose requirement and risk of bleeding complications. Lancet 1999;353:717-3.

ALBERS G, EATON D, SACCO RL, TEAL P. Antithrombotic and thrombolytic therapy for ischemic stroke. Chest 1998; 114:683S-98S.

ANTIPLATELET TRIALISTS' COLLABORATION. Collaborative overview of randomized trials of antiplatelet therapy. I. Prevention of death, myocardial infarction, and stroke by prolonged antiplatelet therapy in various categories of patients. Br Med J 1994; 308:235-46.

BERGE E, ABDELNOOR M, NAKSTAD PH, et al. Low molecular-weight heparin versus aspirin in patients with acute ischaemic stroke and atrial fibrillation: a double-blind randomized trial. Lancet 2000;355:1205-10.

CAIRNS JA, THÉROUX P, LEWIS HD, et al. Antithrombotic agents in coronary artery disease. Chest 1998; 114:611S-33S.

COLLER BS. Platelet GPIIb/IIIa antagonists: the first anti-integrin receptor therapeutics. J Clin Invest 1997;100:55-60.

COLLINS R, PETO R, BAIGENT C, SLEIGHT P. ASPIRIN, heparin, and fibrinolytic therapy in suspected acute myocardial infarction. N Engl J Med 1997; 336:847-60.

GIANETTI J, GENSINI GF, DE CATERINA R. A cost-effectiveness analysis of aspirin versus oral anticoagulants after acute myocardial infarction in Italy: equivalence of costs as a possible case for oral anticoagulants. Thromb Haemost 1998; 80:887-93.

HIRSH J, DALEN JE, DEYKIN D, et al. Oral anticoagulants: Mechanism of action, clinical effectiveness and optimal therapeutic range. Chest 1998;114:445-69.

JACKSON MR, CLAGETT GP. Antithrombotic therapy in peripheral arterial occlusive disease. Chest 1998;114:666S-82.

PATRONO C. Aspirin as an antiplatelet drug. N Engl J Med 1994;330:1287-94.

PATRONO C. ROTH GJ. Aspirin in ischemic cerebrovascular disease: How strong is the case for a different dosing regimen? Stroke 1996; 27:756-60.

PATRONO C. COLLER BS, DALEN JE, et al. Platelet-active drugs: The relationship among dose, effectiveness, and side effects. Chest 1998; 114:470S-88.

TAYLOR DW, et al. Low-dose and high-dose acetysalicylic acid for patients undergoing carotid endoarterectomy. Lancet 1999; 353:2179-84.

VOECKHEIMER DA, BADINON JJ, FUSTER V. Platelet glycoprotein IIb/IIIa receptor antagonists in cardiovascular diseases. JAMA 1999; 281:1407-14.

75

Drugs for the immune system

Torsten Witte, Reinhold E. Schmidt

The immune system has evolved to discriminate self from nonself. It can mount a destructive response against pathogens but normally does not react against self components. The major site where precursor cells of the immune system are located is the bone marrow. Cells of the immune system differentiate into granulocytes, monocytes, and lymphocytes. The lymphocyte compartment is divided into three populations: B-lymphocytes mature in the bone marrow and lymphatic organs; T-lymphocytes migrate and differentiate in the thymus; and natural killer (NK) cells function as immune surveillance of tumors and virus-infected cells. The cells of the immune system are found both in the peripheral blood and lymphatic organs such as the spleen, lymph nodes, thymus, and mucosae.

Defense mechanisms generally can be divided into innate and adaptive immunity. *Innate immunity* is part of the first-line defense against pathogens or tumor cells. The system consists of barriers to pathogens such as the epithelium, acidic pH in the stomach, and mucous membranes or cilia removing pathogens mechanically; soluble factors in the serum such as components of the complement cascade, cytokines, and chemokines; and finally, cells that are able to kill virus-infected targets immediately, such as NK cells or phagocytes (i.e., granulocytes and macrophages). *Adaptive* or *acquired immunity* develops over a period of several days after the first encounter with an antigen. There are several components of adaptive immunity. Antigen-presenting cells take up and present antigens of a pathogen. T-lymphocytes recognize these antigens on antigen-presenting cells and proliferate. B-lymphocytes recognize soluble antigens without the need for antigen-presenting cells and proliferate, provided they get help from activated T-cells.

The lymphocyte compartment consists of three populations: T-lymphocytes, B-lymphocytes, and NK lymphocytes (Tab. 75.1). T-cells are characterized by expression of the T-cell receptor (TCR), which can bind to antigens presented on cells expressing molecules of the major histocompatibility complex (MHC). The T-cell receptor is a heterodimer formed by two chains. Most T-cells use an α and a β chain; a minority only express a TCR formed by a γ and a δ chain. Each chain contains a highly variable domain that can interact with peptides presented on MHC

Table 75.1 Cells of the immune system and their functions

Cell line	Function
T-lymphocyte	Activation of B cells (T-helper cell) defense against tumor and virus-infected cells (cytotoxic T-cell)
B-lymphocyte	Production of antibodies, presentation of antigens
NK lymphocyte	Defense against tumor and virus-infected cells
Monocyte/macrophage	Phagocytosis of bacteria, presentation of antigens
Neutrophil granulocyte	Phagocytosis of bacteria
Eosinophil granulocyte	Defense against parasites, allergic reactions
Basophil granulocyte	Allergic reactions

molecules. The extremely high degree of variability gives rise to a wide variety of TCR specificities. The TCR is associated with the CD3 complex, consisting of a γ, a δ, two ε, and two ξ chains. On ligation of the TCR, a signaling cascade is started that involves phosphorylation of the ξ and ε chains and subsequent recruitment and phosphorylation of the tyrosine kinases lck and fyn and later zap 70 and leads to activation of the T-cell.

T-lymphocytes are generated in the bone marrow but develop in the thymus. In the thymus they undergo a process of negative and positive selection. T-cells expressing TCRs that recognize self antigens in the thymus are negatively selected and die. On the other hand, T-cells expressing TCRs that recognize mutants of self peptides will be positively selected and survive. This process ensures that only T-cells that will not react with self antigens will survive and provides protection against autoimmunity.

The T-cell population is divided into two subsets characterized by the expression of different cell surface molecules: CD4 is expressed on T-helper cells and CD8 on cytotoxic T-cells. The TCR of CD4+ T-cells recognizes antigen presented on MHC class II molecules. MHC class II molecules are surface heterodimeric molecules composed of a 34-kDa α chain and a 29-kDa β chain. Both chains form a peptide-binding groove on which the antigenic peptides are bound and presented to the T-cells. Antigens presented in the groove are derived from proteins taken up and subsequently digested by antigen-presenting cells (APCs). MHC class II molecules are constitutively expressed by so-called professional APCs such as B-cells, dendritic cells, monocytes, and macrophages. In addition, MHC class II molecules can be expressed by almost any other activated cell of the immune system. There are three major categories of MHC class II molecules (HLA-DR, -DQ and -DP) with an extensive polymorphism within these categories. Therefore, the expression of MHC class II molecules varies among individuals.

The TCR of CD8+ T-cells recognizes antigens presented on MHC class I molecules. This cell surface protein consists of a highly polymorphic α chain and β_2-microglobulin. The α chain forms the peptide-binding groove between its α_1 and α_2 domains. MHC class I molecules present octa- or nonapeptides to the TCR, usually derived from proteins synthesized within the antigen-presenting cells. They form complexes with MHC class I molecules in the cytoplasm and are transported to the cell surface via the endoplasmic reticulum. The peptides are normally derived from viruses or bacteria. MHC class I molecules are expressed by all the cells of the body. There are three major categories of MHC class I proteins termed HLA-A, -B, and -C. Within every class there are a variety of different alleles, so the expression patterns of these antigens are highly variable among different individuals.

B-lymphocytes and immunoglobulins

B-cells develop in the bone marrow and home to lymphoid organs such as the spleen and lymph nodes. They are characterized by the expression of the B-cell receptor (BCR), a surface immunoglobulin. On further maturation, B-cells differentiate to plasma cells. These cells produce a soluble immunoglobulin. There are five classes of immunoglobulins: IgM, IgG, IgA, IgE, and IgD (Tab. 75.2). Immunoglobulins are composed of two disulfide-linked heavy chains and two light chains that are disulfide-linked to the heavy chains, except from IgM, which is composed of 10 of each unit. Every immunoglobulin contains a variable region formed by the variable part of the heavy and light chains and a constant domain. The variable regions are formed by random rearrangements leading to a high degree of variability. The whole repertoire of antibodies contains approximately 10^{11} specificities.

Surface immunoglobulins and secreted Ig are products of alternative splicing of the Ig heavy chain. After binding of antigen to surface Ig, a signal is transmitted via the

Table 75.2 The functions of immunoglobulins

Immuno-globulin	Average (g/l) serum level	Function
IgM	1.5	Early immune response, initiation of the complement cascade
IgG	13	Late immune response, binding to Fc receptors
IgA	4	Secretory immunoglobulin, defense in the respiratory and digestive tract
IgE	0.00005	Defense against parasites, allergic reactions
IgD	0.03	Unknown

associated Ig-α and Ig-β transmembrane proteins. Clonal expansion occurs, and B-cells differentiate to plasma cells. During this process, somatic hypermutation takes place that leads to the formation of antibodies with a slightly altered variable region. Antibodies with higher affinities may be generated. In the primary immune response, IgM is produced. Later on, isotype switching occurs and other isotypes, mainly IgG, are formed.

Isotype switching is largely directed by T-helper cells and cytokines. B-cells internalize antigen via their surface immunoglobulin. The antigen is hydrolyzed and presented on MHC class I to the T-helper cell. The T-cell recognizes the antigen via the TCR, and the T-helper cell releases cytokines that direct the manner of isotype switching. In addition to T-cell-dependent stimulation, B-cells also can be stimulated independently of T-cells by specific antigens. These antigens include lipopolysaccharides and other proteins.

NK cells

NK cells are characterized by the expression of an NK receptor. In addition, they coexpress Fc receptor III (CD16). NK cell precursors originate from the bone marrow. They are probably related to precursors of the T-lymphocytes but do not mature in the thymus. Their ontogeny is still unclear. NK cells circulate in the blood and recognize target-cells via various NK cell receptors that bind to MHC class I molecules expressed on the target-cells. Most NK receptors deliver a negative signal into the cell that inhibits the cytolytic machinery of the NK cell and thus protects the target from destruction. However, invaders or tumor cells expressing different MHC molecules are not recognized by NK receptors and are not protected. The NK cells lyse these invaders and therefore form an important part of the first-line defense against virus-infected and tumor cells.

Phagocytes

Monocytes and macrophages

Monocytes circulating in peripheral blood and macrophages present in various organs are potent phagocytes. They contain lysosomes filled with lytic enzymes. They recognize opsonized bacteria via Fc and complement receptors. The bacteria are phagocytosed and, after ingestion, lysed by fusion of the phagosomes with the lysosomes. Peptides derived from the lysed bacteria are presented on MHC class II molecules expressed on the surfaces of monocytes and macrophages. Therefore, monocytes and macrophages are the most potent antigen-presenting cells together with B-cells and dendritic cells.

Granulocytes

There are three types of granulocytes named *neutrophil, eosinophil,* and *basophil granulocytes.* Neutrophil granulocytes are the most important-cells of this group, representing the most abundant immune cell of the peripheral blood. They are able to phagocytose bacteria and lyse them. In contrast to monocytes, they express MHC class II molecules only when activated and are not potent antigen-presenting cells.

Eosinophil granulocytes play a minor role in the defense against bacteria. Their physiologic role appears to be defense against parasites such as helminths. They contain various helminthotoxic substances and are found mainly in the skin and mucous membranes. They are a minor population in peripheral blood, but their number increases on allergic reactions.

Basophil granulocytes circulate in small numbers in peripheral blood and can enter tissues in allergic type I and IV reactions. Basophil granulocytes can produce cytokines such as interleukin 4 (IL-4) and IL-5. On activation via crosslinking of Fc-ε receptors, they degranulate and release histamine, inducing allergic reactions (see Tab. 75.1).

Cytokines

Cytokines are peptides that are released by cells of the immune system. They bind to other cells that express the respective cytokine receptors and exert a variety of effects. A very large number of cytokines have been described. Many cytokines are growth and activating factors. The most important example is IL-2, which is produced by T-cells. It activates and increases the proliferation rate of T- and NK cells as well as B-lymphocytes. Other cytokines are growth and differentiation factors such as the colony-stimulating factors (CSFs) and IL-3.

Proinflammatory cytokines such as type I interferon (IFN), tumor necrosis factor alpha (TNF-α), IL-1, and the chemokines activate cells of the immune system on infection but also may augment autoimmune reactions (Tab. 75.3). Cytokines bind to cytokine receptors expressed on the targeT-cells. Some of the cytokine receptors are detected in serum as soluble products and can antagonize the cytokine effect (see Chap. 51).

Intracellular signal transduction

Binding of a ligand to a cell surface receptor transmits a signal into the cell. Intracellularly, a cascade of metabolic pathways is initiated that finally activates or inhibits gene

Table 75.3 The functions of clinically relevant cytokines

Cytokine	Producing cells	Effect of the cytokine
IL-1	Monocytes, macrophages	Proliferation of lymphocytes, secretion of IL-2, IL-4, IL-6, potent proinflammatory effect
IL-2	T-cells	Proliferation of lymphocytes, activation of T and NK lymphocytes
IFN-α	Leukocytes	Antiproliferative and antiviral effect
IFN-β	Fibroblasts, epithelial cells	Antiproliferative and antiviral effect
IFN-γ	T and NK lymphocytes	Antiproliferative effect (treatment of chronic granulomatous disease)
TNF-α	Macrophages, monocytes, T-cells, mast cells	Activation of granulocytes, proinflammatory effect, protein and lipid catabolism
GM-CSF	T-cells, monocytes, macrophages, endothelial cells, fibroblasts	Growth and differentiation of granulocytes and macrophages
G-CSF	Monocytes, macrophages, endothelial cells, fibroblasts	Differentiation of granulocytes
M-CSF	Monocytes, macrophages, endothelial cells, fibroblasts	Differentiation of monocytes and macrophages

transcription. Although several hundred different receptors are expressed on cells of the immune system, many of these receptors use the same intracellular signal transduction pathway. To date, intracellular signal transduction pathways involving tyrosine, serine, or threonine kinases have been described. Signaling via the TCR induces phosphorylation of the associated CD3 proteins ζ and ε and subsequently zap 70. Further on, phosphatidylinositol phospholipase C-γ_1 is phosphorylated and activates two pathways, the protein kinase C/ras pathway and the inositol pathway, releasing intracellular calcium. Both pathways induce activation of the protein NFAT that regulates gene transcription. Several enzymes involved in the signaling cascade can be influenced by immunosuppressants.

Complement

The complement system consists of plasma proteins, normally present in an inactive state. Challenge with certain bacteria can activate a cascade of reactions (the alternative complement pathway) that starts with activation of the complement component C3 and results in generation of a complex of complement proteins C5-C9, which are able to lyse the invaders. In addition, immune complexes can activate the complement system via the classic pathway. Here, complement components C1, C4, and C2 are used to activate C3 for the catalysis of C5-C9 activation and formation of the membrane attack complex (MAC). This complex is able to lyse cells bound by immune complexes.

Cleavage of C3 results in the formation of two products, C3a and C3b. C3a is an inducer of mast cell degranulation, whereas C3b can bind to the surface of targeT-cells and is the ligand of a complement receptor expressed on leukocytes. Binding of C3b results in opsonization of the target cell and facilitates the immune response of leukocytes against invaders.

Substitution of components of the immune system

Immunodeficiencies

Immunodeficiencies can be divided into humoral and cellular immune defects. Within these groups, primary and secondary deficiencies are distinguished. Secondary immunodeficiencies occur due to other diseases affecting the immune response such as reduction of CD4+ T-cells due to HIV infection and impairment of formation of immune cells due to bone marrow infiltration by a malignant disease such as lymphoma. Common variable immunodeficiency (CVID) is an example of a primary humoral immunodeficiency, and it is characterized by a reduction or lack of immunoglobulin classes or subclasses. The disease usually presents in late childhood or in adults. Patients suffer from recurrent bronchitis, sinusitis, and pneumonia. Selective IgA deficiency is the most common immunodeficiency, with a prevalence of 1 in 300 persons. Affected patients rarely suffer from severe infec-

tions. In the hyper-IgM syndrome, T-cells of the patients do not express CD40. Therefore, T-helper cells cannot induce the switch from IgM to other immunoglobulin classes (see above). The serum of such patients usually contains elevated concentrations of IgM but no or reduced concentrations of the other immunoglobulin classes. X-linked agammaglobulinemia and μ heavy-chain deficiency are other rare humoral immunodeficiencies. In affected patients, the development of B-cells from pre-B-cells is impaired. Therefore, no or few B-cells and reduced or absent immunoglobulins are found. Patients with humoral immunodeficiencies normally present with recurrent bacterial infections of the respiratory tract. In patients with recurrent severe infections, a substitution therapy with immunoglobulins is indicated.

Cellular immunodeficiencies

The clinical presentation of cellular immunodeficiencies depends on the type of the immune cell affected. T-lymphocyte deficiencies are characterized by recurrent respiratory tract infections predominantly with atypical pathogens such as *Pneumocystis carinii* and recurrent mucocutaneous candidiasis. Infection with HIV is the most important acquired deficiency affecting CD4+ T-helper cells. Severe combined immunodeficiency (SCID) is a hereditary form of a T-cell defect and can be caused by several gene mutations. SCID becomes evident during the first months after birth and is treated either by bone marrow transplantation or by genetic enzyme replacement.

Defects of the phagocyte system are characterized by recurrent infections, frequently by *Staphylococcus aureus* and *Candida*. Chronic granulomatous disease (CGD) affects granulocytes and can be caused by several recessive gene defects. The genes encode for proteins that play a role in the oxidative killing pathway for ingested microorganisms. There is no specific therapy, but the rate of severe infections can be reduced by prophylactic antibiotic therapy with cotrimoxazole, clindamycin, or oxacillin. In addition, a multicenter trial has shown that continuous administration of IFN-γ reduces the rate of infections and the number of days of hospitalization (see below).

Treatment with immunoglobulins

Immunoglobulins are pooled from plasma obtained from at least 1000 donors, thus achieving a broad spectrum of specificities. The immunoglobulins are fractionated using Cohn's ethanol fractionation, pasteurized twice, and precipitated with polyethylene glycol (PEG). Because of these purification steps, the virus safety of the immunoglobulin preparations is very high. Normally, more than 95% of the fractionated immunoglobulins are of the IgG class. Some preparations are enriched for IgM.

Historically, immunoglobulins were administered intramuscularly, but today, immunoglobulins are given iv, allowing the substitution of large amounts of IgG. For substitution therapy in humoral immunodeficiencies, 10 to 20 g of immunoglobulin is applied every 3 to 4 weeks. In order to prevent aggregation of IgG, the immunoglobulin preparations are either pepsin- or plasmin-cleaved or dysaggregated at an acidic pH or chemically modified with β-propiolactone. The half-life of most commercially available immunoglobulin preparations treated with acid or β-propiolactone is approximately 3 weeks (range 2-7 weeks). Plasmin- and pepsin-treated preparations have shorter half-lives of 10 to 20 and 2 days, respectively.

The most frequent adverse events observed during immunoglobulin infusions are allergic reactions, chills, fever, rash, and hypotension. Allergic reactions can be caused by antibodies against IgA present in extremely low amounts in the preparations. Furthermore, the IgG fraction can aggregate and bind components of the complement system, causing anaphylactic reactions. Large doses of immunoglobulins (more than 1 g/kg) rarely can cause aseptic meningitis, a condition that resolves spontaneously. In order to avoid major adverse reactions, the infusion rate of immunoglobulins should be low at the start, e.g., 30 ml per hour, and gradually increased up to a maximum of 200 ml per hour. Previously, a few transmissions of non-A, non-B hepatitis were reported. In 1994, after a number of cases of hepatitis C infection were caused by an immunoglobulin preparation, an additional solvent-detergent step was added to the purification protocol; since then, no more cases of viral transmission have been reported.

Substitution therapy is performed in patients with primary (CVID, agammaglobulinemia, etc.) or secondary (lymphoma, AIDS, etc.) humoral immunodeficiencies suffering from an increased number of severe infections. There is no strict schedule, but as a rule of thumb, a serum IgG concentration of more than 4 to 5 g/liter should be achieved, with infusions being performed every 3 to 4 weeks. Doses of immunoglobulins should be individually tailored, based on the number and severity of infections under substitution therapy. Since patients suffering from IgA deficiency are more likely to develop allergic reactions against IgA in the preparations, selective IgA deficiency is a contraindication to substitution of immunoglobulins. No harmful effects have been observed during pregnancy or lactation. Following administration of immunoglobulins, live vaccinations should be given only after an interval of at least 3 months. Antibodies present in the immunoglobulin preparations may otherwise impair multiplication of the organism used for vaccination and prevent the success of the vaccination.

High-dose immunoglobulin therapy

High-dose immunoglobulin therapy has been established as a successful treatment of Kawasaki's syndrome in children and for intervention in idiopathic thrombocytopenic purpura (ITP). For the treatment of ITP, high-dose immunoglobulins are applied in emergency situations with acute bleeding, in pregnancy, and preoperatively to elevate platelet counts. Further indications can be the treatment of autoimmune hemolytic anemia and severe forms of systemic lupus erythematosus and vasculitis. The mechanism of action of high-dose immunoglobulin therapy is not entirely clear. High concentrations of immunoglobulins block the Fc receptors expressed on cells of the reticuloendothelial system. Therefore, autoantibody-bound cells are not recognized and are destroyed by these cells. In addition, the immunoglobulins administered may contain or induce anti-idiotype antibodies that suppress B-cells producing autoantibodies. For high-dose immunoglobulin therapy, either 1 mg/kg of the immunoglobulins is administered on each of 2 days or 0.4 mg/kg on each of 3 to 5 consecutive days. The side effects are identical to the side effects observed on immunoglobulin infusion in substitution therapy.

Cytokine therapy

The complexity of the immune system requires the use of a wide array of signals that can adapt the immune system to different conditions of defense. So far, of the large number of cytokines described, the interferons and IL-2 have reached clinical use.

The interferons, biologically active molecules, can be divided into type I and type II interferons. The family of type I interferons consists of IFN-α and IFN-β. IFN-α is mainly produced by leukocytes, whereas IFN-β is formed by fibroblasts and epithelial cells. IFN-α and IFN-β share the same receptor and are potent biologic response modifiers with antiviral, antitumoral, and antiproliferative activity. IFN-γ binds to a different receptor.

IFN-α Two forms of recombinant IFN-α (IFN-α2a and IFN-α2b) have been approved for a variety of clinical indications. These include malignancies such as hairy cell leukemia, chronic myelogenous leukemia (IFN-α2a only; see Chap. 63), adjuvant therapy for malignant melanoma (IFN-α2b only; see Chap. 55), and viral diseases such as hepatitis B and C (see Chap. 40), AIDS-related Kaposi's sarcoma, and condyloma.

The dose of IFN-α depends on the indication. For the treatment of hairy cell leukemia, 3×10^6 units of IFN-α is injected subcutaneously three times a week. For the treatment of chronic hepatitis B and C, 3 to 5×10^6 units of IFN-α is injected subcutaneously three times a week. Malignant melanoma and Kaposi's sarcoma are treated with of 20 to 30×10^6 units/m^2 of IFN-α administered iv on 5 days per week. Later on, maintenance therapy with 10×10^6 units of IFN-α injected subcutaneously three times a week can be performed. Side effects include flu-like symptoms, fatigue, anorexia, and depression, which may be mild or severe. Flulike symptoms (i.e., fever, myalgia, headache, nausea) always accompany the first injections of IFN-α. They begin 2 to 6 hours after injection and resolve within 24 hours. These symptoms can be relieved by prophylactic coadministration of paracetamol and normally tend to become milder after the first few weeks of treatment (see Chap. 51). If the side effects are not tolerable, a dose reduction of 50% is performed.

IFN-β IFN-β is applied in the treatment of multiple sclerosis. A recombinant form of IFN-β1b (Betaseron) was shown to reduce relapse rates in patients with relapsing-remitting multiple sclerosis. Patients are treated with 8 × 10⁶ units every second day. Administration of IFN-β is associated with side effects comparable with those observed after injection of IFN-α. These side effects include fever, chills, myalgias, arthralgias, and other flu-like symptoms beginning 2 to 6 hours after injection and resolving within 24 hours of injection. Transient worsening of preexisting symptoms of multiple sclerosis and depression also occur infrequently. Simple management strategies can be used to minimize these reactions, including patient education, tailoring the dose and time of administration of IFN-β, and prescribing appropriate combinations of antipyretic drugs (paracetamol), nonsteroidal anti-inflammatory drugs (NSAIDs), and steroids. Side effects tend to diminish with treatment.

IFN-γ Endogenous IFN-γ is a 166-amino-acid protein encoded by a single gene on chromosome 12. Recombinant human IFN-γ is purified from *Escherichia coli* as a monomer consisting of only 139 amino acids. IFN-γ has antiviral, immunomodulatory, and antiproliferative activity. Evidence that recombinant IFN-γ can enhance phagocytic oxidative metabolism led to its evaluation for use in the treatment of chronic granulomatous disease (CGD). In CGD, diminished or absent neutrophil NADPH oxidase function leads to recurrent pyogenic infections and granuloma formation. Short-term prophylactic use of recombinant human IFN-γ (rIFN-γ1b) reduced the risk of serious infection in CGD patients by 67%. Therefore, IFN-γ has been approved because of its immunomodulatory activity for the treatment of CGD. The recommended dosage in CGD-afflicted children whose body surface area is greater than 0.5 m² is 50 μg/m² given by subcutaneous injection three times a week for life. Clearance after intramuscular or subcutaneous administration fits a two-compartment model. The half-life is 3.5 to 7.5 hours, and bioavailability is 89%.

Adverse effects of recombinant IFN-γ in patients with CGD consist of fever, chills, headache, diarrhea, flulike

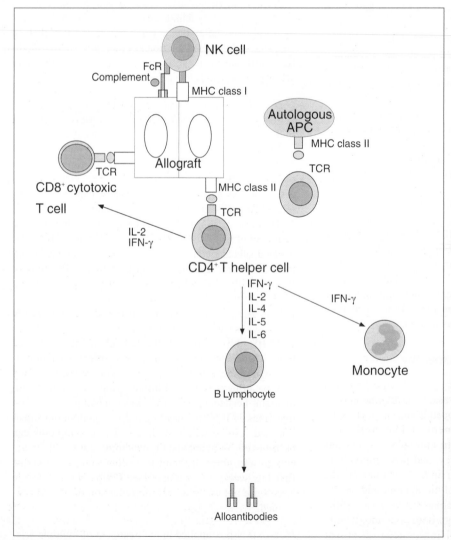

Figure 75.1 Mechanisms of rejection of an allograft. Graft rejection is initiated by CD4⁺ T-helper cells. Antigen-presenting cells (APCs) from the host can present processed foreign antigens derived from the allograft on MHC class II molecules and activate CD4⁺ T-helper cells of the host. Alternatively, CD4⁺ T-cells can directly interact with MHC molecules of the graft in an allogeneic reaction. The activated CD4⁺ T-cells produce cytokines that stimulate CD8⁺ T- cells. The cytotoxic cells recognize foreign antigens of the allograft presented on MHC class I molecules and lyse cells of the allograft. Furthermore, cytokines produced by the T-helper cells activate B cells. These B cells proliferate and differentiate to antibody-producing plasma cells. The antibodies are directed against proteins of the allograft. Cells of the allograft, bound by an antibody, are destroyed either by complement or by Fc receptor-expressing cells such as NK cells, granulocytes, or macrophages. Cytokines produced by T-helper cells also stimulate and attract monocytes that differentiate to macrophages and migrate into the allograft, where they promote an inflammatory reaction. In addition, cells of the allograft can be recognized and lysed by NK cells without prior sensitization.

illness, erythema, and loss of appetite and weight. These side effects generally are mild. Therefore, rIFN-γ is a safe and effective adjunctive therapy for reducing the frequency and severity of serious infections and days of hospitalization in CGD patients. Treatment with IFN-γ is very expensive but, because of the reduction of hospitalization in CGD patients to approximately 33%, nevertheless cost-efficient.

IL-2 IL-2 is an important cytokine that activates T- and NK cells, both cell groups that recognize and destroy tumor and virus-infected cells. Because of its potential antitumor effect, IL-2 was used initially to activate peripheral blood cells obtained by leukopheresis from cancer patients. The activated lymphokine-activated killer (LAK) cells were reinfused into the patients. The patients received IL-2 iv to continue the activation stimulus. In the initial study, responses were observed in 44% of patients resistant to conventional chemotherapy. Since the generation of LAK cells is laborious and expensive, trials with administration of IL-2 alone without prior generation of LAK cells were performed. IL-2 therapy was shown to have an effect in patients with malignant melanoma and renal cell carcinoma, although the combination of LAK cells and IL-2 may be more efficient than IL-2 alone.

IL-2 is infused continuously over 5 days. Every day, 18×10^6 units/m^2 of IL-2 is administered. After an interruption of 2 to 6 days, the infusion is repeated. Then therapy is stopped for 3 weeks. This whole cycle is repeated at least one more time (see Chap. 51).

Side effects of IL-2 therapy may be severe. The major dose-limiting toxicity of IL-2 therapy is the vascular leak syndrome (VLS), characterized by an increase in vascular permeability accompanied by extravasation of fluids and edema. Symptoms of VLS include fluid retention, peripheral edema, pleural and pericardial effusions, ascites, anasarca, and in severe form, signs of pulmonary and cardiovascular failure. Neurologic side effects consist of depression, hallucinations, agitation, neuropathy, convulsions, and paresthesias. Gastrointestinal (GI) side effects such as nausea and vomiting, diarrhea, and obstipation are frequent. Furthermore, oliguria, elevated liver enzymes, hyperglycemia, arrhythmias, anemia, thrombocytopenia, leukopenia, and eosinophilia may be observed.

Due to the toxicity of high-dose IL-2, other schedules are being examined. Recent studies compared high-dose (720 000 IU of IL-2/kg) and low-dose (72000 IU of IL-2/kg) IL-2 administered every 8 hours for up to 15 consecutive doses. Furthermore, schedules of sc applied IL-2 (week 1: 250 000 IU/kg/day for 5 of 7 days; weeks 2-6: 125 000 IU/kg/day for 5 of 7 days) were evaluated. Low-dose iv and sc IL-2 induced significantly less hypotension, thrombocytopenia, malaise, pulmonary toxicity, and neurotoxicity, but it is not clear yet whether low-dose therapy is as efficient as high-dose therapy.

Monoclonal antibodies

In recent years, numerous monoclonal antibodies have been developed to treat malignancies. One approach is to develop antibodies against antigens expressed on tumor cells such as CD19, CD20, or CD22 on B-cell lymphomas. In order to enhance the antitumor activity of monoclonal antibodies, they have been conjugated with toxins. The generation of bispecific antibodies is another promising approach. Thus, an antibody directed against the NK cell antigen CD16 and the Hodgkin's disease-associated CD20 antigen has been developed (see Chap. 63). Side effects, e.g., fever, pain, and skin rash, are mild. However, some patients develop antimurine antibodies. Currently, attempts are being made to generate human antibodies, which should not be immunogenic. The efficacy of an antitumor antibody can be enhanced by coadministration of IL-2, inducing NK cells that kill the antibody-bound tumor cells via antibody-dependent cellular cytotoxicity (ADCC).

Immunosuppression

Suppression of the immune system is indicated in autoimmune disorders and after organ or bone marrow transplantations in order to avoid rejection of the transplant by the immune system due to recognition of foreign antigens. Because the immune system recognizes foreign antigens, noncompatible organs transplanted into an immunocompetent host will be rejected. Antigens determining compatibility of transplants are called *histocompatibility antigens* and are expressed on the surface of the donor organs. They are divided into major and minor histocompatibility antigens. Major histocompatibility (MHC) antigens consist of class I and class II antigens, as discussed earlier. Minor histocompatibility antigens are scattered throughout the genome and have not been characterized completely.

Graft rejections are divided into acute and chronic rejections. *Acute rejection* takes place within 1 month of transplantation, whereas *chronic rejection* is a slow process extending over weeks or months that usually starts months after transplantation. The cellular response in graft rejection is initiated by T-lymphocytes and NK cells. CD8+ cytotoxic T-cells and NK cells attack cells of the transplant organ directly. CD4+ T-helper cells produce cytokines that recruit macrophages and activate B-cells. The B-cells produce antibodies directed against antigens of the graft. The antibodies bind to these antigens and induce antibody-dependent cellular cytotoxicity (ADCC) as well as complement-mediated lysis (Fig. 75.1). Neutrophils appear in the late phase of graft rejection and remove the cellular debris.

In order to reduce the likelihood of graft rejections after allogenic transplantations, MHC-compatible donors are used, preferably relatives of the hosts; to prevent rejection of not completely compatible organs, immunosuppressive therapy is necessary. Triple therapy consisting of a combination of cyclosporine, azathioprine, and corticosteroids (glucocorticoids) is the protocol currently used. Recently, other immunosuppressive drugs have been introduced that ultimately may change this immunosuppressive approach.

Glucocorticoids Glucocorticoids have a variety of immunomodulating effects. Glucocorticoids are hydrophobic substances that diffuse into cells and bind to the glucocorticoid receptor in the cytoplasm. The complex consisting of glucocorticoid and receptor is translocated into the cell nucleus and binds to glucocorticoid response elements in the DNA. Expression of most genes bound by the complex is activated. Transcription of many genes coding for key elements in the immune response is reduced. Thus, the transcription of such cytokines as IFN-γ, TNF-α, IL-1, IL-2, IL-6, and IL-8 is affected. Although the number of circulating neutrophils is enhanced, glucocorticoids inhibit neutrophil migration into sites of inflammation. Furthermore, the activation of neutrophils is reduced. Glucocorticoids reduce the number and function of monocytes and macrophages. Expression of MHC class II and Fc receptors is decreased. T-cell activity is impaired by reduction of IL-2 production.

Owing to their wide variety of immunosuppressive and immunomodulating effects, glucocorticoids are applied in the treatment of a number of diseases such as autoimmune and rheumatologic conditions, as well as for dermatologic and allergic problems. They are also used for the prevention and treatment of rejection of organ grafts.

Glucocorticoids can be divided into short-, intermediate-, and long-acting substances on the basis of their half-life in plasma. For immunosuppressive therapy, usually prednisone or prednisolone is applied. For prevention of graft rejection, steroid doses of 10 to 20 mg/kg are applied on the day of transplantation. The dose is tapered from 1 to 2 mg/kg on the second day to 0.3 mg/kg after 3 months and finally to a maintenance dose of 0.15 to 0.3 mg/kg per day after a further 3 months. On acute graft rejection, 500 to 1000 mg of prednisolone equivalents is injected intravenously each day for 2 to 3 consecutive days. Then the dose is reduced by 50% every 3 days.

Because of the side effects of glucocorticoids, particularly osteoporosis, long-term treatment should be performed with doses as low as possible. In order to prevent osteoporosis, vitamin D and calcium or thiazide diuretics may be given orally to patients treated with glucocorticoids (see Chap. 46). However, it is rather doubtful if these measures influencing calcium metabolism and excretion are really effective. Recently, bisphosphonates have been shown to reduce the rate of vertebral fractures and are recommended in severe osteoporosis.

Glucocorticoids should not be given in an immunosuppressive dose to patients suffering from severe infections. In addition, patients treated with an immunosuppressive drug should not receive live vaccinations. Glucocorticoids are still among the most potent and most widely used immunosuppressive drugs. If administered correctly, they are safe and comparatively inexpensive.

Azathioprine Azathioprine is an imidazolyl derivative of 6-mercaptopurine that was first synthesized in the early 1950s. It has been the most important immunosuppressive drug for the prevention of graft rejection next to corticosteroids since its first application in a clinical trial in 1961. Initially, azathioprine was combined with high-dose glucocorticoids. However, severe side effects were observed. From 1977 on, several trials showed that azathioprine was as effective in the prevention of graft rejection in combination with low-dose as with high-dose glucocorticoids. Therefore, until the introduction of cyclosporine, the combination of azathioprine with low-dose glucocorticoids became the generally accepted standard protocol for the prevention of graft rejection.

Orally administered azathioprine is cleaved to 6-mercaptopurine through hepatic metabolism. Both substances are cleared rapidly from the blood and are methylated or oxidized in the liver and in erythrocytes. The metabolites including 6-mercaptopurine are incorporated into developing DNA and inhibit de novo purine synthesis. Therefore, azathioprine is antiproliferative and affects predominantly rapidly dividing cells such as precursor cells in the bone marrow.

The dosage of the drug depends on the indication. For renal transplantation, a starting daily dose of 3 to 5 mg/kg is given orally from the day of transplantation. After 2 months, the dose is reduced to a maintenance level of 1 to 3 mg/kg daily. For autoimmune diseases, azathioprine is applied as a single dose of 1 to 2.5 mg/kg per day from the start of therapy. In order to avoid an increased rate of infections, the number of leukocytes should not be less than 3000/µl. The therapeutic response generally is seen 4 to 8 weeks after the start of therapy.

Azathioprine is well absorbed after oral administration. C_{max} is reached 1 to 2 hours after oral administration, and the serum half-life of azathioprine and its metabolites is approximately 5 hours. Both azathioprine and mercaptopurine are moderately bound to serum proteins (30%). Metabolites that are functionally inactive are excreted into the urine. In acute kidney transplant rejection with severely impaired renal function, a dose reduction of azathioprine to less than 1 mg/kg per day is recommended.

A large fraction of azathioprine is inactivated to 6-thiouric acid by xanthine oxidase, a pathway inhibited by allopurinol (see Chap. 71). Patients receiving azathioprine should not take allopurinol; if this is absolutely required, the dose of azathioprine must be reduced to 25%.

The most important side effects of azathioprine affect the hematologic and gastrointestinal systems. In patients receiving high doses of azathioprine after renal transplantation, leukopenia and/or thrombocytopenia is observed in more than 50%. Leukocyte numbers of less than 3000/µl require a dose reduction. As a consequence of leukopenia, infections appear in 20% of patients after renal transplantations. Between 10 and 15% of patients suffer from nausea and vomiting. Frequently these symptoms can be relieved by splitting azathioprine into three daily doses. Hepatotoxicity, manifested by elevation of liver enzymes and bilirubin, may require dose reduction or withdrawal of azathioprine. Hypersensitivity pancreatitis, skin rashes, alopecia, diarrhea, fever, and hepatic venoocclusive disease are rare adverse reactions. The rate of lymphoproliferative diseases may be slightly elevated after long-term therapy. Although there are no well-controlled studies of administration of azathioprine in pregnancy, several case reports suggest that the drug can damage the fetus. Since low concentrations of azathioprine and its metabolites are also found in breast milk, the drug should not be used by nursing mothers. Furthermore, azathioprine is contraindicated in patients with severe depression of bone marrow and liver function.

In order to control possible side effects of azathioprine, the whole blood count, serum transaminases, gamma GT, alkaline phosphatase, and serum creatinine levels must be checked once a week until the eighth week of therapy and then once a month.

The most important drug interaction in addition to that with allopurinol (see above) is with inhibitors of angiotensin-converting enzyme, reported by inducing leukopenia.

Cyclosporine Cyclosporine was introduced into clinical practice in 1978. In numerous trials it was tested as monotherapy for the prevention of graft rejection. However, high doses of cyclosporine were needed, and the side effect profile was severe. Therefore, cyclosporine A (CsA) was used either in combination with low-dose glucocorticoids, replacing azathioprine, or in a triple therapy with low-dose glucocorticoids and azathioprine. Triple therapy is still the standard treatment for the prevention of graft rejection and is accepted worldwide.

CsA is a cyclic peptide consisting of 11 amino acids that is produced by the fungus *Tolypocladium inflatum.* The immunosuppression induced by CsA is directed specifically against TCR-mediated signaling in lymphocytes. The signaling cascade in T-cells after ligation of the TCR involves intracellular release of Ca^{2+}, which binds to calmodulin. Ca^{2+}/calmodulin forms a complex with the

phosphatase calcineurin, which in turn binds to several isoforms of the so-called immunophilins. The complex dephosphorylates the cytosolic transcription factor NFATc, which translocates into the nucleus and forms an active transcription factor together with NFATn. The resulting factor starts transcription of the IL-2 gene. CsA binds the immunophilin cyclophilin A. This complex binds to calcineurin. The complexed calcineurin can no longer be activated by calcium, and therefore, NFATc cannot be dephosphorylated. CsA inhibits all genes that are activated by NFAT (Fig. 75.2). These genes include the IL-2 gene but also the genes for IL-4 and CD40 ligands, important for B-cell adjuvant effect. In addition, messenger RNA expressions of GM-CSF, TNF-α and IFN-γ are inhibited.

CsA is administered orally twice daily. It also can be given intravenously. After oral administration, approximately 35% of the dose is absorbed in the small intestine; metabolite excretion is predominantly biliary and to a lesser extent urinary. After oral administration, C$_{max}$ occurs after 3 to 4 hours, and the half-life is approximately 24 hours. Absorption depends on the drug's solubility in intestinal chyme, intestinal transit time, and the composition of bile salts. Therefore, bioavailability is extremely variable. In order to optimize effects and reduce the side effects of therapy with CsA, trough levels are measured routinely. Since 70% of CsA in the peripheral blood is located within erythrocytes and leukocytes, whole blood and not serum samples should be used for measuring drug concentrations. Usually, blood samples are drawn before

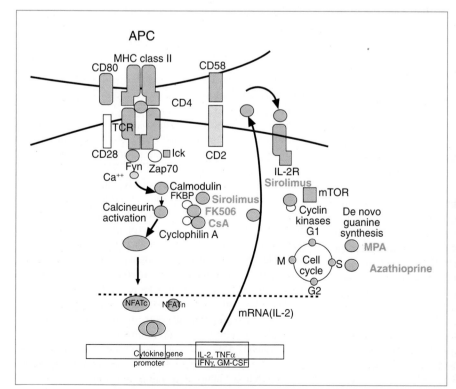

Figure 75.2 Receptor signaling and action of immunosuppressants. Recognition of a cognate antigen expressed on MHC class II molecules by a TCR expressed on a CD4+ T-helper cell and simultaneous binding of coreceptor molecules induce Ca^{2+} release. The complex of Ca^{2+} and calmodulin activates calcineurin. This activation can be blocked by CsA and tacrolimus (FK506). The further signaling cascade involves activation of NFAT and induction of various genes coding for cytokines. Released IL-2 can bind to IL-2 receptors expressed on T and NK cells. The IL-2-induced proliferation can be blocked by sirolimus. Furthermore, the cell proliferation can be inhibited by MPA or azathioprine.

intake in the morning. A new oral formulation (Neoral) has somewhat improved blood level variability.

So far there is no general agreement about optimal trough levels of CsA to be achieved after transplantations. Most authors suggest that concentrations should be higher in the first months after transplantations than in later maintenance therapy. Thus trough levels between 150 to 300 ng/ml are recommended for the first month or by some authors for a year after transplantation, in combination therapy with glucocorticoids and azathioprine. Later on, trough levels between 150 and 200 ng/ml are recommended, and 1 to 2 years after transplantation, maintenance levels between 100 and 200 ng/ml are recommended. In order to achieve trough levels between 100 and 200 ng/ml, usually a dose of 3 to 5 mg/kg per day divided into two daily doses is applied orally. Because of the extreme variability in bioavailability, trough levels have to be controlled once a day during the first weeks of treatment and later once a week.

In order to monitor the concentration of CsA in whole blood, various methods can be employed. FPIA (Abbott Tdx) is the fastest but also the most expensive. Alternatively, HPLC and an RIA methods can be used.

Hepatic metabolism of CsA depends mainly on cytochrome P450 3A4. Therefore, all drugs influencing the activity of this CYP isoform can alter the blood concentration of CsA. Oral antimycotics, particularly ketoconazole, decrease the hepatic metabolism and increase the blood concentration of CsA. Concomitant treatment with ketoconazole therefore requires a dose reduction of up to 85% (see Chaps. 6 and 41). Other drugs influencing hepatic metabolism of CsA are listed in Table 75.4.

Nephrotoxicity is the most important side effect of CsA. Therefore, CsA should not be administered with other potentially nephrotoxic drugs. These include antibiotics such as aminoglycosides, trimethoprim, and amphotericin B. Nephrotoxicity is characterized by an elevation of serum creatinine and urinary protein concentrations. Acute nephrotoxicity in the early stages after transplantation due to elevated blood levels of CsA is reversible after dose reduction. Chronic nephrotoxicity may be irreversible. The pathogenesis of nephropathy is still unclear. The appearance of hypertension may be related to nephropathy. Uncontrollable hypertension may require withdrawal of CsA therapy.

Hepatotoxicity with a slight elevation of serum transaminases or bilirubin is frequently observed in the early course of therapy when high doses are applied. Dose reductions usually solve the problem; severe or persistent cholestasis may require withdrawal of CsA.

Other side effects include hyperlipidemia, hirsutism, neuropathy, gingival hyperplasia, nausea, vomiting, and diarrhea. Cardiotoxicity and neuropathy with tremor and paresthesia require the withdrawal of therapy. Headaches, hyperkalemia, hyperuricemia, anemia, edema, thrombocytopenia, and muscular cramps are rare side effects. CsA increases the susceptibility to infections controlled by T-lymphocytes. Therefore, patients treated with CsA have a

Table 75.4 Drug interactions of CsA and tacrolimus

Drugs increasing the blood concentration of CsA and tacrolimus	Drugs decreasing the blood concentration of CsA and tacrolimus
Azole antifungals (see Chap. 41)	Phenytoin, rifampin
Macrolide antibiotics	Barbiturates
Doxycycline	Carbamazepine
Calcium antagonists	Metimazole
Propafenone	Octreotide
Oral contraceptives	Sulfadimidine (iv)
Metoclopramide	Trimethoprim
Allopurinol	Nafcillin
Amiodarone	

higher incidence of *Pneumocystis carinii* pneumonia (see Chap. 42) and cytomegalovirus infections. At some centers, routine prophylactic treatment with cotrimoxazole is applied.

In order to control possible side effects of CsA, weekly determinations of serum creatinine level, liver enzymes, whole blood count, uric acid level, serum electrolyte levels, blood pressure, body weight, and urinalysis have to be performed in the early phases.

CsA is probably not teratogenic, but no controlled studies are available that have monitored the safety of the drug in pregnancy.

Tacrolimus (FK506) Tacrolimus is a neutral macrolide isolated from *Streptomyces tsukubaenis*. FK506 is a hydrophobic substance whose molecular structure is unrelated to CsA. Nevertheless, both drugs act similarly. FK506 binds to FK506-binding protein (FKBP), another member of the immunophilin family. The complex FK506/FKBP binds to calcineurin, which cannot be activated by calcium. Thus the dephosphorylation of NFAT is inhibited (Fig. 75.2). FK506 inhibits the transcription of the same genes as CsA (IL-2, IL-4, CD40 ligand, GM-CSF, TNF-α, and IFN-γ). Compared with CsA, FK506 is 10 to 100 times more potent in inhibiting T-cell proliferation in vitro.

Similar to CsA, the pharmacokinetics of FK506 varies considerably interindividually. FK506 is metabolized by CYP 3A4 in the liver, and therefore, blood levels are influenced by the same drugs (Tab. 75.4). Hepatic dysfunction leads to accumulation of FK506.

The side effects of FK506 are related to drug concentration. Therefore, the desired blood concentration has to be monitored using an ELISA, microparticle enzyme assay (MEIA) or HPLC. Usually, trough levels of 20 ng/ml are desirable up to 10 days and 15 ng/ml up to 3 months after transplantation. Maintenance concentrations are normally between 10 and 15 ng/ml. In order to achieve these concentrations, tacrolimus is administered at doses ranging from 0.03 to 0.30 mg/kg/day (average approximately 0.10-0.15 mg/kg/day). The oral bioavailability of tacrolimus is approximately 15%, but it shows considerable interindividual variation. The volume of distribution is 0.93 l/kg. The C_{max} is reached 2 hours after oral application.

Adverse effects of tacrolimus and CsA are very similar. However, induction of diabetes mellitus and neuro- and nephrotoxicity are more common with tacrolimus. FK506 is directly glomeruloconstrictive and reduces renal perfusion and glomerular flow. Neurologic symptoms are observed in 10% of the patients and include seizures, psychosis, aphasia, tremors, headaches, insomnia, and depression. Furthermore, hypertension, hirsutism, hyperlipidemia, gastrointestinal symptoms, and gingival hyperplasia may be observed in addition to disturbances of electrolyte balance, elevation of liver enzymes, anemia, and thrombocytopenia. Cardiomyopathies may occur rarely. Like CsA, tacrolimus enhances the risk for infections. Owing to its potential nephrotoxicity, tacrolimus should not be coadministered with other potentially nephrotoxic drugs. In addition, simultaneous application of tacrolimus and NSAIDs seems to be associated with an increased risk of nephrotoxicity. Most side effects of FK506 resolve after dose reduction.

In order to detect possible side effects under therapy with tacrolimus, initially daily determinations of plasma concentrations, blood pressure, ECG, serum electrolyte levels, glucose level, creatinine level, whole blood count, liver enzymes, and clotting should be performed. Later on, these controls may be performed weekly to monthly.

Although it has not been proven that tacrolimus can damage the fetus, treatment of pregnant and nursing women should be avoided unless absolutely required. Woman of childbearing age should receive an adequate contraceptive during treatment. Tacrolimus decreases plasma concentrations of glucocorticoids and estrogens. Therefore, the efficiency of oral contraceptives is decreased.

Tacrolimus has been evaluated as an immunosuppressive agent in patients with bone marrow and solid organ transplants, particularly for kidney and liver transplantations. In prospective trials evaluating patient and graft survival after kidney and liver transplantation, tacrolimus was equivalent or more effective than CsA. In addition, the steroid-sparing effect of tacrolimus was better compared with CsA. FK506 has been demonstrated to reverse advanced cellular rejection in kidney transplants; 74% of patients with refractory rejection of the renal allograft under treatment with CsA had a remission under subsequent treatment with FK506. On the other hand, the profile of side effects of tacrolimus appears to more severe than that of CsA. Therefore, although tacrolimus is at least as effective in prophylaxis of acute and chronic graft rejection as CsA, also in view of the markedly high costs, it is currently used as a rescue therapy, substituting for CsA after episodes of graft rejection.

Methotrexate Methotrexate is an antifolate that inhibits the enzyme dihydrofolate reductase. Enzyme inhibition results in accumulation of inactive oxidized folates and stops synthesis of nucleotides. Because of this mechanism of action, methotrexate kills proliferating but not resting cells and affects all cells of the immune system (see Chap. 44). Methotrexate is used for the prevention of graft rejection but is widely considered an alternative therapy, to be used only if the classic triple therapy has failed. Doses of 7.5 to 25 mg of methotrexate are applied once a week either iv, im or po. Exanthema, loss of hair, nausea, vomiting, elevated transaminases, and susceptibility to infections are frequent side effects. Interstitial pneumonitis and liver fibrosis, as well as cirrhosis, are rare but severe side effects. In addition, leukocytopenia, thrombocytopenia, and anemia, stomatitis, impaired renal function, depression, headaches, and vasculitis may occur. In order to control possible side effects of methotrexate, whole blood count and alkaline phosphatase, γ GT, transaminases, and creatinine levels should be determined once a week in the first month, once every other week in the second and third months, and once a month later on. Gastrointestinal side effects can be reduced by coadministration of methotrexate with folic or folinic acid. Since methotrexate is teratogenic, pregnancy is a contraindication.

Mycophenolate mofetil Mycophenolate mofetil (MMF) is an ethyl ester of mycophenolic acid that is absorbed after oral administration and hydrolyzed to mycophenolic acid (MPA), the active metabolite. MPA reversibly and noncompetitively inhibits inosine monophosphate dehydrogenase (IMPDH), the rate-limiting enzyme in the de novo synthesis of guanine nucleotides in T- and B-cells. All other cells synthesize purines preferentially by the salvage pathway via hypoxanthine-guanine phosphoribosyl transferase (HGPRT) (see Chap. 71), which is not affected by MPA. MPA causes the depletion of guanosine monophosphate and inhibits DNA synthesis. Therefore, it blocks proliferation of T- and B-cells as well as antibody formation by B-cells, whereas all other cells are affected only to a minor extent. In vitro, MPA also inhibits synthesis of glycoproteins and therefore may be able to affect adhesion molecules expressed on all cells of the immune system.

The optimal dose with regard to side effects and prophylactic treatment of graft rejection is 2 g per day. After oral administration, MMF is rapidly and almost completely absorbed. Hydrolysis to MPA is rapid, and MMF itself is not detected in plasma. MPA is almost completely bound to albumin in serum. The half-life of MPA is approximately 16 hours, the major route of clearance of MPA and mainly glucuronate metabolites being urinary. Impaired renal function requires a dose reduction of MMF.

The most common side effects of MMF are gastrointestinal problems such as vomiting and diarrhea and infections. Furthermore, fever, headaches, myalgia, anemia, thrombocytopenia, hypertension, electrolyte disturbances, edema, insomnia, and tremor are observed. Other side effects such as lymphoproliferative diseases, elevation of liver enzymes, or gingivitis are rare.

MMF both prevents and reverses rejection of allografts. Owing to its antiproliferative effect (similar to azathioprine), it is a promising candidate to replace azathioprine in combination with glucocorticoids and CsA. In prospective trials, MMF was significantly superior to azathioprine in triple therapy with regard to prevention of renal graft rejection. In addition, MMF was effective in the treatment of acute rejection of renal allografts. In a controlled trial, MMF reduced graft loss and death in combination with CsA more effectively than pulsed glucocorticoids. Currently, MMF is approved for the prevention of acute renal allograft rejection when given in combination with CsA and glucocorticoids. Several studies concluded that it is effective in the treatment of refractory and chronic rejection of other transplanted organs as well. MMF is also applied as an immunosuppressant in phase I/II trials in autoimmune disorders such as systemic lupus erythematosus (SLE) (see Chap. 47).

Sirolimus and SDZ-RAD [rapamycin and 40-O-(2-hydroxyethyl)-rapamycin] Rapamycin (Sirolimus) is a hydrophobic macrolide antibiotic isolated from *Streptomyces hygroscopicus*. It is structurally closely related to tacrolimus but acts at a different site. It binds in fact the immunophilin FKBP and may interfere with tacrolimus action. In contrast to tacrolimus, the complex involving rapamycin does not bind to calcineurin. Instead, it binds to intracellular targets not clearly defined and called *TOR* (target of rapamycin). TOR is probably a phosphatidylinositol kinase critical for signaling via cytokine receptors such as the IL-2 receptor. During T-cell mitogenesis, IL-2 signaling activates cyclin E/cyclin-dependent kinase 2 (Cdk2) complexes. IL-2 allows Cdk activation by causing the elimination of the Cdk inhibitor protein p27Kip1, prevented by rapamycin. Also, the induction of the Cdk inhibitor p21 by IL-2 is blocked by rapamycin.

Rapamycin is an inhibitor of signaling from growth factor receptors. In contrast to FK506 and CsA, production of IL-2 is not affected. Therefore, FK506 and CsA affect production of cytokines necessary for T-cell activation, whereas rapamycin blocks the reaction to IL-2 and thus inhibits activation and proliferation of T-cells.

The oral bioavailability of rapamycin is low. After single oral doses of 3 to 15 mg/m^2, the peak plasma level is reached after approximately 1.4 hours, and the terminal half-life is 62 hours. The oral volume of distribution is very large, i.e., approximately 12 l/kg. All parameters vary considerably interindividually.

Recently, a rapamycin analogue (SDZ-RAD) with a better oral bioavailability has been developed. Like rapamycin, SDZ-RAD inhibits growth factor-driven cell proliferation. SDZ-RAD is effective in in vivo models when given orally in doses ranging between 1 and 5 mg/kg per day. Although its in vitro activity is generally about two to three times lower than rapamycin, SDZ-RAD is at least as active in vivo as rapamycin due to better bioavailability.

The side effect profiles of rapamycin and SDZ-RAD are not entirely clear yet. Generally, these agents appear to be well tolerated. Preliminary trials suggest that they may cause thrombocytopenia, and hyperlipidemia occurs in a majority of treated patients, advising use of a lipid-lowering medication. In addition, toxic effects on the kidney and gastrointestinal and central nervous systems have been reported in animal studies.

Rapamycin so far has only been applied in phase I/II trials to replace azathioprine as an immunosuppressant after organ transplantations. Owing to its unique mode of action, rapamycin is expected to work in adjunct therapy combined with CsA. Animal models have reported synergism of rapamycin and tacrolimus in prolonging survival of allografts. However, this combination has not been studied in humans because rapamycin and tacrolimus may be antagonistic due to their common binding to FKBP. More recently, its addition to combination therapy with CsA and glucocorticoids substantially reduces the rate of acute rejections of renal allografts. STZ-RAD may have unique effects suppressing graft vascular disease. The early results show that especially SDZ-RAD is an interesting new immunosuppressive drug that may prolong long-term graft function.

15-Deoxyspergualin 15-Deoxyspergualin is a synthetic analogue of spergualin produced by *Bacillus laterosporus*. It is absorbed only minimally after oral administration and has to be injected intravenously.

15-Deoxyspergualin exerts an immunosuppressive activity by inhibiting growth and differentiation of cytotoxic T- and B-cells. It has been suggested that the drug stops IL-2–induced blast formation and proliferation. 15-Deoxyspergualin binds to the intracellular protein Hsc70 that participates in the transport of proteins from the cytoplasm to the nucleus and can be thus blocked. In contrast to CsA and tacrolimus, 15-deoxyspergualin does not block IL-2 production. Instead, it suppresses induction of cytotoxic T-lymphocytes.

So far, 15-deoxyspergualin has only been examined in phase II trials with regard to its efficacy in the treatment of acute rejection of renal allografts. In these studies, 15-deoxyspergualin displayed promising results. 15-Deoxyspergualin was administered in a dose of 3 or 5 mg/kg per day for 7 days following the onset of rejection by intravenous infusion each day over 3 hours. The side effect profile was mild, with nausea, gastrointestinal symptoms, and reduced white blood cell and platelet count. All side effects reversed about 3 weeks after the end of the treatment.

Owing to its efficacy in reversing acute renal graft rejection and its mild side effect profile, 15-deoxyspergualin will now be examined for other indications such as use in combination therapy with CsA and glucocorticoids to prevent graft rejection.

Antilymphocyte globulins Administration of CsA to oligoanuric patients after renal allograft transplantation is associated with prolongation of acute tubular necrosis. Acute tubular necrosis is the major reason for a delayed function of the renal allograft and may be responsible for increased graft failure. Therefore, protocols have been developed to avoid the early use of CsA in oligoanuric patients. Instead, polyclonal antilymphocyte globulins have been applied. These immunoglobulins are purified from peripheral blood of horses or rabbits immunized with human lymphocytes. After infusion of these antisera into humans, the number of circulating lymphocytes is reduced dramatically. This effect is due to binding of the polyclonal antibodies to the lymphocytes and subsequent complement-mediated lysis or antibody-dependent cellular cytotoxicity. In addition, the function of the remaining lymphocytes is affected because functionally relevant cell surface molecules are blocked by the antibodies.

The basic immunosuppressive regimen after renal allograft transplantation involving antilymphocyte globulins (ALG) consists of a combination with glucocorticoids and azathioprine. For therapy of acute graft rejection, 3 to 5 mg/kg of the rabbit antiserum is applied intravenously every day over 4 to 6 hours. For prophylaxis of graft rejection, 1.25 to 2.5 mg/kg of the rabbit antiserum is administered. The therapy is limited by the development of neutralizing antibodies against the horse or rabbit immunoglobulins and normally can be continued for 10 to 14 days and rarely for up to 3 weeks. Since foreign proteins are applied, severe anaphylactic reactions can develop. Furthermore, hemolytic anemia and thrombocytopenia and gastrointestinal side effects such as nausea, vomiting, and diarrhea can occur. Opportunistic infections are frequent.

Therapy with antilymphocyte globulins has not been shown to bring any benefit over the classic triple therapy in patients with good initial function of renal grafts and therefore should be reserved for oligoanuric patients. In addition to application in these patients, antilymphocyte globulins also can be used for treatment of acute graft rejection. Antilymphocytes globulins also have been applied successfully in the treatment of aplastic anemia.

Monoclonal antibodies Monoclonal antibodies (MABs) directed against the pan-T-cell antigen CD3, a complex associated with the TCR, are applied in early acute rejections of solid transplant organs. The monoclonal antibody Orthoclone OKT3 recognizes the CD3 ε unit of the CD3 complex. Binding of the antibody inhibits the effector function of T-cells and reduces the number of peripheral blood T-cells. Most schedules combine CD3 MABs with azathioprine and glucocorticoids.

Daily doses of 5 mg of the antibody (Orthoclone OKT3) are injected intravenously over 10 to 14 days. The goal of the treatment is to reduce the number of CD3+ T-lymphocytes substantially, possibly to less than 10% of the peripheral blood lymphocytes.

At the beginning of therapy, binding of the MABs to CD3 stimulates T-cells and induces cytokine release. Most patients therefore develop severe side effects 30 to 60 minutes after injection, consisting of fever, chills, nausea and vomiting, dyspnea, pulmonary edema, gastrointestinal side effects, headache, and thoracic pain. These adverse reactions are observed primarily after the first injection and are caused by cytokine release of T-lymphocytes, activated by the injection of CD3 antibodies. Adverse reactions can be relieved by coadministering glucocorticoids with the first antibody injection. On the first day of treatment, prednisolone (8 mg/kg) should be

Table 75.5 Characteristics of immunosuppressants

Drug	Mechanism of action	Major side effects
Glucocorticoids	Inhibition of gene transcription of proinflammatory cytokines and arachidonic acid	Osteoporosis, diabetes mellitus, aseptic bone, necrosis, Cushing disease
Cyclosporine	Inhibition of calcineurin and IL-2 production	Nephropathy, hypertension, neuropathy, gingival hyperplasia, tremor
Tacrolimus	Inhibition of calcineurin and IL-2 production	Nephropathy, hypertension, diabetes mellitus, neuropathy
Rapamycin (Sirolimus)	Inhibition of cell cycle progression	Thrombocytopenia, gastrointestinal disorders, hyperlipidemia
Azathioprine	Inhibition of de novo purine synthesis	Anemia, leukopenia, nausea, elevation of liver enzymes
Methotrexate	Inhibition of DNA synthesis	Pulmonary and liver fibrosis, anemia, leukopenia, thrombocytopenia, gastrointestinal disorders
Mycophenolate mofetil	Inhibition of de novo purine synthesis of lymphocytes	Gastrointestinal disorders, anemia, thrombocytopenia
Mizoribine	Inhibition of de novo purine synthesis of lymphocytes	Gastrointestinal disorders, bone marrow suppression
15-Deoxyspergualin	Inhibition of growth and differentiation of cytotoxic T and B cells	Gastrointestinal disorders
Anti-CD3 antibodies	Depletion of T cells	Anaphylactic reactions, gastrointestinal disorders, anemia, thrombocytopenia, infections, pulmonary edema, fever
Antilymphocyte globulins	Depletion of T cells	Anaphylactic reactions, gastrointestinal disorders, anemia, thrombocytopenia, infections

administered intravenously 1 to 4 hours before application of the MABs. The dose of glucocorticoid can be reduced to 250 mg on days 2 and 3 and then further on depending on the degree of the side effects. Because of possible pulmonary edema and anaphylactoid reactions, the first injections should be carried out on an intensive care ward.

Furthermore, neuropsychiatric side effects with encephalopathy, hallucinations, and paralysis can occur. Hematopoietic side effects consist of leukopenia, thrombocytopenia, and anemia.

Reduction of T-cells predisposes patients to infection with cytomegalovirus. Therefore, ganciclovir is coadministered prophylactically during treatment with OKT3 at many centers. Several studies have suggested that treatment with MABs increases the incidence of lymphoproliferative diseases.

Since the MAB is derived from the mouse, repeated injections induce formation of neutralizing antimouse antibodies. These will block the effect of the injection of CD3 antibodies and may cause hypersensitivity reactions. Development of neutralizing antibodies limits the therapy to 14 days. A repeat of the treatment after a second episode of graft rejection would not have an effect and may induce anaphylactic symptoms.

A prior hypersensitivity to mouse immunoglobulins represents a contraindication to CD3 therapy. Furthermore, an infection has to be ruled out before the OKT3 injection is started. Moreover, since this therapy can cause pulmonary edema, patients should be in fluid balance. If necessary, dialysis or ultrafiltration should be performed prior to OKT3 injection.

OKT3 therapy is an effective way to treat acute graft rejection. Approximately 90% of acute rejections can be treated effectively. However, because of the severe side effects, it is only recommended when other therapies of acute graft rejection such as glucocorticoids have failed.

In animal models, MABs against the T-helper cell antigen CD4 have been shown to abrogate acute rejection. Future studies will have to prove if such antibodies and possibly further antibodies directed to other T-cell antigens will exert an immunosuppressive effect.

The administration of soluble cytokine receptors is a further method of immunosuppression. Recently, a recombinant human TNF receptor linked to the Fc portion of human IgG_1 has been developed (etanercept, see Chap. 45). In patients with rheumatoid arthritis up to 16 mg/m^2 of the protein sc twice weekly for 3 months reduced the inflammatory activity significantly. Only mild side effects consisting of upper respiratory tract symptoms were observed (see Chaps. 44-45). No antibodies against the constructs were detected in the patients.

Suggested readings

BURKE J, PIRSCH J, RAMOS E, et al. Long-term efficacy and safety of cyclosporine in renal transplant recipients. N Engl J Med 1994;331:358-63.

EUROPEAN MYCOPHENOLATE MOFETIL COOPERATIVE STUDY GROUP. Placebo-controlled study of mycophenolate mofetil combined with cyclosporine and corticosteroids for prevention of acute rejection. Lancet 1995;345:1321-5.

GALLANT-HAIDNER HL, TREPANIER DJ, FREITAG DG, YATSCOFT RW. Pharmacokinetics and metabolism of sirolimus. Ther Drug Monit 2000;22:31-35.

INTERNATIONAL CHRONIC GRANULOMATOUS DISEASE COOPERATIVE STUDY GROUP. A controlled trial of interferon gamma to prevent infection in chronic granulomatous disease. N Engl J Med 1991;324:509-16.

JORDAN ML, NARAGHI R, SHAPIRO R, et al. Tacrolimus rescue therapy for renal allograft rejection: five years experience. Transplantation 1997;63:223-8.

KAHAN BD, WONG RL, CARTER C, et al. A phase I study of a 4-week course of SDZ-RAD (RAD) in quiescent cyclosporine-prednisone treated renal transplant recipients. Transplantation 1999;68:1100-6.

LINDHOLM A, KAHAN B. Influence of cyclosporine pharmacokinetics, trough concentrations, and AUC monitoring on outcome after kidney transplantation. Clin Pharmacol Ther 1993;54:205-18.

ROSENBERG S, LOTZE M, MUUL L. Observations on the systemic administration of autologous lymphokine-activated killer cells and recombinant interleukin-2 to patients with metastatic cancer. N Engl J Med 1985;313:1485-92.

ROSTAING L, CHABANNIER MH, MODESTO A, et al. Predicting factors of long-term results of OKT3 therapy for steroid resistant acute rejection following cadaveric renal transplantion. Am J Nephrol 1999;19:634-40.

SIBLEY W, EBERS G, PANITCH H. Interferon beta-1b is effective in relapsing-remitting multiple sclerosis. I. Clinical results of a multicenter, randomized, double-blind, placebo controlled trial. Neurology 1993;43:655-61.

SIGAL NH, DUMONT FJ. Cyclosporin A, FK-506, and rapamycin: Pharmacologic probes of lymphocyte signal transduction. Annu Rev Immunol 1992;10:519-60.

SLAKEY DP, JOHNSON CP, CALLALUCE RD, et al. A prospective randomized comparison on quadruple versus triple therapy for first cadaver transplants with immediate function. Transplantation 1993;56:827-31.

SOLLINGER H. Mycophenolate mophetil for the prevention of acute rejection in primary cadaveric renal allograft recipients. Transplantation 1995;60:225-32.

SORENSEN RU, POLMAR SH. Efficacy and safety of high dose immune globulin therapy for antibody deficiency syndromes. Am J Med 1984;76:83-90.

U.S. MULTICENTER FK506 LIVER STUDY GROUP. A comparison of tacrolimus (FK506) and cyclosporine for immunosuppression in liver transplantation. N Engl J Med 1994;331:1110-5.

Skin

76

Major skin disorders

Vladimir Čajkovac

The diagnosis of skin disorders is based on family history (e.g., hereditary dermatoses, endocrine and metabolic diseases, and disposition to allergic diseases), profession, and habits, vital functions, etc. (e.g., smoking, alcohol intake, sleep patterns, appetite, and sexual practices). Many skin diseases can then be diagnosed by physical examination alone.

Nails and hair should be examined carefully. It is necessary to be familiar with the primary and secondary lesions and their arrangements and distribution. Lesions can be monomorphic or polymorphic. If changes are symmetrically distributed, one speaks of exanthema, and one speaks of enanthema if the changes are on the mucosa. Primary lesions are macules, papules, nodules, vesicles, bullae, pustules, wheals (hives), and telangiectasias. Secondary lesions are scales, crusts (scabs), erosions, ulcers, excoriations, lichenification, atrophy, and scars.

Vesiculobullous dermatoses

The pemphigus group

Acantholysis in the epidermis is the cause of bullous changes of the skin and mucous membranes in this autoimmune disease. Acantholytic cells, the so-called pemphigus cells, can be found by the Tzanck test - smears taken from the base of a bulla. Autoantibodies localized on the surface of the prickle cells are responsible for the acantholysis. Such autoantibodies can be shown by direct and indirect immunofluorescence (DIF and IIF) tests in the intercellular spaces as well as in the patient's sera.

Systemic treatment of serious cases of blistering is 200 to 250 mg per day of prednisolone or equivalent. In less serious cases 120 to 200 mg and in mild forms 80 to 120 mg is given until remission. Maintenance doses are usually 5 to 15 mg prednisolone or equivalent. Intralesional administration of glucocorticoids is useful in the treatment of localized disease. Combinations with immunosupressive drugs are recommended: azathioprine in the initial phase, 50 to 250 mg daily; methothrexate, 25 to 30 mg iv or po weekly; as well as cyclosporine, 6 to 8 mg/kg.

The so-called pulse therapy with high, short-lasting doses of glucocorticoids, 100 to 150 mg dexamethasone iv 3 days a month, and cyclophosphamide, 500 to 15 000 mg iv in intervals of 2 to 4 weeks, for 6 months is also used. Combinations of glucocorticoids and preparations of gold intramuscularly or by mouth are effective as well. In the most serious cases that do not respond to therapy, plasmapheresis with high doses of steroids can be tried.

Ideal treatment is with pyoctanine 0.1 to 0.5% aqueous solution, silver sulfadiazine, and potassium permanganate baths. Washing of the oral cavity with antiphlogistics and anesthetics can decrease pain. The application of betamethasone valerate as a "spread dressing" is soothing for an extensively blistered skin.

The pemphigoid group

Bullous dermatoses with a similar clinical picture to pemphigus vulgaris have bullous or vesicular changes with subepidermal separation and without acantholysis and pemphigus cells. Subepidermal separation is caused by autoantibodies directed against specific components of the basement membrane.

For bullous pemphigoid, a systemic prednisolone treatment with 40 to 100 mg per day or equivalent followed after several weeks by a maintenance dose is used. Combination with azathioprine, 100 to 150 mg per day and later 50 to 100 mg per day, may be useful. Methothrexate, 15 to 30 mg iv, can be given once weekly, followed by 5 to 10 mg po in intervals of 12 hours, three times weekly alone or in combination with steroid. In milder cases, dapsone, 50 to 150 mg daily, alone or combined with steroids, 20 to 30 mg of prednisolone equivalent. In the most severe cases, plasmapheresis has been used.

Topical treatment disinfectants (e.g., pyoctanine, brilliant green, povidone-iodine), antibiotic ointments, and antiseptic baths or corticosteroid creams can be evaluated in mild cases. For cicatricial pemphigoid, a combination of glucocorticoids with immunosupressives (azathioprine or cyclophosphamide) is given. Dapsone, 50 to 200 mg per day, isotretinoin, acitretin, and cyclosporin, 2.5 to 5 mg/kg, have been used in the most severe cases.

Dermatitis herpetiformis (Duhring's disease)   It is a benign, chronic, symmetric dermatosis with polymorphic changes of the skin that cause a feeling of burning and itching and the appearence of herpetiform blisters. Often a gluten-sensitive enteropathy coexists. There is a hypersensitivity to halogens. It is necessary to avoid medicaments and foods containing iodine, e.g., seafood. Therapy is dapsone in a dose of 100 to 150 mg per day. The danger of hematologic changes should be observed, and a complete blood count (CBC) should be done regularly. Antibiotics may be used, if necessary, in combination with a gluten-free diet. Topical treatment is by zinc lotion, liquor carbonis detergens, ichthammol 5 to 10 %, glucocorticoids, and tar baths.

Erythematous, erythematosquamous, and papular dermatoses

Erythema multiforme (exudativum)

It is an acute dermatosis with the features of a hypersensitivity reaction. Mild (minus) forms are relatively common, especially in the spring and autumn. More serious forms (Stevens-Johnson syndrome) are rare and usually accompanied by severe general symptoms. Causes are infections, drugs (e.g., antimicrobials, sulfonamides, phenytoin, pirazolone derivatives, barbiturates, and phenotiazines), malignant tumors (especially lymphomas and carcinomas), and autoimmune diseases (e.g., systemic lupus erythematosus, polyarteritis nodosa, and Wegener's granulomatosis). Skin changes are typical. Annular, macular, and papular areas and urticaria-like lesions are seen most often on the hands. Central vesicles or livid erythema is surrounded by a concentric pale and then red ring. Mucosal changes are present in up to 60% of patients. In severe forms, purulent discharge from the eyes and mouth can be seen.

It is important to identify and eliminate the underlying causes. Mild cases can be treated symptomatically with antihistamines, analgesics, topical glucocorticoids, and topical antipruritic or antibiotic preparations; in patients in whom the oral cavity is involved, 1.5% aqueous hydrogen peroxide mouthwash is used. Oral acyclovir may be effective in the prophylaxis of recurrent postherpetic erythema multiforme. Patients with severe forms must be hospitalized, preferably in burn units.

Erythema nodosum

It is an acute polyetiologic dermatosis characterized by eruption of cutaneous-subcutaneous nodules that are painful predominantly in the pretibial region. The main causes are streptococcal infection, tuberculosis, sarcoidosis, *Yersinia* infections, toxoplasmosis, other infections, Crohn's disease, certain drugs, and sepsis. Treatment should be addressed to the underlying cause. If an underlying streptococcal infection is suspected, long-term penicillin (at least 1 year) is beneficial. Bed rest (elevated legs), analgesics (aspirin), and potassium iodide 300 to 600 mg per day by mouth for a period of 2 days to 3 to 4 weeks are given. In more serious cases, glucocorticoids 30-60 mg per day of prednisone or equivalent are used for 1 to 2 weeks. Topically, corticosteroid creams under occlusive dressings or intralesional injections are used.

Psoriasis

It is a chronic inflammatory proliferative epidermal disease. The clinical presentation can be either acute exanthematic or chronic stationary, characterized by dry, well-circumscribed, silvery scaling papules and plaques of various sizes. Lesions can be limited to a small number of foci or confluent in bigger ones or be generalized. Nails are involved in more than 50% of patients. The disease can be associated with arthropathy. Atypical cases are not rare.

The course of the disease is variable. About 2 to 4 % of the white population and far fewer blacks are affected. It is one of the most common dermatoses. A family history (30%) indicates the significance of genetic factors. In psoriatic patients, the histocompatibility antigen HLA-Cw6 is most strongly associated with psoriasis, and the coexistence of HLA-B17 or -B27 is linked with more severe skin disease. A great number of other factors can provoke the disease: physical (e.g., ultraviolet light, X-rays), vaccinations, drugs (e.g., lithium, beta-blockers, nonsteroidal anti-inflammatory drugs), infection (e.g., *Streptococcus*), surgery, tattoos, burns, and many others. Many inflammatory dermatoses involving the epidermis (e.g., impetigo contagiosa, candidiasis, herpes zoster infection) also can be responsible.

Topical treatment has the purpose of inducing flattening or clearing of lesions. For this purpose, salicylic acid 3 to 20% in petrolatum is still used. Dithranol (anthralin) 0.1 to 4% (stains the skin brown) and tar (coal tar 2-5% paste, stains bed clothing) are used, possibly in combination with ultraviolet (UV) radiation. Powerful steroids (betamethasone valerate 0.1%, fluocinolone acetonide 0.025%, clobetasone propionate 0.05%) applied twice or thrice daily, possibly overnight or over 24 hours, under polyethene occlusion delay evolution in most lesions.

Calcipotriol (cream or ointment applied once or twice daily, maximum of 100 g weekly), a vitamin D analogue, has been introduced recently. Vitamin D regulates keratinocyte proliferation and inhibits cytokine production.

The effect of phototherapy (ultraviolet B) is based on the inhibitory effect on increased DNA synthesis in psoriatic epidermis. It is the most rapid and effective means of inducing remission in mild to severe disease, and sometimes it is used after previous photosensitization with psoralens. Methoxsalen is supplied in capsules and is given in doses of 0.5 mg/kg taken 1.5 to 2 hours before ultraviolet A (UVA) exposure. A lotion containing methoxsalen also is available for topical application. It can be diluted for bathwater delivery, a method that produces low systemic psoralen levels. Intralesional corticosteroids injected beneath isolated chronic plaques cause involution within 7 to 10 days and last several months.

Systemic treatment is necessary in severe or recalcitrant cases. Glucocorticosteroids have only a symptomatic effect. After discontinuation, recurrences may be seen in about 80% of patients. Steroids are indicated in generalized psoriasis, pustular psoriasis, psoriatic erythroderma, and psoriatic arthritis, as well as in cases of generalization and cases refractory to phototherapy or cytostatics. Steroid therapy starts with a middle dose (40-80 mg/d of prednisone or equivalent). After improvement, the dose should be reduced.

Cytotoxic drugs may be given to decrease the accelerated epidermopoesis. Because of the much higher risk of side effects with this kind of therapy, it should be tried only if other approaches, e.g., phototherapy, cannot be used. The main indications for the use of cytotoxic drugs are generalized vulgar or pustular psoriasis, arthritis psoriatica, and psoriasis resistant to other therapies.

Methotrexate (see Chap. 44) orally or im should be used for treatment of severe cases refractory to less dangerous therapies. It is given weekly as a single dose or split into two daily doses (12 hours apart) for 24 to 36 hours weekly. An initial test dose of 5 to 7.5 mg is given with careful laboratory monitoring (CBC and liver function tests 5-6 days after treatment). The dose is increased as necessary in 2.5- to 5-mg increments weekly, with final doses ranging from 7.5 to 30 mg per week. The goal is to control but not totally eradicate the skin lesions.

Antibiotics are given in generalized pustular psoriasis, e.g., cloxacillin 500 mg qid for several weeks. In pustular palmoplantar psoriasis and generalized pustular psoriasis, retinoids (acitretin 10-50 mg daily in a single dose for 2-4 weeks; then, according to the effect, 25-50 mg daily) can be indicated. Careful monitoring of side effects is necessary (e.g., liver toxicity, hyperlipoproteinemia, loss of hair, and dryness of mouth). Because of proven teratogenicity, contraception is mandatory. Excretion of acitretin from the body is extremely slow.

Cyclosporine in the dose 3 to 6 mg/kg causes dramatic clearing of widespread psoriasis. The drug selectively inhibits T-helper cell production of interleukin-2 while allowing an increase in suppressor T-cell populations (see Chap. 75). Psoriasis is associated with increased T-helper to suppressor T-cell ratios and decreased suppressor T-cell activity.

Sulfasalazine (3.0 g daily for 8 weeks) has proven to be safe alternative to more toxic oral therapies.

There is no consistently effective therapy for psoriatic involvement of the nails. Removal of subungual debris must be undertaken (urea 40% ointment); then corticosteroids or fluorouracil 1% solution should be applied. Acitretin also can improve the affected nails.

Pityriasis rubra pilaris

It is a chronic inflammatory erythematous keratotic dermatosis characterized by tiny acuminate, reddish brown follicular papules topped by central horny plugs in which hairs are embedded, along with yellowish-pink scaling patches. Hyperkeratoses of the palms and soles have a tendency to fissure. Therapy includes vitamin A 150 000 to 300 000 units orally daily up to several months (maximum 3). Either isotretinoin or acitretin, both in a dose of 0.5 mg/kg, is given for several weeks. These agents can be combined with fluorinated steroids (triamcinolone or betamethasone in doses 20-40 mg prednisone equivalent) po or topically under an occlusive dressing. Urea 5 to

10% or tretinoin 0.005% or more is also used. Phototherapy should be avoided because of its irritating effect.

Lichen (ruber) planus

It is a subacute or chronic progressive inflammatory pruritic dermatosis sometimes involving the oral and genital mucosa and characterized by angular, umbilicated, flat-topped violaceous papules and itching. The phenomenon of striation (Wickham's striae) is especially visible on mucous membranes. It is caused by drugs (e.g., synthetic antimalarials, gold salts, and isoniazid), autoimmune diseases (e.g., systemic lupus erythematosus and primary biliary cirrhosis), and graft-versus-host disease reactions. Most often no treatment is necessary. For hypertrophic lesions, low-potency topical steroids are used with an occlusive dressing; cryotherapy with CO_2 or liquid nitrogen is used if necessary. Oral steroids are given if large areas of skin are involved.. Steroids can be applied intralesionally as well. Itching can be suppressed topically by zinc oxide paste with 5% of coal tar or ichthammol and systemically by H_1 antagonists (see Chap. 77).

Pyodermas

A *pyoderma* is a purulent infection of the skin. Preceding cutaneous lesions, obesity, immunosuppression, white cell drug function, and diabetes are predisposing conditions. Various forms or pyodermas and their therapies are presented in Table 76.1.

Diseases caused by mycobacteria

Tuberculosis cutis comprises a number of cutaneous diseases caused by *Mycobacterium tuberculosis* that differ clinically and prognostically. The causative organism has various characteristics, and the immunologic status of the patient as well as skin factors may have a significant impact. The general principles of antituberculous therapy are valid.

Leprosy (Hansen's disease)

Leprosy is a chronic, progressive infectious disease of low contagiosity caused by *M. leprae*. Acute exacerbations are possible. The disease can cause serious mutilations. Leprosy is a disease of tropical and subtropical regions and is seen only rarely in other parts of the world.

Treatment_____

Depending on the start of therapy, healing is possible. Dapsone 50 to 100 mg is given as a single dose (WHO recommends 100 mg daily, maximum of 200 mg). Rifampin 10 mg/kg is given daily (minimum of 450 mg, maximum of 750 mg) for 6 to 12 weeks, possibly life-

Table 76.1 Various forms of pyodermas and their therapy

Form/Definition	Causative organism	Therapy
Impetigo contagiosa *Definition*: Contagious p. caused by inoculation of *Staph.* or *Strep.* into superficial cutaneous abrasions or compromised skin. Discrete fragile vesicles with erythematous border that become pustular and rupture	*Streptococcus hemolyticus* *Staphylococcus aureus*	**Topical**: Soap + water (prevention); removing of crusts, clioquinol 1-3% ointment, antibiotics (esp. neomycin), risk of sensitization. Mupirocin 2% cream tid for 7-10 days **Systemic**: A group streptococci: 200 000 IU phenoxymethylpenicillin tid. *S. aureus*: 2-3 g oxacillin in 4-6 single doses. Nursed children older than 3 months, 1 g per day in 4 doses.
Impetigo contagiosa staphylococcica (staphylococcal pemphigoid of the newborn)	*Staphylococcus aureus*	Up to 3 months, 50 mg/kg per day. In allergic patients, erythromycin 1 g per day in 2 doses, azithromycin. Nursed and small children, 30-50 mg/kg macrolids in 3-4 doses
Bulla repens	*Staphylococcus aureus*, rarely *Streptococcus*	**Topical**: Opening of bullae, clioquinol, mupirocin **Systemic**: Usually not necessary. In children, PRP, possibly macrolides
Ostiofolliculitis (impetigo Bockhardt) *Definition*: Superficial folliculitis marked by formation of small purulent pustules at the orificies of the pilosebaceous glands	*Staphylococcus aureus*	**Topical**: Opening of bullae, povidone-iodine, clioquinol 0.5%, mupirocin **Systemic**: Antibiotics according to sensitivity
Folicullitis simplex barbae	*Staphylococcus aureus*, rarely others	**Topical**: Disinfectants, clioquinol, 70% depilation **Systemic**: Antibiotics according to sensitivity
Gram-negative folliculitis *Definition*: Superinfection complicating long-term systemic antibiotic treatment of acne vulgaris, particularly tetracyclines	*Enterobacter, Klebsiella, Escherichia coli Proteus*	**Topical**: Disinfectants in solution. Benzoyl peroxide 3-5% **Systemic**: Isotretinoin 0.5-2 mg/kg during 12-20 weeks. Alternatively, systemic administration of antibiotics, e.g., first- or second-generation cephalosporins (parenteral)

(PRP = penicillinase-resistant penicillins [e.g., oxacillin, cloxacillin, etc.])

long. Rifampin can be given for 4 to 6 weeks and then changed to dapsone.

Diseases caused by fungi and yeasts

The dermatophyte (or ringworm) fungi are a distinct and unique class. They live in the human host in the superficial layers of the epidermis, nails, and hair. For all forms of skin mycoses, the term *tinea* has been accepted. Tinea capitis is caused by species of the genuses *Trichophyton* and *Microsporum*. For practical reasons, tinea capitis is divided into three types: superficial and deep trichophytosis, microsporosis, and favus.

Trichophytosis barbae, faciei et corporis

These forms of tinea can be caused by *T. mentagrophytes, Epidermophyton floccosum,* and *T. rubrum,* whereas onychomycoses (*T. unguium*) are caused mostly by *T. rubrum* and *T. mentagrophytes.* An exact diagnosis is essential, and treatment depends on localization, acuteness, and

deepness of the infection. Prophylactic measures are important - avoidance of heat, moisture, and maceration.

A great number of topical products are available on the market, mostly creams, gels, and solutions. Specific antifungal agents (see Chap. 41) are mainly derivatives of azoles. They are the imidazoles (e.g., clotrimazole, econazole, miconazole, oxiconazole, sulconazole, and many others) and a triazole (i.e., terconazole). The allylamines include naftifine and terbinafine and the pyridone derivative cyclopyroxolamine. Amorolfine is a morpholine. Thiocarbamates include tolnaftate and tolciclate, which are active only against dermatophytes, whereas all others are active against dermatophytes, yeasts, and molds. Nonspecific topical agents include Whitfield's ointment, gentian violet, compound undecylenic acid, Castellani's paint (carbol-fuchsin solution), potassium permanganate, selenium sulfide, and urea preparations.

Azole or allylamine creams and solutions should be applied twice daily for at least 4 weeks to decrease the relapse rate. Thick hyperkeratotic lesions such as on the palms and soles may require keratolytic agents such as salicylic acid. Combination of a keratolytic agent under occlusion overnight and an antifungal agent during the day is useful. Whitfield's ointment at half or full strength is another effective keratolytic. Aluminum chloride hexahydrate 20% applied twice daily for 7 to 10 days is useful in interdigital tinea pedis.

Systemic therapy can be carried out with griseofulvin, which is effective against all dermatophyte fungi but not against yeast (i.e., *Candida*) or molds. The drug enters the epidermis by diffusion from the extracellular fluid, reaching higher concentrations in the horny layer than in serum. It is deposited in the newly formed nails but does not diffuse through the nail bed. Onychomycoses must be treated longer. For tinea pedis, 660 to 750 mg griseofulvin is given daily for 3 months; for infections of non-hair-bearing skin regions, 330 to 375 mg is given daily for 3 to 4 weeks. Tinea capitis caused by *T. tonsurans* requires administration for 6 weeks or longer (children: 10-11 mg/kg). Tinea caused by *Microsporum* responds to 250 to 500 mg or 1.5 to 2.0 g griseofulvin as a single dose, which may be repeated in 3 to 4 weeks. Griseofulvin should not be given to hepatic or renal patients, and its main side effects are nausea and headache. It is a potent inducer of liver microsomal enzymes.

Itraconazole and fluconazole are broad-spectrum systemic antifungal agents (see Chap. 41). Itraconazole 100 mg is given daily over 2 weeks for palmar and plantar localization and may be continued for up to 4 weeks. Fluconazole 50 mg is given daily over 2 to 7 weeks. These agents should not be given to patients with liver disorders. Side effects are minor; most frequent are headache and nausea, but peripheral neuropathy and hepatotoxicity are possible. Both agents inhibit hepatic microsomal enzymes, thus potentially causing severe interactions. Ketoconazole 2.5 to 5 mg/kg for children and 200 mg daily for adults for 2 months also inhibits microsomal enzymes (see Chap. 41). Terbinafine is particularly useful in onychomycoses. It is given in a daily dose of 250 mg for 2 to 6 weeks, longer in nail infections. Side effects include abdominal discomfort, nausea, diarrhea, headache, taste disturbances, and erythema multiforme.

Onychomycoses In onychomycoses, treatment may be difficult because of reduced penetration of the drug through the nail keratin. A systemic therapy in addition to the topical one is mandatory. Therapy should last longer than in cases of tinea of the skin or scalp, and cure is verified by microscopic loss of mycelial elements and a negative sensitivity test. All the systemic drugs mentioned earlier (e.g., griseofulvin in a daily dose of 660 mg for 2 to 3 months and, for toenails, even 12 to 18 months) can be used. Before eventual avulsion of the nails, their softening with 20% urea should be tried.

Candidiasis

It is a mycosis caused by the yeast of genus *Candida*. It can affect the skin, mucosa, internal organs, and organ systems (digestive tract or lungs). It can cause a sepsis or endocarditis. Most people have *C. albicans* as a saprophy-

te in their saliva and their feces, and when predisposing factors are present (e.g., immunosuppression, AIDS, X-ray therapy, long-term therapy with broad-spectrum antibiotics, as well as certain metabolic diseases such as uncontrolled diabetes mellitus), *Candida* becomes a pathogen.

Stomatitis candidomycetica (thrush) It appears in neonates and persons with poor oral hygiene, edentulous persons, or persons with poorly fitting dental prostheses, as well as in immunosupressed patients (e.g., AIDS). Topical 2% miconazole gel, once or twice weekly, generally is useful. Nystatin oral suspension (4-6 ml, 400 000-600 000 units, qid) and amphotericin B (as a rinse, 80 ml/kg) are alternatives. Moreover, amphotericin B lozenges qid, clotrimazole buccal troches, and gentian violet 0.25 to 2% may be used. Amphotericin B is ineffective against dermatophytes. Systemic treatment with oral fluconazole 50 to 100 mg daily can be given for 7 to 14 days (see Chap. 41).

Genital candidiasis It presents as vulvovaginitis in women and balanitis in men. Most common causes are diabetes mellitus and medications with hormonal drugs (e.g., estrogens). Vulvovaginitis candidomycetica also can appear in healthy pregnant women. Therapy consists of removal of predisposing factors. In vulvovaginitis, clotrimazole 500 mg daily is applied topically; alternatively, nystatin genital cream can be used qd or bid. If the topical therapy is ineffective, fluconazole 150 mg should be given po. A single daily dose of 400 mg itraconazole cures up to 80% of acute vulvovaginal candidiasis. In cases of balanitis, a mild solution of potassium permanganate or gentian violet 0.1 to 0.5% aqueous solution topically should be tested.

Candidiasis interdigitalis (erosio interdigitalis candidomycetica) It may appear in housekeepers, some construction workers, and athletes (athlete's foot). Therapy includes 0.5% gentian violet solution, lotio alba with clioquinol 0.5%, and topical polyenes or azoles (clotrimazole).

Candidiasis intertriginosa It occurs in obese people, especially diabetics, and has a chronic course. Therapy consists of keeping intertriginous spaces dry. Painting with 0.5% gentian violet solution or 0.5% clioquinol in zinc lotion is generally effective. Nystatin powder, amphotericin B, and imidazole derivatives are alternatives.

Diaper dermatitis (diaper rash) It is the result of a constant adverse local enviroment. It should be treated by observing hygienic measures and keeping the area dry. Therapy is similar to that for intertriginous forms of candidiasis, i.e., nystatin cream with clioquinol 0.5% in zinc oil. Concomitant oral and intestinal candidiasis may be treated with nystatin or amphotericin B 1 mg po for 14 days.

Folliculitis candidomycetica It may occur in the beards of adult men. Therapy involves crust removal with 5%

salicylic acid in petrolatum, wet potassium permanganate or clioquinol dressings, followed by an antimycotic solution or cream. If *Candida* is found in the oral cavity or in the feces, oral therapy with nystatin or amphotericin B generally is effective.

Chronic mucocutaneous candidiasis It is an infection resistant to therapy. It occurs on the skin and mucous membranes and is mostly associated with a number of immunologic defects. If the gastrointestinal tract is involved, oral therapy is with nystatin or amphotericin B; the latter also may be given as an intravenous infusion (liposomal formulation). Miconazole (iv), ketoconazole, and fluconazole (also iv) are alternatives.

Pityriasis versicolor (tinea versicolor)

It is a chronic folliculitis caused by the lipophilic yeast Pityrosporum orbiculare (Malassezia furfur). Typical changes are follicular yellowish-brown to dark brown papules in different phases of development, usually on the trunk. Sometimes a mild itching is present. Therapy is mainly topical; painting with a 50% solution of propylene glycol in water, initially twice daily, later twice weekly, for 3 weeks is usually effective. Shampoos containing selenium sulfide are also effective. Broad-spectrum antifungal drugs, e.g., econazole cream and ketoconazole shampoo, can be used as well. Systemic ketoconazole (200 mg po for 5-10 days), itraconazole (200 mg for 5-7 days), and fluconazole (400 mg as a single oral dose) are also used. Recurrences are common.

Skin diseases caused by viruses

Viruses are causative organisms of a number of dermatoses. Skin changes are either a direct consequence of infection by a dermatotrophic virus (e.g., warts, mollusca contagiosa), or they develop during a systemic viral disease (e.g., varicella).

Common warts (verrucae vulgares) are caused by the human papillomaviruses (HPV). Warts often appear on the distal parts of the extremities, particularly in atopic children. The initial lesion is a pinhead papule with a normal skin color. Changes gradually increase and become keratinized on their surface. Daughter warts can develop by autoinoculation. Common warts also can appear on the mucous membranes. In patients with an inborn or acquired defect of immunity, dissemination can occur (verrucosis generalisata). Cryosurgery with liquid nitrogen is the therapy of choice. Light electrodesiccation and curettage and keratolytic therapy (with paints such as 5-20% salicylic acid and 5-20% lactic acid in flexible collodion) are also used. Alternatives are cantharidin (a mitochondrial poison derived from the blister beetle *Cantharis vesiccatoria*), which causes changes in cell membranes, epidermal cell dyshesion, acantholysis, and blister formation, and podophyllum resin (a cytotoxic agent that arrests mitosis in metaphase), which is used primarily for condyloma acuminata.

Verrucae planae juveniles (flat juvenile warts)

It occur very often in children and adolescents. They occur suddenly and in large numbers on the backs of the hands, in the temporal region, and on the face and forearms. Papules are round or oval, rarely polygonal, and grayish- yellowish or yellowish-brown in color. Treatment consists of short application (5-15 s) of liquid nitrogen.

Condylomata acuminata (genital warts)

Genital warts are located in intertriginous regions, most often on the genitals or in the perigenital or perianal region. Clinically they resemble cauliflowers and can reach the size of a fist. Therapy consists of topical use of 25% podophyllum resin (weekly painting), provided that a thin covering of petrolatum around the lesion before therapy is ensured. Liquid nitrogen therapy must be repeated every 2 to 3 weeks. Interferon (intralesionally, 106 units into each lesion 3 times a week for 3 weeks) is also efficacious but expensive.

Herpes simplex

The causative organism is *Herpesvirus hominis* type 1 (HSV-1) or type 2, a caryotropic DNA virus (Tab. 76.2). HSV-1 attacks the skin and mucous membranes, whereas HSV-2 is the primary cause of genital herpes. Primary infections caused by HSV are gingivostomatitis herpetica (stomatitis aphthosa), vulvovaginitis herpetica, meningoencephalitis herpetica, herpes sepsis of the newborn, eczema herpeticatum, keratoconjunctivitis herpetica, and primary herpes simplex of the skin or mucosa with a serious general course. Secondary infections are herpes simplex recidivans, herpes genitalis, herpes genitalis recidivans, keratoconjunctivitis herpetica recidivans, and eczema herpeticatum.

Herpes infections present a special problem in human immunodeficiency virus (HIV)-positive patients. Such infections are characterized by a tendency to dissemination with possible complications - encephalitis, eczema herpeticum, and herpetic sepsis.

Herpes zoster (shingles)

It is a secondary infection with or a reactivation of a varicella-zoster infection. Typical cases are characterized by an eruption of vesicles grouped on an erythematous base inside one or more cutaneous dermatomes. Localization of importance is that in the region of innervation of the trigeminal nerve (e.g., zoster ophthalmicus, maxillaris, mandibularis). An especially serious form is zoster necrotisans, which is seen usually in patients suffering from malignant tumors (e.g., leukemias, Hodgkin's disease).

Treatment of herpes zoster is by symptomatic analgesic and anti-inflammatory drugs and anti-infective agents. Intravenous acyclovir has been proven to be effective in both localized and disseminated zoster. Administered iv, it decreases duration of pain and shortens the time of healing. In immunocompromised patients, it also can prevent or abort dissemination. Oral

Table 76.2 Forms of herpesvirus infections and their therapy

Infection	Primary forms
Gingivostomatitis herpetica	**Topical:** Acyclovir q3h disinfectants (pyoctanine 0.2-0.5% in aqueous solution) **Systemic:** In serious cases, acyclovir iv (500 mg/m² q8h in infusion). Nursed children < 3 months, children over 12 years, and adults with normal immune status, 5 mg/kg; in encephalitis, 10 mg/kg 5 times daily, at least 5 and up to 10-14 days if necessary. Prophylactic oral acyclovir 200-400 mg bid. Gancyclovir and famcyclovir as well as foscarnet (for acyclovir-resistant cases) are also effective but expensive. In secondary bacterial infections, antibiotics according to the sensitivity test and NSAIDs
Vulvovaginitis herpetica	**Systemic:** Acyclovir as in stomatitis aphtosa. Analgesics and NSAIDs
Herpetic sepsis of newborn	**Topical:** As in gingivostomatitis **Systemic:** Acyclovir (contraindicated in pregnancy), immunoglobulins
Eczema herpeticatum	**Topical:** Zinc lotion with 0.5% clioquinol **Systemic:** Acyclovir iv 5-8 days, if necessary by mouth, too. In secondary infections while waiting sensitivity results, erythromycin 500 mg tid or qid
Infections	Secondary forms
Herpes simplex Herpes simplex in loco recidivans	**Topical:** Astringents, pastes. At the beginning, steroids (creams). In case of vesiculation, 0.5% clioquinol as lotion. If crusts are present, antibiotic ointments with antiseptics. Virustatics: Acyclovir, idoxiuridine, and vidarabine are of unproven value **Systemic:** Symptomatic. In serious cases, acyclovir po and iv if necessary (strains resistant to acyclovir already exist)

(NSAIDs = nonsteroidal anti-inflammatory drugs.)

acyclovir (800 mg every 4 hours for 7-10 days), if started within the first 24 to 48 hours, shortens the time to lesion crusting, healing, and cessation of pain; reduces new lesion formation, and favorably influences the post-zoster neurologic symptoms. Famcyclovir 500 mg is given tid for 7 days.

The efficacy of high-dose vitamins B_1, B_6, and B_{12} has not been proven. In extremely serious cases, the use of steroids is justified. After regression of vesicles, a fast regression of inflammatory changes and pain occurs. Postzoster neuralgias can persist for a long time after regression of skin manifestations, and there is no favorable effect of steroids. Topical therapy depends on the phase of the disease. In early cases, zinc lotion with 0.5% clioquinol is effective. Acyclovir 5% in polyethylene glycol every 4 hours for 10 days promotes healing of localized zoster in immunocompromised patients. However, it is ineffective in reducing pain. Burrow's solution compresses are useful when lesions are crusted and/or infected. Intralesional injections of corticosteroids and/or anesthetics decrease pain during the acute disease. Postherpetic neuralgia persisting longer than 1 month occurs in up to 15% of patients. Capsaicin cream (which depletes and prevents reaccumulation of substance P) applied up to four times daily reduces pain.

Diseases caused by parasites

Scabies

Scabies is caused by a mite *Sarcoptes (Acarus) scabiei*. The female digs tunnel-like burrows in the stratum corneum of the epidermis, laying 2 to 3 eggs a day for a few weeks. The larvae hatch from the eggs and change into nymphes and finally into sexually mature mites. This process lasts for about 3 weeks. Scabies is transmitted by close contact, e.g., in a bed or by sexual intercourse, in camps and schools and in places with poor sanitary conditions. The main symptom is severe itching. Places of predilection are the interdigital spaces of the hands and feet, the elbows, the anterior axillary folds, the areolae of the breasts, the penis, and the ankles. A bacterial superinfection is possible. General rules of treatment are as follows:

Change and boil bed and body linen. Clothing should not be used for 4 days, and if possible, it should be dry-cleaned.

Rub drug (cream or lotion) into the entire skin from the neck down. Approximately 30 to 60 g or 60 to 120 ml is required to cover the trunk and extremities of an average adult; after 24 to 48 hours, the emulsion should be washed off in a bath or shower, and the procedure should be repeated.

Permethrin 5% cream applied for 8 to 12 hours and then washed off, repeated 1 week later if necessary, is more effective and less dangerous than lindane. Lindane (gamma-benzene hexachloride) is not used any more. Percutaneous absorption can cause adverse central nervous system effects. Lindane is especially contraindicated in pregnancy and in small children. Less toxic drugs (especially for children) are 20 to 25% benzyl benzoate, 10% crotamiton, and precipitated 6% sulfur. Itching, if severe, can be treated topically with H_1 antagonists or corticosteroids. The latter can be given orally as a short, tapering course (7-10 days).

Pediculosis

Pediculosis capitis (head louse) The causastive organism is the louse *Pediculus capitis.* Transmission is from person to person. Insufficient hygienic measures favor the spread of lice in hair. The changes are localized mainly to the scalp. Very rarely the beard and pubic region can be involved. Pyrethrins are the treatment of choice. These compounds interfere with neural transmission, leading to paralysis and death of the parasite. Piperonyl butoxide potentiates their insecticidal action up to 10 times. Medication is applied for 12 minutes and then rinsed off. These agents kill lice in 10 to 23 minutes (lindane in 3 h). Permethrin has 70 to 80% ovicidal activity and leaves an active residue on the scalp. The cream is applied, allowed to soak for 10 minutes, and then rinsed off with water. Lindane is less effective than pyrethrins or malathion. Shampoo is used for *P. capitis* and *pubis,* and cream and lotion are used for treating scabies and all forms of pediculosis. Up to 10% of topically applied drug can be absorbed through the skin. Most side effects including aplastic anemia are the consequence of improper use. Malathion 1% lotion has ovicidal effects (95%) in 5 minutes.

Pediculosis vestimenti (body louse) It is caused by *P. vestimenti* and can be a vector for rickettsial diseases: louse-borne and mite-borne typhus, Wolhynia fever, Q fever, African tick tiphus, and recurrent fever. On the skin, numerous red wheels appear as well as nodes with intense itching; the skin is soon covered with the effects of scratching, and a secondary pyodermization occurs. In some places hypo- and/or hyperpigmentation can be seen. Treatment involves boiling of clothes or powdering of the skin with contact insecticides. Skin changes are treated according to their acuteness and secondary pyodermization.

Pediculosis pubis (phthiriasis) The causative organism is a louse, *P. pubis* (*Phthirus pubis*). The disease is transmitted by a close contact, very often sexual, but also by bed clothes. Predilectional sites are regions with apocrine sweat glands (i.e., pubic and axillary regions), in hairy people on the abdomen and chest, and in small children on the scalp, eyebrows, and eyelashes. The treatment is the same as for the head lice.

Seborrheic dermatoses

Acne vulgaris is a common self-limited multifactorial disorder of sebaceous follicles. The disease is characterized by increased sebum production and abnormal keratinization in follicles with comedones, proliferation of *Propionibacterium acnes* (which produces peptides that are chemoattractant for polymorphonuclear leukocytes), inflammatory papules, pustules, and nodular abscesses with the formation of scars. High levels of androgens and heightened end-organ responsiveness of the sebaceous glands are implicated. Based on the clinical picture and the intensity of changes, acne comedonica, acne papulopustulosa, and acne conglobata as well as various acneiform eruptions of other etiologies can be distinguished.

Treatment is directed to a reduction in sebum production, removal of existing comedones and prevention of appearance of new ones, suppression of *P. acnes,* and prevention of scarring (decreasing the inflammatory reaction to follicular rupture). Seborrhea can be suppressed by estrogens (e.g., oral contraceptives), antiandrogens (e.g., prednisone 5-7.5 mg per day, spironolactone 50-200 mg per day), and isotretinoin (0.5-1 mg/kg). Prednisone is useful in female patients with severe acne who have adrenal gland overproduction of androgens.

Acne comedonica Tretinoin cream, gel, or solution 0.01 to 0.1% and benzoyl peroxide 3.5 or 10% gel as well as azelaic acid 20% cream are used. Tretinoin can be combined with salicylic acid. An artificial or natural ultraviolet (UV) radiation is helpful. Mechanical removal of comedones may prevent inflammatory progression.

Acne papulopustulosa Therapy begins with peeling as in acne comedonica, and in the case of papules and pustules, topical (e.g., tetracyclines, erythromycin, or clindamycin) and systemic (e.g., tetracycline, erythromycin) antibiotics are given. Minocycline is given in smaller doses (50 mg 1-2 times qd or bid for up to 6 months or longer). Tetracycline is given at 500 mg tid for a few weeks, then 500 mg bid, and finally 500 mg qd or even 125 mg qd for months if necessary.

Acne conglobata Therapy begins with degreasing and peeling with tretinoin and benzoyl peroxide. Antibiotics in high doses are given systemically (clindamycin up to 3 g/d). Bigger incisions cause scars and should be avoided. Intralesional corticosteroids can be injected, diluted with saline or anesthetics (1:2-4). With tetracyclines, dapsone 50 to 100 mg qd for weeks and months can be administered. Contraindications for isotretinoin therapy are pregnancy and lactation. Teratogenic effects (e.g., hydro- and microcephalus, malformations of the ears, microphthalmos, and cardiovascular malformations) are well known.

After a longer period of treatment and regression of inflammatory changes, the correction of scars may be necessary. Zinc salts by mouth (50 mg tid) in the form of zinc orophate or aspartate taken over several months sometimes have a good effect in inflammatory forms of acne. Phototherapy of inflammatory forms of acne also may have a favorable effect: UVA radiation or combined UVA/UVB. UVB radiation has no comedolytic effect. Photochemotherapy (PUVA) is not recommended.

Rosacea (acne rosacea) Rosacea is a chronic disorder of unknown etiology that affects the central face and neck. Localized papules and pustules with livid erythema and telangiectasias are typical. Hypertrophy of the connective tissue as well as of sebaceous glands may occur on the nose (rhinophyma). There is no correlation between sebum secretion and severity of rosacea. Lesional blood flow is three to four times that of controls.

The same rules as in the treatment of acne conglobata should be applied. Tetracyclines by mouth are very effective; tetracycline HCl or oxytetracycline have the same efficacy as minocycline. Starting dose for tetracycline is between 1000 and 1500 mg daily. Minocycline, which can cause photosensitivity, is given 50 mg twice daily up to 200 mg daily. After improvement, the dose is reduced. In long-term therapy, monitoring of side effects is necessary. Tetracyclines are the therapy of choice if the eyes are involved (rosacea keratitis). Metronidazole 200 mg bid is as effective as the tetracyclines. The best results occur in the most serious forms of rosacea (rosacea conglobata) and are achieved with monotherapy with isotretinoin in a daily dose of 0.2 to 1.0 mg/kg; remission may last for years.

All irritating substances must be avoided, such as strong soaps and alcoholic tinctures. Antibiotics such as erythromycin, clindamycin, and the tetracyclines 0.5 to 2% gel or emulsions of the oil/water type can be applied topically, or alternatively, topical therapy with metronidazole (0.75-2% in a basic vehicle), overnight ichthammol paste, or sulfur or zinc lotion with 3 to 5% of ichthammol may be tried. A massage is recommended in milder, erythematous cases in the morning and in the evening to achieve better lymph drainage.

Dermatitis perioralis (periorificial, perioral dermatitis) It is a distinct clinical entity often confused with rosacea, seborrheic dermatitis, or acne. Clinically, it is characterized by localized perioral small spherical, spiked papules, papulovesicles, and papulopustules with diffuse redness of the skin, mainly in young women. Provocative factors include hypersensitivity to cosmetics and fluorinated toothpastes and fluorinated corticosteroids, light, and certain hormones (e.g., oral contraceptives). Treatment is by oral tetracyclines (tetracycline HCl or minocycline): the first week 500 mg tid; the second week 250 mg bid, and from the third to sixth week 250 to 500 mg qd. If necessary, a maintainence dose can be continued for many months. In more severe cases, isotretinoin is given in smaller doses of from 0.05 to 0.2 mg/kg for 8 to 12 weeks, but this is contraindicated in pregnant women or those of childbearing age. It is necessary to avoid all irritating substances, cosmetics, and steroids.

Dermatitis seborrheica (eczema seborrhoicum) and dandruff (pityriasis sicca) These entities are cause a scaling of the scalp, often associated with itching. Seborrheic dermatitis is an inflammatory, erythematous eruption that occurs primarily in seborrheic areas (i.e., scalp, face, and trunk). Dandruff is a noninflammatory increased scaling of the scalp – a more active end of physiologic desquamation. Treatment consist of local (shampoo) or systemic applications of antimycotics, e.g., ketoconazole or itraconazole. Antibiotics are used according to sensitivity only in the case of a concomitant secondary bacterial infection.

Shampoos of 0.5% selenium sulfide (2-3 times a week for up to 10 minutes), zinc pyrithione 1 to 2%, salicylic acid-sulfur shampoos, tar shampoos, and nonmedicinal shampoos with surfactants and detergents remove scales and decrease desquamation for about 4 days. Ketoconazole is effective against *P. ovale* when given orally (200 mg per day) or topically (2% cream applied bid or as a 2% shampoo). Lesions on other areas respond

to corticosteroid cream (hydrocortisone 1% applied 1-3 times per day). Seborrheic blepharitis can be treated with sulfacetamide 10% alone or with prednisolone 0.2% or phenylephrine 0.12% suspension. Isotretinoin (5-10 mg per day) suppresses sebaceous glands.

Dermatitis seborrheica neonatorum (seborrheic dermatitis of the newborn) It occurs rarely and is probably caused by endogenic stimulation by maternal androgens. Emphasis is placed on skin colonization with *C. albicans.* The skin must be kept dry and the inflammation controlled. Lesions respond rapidly to corticosteroid creams, e.g., hydrocortisone 1% cream three times daily. Aerosols and lotions are applied to hairy areas. Scales are removed from the scalp with 2% salicylic acid in the olive oil. Body lesions are treated with zinc lotion with 5% of clioquinol, whereas intertriginous regions are treated with clioquinol zinc oil (0.5%). Steroids combined with antibiotics are used in secondary infections. In *Candida* infections, amphotericin B locally, nystatin, and ketoconazole are also effective.

Dermatitis nummularis (nummular dermatitis) It presents as disseminated eczematoid, itching coin-shaped plaques, usually sharply limited with a tendency to oozing and crusting. Etiopathogenesis includes reaction to topical irritants and manifestation of xerosis and emotional stress. H_1 antagonists diminish anxiety and itching. Dressings with steroidal ointments and creams possibly with neomycin or clioquinol can improve the exudative phase. Pastes with clioquinol 0.5%, ichthammol 2%, or tar 0.5 to 3% then may be used. UV radiation is also helpful as well as Burrow's solution compresses for 20 minutes three times daily, tar compounds, and phototherapy. Corticosteroids are applied intralesionally.

Alopecia

The alopecias can be focal, diffuse, or total. Various forms of alopecias can appear in single phases of the hair cycle – alopecia of a late type or alopecia of an early type. The phase of the hair cycle is determined by means of a trichogram. This is important for treatment (Tab. 76.3).

Sexually transmitted diseases

Syphilis

Syphilis is a chronic infectious disease transmitted mainly by sexual intercourse. Diagnosis is made by detection of *Treponema pallidum* in dark-field microscopy. Primary syphilis (from the moment of infection until the end of the eighth week) is followed by a secondary (resolutive) phase, from the eighth week until the third year after infection, when a latent phase begins without any signs of infection. This phase can last from 2 years until the end of life; in the third period (destructive), all organs and tissues can be affected. So-called metasyphilis can appear after many years, as a result of anergy of the body and is characterized by the appearance of tabes dorsalis and/or

Table 76.3 Kinds of alopecia and their treatment

Kind	Therapy
Atrichia Cicatricial alopecia	None
Atrophic alopecia (pseudopelade)	**Topical**: Intralesional triamcinolone, glucocorticoids possibly under occlusion **Systemic**: Antimalarials, isoniazid, dapsone, NSAIDs
Alopecia androgenetica in men (male-pattern baldness)	**Topical**: Estrogens (17α-estradiol), minoxidil 2% solution (also with tretinoin), surgery **Systemic**: Finasteride (see Chap. 18)
Alopecia androgenetica in women	**Topical**: Estrogens and steroids. Minoxidil **Systemic**: Antiandrogens (cyproterone acetate) in combination with ethinyl estradiol during 21days with a pause of 7 days
Reversible alopecia	**Systemic**: According to the disease (infection, drugs, chemicals, sideropenia)
Alopecia areata (circumscript immunologically mediated)	**Topical**: Glucocorticoids possibly under occlusive dressing or intralesionally at 4-6-week intervals. Topical sensitizers such as dinitrochlorobenzene and diphencyprone. Dithranol, PUVA (decreases the subset of T lymphocytes). Minoxidil **Systemic**: Cyclosporin (6 mg/kg per day)

(NSAIDs = nonsteroidal anti-inflammatory drugs.)

progressive paralysis. Diagnoses of various phases of the disease are verified by serologic tests (VDRL, FTA-ABS, ITP, and TPHA).

Penicillin is still the drug of choice. An effective serum concentration is 0.03 IU/ml. It acts only in the phase of division of treponemas. Generation time for treponemas is 30 to 33 hours; active concentrations of penicillin have to be maintained during 7 to 10 generation times, i.e., 10 to 15 days.

The recommendations of the World Health Organization (WHO) are as follows: all manifestations of syphilis during the first year after infection must be treated with two 2 400 000-IU benzathine penicillin injections with an interval of 7 days or 1 200 000 IU procaine penicillin daily for 14 days. All manifestations after 1 year are treated with three injections of 2 400 000 IU benzathine penicillin with intervals of 7 days or 1 200 000 IU daily for 21 day. If a

hypersensitivity to penicillin exists, erythromycin is given in doses of 500 mg qid for 30 days or chlortetracycline or oxytetracycline at the same doses. Antimicrobial therapy frequently causes degenerating treponemas to release lipopolysaccharides that result in the Jarisch-Herxheimer reaction (occurring in 65-90% of patients), which is an acute febrile reaction that occurs usually within 24 hours and often is associated with headache, myalgias, and a flareup of rashes. It subsides within 16 hours and besides neurologic disorders in patients with high cerebrospinal fluid cell counts (e.g., hemiplegia, seizures), it causes only anxiety. Antipyretics are the only therapy.

Ulcus molle

Ulcus molle (chancroid, soft sore) is transmitted only by sexual intercourse. The causative organism is gram-negative *Hemophilus ducreyi.* The disease is seen most often in tropic and subtropic regions but can occur all over the world. It occurs 5 to 20 times more often in men than in women. Incubation is 2 to 4 days, after which the primary lesion appears. It has a variable course. Diagnosis is established by microscopic detection of the causative organism on Giemsa's or Gram's stain. Smears are positive in less than 50% of patients. Therapy involves azithromycin 1 to 2 g po in a single dose, ceftriaxone 250 mg in a single dose, ciprofloxacin 500 mg po tid for 3 days, or erythromycin 500 mg qid for 7 days. Fluctuant nodes should not be drained or incised but aspirated through the (healthy) skin.

Gonorrhea

It is an acute infectious disease of the epithelium of the urethra, cervix, rectum, pharynx, or eyes. It is caused by the gram-negative diplococcus *Neisseria gonorrhoeae.* Humans are the only host of *Neisseria,* and infection occurs by direct contact of mucous membranes, most often during sexual intercourse. Incubation takes 2 to 5 days. Diagnosis is based on direct finding of intracellular gram-negative gococci in smears of an urethral exudate. The clinical picture differs between women and men as well as possible complications. In women, endometritis, cervicitis, and salpingitis (with sterility) are observed, and in men, prostatitis, vesiculitis, funiculitis, and epididymitis are seen. The choice of the treatment regimen depends on many factors, the most important of which is the local level of resistance to antimicrobials. Because of this, penicillin is not the drug of choice, but in the case of proven sensitivity, amoxicillin 2.0 to 3.0 g (plus probenecid 1 g) is given in a single dose.

Uncomplicated infection in adults and adolescents The recommended drugs are ceftriaxone 125 mg im, cefixime 125 mg po, ciprofloxacin 500 mg po, ofloxacin 400 mg po, or spectinomycin 2 g im all in a single dose. Since none of the agents mentioned will eradicate *Chlamydia trachomatis,* which can be detected in up to 30% of men and up to 50% of women infected with *N. gonorrhoeae,* a concurrent therapy to eradicate this microorganism is also recommended. The following may be used: doxycycline 100 mg bid for 7 days or azithromycin 1.0 g in a single oral dose. This new macrolide antibiotic is effective, often for short-term therapy, but its cost is considerably greater than that of erythromycin or doxycycline. Other regimens for *C. trachomatis* include ofloxacin (600 mg), cotrimoxazole (960 mg), and sulfafurazole (2.0 g) all given for 7 days.

Gonococcal conjunctivitis in adults Therapy is with ceftriaxone 1.0 g intramuscularly in a single dose with lavage of the infected eye with saline.

Disseminated infections These need multiple-dose treatments 24 to 48 hours longer than after improvement begins. Agents of choice include ceftriaxone 1.0 g im or iv qd, spectinomycin 2.0 g im bid, and cefotaxime 1.0 g iv tid.

Complicated gonococcal infections (pelvic inflammatory disease) These can be controlled with ceftriaxone 1.0 to 2.0 g intravenously twice daily for 10 days. For endocarditis, treatment must continue for at least 28 days.

Infections in children who weigh 45 kg or more Children weighing more than 45 kg should be treated with adult regimens. Patients under 17 years of age should not receive quinolones, and those under 9 years of age should not receive tetracyclines. Children who weigh less than 45 kg should receive ceftriaxone 125 mg intramuscularly or spectinomycin 40 mg/kg.

Neonatal patients with gonococcal ophthalmia must be hospitalized because of the danger of perforation and blindness.

Chlamydia urethritis

Treatment is doxycycline 100 mg bid for 7 days. Azithromycin 1 g in a single dose is more convenient but more expensive.

Lymphogranuloma venereum (lymphopathia venerea)

It is a systemic sexually transmitted disease with a transitory primary lesion followed by suppurative lymphangitis and serious local complications. The causative organism is *C. trachomatis.* The disease has three stages (i.e., primary lesion, buboes, and anogenitorectal ulcers). Incubation is less than 14 days, rarely longer. The diagnosis is difficult. The complement fixation test becomes positive within 1 month. Fluorescein-tagged monoclonal antibodies recently have been used for detection of chlamydial antigens. Doxycycline 100 mg bid or erythromycin 500 mg qid should both be used for 21 days. The lesion should be aspirated, not incised. Surgery may be necessary for relieving strictures and fistulas.

Trichomoniasis

Infections of the urogenital tract may be caused by *Trichomonas vaginalis.* The disease is relatively frequent and is transmitted by sexual intercourse as well as by towels, sponges, etc. Incubation is 21 days. In men the disease manifests as urethritis and in women as colpitis. The causative organism is visualized on a wet mount. Monoclonal antibody staining detects 77% of wet-mount-negative cases. Metronidazole 2.0 g is effective in a single dose or at 250 mg tid for 6 days. If this is unsuccessful, 500 mg is given bid for 7 days. Simultaneous treatment of the sexual partner(s) is mandatory. In the case of metronidazole resistance, tinidazole 2.0 g should be tested.

Suggested readings _____

ANONYMOUS. Drugs used in skin diseases, WHO Model Prescribing Information. Geneva, WHO, 1997.

ARNDT KA. Manual of dermatologic therapeutics, 5th ed. Boston: Little, Brown, 1995.

BERT-JONES J, HUTCHINSON PE. Modern treatment of warts: cure rates at 3 and 6 months. Br J Dermatol 1992;127:262-5.

BOWSKER D. Post-herpetic neuralgia in older patients. Drugs Aging 1994;5:411-8.

COREY L, SPEAR PG. Infections with herpes simplex viruses (first of two parts). N Engl J Med 1986;314:686-91.

COREY L, SPEAR PG. Infections with herpes simplex viruses (second of two parts). N Engl J Med 1986;314:749-57.

GRUPTA AK, EINASSON TR, SUZUNVERBELL RC, SHEAR NH. An overview of topical antifungal therapy in dermatomycoses. Drugs 1998;55:645-74.

GUZZO C, et al. Dermatology. In: Hardman JG, Lumbird LE (eds). Goodman & Gilman's Pharmacological basis of therapeutics, 9th ed. New York: McGraw-Hill, 1996:1591.

HALL RP. The pathogenesis of dermatitis herpetiformis: recent advances. J Am Acad Dermatol 1987;16:1129-44.

HUFF JC, WESTON WL, TONNESEN MG. Erythema multiforme: a critical review of characteristics, diagnostic criteria and causes. J Am Acad Dermatol 1983;8:763-75.

THIERS, BH (ed). Office dermatology. Part 1. Med Clin North Am 1998,82:481-720.

TOYODA M, MOROHASHI M. An overview of topical antibiotics for acne treatment. Dermatology 1998:196:130-34.

WAGSTAFF AJ, FAULDS D, GOA KL. Acyclovir: a reappraisal of its antiviral activity, pharmacokinetic properties and therapeutic efficacy. Drugs 1994;47:153-75.

CHAPTER 77

Allergic skin reactions

Vladimir Čajkovac

Atopy

Atopy is an inherited disposition to allergic diseases of the skin and mucous membranes (e.g., atopic eczema, hay fever, bronchial asthma). In such patients, reagins, cytotropic antibodies that bind to mastocytes or basophilic leukocytes, can be found. These reagins are immunoglobulin E (IgE), and they can be detected by the RAST and RIST methods. Immune reaction is of the immediate type (type I, according to Gell and Coombs).

Atopic dermatitis (neurodermitis, atopic eczema) is a chronic itching superficial inflammation of the skin that often occurs familiarly. Recently, it was found that the allergen-specific IgE antibodies bound to epidermal Langerhans cells react with corresponding contact allergens – which reach the skin from outside – causing the delayed type reaction (type IV, according to Gell and Coombs) (Tab. 77.1). The disposition to atopy with increased production of humoral antibodies (IgE) after contact with allergens is inherited. The inheritance is polygenic, depending partially on the HLA complex. Many other factors may play a role in atopy (e.g., infections, stress, emotional disturbances, etc.). Frequently atopy is associated with other allergic diseases (e.g., asthma, rhinitis allergica, conjunctivitis allergica). Vitiligo, ichthyosis vulgaris, sebostatic changes of the skin, and alopecia areata are frequent accompanying features. Atopy typically involves the antecubital and popliteal spaces, face, neck, and hands.

The etiopathogenesis is unknown. High levels of cyclic AMP phosphodiesterase can be found in leukocytes. The disease may appear in nursing children and has a variable course. In early childhood it is characterized by inflammatory exudative changes (i.e., redness, vesicles, and crusts) and later by more inflammatory proliferative changes (i.e., lichenoid papules and lichenification).

Treatment

Treatment depends on the clinical picture. It is indicated in exudative eczematous changes in nursing children. Avoidance of precipitating factors is most important. In cleaning of the skin, it is necessary to avoid alkaline soaps.

Table 77.1 Hypersensitivity reactions: the Gell and Coombs classification

Type I Allergens combine with specific IgE antibodies that are bound to membrane receptors on tissue mast cells and blood basophils. Potent vasoactive and inflammatory mediators are released - preformed (histamine and chemotactic factors) or newly generated (leukotrienes and platelet-activating factor). They cause vasodilatation, increased capillary permeability, glandular hypersecretion, smooth muscle spasm, and tissue infiltration with eosinophils and other inflammatory cells. Disorders belonging to this group are atopic diseases (including atopic dermatitis, which is a chronic disease) and systemic anaphylaxis

Type II Cytotoxic reactions resulting when an antibody reacts with antigenic components of the cell or tissue elements or with an antigen or hapten coupled to the cell or tissue. Cytotoxic cells may be activated (killer cells) to produce antibody-dependent cell-mediated cytotoxicity. Complement activation is usually involved through C3 (with phagocytosis of the cell). If the whole complement system is activated, cytolysis and tissue damage occur. Examples of diseases with this mechanism are Goodpasture syndrome, myasthenia gravis, and hyperthyroidism

Type III Immune-complex reactions resulting from deposition of soluble circulating antigen-antibody immune complexes in vessels or tissue. Immune complexes activate complement, and the resulting sequence of events causes polymorphonuclear cell migration and release of proteolytic enzymes and permeability factors in tissues producing acute inflammation. The proportion of antigens and antibodies in the immune complex determines the consequences of this reaction – rapid precipitation or phagocytosis by macrophages. Immune complexes play a role in serum sickness, lupus erythematosus, rheumatoid arthritis, hypersensitivity pneumonitis, acute glomerulonephritis, and many others

Type IV Delayed, cell-mediated hypersensitivity reaction caused by sensitized T-lymphocytes after contact with a specific antigen. Circulating antibodies are not involved. The sensitized T-lymphocytes may cause immunologic injury by direct toxic effect or through the release of lymphokines The cytokines released from activated T-lymphocytes include factors affecting the activity of macrophages, neutrophils, and lymphoid killer cells. Examples of clinical conditions in which type IV reactions seem to be important are contact dermatitis, some forms of drug sensitivity, thyroiditis, and granulomas due to intracellular organisms

In bacterial infections, antibiotics according to sensitivity tests and in acute viral infections hyperimmune gammaglobulin and virustatics (e.g., acyclovir) are indicated. If *Pityrosporon ovale* infection is suspected of causing a relapse, itraconazole cream is added for a short time.

A satisfactory result has been achieved with long-acting H_1 antagonists such as astemizole, loratadine, or fexofenadine (Tab. 77.2). In nursing children, antihistamines are given in the form of a syrup, preferably in the evening. In patients with neurotic symptomatology, treatment with benzodiazepines (e.g., oxazepam or diazepam) is indicated. Medication should be continued for at least 4 to 6 weeks. Oral glucocorticosteroids at medium to high doses (about 40 mg prednisolone or equivalent) on alternate days are given as a last resort in relapses. After that, the dose is reduced. Combinations with antihistamines also may be useful.

Alcoholic solutions, gels, and lotions should not be used because of their drying effect, except in patients with stronger inflammatory reactions. Semifatty and fatty vehicles (i.e., creams and ointments) generally are preferred. At the beginning of treatment, halogenated glucocorticoids may be given to decrease the inflammatory changes (e.g., betamethasone, halcinonide, fluocinolone, or fluocinonide). In more severe, exudative changes, good results are achieved with glucocorticoid ointments with humid occlusive dressings. Adverse effects may be observed (e.g., adrenal supression) after long-term application of halogenated glucocorticoids on large surfaces, especially in children. Loss of effect of topical steroids can be avoided by periodically interrupting continuous use for a week or more. In the case of more severely infiltrated and lichenified regions, application of tar for 5 to 8 weeks in the form of painting with liquor carbonis detergens or a stone tar in a soft paste is effective.

During the use of glucocorticoids, it is always necessary to look for potential adrenal suppression and the occurrence of various complications, such as bacterial and mycotic infections (candidiasis). Baths with extracts of cereal and oat pollard with added oil are used frequently. Subsequent greasing of the skin is important (wet skin) with ointments. Both oral and topical sodium cromoglycate (a mast cell stabilizer) is effective. Recently, cyclosporine use has improved severe atopic dermatitis considerably. In generalized cases, ultraviolet A (UVA) or a combination of UVA with UVB is used. No special diet is necessary, but a transitory hypersensitivity to eggs and milk products can

Table 77.2 H_1 receptor antagonists

Class and name	Duration of action (h)	Form	Daily dose
First generation			
Ethanolamines			
Clemastine fumarate	12-24	Tablets, liquid (elixir)	2×1 mg
Diphenhydramine HCl	4-6	Tablets, liquid, injection, topical	50-75 mg
Dimenhydrinate	4-6	Tablets, injection	50-100 mg
Alkylamines			
Chlorpheniramine maleate	4-6	Tablets, liquid, injection	24 mg po; sc, im 40 mg
Brompheniramine maleate	4-6	Tablets, liquid (elixir), injection	24-48 mg po; 5-20 mg
Piperazines			
Hydroxyzine HCl	6-24	Tablets, liquid (syrup), injection	25-100 mg
Cyclizine HCl	4-6	Tablets, injection	50-150 mg
Meclizine	12-24	Tablets	50 mg
Phenothiazines			
Promethazine HCl	4-6	Tablets, liquid, injection, suppositories	25 mg
Piperidines			
Cyproheptadine HCl	6-8	Tablets	12-24 mg
Second generation			
Piperidines			
Astemizole[1]	24	Tablets	10 mg
Loratadine	24	Tablets	10 mg
Fexofenadine	12-16	Capsules	120-180 mg
Alkylamines			
Acrivastine	6-8	Tablets	8 mg
Piperazines			
Cetirizine HCl	12-24	Tablets	5-10 mg

[1]Astemizole was recently withdraw in many countries because of dangerous interaction potential.

exist. Because of the possible role of essential fatty acids in the etiopathogenesis of atopic dermatitis (deficit of Δ6-desaturase), a diet enriched with Δ-6-linoleic acid may be advisable. Fingernails should be kept short to minimize excoriations and infections.

Contact dermatitis (eczema allergicum ex contactu)

This is one of the most frequent dermatoses (5-15 % of all dermatologic patients). It is a manifestation of contact allergy with inflammatory reaction in the epidermis and dermis. Contact dermatitis can be caused by a primary chemical irritant or may be a type IV delayed hypersensitivity reaction with special involvement of the epidermis. Irritants may damage normal skin or irritate an existing dermatitis. Weak irritants are soaps, acetone, and detergents. Allergic contact dermatitis is a delayed hypersensitivity reaction. It may take from 6 to 10 days (for strong sensitizers) to years (weaker ones) for individuals to become sensitized. The patient is sensitized by earlier contacts with allergens, so in repeated contacts an acute, subacute, or chronic eczema appears. Important factors in the etiology are contact sensitization, genetic predisposition, and diseases such as diabetes mellitus, hyperthyroidism, acrocyanosis, and cutis marmorata. The process of sensitization starts by contacting the allergen on the skin surface and ends by proliferation of allergen-specific T-lymphocytes in lymph nodes and by their appearence in the circulation, after which they can reach the skin again.

Contact allergens generally are substances of low molecular weight (<1000). High-molecular-weight substances such as proteins are less frequent sensitizers. Very frequent allergens are derivatives of benzene (e.g., dinitrochlorobenzene, paraphenylenediamine, and some sulfonamides), extracts of some plants, ether oils, and some antibiotics. Many cosmetics can act as sensitizers (e.g., hair dyes, lipsticks, toothpastes, and various lotions) as well as jewelry; among plants, *Primula obconica* and *Rhus toxicodendron* (poison ivy, and others) are common sensitizers. Photoallergic and phototoxic contact dermatities must be differentiated from photosensitivity reactions to systemic drugs. They require exposure to light following topical application.

Treatment

Etiologic treatment is possible in cases in which the allergen is known. In the photoallergic or phototoxic variety, strict avoidance of light exposure is mandatory. Otherwise, treatment depends on the stage of eczema localization and possible combination with other dermatoses (eczema pyodermisatum).

Topical treatment is based on the application of a suitable vehicle. Some vehicles themselves can cause allergic sensitization, however. Glucocorticoids are used in the chronic local therapy of eczema. They are very effective (except in the blistering phase) and can shorten the duration of the acute phase. Therapy usually starts with betamethasone dipropionate or fluocinolone 0.02% with the applica-

tion of occlusive dressings. Corticosteroids only have a symptomatic effect, and recurrences are seen often. Tars (pix lithantracis or ichthammol) may be added for the treatment of lichenified changes. The combination of tars with corticosteroids is also effective. Patients should be warned to avoid sunlight or radiographs.

Antimicrobials are used in bacterial or mycotic superinfections, often in the form of dressings (argentum nitricum or chinosol 0.1%). Brilliant green as well as gentian violet are used in infected eczema of intertriginous areas. In secondary mycotic infections, antimycotics, possibly combined with corticosteroids (e.g., hydrocortisone-miconazole, triamcinolone-econazole), may be used. Salicylic acid has mild keratolytic and antimicrobial properties and may improve penetration of corticosteroids, especially in hyperkeratotic changes of the palms and soles. Urea has similar properties and usually can be given in 10% concentration, combined with steroids.

Systemic therapy with glucocorticoids is indicated only in disseminated disease. Duration of therapy should be as short as possible (1-6 weeks). The starting daily dose is 40 to 60 mg prednisolone or equivalent. In children, the starting dose is 1 to 2 mg/kg. Long-term therapy, not above 75 mg per day of prednisolone or equivalent, is indicated only in persistent, refractory relapsing dyshidrotic eczema. Retinoids are given in hyperkeratotic rhagadiform eczemas of the palms and soles. The initial dose of acitretin is 30 mg per day, soon to be decreased to 10 mg per day. Antihistamines (H_1 blockers) are useful only to reduce itching. Even antihistamines may act as an allergen. The therapeutic effect of calcium salts is not proven.

Allergic urticaria (hives)

Local wheals and erythema in the dermis characterize the most frequent form of urticaria. It occurs more often in women than in men and is most common between 20 and 40 years of age. Allergens may be drugs, certain food additives, inhalants, insect stings or bites, microbial antigens in infections, metabolic disturbances, autoantigens (e.g., malignant tumors, autoimmune diseases), and even emotional factors. The cause often remains unknown (idiopathic urticaria).

The immediate-type reaction occurs a few minutes after contact with the antigen of IgE-dependent type I reactions in sensitized patients as a part of an anaphylactoid reaction. The reaction can be associated with bronchospasm or laryngeal edema. Late skin reactions depend on IgE but occur 8 to 36 hours after contact with the antigen. Serum sickness occurs 7 to 11 days after the first exposure to an antigen as part of a type III reaction. The course is acute, chronic intermittent, or chronic recurrent. Diagnosis is established by means of an avoidance test, exposition test, intradermal tests, or a radioallergosorbent test (RAST).

Acute urticaria may last up to 4 weeks. It occurs suddenly as an anaphylactoid immediate reaction (type I) in sensitized patients. It manifests as an eruption of wheals and angioedema, as well as laryngeal edema or bronchial edema, with raised body temperature, nausea, vomiting, and hypotension. The clinical picture is similar to shock. Allergens are drugs, foods, inhalants, and insect stings. All drugs can be an allergen – most often the systemic ones as well as plasma products. Food items are animal proteins (e.g., fish, crabs, lobsters, oysters, meat, and cheeses), strawberries, nuts, lemons, tomatoes, stimulants such as cocoa, wine, and tonic water, as well as inhalants (e.g., pollen, dust, fragrances).

Chronic intermittent urticaria is characterized by recurrent epizodes of acute urticaria that occur repeatedly within periods not longer than 4 weeks, often after years of no symptoms. Allergens often are recognized by the patient. It is an IgE-dependent immediate type I allergic reaction. The allergens are the same as in acute urticaria.

Chronic urticaria is a form of urticaria that lasts longer than 4 weeks. It is common in adults and can last for months to years. Only a small percentage of these cases result from a type I immediate reaction mediated by IgE antibodies. A larger fraction is probably idiosyncratic, and in some cases, immune complexes (type III) play a role. In 30 to 50% of patients, the cause cannot be found. Important factors are drug reactions (e.g., to aspirin), intolerance, inhalatory allergens, pollens, animal hair, house dust, feathers, wool, and cotton.

Endogenous chronic urticaria develops as a consequence of autoantigens, foreign proteins (type I) reactions, immune-complex (type III) reactions (Tab. 77.1). Among responsible factors are gastrointestinal (hyper- or hypoacidity or pancreatic disease) disturbances, intestinal candidiasis, focal infections due to bacteria or parasites, endocrine disturbances, and so on. Psychogenic factors are of questionable importance.

Treatment

Treatment is aimed at removal of the trigger factors. If the cause is not obvious, all nonessential drugs should be stopped until the reaction has subsided. H_1 antagonists are the therapy of choice. Topical therapy consists only of suppression or mitigation of itching with zinc or other lotions, glucocorticoids (lotions or creams), and alcoholic solutions (e.g., menthol 1.0%, thymol 0.5%, or ethanol 60%). Systemic antihistamines block the binding of histamine (present in basophils, mast cells, and platelets) on H_1 receptors of smooth muscles of blood vessels and other cells by competitive inhibition. In addition, by reducing vascular permeability, they may have a mild sedating effect. Several chemical classes of antihistamines show only minor variations in their properties. However, individuals react differently, so different agents have to be tried to find the best regimen (Tab. 77.2). Second-generation H_1 antagonists (e.g., astemizole 10 mg/d, fexofenadine 120-180 mg/d, loratadine 10 mg tid, cetirizine 10 mg/d, and others) are less sedating, but patients must be warned of possible side effects due to drug interactions (see Chap. 6). H_1 antagonist are given, depending on the severity of the urticaria, for

several weeks. Combinations of H_1 and H_2 antagonists (cimetidine) may be tried. The tricyclic antidepresant doxepin (10-50 mg tid) has some effect.

Glucocorticoids can be used for serious cases of urticaria and for life-threatening complications, e.g., edema of the larynx or anaphylactic shock. They are administered intravenously or intramuscularly (in a single dose up to 1000 mg). After that, 40 to 80 mg per day of prednisolone or equivalent by mouth may be necessary. In cases of threatening anaphylactic shock, glucocorticoids must be given iv, after stabilization of blood pressure with epinephrine.

Glucocorticoids should be avoided in chronic urticaria whenever possible. They are not indicated for long-term therapy unless the maintenance dose is under 7.5 mg of prednisolone or equivalent, i.e., below the potentially iatrogenic Cushing dose. Specific hyposensitization is justified only in allergic reactions caused by insect stings (type I reaction). Attention to food additives and salicylates is necessary.

Disodium chromoglycate stabilizes mast cell membranes, inhibits histamine release, and can be given as prophylaxis (see Chap. 28). It acts in bronchial asthma and hay fever when applied as an aerosol powder at 20 mg four times daily. It is used only in cases of chronic urticaria caused by food, whereas it is ineffective for other causes of chronic urticaria. Ketotifen (1-2 mg bid) inhibits mast cell mediators. Because of the "intolerance phenomenon", it is important to remove salicylates as food additives. If present, it is important to treat colonization of the intestine by *Candida albicans* using nystatin 500 000 to 1 million IU three times daily or amphotericin B 100 mg po tid for 5 days.

Other forms of urticaria

Urticarial vasculitis manifests like chronic urticaria but is linked with some internal diseases. It occurs in 1 to 5% patients with chronic urticaria, most often in women. Autoimmune events are thought to be based on vasculitis caused by immune complexes (type III allergic reactions). It occurs in lupus erythematosus and other connective tissue diseases, various types of hepatitis, and cryoglobulinemias. Beside skin changes, arthralgias, and joint edema, myalgias, abdominal pains, polylymphadenopathy, and less frequently, glomerulonephritis may occur. The course is chronic. Treatment is not satisfactory. Antihistamines or prednisone (up to 30 mg per day) have a modest effect. Indomethacin (50-100 mg per day), colchicine (0.6 mg po bid-tid), and dapsone (1-2 mg/kg per day) may be effective. Immunosupressors such as azathioprine and mercaptopurine may be tested. Topical zinc or other lotions and glucocorticoid creams may be useful.

Contact urticaria can be a consequence of immunologic as well as nonimmunologic events. It must be distinguished from the acute allergic urticaria caused by allergy to bees and wasps. Histamine release can cause an immediate type I reaction (IgE-mediated reaction). It can be caused by animal allergens (e.g., bee venom, wasp venom, animal hair, and caterpillar hair), plant allergens, fish, drug contacts, cosmetics, iodine, cobalt, Peru balsam, latex, and ammonium persulfate. Treatment involves avoidance of toxic or allergic contacts, systemic H$_1$ antihistamines (if necessary oral), and then local glucocorticoids.

Physical urticaria is caused by physical stimuli (e.g., cold, sunlight, heat, or mild trauma). In most cases there is no atopy or allergy. Cold urticaria is the most frequent. It can appear as an autosomal dominant inherited of immediate or delayed type of sensitivity, or it can be transferred passively with serum that contains specific IgE. In some patients, IgG and IgM autoantibodies have been found. Treatment is with oral H$_1$ antihistamines, also taken before cold exposure. Cyproheptadine (12-24 mg per day) is most useful in cold urticaria, but prednisone should be given in severe light eruptions. In the case of photosensitivity, protection is indicated.

Pressure urticaria (urticaria mechanica) is caused by pressure. It has a clinical picture very similar to angioedema. It can be associated with other forms of recurrent urticaria. Treatment consists of systemic high doses of H$_1$ antihistamines or psychotropic medications (doxepin 10-50 mg po tid).

Cholinergic urticaria (sweat urticaria) is mediated by acetylcholine. It is triggered by heat, exercise, change in temperature, or emotions. Small wheals on erythematous areas are detected, probably related to an increased sensitivity to acetylcholine. Intracutaneous acetylcholine injections (or of 1/1000 pilocarpine) are diagnostic. It is an immunologic type I IgE-dependent reaction, and it is important to exclude (all) psychosomatic disturbances. Parasympatholytics, ergotamine alkaloids, and hydroxyzine 10 mg tid and then every day as a maintenance dose are effective.

Nonimmunologic urticarias provoked by drugs are caused most commonly by anesthetics, anticholinergics, plasma expanders, contrast media, and nonsteroidal anti-inflammatory drugs (NSAIDs). As in cases of acute urticaria, treatment is guided by the severity of symptoms, including anaphylactic shock.

Angioedema

Quincke edema (angioneurotic edema) is an acute, circumscribed swelling of the skin involving both dermis and subcutaneous tissue. It occurs mostly in young women. Hereditary factors are not known, and it is not related to atopy. Generally, it is assumed to be an expression of an allergic immediate type I reaction. Occasionally, it occurs together with acute or chronic intermittent urticaria or as a symptom of an anaphylactic reaction. Edema of the larynx or glottis can be present. Causative factors are food and food additives, inhalatory allergens, and plant allergens. It is also an expression of pseudoallergy (intolerance or idiosyncrasy), particularly to salicylates. A relationship with gastrointestinal, endocrine (thyroid), or psychosomatic factors has been discussed. The course is acute as a part of an anaphylactoid type I reaction or intolerance, chronic recurrent as idiopathic angioedema, or chronic as an allergic cutaneous reaction followed by a chronic urticaria. Treatment is the same as for urticaria (see above).

Hereditary angioedema is a rare disease characterized by subcutaneous edema associated with gastrointestinal symptoms. It is an autosomal dominant genetic disease occurring in 0.4% of patients with urticaria and angioedema, beginning before the age of 15 years, more often in women. In 85% of patients, a deficiency or absence of C1 esterase inhibitor is detected, and in 15%, function of this gammaglobulin is altered. The C1 esterase inhibitor antagonizes the formation of kinins, active Hageman factor, kallikrein, and plasmin. Malfunction may be present despite immunochemical existence of the protein. The clinical picture is characterized by skin tension without itching. Patients may have 1- to 2-day abdominal attacks with vomiting and pain similar to an acute abdomen. This is probably a consequence of acute edema of the intestinal wall. The most serious complications are laryngeal edema with asphyxia. Sometimes lupus erythematosus or lymphosarcoma coexist.

Treatment

H$_1$ antihistamines and glucocorticoids have a modest or no effect. An acute attack is treated with parenteral epinephrine. Fresh plasma (400-2000 ml) contains sufficient concentrations of the C1 inactivator (3000-6000 units). These agents can be given for prevention before surgery. An effective prevention of an acute attack can be achieved with high doses of antifibrinolytic drugs, e.g., ε-aminocaproic acid 1 to 1.5 g bid or tranexamic acid 12 to 25 mg/kg tid. Danazol (200-600 mg per day) and stanozolol (2 mg tid) are the most valuable anabolic steroids in the prophylaxis of an acute attack. The initial dose should be higher, followed by slow reduction until the maintenance dose is achieved, generally for danazol 250 mg every other day. This therapy prevents the development of acute edema and can improve the synthesis of C1 esterase inhibitor and C4 toward normal.

Suggested readings _____

ABEL EA, FARBER EM. Atopic dermatitis, eczema and ichthyosis. Sci Am Med 1994;2:1-9.

ANONYMOUS. WHO Model prescribing information, drugs used in skin diseases. Geneva, WHO, 1997.

ARNDT KA. Manual of dermatologic therapeutics. Boston: Little, Brown, 1995.

GUZZO CA, LAZARUS GS, WERTH VP. Dermatological pharmacology. In: Hardman JG, Limbird LE eds. Goodman & Gilman's The pharmacological basis of therapeutics, 9th ed. New York: McGraw-Hill, 1996:1593-616.

KENNARD CD, ELLIS CN. Pharmacologic therapy for urticaria. J Am Acad Dermatol 1991;25:176-87.

LEE M. The role of corticosteroids in dermatology. Austr Prescrib 1998;21:9-11.

Topical therapy

Vladimir Čajkovac

Many skin diseases can be treated with topical therapy, whereas a number of them require systemic therapy as well. The goals of topical therapy are to cleanse, debride, and protect the skin; to inhibit or neutralize causative agents (e.g., infections or infestations); to relieve symptoms (e.g., itching, burning, or pain); and to reduce inflammation and promote healing. All these effects should take place without systemic absorption of the active agent.

Topical therapy depends on the pharmacodynamic action of the drug chosen as well as on the physical action of the vehicle (base or carrier) in which the drug is incorporated. The choice of an active agent depends on the clinical picture of the dermatosis, on the phase of the disease (i.e., acute, subacute, or chronic), and on the type of the skin (i.e., seborrheic, sebostatic, or normal). Vehicles have many pharmaceutical forms (e.g., dressings, powders, lotions, aerosols, sprays, creams, and ointments). Indications and contraindications for the application of topical agents are different, and the possible side effects are either cutaneous or systemic (e.g., of the local application of glucocorticosteroids). Often local therapy with the vehicle alone is sufficient without the addition of other pharmacologically active substances (e.g., dressings of cold water in simple inflammatory changes of the skin with oozing and neutral powders in acute dermatitis without oozing).

The suitability of the pharmacokinetics of drugs applied topically depends on the rate of percutaneous absorption and on subsequent penetration of the drug through the structures of the skin. After topical application on the skin, the methods of penetration can be different (e.g., intercellular, transfollicular, and probably transcellular). The intact skin is practically impermeable. The rate of penetration is inversely proportional to the thickness of the epidermis. Palms and soles are less permeable than other regions of the body.

Regions with many follicles (e.g., scalp, forehead, and retroauricular region) allow a much greater rate of penetration, which indicates that the cutaneous adnexa can be important for skin penetration. Percutaneous absorption depends further on the size of drug molecules applied, their lipo- or hydrosolubility, the concentration on the skin, and the degree of hydration of the stratum corneum. Nonpolar (lipid-soluble) compounds are absorbed better than polar (water-soluble) compounds. The rate of penetration can be intensified considerably by occlusive dressings.

Types of topical treatments

Wet dressings

These dressings act antiflogistically by cooling and drying, making possible the drainage of secretions. Impermeable (closed) dressings retain heat, prevent evaporation, cause hyperemia, and are indicated in cases where ripening of some process is desirable. Indications for wet dressings are acute inflammations in the phase of oozing and crusting. Wet dressings should be removed, remoistened, and reapplied every 10 to 15 minutes for 30 to 120 minutes tid.

If necessary, various pharmacologically active ingredients can be added (e.g., astringents, antiseptics, disinfectants and cleansers, antimycotics, antibiotics, corticosteroids, etc.), as can silver nitrate 0.1 to 0.5%, aluminium acetate, Burrow's solution, potassium permanganate, copper and zinc sulfates, and camphor solution. Dressings with 0.9% saline are often used.

Baths

Baths are used in the treatment of widespread eruptions. It is possible to add various other ingredients, such as potassium permanganate, oil, starch, and others. They can be warm (31-35 °C) and hot (36-40 °C). The tub should be half full, and the exposure should be limited to 30 minutes. Baths clean crusts, any ointments remaining, and so on. They may be very soothing, antipruritic, and antiinflammatory. Salty baths are used in the therapy of hyperkeratotic dermatoses, and baths with added photosensitizer (psoralen) are used in some forms of psoriasis and circumscribed scleroderma.

Medical shampoos

These are preparations used for cleansing. Beside detergents (which wash the hair and scalp), they contain healing substances. These are selenium disulfide, colloid sulfur, coal tar (effective in managing seborrhoic dermatitis, psoriasis, and dandruff), antimycotics (e.g., ketoconazole), pediculocides (e.g., pirethrin) and zinc pyrithione (effective in managing dandruff, seborrheic dermatitis, and tinea versicolor).

Solutions

Solutions of active substances in ethanol, isopropanol, and other organic solvents (in dermatotherapy called *tinctures*) are indicated in chronic infiltrative and lichenified lesions to which an ointment is applied later.

Varnishes

Varnishes are nongreasy preparations that are applied locally and form a thin membrane on the skin. They are used when a strictly localized action is desirable (e.g., collodium elasticum with keratolytics).

Emulsions

Emulsions are dispersions of two or more liquid substances that do not mix. Emulsions of the type O/W (oil in water) and W/O (water in oil) are differentiated. The latter is a better lubricant. The application of emulsions in dermatotherapy is very common. Cholesterol, lanolin alcohols, and triethanolamine stearate are used as emulsifying agents. Type O/W emulsions have a cooling effect. Emulsions are applied in all phases of inflammation.

Shake lotions

These lotions are suspensions of mineral powders in a liquid. To retain them on the skin, glycerol is usually added. Because of their physical properties, their action is keratoplastic and astringent, and they are indicated in subacute inflammatory dermatoses prone to recurrences. They should not be given in dermatoses with strong exudation, nor should they be applied to hairy regions, because removal is difficult. In shake lotions, various other substances can be present (e.g., antiparasitics, antiseborrheics, and antiseptics) as well as zinc oxide, glycerol, ichthammol, menthol, and resorcinol.

Ointments

Ointments consist of water droplets suspended in oil (W/O) or a fine base such as petrolatum. They contain crude or liquid active ingredients. Ointments may be soluble in water, emulsified with water, and insoluble in water. Ointments usually consist of triglycerides, fatty acids, fatty oils, waxes, lanolin, paraffin, and silicone oils. They can contain emulsants and generally are used in the treatment of dry skin.

Creams

Creams are semisolid emulsions of oil in water. Their viscosity depends on the proportion of water. Creams may be greasy (type W/O), washable (type O/W), or of a mixed type. Type W/O is best for application on a dry and lichenified skin and for softening hyperkeratotic changes. Type O/W and the mixed type have cooling properties and are easily washable from the skin. Creams are used in the treatment of oozy dermatoses and in seborrheic skin.

Gels

Gels are transparent, colorless systems that liquefy on contact with the skin. They contain essential macromolecular substances (e.g., tragacanth, alginates, or cellulosa derivatives), moisturizers (e.g., glycerol, sorbitol, or propyenglycol), preservatives, and various other molecules. They are best applied on hirsute parts of the body and scalp and act as emollients; they protect and cool the skin.

Pastes

Pastes are mixtures of powder and ointment. Hard pastes contain more than 50% powder, and soft ones contain less than 50% powder. They are generally used as bases for drugs that have to act on a limited region in the subacute phase of inflammation in superficial, inflammatory processes. Zinc oxide paste is part of practically all pharmacopoeia.

Powders

Powders are used infrequently today, generally as a protection of the skin from friction in intertriginous areas. Their action is limited to the most superficial parts of the skin. Powders are used in subacute inflammatory processes primarily for intertriginous areas. Various active substances can be added.

Drug groups used in dermatology

Glucocorticoids

Glucocorticoids are used widely as a topical therapy in dermatology because of their anti-inflammatory properties and ability to inhibit cell division. They are rarely irritating or sensitizing, and application is easy. Combination with other agents and bases is possible. Their potency is quite variable (Tab. 78.1). Compared with systemic administration, topical use of steroids causes fewer side effects. However, side effects of topically applied corticosteroids (especially fluorinated ones), such as the development of striae, atrophy, teleangiectasia, hirsutism, and skin redness, must be mentioned. In long-term use, especially under occlusive dressings over greater regions, systemic resorption can occur with systemic consequences. Intralesional administration is also possible (e.g., for acneic cysts, psoriatic plaques, and keloids). Topical steroids are indicated in dermatoses such as subacute and chronic contact dermatites, intertriginous and nummular dermatites, and many other pruritic dermatoses of various etiologies. Their action is rarely etiologic, so therapy has to be changed as soon as possible after establishing etiology.

Antimicrobial agents

Local application of antibiotics is justified only in cases where a close contact with microorganisms can be established. This is the case with impetigo or superficial folliculitis caused by *Streptococcus pyogenes*. In deeper infections, such as furuncles or abscesses, local application is not effective, and a systemic route must be chosen after appropriate sensitivity tests. Nonsystemic antimicrobial agents may be used safely topically; among these are

Table 78.1 Classification of topical corticosteroids

Potency	Topical corticosteroid	Formulation
Ultrahigh	Clobetasol propionate	Cream 0.05%
	Diflorasone diacetate	Ointment 0.05%
High	Amcinonide	Ointment 0.1%
	Betamethasone dipropionate	Ointment 0.05%
	Desoximetasone	Cream or ointment 0.025%
	Fluocinonide	Cream, ointment, or gel 0.05%
	Halcinonide	Cream 0.1%
	Betamethasone dipropionate	Cream 0.05%
	Betamethasone valerate	Ointment 0.1%
	Diflorasone diacetate	Cream 0.05%
	Triamcinolone acetonide	Ointment 0.1%
Moderate	Desoximetasone	Cream 0.05%
	Fluocinolone acetonide	Ointment 0.025%
	Fludroxycortide	Ointment 0.05%
	Hydrocortisone valerate	Ointment 0.2%
	Triamcinolone acetonide	Cream 0.1%
	Betamethasone dipropionate	Lotion 0.02%
	Betamethasone valerate	Cream 0.1%
	Fluocinolone acetonide	Cream 0.025%
	Fludroxycortide	Cream 0.05%
	Hydrocortisone butyrate	Cream 0.1%
	Hydrocortisone valerate	Cream 0.2%
	Triamcinolone acetonide	Lotion 0.1%
Low	Betamethasone valerate	Lotion 0.05%
	Desonide	Cream 0.05%
	Fluocinolone acetonide	Solution 0.01%
	Dexamethasone sodium phosphate	Cream 0.1%
	Hydrocortisone acetate	Cream 1%
	Methylprednisolone acetate	Cream 0.25%

(Source: WHO, 1997.)

mupirocin, bacitracin, gramicidin, tyrothricin, and polymyxin. These rarely sensitize the skin. However, with the topical use, the development of resistant strains of microorganisms is also possible. Among macrolides, erythromycin and clindamycin may be used topically, and among aminoglycosides, neomycin, framycetin, and fucidin may be used.

Virustatics

Acyclovir can be given topically. Indications are herpes simplex labialis and herpes simplex genitalis with itching. If applied early enough, the drug can shorten the duration of disease. Tromantadine hydrochloride as 1% cream can be given at the beginning of herpes simplex and herpes zoster lesions (see Chap. 40). Idoxuridine 0.2% ointment and 0.5% lotion, vidarabine 3% ointment, and trifluridine 1% solution are used in herpetic keratitis. Foscarnet sodium 2% cream is used in the treatment of condylomata acuminata. It can shorten the vesiculation period in herpes labialis but not in herpes genitalis.

Antimycotics

The first topical antimycotics were polyenes, e.g., amphotericin B (also for systemic application) and nystatin. Allylamines are effective in the topical treatment of various forms of tinea; among them are tolnaftate, naftifine, and terbinafine as creams, gels, or suspensions. Azoles are broad-spectrum antimycotics. This group includes miconazole, clotrimazole, econazole, itraconazole, ketoconazole, oxiconazole, and sulconazole (see Chap. 41). A hydroxypyridone cyclopiroxolamine cream or powder given as 8% solution is used in the therapy of onychomycoses. It is unrelated to other agents but has a similar spectrum to the azoles. Amorolfin in the form of a nail polish also is used for the treatment of onychomycoses. There are a number of nonspecific over-the-counter preparations such as Whitfield's ointment (benzoic 12% + salicylic 6% acid), potassium permanganate, Castellani's paint (carbol fuchsin solution), selenium sulfide 2.5% lotion, gentian violet 0.5 to 3%, sodium thiosulfate 25%, preparations containing undecylenic acid cream, powder, urea, and zinc pyrithione.

Antiparasitics

Antiparasitics are used in the therapy of pediculosis and scabies. A classic drug from this group is g-benzenehexachloride (lindane), which kills lice in the scalp and hair of the pubis. Especially in children, due to systemic resorption, it can cause adverse central nervous system effects. Benzyl benzoate 20 to 25% and crotamiton are effective for scabies. The former should be avoided in individuals with asthma. Malathion (0.5% lotion, 1% powder) is effective in pediculosis. Pyrethroids are an alternative. They are active against lice, ticks, mites, and fleas, but they are contraindicated in nursing children and during lactation. Permethrin 5% cream has a broad insecticidal activity, and because of its low toxicity, it can be used in pregnancy and infancy.

Insect repellents

These are preparations against insects, particularly useful in tropical regions, where malaria may exist. In this group, the most important is diethyltoluamide in the form of a spray, milk, or stick, followed by ethyl hexanediol, benzyl benzoate 5% emulsion, and permethrin 0.5% spray. There are preparations with multiple ingredients. Dimethylcarbamate can repel ticks from clothing.

Sunscreens

Sun protection factors (sunscreens) are used as an essential defense for persons sensitive to sunlight. Such people become easily ill from photodermatoses or from dermatoses that are light sensitive (e.g., lupus erythematosus or porphyrias). Long exposure to sunlight can be followed by the development of solar keratoses, lentigo, angiomas, and teleangiectasias, as well as by various skin tumors (e.g., carcinomas and melanoma). Ultraviolet B (UVB) rays are more harmful and are primarily resposible for causing malignant tumors. UVA rays are responsible for premature aging of the skin. As UVA sunscreens, benzophenones may be used; UVB screens include para-aminobenzoic acid preparations, cinnamates, and salicylates. Some are frequently combined. Products containing titanium dioxide as a physical blocker reflect and scatter UV rays.

Antihistamines

Antihistamines for local application can be used in cases of insect stings or bites on smaller surfaces and only for a short time (e.g., promethazine, chlorpheniramine, and doxepin). Previous concerns about antihistamine-induced contact dermatitis could not be verified in recent studies. Antihistamines are also incorporated in some topical antipruritic lotions.

Anhidrotics

A number of agents is used in the treatment of hyperhidrosis. Glutaraldehyde solution three times weekly for 3 weeks, methenamine in the form of a stick or solution (which hydrolyzes to ammonia and formaldehyde), and aluminum compounds (aluminum chloride hexahydrate) can block the sweat gland canals. The anticholinergic propantheline bromide is suitable for local application. Iontophoresis with tap water is simple and cheap. General hygienic measures should not be forgotten.

Photosenzitizers inducing hyperpigmentation and repigmentation

Methoxsalen 1% lotion applied locally induces hyperpigmentation and repigmentation. Used systemically (capsules) like trioxsolen tablets, it is a part of PUVA therapy of psoriasis vulgaris and vitiligo. For the treatment of vitiligo, dihydracetone is used for "tanning" the involved areas of the skin. In the treatment of hyperpigmentation, hydroquinone cream, gel, or solution and monobenzone 20% ointment are used. They can cause local sensitization.

Antipruritics

The pathophysiology of itching is not completely understood, and it is difficult to develop effective antipruritic drugs. The *WHO Model Prescribing Information on Drugs Used in Skin Disease* lists anti-inflammatory and antipruritic drugs together: betamethasone (ointment or cream 0.1%), calamine lotion, hydrocortisone (ointment or cream 1%), prednisolone, chlorpheniramine, and other antihistamines. Tars (e.g., coal tar solution 3-10%) are used as well; they are a mix of approximately 10 000 various chemicals. Other substances used are menthol 0.25 to 2%, pramoxine (often with hydrocortisone), methyl salicylate, oils (e.g., clove, turpentine), and a product of cayenne pepper, capsaicin oleoresin. In long-term treatment, all these preparations under the influence of

UV light may be carcinogens.

Local anesthetics

Pain travels to the brain along nerves, the action potential being propagated by sodium ion flow into and potassium ion flow out of the axon. Local anesthetics block the conduction by interfering with opening of the sodium channel. Two groups of agents are used: the amide-type agents includes lidocaine, bupivacaine, dibucaine, prilocaine, and others. To the ester-type agents belong tetracaine, procaine, and benzocaine. Other agents used for the same indication are benzyl alcohol, methyl chloride spray, dicyclomine HCl, and pramoxine HCl. The EMLA (entectic mixture of local anesthetics) contains 2.5% lidocaine and 2.5% prilocaine in an O/W emulsion. EMLA should be applied 1 hour prior to a procedure under occlusion. Capsaicin also can be used as an anesthetic.

Keratolytics

Keratolytics are used for the treatment of hyperkeratotic dermatoses. Urea-containing preparations (10% ointments and cream) have a moisturizing and softening effect. They help in maintaining hydration of the skin. The effect of urea can be intensified by adding corticosteroids (hydrocortisone 1%). Salicylic acid is a classic keratolytic. It has antimicrobial and antiproliferative activity. It can be combined with various other substances such as glucocorticoids, antibiotics, antimycotics, etc. Benzoyl peroxide is a strong oxidant. It can sensitize and is suspected of being carcinogenic. Many lotions and creams containing benzoyl peroxide are used in acne therapy. Azelaic acid 20% cream is recently a favored substance in acne therapy. It posesses antimicrobial (*Pityrosporon ovale*) and desquamative properties and favors the conversion of testosterone to 5α-dihydrotestosterone. Tretinoin gel or cream 0.1 to 0.025% acts primarily on the keratotic content in altered hair follicules. Skin irritation is frequent, and treatment may have to be discontinued as a result.

Cytostatics

Cytostatics are seldom applied topically in dermatotherapy. Podophyllin in 25% solution in absolute alcohol acts in cell metaphase. It is used for the treatment of condyloma acuminata. It can cause peripheral neuropathy and in pregnant women fetal death. 5-Fluorouracyl is a synthetic pyrimidine antagonist. As a cytostatic it inhibits the activity of thymidylate synthetase. It can be used in treating basaliomas, senile keratoses, and Bowen's disease. Bleomycin 0.5 to 1.0 units/ml is used intralesionally in the treatment of warts.

Antipsoriatics

A range of various substances can be used in the treatment of psoriasis. Two of them are important in the topical therapy. Anthralin (dithranol) reduces epidermal mitotic activity, interfering with mitochondrial DNA or cellular enzymes. It is incorporated in a paste or ointment with salicylic acid. Applied on the skin as a reservoir, it allows considerable systemic resorption. In the skin an oxidative degradation of anthralin takes place, and the substance and metabolites are eliminated in feces and urine. Anthralin is prescribed at concentrations of 0.05 to 4 % in petrolatum with 1 to 3% salicylic acid. It can cause a severe dermatitis and stains the skin and dressings.

Calcipotriol 0.005% ointment is a synthetic vitamin D_3. Its mechanism of action involves induction of terminal differentiation of keratinocytes and inhibition of keratinocyte production. It differs from other vitamin D_3 analogues in that it has a lesser interference with calcium metabolism. For safety reasons, it should never be applied on more than 30% of the skin surface. Liver and kidney impairment contraindicate this treatment.

Skin ulcers

Ulcers, especially hypostatic ones, are a problem in dermatotherapy. Three phases should be distinguished: cleaning, granulation, and epithelialization. For these purposes, a number of synthetic dressings exist, including alginates, films, foams, hydrocolloids, hydrogels, laminates, and polysaccharides (dextramonomer). Cleaning the ulcer can be done with normal saline solution, hydrogen peroxide, or a solution of potassium permanganate. Sometimes slough must be removed surgically or by proteolytic enzymes, urea cream, or exudate-absorbing substances. Topical antibacterials applied to ulcers carry the risk of contact sensitivity that may delay ulcer healing. The most important part of treatment is constantly changing dressings, dictated by pain and/or discharge. If pain and/or discharge is absent, the ulcer can be occluded for days or weeks. Bandages should be applied on top to reduce edema. Oxygen therapy (hyperbaric) is still investigational, and special wound-healing agents (e.g., artificial skin) or 20% benzoyl peroxide emulsion can be used for the same purpose. Silver nitrate facilitates granulation, and moisture facilitates healing.

Suggested readings

ANONYMOUS. Drugs used in skin disease, WHO Model Prescribing Information. Geneva: WHO, 1997.

ARNDT KA. Manual of dermatologic therapeutics, 5th ed. Boston: Little, Brown, 1995.

CZARNETZKY BM. Vitamin D3 in dermatology: a critical appraisal. Dermatologica 1989;178:184-8.

DANIEL RC. Traditional management of onychomycosis. J Am Acad Dermatol 1996;35(suppl):S21-5.

GUPTA AK, EINASSON TR, SUMMERBELL RC, SHEAR NH. An overview of topical antifungal therapy in dermatomycoses Drugs 1998;55:645-74.

HAY RJ. Antifungal drugs in dermatology. Semin Dermatol 1990;9:309-17.

KEMENY L, RUZICKA T, BRAUN-FALCO O. Dithranol. A review of the mechanism of action in the treatment of psoriasis vulgaris. Skin Pharmacol 1990;3:1-20.

New areas of drug development

Beate M. Henz

In the past, major advances in the pharmacologic treatment of skin diseases have taken place mostly in the context or as a consequence of developments and discoveries in other specialties. Examples include the coincidental improvements observed in patients with psoriasis and acne during retinoid treatment and in patients with psoriatic arthritis during cyclosporine A (CsA) therapy. The major reason for this lack of direct drug development for skin diseases is their largely unclarified pathogenesis and the lack of animal models for testing new drugs.

When the literature is searched for promising new treatment modalities, one finds a striking plethora of immunomodulatory drugs for dermatologic indications such as psoriasis, atopic and contact eczema, urticaria, diverse autoimmune and allergic diseases, and skin cancer, particularly melanoma. For infectious diseases, new drugs represent primarily improvements in already available agents, and for genetic diseases, gene therapy is being discussed but has so far not been implemented. This chapter therefore focuses on novel immunomodulatory therapy of dermatologic diseases.

Cyclosporine and related drugs

The discovery of the fungal peptide cyclosporin A (CsA) was of fundamental importance to the progress of modern organ transplantation. Its main mechanism of action involves an inhibition of cytokine and growth factor production, particularly interleukin-2 (IL-2)-dependent lymphocyte proliferation (see Chap. 75).

Indications for CsA treatment in dermatology include severe psoriasis and psoriatic arthritis, severe atopic dermatitis, treatment-refractory chronic and physical urticaria, and a long list of more rare diseases with associated well-recognized or putative immune pathology (Tab. 79.1). Although CsA inhibits mediator release from mast cells, it does not inhibit mast cell proliferation and is thus not useful in the treatment of mastocytosis.

Cyclosporin A has been studied extensively in the past in an oil-in-water emulsion formulation, but more recently, a microemulsion with improved bioavailability has

become available. In a recent double-blind study design, this preparation proved to be slightly more effective and more rapid in onset of action than the old formulation. Furthermore, it induced a marked improvement even in psoriatic patients previously unresponsive to CsA.

The dosage of cyclosporin A used in dermatologic indications is low and, in fact, should be kept as low as possible because of potential adverse effects, with dose ranges between 3 and 5 mg/kg per day for adults and up to 6 mg/kg for children. In carefully controlled clinical studies, hardly any adverse effects were observed, even in children and on treatment for up to 1 year. Relapse is observed in most children with atopic eczema, however, within 1 to 38 months after cessation of treatment.

The potential acute nephrotoxic effects, as well as the long-term effects in terms of enhancement of carcinogenesis due to immunosuppression, limit the extensive use of

---

Table 79.1 Dermatologic diseases shown to be responsive to cyclosporine and other immunosuppressive agents

Major indications
Psoriasis[1]
Psoriatic arthritis[1]
Atopic eczema[1]
Acrodermatitis continua suppurativa
Autoimmune blistering diseases (pemphigus vulgaris, bullous pemphingoid, epidermolysis bullosa acquisita)
Chronic and physical urticaria[1]
Generalized lichen planus[1]

Rare diseases
Pyoderma gangrenosum
Scleroderma/morphea
Pustular psoriasis[1]
Behçet's disease
Prurigo nodularis
Lupus erythematosus
Granulomatous diseases
(granuloma anulare, sarcoidosis)
Vitiligo
Alopecia areata

[1]Indicated only in severe, recalcitrant disease.

this drug. Total dose reduction is thus desirable by keeping the daily treatment at the minimal effective level, restricting treatment to short courses, or capitalizing on the very distinct adverse effect profile of CsA and retinoids or vitamin D3 derivates by using CsA together with topical vitamin D3 or systemic retinoids at lower dosages, as recently reported to be successful for the latter combination in psoriasis. Topical formulations of CsA aimed at decreasing the risk of systemic toxicity would be another alternative, but these proved to be rather ineffective, most likely due to poor penetration of the CsA molecule through the epidermal barrier.

Tacrolimus (FK506)

This more recently developed drug is also used primarily in transplantation medicine, with immunosuppressive properties 10 to 100 times greater than cyclosporin A and with a similar mode of action and side-effect profile. Since the molecule is much smaller than cyclosporin A, it was recently tested topically and found to be highly effective in atopic eczema in a double-blind multicenter study using a 0.03 to 0.3% ointment base. No serious adverse effects were observed.

Apart from another study showing efficacy of the drug in contact eczema, further dermatologic indications have not been explored as yet.

Other immunomodulatory drugs targeted for organ transplantation

Rapamycin differs in its mechanism of action from cyclosporin A and FK506 in that it induces intracellular signaling independent of calcium, although it also binds to immunophilin. Because of its high toxicity, this drug has not been studied so far in psoriasis or atopic eczema. In combination with CsA, however, it has been shown to induce 27-fold higher immunosuppressive effects, and both drugs might thus cause fewer side effects when used in combination at lower doses in a clinical setting. Thus far, no clinical studies have been published on the efficacy in psoriasis or atopic eczema.

Leflunomide is a crotonic acid amide with proven efficacy in organ graft rejection, autoimmune disorders, and rheumatoid arthritis (see Chap. 48). Like other newer approaches to immunosuppression in organ transplantation (mycophenolate mofetil, HLA-derived peptides), no published data are available on its effects in skin diseases.

Vitamin A derivatives (retinoids)

In agreement with observations in patients with vitamin A deficiency, chemically modified vitamin A derivatives were developed for the treatment of cancer and disorders of keratinization. The resulting drugs provided a major unprecedented advancement in the treatment of ichthyoses and severe acne. More recently, all-*trans* retinoic acid (ATRA) proved highly effective in the treatment of acute promyelogenous leukemia of adults, but in cutaneous T-cell lym-

phoma, it was inferior in combination with interferon-(IFN-α) compared with ATRA plus psoralen-enhanced ultraviolet A (UVA) light treatment.

The effects of retinoids on the immune system, as evidenced by efficacy in enhancing resistance against infections in malnourished children and maturation of B-cell function in infants with common variable immunodeficiency, received further support from recent findings that retinoids inhibit initiation of immunoglobulin E (IgE) synthesis at the germ line level. This activity is mediated primarily via the nuclear RARα receptor. These drugs thus might be useful in normalizing the supposedly immature and imbalanced immune system in patients with atopic dermatitis. Although retinoids also modulate mast cell proliferation in vitro, they proved in my hands to be ineffective, however, in adult-onset mastocytosis (unpublished own observations).

Recently, liarozole, an inhibitor of retinoic acid metabolism, has been tested for the first time in a double-blind study in psoriasis patients, and the drug was as effective with a similar adverse-effect profile. Since liarozole raises the intrinsic level of ATRA, however, it has no advantage over synthetic retinoids with regard to teratogenicity.

Vitamin D_3 and derivatives

These molecules act via the same nuclear receptor family as glucocorticoids and retinoids and, accordingly, have a broad range of pharmacologic and immunologic activities. They were targeted originally for the systemic treatment of osteoporosis and accidentally were found to be beneficial in patients suffering concomitantly from psoriasis. Because of the potential systemic toxicity, topical formulations (e.g., calcipotriol, tacalcitol) were developed for the treatment of plaque psoriasis, with good efficacy. More recently, derivatives with a higher in vitro efficacy at suppressing keratinocyte proliferation have been evaluated. Thus, 1,25-dihydroxy-2-oxocalcitriol has been tested in a 25 and 50 mg/g ointment base in a left-right comparison in plaque psoriasis and showed slightly more favorable results vs. calcipotriol.

New drugs in allergic diseases

Conventional drug development in allergy has been aimed primarily at control of symptoms. H_1 receptor-blocking antihistamines are a classic group of such agents with high efficacy against mast cell-dependent histamine action. Newer antihistamines are being developed to improve the adverse-effect profile, particularly regarding drowsiness and potential cardiotoxic effects. Recent evidence is also emerging suggesting that H_1 antagonists have distinct efficacy and adverse-effect profiles, as shown for azelastine versus cetirizine. Of particular interest is the anti-inflammatory activity of this group of compounds, which seems to be due to inhibition of mediator release from mast cells and basophils. Thus, loratadine and azelastine also are effective in inhibiting tumor necrosis factors-α (TNF-α) and IL-8 release from mast cells in vitro, and loratadine has similar effects on peripheral blood cells after in vivo treatment (unpublished own data).

Despite major efforts, drugs aimed at mediators other than histamine in immediate-type allergic reactions have been disappointing. This holds in particular for platelet-activating factor (PAF) antagonists. Leukotriene antagonists (e.g., montelukast, zafirlukast), however, have been shown recently to be active in the treatment of asthma (see Chap. 28). They have not yet been studied in dermatologic allergic diseases or atopic eczema, although a recent report of induction of urticaria in aspirin-sensitive patients makes their usefulness in urticaria therapy doubtful.

Additional newer immunomodulatory drugs are intravenous immunoglobulin (IVG) and interferons (IFNs). The mechanism of action of IVG is unclear, but it is thought to involve interference with IgG binding to Fc receptors on macrophages and with the anti-idiotype network (see Chap. 75). Treatment is effective in autoimmune vasculitis and chronic idiopathic urticaria, but use is limited by the high cost of the preparation.

IFNs have been studied extensively in various dermatologic conditions but has been proven to be of value in only a few. Thus IFN-α seems effective in some very severely affected children with atopic eczema, and selected patients with mastocytosis seem to benefit, particularly those with associated osteoporosis.

In atopic eczema, newer approaches also involve treatment with Chinese tea, which according to a recent analysis contains corticosteroids to explain part of its action, and linoleic acid-containing preparations, only effective in moderately affected individuals on long-term therapy.

Newer efforts in drug development for allergic diseases aim at modulating the basic allergy-related immune response either via inhibition of IgE synthesis (e.g., IL-4 inhibition) or by blockade of the binding of allergens to receptors on mast cells, basophils, or T-lymphocytes. Thus far, only T-cell epitope peptides have proven to be effective during hyposensitization therapy of bee venom-allergic patients, but peptides inhibiting FceRI binding have so far been disappointing.

New drugs in melanoma therapy

Among skin tumors, melanoma is both the most life-threatening and the most treatment-refractory malignant disease. A promising new cytostatic drug, temozolomide, was studied recently in advanced melanoma, but it proved to be only slightly more favorable than the "golden standard" dacarbazine (DTIC). Its usefulness in an adjuvant setting or in patients with melanoma brain metastases has not yet been clarified. On the other hand, high-dose IFN-α therapy has been shown recently to be of value as an adjuvant in high-risk cutaneous melanoma after resection of the primary tumor.

In patients with generalized metastases, gene therapy using tumor cells transfected with cytokine genes (e.g., IL-2, IL-7, IL-12, and GM-CSF) has been attempted recently, with the aim to induce cytotoxic or killer lymphocytes. Thus far, results are not encouraging. An exception is a recent study in which dendritic cells were cultured in vitro from patient peripheral blood with immunologic "education" of these cells against melanoma antigens. The results were most encouraging, including remissions in patients with brain metastases. Taken together, these novel experimental approaches will have to stand the test of time, with evaluation of many more patients, although they raise hopes of conquering these extremely difficult therapeutic challenges.

Suggested readings

FRY L. Immunosuppressive drugs. In: Bos JD, ed. The skin immune system, 2nd ed. Boca Raton, CRC Press, 1997, chap 40, 629-39.

HENZ BM, METZENAUER P, O'KEEFE E, ZUBERBIER T. Differential effects of new generation H1-receptor antagonists in pruritic dermatoses. Allergy 1998;53:180-3.

KIRKWOOD JM, STRAWDERMAN MH, ERNSTOFF MS, et al. Interferon alpha-2b adjuvant therapy of high-risk resected cutaneous melanoma: the Eastern Cooperative Oncology Group trial EST 1684. J Clin Oncol 1996;14:7-17.

KOO J. A randomized, double-blind study comparing the efficacy, safety and optimal dose of two formulations of cyclosporine (Neoral and Sandimmun) in patients with severe psoriasis. Br J Dermatol 1998;139:88-95.

MÜLLER U, CEZMI AA, FRICKER M, et al. Successful immunotherapy with T-cell epitope peptides of bee venom phospholipase A2 induces specific T-cell anergy in patients allergic to bee venom. J Allergy Clin Immunol 1998;101:747-54.

NESTLE FO, ALIJAGIC S, GILLIET M, et al. Vaccination of melanoma patients with peptide- or tumor lysate-pulsed dendritic cells. Natl Med 1998;4:328-32.

O'DONNELL BE, BARR RM, KOBZA BLACK A, et al. Intravenous immunoglobulin in autoimmune chronic urticaria. Br J Dermatol 1998;138:101-6.

OHNISHI-INOUE Y, MITSUYA K, HORIO T. Aspirin-sensitive urticaria: provocation with a leukotriene receptor antagonist. Br J Dermatol 1998;138:483-5.

RUZICKA T, BIEBER T, SCHÖPF E, et al. A short-term trial of tacrolimus ointment for atopic dermatitis. N Engl J Med 1997;337:816-21.

SCHADENDORF D. Novel strategies in the treatment of melanoma. Z Hautkr 1997;72:175-83.

STADLER R, OTTE HG, LUGER T, et al. Prospective randomized multicenter clinical trial on the use of interferon alpha-2a plus acitretin versus interferon alpha-2a plus PUVA in patients with cutaneous T-cell lymphoma (CTCL) stage I and II. Blood 1998;92:3578-81.

TOUBI E, BLANT A, KESSEL A, GOLAN TD. Low-dose cyclosporine A in the treatment of severe chronic idiopathic urticaria. Allergy 1997;52:312-6.

WORM M, KRAH JM, MANZ RA, HENZ BM. Retinoic acid inhibits CD40-IL-4 mediated IgE production. Blood 1998;92:1713-20.

ZAKI I, EMERSON R, ALLEN BR. Treatment of severe atopic dermatitis in childhood with cyclosporine. Br J Dermatol 1996;135(suppl 48):21-4.

ZONNEVELD IM, DE RIE MA, BELJAARDS RC, et al. The long-term safety and efficacy of cyclosporine in severe refractory atopic dermatitis: a comparison of two dosage regimens. Br J Dermatol 1996;135(suppl 48):15-20.

Drug abuse

Definition of drug dependence

Pier Francesco Mannaioni, Marco Moncini

Pharmacologic definition of substance of abuse

A vast number of terms have been used both in the lay press and in scientific reports to identify the interplay between a drug and a subject beyond the correct use of a drug to treat and cure a disease under medical prescription. The terms include *drug addiction, drug abuse, drug habituation, abuse liability,* and *addiction.* In defining drug dependence, it is therefore paramount to understand what is meant by *dependence, addiction,* and *abuse.*

Dependence is "a state of psychic or physical dependence, or both, on a drug, arising in a person following administration of that drug on a periodic or continuous basis." The characteristics of such a state will vary with the agent involved. Since 1964, the terms *drug addiction* and *drug habituation* have been replaced by *drug dependence,* according to the recommendation of the World Health Organization Expert Committee on Addiction Producing Drugs, which issued the preceding definition. The cues for understanding drug dependence, as defined above, are the periodic or continuous administration of the same (or closely related) drug in such a way as to produce psychicologic and/or physical dependence. There are, however, authors who stick on the term *addiction,* defined as "a behavioral pattern of drug use characterized by overwhelming involvement in the use of a drug (compulsive use), the securing of its supply, and a high tendency to relapse after withdrawal."

The term *drug abuse* is a social judgment. A drug abuser is a subject who uses an illegal substance (e.g., heroin, cocaine) or a legal substance in amounts that others consider excessive (e.g., ethanol) or a legal substance in any amount (e.g., tobacco).

Abuse (or *addiction*) *liability* is a pharmacologic term to signify a drug's potential for inducing addictive behavior. In clinical practice, the DSM-III-R has set up the diagnostic criteria for psychoactive substance dependence (Tab. 80.1).

Putting together the specific cues to understanding the preceding definitions, the question arises as to how to define the continuous or periodic use of a drug. What is meant by psychologic and physical dependence, by drug-seeking behavior, by compulsive relapse, by differential social judgment, and by the differential capacity of a drug to induce drug dependence?

In terms of both clinical features and neurobiology, *drug dependence* may be defined as "a social, chronic, relapsing illness produced by the periodic or continuous use of a drug endowed with certain characteristics". At least two of the following characteristics must be met by a drug [for it] to be considered capable of producing drug dependence: (1) tolerance, (2) psychologic dependence, (3) physical dependence, (4) social dependence, (5) psy-

Table 80.1 DSM-III-R diagnostic criteria for psychoactive substance dependence

At least three of the following:

1. Substance often taken in larger amounts or over a longer period than the person intended
2. Persistent desire or one or more unsuccessful efforts to cut down or control substance use
3. A great deal of time spent in activities necessary to get the substance, taking the substance, or recovering from its effects
4. Frequent intoxication or withdrawal symptoms when expected to fulfill major role obligations at work, school, or home, or when substance use is physically hazardous
5. Important social, occupational, or recreational activities given up or reduced because of substance use
6. Continued substance use despite knowledge of having a persistent or recurrent social, psychological, or physical problem that is caused or exacerbated by use of the substance
7. Marked tolerance: need for markedly increased amounts of the substance (i.e., at least a 50% increase) to achieve intoxication or desired effect, or markedly diminished effect with continued use of the same amount
8. Characteristic withdrawal symptoms
9. Substance often taken to relieve or avoid withdrawal symptoms

Some symptoms of the disturbance have persisted for at least 1 month or have occurred repeatedly over a longer period of time

Note: The items 8 and 9 may not apply to *Cannabis,* hallucinogens, or phencyclidine.

chotoxic reactions to overdose, (6) psychotoxic reactions to withdrawal, [and] (7) concomitant illnesses".

Tolerance is "... an adaptive state characterized by diminished response to the same quantity of drug or by the fact that a larger dose is required to produce the same degree of pharmacodynamic effect." There are many kinds of tolerance, and they can be classified as innate tolerance, acquired acute tolerance, and acquired chronic tolerance. *Innate tolerance* reflects a number of genetic or acquired factors that explain the difference in the initial response in terms of species, sex, age, diet, state of health, and previous exposure. The rabbit experiences no harm from eating *Atropa belladonna* shrubs because this animal species is provided with specific atropine esterases. Chinese and North African populations may have more adverse effects than Caucasians from drinking the same amount of alcohol because they have reduced alcohol dehydrogenases (inverse tolerance).

Acquired acute tolerance (tachyphylaxis) involves a sudden decrease in the effect of a drug, which fades after the second or third administration, as a result of depletion of endogenous substances that indirectly produce the pharmacologic effect. The reward of amphetamines is due, at least in part, to the release of catecholamines at the presynaptic level. A second administration of amphetamine after a short time (30-60 minutes) will be ineffective because the previously released mediators were not resynthesized.

The most common form of tolerance is *acquired chronic tolerance*. There are two kinds. Metabolic, or kinetic, tolerance reflects the organism's increased ability to metabolize the drug such that the concentration of drug in contact with the sites of action is reduced. This is one of the distinguishing features of the dependence induced by ethanol, barbiturates, and the benzodiazepines. Cellular, or pharmacodynamic, tolerance represents a decreased sensitivity of the drug-sensitive physiologic system to a given drug concentration. Cellular tolerance signifies an adaptive change in the brain meant to maintain homeostasis. Among the possible mechanisms is receptor desensitization or downregulation, either limited to ligands of one receptor type or involving other receptors that converge to the same signal-transduction pathway or ion channel. This kind of tolerance is produced by opioids, ethanol, barbiturates, and the benzodiazepines.

Acquired chronic tolerance, both pharmacokinetic and pharmacodynamic, has the following characteristics: (1) many, but not all, drugs induce tolerance, (2) tolerance may develop to some, but not all, actions of a drug, (3) tolerance may develop unaccompanied or accompanied by physical dependence, (4) tolerance may arise to drugs that do not induce physical dependence, (5) tolerance begins to decline on withdrawing the drug but its effects may still be detectable a long time thereafter, (6) small doses of a drug are able to produce tolerance to larger doses of the same substance, and (7) tolerance may be produced in isolated organs or cells.

The interplay between tolerance and the other distinguishing features of drug dependence (i.e., physical dependence, drug-seeking behavior) is complex. Marijuana and lysergic acid diethylamide (LSD)–like drugs produce striking tolerance and no physical dependence. With opioids, tolerance preferentially develops to certain effects, being overt for psychic and analgesic effects and less evident for smooth muscle relaxation. Tolerance develops to the euphoric effect of cocaine, whereas a reverse tolerance/sensitization is produced toward psychosis and to choreic movements. Whether tolerance is required for physical dependence is unclear. However, understanding tolerance would help to explain why addicts survive to dose ranges that would have killed nontolerant subjects.

Psychic or psychogenic dependence traditionally has been recognized as another important feature of drug dependence. Psychic dependence may be accompanied by physical dependence (as in the case of the opioid and ethanol-barbiturate types of addiction). It may not be present at all (as in the case of dependence on pentazocine) where there is only physical dependence. It also may exist without physical dependence, as in the case of use of cocaine, marijuana, and hallucinogenic drugs.

The Expert Committee on Addiction-producing Drugs of the World Health Organization has defined *psychic dependence* as "... a state of discomfort produced by withdrawal of a drug... The discomfort may consist of a non-specific and ill-defined dissatisfaction giving rise to a desire (ranging from a mild wish to intense craving) for the perceived effect of the drug." Subjective feelings of psychic irritability, particularly toward the idea of a possible relapse, are characteristic of psychic dependence.

Physical dependence represents a physiologic and biochemical adaptation to the presence of an addicting drug so that the organism is normal while drug concentrations are maintained. Removal of the drug unmasks an underlying pathophysiology. The "withdrawal syndrome" is often characterized by effects opposite to the acute pharmacologic actions of the drug itself. These disturbances are all relieved dramatically by reestablishing an effective drug concentration.

Besides physical and psychic dependence, social dependence is difficult to overcome when treating drug addiction. *Social dependence* may in fact be defined as an adaptation of the individual to his/her new condition. He joins peer groups using marijuana, heroin, or alcohol as their cultural basis. In the case of alcohol, delirium tremens is an expression of physical dependence and can be cured by specific pharmacologic interventions. The psychologic dependence also may be abated by specific psychologic interventions. However, when the patient finally returns to normal life, he realizes that he no longer has any friends because his or her group was based on alcohol use (social dependence).

Tolerance and physical dependence by themselves do not imply "addiction." Tolerance, physical dependence, and withdrawal are biologic phenomena that can be produced in any human being who takes certain medicines repeatedly. A hypertensive patient may develop tolerance to β-blockers or to adrenergic agonists of the α_2 type and also experience a withdrawal syndrome when the medication is stopped abruptly, consisting in a rebound of high blood pressure (see Chap. 23).

Besides tolerance and physical dependence, drug-seeking behavior and craving are of paramount importance in understanding drug dependence. A standard explanation for substance abuse implies that abusers became caught up in a vicious cycle of drug administration, tolerance, physical dependence, withdrawal, and readministration. The substance abuser was believed to self-administer abusable substances on a negative basis, i.e., to ward off the negative physical consequences of drug withdrawal. This may be the case in hard-core continuous heroin self-administration but does not explain the initial self-administration and periodic use of heroin (nowadays the most common pattern). More recently, emphasis has been placed on the possibility that abusable substances may have powerful positively enforcing properties.

Drug-seeking behavior and craving (defined as "a subset of desires or urges that have crossed a subjective threshold of intensity") originate from the effect of all the abusable drugs on the brain reward mechanisms, on which they act as positive reinforcers.

There are several classes of self-administered drugs, all of them acting on the central nervous system (CNS). On the basis of the pharmacologic actions on the CNS, self-administered drugs can be grouped under three broad categories:

• *stimulants* are drugs that stimulate the CNS and cause an elevation of mood (euphoria) and a sense of increased energy and strength. Cocaine, the amphetamines, caffeine, and nicotine produce these effects;
• *psychedelics,* or *hallucinogens,* affect normal perceptive functions of the CNS and induce states of altered perception, thoughts, and feelings that are not experienced otherwise except in dreams or at times of religious exaltation. Lysergic acid diethylamide (LSD), mescaline, psilocybin, and phencyclidine are typical examples. Cannabis products are also included in this group, but only the strong preparations such as hashish and hash oil have distinct psychedelic effects, whereas the weak preparations such as marijuana rather act like sedative-hypnotics;
• *depressants* relieve tension and anxiety; produce euphoria or a feeling of well-being, peace, and contentment; and induce sleep. Depressants include such drugs as alcohol, barbiturates, benzodiazepines, and different opioid drugs (e.g., morphine, heroin, buprenorphine).

Although seemingly diverse, these groups of drugs can be identified by their common ability to serve as positive reinforcers in humans and experimental animals; each of the drugs in these groups has the ability to control behavior in a manner similar to natural positive reinforcers such as food and water. A positive reinforcer is any event or substance that stimulates specialized brain systems, producing a reward that increases the likelihood of repetition of the whole experience. There are natural reinforcers that gain access to the brain reinforcement circuitry by way of the sensory system, such as olfaction, taste, and vision. The reward circuit originates in cells of the midbrain ventrotegmental area (VTA) and projects via the medial forebrain bundle to the nucleus accumbens (NA). VTA cells of the reward circuit are dopaminergic, whereas the efferent pathway from the NA is GABAergic.

Accordingly, drug dependence may be redefined as the result of self-administration of drugs that produce positive reinforcement and negative reinforcement. In the case of heroin, the initial self-administration activates the reward circuit by releasing dopamine, which evokes the positive reinforcement through the expected reward.

In terms of the neurobiology of drug dependence, the positive reinforcement is due to the release of dopamine. The negative reinforcement has been accounted for by the neuroadaptations in the second-messenger systems in competent neuronal cells. In NA cells, chronic exposure to opiates, cocaine, or ethanol shows similarities in postreceptor neuroadaptations. Chronic exposure to these drugs decreased levels of inhibitory G-proteins and increased adenylate cyclase, producing an upregulation of the NA cell cAMP pathway.

Beside dopamine and the cAMP system, other brain neurotransmitters come into play for their relation to the addicting drugs. As shown in Table 80.2, each family of addicting drugs mimics or blocks a particular neurotransmitter in the brain. The barbiturates, benzodiazepines, and ethyl alcohol enhance the action of γ-aminobutyric acid (GABA), and they have been shown to enhance GABA binding through a specific interaction with the GABA (A) receptor complex. Cocaine and the amphetamines block the reuptake of catecholamines at synapses, thus increasing local concentrations and enhancing the neurotransmitter effects; a putative site of action of cocaine on a dopamine transporter was identified recently. Morphine derived from heroin mimics the actions of one or another endogenous opioid, preferentially binding to and activating the μ type of opioid receptor. Nicotine activates the nicotinic type of acetylcholine receptor in brain, caffeine is an antagonist of adenosine receptors, and tetrahydrocannabinol (THC), the active ingredient of *Cannabis,* mimics the effect of endocannabinoid anandamide on the THC1 receptor in the brain.

However, the paradigm of the neurobiology of drug dependence as described earlier may be reductive and misleading. Assuming dopamine as the sole mediator of the positive reinforcement is not entirely tenable, since other transmitters are released on acute administration of addictive drugs (e.g., serotonin, histamine), and destruction of dopamine terminals fails to influence the development of heroin dependence. The upregulation of the cAMP pathway is shared by neuronal cells activated by different transmitters. The interaction between the addicting drugs and the brain neurotransmitters, as shown in Table 80.2, is only preferential. For example, ethyl alcohol also interacts with serotonin and NMDA receptors; heroin is supposed to act after activation to 6-acetyl-morphine and to morphine β-glucuronide, acting on a novel subtype of opioid receptor; and cocaine increases the turnover of histamine in NA cells.

The biologic basis of drug dependence has not yet been explained satisfactorily. Any hope for a specific pre-

Table 80.2 Neurobiologic substrates for acute reinforcing effects of drugs of abuse

Drug of abuse	Neurotransmitter	Sites
Cocaine and amphetamines	Dopamine Serotonin	Nucleus accumbens, amygdala
Opiates	Dopamine Opioid peptides	Ventral tegmental area, nucleus accumbens
Nicotine	Dopamine Opioid peptides?	Ventral tegmental area, nucleus accumbens, amygdala?
THC	Dopamine Opioid peptides?	Ventral tegmental area

(THC = tetrahydrocannabinol.)

ventive or therapeutic intervention based on neurobiologic knowledge is unlikely to be fulfilled. However, this fact should constitute a strong argument for continued experimental, clinical, and epidemiologic analyses of the nature of drug dependence.

Clinical presentation and laboratory diagnosis

A technical discussion of the clinical presentation of the different types of drug dependence is given in chapters that follows; however, some general outlines can be drawn. In the case of opioids, medical care is sought as a consequence of overdose (i.e., an excess of agonists on receptors) or of withdrawal (i.e., a lack of agonists and the interaction of neurotransmitters with upregulated receptors). A third possibility exists in the case of heroin addicts asking for detoxification while in good standing.

The same clinical presentation is shared by alcoholics, who seek care when acutely intoxicated, when suffering the different stages of alcoholic withdrawal, or when they ask for treatment while in good standing.

Cocaine addicts seldom require care, since the use/abuse of snorted cocaine hydrochloride is wisely titrated. Similarly, the clinical presentation of the use/abuse of *Cannabis* derivatives is of little concern, although the diffusion of marijuana smoking is as high in European as in American youths.

Different testing systems are available for identifying drugs in urine, which is preferentially analyzed over blood. Testing of hair, meant to detect drugs used days to months earlier, is limited to forensic cases. Thin-layer chromatography requires 3 to 4 hours to perform and is relatively insensitive. More sensitive are immunoassays, which include enzyme immunoassay, radioimmunoassay, and latex agglutination inhibition assay. Of these, the enzyme multiplied immunoassay technique (EMIT) is the most widely used. It is advisable to confirm any positively screened sample with gas chromatography and/or mass spectrometry, which are more sensitive and more specific but also more expensive and time-consuming.

Urine can be positive for cannabinoids several days after a single casual use of marijuana, and the major metabolite of cocaine, benzoylecgonine, is detectable for several weeks in the urine. This fact has to be kept in mind when establishing the clinical diagnosis of drug dependence.

Short- and long-term risks

The acute and chronic effects of the different drugs of abuse and the consequent risks are not similar.

Cocaine and amphetamines

Cocaine hydrochloride is generally used by snorting or by intravenous injections (alone or in combination with heroin, i.e., a "speed ball"). Cocaine free base ("crack" cocaine) may be smoked because it is resistant to the high temperature realized during the pyrolysis of smoked tobacco. Cocaine produces a brief enhancement of mood (euphoria); feelings of excitement and increased energy and muscular strength; an increase in cardiac and pulse rates, respiratory rate, blood pressure (risk of heart attack), and body temperature; a temporary increase in libidinal drive and sexual performance; and a decrease in appetite. Cocaine exerts its reinforcing action by blocking neuronal reuptake of the excitatory neurotransmitters dopamine and norepinephrine, thereby increasing synaptic concentrations in specific brain areas.

The acute effects of amphetamines (such as benzedrine, dexedrine, methylamphetamines, and methylen-dioxy-methamphetamine, MDMA, "ecstasy") are similar to those of cocaine but also persist for a longer time. Amphetamines parallel cocaine in their capacity to increase synaptic concentrations of dopamine and norepinephrine, but they cause this increase by stimulating their release from intraneuronal stores and by blocking their inactivation by monoaminoxidases. MDMA ("ecstasy") is also known to interact with serotoninergic neurons, producing the depletion of serotonin in the raphe of experimental animals. The short-term risks of amphetamine abuse are similar to those of cocaine, especially in the induction of toxic psychosis.

As far as the long-term risks of amphetamine abuse are concerned, recent evidence suggests that amphetamines induce degeneration and death of dopaminergic and serotoninergic neurons through an oxidative stress. Accordingly, the released dopamine and serotonin would be oxidized in the neuronal cleft to 6-hydroxy-dopamine (6-OH-DA) and to 5-6-dihydroxytryptamine (5-6-DHT). 6-OH-DA and 5-6-DHT undergo specific reuptake into the presynaptic terminals, where they are activated to neurotoxic free radicals by a Fenton reaction.

Cannabinoids

The psychoactive nature of *Cannabis* is due to the presence of delta-9-tetraydrocannabinol (THC) in concentrations from 1 to 2% (bhang), 5% (ganja, marijuana), and 10 to 20% (hashish or charas). These substances generally are smoked and sometimes are taken orally, particularly in Oriental countries. Ordinary-grade marijuana produces an increased sense of well-being (euphoria), accompanied by feelings of relaxation and sleepiness when subjects are alone. When users can interact, sleepiness is less pronounced, and there is often spontaneous laughter and garrulity. Short-term memory is impaired, and the capacity to carry out tasks requiring multiple mental steps deteriorates, the effect being called *temporal disintegration* or *amotivational syndrome*.

Opioids

Heroin is the most notorious of all abused drugs, generally used by intravenous administration or by snorting and smoking. Heroin produces a warm flushing of the skin, tingling sensations running up and down the limbs, and sensations in the lower abdomen described by addicts as similar in intensity and quality to sexual orgasm.

The short-term risk of heroin abuse entails the overdose (e.g., coma, miosis, bradypnea) and the withdrawal syndrome. The long-term risks are difficult to relate to heroin itself or to noninfectious or infectious complications. Among the noninfectious complications, the nonoverdose sudden death, asthma, and the syndrome of fever, myalgia, and periarthritis are the most common. In some patients, coma and death are difficult to explain on the basis of true overdose. Both asthma and the nonoverdose sudden death have been accounted for by a massive release of histamine.

Possible treatment approaches

A drug abuser may be treated for overdose, for withdrawal, for medical or neurologic complications, or for addiction itself (detoxification and antirelapse programs). A point worth emphasizing is how inefficient unimodal approaches are. In fact, drug abusers do not limit themselves to one agent but develop a sometimes stereotyped trend that starts with a single drug of abuse and moves toward polydrug abuse. Heroin addicts frequently became successfully maintained on methadone and then became alcoholic or addicted to cocaine.

The efficacy of treatment must be evaluated not only focusing on whether clients have stopped using drugs but also on other outcome measures such as (1) decreased level of illegal activity, (2) increased employment and less dependence on social service agencies, (3) improved social and family functioning, (4) improved psychologic functioning, and (5) decreased mortality and improved physical health.

Four program features are of greatest importance in designing and implementing treatment programs:
1. The period of intervention must be a lengthy one, since drug dependence is typically a chronically relapsing condition requiring several rounds of treatment, except in a minority of cases.
2. Programs must provide a significant level of structure initially, such as a residential stay in a hospital or in a controlled inpatient setting or a very closely monitored outpatient setting.
3. Programs must be flexible. In a methadone maintenance program, intermittent drug use does not automatically disrupt the individual's program plan and should be dealt with on an individual basis.
4. Any intervention program must undergo regular evaluation to determine its level of effectiveness and to establish the need for any change.

Suggested readings _____

GOLDSTEIN A. Molecular and cellular aspects of the drug addiction. Berlin, Heidelberg, New York, London: Springer-Verlag, 1989.

LOWINSON JH, RUIZ P, MILLMAN RB. Substance abuse. A comprensive textbook. Baltimore, Hong Kong, München, Philadelphia: Williams and Wilkins, 1992.

WATSON RR. Drug abuse treatment. Totowa (NJ): Humana Press, 1992.

Opioids

Pier Francesco Mannaioni, Marco Moncini

The poppy has been harvested for its opioid content for more than 6000 years, and it was used for analgesia in ancient Assyrian and Egyptian medicine. In Europe, Paracelsus formulated laudanum (tincture of opium) in the middle of the sixteenth century, and eighteenth-century physicians recognized its dependence potential. In the nineteenth century, opium was commonly present in over-the-counter remedies such as Dover powder. The invention of the hypodermic needle, the extraction of morphine from the poppy, and the introduction of heroin in 1890 as a "nonaddictive" opioid for treating morphine dependence and as an over-the-counter antitussive facilitated the spread of opioid dependence all over the world. In 1914, the Harrison Narcotics Act in the United States curtailed a physician's right to give opioids to addicts and banned their nonmedical availability. Whether the Harrison Act led to a decrease in opioid addiction is uncertain.

The epidemic spread of opioid addiction in the United States began in the 1950s. In 1967, the number of opioid addicts known to the authorities had reached 108 424; a higher figure (i.e., 250 000-310 000) was proposed in 1972. English figures for this phenomenon were in marked contrast, where confirmed addicts had only reached 2944 in 1972, a low number, even though considerably higher than the 437 registered addicts in 1960.

At the present time, the figures for the prevalence of opioid addiction in the United States, as reported in the last Community Epidemiology Working Group (CEWG) in a yearly report issued by the National Institute of Drug Abuse (NIDA), are as follows: for the New York urban area, where opioid addiction is thought to be at its highest levels, in the year 1993: 793 deaths involving heroin, 11351 heroin Emergency Department mentions, 12 936 state-funded treatment admissions, and 24 595 heroin arrests.

In Italy, the latest accounts of heroin addiction come from the number of subjects enrolled in therapeutic communities (22 434 in 1996) and in social service agencies (90 577 in 1996). The nationwide mortality rate was 1551 deaths in 1996. Both figures, when corrected for the percentage of actual heroin addicts asking for intervention in therapeutic communities or from social services (about 5-10% of the real population) and for age-related mortality rate (i.e., the number of heroin-related deaths in the population 15-30 years of age), rank the incidence of the disease as 3.3 to 5.4 per 1000 persons and heroin as the fourth leading cause of death in youngsters, a higher toll than viral diseases.

In the case records of the Toxicological Unit of Florence University, the age distribution for this disease indicates that the period of major epidemic incidence is adolescence and early youth. However, a trend toward shifting the incidence to the third and fourth decades is now apparent.

Opioid dependence is at present mainly a male phenomenon. The female population is represented by 16 to 21% of US cases and by 35% of the Italian cases.

Heroin is the drug of choice among opioid addicts. In 1966, 70.2% of US addicts used heroin, 6.8% morphine, 6% hydromorphone (Dilaudid), 6.8% paregoric, 4.1% codeine, 4.1% meperidine, and 0.8% methadone. The gradual substitution of morphine by heroin is also evident in Italian observations, which are analogous to the data presented for England (309 addicts to morphine and 122 to heroin in 1960 as opposed to 295 addicts to morphine and 2321 addicts to heroin in 1970).

The social extraction of opioid addicts in Italy is not easily compared with data from US surveys because of the cultural and social differences between the two countries. Italian data are in contrast with some US epidemiologic surveys. Data collected in the US for 1965 indicate a prevalence of the phenomenon (71.2%) among the black and hispanic populations, emphasizing that drug addiction is one of the aspects of social hardship. Our data for Tuscany show a more homogeneous distribution of the phenomenon and include opioid addicts coming from families of white-collar workers (38%), industrialists, executives, and professionals (32%), as well as the underemployed and unemployed (14%). This distribution can be further explained by the fact that the major epidemiologic areas are all urban, where these classes are prevalent, in comparison with rural areas.

An examination of schooling levels in opioid addicts reveals that 25% have completed primary school, 50% lower middle school, 26% upper middle school, and 1.6% university. These data are particularly close to the results of US surveys, which indicate that 52% of drug addicts have attended the equivalent of the Italian lower middle school, 27% have attended the upper middle or secondary school, while 11% have reached university level.

The alleged motivations leading to heroin addiction in 150 patients show that a high percentage of addicts (82%) identify the initial cause of addiction as a general curiosity as to the effects or a casual social experience with peers. As far as gateway drugs are concerned, Italian data are comparable with those reported elsewhere. In England, 87% of a population of 80 heroin addicts had begun to abuse heroin starting with *Cannabis indica* derivatives. In the Italian cases, 59% had begun in the same way.

To sum up the epidemiologic features, the typical opioid addict in our cultural environment is young, usually male, living in an urban area, and physically and psychologically dependent on intravenous heroin. He comes from various social groups and is usually unable to define clearly the motivations for his heroin addiction. He belongs to a cultural group that does not recognize any specific ideology and usually begins to drift toward heroin through the use of other habit-forming substances.

Pathophysiology

The neurobiology of opioid addiction has been at issue for many years both in experimental animals and in isolated cells and may help to understand opioid (heroin) dependence in humans. In experimental animals, opioids activate the reward circuit in the brain responsible for positive reinforcement. A *positive reinforcement* is any event that stimulates specialized brain systems to produce a reward that increases the likelihood of repetition of the whole experience. The reward circuit originates in cells of the midbrain ventrotegmental area and projects via the medial forebrain bundle to the nucleus accumbens. Ventrotegmental area cells of the reward circuit are dopaminergic, whereas the efferent pathway from nucleus accumbens is GABAergic. In the experimental animals, the initial self-administration of any opioid activates the reward circuit by releasing dopamine, which evokes positive reinforcement through the expected reward (place preference, increase in self-administration). In humans, parenteral opioids (heroin) produce an ecstatic feeling lasting about 1 minute and often compared with orgasm but usually referred to the abdomen, followed by a dreamlike, pleasant drowsiness. In both experimental animals and humans, marked tolerance develops to the positive reinforcement given by the opioids, which can be reached only by significantly increasing the doses.

The usual analgesic dose of morphine is 10 mg. The equivalent dose of heroin (diacetylmorphine) is 1 to 5 mg, due to its most rapid effect. When tolerance has not developed, the acute administration of doses of morphine or heroin several times greater produces severe depressant effects. When tolerance has developed, high doses of opioids not only do not produce depressant effects but also become necessary for maintenance of homeostasis in those tissues which develop tolerance. For morphine, a dose of 80 mg per day is considered a "light addiction," and such a dose, eight times the therapeutic dose, is used clinically as a daily maintenance dose. In one heroin-addicted patient, the daily dose was 1080 mg (500-1000 times the initial dose). When heroin is used for maintenance, the chosen dose is 100 to 450 times the analgesic dose.

Chronic, acquired tolerance to opioids may occur either because of a more rapid disposal by metabolism of the drug (acquired dispositional or metabolic tolerance) or because of reduced activity and/or sensitivity of drug receptors. In the case of opioids, the possibility that tolerance is evoked in response to dispositional or metabolic modifications may be ruled out.

Under normal conditions, morphine and heroin are easily absorbed and equally distributed throughout the body. Their pharmacologic action terminates with hepatic metabolism (microsomal *N*-demethylation with formation of a glucuronide), coupled with renal elimination of the newly formed metabolites and of unmodified morphine. The pharmacokinetics of morphine and heroin (absorption, distribution, and metabolism) do not change in the individual who has become tolerant. Similar results were obtained in experimental animals. The only report of a significant change in morphine metabolism related to the development of tolerance shows that chronic administration of morphine produces in the rat a profound diminution in both the analgesic response (tolerance) and the ability of liver enzymes to *N*-dealkylate morphine. On this basis, it has been proposed that the continuous interaction of narcotic drugs with the demethylating enzymes markedly reduces the active metabolizing sites of these enzymes. Similarly, the continuous interaction of narcotic drugs with analgesic receptors also may reduce the active sites on these receptors. If the number of central receptor sites is decreased, this would result in fewer narcotic drug-receptor combinations and a decreased effect. Accordingly, tolerance to opioids is a kind of cellular tolerance, representing a decreased sensitivity of the drug-sensitive physiologic systems to a given drug concentration.

However, it is not known whether tolerance is associated with changes in endorphin concentrations or in the sensitivity of opioid receptors. It is also unknown how opioids specifically affect other neurotransmitter systems and how such actions contribute to reinforcement and tolerance. In fact, besides dopamine, clearly recognized as the mediator of the positive reinforcement, investigators have studied serotonin, acetylcoline, adenosine, glutamate, norepinephrine, and colecystokinin.

Drug-seeking behavior is fueled by positive reinforcement leading to reward and by negative reinforcement that entails avoiding the aversive effect of the withdrawal syndrome. The sudden discontinuation of use of an addicting drug (in this case, any opioid) or the administration of a narcotic antagonist (e.g., naloxone, naltrexone) produces a stereotypical reaction in both humans and experimental animals that have become opioid-tolerant. This reaction is characterized by behavioral and neurovegetative changes that are termed the *withdrawal* or *abstinence syndrome* (Tab. 81.1). Physical dependence on

Table 81.1 Symptoms and signs of opioid withdrawal

Drug craving
Irritability, anxiety
Tearing
Rhinorrhea
Sweating
Yawning
Myalgia
Mydriasis
Piloerection
Anorexia, nausea, and vomiting
Diarrhea
Hot flashes
Fever
Tachypnea
Productive coughing
Tachycardia
Hypertension
Abdominal cramps
Muscle spasms
Erection, orgasm

opioids exists because interruption in their chronic use provokes a deprivation sickness that is an overt manifestation of how modifications in cell functions have taken place during tolerance development. The withdrawal syndrome therefore must be considered as the indirect measure of physical dependence.

The withdrawal syndrome represents the counterpart of the initial effects of opioids. Wherever the initial effects of opioids are sedation and drowsiness, those of sudden discontinuation of opioids in tolerant subjects encompass hyperactivity of the central and peripheral nervous system.

Although incompletely understood, the hyperactivity of the nervous system expressed during opioid withdrawal may be explained by changes induced by the chronic exposure to opioids in the second-messenger system. In neuroblastoma-glioma cells cultured in vitro, it was found that adenylate cyclase (the enzyme that forms cyclic AMP after activation by certain hormones or transmitters) is inhibited by acute exposure to opiates or enkephalin. Over long periods of exposure to morphine or enkephalin, the cells compensate by synthesizing more molecules of the enzyme. As a consequence, higher opioid concentrations are required to produce a decrease in cAMP because the newly synthesized adenylate cyclase molecules make up for those which have been inhibited by morphine. The system at this point appears to be in a state of "tolerance." When drug administration is stopped, all the enzyme molecules become active and synthesize an excess of cAMP. This excess may trigger a sequence of events leading to withdrawal symptoms.

The withdrawal syndrome is an acute phenomenon that begins 4 to 6 hours after the last dose. Besides the acute abstinence, a protracted abstinence has been reported. Protracted abstinence has been observed in animals. Monkeys display signs of acute abstinence for up to sev-

eral months after withdrawal from morphine, and rats have electroencephalographic abnormalities, "wet dog" shakes, fever, hypermetabolism, increased water intake, and drug-seeking behavior for up to a year.

Clinical findings

The opioid addict as a medical patient shows signs and symptoms that occur because of the addiction as such. However, some diseases that are relatively unusual in the general population may occur with increased frequency among opioid addicts, and some relatively common diseases may manifest unusual features in opioid-dependent subjects.

In opioid-dependent subjects, medical care is sought (1) as a consequence of overdose (i.e., an excess of agonists on receptors), or (2) because of withdrawal (i.e., the lack of agonists and the interaction of neurotransmitters with upregulated receptors). Furthermore, opioid addicts may apply for medication (3) seeking detoxification while in good standing, or (4) after hospitalization due to concomitant diseases.

Opioid overdose

Opioid dependence may terminate in an acute high-risk disease – opioid overdose. Although any opioid may produce overdose, the main etiology is represented by intravenous heroin self-administration.

The clinical feature of opioid overdose is characteristic, and the diagnosis of opioid overdose is easy in noncomplicated cases. The "classic triad" of signs includes (1) stupor or coma, (2) respiratory depression, and (3) pinpoint pupils (miosis). Other common signs are the injection marks and the remnants of "homemade" first-aid maneuvers to which the patient has been subjected prior to hospital admission.

The coma shows no signs of asymmetry in reflexes, suggesting a lack of organic cerebral lesions. Reflexes and pain reactivity are consistently depressed or absent. Respiratory depression is characterized by a decrease in number of breaths (one to two breaths per minute) without pathologic appearance of respiratory rhythms (Kussmaul and/or Cheyne-Stokes type breathing). The miosis is very marked and bilateral, and the pupils are completely unreactive to light stimulation. Systemic arterial hypotension and cardiocirculatory failure are observed rarely. The overdose syndrome is usually of long duration, with a time lag of several hours between the act of self-administration and death. During this time, many complications can arise to alter the initial features, making the diagnosis more difficult.

The sudden-death type of heroin overdose, in which death occurs a few seconds after intravenous injection, the needle is found in the vein, and coma may not respond to antagonists, has been accounted for by many causes. Among them are (1) the self-administration of unusually high doses of heroin in tolerant subjects or in subjects who have lost tolerance after detoxification, (2) the decrease of myocardial contractility induced by quinine, often found as an adulterant in street heroin, due to its bitter taste and vasodilating effect, (3) cardiac anaphylactic or anaphylactoid reaction giving rise to lung edema or a lethal arrhythmia, (4) the combination of heroin with other drugs of abuse that markedly potentiate the acute toxicity of heroin.

Blood is the body compartment of choice in which to detect morphine (the metabolite of heroin) to validate the clinical features. In the blood, morphine concentration has a linear relationship with the severity of coma, at least in uncomplicated overdoses.

Acute withdrawal reactions

The acute withdrawal reaction in opioid addicts involves functional changes in a brain center, the locus ceruleus, a noradrenergic neural center concerned with the feelings of alarm, panic, fear, and anxiety. The opioid (i.e., heroin) inhibits the locus ceruleus neurons, and the latter soon become adapted to repeated use of the drug. An abrupt cessation of the drug causes excessive firing of the locus ceruleus neurons, followed by an intense craving for the drug and an outbreak of withdrawal symptoms.

During the first hours of abstinence, no signs or symptoms are observed. Occasional yawning, slight perspiration, rhinorrhea, and lacrimation are likely to appear 6 to 9 hours after the last dose. These symptoms become much more intense in the following hours and are supplemented by midriasis and recurring waves of piloerection ("cold turkey"). Twitching of various muscle groups then begins, and the patient complains of pain in the back and legs and of recurring sensations of hot and cold. About 24 hours later there is complete insomnia, accompanied by a genupectoral position and stereotypical movements (a typical one is to cover oneself with as many blankets as one can find). After 36 hours, the patient is constantly in motion, begins to retch and vomit, and has diarrhea.

During the whole abstinence period, the patient does not feed himself, and as a result of insomnia and fluid loss, he suffers a notable weight loss.

Arterial pressure increases by 15 to 30 mm Hg, and body temperature increases by 1°C. Symptoms reach peak intensity 48 hours after the last dose, remain intense for 50 to 70 hours of abstinence, and then begin to decline. One week later, all the signs have disappeared, even if the patient complains of insomnia, asthenia, and muscular aches and pains for many weeks afterwards.

Detoxification

Opioid-dependent subjects may apply to detoxification and antirelapse programs while in good standing, i.e., not expressing signs and symptoms of overdose or withdrawal. In such patients, the diagnosis of opioid dependence is based on scanty clinical evidence. Severe miosis, cuta-

neous "needle tracks," and the general appearance of the subject may be significant in suspecting opioid dependence.

However, the diagnosis of opioid dependence entails recognition of the molecule and rating of the physical dependence. In fact, the answer to these two diagnostic questions is of paramount importance for the therapeutic decision-making. The nature of the addicting molecule is easily recognized by chemically identifying the molecule in the patient's body fluids. In the chemical evaluation of opioids (by means of the current methodologies, from very simple to very sophisticated), urine examination is preferable to blood because the plasma half-life is shorter than the rate of urinary excretion. The presence of morphine in the urine of a subject at any given concentration does not allow the quantitative diagnosis of physical dependence, which is mandatory to start therapy with agonists or antagonists.

To evaluate a clinically significant and detectable degree of physical dependence, the naloxone precipitation test is useful. The method consists of administering naloxone (0.4-0.8 mg iv) under double-blind conditions and rating the signs and symptoms of the evoked withdrawal according to one of the common scoring system. In this way, it has been possible to separate alleged addicts into one group that responds to naloxone with a positive precipitation test and another group of nonreactors.

The precipitation test has relevant implications in the treatment of narcotic addiction. The group of subjects showing a negative naloxone challenge (i.e., lack of physical dependence) will be treated with narcotic antagonists and/or psychodynamic and rehabilitation techniques in outpatient antirelapse protocols. Those who show a positive naloxone challenge (i.e., actual physical dependence) will be detoxified by means of specific protocols before entering the antirelapse programs.

Concomitant diseases

The final reason that heroin addicts seek medical care is represented by the high incidence of concomitant diseases among the opioid-dependent population. Heroin abuse is associated with both noninfectious and infectious medical complications.

Among the noninfectious medical complications of heroin abuse, rabdomyolysis is frequently associated with opioid overdose that lasts a long time before any medical intervention occurs, and sometimes is related to lower limbs being maintained in the same position in a cold environment. The disease is characterized by an increase in serum lactate dehydrogenase (LDH) and creatine kinase (CK) activities. The subsequent increase in scrum potassium levels is due to the precipitation of myoglobin within the kidney tubules, leading to acute renal failure that necessitates hemodialysis.

Another frequent noninfectious complication of heroin abuse is a sudden transient hyperpyrexia as a result of pyrogens present in the street heroin preparations.

A number of infectious complications are seen in the population of heroin addicts, and the infectious complications can be subdivided in bacterial and viral infections, which may occur separately or concomitantly. Among the bacterial infectious complications, endocarditis is almost always part of the differential diagnosis of fever in opioid abusers. Right-sided bacterial endocarditis has a good prognosis, and septic pulmonary emboli respond to effective antimicrobial therapy. The bacterial endocarditis may be associated with, or preceded by, extended thrombophlebitis. Other frequent infectious complications of bacterial origin are aspiration pneumonia, skin and soft-tissue infections (e.g., cellulitis, cutaneous abscesses), and mycotic aneurysms.

Sexually transmitted diseases (e.g., syphilis, gonorrhea, chancroid) are more frequently associated with crack cocaine abuse than with heroin dependence. The incidence of tuberculosis has increased, however, mainly because heroin abusers are subject to HIV infection a condition that favors the occurrence of tuberculosis.

Treatment

Heroin abusers may be treated for overdose, for withdrawal, for medical or neurologic complications, or for the addiction itself (e.g., detoxification and antirelapse programs; opioid maintenance programs). Naloxone is the drug of choice for treating heroin overdose. Naloxone is a pure and selective antagonist at the μ receptors. Due to higher affinity at the receptor sites, naloxone is capable of displacing morphine (the active metabolite of heroin) from receptors and of shielding unoccupied receptors from further occupation by morphine. It is administered by iv infusion (or by im route when venous access is not available) at an initial dose of 0.4 mg, to be repeated up to resolution of the signs of overdose. Once the signs of overdose have subsided, careful monitoring of the patient is mandatory. In fact, the half-life of the antagonist is many times shorter than that of the agonist, making it possible that after awakening by means of the initial administration, the patient will return to a comatose state, rendering a further administration of the antagonist necessary. Naloxone therapy for opioid overdose does not entail any side effects, except the precipitation of withdrawal after awakening from coma in severely addicted patients.

The drug of choice for treating opioid withdrawal syndrome is clonidine. Clonidine at oral doses of 0.15 to 0.60 mg reduces many of the autonomic components of the opioid withdrawal syndrome, although restlessness and muscle aches are not entirely suppressed. Clonidine acts by binding to adrenergic α_2 autoreceptors in the brain (e.g., locus ceruleus) and spinal cord. The locus ceruleus is hyperactive during opioid withdrawal. Orthostatic hypotension and dizziness are the main side effects of clonidine therapy.

Opioid addicts also may be treated for the addiction itself while in good standing (i.e., in the absence of opioid overdose or of opioid withdrawal syndrome). This cohort of heroin addicts may be subdivided on the basis of their response to naloxone challenge. Subjects with a negative naloxone challenge (i.e., in the absence of physical dependence) may be enrolled in the naltrexone protocol, with or without the support of vocational rehabilitation, psy-

chotherapy, and drug-free communities. Naltrexone is a pure and selective antagonist at the μ receptors, which differs from naloxone in that it is 50 times more potent as an antagonist, is orally effective, and is long lasting due to generation of β-hydroxylated active metabolites. In the absence of physical dependence, whether initial or acquired after detoxification, naltrexone administration at oral doses of 50 mg per day (daily administration of 50 mg or thrice-weekly administration of a total 300 mg) blocks the heroin effect for more than 24 hours, abating the positive reinforcement of opioid self-administration. However, naltrexone does not block the craving and is recommended for intermittent use in highly motivated patients who are otherwise drug-free and receiving appropriate supportive therapy. Long-term opioid abstinence seems to require at last 3 months of continuous naltrexone. Chronic naltrexone administration has been claimed to induce liver damage, to reduce food intake, to inhibit liver microsome enzymes, and to alter neuroendocrine responses. Careful evaluation of the side effects has substantiated sporadic increases in serum transaminases and prolactin levels.

Subjects with a positive naloxone challenge (i.e., in the presence of physical dependence) may be enrolled in detoxification protocols or harm-reduction protocols. The difference between these two modalities lies in the fact that the aim of the first is to reach a stable drug-free state, while the second is meant to check the disease, both on social and toxicologic grounds

The techniques of detoxification stretch from substitution with and tapering of methadone to the most recent ultrarapid opioid detoxification (UROD). The different modalities of detoxification must be tailored to the subject's physical and psychologic state, after an informed consent, preferentially enrolling the family. The modalities also must be weighed according to the cost-benefit ratio.

To reach the initial drug-free state (i.e., to remove the physical dependence), the following withdrawal schedules are available:

• *Substitution with and tapering of methadone.* This technique entails the administration of methadone at an oral dose consistent with the score on the naloxone challenge and the tapering of the initial dose up to the drug-free state. According to Food and Drug Administration (FDA) guidelines for narcotic detoxification, short-term narcotic detoxification cannot exceed 30 days, and long-term detoxification should not exceed 180 days. The protocol may be implemented in both inpatient and outpatient settings, according to the initial dose of methadone. The daily dose of methadone must be taken in the presence of experienced personnel, at least at the beginning of the tapering period, in exchange for a urine sample to be analyzed for the presence of substances of abuse other than methadone. In the case of repeated presence of such substances, the subject is considered ineligible to continue the protocol. In the case of repeated clean urinalyses, take-home privileges for methadone administration may be granted. The advantage of the methadone protocol is that the drug is orally effective, long acting, and associated with a smooth withdrawal. However, the slow detoxification is relatively expensive and includes the disadvantage of exposing the subject to more temptations to use, causing a relatively high dropout rate.

• *Detoxification techniques not making use of methadone.* All the nonsubstitution techniques for narcotic detoxification are based on the observation that heroin addicts very quickly lose their physical dependence when challenged with repeated doses of an antagonist. The first administration of naloxone will produce a full-blown abstinence syndrome, whose intensity will fade away with the following doses, up to a negative naloxone challenge, showing the loss of physical dependence in 2 to 3 days. Obviously, this technique is highly demanding because of the intense discomfort of the evoked abstinence syndrome ("cold turkey"). However, this approach has been proposed whenever the discomfort of the abstinence syndrome is partially abated by the contemporary administration of drugs meant to check the severity of antagonist-induced abstinence, as in the following:

1. *withdrawal from opioids using clonidine hydrochloride.* In this protocol, the abrupt withdrawal from the opioid does not produce an overt abstinence syndrome because the subject is treated with clonidine. Both outpatients and inpatients are treated with an initial dose of clonidine of 0.3 to 0.4 mg daily, and this is increased up to 1.2 mg daily in 4 days. The dose is maintained for 5 additional days and is reduced by 0.2 mg per day from day 11 to completion. The use of clonidine as an alternative to gradual methadone reduction provides a shorter time to detoxification but relatively more discomfort in terms of partial reduction in the signs and symptoms of opioid abstinence, especially during the first 2 days. Clonidine has to be used with caution in subjects with hypotension or in those receiving antihypertensive medications. Exclusions include subjects who have used tricyclic antidepressants within the past 3 weeks and those with a history of cardiac arrhythmias;

2. *clonidine-naloxone rapid withdrawal.* This protocol involves administration of clonidine hydrochloride at a total daily dose of 0.9 to 1.2 mg in four divided doses for the first 2 days. The dose is maintained on days 3 and 4, when naloxone is also administered im at a total daily dose of 1.2 to 1.6 mg in four divided dose. No medication is provided on day 5. On day 6, a negative naloxone challenge indicates the loss of physical dependence and the drug-free condition. The protocol is usually well accepted by motivated opioid addicts seeking the drug-free state in a short time. Disadvantages include the incomplete protection afforded by clonidine against the opioid abstinence syndrome, which may be precipitated in some subjects by the first administration of the narcotic antagonist;

3. *clonidine-naltrexone rapid withdrawal.* This method is similar to the preceding technique and uses the known ability of naltrexone to produce immediate withdrawal from an opioid as it displaces the opioid from the endogenous receptor. When clonidine is used as pretreatment, the symptoms of opioid withdrawal are substantially relieved. Increasing oral daily doses of clonidine (up to 1.2 mg) are given on days 1 and 2, in combination with an oral naltrexone dose of 12.5 mg on day 1 and 25 mg on day 2. On days 3 through 5, the total dose of clonidine is tapered by 0.2 to 0.4 mg per day, and that of naltrexone is increased to 50 mg per day. The advantages of this protocol are use of the antagonist by the oral route and completion of the program at a daily dose of naltrexone of 50 mg, which allows the subject to enroll immediately into an antirelapse protocol;

4. *ultrarapid opioid detoxification (UROD).* In an attempt to reduce the duration of detoxification as much as possible, a more invasive approach has shortened the detoxification time to a few hours. This has involved the simultaneous iv administration of the opioid antagonist naloxone during iv sedation with the benzodiazepine midazolam. A further extension of this protocol entails the intragastric administration of the opioid antagonist naltrexone to patients fully anesthetized with midazolam and fentanyl. Patients undergoing this protocol were able to start naltrexone maintenance therapy within hours of completing detoxification. However, this approach may involve some medical risk from anesthesia that is not a part of the other approaches and casts some doubt about the cost-benefit ratio.

To summarize, opioid addicts with a positive naloxone challenge may be detoxified using one of the detoxification techniques just described (i.e., methadone substitution and tapering; detoxification with clonidine alone or in association with naloxone and naltrexone; the use of naloxone and naltrexone in heavily sedated or anesthetized patients). Once the drug-free state has been reached, the detoxified addict must face the problem of how to maintain the drug-free condition. In fact, craving is not hampered by the detoxification techniques, and this represents an impending risk to relapse. Former addicts who try to maintain abstinent without any vocational, psychosocial, or pharmacologic assistance have a very high rate of relapse. The rate of relapse decreases significantly when detoxified addicts enroll in the naltrexone maintenance protocol or apply to drug-free therapeutic communities.

The naltrexone protocol has been described previously for opioid addicts lacking physical dependence. Here we want to add that the major problem of naltrexone maintenance is compliance. Unlike opioid agonists, naltrexone does not produce opioid agonist-like effects, nor does it attenuate craving. Compliance may be increased by combining naltrexone therapy with psychotherapy.

Drug-free communities are fundamental aids to maintaining the drug-free state in detoxified addicts. However, such communities reach only a small percentage of abusers, are relatively costly, and the relapse rate is still present after patients leave a program.

The harm-reduction protocols are based on the premise

that opioid abuse is a chronic metabolic disorder that needs a substitution for a patient's endogenous deficiency. Legalized morphine or heroin, practiced in United States, UK, and Switzerland, demonstrated that a stable daily dose of heroin or morphine is compatible with social productivity. However, heroin must be taken two or three times daily, oral efficacy requires very high doses, and users vary widely in what they consider the optimal dosage, leading to frequent illicit supplementation. Moreover, morphine and heroin strongly reduce the immunologic response, especially impairing the "natural killer" (NK) lymphocyte activity, a harmful side effect considered to be responsible for the high incidence of viral and bacterial infections among opioid abusers. These effects are not shared by methadone, which is definitely the drug of choice in harm-reduction protocols. The advantages of methadone over morphine and heroin are (1) better absorption by the oral route, (2) once-daily administration in comparison with three to four administrations of morphine or heroin needed to keep the addict in a stable, "straight" physical and psychologic state, and (3) lack of immunosuppressive activity. The goal of methadone maintenance treatment is rehabilitation, not abstinence. To achieve this goal, the great majority of patients must continue maintenance therapy indefinitely, at adequate doses. The definition of methadone dose in the harm-reduction protocols is controversial. Some workers advocate not exceeding a daily dose of 40 mg. Others advocate tailoring the methadone dose in an ascending manner, up to the very high doses of 120 to 200 mg per day. With this schedule, methadone is provided for positive-reinforcement effects on the circuitry of the "pleasure brain." Controversy also centers around whether reaching a blood concentration of 200 ng/ml is really necessary for effective blockade.

Besides any moral posturing on methadone maintenance, major social and medical drawbacks of methadone maintenance include its potential diversion to street use and the possible adverse effects of methadone maintenance on children born of treated mothers. The harm-reduction protocol using methadone maintenance is easily implemented in an outpatient setting. Daily doses of methadone are given, usually in exchange of urine samples to be analyzed for the presence of substances of abuse other than methadone. Different levels of enforcement are provided in the case of repeated dirty urine samples. Take-home doses are usually given to patients in good standing. Notwithstanding the many criticisms, methadone maintenance therapy, developed in the 1960s, is still the standard treatment to which all other opioid maintenance approaches are compared.

Other approaches to opioid maintenance treatment involve the use of L-acetylmethadol (LAAM) and buprenorphine. LAAM is a derivative of methadone that acts as a pure agonist at the μ-receptors. LAAM is much longer acting than methadone, with the ability to suppress the symptoms of opioid withdrawal for more than 72 hours. The long duration of action is due to the production of two active metabolites: L-noracetylmethadol and 1-dinoracetyl-methadol, both more potent than the parent compound and possessing a longer pharmacologic half-life.

LAAM maintenance therapy has the following advantages over methadone maintenance: LAAM is typically administered every other day or three times weekly. This may be useful in patients who are unable to come to the clinic on a daily basis, such as the majority of methadone-maintained patients. The schedule also allows for a significant decrease in the expenditures for services and allows for the enrollment of more subjects. Unlike methadone, patients do not experience a "rushlike" effect after administration. This property may be useful in patients who wish to minimize their ability "to feel the drug."

Disadvantages over methadone maintenance include lack of any positive reinforcement, which decreases the initial compliance. Stabilization onto an effective dose of LAAM takes longer than with methadone owing to the longer period of time required for the accumulation of its long-lived metabolites. The protocol is implemented on an outpatient basis using an induction schedule starting from an oral daily dose of 20 mg to be incremented up to the maximum of 60 mg three times weekly.

Buprenorphine is a synthetic derivative of thebaine that has partial agonist activity at μ-receptors and, at higher doses, opioid antagonist activity. Buprenorphine is given sublingually on a daily basis or on a thrice-weekly schedule because of its long half-life. The sustained action of buprenorphine is also due to its slow dissociation from opioid receptors.

Buprenorphine has the following advantages over methadone maintenance: the ability to administer the medication on a thrice-weekly schedule, a lower abuse potential and a milder withdrawal syndrome than full agonists such as methadone or LAAM, a relative safety from overdose due to a dose-dependent shift from agonistic activity to antagonistic activity that flattens the dose-response curve on respiratory depression at high doses, the unique possibility to initiate a substitution program at low doses (maintenance with an agonist) and to switch to a nonsubstitution program at high doses, at which the drug is endowed with antagonistic activity, and a reduction in cocaine use in opioid abusers who also self-administer cocaine.

Disadvantages over methadone maintenance include the sublingual route of administration, which makes it more difficult for the therapist to see if the drug is really ingested; a rather widespread abuse by the intravenous route by dissolving one or more 0.1 mg tablets in water and injecting the solution iv; and the relatively higher cost of the raw material.

The protocol with buprenorphine is easily implemented on an outpatient basis. More debatable is the choice of the dose, which has been reported to extend from 1.5 mg daily to suggested maintenance doses of 16, 16, and 40 mg on Monday, Wednesday, and Friday.

In conclusion, detoxification is not the only treatment necessary for stable abstinence, but it may be viewed as only the first step in the long process of remaining off illicit drugs. Harm-reduction protocols are also useful in the realm of flexible programs in which patients can move at their optimal rates from methadone substitution to total abstinence and back to methadone substitution or other programs if relapse occurs.

Suggested readings

AXELROD J. Cellular adaptation in the development of tolerance to drugs. In: Wikler A, ed. The addictive states. Baltimore: Williams & Wilkins, 1968;247-64.

BALL JC, CHAMBERS CD. The epidemiology of drug addiction in the USA. Springfield: Charles C Thomas, 1970.

BEST SE. OLIVETO AH KOSTEN TR. Opioid addiction: recent advances in detoxification and maintenance therapy. Drugs 1996;6:301-14.

BRECHER EM. Licit and illicit drugs. Boston: Little, Brown, 1972.

BRUST JCM. Neurological aspects of substance abuse. Stoneham: Butterworth-Heinemann, 1993.

COLLIER OJ. Tolerance, physical dependence and receptors: a theory of the genesis of tolerance and physical dependence through drug-induced changes in the number of receptors. Adv Drug Res 1966;3:171-88.

CORSSEN G, SKORA IA. "Addiction" reaction of cultured human cells. JAMA 1964;187:92-6.

COX BM, GINSBURG M. Is there a relationship between protein synthesis and tolerance to analgesic drugs? In: Scientific Basis of Drug Dependence. London: J&A Churchill, 1969.

KLEBERT HD. Detoxification. In: Gabbard GO, ed. Treatment of psychiatric disorders. Washington: American Psychiatric Press, 1995; 744-56.

LESHER GA, SPRATTO GR. Brain and plasma concentration of morphine during the development of physical dependence and tolerance. J Pharmacol Pharamacother 1976;28:843-4.

MANNAIONI PF. Clinical pharmacology of drug dependence. Padova: Piccin, 1984.

MONCINI M, GIRALDI M, MANNAIONI PF, MASINI E. Incidence and evolution of HIV infection in a cohort of heroin addicts admitted to the Hospital Toxicology Unit in Florence from January 1991 to December 1996. Boll Farmacodep Alcoholism 1998;3:44-50.

RASOR RW. Narcotic addiction in young people in the United States. In: Wilson WCM, ed. Adolescent drug dependence. New York: Pergamon Press, 1968.

Hypnotics

J. M. Ad Sitsen

The class of drugs usually referred to as hypnotics includes a number of agents for which the terminology has not been clearly established. The hypnotic effects of many such drugs are on a continuum with sedative effects and to some degree also with anxiolytic effects. They cover a wide spectrum of pharmacologic agents, and the terminology implies more specificity than seems justified on the basis of the pharmacologic properties. The class of sedative/hypnotics shows substantial overlap with the class of drugs commonly referred to as anxiolytics.

Chemically and pharmacologically, these drugs can be classified into (1) benzodiazepines and pharmacologically related agents acting on the benzodiazepine receptor, (2) barbiturates, and (3) miscellaneous, including older drugs such as meprobamate, chloral hydrate, glutethimide, and methaqualone.

The pharmacology of these three compounds is not equally well understood. That of the benzodiazepines is probably best understood, and that of the miscellaneous group least.

The benzodiazepines include widely prescribed compounds such as diazepam, oxazepam, flunitrazepam, and many others. They bind at the so-called benzodiazepine receptors that are part of the γ-aminobutyric acid (GABA) receptor complex. This receptor complex involves the GABA receptor, which has a major role in inhibitory mechanisms of brain function. Detailed studies including receptor cloning have shown that the benzodiazepine receptor (and the barbiturate receptor; see below) are contained within the multisubunit GABA (A) receptor–ion chloride channel complex. GABA (B) receptors play different and largely unrelated roles, controlling mainly skeletal muscle spasticity. Benzodiazepines bind to an allosteric site distinct from the GABA receptor but require integrity of the GABA receptor function to increase inhibitory synaptic activity. Binding of benzodiazepines to the GABA receptor complex facilitates the activity of GABA to open the chloride ion channels, resulting in enhanced inhibitory activity. Slight variations in receptor structure occur in different brain regions and account for differences in efficacy of individual benzodiazepines as to sedative, anticonvulsant, and anxiolytic properties. An often underestimated effect of the benzodiazepines is their skeletal muscle-relaxing effect, which may lead to falls and fractures, particularly in elderly patients.

Many different benzodiazepines are being used. Their pharmacodynamic differences are small, although it has been claimed that some benzodiazepines, in particular alprazolam, have antidepressant properties. The major differences concern the pharmacokinetic properties, such as the plasma half-life and the formation of pharmacologically active metabolites. In particular, the benzodiazepines with short plasma half-lives are prone to causing withdrawal symptoms.

Zolpidem and zopiclone are chemically not related to the benzodiazepines but their pharmacologic effects to some extent resemble those of the benzodiazepines (see Chap. 15). Their main indication is insomnia, and withdrawal or rebound symptoms may be less problematic with these compounds than with the benzodiazepines.

The barbiturates have the barbituric acid ring in common. They have been and are to a very limited extent still being used as hypnotics and antiepileptics. Closely related thiobarbiturates are still used as intravenous anesthetic agents. Many different barbiturates have been used as hypnotics, including such compounds as pentobarbital, amobarbital, and hexobarbital. Phenobarbital is being used mainly as an antiepileptic drug (see Chap. 10). Barbiturates bind to a site contained in the GABA receptor complex adjacent to the chloride ion channel that is distinct from the benzodiazepine receptor. Some barbiturates have GABA-mimetic effects (in particular the hypnotic barbiturates), i.e., a direct action on the chloride ion channels, whereas other barbiturates have GABA-potentiating effects (in particular the anticonvulsant barbiturates), i.e., prolonging the opening of the chloride ion channels achieved by a given amount of GABA. Barbiturates vary widely in their pharmacokinetic properties. Most of them are metabolized by cytochrome P450 enzymes in the liver and, after conjugation with glucuronic acid, are excreted by the kidneys. Some ultra-short-acting compounds are used as intravenous anesthetic agents.

The miscellaneous group of compounds is chemically heterogeneous and includes a number of older compounds. The pharmacologic properties of this group are less well understood than those of the benzodiazepines and the barbiturates and will be reviewed only briefly.

Chloral hydrate is converted in vivo to its active metabolite, trichloroethanol. The pharmacologic properties of this compound resemble those of ethanol, which are not well defined. Ethanol may affect the function of ion channels and appears to have both inhibitory and facilitatory effects, resulting in depression of the central nervous system (CNS). Benzodiazepines and barbiturates have additive suppressive effects on the brain, suggesting that all three groups of compounds share a common mechanism of action, possibly through the GABA receptor complex.

Glutethimide is chemically distinct from the barbiturates, but its pharmacologic properties resemble those of the barbiturates. In addition, it exhibits strong anticholinergic activity. The pharmacologic properties of the anxiolytic drug meprobamate are to some extent similar to those of the benzodiazepines. Methaqualone possesses sedative, anticonvulsive, local anesthetic, and antispasmodic activity. Its pharmacologic properties seem to be related to those of the barbiturates.

Epidemiology

Almost by definition, epidemiologic data on drug abuse are scarce and unreliable. Nevertheless, there seems to be agreement that abuse of hypnotics such as the benzodiazepines, barbiturates, and related compounds is widespread. In general terms, there are now indications that genetic influences in drug use disorders are present.

Since their introduction, the benzodiazepines have been prescribed on an unprecedented scale. They appeared to be much safer than the previously used barbiturates and therefore have almost completely replaced the barbiturates. Barbiturate use by adolescents has increased gradually in the past several years, but few adolescents use this class of drugs regularly. These sedatives are used most often to treat unpleasant effects of illicit stimulants. Many young people seem not to be aware of the significant danger and toxicity of this class of compounds. Focus is therefore mainly on the benzodiazepines.

The widespread legitimate use of the benzodiazepines has led to the erroneous impression that they have a relatively high abuse liability among recreational drug abusers. Two different types of problematic benzodiazepine use have been recently distinguished, i.e., recreational abuse and chronic quasi-therapeutic use. The characteristics of these two types of use can be summarized as follows. Recreational abuse occurs often in a pattern of polydrug abuse (with opioids or alcohol), and high doses are used either chronically or intermittently to achieve alcohol-like intoxications. The source of the benzodiazepines is often illicit. Its incidence is relatively rare (but by no means trivial) relative to the rate of prescription but similar to abuse of other illicit substances such as opioids or cocaine. Benzodiazepines used include diazepam, temazepam, triazolam, and flunitrazepam. Most abuse of these benzodiazepines is via the oral route, but abuse via the intravenous route has been reported from several countries. Associated problems include involvement in the illicit drug culture with associated legal and health risks, memory impairment, risk of accidents, and the occurrence of withdrawal symptoms.

Chronic quasi-therapeutic use is characterized by long-term use by patients that is inconsistent with accepted medical practice, e.g., the nightly use of triazolam as a hypnotic or the daily use of lorazepam as an anxiolytic for years despite physician recommendations to the patient that medication be stopped. This type of use occurs relatively often in elderly patients, patients with chronic pain, and patients with a history of alcohol or drug abuse. Patients may report unsuccessful attempts to cut down the use and continue the use to relieve or avoid withdrawal. The source of the benzodiazepines is often licit, but deception to obtain the drug is not uncommon. This type of use is relatively prevalent relative to the rate of prescription. Associated problems include memory impairment; risk of accidents, falls, and hip fractures in the elderly; and the occurrence of withdrawal symptoms.

According to a community survey conducted in the United States in 1991, approximately 4% of the population sampled had ever used sedatives for nonmedical purposes, approximately 1% had done so in the last year, and approximately 0.4% had done so in the last month.

Clinical findings

The intoxication syndromes induced by sedative, hypnotic, and/or anxiolytic compounds are largely similar and to a large extent resemble alcohol intoxication.

Benzodiazepine intoxication causes mainly sedation but may be associated with behavioral disinhibition that may result in hostility or aggression. Only at very high doses may coma, respiratory depression, or hypotension occur. Low doses of barbiturates and related compounds cause a clinical syndrome of intoxication that is indistinguishable from alcohol intoxication, including sluggishness, incoordination, slowness of speech and comprehension, faulty judgment, disinhibition, etc. With overdose, barbiturates are lethal because of their induction of respiratory depression. Similar clinical syndromes are induced by glutethimide, meprobamate, and chloral hydrate. Methaqualone is different in that with overdose it induces restlessness, delirium, hypertonia, convulsions, and eventually, death. In contrast to barbiturate and similar compounds, it rarely causes respiratory or cardiovascular depression.

The Diagnostic and Statistical Manual of Mental Disorders, 4th edition (DSM-IV), gives the following diagnostic criteria for sedative, hypnotic, or anxiolytic intoxication:
1. Recent use of a sedative, hypnotic, or anxiolytic.
2. Clinically significant maladaptive behavioural or psychological changes (e.g., inappropriate sexual or aggressive behaviour, mood lability, impaired judgment, impaired social or occupational functioning) that developed during, or shortly after, sedative, hypnotic, or anxiolytic use.
3. One (or more) of the following signs, developing during, or shortly after, sedative, hypnotic, or anxiolytic use:
   • slurred speech;
   • incoordination;

- unsteady gait;
- nystagmus;
- impairment in attention or memory;
- stupor or coma.

4. The symptoms are not due to a general medical condition and are not better accounted for by another mental disorder.

The long-term use of sedatives, hypnotics, and anxiolytics rapidly induces tolerance, i.e., a decrease in the effects of administration of identical doses. This tolerance may be pharmacodynamic in nature (i.e., the effector cells adapt to the presence of the substance, for example, by means of receptor downregulation) or pharmacokinetic in nature (i.e., the metabolism of the substance is enhanced due to enzyme induction). The latter occurs mainly with long-term use of barbiturates and some other nonbenzodiazepine sedatives, whereas the former (presumably among others downregulation of GABA (A) receptors) is common with both the benzodiazepines and the barbiturates. Because of this tolerance, the clinical picture after long-term use may be quite different from that observed after acute overdosage referred to earlier. Effects may be more subtle and require more careful observation and laboratory investigations.

Acute discontinuation of the use of benzodiazepines, barbiturates, and related compounds may result in a discontinuance syndrome. The benzodiazepine discontinuance syndrome consists of return of the original symptoms (recurrence), worsening of these symptoms (rebound), or occurrence of new symptoms (withdrawal). Depending on the individual compound used, the daily dose, and duration of use, the clinical picture may include one or more of the following symptoms: disturbances of mood and cognition (e.g., anxiety, apprehension, dysphoria, pessimism, irritability, obsessive rumination, paranoid ideation), disturbances of sleep (e.g., insomnia, altered sleep-wake cycle, daytime drowsiness), physical signs and symptoms (e.g., tachycardia, high blood pressure, hyperreflexia, agitation, restlessness, tremor, myoclonus, muscle and joint pain, nausea, coryza, sweating, ataxia, tinnitus, grand mal seizures), and perceptual disturbances (e.g., hyperacusia, depersonalization, blurred vision, illusions, hallucinations).

The severity of the discontinuance syndrome of barbiturates depends on the daily dose and duration of use. At low doses (e.g., 400 mg pentobarbital per day), paroxysmal electroencephalographic (EEG) changes may occur; higher daily doses result in more severe symptoms such as anxiety, insomnia, anorexia, tremor, delirium, and EEG changes. Still higher doses may lead to apprehension, tremors, myoclonic jerks, grand mal seizures, postural hypotension, anorexia, vomiting, and EEG changes.

Laboratory findings

Confirmation of suspected abuse of benzodiazepines, barbiturates, and related drugs can now be obtained relatively easily by screening of urine or plasma for the presence of these drugs and their metabolites. Sensitive methods for such screening are available for a wide variety of such drugs. A negative screening in the presence of clinical indications for abuse should be viewed with scepticism; patients may be aware of screening programs and arrange for negative urine tests.

Short- and long-term risks

Benzodiazepines have been and still are prescribed and used on an unprecedented scale. Their dependence potential has been known for quite some time. The occurrence of withdrawal reactions also has been recognized since the 1980s. Their long-term use is by no means rare. Thus, it appears that the medical risks related to the short- and long-term therapeutic use of benzodiazepines are small. The main risks are the development of clinically significant maladaptive behavior or psychologic changes. Memory impairment is also a prominent feature. Acute overdoses of benzodiazepines are only very rarely lethal. Traffic accidents resulting from the use of psychoactive drugs including benzodiazepines are being seen increasingly and are a cause for concern. Similar considerations apply to the other sedative/hypnotic drugs discussed earlier. One major exception is the risk of overdose. The barbiturates and a number of related sedative/hypnotic drugs are very dangerous at overdose and potentially lethal.

Treatment

Treatment of acute overdoses of sedative/hypnotics involves gastric lavage, activated charcoal, and careful monitoring of vital signs and CNS activity. If necessary, mechanical ventilation should be provided. Treatment of acute benzodiazepine overdose may be supported by the careful and judicious use of the benzodiazepine receptor antagonist flumazenil. Two dosing regimens can be followed:

1. an initial bolus dose of 0.3 mg, followed by 0.1 mg every 60 seconds until the patient has regained a reasonable degree of consciousness; maximum dose is 2 mg. If severe sedation occurs again, another bolus of 0.3 mg can be given;
2. an intravenous infusion delivering 0.1 to 0.4 mg per hour depending on the degree of respiratory depression.

The basic principle underlying the safe withdrawal of sedative/hypnotics is gradual tapering of the drugs. If daily doses of (therapeutic) benzodiazepines are known, the tapering protocol usually can be calculated easily, e.g., weekly reductions of 10 to 25% of the daily dose. In the case of barbiturates, the daily dose is usually less well known, and the administration of a test dose to determine tolerance may be indicated. Alternatively, the equivalent hypnotic dose of phenobarbital is calculated based on the dose of barbiturate or other sedative drug the patient reports taking. It may be necessary to also take into account any alcohol the patient may be consuming. Subsequently, daily dose reductions are made every few days. This method has disadvantages, however, because published equivalencies are only approximations and patient metabolic (pharmacokinetic) and pharmacodynamic adaptations may vary widely. Cross-tolerance between various anxiolytics and sedative/hypnotics is not

complete. Finally, another method involves using loading doses of phenobarbital until clinical symptoms are present (e.g., nystagmus, drowsiness, ataxia, dysarthria, and/or emotional lability), followed by gradual tapering of the daily dose.

Psychologic interventions may be needed. Sometimes psychiatric care is necessary for recurring anxiety or unmasked depressive disorders. Long-term outcome is uncertain.

Suggested readings

AMERICAN PSYCHIATRIC ASSOCIATION. Diagnostic and statistical manual of mental disorders, 4th ed. Washington: American Psychiatric Association, 1994.

BUSTO UE, SELLERS EM. Anxiolytics and sedative/hypnotics dependence. Br J Addiction 1991;86:1647-52.

BUSTO U, SELLERS EM, NARANJO CA, et al. Withdrawal reactions after long-term therapeutic use of benzodiazepines. N Engl J Med 1986;316:854-9.

GRIFFITHS RR, WEERTS EM, Benzodiazepine self-administration in humans and laboratory animals: implications for problems of long-term use and abuse. Psychopharmacology 1997;134:1-37.

HUTCHINSON MA, SMITH PF, DARLINGTON CL. The behavioral and neuronal effects of the chronic administration of benzodiazepine anxiolytic and hypnotic drugs. Progr Neurobiol 1996;49:73-97.

ISACSON D. Long-term use benzodiazepine: factors of importance and the development of individual use patterns over time: a 13-year follow-up in a Swedish community. Soc Sci Med 1997;44:1871-80.

ITO T, SUZUKI T, WELLMAN SE, HO IK. Pharmacology of barbiturate tolerance/dependence: GABA(A) receptors and molecular aspects. Life Sci 1996;59:169-95.

LADER M. Dependence on benzodiazepines. J Clin Psychiatry 1983;44:121-7.

MINTZER MZ, GUARINO J, KIRK T, et al. Ethanol and pentobarbital: comparison of behavioral and subjective effects in sedative drug abusers. Exp Clin Psychopharmacol 1997;5:203-15.

MORGAN WW. Abuse liability of barbiturates and other sedative-hypnotics. Adv Alcohol Subst Abuse 1990;9:67-82.

PRATT JA, BRETT RR, LAURIE DJ. Benzodiazepine dependence: from neuronal circuits to gene expression. Pharmacol Biochem Behav 1998;59:925-34.

SIMPSON D, BRAITHWAITE RA, JARVIE DR, et al. Screening for drugs of abuse (II): cannabinoids, lysergic acid diethylamide, buprenorphine, methadone, barbiturates, benzodiazepines and other drugs. Annu Clin Biochem 1997;34:460-510.

TSUANG MT, LYONS MJ, EISEN SA, et al. Genetic influences on DSM-III-R drug abuse and dependence: a study of 3327 twin pairs. Am J Med Genet 1996;67:473-7.

Amphetamines and cocaine

Lisa H. Brauer, Roy Stein, Harriet de Wit

The amphetamines and cocaine are among the most widely abused drugs in the world, with significant and problematic use reported in the United States, Australia, western Europe, Japan, the Philippines, the Republic of Korea, and Thailand. In the United States, stimulants are among the drugs most frequently included in emergency room episodes and medical examiner reports. Abuse of these drugs has been extremely difficult to treat and carries with it the potential for substantial morbidity and mortality. Thus, stimulant abusers likely will continue to come to the attention of medical professionals, either in emergency departments or in primary care settings. A brief overview of the characteristics and management of the medical and psychiatric sequelae of stimulant use and abuse will focus on the prototypical psychomotor stimulants amphetamine and cocaine but, where relevant, also will discuss the "designer drugs" [e.g., methylenedioxymethamphetamine (MDMA, ecstasy) and methylenedioxyamphetamine (MDA)]. The term *stimulant* refers to the effects common to drugs of this class, and individual drug names will be used where differences exist.

Stimulant drugs generally are used recreationally in low to moderate doses for their acute mood-altering, anorectic, and performance-enhancing effects. These doses produce feelings of well-being, arousal, euphoria, enhanced alertness and self-esteem, increased sexuality and mental clarity, and reduced social inhibitions and anxiety. Behaviorally, they can enhance psychomotor performance, especially performance that has been degraded by sleep deprivation or fatigue. Physiologically, stimulants produce sympathomimetic effects, including increased heart rate, blood pressure, body temperature, and pupil size and reduced appetite and eating. Although most recreational stimulant users do not escalate to problematic use, a significant number of individuals use stimulants in higher doses or with increasing frequency to achieve a more intense euphoria. The transition to problematic use typically results from increased access to the drug and from the use of a route with a higher abuse liability (e.g., iv, smoked). The use of higher drug doses in an effort to achieve a greater euphoria can have dangerous consequences because tolerance may not develop at the same rate to the mood-altering and physiologic effects of the

drug. The user thus may experience additive sympathomimetic effects and elevated plasma levels that can lead to significant toxicity. Adverse psychiatric and sympathomimetic effects also may result from sensitization to these drug effects, which have been documented after intermittent stimulant use.

Chronic or high-dose use of stimulants produces a number of negative mood effects in addition to euphoria, including irritability, grandiosity, depression, dysphoria, agitation, insomnia, paranoia, and a psychotic syndrome that can be indistinguishable from schizophrenic psychosis. Stereotypical behavior is sometimes observed following high-dose use of stimulants. Chest pain and headache also may accompany high-dose stimulant use. Hyperthermia and cardiovascular effects can be life-threatening in acute overdose situations (see below).

The "designer drugs", such as MDMA and MDA produce stimulant-like subjective and physiologic effects, as well as some unique effects. Acute doses produce increased self-awareness, sensuality, and spirituality; facilitated social interactions, including empathy toward and connection with others; increased awareness of sensations; and in some instances, perceptual distortions often classified as visual hallucinations. Related to these effects, there has been some limited, and controversial, use of these drugs as adjuncts to psychotherapy. The designer drugs also cause anxiety, nausea, and insomnia. Although chemically related, MDMA and MDA differ in their hallucinogenic properties, with methylenedioxymethamphetamine having lesser psychotomimetic effects than methylenedioxyamphetamine. Frequently reported physiologic effects of these drugs include increases in blood pressure and heart rate, diaphoresis, blurred vision, dry mouth, anorexia, and tremor, as well as trismus and bruxism.

In abusers, cocaine is generally used in binges lasting from several hours to several days (average, 12 hours), during which the drug is ingested several times per hour. The binge typically ends when the user is exhausted or the supply of drug runs out. During the binge, the user is intensely focused on the euphoria to the exclusion of other reinforcers (e.g., social interactions) and despite negative psychosocial consequences. The frequency and pattern of drug administration are related to the pharmacokinetics of cocaine. Its half-life is very short, approximately 60 to 90 minutes, and the euphoric effects dissipate even sooner due to the development of acute tolerance. The half-life of the amphetamines is 4 to 10 times longer than of cocaine; amphetamine binges typically last more than a day, and drug administration is much less frequent, with several hours between doses. Little information exists on the use patterns associated with MDMA and MDA, but it is generally believed that these drugs are used with less regularity and in more circumscribed contexts than amphetamine and cocaine (e.g., in psychotherapy or at "rave" parties).

Definition of substances

Amphetamine is a phenylpropylamine that increases synaptic concentrations of the catecholamines and serotonin via release of catecholamines from vesicular pools into the synapses, blockade reuptake, and inhibited monoamine oxidase. As a result of these actions, amphetamine potentiates and prolongs the synaptic effects of catecholamines in several brain areas, including the ventral tegmental area, the locus ceruleus, and the raphe nuclei. The effects of amphetamine on dopamine concentrations in brain reward pathways (i.e., mesolimbic and mesocortical areas) are believed to underlie its rewarding effects.

Cocaine is a benzoic acid ester derived from the leaves of the *Erythroxylon coca* plant indigenous to South America. It prolongs the effects of extravesicular catecholamines and serotonin by blocking their reuptake. The rewarding properties of cocaine are also thought to be related to its enhancement of dopaminergic activity. In addition to its psychoactive effects, cocaine has local anesthetic effects, which may contribute to its cardiovascular and central nervous system (CNS) toxicity.

MDMA and MDA are ring-substituted amphetamines that share structural chemistry and pharmacology with both hallucinogens and amphetamine.

MDMA and MDA cause release of vesicular monoamine neurotransmitters and block their reuptake. Although release of dopamine is one of the neurochemical effects of these drugs, their effects on serotonin release also appear to contribute substantially to their psychoactive effects.

Clinical findings

Individuals exhibiting stimulant abuse or dependence may come to clinical attention with either acute or chronic manifestations. Acute presentations, typically encountered in Emergency Departments, include stimulant intoxication, withdrawal, and various physical and psychiatric complications. Patients with chronic stimulant use seek routine medical attention for a broad range of medical and psychiatric conditions caused or exacerbated by their drug use. In both settings, patients are often reluctant to acknowledge their drug use; furthermore, many are unaware of the connection between their symptoms and drug use and thus do not mention it. A high index of clinical suspicion, coupled with familiarity with the range of acute and chronic manifestations of stimulant abuse and appropriate diagnostic skills, is therefore necessary to detect stimulant abuse and offer intervention.

Symptoms and signs

Acute intoxication and overdose

The behavioral symptoms of acute stimulant intoxication include agitation and irritability, restlessness, hyperactivity and dyskinesias, impaired judgment, grandiose and delusional thinking, aggressive and impulsive behavior, and hypersexuality. Symptoms of paranoid psychosis with auditory hallucinations have been reported following chronic high-dose use of both the amphetamines and cocaine. Patients also may show evidence of malnutrition and suicidal or homicidal tendencies. Psychotic symptoms associated with high-dose cocaine usually remit in hours, whereas amphetamine psychosis may last for days or weeks. Concurrent with these psychotic symptoms, patients may engage in deviant, illegal, or destructive behavior.

Physiologic symptoms of acute stimulant intoxication include hypertension, tachycardia, hyperpyrexia, tremor, diaphoresis, midriasis, increased respiration, muscle twitching, dizziness, seizures, rhabdomyolosis, and hyperreflexia. In severe cases, convulsions, cerebral infarction, cardiac arrhythmias, and ischemia also may be observed. Hyperthermia, convulsions, and cardiac arrhythmias are potentially the most lethal consequences of stimulant overdose. The risk of convulsions appears to be greater with cocaine than with the amphetamines. Death from stimulant overdose can result from heart attacks, peripheral autonomic catecholamine excess, or respiratory depression.

In addition to the behavioral and physiologic effects of stimulants described earlier, complications may arise from factors related to drug-associated behaviors. Use of stimulant drugs is associated with violent and aggressive behavior, coupled with impaired judgment and impulse control, that can have devastating consequences. In addition, stimulant use often occurs in the context of promiscuous sexual behavior and needle sharing, increasing the risk of human immunodeficiency virus (HIV) infection, other sexually transmitted diseases, and hepatitis. The risk of infection of intravenous drug use is augmented by the direct immunosuppressive effects of these drugs. Intranasal cocaine creates the potential for rhinitis and/or septal necrosis, as well as loss of sensitivity to odors, and smoked cocaine use has been associated with pneumomediastinum and cervical emphysema. Complications also may result from adulterants used in drug manufacture or administration. Intravenous use of methamphetamine is sometimes associated with lead poisoning related to the procedure used for synthesis, and other added drugs or sugars can increase the risk of infection. The use of stimulant drugs during pregnancy has been associated with a number of complications, including preterm labor, placental abruption, and spontaneous abortion, as well as anatomic and neurophysiologic abnormalities in the offspring (e.g., fetal cerebrovascular accidents, intrauterine growth retardation). Poor obstetric care and nutrition, as well as concurrent use of other drugs, may exacerbate the obstetric and perinatal effects of stimulants. Finally, cocaine, amphetamines, and the designer drugs have been shown to produce neuronal destruction and long-lasting decreases in monoamine concentrations in laboratory animals, even after single doses.

Substance abuse and dependence

Patients reporting frequent and/or problematic drug use should be evaluated for drug dependence using criteria described earlier in Chapter 80 and outlined in the *Diagnostic and Statistical Manual of Mental Disorders* (DSM-IV). Careful assessment is critical, since both behavioral and pharmacologic treatment strategies may differ for different diagnoses. In this regard, a thorough review of the patient's medical records and collateral reports, where available, is useful.

Chronic stimulant abuse produces a number of common medical and psychiatric complaints that need to be recognized. Hypertension, episodic chest pain, insomnia, mood disturbances, anxiety, paranoia, and sexual dysfunction can all be induced by stimulant use; any of these complaints should prompt consideration of this condition in the differential diagnosis. The possibility should be pursued by a tactful, nonjudgmental, but direct inquiry about drug use, along with seeking confirmation through collateral history and urine drug testing, depending on the level of suspicion. The clinician needs to guard against stereotypical notions about what sort of patient might – or might not – engage in abuse of cocaine, amphetamine, or other stimulants. Even subtle expression of moralistic, accusatory attitudes toward drug use and users is likely to thwart efforts at detection and treatment intervention.

Patients using stimulants at high doses or on a chronic basis may experience a withdrawal syndrome on cessation of use. Clinical observations with outpatients suggest that there are three phases of abstinence: a crash, withdrawal, and extinction. The "crash" occurs immediately on cessation of prolonged drug use and is characterized by intense drug craving, hypersomnolence, and hyperphagia. Affectively, patients experience extreme depressive symptoms along with anxiety and agitation. Patients may use other drugs, including opiates and alcohol, to offset some of the effects of the crash and to titrate mood. The affective symptoms during this period are often difficult to distinguish from major depression, and patients need to be monitored carefully for suicidality during this phase.

After remission of the crash, usually in several days, behavioral symptoms of drug withdrawal typically are observed. Drug withdrawal is associated with decreases in energy (anergia) and experience of pleasure (anhedonia). These symptoms typically persist and increase for several days and often contribute to early relapse into binge use. Dysphoria and anhedonia generally remit if the patient is able to maintain abstinence for at least 6 weeks. The final phase, extinction, occurs gradually in patients who have managed to remain abstinent despite the presence of drug-associated cues and situations. Clinicians are reminded that a number of factors can influence clinical presentation of drug-related symptoms, including patterns and route of drug administration, comorbid psychiatric diagnoses, concurrent use of other drugs, and particular drug used. Symptomatology also may vary at different time points in the same user, as acute and phasic symptoms overlap.

Diagnostic procedures

Patients with symptoms of acute drug intoxication or overdose should be evaluated with a standard battery of diagnostic tests, including an electrocardiogram (ECG), chest radiograph, urine or blood drug screen, blood or saliva alcohol concentration, urinalysis, complete blood count, and liver enzyme determination. Urine drug testing for cocaine actually assays for the metabolite, benzoylecgonine, ordinarily detectable for 48 to 72 hours after the last cocaine use. There are reports of sustained positive assays after as long as 30 days of abstinence in chronic very high-dose cocaine addicts. For amphetamine, patients typically test positive for at least 7 days after drug use but may test positive for several weeks. Currently available toxicology screens are neither sensitive nor specific for the presence of designer drugs.

Frequently observed laboratory abnormalities related to stimulant overdose include: leukocytosis, increased blood sugar, creatine phosphokinase, sodium, chloride, and blood urea nitrogen; increased serum phosphate, uric acid, potassium, and decreased bicarbonate. Laboratory results should be assessed in the context of a complete history, including medical, psychiatric, and psychosocial information, to be confirmed by collateral reports. Once stabilized, patients with stimulant abuse should undergo testing for HIV and hepatitis B and C infection; skin testing for tuberculosis also should be considered. While the risk of HIV infection and viral hepatitis is highest in needle-sharing intravenous drug users, the strong association between stimulant abuse generally and high-risk sexual behavior warrants screening of all stimulant abusers.

Possible approaches to treatment_____

Acute intoxication and overdose

No specific pharmacologic treatments for acute stimulant intoxication exist; treatment is symptomatic and supportive, with an emphasis on stabilizing patients. Patients presenting with evidence of severe stimulant overdose, such as marked hypertension or tachycardia, chest pain, cardiac arrhythmia, respiratory distress, hyperthermia, delirium, coma, or seizures, should receive aggressive medical monitoring, with attention to airway maintenance and immediate access to intensive cardiorespiratory support. Intoxication with multiple substances (e.g., alcohol, opiates, benzodiazepines), as well as other metabolic and structural causes of altered mental status, always should be considered. The medical management of the many specific acute complications of stimulant overdose is beyond the scope of this chapter. Certain features unique to stimulant intoxication, however, deserve emphasis.

Psychomotor agitation or anxiety without autonomic sequelae should be managed with short-term administration of a benzodiazepine or short-acting barbiturate; however extended use of sedative-hypnotic or anxiolytic agents should be avoided because of their liability to produce abuse or dependence in this clinical context. Severe or persistent psychotic symptoms can be treated with conventional antipsychotic medication, but this approach is not uniformly recommended due to the potential for haloperidol and related drugs to lower seizure threshold and to induce dystonia and hyperthermia. Low doses of high-potency neuroleptics are suggested, accompanied by monitoring of body temperature and neuropsychiatric status. In milder cases, patients may respond to reassurance and placement in a quiet, nonthreatening environment.

Hyperthermia is a common component of fatal stimulant overdose and, if left untreated, can lead to respiratory distress, acute renal failure, and coma. Body temperatures greater than 40 °C are predictive of poor prognosis. In extreme cases, physical cooling may not be effective. Muscle paralysis may be necessary using pancuronium (with proper ventilatory support) or dantrolene.

Hypertension, if mild or moderate, should not be treated. However, if diastolic blood pressure reaches 110 mm Hg or greater, treatment with alpha- or combined alpha- and beta-blockers, vasodilators, or calcium channel blockers can be used. Drugs that act quickly, can be given iv, and can be titrated easily, including nitroprusside, are optimal in this situation. The use of sublingual nifedipine, obtained by puncturing the capsule, also has been advocated as a means to quickly lower blood pressure. β-adrenergic blockers such as propranolol probably should not be used in the setting of stimulant intoxication unless accompanied by the administration of an α-adrenergic blocker. There is evidence that β-blockade following stimulant overdose may result in excessive, unopposed α stimulation resulting in coronary vasospasm.

Stimulant-induced seizures should be treated with diazepam or barbiturates. Rhabdomyolysis should be managed with urine alkalinization with sodium bicarbonate, in combination with either mannitol or furosemide. Although drug elimination can be increased through urine acidification, rhabdomyolosis decreases the safety of this option.

Patients experiencing cocaine overdose typically improve within the first 24 hours, although some symptoms (e.g., sleep disturbances, tachycardia, anorexia, and tremor) may persist for several days. Symptoms may be more prolonged after amphetamine overdose. Drug-related deaths typically occur early in the course of overdose, from cardiac arrhythmias, myocardial infarction, cerebrovascular complications, or hyperthermia. With respect to methylenedioxymethamphetamine polymorphic

responses to drug intoxication should be expected. MDMA is metabolized by CYP2D6 (see Chap. 6) and poor metabolizers are particularly prone to severe side effects consequent to the interaction with the numerous CYP2D6 substrates.

Substance abuse and dependence

While acute intoxication generally can be managed successfully with intensive medical support, treatment of the underlying stimulant dependence remains a challenge. Abstinence rates for nonpharmacologic treatment generally range from 20 to 40% after 1 year. Viewed as a solitary measure of treatment outcome, such abstinence rates are sometimes regarded as evidence that treatment is ineffective. However, stimulant dependence is more productively viewed as a chronic disease with relapses and remissions, in which treatment outcome is measured not just in absolute terms of use versus abstinence but also with regard to the amount and frequency of use, extent of adverse physical, psychologic, and social consequences, and functional status in each of these domains. In this biopsychosocial perspective, currently available treatment of stimulant dependence is of substantial benefit. It is crucial to emphasize complete abstinence not only from stimulants but also from other illicit drugs and from alcohol in working with the individual patient. Use of even small stimulant doses in the dependent patient can serve as a powerful trigger for drug craving and also perpetuates the patient's association with drug-taking behaviors, environments, and social circles. Use of alcohol or cannabis is frequently cited as a precipitant of relapse to stimulant dependence, most likely through disinhibition and diminished attention to the negative consequences of resuming stimulant use.

Cognitive behavioral and motivational enhancement therapy can have a positive impact in motivating and assisting patients to achieve abstinence and avoid relapse. Contingency contracting and incentive therapies are specific behavioral therapies that have shown promise. Although general drug abuse treatment principles apply to stimulant abuse, some features of stimulant abuse are unique, and tailored programs should be sought out whenever possible. Outpatient treatment should be considered the first option, since 30 to 90% of patients achieve abstinence while in outpatient treatment, and stimulant withdrawal does not have physiologic sequelae that require medical management. Hospitalization is indicated for patients with a serious medical or psychiatric disorder; those with acute suicidality, homicidality, or uncontrolled aggressive or agitated behavior; and those who have concurrent dependence on other drugs, necessitating supervised withdrawal. It is important to distinguish concurrent abuse of other drugs (i.e., use only in combination with stimulants in order to titrate mood or withdrawal effects) from dependence on those drugs (which may develop in the course of stimulant addiction). Inpatient treatment is also indicated for patients who have been unable to maintain abstinence while participating in outpatient treatment. This is often the case for patients who have used stimulants chronically via the intravenous or smoked routes and for those lacking social support.

Behavioral and psychologic treatment efforts aim to assist patients to achieve and maintain abstinence and to prevent relapse. Intensive treatment is required, including multiple weekly contacts and frequent urine drug testing, in combination with patient education on the dangers of stimulant use and the role of drug use in their lives. Family counseling and individual psychotherapy also may be employed, and self-help groups can be useful in providing role models of recovery and a forum for discussing the patient's drug use and reasons for wanting to quit. Relapse prevention involves the identification of individuals, environments, mood states, and other drug-related cues likely to increase craving and the possibility of relapse. This phase of treatment involves the development of strategies to minimize exposure to high-risk situations and to resist using drugs when such situations cannot be avoided. Relapse prevention also promotes strategies to prevent progression of a limited "slip" into a full-blown relapse. Patient participation in abstinence-oriented mutual self-help groups, such as Narcotics Anonymous, should be strongly encouraged in almost all cases.

Pharmacotherapy is aimed primarily at reducing drug craving and withdrawal symptoms and managing concurrent psychiatric or substance abuse disorders that may have an impact on abstinence. More than 30 agents have been explored for benefit as adjuncts to psychosocial treatment of stimulant dependence, but none has demonstrated clinical utility. Dopamine agonists studied include bromocriptine, amantadine, pergolide, L-DOPA, mazindol, and methylphenidate. Although bromocriptine, a postsynaptic D_2 dopamine receptor agonist, reduces craving for cocaine and/or psychiatric symptoms associated with discontinuation of cocaine use, its long-term success in treatment is poor, and the drug is not well tolerated. Amantadine and methylphenidate have been shown to reduce craving for cocaine in some, but not other, studies; methylphenidate decreased cocaine use in some cocaine abusers with attention deficit disorder but not in subjects without this diagnosis. Tricyclic antidepressants, most notably desipramine, also have been explored for their effects on affective symptoms resulting from abstinence from cocaine. In general, however, these agents have produced only modest effects in maintaining abstinence, and some have produced side effects that limit their utility. Other agents such as opioid antagonists and mixed agonist-antagonists, the anticonvulsant carbamazepine, and the selective serotonin reuptake inhibitors, including fluoxetine, have shown promise in preliminary studies but await confirmation from large-scale controlled clinical trials.

Suggested readings

BRAUER LH, AMBRE J, DE WIT H. Acute tolerance to subjective but not cardiovascular effects of D-amphetamine in normal, healthy volunteers. J Clin Psychopharmacol 1996;16:72-6.

BUCHANAN JF, BROWN CR. "Designer drugs": a problem in clinical toxicology. Med Toxicol Adverse Drug Exp 1988;3:1-17.

DE LA TORRE R, et al. Fatal MDMA intoxication. Lancet 1999;353: 593-8.

DIXON SD. Effects of transplacental exposure to cocaine and methamphetamine in the neonate (specialty conference). West J Med 1989;150:436-42.

GAY GR. Clinical management of acute and chronic cocaine poisoning. Ann Emerg Med 1982;10:562-72.

GAWIN FH, ELLINWOOD EH. Cocaine and other stimulants: actions, abuse and treatment. N Engl J Med 1988;318:1173-82.

KARAN LD, HALLER DL, SCHNOLL SH. Cocaine. In Frances RJ, Miller SI, eds. Clinical textbook of addictive disorders. New York: The Guilford Press, 1991:121-45.

KLEBER HD. Pharmacotherapy, current and potential, for the treatment of cocaine dependence. Clin Neuropharmacol 1995;18(suppl 1):S96-109.

KOOB GF, BLOOM FE. Cellular and molecular mechanisms of drug dependence. Science 1988;242:715-23.

LANGE RA, CIGARROA RG, FLORES ED. Potentiation of cocaine-induced coronary vasoconstriction by beta-adrenergic blockade. Ann Intern Med 1990;112:897-903.

MACK RB. The iceman cometh and killeth: smokable methamphetamine. NC Med J 1990;51:276-78.

MENDELSON JH, MELLO NK. Management of cocaine abuse and dependence. N Engl J Med 1996;334:965-72.

SEIDEN LS, SABOL KE, RICUARTE GA. Amphetamine: effects on catecholamine systems and behavior. Ann Rev Pharmacol Toxicol 1993;32:639-77.

STEIN RM, ELLINWOOD EH. Diagnosis and treatment of stimulant dependence. In: Dunner DL, ed. Current psychiatric therapy, vol II. Philadelphia: WB Saunders, 1997:139-47.

STEIN RM, ELLINWOOD EH. Medical complications of cocaine abuse. Drug Ther 1990;20:40-50.

STITZER ML, WALSH SL. Psychostimulant abuse: the case for combined behavioral and pharmacological treatments. Pharmacol Biochem Behav 1997;57:457-70.

TUCKER GT, LENNARD MS, ELLIS SW, et al. Demethylation of methylenedioxymethamphetamine ("ecstasy") by debrisoquine hydroxylase (CYP2D6). Biochem Pharmacol 1994;47:1151-6.

Cannabis

Irma B. Adams

Cannabis has long been used medicinally in China, the Middle East, and South America to treat a wide variety of conditions. The earliest reference to the medicinal properties of cannabis dates from 2700 B.C. in China. The euphoric and intoxicating properties of cannabis were discovered in India between 2000 and 1400 B.C., and these properties have led to the widespread use and abuse of cannabis. Worldwide estimation of cannabis use is 200 to 300 million people. The psychoactive constituents in cannabis are classified as *cannabinoids*. This class of substances produces a distinct combination of effects that do not fit traditional pharmacologic classification.

Cannabis is a term that refers to components of the plant *Cannabis sativa*. Cannabinoids are found in all parts of both male and female plants. The highest concentration of these psychoactive ingredients is found in the flowering tops, followed by the leaves, with smaller amounts of cannabinoids in the stems and roots. The canabinoid content varies depending on the climate, cultivation techniques, type of plant, and soil. The plant in western countries is most commonly cut, dried, and incorporated into cigarettes with or without tobacco. This plant preparation is know as *marijuana*. Hashish is prepared from resin extracted from the plant and is more potent. Products from the cannabis plant also can be chewed, eaten in baked goods, or smoked in a waterpipe.

Definition of substances

The cannabis plant contains approximately 400 chemicals, of which about 60 are cannabinoids. The term *cannabinoid* refers to the C21 compounds present in the plant and includes their transformation products. The principal psychoactive constituent of the plant is $(-)$-*trans*-Δ9-tetrahydrocannabinol (THC). During the late 1960s, the average THC content was 1.5% in cannabis plants confiscated in the United States. By the mid-1980s, levels had doubled to about 3%. Recent emphasis on genetic crossbreeding and indoor hydroponic cultivation techniques have led to cannabis plants with THC concentrations as high as 20%. While it is currently unknown what effects these potent THC levels will have on patterns of cannabis use and health consequences in the future, average THC levels in confiscated cannabis remain in the 3% range.

Smoking is the preferred route of administration in western countries. Following inhalation, THC is absorbed into the bloodstream and extensively metabolized by the liver. One of the metabolites, 11-hydroxy-THC (11-OH-THC), is more potent than THC, yet it is not nearly as abundant following smoking. Metabolism results in many inactive metabolites, including 11-nor-carboxy-9-THC (THC-COOH). Blood levels of THC rise rapidly and peak prior to the end of smoking and then quickly decrease. Levels of 11-OH-THC are lower than THC levels and peak at the end of smoking. THC-COOH is detected minutes after smoking, and levels plateau for an extended period. In an experienced user, drug effects are experienced after a few inhalations. Acute peak psychologic effects, which are dose-dependent, appear between 30 and 60 minutes. Establishing a relationship between blood levels of THC or its metabolites and level of impairment is difficult. Immediately after smoking, blood levels are high, whereas drug effects are low; the situation reverses at later times. Cannabis can be taken orally in various preparations. The absorption rate of THC is slower and more variable by this route, yet the duration of action is longer. Peak effects are delayed 3 to 4 hours after ingestion and last for 6 to 8 hours. Concentrations of 11-OH-THC in the blood are higher after oral ingestion. Owing to their high lipophilicity, cannabinoids are sequestered in lipid-rich tissues and then released slowly and unevenly, thereby producing a long elimination rate. Estimates of elimination range from 18 hours to 5 days from a single cannabis cigarette; variability is due to assay sensitivity and timing of blood measurements.

It is now recognized that cannabinoids produce their psychoactive effects through a very specific central action. Development of highly potent THC analogues led to the identification of a specific cannabinoid receptor in the brain. Binding to this receptor is limited to psychoactive cannabinoids. The distribution of this central cannabinoid receptor is similar in several mammalian species and is located neuronally. Autoradiographic distribution studies have revealed that some correlation exists between the density of receptor location and the effects of cannabis. High numbers of receptors occur in the basal ganglia (e.g., enteropeduncular nucleus, globus pallidus, lateral caudate putamen, and substantia nigra pars reticulata) and the molecular layer of the cerebellum, which may explain cannabinoid interference with movement. Cannabinoid effects on cognition and memory could be due to receptor locations in cell layers in the cortex and hippocampus. Cannabinoid receptors are also associated with regions mediating brain reward. Low levels of receptors are found in the brain stem, hypothalamus, corpus callosum, and deep cerebellar nuclei. The sparse number of receptors in brain stem areas involved in cardiovascular and respiratory functioning is consistent with the lack of lethality of cannabis. A peripheral cannabinoid receptor that is structurally distinct from the central cannabinoid receptor has been identified in macrophages in the spleen and peripheral blood lymphocytes. While the role of the peripheral receptor is presently unknown, cannabinoids are known to inhibit the immune system.

Recently, an endogenous compound that binds to the cannabinoid receptor has been identified. Anandamide (arachidonylethanolamide) is a fatty acid-derived compound that is structurally quite dissimilar from THC. Anandamide in animal and other in vitro models produces effects similar to THC, although with reduced potency. Pathways for the synthesis and degradation of anandamide have been demonstrated. The existence of a receptor, endogenous ligand, and biosynthetic and degradative pathways leads to the postulation of a possible "cannabinoid" neurochemical system. The physiologic role of anandamide and its interaction with other neurochemical systems in the brain remain unclear. The recent discovery of cannabinoid receptor antagonists (SR 141716A and others) should provide a tool for elucidating the role of anandamide and cannabinoids in the central nervous system and peripheral sites.

Epidemiology

Cannabis is the most widely used illicit drug worldwide; in fact, in many countries cannabis ranks only behind the consumption of alcohol and cigarettes. Epidemiologic studies of patterns of cannabis use are more complete in developed countries and were undertaken as cannabis use became more widespread among adolescents and young adults. Recently, developing countries have started conducting studies as well. Since cannabis is an illegal substance, users contacted in surveys are less likely to participate and give truthful responses. Therefore, studies must be designed carefully to allow inferences about trends of illegal drug use.

Cannabis is the most commonly used illicit drug in European countries. In 1994, the prevalence of lifetime use (i.e., tried cannabis at least once) ranged from 40% in Denmark between the ages of 16 and 44 years to 14% among 12- to 59-year-olds in the United Kingdom. Surveys indicate that current use is increasing. Drug use data have been collected regularly for 20 years in the United States. In 1992, 33% of the national household sample reported having tried cannabis at least once in

their lifetime, 9% had used it in the past year, and 4% were current users. Lifetime rates were the highest in the 26- to 34-year age group, which reported that 59% had used cannabis at least once. Discontinuation rates were high, and weekly use was uncommon. Overall, 9% of men and 6% of women used cannabis weekly; however, a peak prevalence of 21% was reported among those aged 12 to 17 years. After a steady decline of cannabis use in the 1980s, recent surveys indicate an abrupt rise in use among adolescents. The recent upturn comes at a time where there is a decline in social disapproval of cannabis and in perceived risks, lower public attention to cannabis, and an increase in prodrug messages in popular culture. Current levels of use are still much lower than the peak periods of use, though rates of use are higher in the United States than in Europe.

Several Canadian studies of school-aged children have shown trends similar to those in the United States, with a rise in the use of cannabis in the 1970s followed by a decline throughout the 1980s and then an increase in overall rates within the past few years. However, the rates of use are lower than in the United States. In a 1994 survey conducted by Health Canada consisting of 12,155 persons aged 15 years or older, 28.2% reported lifetime use of cannabis, with 7.4% of the sample reporting use within the past year. Prevalence of current use was related to age, with 26.1% of those aged 15 to 17 years currently using cannabis, whereas 1.4% of those aged 45 to 54 years currently were users. Men were twice as likely to use cannabis than women. Cannabis use in Australia is also widespread. In a national household survey of adults conducted in 1993, 33% of total respondents reported lifetime use, whereas 72% of young adults aged 20 to 24 years had used cannabis at least once.

Survey data suggest that cannabis use has increased in the last decade in Europe, Australia, Canada, and the United States. Use is related to sex and age. Men are more likely to use cannabis than women, and use is more prevalent among young people. Current use was much lower than lifetime use, which indicates high discontinuation rates. Great debate regarding the legalization of cannabis is currently underway in many countries, with proponents of legalization arguing that the consequences of incarceration outweigh the potential adverse effects of cannabis use on health.

Although cannabis is used throughout the world for medicinal, religious, or recreational purposes, limited survey data are available in many parts of the world. Often these data provide only an indication of overall levels of use. Frequently, survey methods are not reported or standardized, rate results are only summarized, sex-specific rates are not reported, and teenage levels of use are underreported. The limited data on cannabis use in African, Asian, and Central and South American countries suggest that these countries have lower rates of lifetime use than many western countries. For example, a 1993 school survey from Brazil reported lifetime use rates of 5.3%. Similar low lifetime rates were found in three northern Indian states and southern India. Use levels are not available from other Asian countries.

Cannabinoids produce a variety of acute psychologic, perceptual, and physical effects in humans, as summarized in Table 84.1. The psychologic effects vary depending on the route of administration, quantity smoked or ingested, environment, experience of the user, and individual susceptibility to cannabis. Cognitive ability, mood, senses, perception, memory, and motor coordination are all affected after smoking a cannabis cigarette containing 2% THC or after orally consuming 20 mg THC. Cannabis users typically experience a "high" that is described as a state of euphoria and an increased sense of well-being. Users often display uncontrollable and spontaneous laughter and increased sociability on interaction; feelings of sleepiness and relaxation are more pronounced when alone. Cannabis heightens sensitivity to external visual and auditory stimuli, thereby brightening colors and enhancing music. THC alters time perception by producing an overestimation of elapsed time. Short-term memory may be impaired, and users sometimes have difficulty in completing goals that require multiple mental steps. Associated with altered time perception and memory impairment is *temporal disintegration,* which is defined as difficulty in retaining and coordinating memories relevant to a task the user is pursuing. Impairment is demonstrated in many psychologic tests depending on the complexity of the test and size of the cannabis dose. Users later experience relaxation and a dreamlike state with drowsiness and sometimes depression. Less experienced users have fewer of the subjective effects and more motor and cognitive impairment. At higher doses, acute effects include hallucinations, paranoia, and delusions. Depersonalization and confused thinking become more pronounced. Anxiety and sometimes panic replace drug-induced euphoria. A toxic psychosis involving hallucination can result acutely from very high doses or after months of use.

Table 84.1 A description of acute psychologic, perceptual, and physiologic effects and short- and long-term risks of cannabis

Acute psychologic and perceptual effects

State of euphoria
Increased sense of well-being
Spontaneous laughter
Increased sociability with interaction
Sleepiness and relaxation more pronounced when alone
Heightened sensitivity to external visual and auditory stimuli
Altered time perception

Acute physiologic effects

Conjunctiva reddening
Increased heart rate
Orthostatic hypotension at high doses
Dry mouth and throat
Increased consumption of food
Alterations of motor control with decreased balance and stability
Impairment of simple motor tasks and reaction times at high doses

Short-term risks

Impairment of learning ability
Possible short-term memory impairment
Reduced psychomotor performance
Possible carryover effect

Long-term risks

Impairment of organization of complex information
Reduced ability to filter out irrelevant information and focus attention
Delayed speed of information processing
Impairment may not be reversible
Worsened symptoms of schizophrenia
Higher prevalence of acute bronchitis, injury to the air ways, and lung inflammation
Impaired lung immune defense
Impaired fetal growth, reduction in birth weight and length of gestation

---

Clinical findings

Symptoms and signs

Acute cannabis intoxication results in several physiologic manifestations. Cannabis consistently affects the cardiovascular system and characteristically causes conjunctivae to redden due to dilatation of blood vessels and increased heart rate with accompanying peripheral vasodilatation. THC also produces orthostatic hypotension at higher doses and decreased platelet aggregation. Cannabis smokers report dry mouth and throat. Cannabis use increases the consumption of food. Other symptoms of cannabis intoxication include alterations of motor control with decreased balance, stability, and muscle strength and increased hand tremors. At higher doses, simple motor tasks and reaction times are impaired. Tremors, muscle weakness, and increased deep tendon reflexes may be observed.

When identifying a patient for cannabis abuse or dependency, risk factors for drug use and symptoms of drug use should be assessed. Risk factors for cannabis use include personal and family history of alcoholism or other drug use, psychiatric and emotional disturbances, including mood disorders, and cognitive disabilities. Physical signs of cannabis use may include increased heart rate and reddened conjunctiva. However, heart rate increases are often unnoticed, and eye irritation may be masked with eye drops. Other physical symptoms, such as pulmonary or reflex changes, are often absent. Usually, diagnosis depends on changes in behavioral or cognitive areas. These changes are more likely noticed by family members and friends. Urine testing will only demonstrate use within the past few days. Individuals dependent on cannabis become preoccupied with obtaining and using cannabis, often attempt to abstain from use, and then relapse and deny having a problem. Cannabis abuse can be described as use almost every day, several times a day for a month. Cannabis dependence is defined by *Diagnostic and Statistical Manual of Mental Disorders* (DSM-IV) criteria as specified by the American Psychological Association.

Dependence is generally characterized by the failure of the individual to reduce his/her use even though he wishes to do so, foregoing normal daily activity to use cannabis, and spending considerable time obtaining cannabis.

Short-term risks

A great deal of concern exists over the possible health consequences of cannabis use due to the large number of users, especially among the young population (see Tab. 84.1 for short- and long-term risks). Ascertaining toxicity from short- and long-term cannabis use in humans is difficult for several reasons. Health studies predominantely have been performed in animals, and extrapolating results to humans is complicated. Most studies have concentrated on young people in excellent general health. Often cannabis is used in combination with alcohol and other drugs. Furthermore, the vast majority of studies have been conducted using cannabis with under 5% THC content. Thus the result of using cannabis with higher THC contents is unknown.

Cannabis can impair short-term memory, as measured in free recall of previously learned items, when cannabis is used during the learning and recall periods. Cannabis impairs the capability of learning, including the associative process, by increasing uncommon associations; thus cognitive development is affected. Psychomotor performance is reduced, as measured in a wide variety of tests, such as motor coordination, handwriting, digit substitution, divided attention, and various types of operant tasks. These decrements are more pronounced as the difficulty of the task increases.

Cannabis use can lead to impaired performance of complex tasks the day after smoking, thus producing a carryover effect. This carryover effect is of particular concern for people responsible for performing complex cognitive and behavioral tasks. Impairment in operating an aircraft simulator has been demonstrated in pilots 24 hours after smoking a single cannabis cigarette of a moderate dose. Yet subjects were unaware of any effects on their performance or alertness.

The risk of having a motor vehicle accident increases on driving when intoxicated with cannabis, although the extent that cannabis impairs driving performance is not known with certainty. THC does affect tracking, reaction time, divided attention, and vigilance or sustained attention tests. Drivers under the influence of THC in actual driving tests tend to overestimate the level of impairment and compensate by concentrating on driving and/or driving slowly. However, compensation becomes problematic when impaired drivers are presented with unanticipated events.

Long-term risks

Since one of the well-known acute effects of cannabis is to impair cognitive functioning, it has long been suggested that chronic cannabis use may cause lasting cognitive and memory impairments. Assessing the chronic effects of cannabis on cognitive functioning is difficult because many factors other than drug use must be controlled, including determining levels of cognitive impairment that might have preceded drug use, taking into account the effects of multiple drug use, and determining the frequency and duration of drug use. Earlier research was insufficient to conclude that long-term use produces lasting gross impairment. Recent research that uses improved test procedures and electrophysiologic methods provides evidence that cannabis produces complex and subtle impairments that are related to the duration of cannabis use. Impairments appear specific to higher cognitive functions, such as the organization and integration of complex information that involves attention and memory processes. Cannabis slows information processing and reaction time. The number of years of cannabis use impairs the ability of the brain to filter out irrelevant information at an early stage of processing and to focus attention. The speed of information processing is delayed with frequency of use but is not affected by duration of use. An impaired mode of information processing could cause distractibility and impairment when concentration and attention are required. The reversibility of the impairments are unknown.

Great interest has been generated in the effects of cannabis on adolescent development and educational performance and production of an "amotivational syndrome." A modest statistical relationship may exist between cannabis and other illicit drug use and poor educational performance. Individuals who already have a learning disability are more susceptible to memory disruptions. However, attempts to verify the existence of an amotivational syndrome specifically resulting from cannabis use have failed. Clearly, cannabis should be avoided in those considered "at risk".

Identification of a specific cannabis psychosis even in chronic, heavy users has not been clearly defined. Cannabis does appear to worsen symptoms of schizophrenia. Acute panic attacks, paranoid states, and toxic delirium are rare. No specific brain damage has been identified in humans, although possible ultrastructural damage has been found in animals.

Cannabinoids may aggravate preexisting conditions such as angina and congestive heart failure. Hypotension and bradycardia result from prolonged exposure to cannabinoids. Heavy smokers experience similar problems to cigarette smokers, including symptoms resembling chronic bronchitis and a higher prevalence of acute bronchitis. Long-term cannabis smoking produces injury to the epithelial lining of the airways and causes lung inflammation. The lung's immune defense is impaired by chronic cannabis smoking; alveolar macrophages have altered morphology, and T-cell lymphocyte counts are lower.

Studies have been performed to assess the effects of cannabis on the immune system, pregnancy, and cell chromosomes. With efforts to use either cannabis or synthetic cannabinoids for therapeutic purposes, the potential effects on the immune system should be considered, especially in patients with a compromised immune system. Immune studies in animal and cell culture models have demonstrated that cannabinoids act as immunomodulators. However, some of these effects can be produced by nonpsychoactive cannabinoids, suggesting a non-receptor-mediated mechanism. The health impact of cannabis on the immune system in humans is unclear.

Cannabis use during pregnancy impairs fetal growth and leads to a reduction in birth weight and length of gestation. Long-term neurobehavioral effects of prenatal exposure are subtle, and results from prenatal exposure studies suggest that the mental growth of the child may be affected to an extent. Children of cannabis users by the age of 4 had reduced verbal ability, memory, and attention and increased impulsiveness, although these effects are subtle. Effects of cannabinoids on chromosomes and cell metabolism are often contradictory and presently are inconclusive.

Although tolerance has been observed in many animal models, the development of tolerance in humans generally occurs in heavy, long-term users of cannabis. Tolerance develops in different degrees to a variety of THC's effects, including cannabinoid-induced decreases in cardiovascular and autonomic functions, increases in intraocular pressure, sleep disturbances, and mood changes. Tolerance develops quickly to the tachycardiac effects of cannabis. Results are less conclusive for behavioral tolerance in moderate users. High doses taken for long periods of time do result in the development of tolerance to the subjective effects of THC.

Most drugs used for recreational purposes produce some form of psychologic and physiologic dependence. The development of tolerance frequently occurs in conjunction with dependence. If one is dependent on a drug, withdrawal symptoms result when the drug is not taken. The most prominent symptoms on cessation of cannabis are increased irritability and restlessness. Other symptoms, although variable, include insomnia, anorexia, increased sweating, mild nausea, increased body temperature, weight loss, and hand tremor. Although it is established that chronic cannabis use does not result in severe withdrawal symptoms, cannabis dependence does develop for a substantial number of people. The probability of becoming dependent increases linearly with frequency and quantity of use. Interestingly, adolescents are more likely to become dependent than adults. A 1994 study from the United States found that of those who had reported lifetime cannabis use, 9.2% developed dependence. Recent reviews have found that of those who have used cannabis more than a few times, 20 to 30% may develop dependence.

Possible approaches to treatment

In previous years, few cannabis users sought treatment, and only a small number of treatment outcome studies have been performed. The lack of treatment probably reflects the belief that since cannabis is often used in combination with other drugs, treatment for polydrug abuse encompasses and treats cannabis users. One study examined two approaches to treatment: the relapse-prevention (RP) model and a social support (SS) group. The RP treatment provides cognitive and behavioral coping training; SS intervention relies on group support and discussion for help. No differences were noted for the two treatments in abstinence rates or days of cannabis use. For both treatments, days of use per month were reduced significantly at follow-up dates. At 30 months after treatment, rates of abstinence were 28%. Thus, individuals attempting to discontinue use can do so with minimal intervention and respond well to several types of treatments, although large relapse rates are observed that are comparable with those of other groups of drug abusers. Brief individual intervention programs are more cost-effective, especially for individuals who are motivated to change. Withdrawal management is important in treating cannabis dependence, although specific strategies for cannabis need further development. Further research also is required to develop more effective treatment programs to decrease relapse rates. At present, there are no therapeutic agents available to assist those who are unresponsive to behavioral and psychologic interventions.

Suggested readings

ADAMS IB, MARTIN BR. Cannabis: Pharmacology and toxicology in animals and humans. Addiction 1996;91:585-614.

AMERICAN PSYCHIATRIC ASSOCIATION (APA). Diagnostic and statistical manual of mental disorders, 3rd ed. Washington: American Psychiatric Press, 1987.

ANTHONY JC, WARNER LA, KESSLER RC. Comparative epidemiology of dependence on tobacco, alcohol, controlled substances and inhalants: basic findings from the National Comorbidity Survey. Exp Clin Psychopharmacol 1994;2:2447-68.

BUDNEY AJ, KANDEL DB, CHEREK DR, et al. College on Problems of Drug Dependence Meeting, Puerto Rico, June 1996. Marijuana use and dependence. Drug Alcohol Depend 1997;45:1-11.

CHAIT LD, PIERRI J. Effects of smoked marijuana on human performance: a critical review. In: Murphy L, Bartke A, eds. Marijuana/Cannabinoids: neurobiology and neurophysiology. Boca Raton: CRC Press, 1992:387-423.

HALL W, SOLOWIJ N, LEMON J. The Health and Psychological Effects of Cannabis Use. Australian National Task Force on Cannabis, National Drug Strategy Monograph No 5, Melbourne, 1994.

HOLLISTER LE. Marijuana and immunity. J Psychoact Drugs 1988;20:3-8.

MECHOULAM R, HANUS L, MARTIN BR. The search for endogenous ligands of the cannabinoid receptor. Biochem Pharmacol 1994;48:1537-44.

SCHWARTZ RH. Identifying and helping patients who use marijuana. Postgrad Med 1989;86:91-95.

WIESBECK GA, SCHUCKIT MA, KALMIJN JA, et al. An evaluation of the history of a marijuana withdrawal syndrome in a large population. Addiction 1996;91:1469-78.

ZWEBEN JE, O'CONNELL K. Strategies for breaking marijuana dependence. J Psychoact Drugs 1992;24:165-71.

85

Anabolic steroids

Paolo Palatini, Franco Giada

Anabolic steroid use by athletes in an attempt to enhance athletic performance represents the most widespread form of doping at all levels of athletic competition. These drugs were first used in the Eastern European countries in the 1950s. Their use subsequently spread to the United States and then worldwide. Anabolic steroids were used initially by elite weight lifters and bodybuilders, but they were adopted subsequently by professional athletes in various sports and even by amateurs. In 1976, anabolic steroids were banned by the International Olympic Committee, but their use continued to grow in magnitude, chiefly among bodybuilders with the specific purpose of improving their outward physical appearance.

Definition of substances

Androgenic activity is shared by many 19-carbon steroidal compounds. The most potent naturally occurring androgen in man is testosterone, which in the circulation serves as a prohormone for the formation of 5-reduced androgens and in particular of dihydrotestosterone, which is responsible for most androgenic actions. Testosterone is secreted by the testis and to a lesser extent by the adrenal cortex. In addition, small amounts of testosterone are secreted by the ovary in women.

Testicular growth, spermatogenesis, and steroidogenesis are regulated by the pituitary gonadotropin luteinizing hormone (LH) and follicle-stimulating hormone (FSH). The actions of the gonadotropins are mediated by cyclic adenosine monophosphate (cAMP), which increases the activity of the enzymes promoting steroidogenesis, thereby favoring testosterone synthesis. Through their action on the hypothalamus and pituitary, androgens regulate gonadotropin secretion with a feedback mechanism.

Dihydrotestosterone binds to the intracellular androgen receptor protein, and the dihydrotestosterone-receptor complex enhances the RNA and specific protein synthesis in the nucleus. A number of other weaker steroids, such as androstenedione, dehydroepiandrosterone, and androsterone, have been described, but their real efficacy in vivo has been questioned.

Testosterone in plasma is bound to a specific globulin, called *sex hormone-binding globulin,* or to albumin and other plasma proteins. Only 2% of dihydrotestosterone

circulates as free hormone and is thus biologically active. Besides being transformed to dihydrotestosterone, testosterone can be aromatized to estradiol, whose role in males has never been defined. Testosterone is inactivated primarily in the liver, where it is converted to androsterone and etiocholanone. Following administration of radiolabeled testosterone, about 90% of the radioactivity appears in the urine and 6% in the feces.

Testosterone synthesis is of crucial importance during three periods of life: the phase of embryonic development in which sexual differentiation takes place, the neonatal phase, and the time of male puberty, when androgens promote the increase in height and skeletal musculature and the development of secondary sex characteristics, spermatogenesis, and sexual behavior. Testosterone also has nitrogen-retaining effects, which promote protein synthesis in skeletal muscles and increase body weight. The anabolic action of androgens is mediated by the receptor that mediates the actions of the hormones in other target tissues. These effects are greater in the hypogonadal male and smaller and shorter lasting in the normal adult. Other testosterone effects include erythropoiesis stimulation, calcium retention, and protein matrix synthesis in the bones.

Anabolic steroids   Testosterone cannot be used as an effective therapeutic agent, either as an oral or as a parenteral preparation. Oral administration is followed by rapid absorption, metabolization, and excretion with mild pharmacologic effects. Testosterone injected as a solution in oil is rapidly metabolized and also has little effect. Testosterone esters injected im in oil are absorbed more slowly and thus facilitate the administration of effective dosages. Other changes in the molecule alter the time course of metabolization. As a result, many synthetic androgens have longer half-lives than testosterone. For this purpose, three main chemical modifications of the molecule have been made. Esterification of the 17-hydroxyl group makes the molecule more soluble in the lipid vehicles, slowing the release of the substance into the circulation and thereby prolonging and potentiating the action. Such esters thus can be administered by parenteral injection every 1 to 3 weeks. Alkylated derivatives (at the 17 position) are effective when administered orally because they are catabolized slowly by the liver. Unfortunately, these drugs have significant hepatotoxicity.

Jaundice is a frequent clinical feature with alkylated derivatives, due to stasis and accumulation of bile in the biliary capillaries, limiting their clinical use. Other changes in the steroid structure were aimed at slowing the rate of inactivation, altering metabolism, and increasing power.

Another goal of researchers was that of producing synthetic compounds with anabolic properties but devoid of androgenic effects. However, no synthetic anabolic steroid proved to be free of androgenic activity. This is not surprising because the anabolic and androgenic effects are mediated by a single receptor.

The most widely used anabolic steroids are the long-lasting ester derivatives, administered as parenteral preparations.

There is no doubt that hypogonadism is the clearest therapeutic indication for androgen administration. In this clinical condition, the anabolic steroids administered at physiologic doses represent first-choice therapy. Less clear indications are catabolic states in debilitated (e.g, AIDS) or elderly individuals and stimulation of erythropoiesis in refractory anemias associated with failure of the bone marrow or renal failure. Androgenic therapy also has been tried in hereditary angioneurotic edema, pituitary dwarfism, carcinoma of the breast, and osteoporosis.

Epidemiology

Over 1 million people use anabolic steroids in the United States, including many adolescents. Among high school students, the percentage of anabolic steroid users is 1 to 3%, and in a European study, 42% of bodybuilders investigated with antidoping tests turned out to be anabolic steroid users. The widespread use of anabolic steroids among athletes and youngsters appears today to be a significant public health problem.

Anabolic steroids are currently used by athletes as a self-prescription or are given by coaches and even team physicians. These drugs usually are taken as a cyclic therapy for 8 to 12 weeks with washout periods lasting 6 to 10 weeks. Anabolic steroid dosage is increased progressively during the first weeks and then decreased gradually up to the end of the cycle. Two or more compounds are frequently taken (so-called stacking phenomenon) in an attempt to attain maximum benefits and minimal side effects, but the real advantage of this approach has never been demonstrated.

The dosage employed by athletes varies considerably in relation to the sport practiced. It is relatively low in cyclists, who use anabolic steroids only to prevent the catabolic effects of intense physical activity, and much higher in bodybuilders, who take them for aesthetic purposes, to increase the muscle mass and reduce subcutaneous fat. Dosages 10 to 100 times higher than those currently used for therapeutic purposes have been reported in bodybuilders (Tab. 85.1). Women take lower doses than men.

Most of the athletes who use anabolic steroids obtain them through the "steroid underground," through physicians' prescriptions, or directly from pharmacists. The easy access of athletes to anabolic steroids is worrisome and indicates that many aspects of the problem are poorly understood even by physicians. It is reckoned that the black market for anabolic steroid sales in the United States exceeds $100 million per year.

To mitigate the side effects of the anabolic steroid, some athletes also take other potentially harmful drugs such as diuretics, human chorionic gonadotropin, growth factors, antiestrogens, and antiacne products. Most of the athletes currently taking anabolic steroids are unaware of the nature of these drugs and the risks associated with their use.

Anabolic steroids are used by athletes in the belief that they may enhance athletic performance by increasing muscle mass and strength. There is no doubt that anabolic steroids promote muscle growth in boys and women of all ages and in hypogonadal males. However, very little is known about anabolic steroid effects on muscle development in sexually mature men. The medical-scientific community has, for a long time now, raised doubt as to the real effectiveness of anabolic steroids in healthy adult male athletes to such an extent as to lose their credibility

Table 85.1 Anabolic steroids currently used by athletes

Generic name	Dose used by athletes (mg/week)	Dose used in clinical practice (mg/week)	Route of administration
Testosterone propionate	300-800	50-100	Parenteral
Oxandrolone	70-80	35-70	Oral
Stanozolol	50-100	28-42	Oral
Methenolone enanthate	100-600	50-100	Parenteral
Androstanolone undecilate	50-300	40-160	Parenteral
Ethylestrenol	80-160	20-40	Oral
Methenolone	300-400	300-600	Oral
Testosterone cypionate	200-800	50-200	Parenteral
Testosterone enanthate	200-800	50-200	Parenteral
Nandrolone decanoate	50-200	10-40	Parenteral

among sports participants. Current studies on the ability of the anabolic steroids to increase muscular mass and strength have produced conflicting results. Furthermore, many studies have methodologic biases such as the lack of an adequate control group and the use of anabolic steroid dosages that are less than those currently used by athletes. On the other hand, it would not be ethical to start further studies that foresee administering supratherapeutic dosages of anabolic steroids to healthy subjects. It is most difficult to carry out double-blind investigations given the obvious side effects of anabolic steroids. Another important methodologic question is based on the fact that there are small differences in the parameters employed to evaluate athletic performance. Even if differences are not significant from a strictly statistical point of view, they could be of extreme importance as far as the results in the individual athlete are concerned and therefore not adequately demonstrable in a clinical study.

A first review of the available literature indicated that anabolic steroids do not increase muscular mass and strength. Different conclusions were reached, however, by Haupt and Rovere, who, having reviewed the literature a few years later, found a significant increase in muscular mass and strength following administration of anabolic steroids, provided three conditions were met: the athlete must have undergone intense training before and during the period of drug administration; the athlete must have adhered to a hypercaloric diet with high protein intake; and the modifications in muscle strength must have been evaluated using tests with which the athlete was familiar.

The mechanisms by which anabolic steroids exert their effect lie in their capacity to antagonize the catabolic effect of glucocorticoids released during physical exercise, to determine a positive nitrogen balance, and to stimulate protein synthesis in muscular cells. Furthermore, anabolic steroids would make a more intense and prolonged period of training possible by reducing the sensation of tiredness and increasing aggressiveness. Finally, an important placebo effect cannot be excluded. The increase in body weight and lean mass combined with a reduction in adipose mass described in athletes using steroids is, nevertheless, short lasting and reversible even after a few weeks of withdrawal.

A further controversial point lies in the fact that the ponderable increase observed with the use of anabolic steroids would be too high to be attributable exclusively to a normal hypertrophy of the skeletal muscles. Some authors maintain that water retention and expansion in plasma volume are significant contributors to the weight increase observed with anabolic steroid use. Despite the capacity of anabolic steroids to increase erythropoiesis, no improvements in sports performance of the aerobic type nor in maximal oxygen consumption in athletes using anabolic steroids have been noted.

Antidoping   Currently, the most effective tool for fighting anabolic steroid doping, combined with a thorough information campaign, seems to be the antidoping control, which reveals traces of illegally consumed substances in biologic samples taken from the athletes. The method now widely used in the antidoping laboratories of the International Olympic Committee is the determination of testosterone and its metabolite epitestosterone in urine using gas chromatography and mass spectrophotometry. A testosterone level in the urine samples that exceeds the epitestosterone level by sixfold reveals an exogenous origin of the testosterone. Such an athlete is thus considered positive and subsequently disqualified.

Given the high reliability of the antidoping analysis, athletes tend to avoid using parenteral anabolic steroids with long-acting effects that are present in urine samples for a number of months. They also choose orally administered products with short-lasting effects that show up in urine samples only for a few weeks associated with the so-called masking agents. In order to deal with this type of doping, controls should be carried out not only during competitions but also during periods of training.

Clinical findings

Unwelcome effects have been found both in patients taking pharmacologic doses of anabolic steroids and in athletes taking large supratherapeutic doses. Despite the widespread use of these drugs, most studies have examined the short-term effects of anabolic steroids. The few available data on the effects of long-term anabolic steroid administration are virtually confined to case reports and anecdotal observations. Other possible confounders are the lack of a control group, differences in training habits and diet among subjects taking and not taking anabolic steroids, and the different doses and treatment durations employed by users.

The mechanisms whereby anabolic steroids exert their toxic effects have not been completely clarified. Specific receptors for anabolic steroids have been identified in virtually all human tissues, including the heart and the arterial walls. The androgen receptors in mature men appear to be completely saturated. Thus, the interaction with other receptors such as those for progesterone, estrogens, and glucocorticoids would account for the toxic effects of anabolic steroids. Generally, the toxic effects of anabolic steroids are short lasting and reversible within a few weeks after the agents have been discontinued. However, it should be pointed out that some athletes take anabolic steroids persistently for long periods of time, and the toxic effects thus can be severe and not completely reversible. Moreover, many of the agents that are used are veterinary drugs or other unapproved derivatives for which no safety data are available. All untoward effects are more common in some groups of individuals such as women and adolescents and in subjects who use large doses for long periods of time.

In mature men, anabolic steroid administration is followed by an increase in the plasma level of the metabolites of testosterone estradiol, androstenedione, and dihydrotestosterone. Prolonged anabolic steroid administration causes a hypogonadotropic hypogonadal state characterized by a significant decrease in the LH and FSH plasma levels, sex hormone-binding globulin, and endogenous testosterone. Clinically, an increase in the size and secretion of sebaceous glands becomes apparent with the development of acne and alopecia. Hypotrophy of the testes and abnormalities of spermatogenesis usually occur, thus compromising fertility in the adult male. Prostate hypertrophy, gynecomastia, and enhanced libido and sexual function are other usual effects of anabolic steroid administration. These effects are reversible after the anabolic steroids have been discontinued, but suppression of spermatogenesis may persist for months after drug withdrawal. In the washout period, a pronounced decrease in libido is usually observed.

In adult females, anabolic steroid administration produces an increase in circulating testosterone and carries the risk of causing masculinization. Undesirable manifestations include hirsutism, acne, male-pattern baldness, hypertrophy of the clitoris, prominent musculature, aggressiveness and increased libido, menstrual irregularities, and coarsening of the voice. Although most of these manifestations are reversible, hypertrophy of the clitoris and deepening of the voice are irreversible if treatment is prolonged. During pregnancy, anabolic steroids can cross the placenta and have virilizing effects on a female fetus. In children and adolescents, anabolic steroids produce virilizing effects and serious disturbances of growth and bone development. In fact, anabolic steroids enhance epiphyseal closure, an effect that may persist for several months after drug discontinuation. Other hormonal effects of anabolic steroids include an increase in growth hormone and hypothyroidism with low levels of T3, T4, TSH, and thyroid-binding globulin. Finally, anabolic steroids can increase water and sodium chloride retention, leading to extracellular volume expansion and peripheral edema.

All androgens with 17-alkyl substitutions can cause cholestatic hepatitis, an effect that has not been observed with testosterone esters administered parenterally. Accumulation of bile in the biliary capillaries of the hepatic lobules causes jaundice and an increase in bilirubin, AST, ALT, and alkaline phosphatase in plasma. These abnormalities are usually reversible within a few months. In patients undergoing prolonged treatment with 17-substituted esters for hematologic disorders, peliosis hepatitis and hepatic carcinoma also have been described.

Changes in psychic and sexual behavior frequently occur after anabolic steroid administration. Elevation of mood, with increased initiative, self-confidence, and aggressiveness, a decreased sense of fatigue, and an increased libido have been described in subjects taking anabolic steroids. After drug withdrawal, the low level of endogenous testosterone does not allow the subjects to withstand intense physical performance, since muscle mass and strength decline rapidly, as do self-esteem, libido, and aggressiveness. Apathy, depression, and a renewed need to take steroids in an attempt to maintain high levels of athletic performance and to satisfy the desire to appear in perfect shape are readily transmitted.

Because of this vicious circle, some individuals eventually develop a dependence on the drugs, a condition frequently witnessed in athletes taking anabolic steroids. Recently, a physical dependence on anabolic steroids has been described, similar to that caused by alcohol or opioids. For this reason, several authors claim that anabolic steroid abuse should be treated as genuine drug addiction.

Personality changes ranging from increased irritability to violent and antisocial behavior and even to true psychiatric disorders have been reported. Behavioral abnormalities are usually reversible with drug discontinuation. Recent observations indicate that anabolic steroid use is often associated with abuse of other drugs such as cocaine, heroin, cannabinoids, and tobacco. Anabolic steroid use also has been associated with other abnormal behavioral and social patterns, such as having suicidal thoughts, engaging in unprotected sexual intercourse, driving after drinking alcohol, possessing firearms, etc. HIV infection caused by contaminated syringes has been reported in athletes using parenteral administration of anabolic steroids.

Studies on the negative cardiovascular effects of anabolic steroids are scanty and mostly confined to single case reports. About 30 serious cardiovascular events, chiefly of a thromboembolic nature, have been reported in subjects taking pharmacologic doses of anabolic steroids. Cerebral hemorrhage and thrombosis and transient ischemic attacks are the most serious cerebrovascular events described. In athletes, mostly in bodybuilders taking large doses of anabolic steroids for long periods of time, major cardiac events have been reported, such as myocardial infarction, heart failure, and arrhythmic sudden death. In the majority of these subjects, hypertrophic or dilated cardiomyopathies associated with myocardial fibrosis were found at the autopsy, with no evidence of lesions of the coronary arteries. However, the actual relationship between anabolic steroid administration and cardiac disease was difficult to establish in these isolated observations, and the doses of anabolic steroids were seldom reported owing to subjects' reluctance to admit anabolic steroid use.

The toxic effects of anabolic steroids on the heart can be due to a direct action on the myocardial fibers or to their effect on cardiovascular risk factors, the arterial wall, and coagulation. A contributing effect of intense physical training in determining the anabolic steroid-induced cardiac lesions cannot be excluded either. Animal studies have clearly demonstrated that prolonged anabolic steroid administration can cause hypertension and cardiac enlargement with decreased pump function.

Ultrastructural changes include damage to fibrils, mitochondria, and intercalated disks and an increase in the collagen-elastin ratio in arterial walls. Data obtained from animal studies may not be transferred directly to human beings, and an actual association between anabolic steroid intake and cardiac dysfunctions has never been proved in humans.

Many aspects of the cardiac effects of anabolic steroids have been clarified through echocardiography, although the results obtained by the various studies have not always been consistent. Some authors found increased heart size, left ventricular mass, and wall thickness in subjects taking anabolic steroids, whereas others observed little or no effect. Left ventricular systolic function was not found to be affected by anabolic steroid intake, whereas somewhat conflicting results were obtained on the effects on diastolic function. Isovolumetric relaxation time was found to be prolonged by anabolic steroids in some studies, but this finding was not confirmed by other reports. In conclusion, the main cardiac effects of anabolic steroid use associated with resistance training are an increase in the left ventricular wall thickness and a tendency toward impairment of diastolic function. These changes differ from those usually observed in the athlete's heart, which is characterized by an increase in left ventricular diameter and wall thickness accompanied by an improvement in diastolic function.

The detection of normal coronary arteries after myocardial infarction in athletes taking anabolic steroids raised the question of whether these drugs could cause arterial wall lesions capable of causing coronary vasospasm. In animals, increased peripheral resistance and arterial hyperreactivity to epinephrine were observed after anabolic steroid administration. An abnormal elastin-collagen ratio in the arterial wall and a reduced arterial vasodilatation also have been described. In humans, a decreased vasodilating response to nitric oxide has been reported. The anabolic steroid-induced alterations in plasma lipids and blood pressure could contribute to the abnormal reactivity of the arterial wall.

Interest in the possible thrombotic effects of anabolic steroids has been raised by the observation of thromboembolic events occurring in anabolic steroid users. Increased platelet aggregation and an alteration in the thromboxane-prostacyclin ratio were demonstrated in subjects taking anabolic steroids. As to the effect of anabolic steroids on the hemocoagulative system, conflicting results were obtained. In fact, increases in coagulation, C protein, S protein, and plasminogen are all effects described in subjects taking anabolic steroids. According to some authors, endothelial changes in the arterial wall leading to prothrombotic effects may occur with anabolic steroid use.

An increase in blood pressure often has been reported by athletes taking anabolic steroids. Clinical studies have demonstrated small increases in blood pressure after anabolic steroid administration, and in some studies, no changes were reported. A recent investigation performed with ambulatory monitoring showed no difference in average 24-hour blood pressure between a group of bodybuilders taking anabolic steroids and a group of control bodybuilders. However, an abnormal diurnal pattern was observed in the subjects self-administering anabolic steroids, characterized by a loss of the physiologic nocturnal fall in blood pressure. A similar flattening of the 24-hour curve was described in subjects with secondary forms of hypertension and was associated to a greater degree with cardiovascular complications in primary hypertension. It is likely that hypertension develops only in predisposed subjects. In the studies in which blood pressure increased after anabolic steroid use, it returned to pretreatment levels after drug withdrawal. An aldosterone-like mechanism has been advocated as a possible mediator of the blood pressure increase induced by the anabolic steroids, with water and sodium retention. Another possible mechanism is an increase in peripheral resistance mediated by the sympathetic nervous system. The pressure overload could contribute to the increase in left ventricular mass caused by anabolic steroids.

A body of evidence indicates that anabolic steroids cause important changes in plasma lipids with a decrease in the high-density lipoprotein (HDL)-cholesterol, particularly of the HDL_2 fraction, and an increase in the low-density lipoprotein (LDL)-cholesterol levels. The mechanism whereby anabolic steroids impair the lipid profile is likely to be the increased activity of the hepatic triglyceride lipase (HL, see Fig. 69.2), which promotes HDL degradation. Increased HL activity also could explain the increased production of LDL-cholesterol through an accelerated metabolism of very low density lipoproteins (VLDLs). The atherogenic action of anabolic steroids seems to be mediated also by profound changes in plasma apolipoproteins, such as an increase in apoB levels and a reduction in apoA-I and apoC-III. Lipoprotein changes seem to occur more frequently with oral compounds than with parenteral preparations and tend to disappear after a few weeks of washout. In agreement with previous observations in patients treated with pharmacologic doses of anabolic steroids, recent studies in bodybuilders have shown that these drugs reduce the lipoprotein (a) plasma level, which is independently associated with an increased coronary risk. This protective action could at least partially counterbalance the atherogenic effect of anabolic steroids on plasma lipids. In addition, elevated fasting insulin levels and an impaired glucose tolerance have been reported in athletes self-administering anabolic steroids. However, these changes also seem to be reversible.

Prevention

Although anabolic steroids have few clinical applications, improper use has had widespread repercussions worldwide. Studies on the toxic effects of anabolic steroids, especially as far as their long-term effects are concerned, are still incomplete. The available literature, however, clearly indicates that these drugs have detrimental effects on many organs. Even though no epidemiology of morbid events has been described among anabolic steroid users, it is not possible to exclude the possibility that major toxic effects can emerge in forthcoming years. The use of anabolic steroids therefore should be strongly discouraged for both ethical and health reasons. To prevent anabolic steroid abuse, which nowadays appears as one of the most important problems that plague the athletic community, three types of interventions should be adopted: (1) an increase in antidoping controls, which also should include amateur sporting events and training periods, (2) promotion of a campaign through the mass media especially addressed to youngsters on the harmful effects of anabolic steroid use, and (3) an increase in police controls of the anabolic steroid black market.

Suggested readings

ALEN M, RAHKILA P. Anabolic-androgenic steroids on endocrinology and lipid metabolism in athletes. Sports Med 1988; 6:327-32.

BALDO-ENZI G, GIADA F, ZULIANI G, et al. Lipid and apoprotein modifications in bodybuilders during and after self-administration of anabolic steroids. Metabolism 1990;2:2038.

ELASCHOFF JD, JACKNOW AD, SHAIN SG, BRAUNSTEIN GD. Effects of anabolic-androgenic steroids on muscular strength. Ann Intern Med 1991;115:387-93.

HAUPT HA, ROVERE GD. Anabolic steroids: a review of the literature. Am J Sports Med 1984;12:469-84.

KIBBLE WM, ROSS MB. Adverse effects of anabolic steroids in athletes. Clin Pharmacol Ther 1987;6:686-92.

KLEINER SM. Performance enhancing aids in sport: health consequences and nutritional alternatives. J Am Coll Nutr 1991; 10:163-76.

LABREE M. A review of anabolic steroids: uses and effects. J Sports Med Phys Fitness 1991;31:618-26.

MELCHERT RB, WELDER AA. Cardiovascular effects of androgenic-anabolic steroids. Med Sci Sports Exerc 1995;27:1252-62.

MIDDLEMAN AB, DURANT RH. Anabolic steroid use and associated health risk behaviors. Sports Med 1996;21:251-5.

NIEMINEN MS, RAMO MP, VIITASALO M, et al. Serious cardiovascular side effects of large doses of anabolic steroids in weight lifters. Eur Heart J 1996;17:1576-83.

PALATINI P, GIADA F, GARAVELLI G, et al. Cardiovascular effects of anabolic steroids in weight-trained subjects. J Clin Pharmacol 1996;36:1132-40.

ROCKHOLD RW. Cardiovascular toxicity of anabolic steroids. Annu Rev Pharmacol Toxicol 1993;33:497-520.

URHAUSEN A, HOLPES R, KINDERMANN W. One- and two-dimensional echocardiography in bodybuilders using anabolic steroids. Eur J Appl Physiol 1989;58:633-40.

WILSON JP, GRIFFIN JE. The use and misuse of androgens. Metabolism 1980;29:1278-95.

Emergencies

Emergencies

Wolfgang Voelckel, Gunnar Kroesen

Acute life-threatening disorders that require immediate intervention can be defined as medical emergencies. A wide variety of diseases, trauma, or poisonings may lead to respiratory and cardiocirculatory failure that endangers life or limb. Under these conditions, first-line therapy will be symptomatic and has to be focused on stabilizing vital functions. The term *basic life support* refers to maintaining an open airway and supporting breathing and circulation without the use of equipment other than a simple airway device or protective shield. *Advanced life support* is meant primarily for restoration or stabilization of adequate spontaneous circulation and respiration, which usually requires the establishment of access routes to vital organs, such as endotracheal intubation and intravenous cannulation, and administration of drugs and fluids.

Besides acute lifesaving interventions by basic and advanced life support, emergency medicine focuses on the reduction of pain and stress, as well as on the prevention of permanent disability. Therefore, rapid onset of emergency therapy is essential. A rescue chain from first aid through bystanders to basic and advanced life support provided by general practitioners or professional emergency medical service with adequate transport facilities up to emergency departments in hospitals characterizes the scope of emergency medicine today.

Prehospital emergency medicine

After World War II, physicians became aware of the necessity to provide advanced prehospital medical treatment in emergencies. From the experience of the wars in Korea and Vietnam, several concepts of prehospital rescue management were adapted for civilian emergency medicine. Early onset of therapy in the prehospital period is proven to be effective and lifesaving. Nowadays, rescue systems in industrialized countries are mainly staffed with paramedics, providing advanced life support according to standing orders, which may include some emergency drugs. In central Europe, emergency physicians are involved in prehospital emergency medical service; this philosophy of treatment includes more sophisticated therapies and therefore requires a wide range of drugs and materials (Tabs. 86.1 and 86.2).

Table 86.1 Emergency drugs: the very essentials

Oxygen
Crystalloid infusions
Epinephrine
Nitroglycerin
Morphine (or alternative, if possible, opioid analgesics)
Ketamine
Midazolam (or alternatively, diazepam)
Lidocaine
Furosemide
Glucose

Table 86.2 Possible choices of emergency drugs

Atropine
Activated charcoal
Adenosine
Chlorpheniramine
Dexamethasone
Diazepam
Epinephrine
Fenoterol spray
Furosemide
Colloidal infusion
Haloperidol
Ketamine
Lidocaine
Naloxone
Morphine
Nitroglycerin spray
Acetaminophen suppositories
Phenytoin
Terbutaline
Theophylline
Ringer's solution
Urapidil

Emergency departments

Administration of a specific and causal therapy requires an environment that allows advanced diagnostic procedures (laboratory tests, radiographs, etc.) and the possibility for therapeutic interventions such as surgery or further intensive care treatment. Emergency medical care in hospitals is organized either in specialized emergency departments or as a branch of a referral clinic.

Emergency physicians must be familiar with a wide variety of patients, from children to the elderly; a broad spectrum of emergency situations, trauma, poisonings, and internal or neurologic disorders requires different strategies of therapy. Safety and efficacy must be the criteria by which emergency drugs should be evaluated for use in the field or in the emergency department. A large number of drugs have been introduced to the practice of emergency medicine, sometimes without the benefit of a thoughtful, patient-centered approach. With the increasing attention paid to the economic aspects of medical care, reflection on some key questions may help to characterize the criteria for effective emergency drugs.

Main characteristics of emergency drugs

The "ideal" drug to be used in medical emergencies should come close to possessing the characteristics listed in Table 86.3. It is obvious that only a few drugs match this profile. Route of application will be mainly intravenous endobronchial or sublingual; since iv cannulation may not be established in an emergency situation, alternative routes of drug administration are listed in Table 86.4. As a general rule, drugs that can be given via a peripheral vein also can be given intraosseously, i.e, an access route suitable for all neonatal, pediatric, and even some adult patients.

Table 86.3 Pharmacokinetic, pharmacodynamic, and galenic criteria for a rational choice of emergency drugs

Rapid onset of action
Short half-life
Efficacy
Potency
Broad therapeutic index
Minimal side effects
Ready to use
Temperature stability
Cost effective

Table 86.4 Possible routes of drug administration in medical emergencies

Intravenous
Sublingual
Endobronchial
Intraosseous
Subcutaneous
Intramuscular
Enteral[1]

---

[1]Only under special conditions in conscious patients.

Some drugs are absorbed very rapidly across the bronchial tree and thus may take effect nearly as quickly when administered through an endotracheal tube as when administered iv. With special regard to emergency medicine, among these are naloxone, atropine, diazepam, epinephrine, and lidocaine. Again, the environment of the emergency situation may influence the choice of drugs and the route of application. For example, a trauma patient in a remote, arctic location needs oral replacement of fluids because an iv infusion may freeze instantly.

RESPIRATORY DISORDERS

Acute respiratory insufficiency is defined as any situation in which arterial PCO_2 rises above 50 mm Hg and/or arterial PO_2 falls below 60 mm Hg (see Chap.29). Since these laboratory values may be difficult to obtain in the prehospital setting, clinical observation and physical examination will be essential for the diagnosis of acute respiratory failure. Signs of respiratory distress are nasal flaring (i.e., wide-open nostrils during inhalation), tracheal tugging (i.e., upward movement of the cricoid and inward movement of the lower part of the neck during inspiration), retraction of the intercostal muscles, use of accessory muscles, and paradoxical respiratory movement. Altered mental states result from either hypoxemia or hypercarbia (e.g., drowsiness, unconsciousness). Pain, stress, and trauma may raise oxygen consumption above oxygen delivery and therefore may result in respiratory distress.

Chronic obstructive pulmonary disease (COPD) is a common respiratory disorder in the western world, with an increasing mortality in the last 15 years. Acute decompensation is characterized by marked respiratory distress with cyanosis, tachycardia or cardiac dysrhythmias, and mental alteration. Hypoxemia subsequently may lead to pulmonary hypertension, right-sided heart failure, myocardial infarction, seizures, and possibly death.

Bronchial asthma (see Chap. 28) is characterized by hyperreactive smooth muscles of the trachea, bronchi, and bronchioli. This condition is triggered either by an external allergen or without an objective stimulus, resulting in a reduction in airway diameter to a critical value. Additional swelling of the mucous membranes and plugging of bronchi by secretions lead to the typical pattern of respiratory distress with characteristic wheezing breath sounds.

The immediate relief of hypoxemia with 4 to 5 liters/min oxygen inhalation is essential. There is no rational reason to withhold oxygen because of fear that a possible "hypoxic drive" for breathing may be overruled by the inhalation of oxygen.

Pharmacotherapy focuses on relaxation of the smooth muscles as well as on reduction of swelling and inflammation of mucous membranes.

Fenoterol, a selective β-mimetic agonist at the smooth muscles of the respiratory system, is a possible choice among inhalative agents. Concentrated either in 0.1 or 0.2 mg per push, the aerosol reaches the bronchial mucosa in an amount of 25 to 70%. Within a couple of minutes, the effect of up to two pushes of 0.2 mg each reaches its maximum; a repetitive dose may be given after 5 min.

Cardiovascular side effects, mediated by $\beta1$-receptor activity, may lead to tachycardia and cardiac arrhythmias. Since a K^+ shift to the intracellular compartment is induced by β-mimetic agents, hypokalemia may reach critical values. Blood pressure may decrease, and very rarely, even pulmonary edema may occur or diabetic acidosis may be induced. Since respiratory distress is a life-threatening medical emergency, close clinical observation is essential.

Since an aerosol may not reach distal bronchi in severe airway obstruction, injection of terbutaline may be indicated. Terbutaline (1 mg/ml) can be given sc (0.01 mg/kg) or slowly via the intravenous route in a dosage of 0.25 mg. Owing to the same cardiovascular and metabolic side effects mentioned earlier, close observation of the patient is essential.

Reduction of swelling and inflammation of mucous membranes may be achieved by steroids, the second essential therapeutic choice in the treatment of acute airway obstruction in asthma and COPD. Since different types of steroids differ significantly in concentration and potency of action, the emergency physician should concentrate on one drug. A possible choice may be dexamethasone, with the strongest anti-inflammatory effect. Dexamethasone is approximately 30 times more potent than hydrocortisone (e.g., the equivalent anti-inflammatory dose of 1 mg dexamethasone is 30 mg hydrocortisone). When used for the treatment of acute respiratory disorders, dexamethasone may be administered parenterally or locally as an aerosol. Dosage will be 1 mg/kg of dexamethasone parenterally in severe asthma.

Abdominal discomfort is usually reported during injection. Since gluconeogenesis is induced by dexamethasone, hyperglycemia may occur. In emergency situations, even high doses can be given safely, because the risk of complications can be neglected.

Despite controversies, theophylline is still indicated in severe asthma. Some authors see no additional benefit when inhaled β_2-mimetic and parenteral steroids are available. Theophylline generally mixed with ethylenediamine (aminophylline), is a competitive antagonist at the adenosine receptor, and is a potent inhibitor of the enzyme phosphodiesterase. Intracellular accumulation of cyclic adenosine monophosphate (cAMP) leads to relaxation of smooth airway muscles.

Aminophylline may be given slowly iv at a dose of 240 to 480 mg over 20 min or 5 mg/kg, respectively.

Because of aminophylline's positive inotropic and chronotropic side effects, tachyarrhythmias may occur, and blood pressure may decrease as a result of a vasodilating effect. Central nervous system (CNS) stimulation may result in an altered mental state or even seizures. β-mimetic drugs may enhance the effects of aminophylline, as well as the diuretic effect of furosemide. In patients who are already being treated with aminophylline, the toxic threshold may be decreased, and aminophylline should be administered carefully.

CARDIOCIRCULATORY DISORDERS

The primary source of cardiocirculatory disorders is coronary artery disease, almost always of atherosclerotic origin. This may result into a decreased blood flow in relation to the metabolic demand of the myocardium caused by severe work or stress. Annually, approximately 2.0 to 2.5 million individuals in the United States suffer an acute myocardial infarction (AMI), and about 40% of these patients do not survive. Of those patients who arrive at the hospital alive, up to 25% die within the next 4 weeks as a result of reinfarction or from complications such as arrhythmias. More than 50% of the prehospital scene calls of emergency medical systems are directed to patients with AMI.

Angina pectoris represents a cardiocirculatory disorder due to an oxygen debt of the myocardium (see Chap. 25). Any new jaw or chest pain developing in an older patient, particularly after stress or effort of any type, should be considered to be due to angina or possible myocardial infarction until proven otherwise. In the worst case, ventricular fibrillation occurs, and cardiopulmonary resuscitation (CPR), including defibrillation, should be started immediately. Differential diagnosis of AMI may be performed by administering a vasodilating drug such as nitroglycerin. Coronary artery spasm will loosen in a short time after injection of a vasodilator.

On the other hand, any thromboembolic process occluding a coronary artery will not change. The diagnosis of an AMI is fairly secure if two of the following criteria are present: typical history of chest pain, typical electrocardiographic (ECG) changes, and typical changes of biochemical markers such as the MB fraction of creatine phosphokinase or troponin T.

Acute coronary insufficiency with or without AMI sometimes may cause an abrupt and alarming increase in blood pressure, with levels in the excess of 250/150 mm Hg. This hypertensive crisis is combined with anxiety, diaphoresis, tachycardia, extreme agitation, and confusion. The differential diagnosis has to consider several clinical entities that produce similar symptoms: acute anxiety, acute pericarditis, dissecting aortic aneurysm, pulmonary embolism, biliary colic, pneumothorax, perforated or penetrating peptic ulcer, necrotizing pancreatitis, constrictive pericarditis, and viral or myocardial cardiomyopathy.

General aspects of emergency treatment without drugs refer primarily to defibrillation, positioning of the patient, and oxygen supply. The only goal-directed measure to treat ventricular fibrillation is defibrillation of the heart with an appropriate defibrillator. Under these conditions, the patient lies in a prone position on a stiff, flat surface. If the first cycle of defibrillation is not successful, the patient must be supported by chest compressions and ventilation. Mechanical ventilation should be performed with oxygen (100% or as high as possible) as soon as possible.

Emergency drugs of first choice Epinephrine, a powerful α- and β-agonist, vasoconstricts the entire vasculature. When given during CPR, epinephrine shifts blood toward vital organs such as the heart and brain. This increases coronary perfusion pressure to a threshold that renders successful defibrillation more likely. Thus, epinephrine has to be administered throughout CPR by the emergency system at a dose of 1 mg in an adult every 3 minutes either iv or endobronchially (eb) through a suction catheter in the endotracheal tube. The eb medication should be 3 times the iv dose, i.e., 3 mg every 3 minutes diluted with saline. The single largest dose of epinephrine should not exceed 5 mg in an adult. In a dose of 0.1 mg per adult sc, epinephrine is appropriate to interrupt a status asthmaticus or to treat a severe anaphylactic reaction.

Atropine sulfate is the strongest parasympatholytic agent; in a dose of 0.02 mg/kg to a maximum of 1 mg per patient; it is recommended to treat extreme bradycardia (<40 beats/min), preferably in children. In adults, a dose up to 3 mg per patient is necessary to achieve a tachycardic effect when extreme vagotonia is suspected as a cause of bradycardia (<15 beats/min).

Lidocaine reduces the incidence of ventricular fibrillation when given prophylactically to patients with AMI, although no decrease in mortality is seen. No effective and safe antiarrhythmic drug has been identified that is capable of providing successful adjunctive therapy in ventricular fibrillation. In broad-complex tachycardia, lidocaine is recommended when a pulse can be felt, systolic blood pressure is greater than 90 mm Hg, chest pain and heart failure are absent, and the pulse rate exceeds 150 beats per minute. The recommended dose begins with 50 mg intravenously within 2 minutes and is continued every 5 minutes up to a total of 200 mg.

The administration of an alkalizing agent preferably should be based on the knowledge of both arterial and mixed central venous blood gas analyses. At present, sodium bicarbonate remains the recommended agent for the correction of acidosis. Dosages should be no greater than 50 mmol (50 ml of an 8.4% solution) in the first instance. There is no definite evidence for a specific level of acidosis that requires correction, but as a guide, this may be indicated at an arterial pH less than 7.1, bearing in mind that simultaneous central venous pH is usually 0.1 to 0.3 units lower.

Emergency drugs of second choice The use of orciprenaline is an alternative strategy for transvenous pacing in patients with bradycardia and a history of asystole, a type II atrioventricular (AV) block, any pause greater than 3 seconds, and complete heart block with a wide QRS complex. Administration is performed using an infusion pump starting with a dose of 0.2 ml per minute of a solution with 2.5 mg in 500 ml of saline.

Amiodarone (see Chap. 24) has powerful antiarrhythmic effects in patients with both supraventricular and ventricular arrhythmias. However, its unusual pharmacokinetic profile and its potential for producing toxicity in many organ systems have limited its usefulness. Emergency indication arises when lidocaine does not lead to the required success of a normal sinus rhythm after ventricular tachycardia. The recommended dose is 300 mg over 5 to 15 minutes, preferentially via a central venous line, and then 600 mg over 1 hour.

The pharmacologic treatment of choice for regular supraventricular tachycardias is adenosine; therapy should start with a small dose of 6 mg. Repetition can be given every 1 to 2 minutes, with at least two injections of 12 mg, if necessary.

Dopamine is a sympathomimetic amine and a biologic precursor of norepinephrine and epinephrine. Its main use is to support coronary perfusion pressure and cardiac output in cardiogenic or septic shock, using infusion rates of 2 to 20 micrograms per minute. The infusion rate is increased until arterial pressure and urine flow respond. In CPR, dopamine is useful for supporting arterial blood pressure after restoration of spontaneous circulation. Side effects include tachycardia, tachydysrhythmias, and increased myocardial oxygen demand. Therefore, a combination of dopamine with metoprolol is recommended. Metoprolol is a β_1-receptor blocker without sympathomimetic activity and membrane stabilizing effect (see Chap. 22). It obviously has side effects such as decreases in blood pressure and stroke volume, which must be avoided.

Urapidil favorably inhibits peripheral and postsynaptic α_2- and α_1-adrenergic receptors and decreases central sympathetic activity. It is appropriate for lowering blood pressure under emergency conditions of a hypertensive crisis. It allows careful titration until the desired effect on blood pressure has been reached (see also Chap. 23). The iv injection usually starts with 1 ml (i.e., 5 mg) and is continued every 2 to 4 minutes with 1 ml to a total amount of 5 ml (25 mg) when required. The antidote to cope with an overdose is epinephrine diluted to 100 to 250 micrograms administered as required.

Nitroglycerin is a classic direct vasodilator, used primarily for the relief of angina pain. It also reduces cardiac preload and afterload by peripheral venous and arterial dilatation. Nitroglycerin also dilates coronary vessels and is therefore beneficial in heart failure that is due to myocardial infarction. For acute relief of angina pain, one nitroglycerin tablet or spray push of 0.3 to 0.4 mg administered sublingually, repeated up to three times at 5-minute intervals, has been recommended. This drug also can be administered in the treatment of acute pulmonary edema in an emergency prehospital situation.

TRAUMA, BURNS, AND SHOCK

In industrialized countries, accidents are the leading cause of death for people between 1 and 37 years of age and the fourth leading cause of death overall. Most of the fatalities occur in motor vehicle accidents, but gunshot wounds became the number two killer in the United States. Accidents at home and during work and leisure time also account for a great deal of blunt or penetrating trauma. Closely linked to multiple injuries is the pattern of traumatic, hypovolemic shock. Besides severe brain injury and acute respiratory failure, shock is the main reason for disability and death from trauma. Immediate onset of therapy, including volume replacement, pain therapy, respiratory support, and surgical intervention at the earliest point in time, has been proven to be effective in reducing mortality after trauma.

Shock Shock can be defined as a state of inadequate tissue oxygenation. Focusing on hypovolemic shock, hypotension and tachycardia, as well as signs of a sympathetic reaction, such as vasoconstriction, mental alteration, and sweating, may be the leading symptoms. Clinical signs of hypovolemia may become obvious after a loss of 6 to 8% of intravascular volume. Unfortunately, hypovolemia is frequently underestimated, paticularly in children, because of their ability to maintain normal blood pressure over a long time.

Hypovolemia in burn injury occurs because of fluid loss across the damaged skin and volume shift due to capillary leakage. Blood loss after blunt or penetrating trauma will result in critically low concentrations of hemoglobin. Patients suffering from additional respiratory or cardiocirculatory disorders are endangered from tissue hypoxemia even in an early state of shock. Restoration of tissue oxygenation is the major aim of emergency therapy in shock. Therefore, as first-line therapy, oxygen should be applied to all patients suffering from trauma. In severe shock, patients may require advanced ventilatory support, including intubation and controlled ventilation. For further pharmacotherapy, especially for fluid replacement, two or more intravenous lines must be established. Reduction of pain and stress reduces oxygen demand and therefore may be helpful to prevent tissue hypoxemia.

Emergency fluid management in trauma must be linked closely to the differentiation between uncontrolled and controlled hemorrhagic shock. In uncontrolled hemorrhagic shock, bleeding cannot be controlled without surgical intervention. Aggressive iv fluid therapy is therefore likely to increase bleeding, but sufficient fluid resuscitation is needed to ensure viable survival until hemorrhage is controlled. Thus, a minimal systolic blood pressure of 50 to 70 mm Hg may be tolerated during transport time prior to surgery. In blunt trauma or under the conditions of controlled bleeding, the goals of fluid resuscitation are to optimize intravasal volume and oxygen delivery. In patients with head trauma and prolonged prehospital times, maximal cardiocirculatory stabilization is essential.

Since anemia is tolerated better than hypovolemia, restoration of intravascular volume should be rapid and efficient. There is an ongoing discussion about whether initial fluid resuscitation should include the use of crystalloid or colloid fluids. Outcome after trauma may be influenced more by variables such as age, injury severity, and past medical history than by the choice of resuscitation fluid. Nevertheless, crystalloids and colloids must be considered as essential emergency drugs.

The Advanced Trauma Life Support Recommendations of the American College of Surgeons include the use of

Ringer's solution for the initial resuscitation phase. Since the use of normal saline may cause hyperchloremic acidosis, Ringer's solution can be considered free of adverse side effects. Because of its isooncotic properties, it also serves as an indifferent carrier for further drugs to be administered. To restore normovolemia, the estimated blood loss needs to be replaced with a 3-fold amount of Ringer's solution. In the treatment of burn injury, lactated Ringer's solution is the essential fluid therapy, since capillary leakage may cause severe volume shifting within the first hours after trauma. Therefore, colloid infusion may not be easily reabsorbed from interstitial compartments after restoration of capillary membranes. The amount of fluids that a burned patient will need during the first hours can be calculated using the Parkland formula: 4 ml × body weight (in kilograms) × % of burned body surface area. For example, in a 70-kg patient with 50% body surface burned, 4 ml × 70 kg × 50% = 14,000 ml of fluids would be needed; half this amount needs to be given during the first 8 hours.

Since plasma oncotic pressure is better maintained with colloids, they are more efficient in equivalent intravascular volume expansion than crystalloids. To maintain the same hemodynamic state in critically ill patients, it takes 2 to 6 times less volume of colloids compared with crystalloids. Colloids are characterized by their molecular structure, molecular weight, weight distribution, and concentration in normal saline. Colloids with a molecular weight of less than 50 kDa can be eliminated by renal filtration. Gelatines and hydroxyethyl starch (HES) solutions are the most common colloids. Gelatines are the most inexpensive colloid infusions available and can be infused in unlimited volumes. With a volume effect of 1:1, infusion dosage will closely follow fluid loss. Plasma half-life of gelatines is 2 to 3 hours; elimination is mainly renal. Severe allergic or anaphylactic reactions are possible with gelatine infusions. Gelatines act as osmotic diuretics. In severe renal failure, therefore, gelatines are contraindicated.

Dosage of HES solution should not exceed 20 ml/kg because of the risk of inducing coagulopathy via an effect on factor VIII and von Willebrand factor.

Pharmacokinetic and pharmacodynamic characteristics are closely linked to the average molecular weight and molecular substitution rate of hydroxyethyl groups for glucose. Therefore, the half-life may vary from 6 hours (HES 200/0.5) to more than 24 hours with prolonged hemodilution (HES 450/0.7). All types of HES solutions may cause anaphylactic shock. Interference with blood coagulation limits the maximum volume that may be infused to 20 to 30 ml/kg.

Spinal injury Spinal trauma mainly affects patients from 15 to 35 years of age, often leading to permanent disability. Most cases are a result of car accidents, falls, or contact sports. In patients suffering from multiple trauma, spinal trauma occurs in about 10%. Therefore, any accident involving significant acceleration-deceleration or compression forces should suggest the possibility of spinal cord injury.

Clinical findings will be influenced by the degree and level of spinal trauma. Therefore, victims suffering from spinal cord injury may present almost normal neurologic function together with a complete paralysis and respiratory arrest and cardiocirculatory instability. Hypotension with normal or slow pulse and warm skin is highly suggestive of neurogenic shock.

Further spinal cord damage must be prevented by adequate immobilization. Reduction of pain and stress and administration of oxygen should be part of emergency therapy in every patient suffering from trauma. In patients with acute spinal cord injury, treatment with methylprednisolone improves neurologic recovery. The most likely explanation of the positive effects is suppression of membrane breakdown by inhibiting lipid peroxidation and hydrolysis at the site of injury. Methylprednisolone should be given as a bolus of 30 mg/kg, followed by infusion of 5.4 mg/kg per hour for 23 hours. Medication must be started within 8 hours of trauma.

Due to induction of gluconeogenesis by glucocorticoids, hyperglycemia may occur. Further possible complications may be neglected during this short-term therapy.

PAIN

One of the primary responsibilities of an emergency physician is to relieve the pain and suffering of patients. Frequently, it is very difficult to adequately manage and treat this rather intangible psychophysiologic phenomenon. The *pain threshold* is the degree of pain at which the patient first perceives a painful stimulus that is fairly constant. Understanding the variety and complex aspects of pain and suffering is integral to adequate treatment of the patient.

The sensation of pain in general is classified into sharp, well-localized pain that is conducted along A-delta nerve fibers and dull, diffuse pain that is conducted along C nerve fibers. The first type is associated with bone fractures; with chest pain from MI, aortic aneurysm, or pulmonary embolus; and with any of the other consequences of acute trauma or severe disease. The second type accompanies chronic pain such as from arthritis, lumbalgia, and other chronic pain disorders.

Patients who are well informed as to the nature of their injury or disease are able to cope with their painful experience better than those who are not informed well (see Chap. 9). Some additional practices include immobilization of the painful organ system or extremity. Abdominal pain may be reduced by a supine position with flexed lower extremities in the knees. The traumatized extremities and the vertebral spine may be best immobilized on a vacuum mattress. Patients with rib fractures usually experience good pain reduction by sitting in a chair.

Emergency drugs of first choice Morphine sulfate and the opioids achieve their analgesic effect by stimulating opioid receptors in the midbrain and medulla, resulting in an alteration of the patient's perception of pain. Narcotic analgesics are indicated for acute pain, for moderate to severe pain, and for pain associated with terminal disease. Negative side effects are apathy, dysphoria, decreased level of consciousness, nausea and vomiting, respiratory depression, orthostatic hypotension, and biliary spasm. Morphine generally is used in a dose of 10 mg in an adult patient; piritramide will be used in a dose of 15 mg in an adult patient; and fentanyl for pain relief will be used in a dose of 0.1 to 0.2 mg in an adult patient. The total dosage should be adapted by titration of the drug.

Ketamine has a wide range of action either for analgesia (0.5 mg/kg for adult patients) or for anesthesia. Its large margin of safety is important in the emergency field. The im injection of 5 to 8 mg/kg. produces a complete anesthesia in children. Adults are treated with 1 to 2 mg/kg iv for the induction of anesthesia or for short surgical procedures. Hypersalivation and pseudopsychotic side effects are addressed by combining ketamine with atropine and diazepam (0.5 mg/10 mg). A special indication for the use of ketamine is present in patients with extended burns.

Emergency drugs of second choice Aspirin is the prototype of the nonsteroidal anti-inflammatory drugs (NSAIDs) for mild to moderate pain (see Chap. 9). Under emergency conditions (e.g., treatment of an AMI), inhibition of platelet aggregation is of foremost importance; 300 to 500 mg in an adult patient for acute therapy is the common range.

None of the other NSAIDs is really more effective as an analgesic than aspirin. If a patient cannot tolerate the side effects of aspirin, it is possible that one of the other NSAIDs will be a suitable substitute. Acetaminophen (paracetamol), not an NSAID, is a potential alternative owing to its central mode of action.

Hyoscine-*N*-butylbromide is a visceral ganglionic blocker with antimuscarinic activity. Dosage is 20 to 40 mg in an adult patient with acute colic. Atropine is a possible alternative.

Narcotics are necessary for extreme pain relief, e.g., traumatic amputation, severe multiple trauma, status epilepticus, and difficult airway management. The most commonly used emergency narcotic is ketamine (see above).

Thiopental is a barbiturate with a short half-life. Handling of this substance is somewhat complicated because the dry substance has to be dissolved in a solvent. Otherwise, its broad therapeutic dose range is very comfortable, and side effects are rare. In general, a dose of 4 to 6 mg/kg in adult patients is efficacious.

Propofol is a nonbarbituric narcotic. It is not water soluble, but dissolved in oil in a water emulsion, is milky dusty, and contains 10 mg in 1 ml. In general, it has the same properties as thiopental, but it must not be dissolved before use. The single dose required for the induction of anesthesia is 2.5 mg/kg in adults. Bolus doses for maintenance of anesthesia are recommended. Blood pressure monitoring is necessary because a depression of hemodynamic variables may occur.

Etomidate is a carboxylic imidazol derivate; 1 ml contains 2 mg of substance, dissolved in propylene glycol. Under emergency conditions, etomidate does not affect circulatory function, as shown by stable heart rate and blood pressure. The single dose generally used for induction of anesthesia is 0.15 to 0.3 mg/kg in adults. Surgical use is not possible because etomidate has no analgesic activity.

ALLERGY AND ANAPHYLACTIC REACTIONS

In allergy, the immune system is hypersensitive to several substances. Contact with an allergen results in an abnormal immune reaction, triggering mast cell degranulation, and release of mast cell mediators such as histamine, slow-reacting substance, and serotonin. Effects on skin, blood vessels, heart, and lung may lead to clinical symptoms, at times severe. An anaphylactic reaction, the most extreme form, affects the entire body. About 2000 Americans die each year from anaphylactic shock.

Signs and symptoms of anaphylaxis vary in target organs. Skin symptoms include flushing due to peripheral vasodilatation, swelling, edema, urticaria, and pruritus; patients also may suffer from bronchoconstriction-mediated dyspnea. Anaphylactic shock is caused by peripheral vasodilatation, capillary leakage, decreased myocardial contractility, and tachycardia. Gastrointestinal symptoms may include cramps, diarrhea, nausea, and vomiting. Stress and inadequate cerebral perfusion may result in headache, dizziness, and confusion.

Anaphylactic shock is an acute, life-threatening situation that requires immediate treatment. Airway management includes administration of oxygen, topical application of epinephrine by a metered-dose inhaler, and possibly endotracheal intubation. Since severe intravascular hypovolemia is caused by vasodilatation and capillary leakage, at least one large-bore iv line must be established.

The drug of choice in the management of an anaphylactic reaction is epinephrine. Because of epinephrine's -adrenergic properties, vasoconstriction elevates blood pressure and coronary blood flow. Bronchospasm as well as myocardial contractility is improved by its α-adrenergic effects.

In severe anaphylactic shock, epinephrine 1:10000 may be given slowly iv while monitoring vital signs. Dosage will be 5 to 10 ml (0.1 ml/kg) 1:10000 epinephrine or 0.01 mg/kg. If an intravenous line cannot be established, epinephrine can be given endobronchially in the same concentration. In mild reactions, 4 to 10 sprays of epinephrine (14 mg/40 pushes) may be given by metered-dose inhaler, or 0.3 to 0.5 ml of 1:1000 aqueous epinephrine can be administered subcutaneously. Since epinephrine is a potent sympathomimetic drug, hypertensive crises and myocardial infarction may be the major risks of this therapy.

Specific antihistamines, acting as antagonists at the H_1 and H_2 receptors, are only useful in the treatment of urticaria and the prevention of glottic edema. Chlorpheniramine may be a possible choice for this purpose (see Chap. 77). Hydrocortisone hemisuccinate also may be of value in mild allergic reactions, although due to a response delay of 1 to 3 hours, it cannot be considered as first-line drug.

NEUROLOGIC DISORDERS

Disturbances of behavior, altered mental state, unconsciousness or coma, and seizures are emergency conditions that may require immediate life support and diagnosis. It is essential to exclude extracerebral sources, such as cardiocirculatory failure, hypoxemia or hypercarbia, endocrinologic disorders, and intoxications, before starting a CNS-orientated therapy. Specific neurologic disorders may include status epilepticus, ischemic or hemorrhagic stroke, and violent psychiatric outbursts with disturbed behavior.

Status epilepticus Status epilepticus is defined as more than 30 minutes of continuous seizures or two or more seizures without a period of consciousness in between (see Chap. 10). Aspiration, prolonged hypoxemia, brain damage, fractures, and cardiac muscle necrosis may be life-threatening.

Treatment is aimed at maintaining a free airway and preventing the patient from injuring himself/herself during the clonic phase. Administration of oxygen in high concentrations or assisted ventilation with a bag-valve mask helps to ensure ventilation, and intravenous cannulation allows drug administration. In status epilepticus, treatment has the objective of stopping the seizure. Possible underlying causes such as hypoglycemia or thiamine deficiency must be ruled out first. In emergency treatment, diazepam is the drug of first choice to stop the seizure.

In adult patients, 5 to 10 mg diazepam can be given iv. If a seizure cannot be controlled, an additional dose may be administered after 5 to 10 minutes. Respiratory insufficiency and hypotension may be possible side effects.

If a seizure persists, phenytoin is the drug of second choice in the treatment of status epilepticus. Phenytoin can be given as a slow intravenous infusion or injection of 15 to 20 mg/kg, but the total dosage should not exceed 50 mg per minute; cardiocirculatory monitoring is essential.

Allergic reactions, cardiac arrhythmias, and hypotension are possible side effects of phenytoin when used as an emergency drug. All other adverse effects of phenytoin are related to a long-term use. Every persisting status epilepticus that cannot be handled with the two abovementioned anticonvulsants should be stopped by induction of general anesthesia.

Cerebrovascular emergencies Ischemic and hemorrhagic strokes kill more than 150 000 people annually in the United States and disable approximately 300 000 to 450 000 patients. Stroke is characterized by a neurologic deficit that lasts more than 24 hours. Leading symptoms are weakness, speech disorders, confusion, coma, and specific neurologic deficits. Although blood pressure may reach high values, the use of antihypertensive drugs should be restricted.

Emergency therapy is oriented to the symptoms and consists of ensuring the free airway and additional oxygen administration. In absence of heart failure, diastolic blood pressure should not be lowered below 120 mm Hg. Among drugs of choice, the α_1-adrenergic antagonist urapidil may reduce peripheral vascular resistance and, as a central serotonin antagonist, lead to sympathetic counter-regulation.

An initial iv bolus dose of urapidil should be 0.2 to 1.0 mg/kg. Since antihypertensive therapy should be titrated very carefully, injection must be slow, and the blood pressure must be monitored. Time to onset is about 5 minutes, and plasma half-life is about 35 minutes. Hypotension, tachycardia, and arrhythmias may result from relative overdose. Headache and restlessness are side effects not related to dosage.

Metoprolol and esmolol are β_1-receptor blockers (see Chap. 22) that also may be used to manage hypertension in cerebrovascular emergencies. Both will not cause cerebral vasodilatation or lead to a further rise in intracerebral pressure.

Emergency situations due to disturbed behavior Behavioral disturbance may result in suicide or violence against the environment, family members, or strangers; under these circumstances, emergency physicians may be confronted with these patients. Reasons for erratic behavior may be situational, organic, or psychiatric. As a general rule, care should be taken with psychotic patients who are hearing voices that command them to hurt themselves or others.

Appropriate assessment of the disturbed patient is an important part of treatment. While maintaining a safe distance, the physician may calm the patient down using a verbal approach. If verbal efforts fail, additional pharmacotherapy employing tranquilizers or antipsychotic drugs may be indicated.

Haloperidol (see Chap. 14), a butyrophenone, is a potent, effective, and long-acting drug for the treatment of various psychoses and behavioral disorders; it also has antiemetic properties. When used to treat psychotic symptoms, the dosage is 0.1 to 0.2 mg/kg iv; a maximum dose of 1 mg/kg may be administered.

Extrapyramidal signs such as dystonias and an oculogyric crisis are relatively common. Hypotension with tachycardia, due to α-receptor blockade, is infrequent. Induction of parkinsonian symptoms or a malignant neuroleptic syndrome is a rare side effect.

PEDIATRIC EMERGENCIES

In the industrialized world, about 5% of emergencies occur in pediatric patients, i.e., patients younger than 16 years of age. Trauma and neurologic and internal disorders may account for about 30% each, with respect to the geographic emergency medical service situation. Children are not simply miniature adults; they are anatomically and physiologically different (see Chap. 87). Nearly all pediatric drug dosages are based on the child's weight. Therefore, the preparation of a weight chart in the forefield may help to titrate emergency drugs under the special stress situation of a pediatric emergency. An aid to estimating the weight of a child up to 9 years of age is the following formula: Weight (kg) = [age (in years) × 2] + 9. Emergency drugs in children may be given rectally, by nebulizers, or intraosseously. A strict protocol for the treatment of special emergency situations and a checklist for drug dosage are essential guidelines for the emergency physician. Only a few special drugs are essential for these special patients.

Neurologic disorders in children Seizures in children can vary widely in clinical presentation and underlying causes. About half of all epileptic seizures are due to fever and infection; they are classified as occasional seizures and may be self-limiting within a few minutes. A prolonged seizure or multiple seizures without a lucid interval between them represent a very serious medical emergency and have to be stopped.

The immediate protection of the child from trauma, rapid airway assessing the presence of hypoxemia, applying oxygen, and ruling out hypoglycemia are the most important steps in emergency treatment. Since iv cannulation may not be established in this situation, rectal application of drugs must be considered.

Diazepam is the drug of first choice. As with all benzodiazepines, diazepam enhances GABA-ergic inhibition at the GABA-receptor complex. If an iv line can be established, diazepam should be titrated at a dose of 0.3 mg/kg, up to a maximum dose of 10 mg, by slow infusion until the seizures are controlled. As an alternative, diazepam may be given rectally; by this route of administration, the dosage must be slightly higher (up to 0.5 mg/kg). For application, a no. 10 French pediatric suction catheter can be used. A suppository containing 5 or 10 mg diazepam is also available; the dosage for suppositories is 5 mg for children less than 3 years of age or 15 kg and 10 mg for older children, respectively.

Because diazepam can produce marked respiratory depression, irrespective of the route by which it is given, special attention must be paid to respiratory function and airway. The physician must be prepared to assist ventilation and even to intubate endotracheally and provide respiratory support if necessary.

Under the special condition of a fever-associated seizure, the additional application of an antipyretic such as acetaminophen may be helpful. Acetaminophen has analgesic and antipyretic effects similar to aspirin but with a different mechanism (see Chap.9).

With an average dose of 10 to 20 mg/kg, the route of

application in children is rectal. Because of acetaminophen's hepatotoxic potential, dosages above 50 mg/kg (up to 200 mg/kg per day) should be avoided.

Allergic or anaphylactic reactions are rare; overdosage produces delayed, subacute liver damage. In the United Kingdom, acetaminophen is responsible for approximately 15% of all patients admitted to emergency departments with drug overdoses. Immediate treatment is essential and includes the application of *N*-acetylcysteine with an initial dosage of 150 mg/kg intravenously.

Airway and respiratory emergencies in children Severe respiratory distress, as manifested by tachypnea (respiratory rate as high as 60 to 80 breaths/min), nasal flaring, use of accessory muscles of respiration, and intercostal retractions, are the leading symptoms of a variety of respiratory emergencies in children. The differential diagnosis includes foreign body obstruction of the airway, acute asthmatic attacks or status asthmaticus, bronchiolitis, croup syndrome, and epiglottitis.

The first step in managing upper airway obstruction in the child is to determine the cause rapidly. All treatment regimens are based on the following principles: improvement of oxygenation, initially by administration of oxygen by mask; reduction of fear and stress; followed by specific treatment of the underlying cause. Acute epiglottitis is a life-threatening bacterial infection of the epiglottis that may lead to complete airway obstruction. Therefore, in the case of severe hypoxemia and unconsciousness, bag-valve ventilation with 100% oxygen may be necessary.

Swelling of the mucosa, inflammatory edema, hypersecretion of mucus, and constriction of the bronchi are the leading causes of respiratory distress in asthma, bronchiolitis, and croup syndrome. Pharmacotherapy is aimed at achieving brochodilatation either by bronchial relaxation of the smooth muscle or by reduction of mucosal swelling. Since establishing iv cannulation may be difficult, first-line therapy may well be aerosolized bronchodilators.

Epinephrine can be nebulized by the use of oxygen as the carrier gas into a special face mask. Therefore, this kind of first-line therapy has several advantages: provision of a high inspiratory oxygen concentration, minimally invasive route of application, and direct application at the site of action. Thus, 1 ml (1 mg) of epinephrine can be diluted to 5 ml with saline in the nebulizer. Inhalation should be accompanied by close observation of respiratory and cardiocirculatory function. Since epinephrine is a sympathomimetic amine, its physiologic response is mediated by both α and β receptors.

Since β_2 receptors contribute to the relaxation of the smooth muscles in the bronchial system, selective β_2-agonists have been developed for use in bronchial asthma, thus causing minor β_1-mimetic effects on the heart. Terbutaline, a specific β_2-agonist, can be administered either by a nebulizer or subcutaneously. Terbutaline (1 mg/ml) can be prepared for inhalation in a dose of 0.2 to 0.3 mg/kg in 3 ml of normal saline. In the case of severe asthma, terbutaline can be given subcutaneously in a dose of 0.01 mg/kg. If the patient fails to respond, status asthmaticus should be considered, and this condition may need aggressive therapy with other agents. Further drugs for the treatment of asthma in children will not differ from those for adults (see above).

Fluid management in children Fluid management in children may be difficult for several reasons. Normal vital parameters differ significantly between adults and children. Children may preserve normal cardiocirculatory function even under severe hypovolemia for a long time, but without fluid replacement, irreversible circulatory failure may occur without further warning signs. Because of their small blood volumes, children are in danger of excess transfusion. Normal steady-state requirements for fluids in children are 4 ml/kg per hour. In emergencies, infusion therapy may include crystalloid and colloid fluids; an access route may be either an intravenous line or an intraosseous needle.

Based on the estimated loss of blood volume, the infusion rate of Ringer's lactate should be 15 to 25 ml/kg per hour during the first hour of emergency treatment. If tachycardia persists, infusion of an additional 10 to 20 ml/kg over 5 minutes may be an option. Drug dosage guidelines for infants and children are given in Table 86.5.

POISONING

The incidence and presentation of patients with poisoning are closely linked to the structure of the population and the environment. In more than two-thirds of poisonings, children are endangered by preventable poisonings comprising household products and poisonous plants. Poisoning in adults, usually intentional, accounts for the majority of emergency medical interventions for poisoning. In urban areas, drug overdoses of all kinds are common. Finally, arthropod bites and stings as well as snake bites may cause severe intoxication in the corresponding environments. Since the public is exposed to more than 350 000 different toxic substances, knowledge about poisoning cannot be comprehensive, and a diagnostic approach must include an extensive patient history and physical assessment. Emergency physicians should be familiar with the typical patterns of poisoning in their sphere of action.

Poisoning should be regarded as a possible diagnosis in every medical emergency, especially when assessing possible reasons for unconsciousness. The potential toxic interference with vital functions may result in a variety of clinical signs and symptoms. Common routes for poisoning are ingestion, inhalation, injection, and absorption across the skin.

Management of poisoning follows a five-step program: first, vital organ function must be ensured. Second, the patient must be prevented from further exposure to the poison or, if possible, detoxified. Third, specific antidotes should be administered. Fourth, probes of poison must be sampled for later identification. Fifth, if necessary, the patient should be transported to an emergency department or hospital for advanced treatment, especially for the management of shock, coma, seizures, and dysrhythmias.

After stabilization of vital organ function, pharmacotherapy is aimed at a further reduction in uptake of the poison and at overcoming the toxic effects by providing an antagonist or inactivator of the poison. The first-line drug for all cases of poisoning is oxygen, especially when administered after inhalation of toxic substances. Inhalation of carbon monoxide will cause severe hypoxia, whereas inhalation of chlorine gas will result in acute respiratory failure by irritating mucous membranes.

Gastric emptying and absorption of poison may further reduce uptake after ingestion of a poison. Therefore, if there are no contraindications (Tab. 86.6), induction of vomiting and oral administration of activated charcoal may be indicated if the patient is alert and has an intact gag reflex. In children, induction of vomiting with ipecac syrup may be indicated if treatment starts within 20 to 30 minutes of ingestion. Administration of 15 ml ipecac syrup orally stimulates the chemoreceptor trigger zone in the area postrema and thus the vomiting center. Again,

contraindications to gastric emptying must be considered. Activated charcoal also may be given orally; 20 to 50 g or at least 5 tablespoonfuls can be mixed into a glass of water, providing an approximately 10% solution.

Narcotic overdose of drug addicts has become a common medical emergency in industrialized countries. These narcotic drugs are mainly heroin, morphine, hydromorphone, methadone, codeine, and oxycodone. Overdose may result in respiratory depression, which rapidly may result in apnea; therefore, immediate airway management and ventilatory support are crucial. Since respiratory depression is mediated via the μ_1- and μ_2-opioid receptors in the limbic system, naloxone, an opioid antagonist without intrinsic properties, should be titrated slowly intravenously in a dose of from 0.1 to 1.2 mg. If the naloxone dosage is too high, an immediate onset of action may result in a sudden withdrawal syndrome. An additional dose of 0.2 mg im should be given to ensure a prolonged effect of naloxone and to avoid recurrent coma, since the half-life of the opioid can be longer than the half-life of naloxone (usually 1-4 hours).

Organophosphates are widely used in insecticides and chemical weapons. Organophosphates inactivate acetylcholine, the chemical messenger between synapses of the autonomic nervous system. Therefore, acetylcholine cannot be inactivated and accumulates at the synapses.

Table 86.5 Drug dosage guidelines for emergency treatment of infants and children

Drug	Dosage	Route	Administration and comments
Activated charcoal	< 12 years: 15-30 gm > 12 years: 1 g/kg	po	Mixed with water

Aminophylline	Loading dose: 6 mg/kg
	    if none previously
		iv	Diluted in 30 ml iv fluid and
			    infused over 30 min

Atropine sulfate
  For cardiac arrest
  For organophosphate
    poisoning
	
	0.02 mg/kg/dose
	0.05 mg/kg/dose
		
		iv
		iv
			
			May be given endobronchially
			Half the dosage may be given im

33% dextrose	0.5 g/kg	iv	Infuse slowly through a good, free-flowing iv line
Diazepam	0.3 mg/kg 0.5 mg/kg	iv Rectal	Hypotension and apnea Via catheter or suppository

Epinephrine
  For severe anaphylaxis
  For cardiac arrest
  For severe asthma
	
	1:10,000, 0.1 ml/kg
	1:10,000, 0.1 ml/kg
	1 mg in 5 ml NaCl
		
		iv
		iv
		Inhaler
			
			May be given endobronchially
			Diluted for use in nebulizer

Acetaminophen	10-20 mg/kg	Rectal	
Ringer's solution	15-25 ml/kg/h	iv	Consider push of 10-20 ml/kg over 5 min
Syrup of ipecac	6-9 months: 5 ml 9-12 months: 10 ml 1-12 years: 15 ml >12 years: 30 ml	po po po po	Follow dose with 5 ml/kg water Consider contraindications
Terbutaline	0.01 mg/kg	sc	Given when an asthmatic is not moving enough air to inhale

Table 86.6 Contraindications for Induction of vomiting

Altered mental state, drowsiness, or unconsciousness
Seizures within the last few minutes
Pregnancy
Suspected myocardial infarction
Poisoning with corrosives, hydrocarbons, iodides,
 strychnine

Most common early symptoms of organophosphate poisoning are headache, weakness, paralysis, and hypotension (nicotinic effects). Vomiting, diarrhea, and abdominal cramps will be accompanied by bradycardia and profuse sweating (muscarinic effects). Besides extensive salivation, miosis is the leading clinical sign; seizures and coma with respiratory paralysis may be acute and life-threatening. Since organophosphates may be inhaled, ingested, or absorbed via the skin, decontamination of the patient is essential and should be performed under adequate self-protection. After immediate stabilization of ventilation and circulation, the use of specific antidotes is essential. Atropine can antagonize parasympathetic overstimulation. In addition, anticonvulsant drugs may be necessary.

Atropine in a dose of 2 to 4 mg iv should be given as soon as possible. This dose should be repeated every 5 to 10 minutes until signs of parasympatholytic effects, such as increased pulse rate or dilated pupils, become apparent.

Although the effectiveness of oxime therapy in organophosphate poisoning is still a matter of debate, obidoxime seems most promising. For reactivation of the enzyme cholinesterase, obidoxime can be administered im or iv. Dosage is 600 mg iv, by autoinjector if available, or 250 mg intravenously, followed by an iv infusion of 0.25 to 1 g per 24 hours. Pralidoxime (2-PAH), another oxime, may be an alternative.

DIABETIC EMERGENCIES

In every unconscious patient, hypoglycemia must be ruled out. Patients suffering from diabetes mellitus may present as medical emergencies when their blood sugar level becomes too high (lack of insulin or hypoglycemic agents) or too low (lack of glucose or overdosage of insulin). Hypoglycemia may result in severe coma and brain damage and therefore requires immediate therapy. On the other hand, hyperglycemia and diabetic ketoacidosis develop more slowly and may not endanger life immediately. Accompanied by vomiting, dehydration, and even shock, fluid replacement is the first emergency therapy in this situation.

Hypoglycemia develops rapidly, within a couple of minutes. The signs of cerebral dysfunction due to glucose deficiency are weakness, confusion, ataxic gait, seizures, and coma. An endogenous attempt to fight hypoglycemia is the activation of the sympathetic nervous system, resulting in tachycardia, tremor, dilated pupils, and cold, clammy skin.

In every unconscious patient, a blood sugar test should be performed. If this test cannot be obtained, the patient should be assumed to be hypoglycemic, and glucose should be administered, unless a stroke is suspected.

If the patient is still alert and able to swallow, sugar may be given orally (e.g., a candy bar or sugar water). In unconscious patients, an infusion of glucose 20% or 33% should be given iv. Since higher concentrations of glucose may result in tissue damage or inflammation of peripheral veins, administration should be strictly intravenous in a large vein via a wide intravenous line. Between 50 and 100 ml of glucose 33% should be administered over at least 3 minutes. In the case of hypoglycemic coma, the patient will awake rapidly.

EMERGENCY DRUGS OF THE FUTURE

Some very promising experimental findings in resuscitation research have demonstrated the beneficial effect of vasopressin as an alternative vasopressor in CPR. Furthermore, in patients suffering from severe sepsis, decreased plasma levels of endogenous vasopressin may result in vasoplegia, which may be overcome by vasopressin infusion. In both medical emergencies, the V_1 receptor–mediated increase in vascular tone after infusion of vasopressin results in higher coronary perfusion pressure and vital organ blood flow. In preclinical studies, comparison of vasopressin with epinephrine in CPR showed that vasopressin led to a more rapid recovery of spontaneous circulation.

The main purpose of the emergency medical service is to stabilize circulation, provide airway management, reduce pain or stress, and treat poisoning. Drugs used to treat life-threatening situations should be safe and efficient; other drugs should be evaluated in controlled trials before general use in emergency medical services can be recommended. An individual choice of drugs that addresses local incidence of typical emergency patients will further be influenced by personal experience and the attitude of the medical director of the emergency medical system. Figure 86.1 may help to develop an individual emergency drug list. With increasing attention being paid to the economic aspects of medical care, different generic drugs should be contrasted in terms of cost and duration of storage.

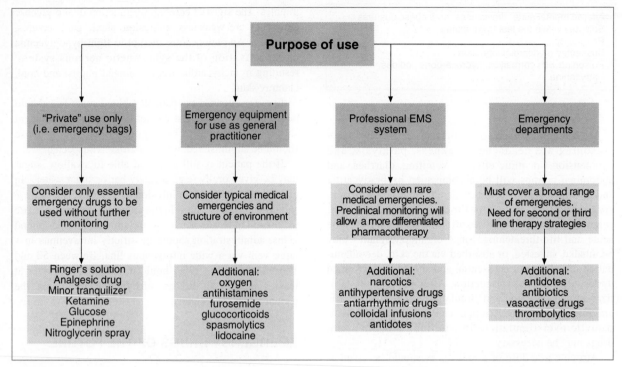

Figure 86.1 Criteria for the choice of emergency drugs.

Suggested readings

ADVANCED LIFE SUPPORT WORKING PARTY OF THE EUROPEAN RESUSCITATION COUNCIL. Guidelines for advanced life support. Resuscitation 1992;24:111-21.

CARDEN NI, STEINHAUS JE. Lidocaine resuscitation from ventricular fibrillation. Circ Res 1956;4:640-52.

CAROLINE NL. Emergency care in the streets. Boston: Little, Brown, 1995.

COMMITTEE ON EMERGENCY CARDIAC CARE, 1991-1994, AND SUBCOMMITTEE ON ADVANCED CARDIAC LIFE SUPPORT, 1991-1994. Textbook of advanced cardiac life support and emergency cardiovascular care programs. Chicago: American Heart Association, 1997.

GOLD HK, LEINBACH RC, SAUNDERS CA. Use of sublingual nitroglycerin in congestive failure following acute myocardial infarction. Circulation 1972;46:839-45.

GOLDBERG LI. Dopamine: Clinical use of an endogenous catecholamine. N Engl J Med 1974;291:707-10.

REICHEK N. Long-acting nitrates in the treatment of angina pectoris. JAMA 1976; 236:1399-402.

WOLFBERG D, VERDILE V, FLINN R. Incorporating drugs and devices into emergency medical service systems. Prehosp Disaster Med 1995;10:189-94.

Drugs and special population groups

Infancy

Ralph E. Kauffman

The definition of infancy in terms of chronologic age is necessarily arbitrary. Nonetheless, infancy is commonly considered to extend through the first 12 months of postnatal life. This is the most rapid period of growth, development, and differentiation of any time during the human life cycle. Weight typically doubles by 6 months of age and triples by the first birthday. Length increases by 50% during the first year. Body surface area doubles by 1 year of age. Surface area relative to body mass is approximately $2^1/_2$ times that of the adult. The respective proportions of body weight contributed by fat, protein, and water change significantly. Total body water decreases from 80% of weight at birth to 60% by 1 year, accompanied by a progressive decrease in extracellular water. The percentage of weight contributed by fat doubles by 5 months of age. The infant becomes ambulatory, develops socialization, and attains rudimentary verbal language during the first year of life.

Major organ systems, including the major organs of drug metabolism and elimination, differentiate, grow, and mature. Liver and kidney weights, relative to body weight, are approximately 10 times in the preschool child what they are in the young adult. Hepatic clearance of many substrates is physiologically decreased during the newborn period, rapidly increases during the first 3 months of life, and reaches adult levels by 1 year. Renal clearance of endogenous as well as exogenous substances follows a similar pattern. These changes have a profound effect on the distribution and time course of drugs in the body, which, in turn, determine age-appropriate doses and dosing intervals.

It is important to remember that infants are not little adults. The dynamic processes of growth, development, and maturation differentiate infants and children from adults. Infants differ from adults in many clinically significant ways, including their response to disease and to therapies applied to treat their illnesses

MATURATION OF DRUG METABOLISM PATHWAYS

Most drugs undergo metabolism in the liver prior to elimination. Drug metabolism is mediated by a number of enzymes, the most prevalent of which are those belonging to the superfamily of cytochrome P450 (CYP) heme-containing enzymes. The most important human CYP enzymes

with respect to the number of drugs metabolized are CYP3A4, CYP2D6, and CYP2C (see Chapter 3). The expression and activity of these enzymes undergo dramatic developmental changes during infancy. The time of maturation is enzyme-specific; e.g., the maturation of various metabolic pathways occurs at different times and at different rates during infancy.

Cytochrome P450 3A (CYP3A) is the most prevalent drug-metabolizing CYP enzyme in the human liver and is responsible for the metabolism of a large number of drugs. The specific form in adult liver is CYP3A4. This isoform is not present in fetal liver. However, an isoform of CYP3A, CYP3A7, is found in fetal liver as early as 6 weeks' gestation. During the first months of postnatal life, CYP3A7 disappears, and CYP3A4, the adult isoform, is expressed. The exact timing of maturation of CYP3A4 is not well described, but activity is thought to approximate adult capacity by 1 year of age.

CYP2D6 normally is not detected in fetal liver. However, during late gestation, CYP2D6 messenger RNA (mRNA) is present, and it increases above adult values during the first week of life. However, enzyme activity is present only after birth. Catalytic activity increases gradually beyond 28 days of age and appears to be mature by 3 years of age. However, the detailed ontogeny of this enzyme is not well defined at the present time.

CYP2C is not found in fetal liver. Postnatal maturation of this enzyme is reflected by changes in phenytoin metabolism, which is catalyzed by CYP2C9. Phenytoin metabolism matures rapidly during the first weeks of life, with a distribution of urinary metabolites similar to adults by 2 to 3 weeks of age. Beyond 6 months, metabolic capacity exceeds that of older children and adults.

Synthetic drug-metabolizing enzymes that catalyze the acetylation, methylation, glucuronidation, and sulfation of drugs also have specific maturation characteristics (Tab. 87.1). Maturation of specific drug-metabolizing pathways can have clinically important implications. For example, the clearance of caffeine, which is used to treat central apnea in infants, increases by threefold during the first year of life. Another example is the analgesic effect of codeine, which depends on CYP2D6-mediated metabolism of codeine to morphine. Codeine is a very poor analgesic in infants because they do not have the capacity to metabolize it to morphine. A third example is the prolonged action of

Table 87.1 Maturation of major drug-metabolizing enzymes

Enzyme	Maturation profile
CYP3A	
CYP3A7	Fetal isoform, unique to the fetus expression extinguished after birth
CYP3A4	Adult isoform, matures during first 2 years of life
CYP2D6	Absent activity in fetal liver; mRNA appears in late fetal life, exceeds adult levels in first week of life; enzyme protein absent in newborns, increases during first month and fully expressed by 3 years
CYP2C	CYP2C8 mRNA detectable in fetal liver, but no catalytic activity; CYP2C9-mediated hydroxylation of phenytoin capacity exceeds adult level beyond 6 months of age
N-acetyl transferase	Low activity in 16-week fetuses; decreased activity during infancy; matures by 2-3 years of age
Thiopurine methyltransferase	Activity 33% adult levels in 15-25-week fetuses; activity >150% of adult activity in newborn erythrocytes with full expression of genetic polymorphism
Glucuronyl transferase	Morphine glucuronidation in fetus 10% of adult; deficient in newborn; various isozymes mature at different times; bilirubin glucuronyl transferase matures during first 7-10 days of newborn life; morphine glucuronidation 20% of adult in newborn, reaches mature levels by 2 years

Table 87.2 Representative developmental changes in drug biodispositon as reflected by drug elimination half-life

Drug	Newborn	Infant	Child	Adult
			$(t_{1/2}$, in hours)	
Amikacin	6		1.6	2.3
Cefotaxime	4	0.8	1	1.1
Clindamycin	3.6	3.0	2.4	4.5
Diazepam	30	10	25	30
Mezlocillin	3.7		0.8	1
Morphine	7.2	4.5	2.9	2
Sulfisoxazole	18	8	8	8
Phenobarbital	80		48	72
Theophylline	30	7.0	3.4	8
Tobramycin	4.6		2	3
Vancomycin	6		2.4	6

morphine because of impaired glucuronyl transferase activity during early infancy. Formation and clearance of morphine glucuronides increase during the first year, approaching adult clearance by 6 months to 2.5 years (Tab. 87.2).

COMMON ILLNESSES OF INFANCY

The discussion of specific illnesses or pathologic conditions in this chapter is limited to several that are most common during infancy. These include fever, acute otitis media, upper respiratory infection, bronchiolitis, and acute infectious gastroenteritis with dehydration. In addition, currently recommended schedules for immunization during infancy are included because preventive treatment through immunization is a major component of medical care for the infant.

Fever

Fever is one of the most common presenting complaints in infants and may be associated with a wide variety of trivial as well as serious illnesses. It usually is secondary to an underlying primary condition. However, fever commonly is viewed as the primary problem by the parent, with the expectation that it must be treated. Although fever typically is perceived as a pathologic condition, it is an integral component of the normal host defense that is triggered by a wide variety of stimuli, the most common in infants being infection. Fever per se is not harmful and actually may be beneficial. The primary reason to treat fever is to provide symptomatic relief of discomfort in the infant.

The febrile response is mediated by the pyrogenic cytokines interleukin 1 (IL-1), IL-6, and tumor necrosis factor (TNF) at the level of the hypothalamus. It involves increased local production of prostaglandin E_2 (PGE_2) and an increase in cyclic adenosine monophosphate (cAMP). The hypothalamic setpoint that regulates body temperature is elevated, leading to physiologic responses that result in increased heat conservation and production until a new steady-state temperature is established.

Methods to decrease febrile body temperature are based on physical facilitation of body heat loss and pharmacologic inhibition of the PGE_2-mediated increase in hypothalamic setpoint. The primary cause of the fever should be treated, when possible. Adequate hydration also is important because fever increases water requirements by 10% for each degree centigrade of temperature elevation. The infant should be lightly dressed to avoid excessive heat conservation. Sponging with tepid water may be used to enhance heat loss by evaporation. However, methods to increase physical heat loss have only a modest and temporary effect unless they are combined with antipyretic medication to also lower the hypothalamic setpoint. The preferred antipyretics belong to the class of drugs known as nonsteroidal anti-inflammatory drugs (NSAIDs). These drugs are thought to exert their antipyretic effect by blocking production of PGE_2 at the level of the hypothalamus.

Paracetamol (acetaminophen) is the antipyretic used most commonly in North America and many European countries. It has been available for more than 30 years but came into widespread use during the early 1980s when the use of aspirin as an antipyretic in infants and children declined as a result of the reported association of aspirin with increased risk of Reye syndrome. Paracetamol is supplied in multiple formulations for children, including a flavored liquid containing 32 mg/ml, chewable tablets containing 80 and 160 mg, respectively, and infant drops containing 100 mg/ml. The drops are supplied with a calibrated dropper for accurate dose administration and are the preferred dosage form for infants. The drops always should be administered with the calibrated dropper. Dosage formulations designed for older children and adults should never be used in infants. The individual dose is 10 to 15 mg/kg and may be repeated every 4 to 6 hours, not to exceed 60 mg/kg per day. Acetaminophen has an excellent safety record when used as directed. Rarely, repeated daily doses in excess of 60 mg/kg have been associated with acute hepatic failure. Acute overdose of paracetamol also causes hepatoxicity.

Ibuprofen also is an effective antipyretic provided in multiple dosage formulations for use by infants and children. Tablets containing 50 and 100 mg, respectively, flavored liquid containing 20 mg/ml, and drops containing 40 mg/ml may be available. As with paracetamol, drops, if available, are the preferred dosage formulation for infants. Infant drops are provided with a calibrated dropper for accurate dosing. The recommended individual dose is 5 to 10 mg/kg, repeated every 6 hours as needed. The antipyretic effect of ibuprofen tends to last longer than that of acetaminophen, although this is not a consistent finding. The antipyretic response occurs more rapidly and is greater in children younger than 3 years compared with older children. In a double blind, randomized study of 84 000 febrile children, the incidence of serious adverse effects associated with ibuprofen and paracetamol was similar. However, ibuprofen should not be given to children who are dehydrated, volume contracted, or have low cardiac output states for other reasons because of the risk of acute renal failure. Most reported cases of renal failure in children due to ibuprofen have been reversible.

Although aspirin is an effective antipyretic, it is not recommended for use in infants and children because it is associated with increased risk of Reye syndrome when taken during certain viral illnesses. The antipyretics dipyrone and phenacetin are no longer available in some countries because of their respective toxicities. Dipyrone (metamizol) is not recommended because of the risk of aplastic anemia (see Chap. 45). Phenacetin has been totally withdrawn because of its association with renal and hepatic toxicity, methemaglobinemia, hemolytic anemia, and neutrapenia.

Other NSAIDs also are effective antipyretics. However, most are not available in dosage formulations that are easily administered to infants. Furthermore, safety experience in infants is greatest with paracetamol and ibuprofen.

Acute otitis media

Acute otitis media has been cited as the most common childhood disorder for which children are brought to the physician's office or emergency department and the leading indication for outpatient antimicrobial use. *Acute otitis media* may be defined as the presence of a middle ear effusion in association with local or systemic signs and symptoms of infection, including otalgia, fever, and upper respiratory tract infection. Approximately 35% of acute otitis media cases are caused by *Streptococcus pneumoniae,* followed by *Hemophilus influenzae* in 30% and *Moraxella catarrhalis* in 10%. The remainder are attributed to upper respiratory viruses. Roughly 35% of *H. influenzae* and 90% of *M. catarrhalis* isolates are β-lactamase producers and, consequently, are resistant to penicillin and ampicillin. More alarming is the worldwide exponential increase in strains of *S. pneumoniae* that are resistant to multiple unrelated antibiotics, including penicillins, cephalosporins, older macrolides, and sulfonamides. The natural course of uncomplicated acute otitis media is one of resolution without antibiotic treatment in 70 to 90% of patients. However, spontaneous resolution is not as frequent, and the incidence of invasive infectious complications is higher in infants less than 2 years of age, in children with recurrent otitis media, and in children with anatomic abnormalities of the ear or upper airway.

Symptomatic relief of the associated pain may be achieved with paracetamol 10 to 15 mg/kg every 4 to 6 hours or ibuprofen 5 to 10 mg/kg every 6 hours. Topical otic preparations containing a local anesthetic such as benzocaine also may be used to provide temporary symptomatic relief.

In North America, antibiotics are prescribed routinely for acute otitis media, whereas in some European countries such as Denmark, Norway, Sweden, and the Netherlands, antibiotics are deferred in children older than 2 years of age unless symptoms persist for more than 2 days. The routine use of antibiotics is being challenged in the US with recommendations that they be prescribed only selectively and with certain criteria in children over 2 years of age because of the rapid emergence of antibiotic-resistant bacterial strains. However, most workers would agree that antibiotics should be prescribed for acute otitis media in infants younger than 2 years of age because of the lower frequency of spontaneous cure and increased risk of serious invasive infections.

There is no objective basis with respect to efficacy for selecting one antibiotic over another. The selection, therefore, should be made on the basis of cost, availability, and patient tolerance. Amoxicillin is the drug of choice for initial treatment. It may be supplied in a suspension containing either 25 or 50 mg/ml. The recommended dose is 50 mg/kg per day in three divided doses. Cotrimoxazole may be used for infants who cannot take amoxicillin. It is supplied in a flavored suspension containing 8 mg trimethoprim and 40 mg sulfamethoxazole per milliliter. The recommended dose is 8 mg/kg trimethoprim and 40 mg/kg sulfamethoxazole daily in two divided doses. Duration of treatment is somewhat arbitrary, ranging from 5 to 10 days.

In children with treatment failure, amoxicillin-clavulanate, azithromycin, or one of the cephalosporins may be prescribed. Azithromycin is administered in a single daily dose, 10 mg/kg the first day and 5 mg/kg for 4 additional days. If multiple antibiotic-resistant *S. pneumoniae* is identified, azithromycin or clindamycin may be used, depending on sensitivity of the specific isolate. The dose of clindamycin is 8 to 12 mg/kg per day in three divided doses for 10 days (see Chap. 38).

Immunization for *H. influenzae* type B has reduced infections due to the typable strains contained in the vaccine but does not induce resistance to nontypable strains. Currently available *S. pneumoniae* vaccines do not induce immunity in infants under 2 years of age and are of no protective value in this age group for acute otitis media due to *S. pneumoniae*.

Upper respiratory tract infections

Infants and young children average between three and eight upper respiratory tract infections annually. The frequency may be higher in infants in day care. Nonspecific upper respiratory tract infections almost always are caused by viruses, the most common being rhinoviruses, coronaviruses, respiratory syncytial viruses, parainfluenza viruses, and respiratory adenoviruses. Secondary bacterial infection is relatively uncommon. Viral upper respiratory tract infection involves inoculation and infection of the upper respiratory epithelium, which is contiguous with the middle ear space and paranasal sinuses. Typical symptoms include nasal congestion, pharyngitis, serous nasal discharge, fever, malaise, headache, anorexia, and cough. Symptoms usually last for 2 to 7 days, although the cough may persist for several weeks.

Acute sinusitis occasionally may complicate a viral upper respiratory tract infection. In the past it was assumed that sinusitis did not occur in infants because the sinuses were not developed. It is now known that the maxillary and ethmoid sinuses are present at birth, whereas the frontal and sphenoid sinuses are only small extrusions of the nasal mucosa. Obstruction of the ostia due to mucosal swelling during an upper respiratory tract infection can result in negative pressure in the sinus, leading to secondary bacterial invasion and infection. Bacteria associated with acute sinusitis are essentially the same as those which cause acute otitis media, e.g., *S. pneumoniae, M. catarrhalis,* and nontypable *H. influenzae*. In addition, *S. pyogenes* and anaerobes are recovered in 2 to 5% of aspirates.

Antibiotics have no place in the treatment of an uncomplicated viral upper respiratory tract infection. Inappropriate use of antibiotics for this indication results in increased colonization with resistant organisms. However, if the infant is likely to have associated acute sinusitis, antibiotics should be prescribed. Amoxicillin is the drug of first choice in children. In locations with a high

incidence of resistant pathogens or in instances of treatment failure, alternative choices include amoxicillin-clavulanate, cotrimoxazole, azithromycin, or loracarbef. With the exception of loracarbef, these drugs have been discussed earlier under otitis media.

The primary treatment of upper respiratory tract infections is symptomatic. This may include antipyretic, decongestant, or antitussive agents, depending on the individual patient's symptoms. Antipyretic use was discussed earlier. Topical sympathomimetic nasal decongestants, such as oxymetazoline, should not be used in infants. Repetitive application of these agents to the nasal mucosa results in tachyphylaxis with rebound vasodilatation and nasal obstruction. Infants tend to be obligate nasal breathers, and bilateral nasal obstruction may result in obstructive apnea. Buffered saline nasal drops or spray may be used to help liquefy nasal secretions and facilitate removal from the nares. Antihistamines have been shown not to be beneficial for nasal congestion, and infants are particularly prone to the anticholinergic side effects of antihistamines. A systemic sympathomimetic decongestant drug such as pseudoephedrine may be used. Products containing pseudoephedrine in infant drops with a calibrated dropper typically contain pseudoephedrine 7.5 mg/0.8 ml. The recommended dose of pseudoephedrine is approximately 1.0 mg/kg every 4 to 6 hours, not to exceed four doses in a 24-hour period. Occasionally, an infant will develop irritability or insomnia because of the stimulating action of pseudoephedrine. In such cases, the dose should be reduced or the drug discontinued. In general, it is advisable to avoid centrally acting cough suppressants in infants because of their increased susceptibility to respiratory depression. In particular, codeine should not be used. If a cough suppressant is used, dextromethorphan is recommended in a dose of 1.0 to 2.0 mg/kg every 4 to 6 hours, not to exceed four doses in 24 hours. The lower dose should be used in younger infants.

Bronchiolitis

A leading cause of hospitalization and emergency department visits in infants beyond the newborn period is bronchiolitis. Bronchiolitis is an inflammation of the bronchiolar small airways caused by viruses, including respiratory syncytial virus, parainfluenza virus type 3, and adenoviruses. It occurs almost exclusively in infants under 2 years of age and results in a marked increase in small airways resistance. The infant characteristically presents with cough, audible wheezing, tachypnea, and respiratory distress. With more severe involvement, the infant may progress to respiratory failure.

In the past, treatment was largely supportive. However, the efficacy of adrenergic bronchodilators for the treatment of viral bronchiolitis has been documented recently. Both salbutamol and epinephrine have been shown to improve clinical scores and oxygenation in infants with bronchiolitis. However, racemic or L-epinephrine has been shown to provide greater improvement than salbutamol in controlled comparison trials.

There is conflicting evidence regarding the efficacy of glucocorticoids. Two controlled trials failed to demonstrate a beneficial effect of dexamethasone. However, a placebo-controlled trial of prednisolone 1 mg/kg per day showed more rapid improvement of symptoms in nonintubated infants and significantly shorter duration of mechanical ventilation and hospital stay in infants who required intubation and respiratory support.

Nonpharmacologic treatment includes adequate hydration and oxygenation. Infants with severe tachypnea may not be able to take adequate fluids enterally and require parenteral fluid replacement. Supplemental oxygen should be given to infants with decreased oxygenation. Infants who progress to impending respiratory failure should be transferred to an intensive care facility, where they can be intubated safely and mechanically ventilated. Initial pharmacologic management should include 3.0 to 5.0 ml of nebulized 1:1000 epinephrine. This may be repeated every 2 to 3 hours for two to three doses. Salbutamol is recommended for subsequent bronchodilator therapy because of its longer duration of action and weaker β-adrenergic effects. Prednisolone 1 mg/kg per day may be administered to infants with more severe symptoms, particularly those with oxygen desaturation and those requiring mechanical ventilatory support.

Croup

Croup, also referred to as *acute spasmodic croup* or *acute laryngotracheobronchitis,* is another common cause of morbidity in infants beyond 6 months of age. It typically occurs in association with a viral upper respiratory tract infection and results from acute edema of the larynx and proximal trachea. The patient presents with acute stridor, hoarseness, and a characteristic barking cough. In more severe cases, life-threatening upper airway obstruction may occur.

Current evidence from controlled clinical studies supports the efficacy of epinephrine and corticosteroids in the treatment of croup. Either racemic or L-epinephrine should be administered as described earlier for bronchiolitis. In addition, a single dose of dexamethasone 0.6 mg/kg may be given either orally or intramuscularly. Alternatively, nebulized budesonide 2 mg may be given twice daily for up to 3 days.

Acute viral gastroenteritis

Acute viral gastroenteritis with emesis and diarrhea is among the most common illnesses of infancy. The causative viruses are rotaviruses, enteric adenoviruses, astroviruses, and caliciviruses. Virtually all children acquire rotavirus infection by 6 years of age. Dominant symptoms are vomiting and secretory diarrhea, although abdominal pain, anorexia, fever, and malaise also may be present. Protective immunity following natural rotavirus infection is inconsistent and frequently incomplete.

The principal threat to the infant suffering from acute viral gastroenteritis is dehydration. Infants are more susceptible to rapid dehydration than adults because of their greater basal fluid and electrolyte requirements per kilogram. A small infant may become significantly dehydrated and acidotic within hours of onset of diarrheal losses.

Approximately 70% of the time dehydration is isonatremic. The primary treatment for the infant with acute gastroenteritis is rehydration and maintenance of fluid and electrolyte balance. In most cases this is best done with an oral rehydration solution (ORS). The World Health Organization ORS contains 111 mmol/l of carbohydrate, 90 mmol/l of sodium, 20 mmol/l of potassium, and 30 mmol/liter of base. Commercially available solutions generally contain 140 mmol/liter of carbohydrate and 45 to 75 mmol/l of sodium. Solutions with 75 to 90 mmol/l of sodium should be used for rehydration therapy and replacement of continuing losses, whereas those with a lower sodium content may be used for maintenance of hydration once the infant is rehydrated. In the presence of mild dehydration, 50 ml/kg should be given within 4 hours. With moderate dehydration, the infant should receive 100 ml/kg over 6 hours. In the presence of vomiting, small quantities of the solution may be given frequently. Nursing infants should be encouraged to breast feed during oral rehydration. Parenteral rehydration should be reserved for infants in shock, with severe dehydration, with severe electrolyte imbalances, with uncontrolled vomiting, with an inability to swallow, or with decreased gut motility.

Antidiarrheal preparations containing drugs such as loperamide, attapulgite, and bismuth subsalicylate should not be given to infants because they have little to offer therapeutically and entail considerable risk of adverse side effects in this age group. In addition, they may mask ongoing fluid losses from the gut, leading to failure to recognize progressive dehydration of the infant and thereby delaying essential fluid replacement therapy.

A safe and effective oral vaccine against rotavirus infection has been developed. This vaccine will markedly decrease infantile diarrheal illness in both the developed and developing worlds.

IMMUNIZATION

Immunization is the cornerstone of cost-effective health care for infants worldwide. Table 87.3 summarizes the current immunization recommendations for the first 18 months of life by the American Academy of Pediatrics.

Table 87.3 Current immunization recommendations for the first 18 months of life by the American Academy of pediatrics

Hepatitis B	Birth, 1-4 months, 6-18 months
Diphtheria, tetanus, pertussis	2, 4, 6, and 15 months
H. influenzae type b	2, 4, 6, and 15 months
Polio	2, 4, and 12 months
Measles, mumps, rubella	12-15 months
Varicella	12-15 months

Suggested readings

AMERICAN ACADEMY OF PEDIATRICS COMMITTEE ON INFECTIOUS DISEASES. Recommended childhood immunization schedule-United States, January-December 1997. Pediatrics 1997; 99:136.

DINARELLO CA. Thermoregulation and the pathogenesis of fever. Infect Dis Clin North Am 1996;10:433-49.

DOWELL SF, MARCY SM, PHILLIPS WR, et al. Principles of judicious use of antimicrobial agents for pediatric upper respiratory tract infections. Pediatrics 1998;101(suppl 1):163-5.

KAUFFMAN RE. Scientific issues in biomedical research with children. In: Grodin MA, Glantz LH, eds. Children as Research Subjects: Science, Ethics, and Law. New York:Oxford University Press, 1994:29-30.

KLASSEN TP. Recent advances in the treatment of bronchiolitis and laryngitis. Pediatr Clin North Am 1997;44:249-61.

KEARNS GL, REED MD. Clinical pharmacokinetics in infants and children: a reappraisal. Clin Pharmacokinet 1989;17(suppl. 1):29-67.

LEEDER JS, KEARNS GL. Pharmacogenetics in pediatrics: implications for practice. Pediatr Clin North Am 1997; 44:55-77.

LESKO SM, MITCHELL AA. An assessment of the safety of pediatric ibuprofen: a practitioner-based randomized clinical trial. JAMA 1995;273:929-33.

McCARTHY PL, KLIG JE, KAHN JS, et al. Fever without apparent source on clinical examination, lower respiratory infections in children, other infectious diseases, and acute gastroenteritis and diarrhea of infancy and early childhood. Curr Opin Pediatr 1997;9:105-26.

MIDtHUN K, KAPIKIAN AZ. Rotavirus vaccines: an overview. Clin Microbiol Rev 1996;9:423-34.

ROSENFELD RM. An evidence-based approach to treating otitis media. Pediatr Clin North Am 1996;43:1165-81.

VAN WOENSEL JB, WOLFS TF, VAN AALDEREN WM, et al. Randomized double-blind placebo controlled trial of prednisolone in children admitted to hospital with respiratory syncytial virus bronchiolitis. Thorax 1997;52:595-7.

Pregnancy

Maurizio Bonati, Antonio Addis

The experience with thalidomide can be said to have laid the foundation for the discipline of clinical pharmacology and for much of our current practices in relation to preclinical toxicology testing of new drugs. The worldwide publicity about the disaster caused by this antiemetic produced a revolution in the way pharmacotherapy is used during pregnancy. Although many drugs and chemicals and a multitude of environmental factors were accused of being human teratogens, only a very limited group of agents has been proven to be teratogenic (Tab. 88.1).

Epidemiologic surveys have determined that between one-third and two-thirds of all pregnant women will take at least one medication during pregnancy, with antimicrobial agents being the most commonly used, followed by antiemetics, tranquilizers, and analgesics. An international survey on 14778 women giving birth in 1148 hospitals from 22 countries shows that most of the mothers (86%) received an average of 2.9 prescriptions during pregnancy. These findings further demonstrate that drug use during pregnancy is not a rare event and needs systematic and continuous monitoring as part of complete care before, during, and after pregnancy. In such a context, an effec-

tive care regimen in pregnancy and the neonatal period has been a milestone in care and has led to the formation of such groups as the Cochrane Library.

This chapter aims to (1) review the principal pharmacokinetic modifications that occur during pregnancy, (2) summarize the treatment of choice for common problems during pregnancy using the most common questions received by a specialized information center, and (3) describe the general principles for drug prescribing and counseling during pregnancy.

PHARMACOKINETIC CONSIDERATIONS

As pregnancy advances, continual physiologic changes occur that may influence the processes of absorption, distribution, and elimination of drugs. Although drug therapy in pregnancy is mostly directed to maternal requirements, it is often carried out without taking into consideration these important modifications. Moreover, as previous studies have determined, most drugs easily cross the placenta, making the fetus an unwanted or even nonbenefit-

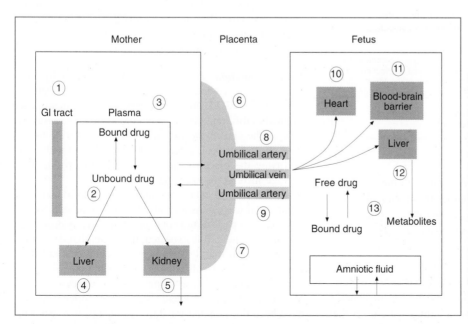

Figure 88.1 Drug disposition in the maternal-placental system. The factors affecting the pharmacokinetics and drug effects on mother and fetus are: (1) altered maternal absorption; (2) increased maternal unbound drug fraction; (3) increased maternal plasma volume; (4) altered hepatic clearance; (5) increased maternal renal blood flow and glomerular filtration rate; (6) placental transfer; (7) possible placental metabolism; (8) placental blood flow; (9) maternal-fetal blood pH; (10) preferential fetal circulation to the heart and brain; (11) undeveloped fetal blood-brain barrier; (12) immature fetal liver enzyme activity; and (13) increased fetal unbound drug fraction.

Table 88.1 Drugs with proven teratogenic effects in humans[1]

Aminopterin,[2] methotrexate	CNS and limb malformations
Angiotensin-converting enzyme (ACE) inhibitors	Prolonged renal failure in neonates, decreased skull ossification, renal tubular dysgenesis
Anticholinergic drugs	Neonatal meconium ileus
Antithyroid drugs (propylthiouracil and methimazole)	Fetal and neonatal goiter and hypothyroidism, aplasia cutis (with methimazole)
Carbamazepine	Neural tube defects
Cyclophosphamide	CNS malformations, secondary cancer
Danazol and other androgenic drugs	Masculinization of female fetuses
Diethylstilbestrol[2]	Vaginal carcinoma and other genitourinary defects in female and male offspring
Hypoglycemic drugs	Neonatal hypoglycemia
Lithium	Ebstein's anomaly
Misoprostol	Moebius sequence
Nonsteroidal anti-inflammatory drugs	Constriction of the ductus arteriosus,[3] necrotizing enterocolitis
Paramethadione[2]	Facial and CNS defects
Phenytoin	Growth retardation, CNS deficits
Psychoactive drugs (e.g., barbiturates, opioids, and benzodiazepines)	Neonatal withdrawal syndrome when drug is taken in late pregnancy
Systemic retinoids (isotretinoin and etretinate)	CNS, craniofacial, cardiovascular, and other defects
Tetracycline	Anomalies of teeth and bone
Thalidomide	Limb-shortening defects, internal organ defects
Trimethadione[2]	Facial and CNS defects
Valproic acid	Neural tube defects
Warfarin	Skeletal and CNS defects, Dandy-Walker syndrome

(CNS = central nervous system.)
[1]Only drugs teratogenic when used at clinically recommended doses are listed. The list includes all drugs proved to affect neonatal morphology or brain development and some of the toxic manifestations predicted on the basis of the pharmacologic actions of the drugs. Data are from Briggs et al.
[2]The drug is not currently in clinical use.
[3]Sulindac probably does not have this effect.

ing drug recipient. On the other hand, with the introduction of modern antenatal diagnostic techniques, the idea of treating the fetus in utero by giving drugs to the pregnant woman has emerged. Maternal and fetal drug responses during pregnancy are influenced by several factors: the changes in absorption, distribution, and elimination of the drug in the mother that are dictated by pregnancy-induced physiologic changes and the placental-fetal unit that affects the amount of a drug that crosses the

placenta, the fraction of a drug metabolized by the placenta, and the distribution and elimination of a drug by the fetus. Although several pharmacokinetic models have been proposed to describe drug disposition in the maternal-placental-fetal unit, in general, two principal changes characterize pregnancy with respect to drug kinetics (Fig. 88.1): the maternal physiologic changes and the effects of the placental-fetal compartment.

Alterations in drug kinetics due to maternal changes

Drug absorption Absorption of enterally administered drugs may be delayed during pregnancy because there is a reduction of intestinal motility resulting in a 30 to 50% increase in gastric and intestinal emptying time. This may be important when one needs to achieve a rapid onset of drug effect because of delayed and lower peak plasma concentrations. On the contrary, for drugs whose absorption depends on the time the drug remains in the intestine, the final amount absorbed may increase. There is a reduction in gastric acid secretions (40% less than in nonpregnant women) together with an increase in mucus secretions, both of which lead to an increase in gastric pH and therefore in buffer capacity. Clinically, this would affect the ionization of weak acids and bases and hence their absorption. Nausea and vomiting, which occur frequently during the first trimester, may be another reason for low plasma drug concentrations. Patients should be advised to take their medication at times when nausea is minimal, usually during the evening.

As cardiac output and tidal volumes increase during pregnancy, hyperventilation and increased pulmonary blood flow occur. These alterations favor alveolar uptake and therefore should be considered when administering drugs by inhalation, although it is (extremely) important to note that for inhalational anesthetics agents, the rate of induction is not necessarily faster because the uptake of these agents depends on both pulmonary equilibrium and tissue distribution kinetics. However, dosage requirements for volatile anesthetic drugs are likely to be reduced during pregnancy, as was demonstrated for halothane, isoflurane, and methoxyflurane.

Drug distribution The plasma volume increases by 50% during pregnancy and may affect the volume of distribution. The increased cardiac output is characteristically distributed to different organs: renal blood flow increases by 50% at the end of the first trimester, and uterine blood flow reaches its peak at term (600-700 ml/min) with 80% perfusing the placenta and 20% the myometrium. The average increase in total-body water is 8 liters, 60% distributed to the placenta, fetus, and amniotic fluid and 40% to maternal tissues. As a result of this volume expansion, a decrease in peak serum concentration of many drugs has been documented. It is expected, therefore, that drugs that are distributed mainly to water compartments and thus have a relatively small volume of distribution will result in the greatest decrease in peak serum concentrations. Moreover, decreased steady-state drug concentrations have been documented for different agents as a result of their enhanced elimination. Drug dosage requirements would be expected to be greater to achieve the same therapeutic effect if these effects were not offset by other pharmacokinetic changes during pregnancy that are discussed later in this chapter.

Protein binding As pregnancy advances, plasma volume expands at a greater rate than the increase in albumin production, creating physiologic dilutional hypoalbuminemia. Moreover, steroid and placental hormones occupy protein-binding sites, thus decreasing protein binding of drugs. The overall effect is a decrease in the binding capacity for albumin and therefore an increase in the unbound ("free") drug. Since the unbound drug is the pharmacologically active drug, pregnant women would be expected to have an increased drug effect. However, enhanced clearance of different agents during pregnancy usually counteracts this effect. For most drugs, the preceding changes do not alter the steady-state concentration of free drug. However, since there is a significant decrease in glycoprotein within the fetus, the free fractions of basic drugs in the developing child are higher. Despite the theoretical risk of toxicity of basic drugs in the fetus, there is no evidence of any clinical significance. Yet clinicians who do not have the means to obtain measurements of an unbound drug may erroneously interpret lower total concentrations of a drug as indicative of a lower free drug measure. Of potential clinical importance is the fact that protein binding of several antiepileptic drugs, including phenytoin, diazepam, and valproic acid, has been shown to decrease toward the last trimester of pregnancy.

Drug elimination Several factors such as the increased secretion of estrogen and progesterone in normal pregnancy may affect hepatic drug metabolism in different ways. For example, while there is an increase in liver metabolism of drugs such as phenytoin, hepatic elimination of other drugs such as theophylline and caffeine is reduced. The preceding changes during pregnancy on hepatic physiology may alter drug metabolism, but their extent can hardly be quantified. The relationship between creatinine clearance and the elimination of drugs excreted mainly by the kidney has been demonstrated for many agents. Since renal plasma flow increases by 25 to 50% and the glomerular filtration rate increases by 50%, drugs that are excreted primarily unchanged in the urine, such as penicillin, digoxin, and lithium, demonstrate enhanced elimination and lower steady-state serum concentrations. However, these changes are clinically insufficient and therefore require no alteration in the dose of the above-mentioned drugs.

The placental-fetal compartment effect

The placenta is no longer considered a barrier to the transfer of drugs from the maternal to the fetal organism. Most drugs cross the placenta by simple diffusion to a greater or lesser extent from as early as the fifth week of embryonic life. Several pharmacokinetic models have

been proposed in an attempt to characterize drug behavior in the placental-fetal unit. When an administered drug readily equilibrates to achieve an even fetal-maternal drug concentration, a single-compartment model may be applied. On the other hand, when the fetal tissue is less easily accessible, thus representing a deep compartment, a two-compartmental model may be more appropriate. Salicylates and diazepam are examples of such a model, for they achieve higher concentrations in fetal plasma than in maternal plasma. Considering the tissue distribution of a drug, two indices may be taken into account: the *absolute transfer ratio* and the *relative transfer ratio*. The first can be regarded as the ability of a drug to get to a tissue (in terms of rate of the process), although it tells us nothing about the time course of the unbound drug concentration to which a tissue (and its receptors) might be exposed. The second index, however, suggests the relative exposure of a tissue to a drug. Such considerations may be important in assessing fetal exposure to different agents on the basis of maternal plasma concentrations. In addition, different physiologic factors such as placental blood flow and differences in plasma protein binding and/or in the acid-base equilibrium of the mother versus the fetus also contribute to the understanding of fetal-maternal drug concentration ratios.

Effect of protein binding Fetal and newborn plasma proteins appear to bind various drugs (e.g., ampicillin and benzylpenicillin) with less affinity compared with maternal plasma proteins. For other drugs (e.g., salicylates), a more extensive binding to fetal than maternal plasma proteins has been documented. Maternal plasma albumin gradually decreases during pregnancy, whereas fetal albumin progressively increases. This dynamic process results in different fetal-maternal albumin concentration ratios at different gestational ages. The fetal albumin concentration reaches its peak at term, when it equals or even exceeds the maternal albumin concentration. This may be clinically important because the free (unbound) drug concentration is an important determinant of drug movement across the placenta. Since only the unbound (free) drug is capable of crossing the placental barrier, drugs such as digoxin and ampicillin that are bound to protein with less affinity reach higher concentrations in the fetus. On the other hand, drugs with high protein binding such as dicloxacillin achieve higher maternal than fetal concentrations.

Differences in pH Non-ionized, highly lipid-soluble molecules penetrate biologic membranes more quickly than less lipid-soluble, ionized molecules. Therefore, the maternal and fetal pH values are important determinants of placental transfer, especially for weakly acidic or basic drugs whose pK_a is close to the plasma pH. Fetal plasma pH is usually slightly more acidic than maternal pH. Consequently, weak bases will be mainly non-ionized and therefore able to easily penetrate the placental barrier. However, after crossing the placenta and making contact with the relatively acidic fetal blood, these molecules will become more ionized. This results in an apparent fall in fetal concentration of the drug and leads to a concentration gradient and therefore a net movement from the maternal to the fetal system. This phenomenon is commonly referred to as *ion trapping*.

Fetal-placental drug elimination There is some evidence that both the human placenta and the fetus are capable of metabolism. All enzymatic processes, including phase 1 (i.e., oxidation, dehydrogenation, reduction, hydrolysis, etc.) and phase 2 (i.e., glucuronidation, methylation, and acetylation) processes have been documented in the fetal liver as early as 7-8 weeks of pregnancy. However, since most enzymatic processes are immature at this stage, their degree of activity is very low, and therefore, their contribution to overall drug-elimination capacity is marginal. On the other hand, the reduced elimination capacity may cause more pronounced and prolonged drug effects in the fetus. The fact that about half the fetal circulation (umbilical vein) reaches the heart and brain directly, bypassing the liver, also may contribute to this effect. Elimination of drugs from the fetus occurs primarily through its diffusion back to the maternal compartment. However, since most metabolites are more polar than their parent compounds, they are less likely to cross the placental barrier. This may result in metabolite accumulation in various fetal tissues. As pregnancy progresses, higher amounts of different drugs are excreted into the amniotic fluid, reflecting maturation of the fetal kidney.

Rate of maternal-fetal drug equilibration Since the primary means of placental drug transfer is simple diffusion, the net transplacental movement of most xenobiotics is proportional to the concentration gradient of the drug across the placenta and the physicochemical characteristics of the xenobiotic and the placental membrane. As with diffusion across other biologic membranes, lipophilic drugs generally cross the placenta more readily than nonlipophilic compounds. Drugs that are non-ionized at the physiologic pH will diffuse across the placenta more rapidly than more basic or acidic compounds. This distinction is not absolute, since some drugs that are ionized at physiologic pH such as valproic acid or salicylate reach the fetus rapidly and efficiently. For most non-ionized, lipophilic compounds, the rate-limiting step that determines placental drug transfer is blood flow. Changes in placental blood flow that may be secondary to pathophysiologic conditions (e.g., pregnancy-induced hypertension, abruptio placenta) or due to pharmacologic effects (e.g., oxytocic drugs, nicotine) can lead to the vasoconstricting effects of these conditions, causing decreased placental perfusion. As opposed to non-ionized compounds, for more polar drugs with lower rates of placental transfer, the rate-limiting step for placental transfer is diffusion. The rate of maternal-fetal drug equilibration is an important determinant in cases where therapeutic fetal drug concentrations need to be achieved as quickly as possible. Clinical examples of such cases are maternal administration of antiarrhythmic agents or antibiotics in order to treat intrauterine fetal arrhythmias or infections. One of the puzzling features of fetal pharmacotherapy of supraventricular tachyarrhythmias with digoxin is the length of time required to achieve control. Even in the

Table 88.2 Questions related to pregnancy received by CRIF[1] during 1998 grouped according to the ATC (Anatomical-therapeutic-chemical) classification system

ATC Group		No. of questions[2]	Percent of questions	Percent of callers[3]
N	Central nervous system (excluding analgesics)	419*	18	33
J	General antiinfectives for systemic use	387	17	30
A	Alimentary tract and metabolism	228	10	18
R	Respiratory system	214	9	17
G	Genito-urinary system and sex hormones	174	8	14
M	Musculo-skeletal system	169	7	13
N02	Analgesics	136	6	11
P	Antiparasitic products	83	4	6
D	Dermatologicals	79	3	6
H	Systemic hormonal prep. (excluding sex hormones)	76	3	6
C	Cardiovascular system	70	3	5
B	Blood and bloodforming organs	55	2	4
S	Sensory organs	34	2	3
V	Various	26	1	2
L	Antineoplastics, immunosupressive drugs	22	1	2
Not drugs (X-rays, echographic examinations, etc.)		147	6	1
Total		2319	100	

[1]CRIF (Regional Drug Information Center, at the "Mario Negri" Research Institute of Milan.)
[2]Selected by pregnancy "yes" or "maybe."
[3]A total 713 callers (57%) asked for information about only one drug, so the sum is more than 100%.

absence of fetal heart failure, conversion to sinus rhythm is not achieved before 7 days and often may take longer in hydropic fetuses. Because of the difficulty in accessing the placenta, human research has been limited by technical and ethical dilemmas, and research has focused on morphologic or biochemical investigations on organs obtained from abortions or on delivery. However, in the last few decades, the in vitro placental perfusion technique has been developed, resulting in more information on the functional performance of the placenta throughout pregnancy.

TREATMENTS OF CHOICE IN COMMON PROBLEMS DURING PREGNANCY

The literature about the risks and benefits of drug treatment in this population is continuously expanding. Most of the clinical pharmacology reviews about the use of drugs during pregnancy discuss the risks and benefits of therapies for mothers following drug classification schemes. It is our opinion that this approach does not correctly address the problems/diseases of the mothers. To be more accurate in reviewing the general guidelines for drug prescription during pregnancy, We would like to analyze this issue from the disease point of view. However, for more detailed information, large collections of data may be found in the "Suggested Readings" at the end of this chapter.

The following problems/diseases have been chosen based on the questions most frequently received by our regional drug information center (Tab. 88.2).

General systemic infections

Information on *urinary tract infections* is frequently requested at any Regional Drug Center (Tab. 88.2). The treatment of choice is the penicillins, some of which cross the placenta, the exceptions being piperacillin and sulbecillin. *Escherichia coli* is the microorganism usually involved in urinary tract infections, and if oral therapy can be tolerated, a dosage of 3 g twice daily of amoxicillin is recommended. Other drugs should be reserved for treatment failures or known penicillin hypersensitivity. The penicillins are safe antibiotics during pregnancy, with no embryo- or fetotoxic effect having been described in large studies. Urinary tract infection therapy always should be preceded by urine culture, and the response should be checked by culture 7 to 10 days after treatment and then monthly or again at 6 months if continuous therapy is given for refractory infections. Where the culture shows that there is some resistance to amoxicillin, the appropriate antibacterial drug should be chosen, keeping in mind that certain agents are relatively or completely contraindicated in pregnancy. Tetracyclines are not recommended during the second half of pregnancy because they can cause discoloration of unerupted teeth and possibly enamel hypoplasia. These drugs also may impair fetal bone growth and so should never be administered during pregnancy. Sulfonamides also may cause hemolytic ane-

mia in infants who are deficient in glucose-6-phosphate dehydrogenase. Therefore, sulfonamides may be a potential cause of kernicterus because of their ability to displace bilirubin from its binding sites on plasma albumin after tranplacental passage. The combination of sulfamethoxazole with thrimethoprim (cotrimoxazole) has not been linked with fetal growth inhibition or teratogenesis. However, because of the anti-folic acid activity of this combination, cotrimoxazole is not considered a drug of first choice during pregnancy. Aminoglycosides cross the placenta and have been associated with the possibility of eighth cranial nerve damage. Congenital ototoxicity has been linked to in utero exposure to streptomycin and kanamycin. However, newer agents, such as amikacin, gentamicin, netilmycin, and tobramycin, have never been associated with this complication or in general with adverse effects in newborns exposed in utero.

Psychiatric and neurologic disorders

A large number of women have psychiatric disorders (e.g., depression) at some time in their lives, most commonly during the childbearing years, and often they require drug therapy. The decision to continue or initiate pharmacotherapy for psychiatric patients during pregnancy is complicated by the need to balance maternal well-being with fetal safety. There is ample evidence that discontinuation of antidepressant drug therapy during pregnancy in patients with medication-responsive illness may be detrimental and may result in high relapse rates. All psychotropic medications diffuse readily across the placenta, so clinicians who care for female psychiatric patients may be faced with the difficult task of making recommendations regarding psychotropic medication use to patients who either are pregnant or wish to conceive.

Depression

An estimated 8 to 20% of women develop clinical symptoms of depression at some time during their lives for which drug therapy is often required. Fluoxetine was approved in the United States for treatment of major depression in 1987 and has become the world's largest selling antidepressant. Due to this trend and the fact that 50% of pregnancies are unplanned, numerous women will be exposed involuntarily to fluoxetine during the first trimester of their pregnancy. The lack of data on fetal safety of fluoxetine has created anxiety among women, their families, and physicians. In 1993, Pastuszak and colleagues published a study comparing 128 pregnant women treated with fluoxetine with 128 controls (exposed to nonteratogenic drugs) and with 74 women treated with trycyclic antidepressants, showing that neither fluoxetine nor tricyclic antidepressants taken during the first trimester were associated with an increased risk of congenital malformations. Recently, Chambers and colleagues reported their cohort of women (162 cases, 225 controls) taking fluoxetine during pregnancy. Despite the fact that this study did not show an increased risk for major malformations, a number of international agencies have decided to caution women against the use of this drug during pregnancy. However, a meta-analytical review of all published studies shows that the use of fluoxetine during first trimester of pregnancy is not associated with measurable teratogenic effects in humans. A recent prospective cohort study investigated the safety of fluoxetine in terms of neurodevelopmental toxicity as well. This study shows that the neurodevelopment of children exposed in utero to fluoxetine is similar to that of controls (exposed to nonteratogenic agents or to other antidepressants) in a large number of domains, including IQ, language development, and behavior. Similar results were obtained when children exposed only during the first trimester were compared with those exposed throughout gestation.

Anxiety

Antepartum exposure to benzodiazepines has been associated with teratogenic effects (e.g., facial clefts, skeletal anomalies) in some animal studies but not others. The risk for cleft palate in the general population is approximately 0.06%. Early human case-control studies found that maternal benzodiazepine exposure increases the risk of fetal cleft lip and cleft palate. Subsequent reports have implicated benzodiazepines as the cause of major malformations, abnormal neurodevelopment, and the possible development of a benzodiazepine syndrome similar to fetal alcohol syndrome. Unfortunately, these studies have no means of controlling for the number of confounding factors. Several prospective cohort studies involving hundreds of benzodiazepine-exposed pregnancies and an equal number of controls failed to show an increased risk of malformations after use of these drugs during the first trimester of pregnancy. These contradictory results have led to considerable controversy surrounding the use of benzodiazepines in pregnancy. Nevertheless, it seems clear that there is a trivial, if any, risk of malformations for newborns exposed to benzodiazepines during the first trimester of pregnancy.

Epilepsy

Epilepsy is a common neurologic disorder with a prevalence of 1%. In most women with epilepsy, seizures are well controlled during pregnancy, but if frequency changes, it is usually for the worse (see Chap. 10). The potential problem in the management of these patients arises from the altered pharmacokinetics associated with pregnancy. In general, peak plasma levels of anticonvulsant drugs fall during pregnancy as a result of the 50% expansion in plasma volume, while steady-state concentrations fall secondary to a decrease in protein binding and an increased clearance. Since most anticonvulsant drugs are acidic or neutral, they are highly bound to serum albumin. Phenytoin and valproic acid are both highly protein bound (approximately 90%). During pregnancy, albumin levels fall, with a corresponding fall in the bound drug. The decrease in plasma protein binding leads

to more free drug available for biotransformation. Thus, the unbound drug levels (free drug) remain relatively constant, but total plasma levels (unbound plus protein-bound drug) fall. It should be remembered that the constant, or even higher, free drug concentration may secure an antiepileptic effect, since it is the free drug that reaches the brain. For practical reasons, most laboratories measure total plasma concentration (bound plus unbound drug) rather than the unbound concentration, which is the pharmacologically active component.

Monitoring total plasma levels of these drugs therefore can be misleading. Only therapeutic drug monitoring that will measure both protein-bound and unbound drug concentrations can be interpreted appropriately. The increase in glomerular filtration rate and renal plasma flow may enhance the clearance of renally excreted drugs such as primidone, gabapentin, and vigabatrin. Carbamazepine is regarded by many as the drug of choice for most forms of epilepsy during pregnancy because of its relatively low teratogenic risk. Phenytoin has been associated with the fetal hydantoin syndrome, particularly with its neurotoxic potential. Both valproic acid and carbamazepine have been shown to cause neural tube defects, and in women using them, a full workup should be performed to rule out this malformation. Phenobarbital has been prescribed much less commonly in recent years because of its tendency to sedate and impair cognitive function.

Cardiovascular disorders

Hypertension

Between 5 and 10% of all pregnancies are complicated by hypertension (see Chap. 23). *Essential,* or *secondary, hypertension* may be discovered in advance and should be suspected if the blood pressure at the first visit exceeds 140/90 mm Hg. *Gestational hypertension* is present when the blood pressure exceeds 140/90 mm Hg after 20 weeks of gestation. *Preeclampsia,* as opposed to chronic hypertension, is a complex clinical syndrome characterized by hypertension, edema, and proteinuria of more than 0.5 g per day that appears after 20 weeks of gestation in previously normotensive women. Preeclampsia may supervene in preexistising or gestational hypertension.

Accumulated data from different studies indicate that pharmacologic treatment decreases the incidence of cardiovascular and cerebrovascular complications only in chronically hypertensive pregnant women with diastolic values above 110 mm Hg. It is unclear whether lowering blood pressure in cases of mild hypertension affects the natural course of disease or the incidence of its complications.

As opposed to chronic hypertension, the chief requirements for successful management of preeclampsia are early diagnosis, close follow-up, and timely delivery. The literature is far from consistent regarding whether antihypertensive therapy is indicated in mild, uncomplicated cases of preeclampsia. While some studies have shown a beneficial effect of antihypertensive therapy on proteinuria, progression to severe disease, and neonatal respiratory syndrome, others have failed to demonstrate any effect. In cases of severe or complicated preeclampsia, on the other hand, antihypertensive therapy is mandatory to ascertain a better maternal and neonatal outcome.

Many agents are available for the treatment of hypertension, but their use during pregnancy should be examined with respect to both maternal and fetal toxicity and teratogenicity. Methyldopa is regarded by many as one of the drugs of choice for maternal hypertension during pregnancy. This is mainly due to its safety profile: a total of 242 newborns exposed during embryogenesis to methyldopa demonstrated no increased incidence of malformations or perinatal complications. Another study showed that 1157 hypertensive pregnancies had no maternal or neonatal adverse effects from methyldopa administration. The mild decrease in systolic blood pressure in methyldopa-treated newborns is considered clinically insignificant.

Like most other antihypertensive agents, hydralazine readily crosses the placenta and achieves fetal serum concentrations equal to or greater than maternal levels. A number of studies have confirmed the lack of association between hydralazine use during gestation (either as monotherapy or with other antihypertensive agents) and congenital malformations. Anecdotal case reports, on the other hand, have linked the use of hydralazine with fetal premature atrial contractions, maternal hypotension, a lupus erythematosus-like syndrome in both the mother and her growth-retarded offspring, and neonatal thrombocytopenia. However, considering the large number of pregnant women treated with hydralazine versus the anecdotal reports of adverse effects, this drug should still be regarded as a first-line agent for antihypertensive therapy during pregnancy.

Calcium channel blockers have been used to treat hypertension and to inhibit premature atrial contractions. A Canadian prospective, controlled study reported the pregnancy outcomes of 78 women with first-trimester exposure to these antihypertensive drugs. There was no increase in the rates of major malformations or perinatal complications in the calcium channel blocker group compared with controls. Maternal hypertension was the most important factor responsible for decreased birth weight observed in the calcium channel blocker group. Nifedipine therapy during the second and third trimesters was shown to be effective in lowering maternal blood pressure without affecting fetal heart rate or blood pressure in different studies. Both the efficacy and low toxicity profiles of nifedipine are expected to result in substantial clinical use of this agent during pregnancy. Based on pharmacokinetic studies demonstrating higher rates of clearance and shorter elimination half-life of nifedipine in preeclamptic patients, a dosing interval of 3 to 4 hours is suggested when rapid-release nifedipine is used during gestation.

Beta-adrenoreceptor blocking agents are used for different indications during pregnancy. There are sufficient data to conclude that β-blockers have no teratogenic effects in humans. However, concern regarding possible perinatal adverse effects has been raised after reports of intrauterine growth retardation, fetal bradycardia, and fetal hypoglycemia related to their use during gestation.

It is important to note that intrauterine growth retardation can be attributed to the underlying maternal disease rather than to β-blocker therapy, a fact that also may explain the discrepancy between different studies that did not control for this variable. Although most neonates have not shown any adverse clinical signs, it is recommended that fetuses exposed in utero to β-blockers be followed closely using serial ultrasounds and that neonates be followed for potential bradycardia and/or hypoglycemia. Data regarding the use of alpha-adrenoreceptor blocking agents during pregnancy are very limited. Although there is no evidence that these agents are human teratogens, more studies and/or clinical experience need to be collected before an evidence-based conclusion regarding their safety during pregnancy can be drawn.

Diuretic therapy is indicated particularly in chronically hypertensive pregnant women with salt-sensitive hypertension or with evidence of left ventricular diastolic dysfunction. Results of nine randomized trials of diuretics in pregnancy have demonstrated a protective effect of these agents against development of preeclampsia; however, diuretic therapy should be discontinued if there is evidence of either preeclampsia or reduced fetal growth.

Both furosemide and thiazide have not been associated with an increased risk of congenital malformations or perinatal complications. Furosemide was not shown to induce diuresis in neonates exposed shortly before birth to the drug. However, no electrolyte abnormalities were recorded. Sporadic cases of neonatal thrombocytopenia and hyponatremia have been reported in association with in utero exposure to thiazides. The human data regarding the use of potassium-sparing agents during pregnancy are very limited.

Angiotensin-converting enzyme (ACE) inhibitors demonstrate a unique pattern of fetotoxicity. Exposure to these agents during the second and third trimesters of pregnancy is associated with development of fetal renal failure leading to intrauterine growth retardation, oligohydramnios, and hypoplasia of skull bones. First-trimester exposure to ACE inhibitors has not been associated with increased risk of structural malformations. As a whole, these data indicate that use of ACE inhibitors should be contraindicated during the second and third trimesters of pregnancy, whereas first-trimester exposure should not be an indication for pregnancy termination.

Respiratory disease

Asthma

Up to 4% of all pregnancies are associated with asthma. As with many diseases, it is not totally clear how pregnancy affects the course of asthma. A combination of nine studies reporting on 1054 pregnancies indicated, however, that 22% of pregnant asthmatic women reported worsening of symptoms and 49% no change. When both symptoms and spirometry measurements were studied in 366 pregnant women in a different study, 35% worsened, 28% improved, and 33% were unchanged. Researchers estimate that 10% of pregnant asthmatic women will have exacerbations during labor and delivery. Suboptimal control of asthma during pregnancy has been associated with adverse outcomes, such as higher rates of prematurity, intrauterine growth retardation, low birth weight, perinatal mortality, and preeclampsia, probably because of fetal hypoxia. Sufficient control of asthma during pregnancy is associated with normal outcome. Current recommendations for maintenance therapy and for managing acute exacerbations are similar for pregnant and nonpregnant patients. These recommendations are based on the fact that no medications used for treating asthma have been found to be human teratogens. Data on albuterol use for asthma during pregnancy are more limited than for tocolysis. Surveys showed that among 1092 newborns exposed to albuterol during the first trimester, no higher number of expected major malformations was found. No data on the safety of other sympathomimetic agents or for ipratropium exist, but there is no reason to believe that they are associated with increased risk.

Use of corticosteroids during pregnancy has been controversial because animal studies show increased risk of cleft palate with high doses. Reports of more than 1000 human pregnancies failed to confirm this, and apparently, corticosteroids have little, if any, effect on development. Use of inhaled glucocorticosteroids is considered safe during pregnancy because of their low bioavailability. Two studies have demonstrated that using inhaled or oral glucocorticosteroids to treat severe asthma during the first trimester was not associated with increased risk of teratogenicity in 101 pregnancies. Risk of premature birth and low birthweight was slightly increased, probably due to the severity of the mothers' disease.

A study of 296 pregnant women indicated that cromolyn sodium was not associated with an increased risk of teratogenicity. Currently, there are no data on the safety of nedocromil during human pregnancy. Use of theophylline for asthma has declined in the 1990s, mainly due to fear of adverse effects and greater use of inhaled and oral glucocorticosteriods. If theophylline is judged necessary during pregnancy, however, it is safe to use.

Gastrointestinal disorders

Gastroesophageal reflux

Gastroesophageal reflux is a common and troublesome disorder during pregnancy. Heartburn affects 30 to 50% of all pregnant women and tends to worsen as pregnancy advances. Some women restrict their meals to once daily due to severe postprandial symptoms; others are forced to sleep upright all night. The main goal of treatment is to relieve the symptoms. Effective acid-suppressing drugs are available now for treating peptic and gastric ulcer, reflux esophagitis, and Zollinger-Ellison syndrome. Data on the safety of acid-suppressing drugs during human pregnancy are, however, scarce.

All H_2 blockers cross the human placenta. Animal reproductive toxicology studies, however, failed to show that any of the H_2 blockers were teratogenic. Of particular note, no consistent animal data prove that cimetidine has antiandrogenic effects in utero. Neither postmarketing surveillance studies conducted by North American drug manufacturers, five anecdotal reports of cimetidine or five of ranitidine exposure during the first trimester, nor record linkage studies and the Michigan Medicaid Surveillance Study (conducted from 1985 to 1992 examining cimetidine in 480 patients, ranitidine in 516 patients, and famotidine in 33 patients) have reported evidence of teratogenicity. There exists only a prospective study on the use of H_2 blockers during pregnancy that involved 178 women exposed during pregnancy compared with controls matched for age, smoking, and heavy alcohol consumption. Most patients ingested ranitidine (71%); others took cimetidine, famotidine, and nizatidine. No increase in major malformations was found following first-trimester exposure to H_2 blockers.

Omeprazole, a proton pump inhibitor, has been shown to be very efficient in treating duodenal and gastric ulcer and is the drug of choice for reflux esophagitis. Although it crosses the placenta, animal studies failed to show drug-induced teratogenicity following doses 250 to 500 times the recommended dose for humans. Human data are scarce and consist of a few published case reports and spontaneous reports to the manufacturer. In these reports there is no consistency in the type of abnormality reported or stage of pregnancy when the mother was exposed to omeprazole. In a prospective cohort study, outcomes of 113 pregnant women exposed to omeprazole during pregnancy, including 101 during organogenesis, were matched with 178 controls showing no significant difference in the incidence of major malformations in their infants. The groups were similar in many ways, including gestational age at delivery, number of preterm deliveries, birth weight, method of delivery, and neonatal health problems.

Cisapride is another widely used drug for gastrointestinal disorders. For this drug as well, the only prospective cohort study came from an international multicenter study of teratology information services that collected data regarding 129 exposures during pregnancy. Eighty-eight women were exposed during fetal organogenesis, and no differences in neonatal and maternal outcomes emerged when compared with matched control groups.

Nausea and vomiting

Nausea and vomiting are common during the first trimester as well as the last period of pregnancy because of physiologic changes. Usually, these symptoms do not require any pharmacologic treatment. However, in some cases antiemetics may be necessary. A doxylamine plus pyridoxine combination was used and studied most widely as a treatment for morning sickness.

Miscellaneous

Analgesics are the topic of some of the most frequently asked questions about symptomatic drug therapy in pregnancy. The drug of choice in pregnancy to treat pain or fever is acetaminophen (paracetamol). When used in therapeutic doses, no teratogenic or adverse effects have been observed. Aspirin also has been used in several conditions during pregnancy (e.g., pain, inflammation, hypertension, preeclampsia and eclampsia, tocolysis) without ever showing evidence of teratogenicity. However, because of its interference with fetal prostaglandin synthesis, which can result in peripartum bleeding, premature closure of ductus arteriosus and central nervous system hemorrhages, aspirin must be taken with caution during the third trimester.

Quite a while has passed now since increasing the intake of folic acid among women planning a pregnancy was shown to prevent neural tube defects. The evidence is conclusive: prevention is effective both for women who have not had a pregnancy in which neural tube defects in the fetus were involved and for those who have. National and international authorities have recommended that women planning a pregnancy should increase their intake of folic acid. The extra folic acid needed for a reasonably protective effect is 0.4 mg a day, twice the current average dietary intake of 0.2 mg. Data originating from clinical trials, observational studies of folate supplementation, studies on dietary intake of folate and neural tube defects (NTDs), studies on dietary counseling and recurrence of NTDs, and studies on folate concentration in serum and red cells have demonstrated the protective effect of this prophylaxis on the first occurrence or recurrence of NTDs. Sadly, most people are still not aware of the importance of folic acid in the prevention of NTDs.

GENERAL PRINCIPLES FOR DRUG PRESCRIBING AND COUNSELING DURING PREGNANCY

Prescribing

The drugs considered dangerous for newborns exposed in utero are few in number (see Tab. 88.1). Nevertheless, there is some doubt that certain drugs, if taken by the mother, can, under certain circumstances, affect the fetus or neonate profoundly, but most drugs probably do not affect it at all.

The following are the recommended guidelines for drug prescribing:

- Take into account that the maternal response to drugs can be modified by pregnancy or the puerpuerium.
- Consider the possibility of pregnancy when prescribing for women of childbearing age.
- During the first trimester of pregnancy, avoid the use of any drug that is not absolutely necessary and proven beneficial.
- After the first trimester, bear in mind that drugs have a potential to affect the fetus or neonate, even its later physiologic and behavioral development.
- Give precedence to older drugs with more documented exposure data regarding pregnant women and newborns exposed in utero.

- Consult the local teratology information service if you have any doubt about any drugs used during pregnancy.

Counseling

Ethical and methodologic problems make the issue of drug use during pregnancy an "orphan" area of controlled clinical data. Animal studies rarely may anticipate the identification of a new teratogenic agent. On the other hand, anecdotal reports regarding new potential teratogens may cause unwanted reactions in the public. A Canadian study demonstrated that pregnant women tend to assign unrealistically high values to the risks associated with their own intake of medications. Misperception of the real risk may lead to unwarranted termination of pregnancies. Even in the literature there are several examples of publications that present data on new potential teratogens that are not confirmed later. This "teratofilia" on behalf of science, which seems to rediscover time after time a new thalidomide, is always a source of panic after media reporting. In the absence of evidence-based studies, many pharmaceutical manufacturers warn the public to minimize or even avoid drug use during pregnancy. With both the unrealistically high perception of teratogenic risk related to drugs and the sometimes incorrect information regarding unfounded teratogenic potential of safe medications, it is not surprising that pregnant women tend to comply less than optimally with drug therapy. During the investigation of low drug serum concentrations during pregnancy, decreases in compliance therefore must be ruled out in addition to the above-mentioned pharmacokinetic changes.

In this context, *information* and *research* play key roles in the rational use of drugs during pregnancy. During the last 10 years, all over the world, specialized information centers (teratology information services) have been implemented for consultation regarding risk exposure during pregnancy. These programs are aimed at informing and counseling and sometimes at following up pregnant women exposed to drugs, chemicals, or radiation during pregnancy. Most of these services provide not only a question and answer service to practitioners and/or patients but also several programs to implement rational drug use during pregnancy (e.g., courses for heath operators, production of informative material, etc.). The collection and recording of data on maternal exposure of women in pregnancy have made it possible to carry out several prospective cohort studies and therefore to study the safety of many drugs. From this point of view, these centers represent a new approach to evaluating the reproductive risks of drugs and chemicals.

CONCLUSIONS

Although it would be ideal if drugs were not needed during pregnancy, they are currently taken both for maternal and fetal therapeutic needs as well as for less rational purposes. Safety is the main requisite for any intervention during pregnancy, but efficacy is also a crucial element of ethics. Unfortunately, the efficacy-safety balance profile of drug use during pregnancy remains undefined. Because the effect a drug has on a pregnant woman and her fetus depends on the type of drug, the amount and length of time for which it is taken, and the stage of the pregnancy during which it is taken, different methods and approach-es should be used to improve knowledge for a rational use of drugs during pregnancy. Thus, from basic to epidemiologic studies, a close relationship between pharmacokinetics, toxicology, teratology, and obstetrics needs to be established in order to provide valuable information in such a particular field. In the end it is important also to remember that clear and comprehensive health (and drug) information should be ensured to all (pregnant) women, in particular when the spectrum of doubts is wide and available information is extremely small.

Suggested readings

BONATI M, TOGNONI G, eds. Health Information Centers in Europe. What is their status? How should they develop? Milano: "Mario Negri" Institute for Pharmacological Research, 1995.

BRIGGS GG, FREEMAN RK, YAFFE SJ. Drugs in pregnancy and lactation, 5th ed. Baltimore: Williams & Wilkins, 1998.

CENTRO REGIONALE DI INFORMAZIONE SUI FARMACI Web site: http://www.irfmn.mnegri.it/mrpm.

COCHRANE LIBRARY. Updated software ed. Oxford, UK, 1993.

HEINONEN OP, SLONE D, SHAPIRO S. Birth defects and drugs in pregnancy. Littleton, Mass.: PSG Publishing Company, 1977.

KOREN G, ed. Maternal-fetal toxicology: a clinicians's guide. 2nd ed. New York: Marcel Dekker, 1994.

KOREN G, PASTUSZAK A, ITO S. Drugs in pregnancy. N Engl J Med 1998;338:1128-37.

LITILE BB. Pharmacokinetics during pregnancy: evidence - based material. Obstet Gynecol 1999;52:858-68.

LARRY C, GILSTRAP, eds. Drugs and pregnancy. Philadelphia: Lippincott Raven Pres Pubs, 2nd ed, 1997.

LOEBSTEIN R, LALKIN A, KOREN G. Pharmakinetic changes during pregnancy and their clinical relevance. Clin Pharmacokinet 1997; 33:328-43.

REPROTOX and SHEPPARD's Catalog of teratogenic

MOTHERISK PROGRAM. Web site: http://www.motherisk.org/.

PACIFICI GM, NOTTIOLI R. Placental transfer of drugs administered to the mother. Clin Pharmacokinet 1995; 28:235-269.

REPROTOX and SHEPPARD's Catalog of teratogenic agents. 1974-1999. Micromedex, Inc.

RUBIN P. Drug treatment during pregnancy. BMJ 1998;317:1503-6.

THEIS JGW, KOREN G. Maternal and fetal pharmacology. In Trevor M, Speight, Nicholas HG, eds. Avery's Drug treatment, 4th ed., Blackwell Science,1997.

The elderly

Pierugo Carbonin, Giuseppe Zuccalà

At present, all western populations are aging populations. The number of individuals over age 65 years has been growing in both absolute and relative terms since 1900. This growth is generally expected to speed up in coming years. The 85+ group is the fastest growing age segment; in Italy, for instance, the number of subjects aged 80+ is expected to double over the next 20 years.

About 90% of older persons take at least one medication; indeed, older persons have been reported to consume on average three to eight different agents daily. According to the database of the Italian Group of Pharmacoepidemiology in Older Persons (GIFA; about 25 000 subjects hospitalized all over Italy in 1988, 1991, 1993, and 1995), the number of drugs administered before hospitalization increased with age, from 2.5 in subjects aged 65 years or less to >3 in patients aged 74+ years; however, the number of drugs increased during hospitalization to 5.6 in younger patients and 6.4 in older patients, respectively. The most frequently administered agents are depicted in Table 89.1.

Apart from the economic impact of such a huge drug consumption, the increased risk of adverse drug reactions (which often present with atypical signs and symptoms) the interference of aging processes with drug kinetics and dynamics, and the peculiar problems regarding the impact of drug therapy on cognitive function, functional ability, and quality of life render clinical pharmacology a complex yet intriguing issue in geriatric medicine.

Age-related alterations in pharmacokinetics and pharmacodynamics

Volume of distribution

Significant alterations in the volume of distribution have been found as a consequence of the age-related modifications in body composition. In fact, the decrease in lean mass and total-body water leads to higher concentrations of many water-soluble agents in older patients so that, for instance, calculations for initial loading doses of most antibiotics must be modified. In this setting, particular attention must be paid to administration of aminoglycosides, since toxicity from these agents is proportional to peak concentrations. On the other hand, the volume of distribution of lipophilic agents such as diazepam, chlordiazepoxide, or thiopental increases with advancing age.

Clearance

The impact of age on hepatic clearance of drugs is as yet undefined. Probably the major age-related difference in hepatic metabolism has to do with benzodiazepines. In fact, many of these agents are converted into desmethyldiazepam, whose elimination half-life approximates 220 hours in older male subjects. Thus chlordiazepoxide, diazepam, chlorazepate, and prazepam are more likely to accumulate in elderly patients, causing excessive sedation and gait abnormalities. These side effects, in turn, may account for the increased risk of hip fracture observed in older subject taking benzodiazepines. Indeed, hepatic metabolism is also involved in transformation of some prodrugs, such as enalapril, into their active forms; thus aging may decrease the concentrations of active metabolites of such agents. However, as pointed out by the more recent studies on cytochrome P-450 isoforms, genetic variations are much more relevant than aging in determining hepatic metabolism of drugs (see Chap. 3).

Table 89.1 Drugs most frequently administered to 24 936 patients (mean age = 69 years) according to the GIFA database

Before admission	Patients (%)	During stay	Patients (%)
Digitalis	22.2	Digitalis	27.6
Nitrates	12.1	H$_2$ antagonists	22.6
Dihydropyridines	11.4	Loop diuretics	21.4
Loop diuretics	10.7	Nitrates	18.6
ACE inhibitors	10.6	Dihydropyridines	21.4
H$_2$ antagonists	9.3	Benzodiazepines	16.8
Benzodiazepines	8.6	ACE inhibitors	15.7
Antiplatelet agents	8.3	Heparin	13.6
Xanthines	4.3	Corticosteroids	12.6
Thiazides	1.7	Insulin	6.5

For these reasons, clearance of drugs undergoing hepatic transformation may be unpredictably changed in the aged. Table 89.2 provides a list of drugs whose clearance is unaffected or moderately affected by age. It is apparent that clearance appears to be essentially independent from the mode of metabolic transformation (type I versus type II reactions). Possibly, conjugations may be more sensitive to age-related changes.

The effects of advancing age on renal clearance of drugs are quite straightforward, since after age 20, a 10% decrease in creatinine clearance has been reported for each 10-year age increase (Tab. 89.3). Data on cross-sectional age differences in creatinine clearance, serum creatinine level, and 24-hour creatinine excretion are provided in Table 89.3.

The dosage of drugs with renal clearance and a narrow therapeutic range, i.e., drugs depending on renal excretory function, particularly digoxin and aminoglycosides, needs to be adjusted for age. In this setting, it should be pointed out, however, that the serum creatinine level per se does not always provide a reliable indicator of creatinine clearance

in older subjects, in whom creatinine synthesis, due to the muscle loss, is reduced.

Finally, a special case is that of drugs undergoing high extraction by the liver (see Chaps. 3 and 6). These include propranolol, verapamil, chlormethiazole, and others. Metabolism of these drugs is both saturable and dependent on liver blood flow, which is reduced in the elderly; the decrease in hepatic blood flow ranges from 12 to 14% (Tab. 89.4). As is clearly evident, kinetic changes occurring with age for drugs of this type are infrequently of elevated clinical significance.

Pharmacodynamics

Despite the relevance of degree of response to drugs in clinical practice, data regarding pharmacodynamics in advanced age are quite sparse and often conflicting. Indeed, clinical responses to single drugs or combinations of drugs usually develop at various levels, which are often unrelated to each other. For instance, the effects of anticholinergic medications on cardiac rhythm seem to be unaffected by age, whereas the effects on the central nervous system are increased in older patients. In a more general sense, older persons show increased rates of adverse effects from many drugs, such as digoxin; however, it is quite difficult to assess whether such effects are simply due to the aforementioned alterations in pharmacokinetics, which might result in altered serum and/or tissue drug levels. Variations in heart rate and blood pressure following the administration of β-blockers have been found to be reduced in older subjects; this has been attributed to the decreased expression of β-adrenergic receptors in older subjects. On the other hand, the hypotensive responses to α-blockers seem to increase with advancing age. Carvedilol (which yields mixed α-and β-blocking effects) has been proved effective in reducing mortality and left ventricular dysfunction in patients with heart failure, yet its use is severely limited in older subjects because of postural hypotension.

Adverse drug reactions

It is widely acknowledged that age is associated with an increased risk of adverse drug reactions (ADRs); however, data regarding the role of aging per se are conflicting. Age is not an independent risk factor for ADRs; rather, the association between increasing age and the occurrence of ADRs is mediated by the use of an increasing number of drugs in the elderly. As mentioned previously, polypharmacy is a common problem among older patients, who consume, on average, from three to eight drugs per day. In this setting, it should be pointed out that drugs may interfere with each other at all pharmacokinetic and pharmacodynamic levels, either directly or by causing pathologies (such as renal failure) that alter drug metabolism or excretion (see Chaps. 3 and 21). Apart from drug interactions, older subjects are simply more likely to consume two or more agents that share similar effects. For instance, combination treatment with antidepressants, antipsychotics, antihistamines, or sedative preparations can easily lead to urinary retention, confusion, or cardiac rhythm abnormalities owing to the anticholinergic effect of all these drugs.

Table 89.2 Relation of age to clearance of drugs cleared by hepatic biotransformation

Drug or metabolite	Initial pathway of biotransformation [1]
Evidence suggesting age-related reduction in clearance	
Antipyrine[2]	Oxidation (OH, DA)
Diazepam[2]	Oxidation (DA)
Chlordiazepoxide	Oxidation (DA)
Desmethyldiazepam[2]	Oxidation (OH)
Desalkylflurazepam[2]	Oxidation (OH)
Clobazam[2]	Oxidation (DA)
Alprazolam[2]	Oxidation (OH)
Quinidine	Oxidation (OH)
Theophylline	Oxidation
Propranolol	Oxidation (OH)
Nortriptyline	Oxidation (OH)
Small or negligible age-related change in clearance	
Oxazepam	Glucuronidation
Lorazepam	Glucuronidation
Temazepam	Glucuronidation
Warfarin	Oxidation (OH)
Lidocaine	Oxidation (DA)
Nitrazepam	Nitroreduction
Flunitrazepam	Oxidation (DA), nitroreduction
Isoniazid	Acetylation
Ethanol	Oxidation (alcohol dehydrogenase)
Metoprolol	Oxidation
Digitoxin	Oxidation
Prazosin	Oxidation

[1] OH denotes hydroxylation and DA dealkylation.
[2] Evidence suggests that the age-related reduction in clearance is greater in men than in woman.
(From Bressler R, Katz MD. Geriatric pharmacology. New York: McGraw-Hill, 1993, p. 48.)

Table 89.3 Cross-sectional age differences in creatinine clearance, serum creatinine level, and 24-hour creatinine excretion

Age (years)	Subjects (n)	Creatinine clearance (ml/min/1.73 m²)	Serum creatinine concentration (mg/100 ml)	Creatinine excretion (mg/24 h)
17-24	10	140.2[1] ± 3.7	0.808 ± 0.026	1790 ± 52
25-34	73	140.1 ± 2.5	0.808 ± 0.010	1862 ± 31
35-44	122	132.6 ± 1.8	0.813 ± 0.009	1746 ± 24
45-54	152	126.8 ± 1.4	0.829 ± 0.008	1689 ± 18
55-64	94	119.9 ± 1.7	0.837 ± 0.012	1580 ± 22
65-74	68	109.5 ± 2.0	0.825 ± 0.012	1409 ± 25
75-84	29	96.9 ± 2.9	0.843 ± 0.019	1259 ± 45

[1]Values indicate mean ± SEM.
(From Bressler R, Katz MD. Geriatric pharmacology. New York: McGraw-Hill, 1993.)

Table 89.4 Comparison of pharmacokinetic parameters of several flow-dependent (high extracted) drugs in young and old subjects

Drug	Old subjects			Young subjects		
	V_d (l/kg)	$t_{1/2}$, (h)	Cl	Vd (l/kg)	$t_{1/2}$, (h)	Cl
Indocyanine green	41.1 ± 5.3	4.7 ± 0.57 (min)	6.1 ± 0.6 (ml/min/kg)	41.6 ± 6.4	3.1 ± 0.3 (min)	7.1 ± 1.2 (ml/min/kg)
Lidocaine	0.85 ± 0.17	2.1 ± 0.14	5.0 ± 1.2 (ml/min/kg)	0.7 ± 0.2	1.5 ± 0.18	5.3 ± 1.5 (ml/min/kg
Nortriptyline	—	45 (23.5-79)	18.8 (l/h) (8.3-38.4)	—	26.8	54 + 24 (l/h)
Propranolol	4.2 ± 0.5	5.6 ± 0.6	9.0 ± 0.9 (ml/min/kg)	3.8 ± 0.3	4.5 ± 0.4	10.6 ± 1.3 (ml/min/kg
Morphine	4.7 ± 0.2	4.4 ± 0.25	12.4 ± 1.23 (ml/min/kg)	3.2 ± 0.3	2.95 ± 0.5	14.7 ± 0.9 (ml/min/kg)

(From Bressler R, Katz MD. Geriatric pharmacology. New York: McGraw-Hill, 1993.)

The "complexity" of aging

Polypathology, polypharmacy, and social inadequacy yield effects on drug treatment far beyond simple interference with pharmacokinetics and pharmacodynamics. Cognitive dysfunction, visual deficits, arthritis, arm paresis, tremor, and dysphagia all can hinder regular consumption of prescribed drugs; in addition many older patients simply cannot sustain the costs of agents needed for long-term treatments. In such cases, drug prescription must meet all the individual needs and deficits; drug treatment has to be fully explained to patients, as well as to caregivers; and tablets should be easily recognized and manipulated (in fact, liquid preparations may be preferred in some instances). In some cases, tablet dispensers labeled with the drug name, hour of administration, and day have proven useful.

Confusion in advanced age represents a common picture when etiology is shared by a host of diseases and pathologic conditions. In some instances, confusion can lead to a diagnosis of dementia, thus excluding older patients from effective, sometimes lifesaving treatments. Older patients with acute myocardial infarction, which often presents with confusion, do not receive thrombolytic treatment because they are thought to be demented. On the other hand, confusion is also a common form of adverse drug reaction in older patients; an example is digitalis toxicity, whose only sign can be disorientation. Thus, the onset of confusion in an older patient always poses a complex diagnostic task for the physician regarding the true etiology. Geriatric assessment can help physicians in disentangling the complex interrelationship between aging, polypathology, polypharmacy, disability, and psychosocial pitfalls.

Multidimensional evaluation also helps the physician to choose appropriate outcomes for drug treatment. In fact, physiologic modifications due to aging, such as those of the cardiovascular system, generally do not need pharmacologic treatment. In the most advanced age segments of the population, the role of mortality as a primary outcome variable becomes uncertain; for instance, in the Baltimore Longitudinal Study on Aging, a definite diagnosis of heart disease was not associated with increased risk of mortality in patients aged 80 years and over. Thus, in many instances, quality of life and functional ability should be considered as primary outcomes of drug treatment. The main areas explored by the various assessment instruments so far developed to quantify both quality of life and the impact of interventions on health-related quality of life (such as the SF-36) include physical functioning, social functioning, pain, mental health, and interference of mood disorders and physical problems with usual daily activities.

Evidence-based medicine in advanced age

Evidence-based medicine requires sound data derived from randomized, controlled trials conducted on representative population samples. However, data regarding the oldest age segments of the population available from intervention trials are sparse and often conflicting. In this setting, many examples are offered by results of trials on thrombolytic therapy for acute myocardial infarction. For instance, the Gruppo Italiano per lo Studio della Streptochinasi nell' Infarto Miocardico (GISSI-1) reported a significant reduction in mortality associated with administration of streptokinase in patients younger than 66 years but not among older participants. Nevertheless, the number of lives saved exceeded 4 per 100 treated in the older group, whereas it was only 2 among younger patients. Also, the Intravenous Streptokinase in Acute Myocardial Infarction (ISAM) trial found a higher mortality among treated older patients as compared with younger participants, but results were not statistically significant because of the insufficient number of older subjects. On the other hand, other studies such as the Anglo-Scandinavian Study of Early Thrombolysis (ASSET) trial or the APSAC International Mortality Study (AIMS) trial found a reduced risk of mortality in older patients with the use of thrombolysis. Owing to comorbidity or disability, older patients are more likely to be excluded from trials, so their number is almost invariably too narrow to allow reliable risk-benefit calculations. Indeed, older patients have been excluded by design from most trials. In addition, in many cases, such as for trials on hypertensive patients, real placebo groups cannot be obtained. Another important issue is represented by the need to consider the absolute rather than the relative risk reduction when examining the results of trials. For example, the relative benefit from reduction in the incidence of stroke in many trials on antihypertensive treatment does not vary according to the event rate, whereas a steep increase is observed in the absolute benefit with increasing event rates. Elderly patients are known to have higher morbidity and mortality after myocardial infarction; thus even small reductions in relative risk obtained with thrombolytic treatment can lead to relevant absolute benefits.

Major issues in geriatric clinical pharmacology

Dementia

Alzheimer's disease (see Chap. 12) represents the most frequent cause of cognitive dysfunction in older subjects. It has been found that over 47% of persons aged 85+ years suffer from such a condition. Therefore, the social and economic benefits of an effective treatment of Alzheimer's dementia (AD) would be huge. So far, only acetylcholinesterase inhibitors have proved effective in patients with mild to moderate cognitive dysfunction. These agents improve cognitive performance in about 25 to 50% of treated patients; some data suggest that they also could delay the onset of behavioral symptoms, which usually lead to institutionalization of demented patients. The effects of acetylcholinesterase inhibitors on patients with other types of dementias, e.g., multi-infarction dementia, have not yet been defined. Tacrine, the first clinically available acetylcholinesterase inhibitor, appears to give better responses in patients with early symptoms, in carriers of the apoE4 allele, and in those who can bear a daily dosage of 80 mg. The second-generation acetylcholinesterase inhibitor donepezil has proven efficacy in AD patients with mild to moderate symptoms; its increased selectivity and prolonged half-life allow a single 5- to 10-mg daily administration. Nausea, vomiting, and diarrhea are the main adverse effects, which usually fade within 2 weeks.

Hypertension

The prevalence of hypertension exceeds 50% among persons aged 65+ years. Some studies, however, suggested the possibility of U- or J-shaped mortality curves with decreasing blood pressure levels, i.e., that excessive blood pressure lowering might increase mortality rates among older subjects. However, further observations indicated that the excess mortality in older subjects with the lowest blood pressure levels was associated with poor cardiovascular health. In the Framingham Study, subjects aged 75+ showed a distinct U-shaped mortality curve, with increased event rates at systolic pressure levels below 120 mm Hg; nevertheless, such an increase could not be noted in subjects free of cardiovascular disease. At present, treatment of hypertension in older patients must be considered mandatory, since large trials have provided evidence that antihypertensive drug therapy reduces incident coronary events, stroke, cardiovascular disease, heart failure, and mortality; however, blood pressure values below 120/90 mm Hg are best avoided in subjects with coronary disease.

Despite the aforementioned limitations in the intervention trials so far conducted, there is enough evidence to consider diuretics and/or β-blockers as first-line treatment. It has been suggested that loop diuretics may be safer than thiazides because of their shorter duration of action and greater natriuresis/kaliuresis ratio; however, such a hypothesis has yet to be proved. Calcium antagonists have been shown to be useful in reducing morbidity, but not total mortality. The controversy regarding safety and efficacy (in terms of long-term survival) of calcium antagonists is still on; however, the main caveats for these agents seem to be represented by the presence of coronary disease (particularly for short-acting nifedipine preparations) and treatment with nonsteroidal anti-inflammatory drugs, which seem to promote gastrointestinal and surgical bleeding. In addition, drugs that may induce or aggravate postural hypotension (such as β-blockers or high-dose diuretics) or associated with increased incidence of cognitive dysfunction (e.g., central α_2-agonists) should be used with caution in older patients.

Heart failure

Despite the improved treatment of hypertension and coronary disease over the last few years, the prevalence and incidence of heart failure are increasing among the oldest age segments of the population; at present, heart failure represents the most commonly diagnosed condition in older patients admitted to acute hospital departments and a major determinant of disability in advanced age. All inotropic agents are not recommended for the long-term treatment of this condition, since they have been found to increase mortality in controlled trials. Antiarrhythmic therapy generally has been associated with decreased survival rates in patients with congestive heart failure; the role of amiodarone is still under evaluation.

Diuretics are the most effective agents currently available for treating congestive symptoms of heart failure; however, they do not seem to affect survival. ACE inhibitors represent the mainstay of chronic treatment for heart failure; they have been proven to decrease both mortality and progression of left ventricular dilatation. Most recently, the angiotensin II receptor blocker losartan has proven more effective than captopril in reducing total mortality in older patients with heart failure; moreover, fewer patients discontinued losartan because of adverse drug reactions as compared with those treated with captopril. A follow up study failed, however, to establish a useful role for losartan in heart failure (see Chaps. 6-27).

The role of digoxin in heart failure with sinus rhythm has long been debated. However, two recent studies provided evidence that the use of digitalis is associated with delayed progression of heart failure, with reduced hospitalization rates; thus, treatment with digoxin has been recommended on an economic basis. The DIG trial definitely has proved the efficacy of digitalis therapy on hospitalization rates and worsening of heart failure in older patients already treated with ACE inhibitors and diuretics (see Chaps. 26-27).

Use of β-blockers, which have proved effective in reducing mortality and disease progression in young and middle-aged patients with heart failure, is not evidence-based in older subjects but may be considered in patients without diabetes, obstructive pulmonary disease, or peripheral vascular disease. Most recently, carvedilol has been used successfully in patients with left ventricular systolic dysfunction, yet its use, due to its α-adrenergic blocking properties, is frequently associated in older patients with postural hypotension.

Osteoporosis

Hip fracture is becoming a crucial health and social problem in western countries. Its incidence increases exponentially with age; in 80-year-old women, the incidence of hip fracture averages 2 per 100 persons per year. A steep increase in the incidence of hip fracture has been reported in Europe, with an 11-fold increase among women and a 7-fold among men over the 1973-1985 period. One-year mortality in older patients with hip fracture ranges between 15 and 30%, and long-term institutionalization is required in 25%. The annual cost of osteoporotic fractures to health services has been estimated at $13 billion in the United States and £750 million in the United Kingdom. Thus, prevention of osteoporosis represents a major challenge to health care systems. Hormone replacement is considered by many authors to be the mainstay of treatment for osteoporosis (see Chap. 46). Oral, transdermal, and parenteral formulations have all been shown to prevent bone loss in menopausal and postmenopausal women and to reduce the risk of fractures, at least in observational studies. The effects of estrogens (conjugated estrogens, 0.625 mg per day; estradiol, 1-2 mg per day; transdermal estradiol, 50 μg per day; estradiol implants, 50 mg twice yearly) and combined estrogen-progesterone preparations are similar (see Chap. 67). Selective estrogen receptor modulators, such as raloxifene, are currently considered as promising alternatives to estrogen treatment. Biphosphonates are effective in reducing osteoclastic bone reabsorption; they can increase spinal bone density by 5 to 8% and femoral neck bone density by 4% with 3-year treatments and reduce the incidence of vertebral fractures by up to 50%. These agents need to be taken 2 or more hours before meals to increase drug absorption. All forms of calcitonin (i.e., porcine, human, salmon, and eel) have been shown to inhibit postmenopausal spinal bone loss, even though at cortical sites. However, the effects on fracture risk have not been definitely proved. Calcium and vitamin D supplementation have been found to reduce bone loss at the femoral neck, spine, and total-body levels and to decrease the incidence of nonvertebral fractures after 3-year treatment in subjects aged 65+ years. The clinical efficacy of sodium fluoride, ipriflavone, and anabolic steroids on the risk of fractures has not been established.

Hypercholesterolemia

The prognostic role of hypercholesterolemia in older patients has been long debated. However, recent data have suggested a beneficial effect of cholesterol lowering with statins on morbidity and mortality in coronary patients aged 65 to 70 years. These agents have proved to be effective and well tolerated; nevertheless, they are expensive, and the cost frequently is not covered by health care systems. Given the increased number of cardiovascular event rates, older patients may achieve a substantially higher absolute risk reduction.

Suggested readings

BERNABEI R, ZUCCALÀ G, CARBONIN PU. Thrombolytic therapy for elderly patients with myocardial infarction. JAMA 1997; 278:1401-2.

BRESSLER R, KATZ MD. Geriatric pharmacology. New York: McGraw-Hill, 1993.

CARBONIN P, ZUCCALÀ G. Inotropic agents in older patients with chronic heart failure: Current perspectives. Aging Clin Exp Res 1996;8:90-8.

CARBONIN P, PAHOR M, BERNABEI R, SGADARI A. Is age an independent risk factor of adverse drug reactions in hospitalized medical patients? J Am Geriatr Soc 1991;39:1093-9.

FOZARD JL, METTER EJ, BRANT LJ. Next steps in describing aging and disease in longitudinal studies. J Gerontol 1990;45:116-27.

GAMBASSI G, CARBONIN P, BERNABEI R. Angiotensin-converting enzyme inhibitors for elderly patients with congestive heart failure. Arch Intern Med 1997;158:97-8.

PAHOR M, CECCHI E, FUMAGALLI S, et al. Association of serum creatinine and age with headache caused by nitrates. Clin Pharmacol Ther 1995;58:470-81.

PAHOR M, CHRISCHILLES EA, GURALNIK JM, et al. Drug data coding and analysis in epidemiologic studies. Eur J Epidemiol 1994;10:405-11.

PAHOR M, GURALNIK JM, GAMBASSI G, et al. The impact of age on the risk of adverse drug reactions to digoxin. J Clin Epidemiol 1993;46:1305-14.

PAHOR M, MUGELLI A, GURALNIK JM, et al. Age and laxative use in hospitalized patients. Aging Clin Exp Res 1995;7:128-35.

PITT B, SEGAL R, MARTINEZ FA, et al. Randomised trial of losartan versus captopril in patients over 65 with heart failure (Evaluation of Losartan in the Elderly Study, ELITE). Lancet 1997;349:747-52.

THE SIXTH REPORT OF THE JOINT NATIONAL COMMITTEE ON PREVENTION, DETECTION, EVALUATION, AND TREATMENT OF HIGH BLOOD PRESSURE. Arch Intern Med 1997;157:2413-46.

VACCARINO V, BERKMAN LF, MENDES DE LEON CF, et al. Functional disability before myocardial infarction in the elderly as a determinant of severity and postinfarction mortality. Arch Intern Med 1997;157:2196-204.

ZUCCALÀ G, PAHOR M, LANDI F, et al. Use of calcium antagonists and need for perioperative transfusion in older patients with hip fracture:observational study. Br Med J 1997;314:643-4.

ZUCCALÀ G, PEDONE C, CAROSELLA L, et al. Optimum dose of digoxin. Lancet 1997;349:1845.

Pharmacoeconomics

CHAPTER

90

Pharmacoeconomics

Thomas D. Szucs

In the past few years, the discipline of pharmacoeconomics has experienced an extraordinary boom within the health care sector. Researchers from a wide range of disciplines have developed new techniques to evaluate the impact of pharmaceuticals on clinical care. Clinicians, pharmacists, economists, epidemiologists, and operations researchers have contributed to the new field of pharmacoeconomics by studying how different approaches to patient care influence the resources consumed in clinical medicine. In front of the basic economic notion that resources are limited and desires, as well as needs, are infinite, pharmacoeconomists try to find solutions to how these resources can be allocated appropriately to maximize the production of health. The common denominator is the search for increased efficiency and effectiveness of health care services and products. Among these efforts, several researchers, especially within the pharmaceutical industry and academia, also have begun to study the economic impact of medicines on health care provision on a micro- and macroeconomic level. This new field of research – pharmacoeconomics – has grown at a tremendous rate, supplying ample evidence of the economic benefits of modern therapeutics.

Not all products, however, have to be subjected to a pharmacoeconomic appraisal. A simple decision tool is displayed in Figure 90.1. This figure takes the two main outcomes of a potential evaluation into consideration: the costs and clinical results or quality of a medical intervention. In circumstances where a drug is more costly and leads to better results, an economic evaluation is advisable. When a drug is available at a lower cost and yields a better outcome, the drug should be accepted. Alternatively, when a more costly drug produces a less favorable outcome, one should reject this drug. Economic evaluations, however, may assist in identifying drugs with worse outcomes that are also cheaper, because this will determine the extent of potential rationalization reserves under the constraints of a limited expenditure ceiling.

THE CHALLENGES OF PHARMACO-ECONOMICS

Despite the methodologic challenges just mentioned, pharmacoeconomic analyses will be critical to the rational allo-

cation of resources by manufacturers, providers, and payers. Many questions can be answered by pharmacoeconomic studies (Tab. 90.1). Effectiveness analysis and outcomes research can help manufacturers allocate research and development funds and make product development decisions. When built into phase III and phase IV studies, cost-effectiveness analyses also can help payers and providers make coverage and utilization decisions and assist the industry in documenting the value of the products it is manufacturing (see Chap. 91). The rational use of new and established technologies is also going to require increased technologic assessment, a better assessment of patient preferences, and more rigorous pharmacoeconomic analyses. The benefit of such assessments, however, certainly will be worth their cost.

Health economics will become one of the most strategic success factors for the pharmaceutical industry in this era of cost containment. The challenge will be not only to meet the requirements of government agencies and payers, who increasingly are asking for economic assessments of commercial products, but also to address the value of medical economics to clinicians. In the future it will be necessary for clinicians to apply the tools of economic analysis both in research and in practice. Instead of waiting for policy analysts, third-party payers, or governmental agencies to hand down decisions about which services are worth the cost, physicians also may become practicing clinical economists. Another approach is to

Table 90.1 The questions that pharmacoeconomic studies can answer

Which drug should be included in the list of services, and which should be eliminated?

What effect will the results of a particular drug have on a patient's quality of life?

Which of several drugs is the most cost-effective?

What are the relative costs and benefits of comparable drugs?

What is the cost per quality year of life saved by using a therapeutic regimen?

What is the best drug for treating a particular condition?

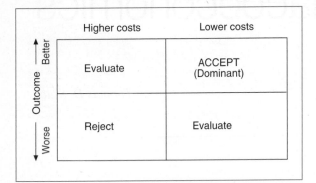

Figure 90.1 Possible outcomes of an economic evaluation.

explore ways in which clinical decisions are influenced by, as well as influence, the cost of care. Clinicians need to integrate economic thinking into their decision making if medical care is to be rational but not rationed. Pharmaceutical companies can contribute significantly to this process by expanding economic research on their products, by providing training and know-how to medical professionals, and by encouraging consumers to acknowledge the validity of such research.

SCARCITY AND HEALTH CARE RESOURCES

The fundamental aim of any health care system is to maximize the health and welfare of the population, but because resources will always be scarce in relation to health care needs, a series of choices must be made. Individuals responsible for allocating resources need to prioritize among competing uses in order to maximize the benefit (or health gain) from any given budget. Prioritization may take place on a health authority level as planners decide on the speciality and service mix they wish to purchase for their residents, or it may take place at the hospital level when decisions are made about the purchase of medical and surgical equipment or medicines. Moreover, at the level of the individual clinician, prioritization can be expected to exert increasing influence as medical audits and other forms of peer review lead toward protocols and clinical guidelines that define what should be done, how it should be done, and for whom it should be done. Economic evaluation provides a decision-making framework that can be used to assist all these decisions.

LIMITATIONS OF PHARMACOECONOMICS

Pharmacoeconomics will not solve all substantive issues, however. For instance, the results of a study may not be conclusive enough to improve the quality of decision making. Or the cost of gathering an extra piece of information may be far more than the extra benefit it gives the decision maker. In addition, it is vital to be aware that health care cannot be rationed using a simple economic calculation. There are always moral and ethical issues for society to take into consideration.

There is also a political danger associated with economic evaluations. They may become the "fourth hurdle" for the registration of new products. Not only may regulators review data about a product's efficacy, safety, and quality, but they also may demand economic efficiency. This is already occurring in some countries (see above).

There are, however, practical problems related to the introduction of a statutory requirement for economic appraisals. They may delay patient access to new technologies and reduce returns to innovators. Because they are expensive and time-consuming, economic appraisals could push costs up. Results may be challenged because there are yet no "gold standards" for conducting economic trials (see below), and many regulatory bodies do not (yet) have the expertise to review economic data. Nonetheless, many countries are moving toward statutory economic evaluations of new health care products, e.g., in the Canadian province of Ontario and in Australia for pharmaceuticals.

TARGETING PHARMACOECONOMIC STUDIES TO DIFFERENT AUDIENCES

Designing a pharmacoeconomic study to address effectively the issues at hand from the perspective of the audience is important to adequately convey the results. In most cases, the pharmacoeconomic analysis is to support choices between alternatives for rational therapy in a particular disease. Rational therapy is in the first instance defined with respect to efficacy. However, results and factors from "real life" settings – the effectiveness of therapy – often differ greatly from those in the carefully controlled setting of the clinical trial, and factors other than efficacy have to be studied. A third dimension to be explored (the pharmacoeconomic one) is the efficiency of the therapy itself with respect to viable alternatives. There are, however, two different meanings for *efficiency:* (1) technical efficiency and (2) allocative efficiency. The *technical efficiency* of an instrument can be crudely defined as its ability to reach effects with the minimum cost possible. With respect to health care, many concerns can be raised about the definitions of effect and cost.

Effects can be intermediate physical outputs such as blood pressure reduction; they can be final physical outcomes such as deaths prevented per years of life saved; they can be final physical outcomes weighed for their utility such as quality-adjusted life-years (QALYs) and HYEs (healthy year equivalents) and they can be physical outcomes translated into monetary terms, also taking into consideration distributional variables. Different outcomes have different implications and a different "appeal" to researchers and decision makers. The same issue can be applied to cost; direct, indirect, and intangible are different categories relating to different aspects of the same events (e.g., treatments, diseases) that have an impact on different dimensions or domains of human life at both an individual and a social level. This point raises the matter of *allocative efficiency.* An allocation of resources can be rated as efficient when its opportunity costs are at the minimum possible level. This has to do with the distribution and redistribution of resources within a system, e.g., society.

Decisions also will be made with respect to specific economic constraints, e.g., budget constraints on the side of the decision maker. Public decision-makers are often concerned with allocative efficiency (i.e., they place resources where they are not only effective but also positively judged), whereas private parties generally are interested in technical efficiency. The choice of perspective may then influence the choice of the type of efficiency and, as a consequence, the type of study.

Depending on the context, both drug and nondrug therapy will need to be considered to quantify costs and benefits. Opportunity costs and the costs and benefits of doing nothing also should be taken into account, as well as the inevitable value judgments involved.

PERSPECTIVE OF THE STUDY

The perspective of the study must be tailored to the audience. The natural audience for such a study is the person who can and/or must make allocative decisions or is involved in the decision-making process, both directly and indirectly (lobbies and pressure groups), especially if the aim of the study is to allocate resources rationally. The perspectives of a pharmacoeconomic study generally fall into one of the following categories. The wider perspective is *society.* Certain minimum standards of care are demanded for all in society, and the consequences eventually fall into the wide field of society. With newer, sophisticated, and increasingly expensive therapies draining society's health care funds, the limits of health care to be provided to an individual will need to be reexamined. For this reason, pharmacoeconomic studies are particularly important: to treat those conditions as efficiently as possible for which safe and acceptable alternative therapies exist so that funds remain to treat threatening, more complex conditions. The problem with this perspective is that it is often too broad. Consequently, it is very difficult to include and compute all costs. In addition, society does not make decisions directly. Moreover, it only makes sense to compute and calculate the costs of an intervention if decisions can be made regarding this phenomenon; otherwise, the economic evaluation is a sterile exercise, since an action cannot be implemented.

Societies tend to organize themselves into *states* and *governments,* and these constitute other perspectives for pharmacoeconomic evaluations. Unfortunately, states and governments are generally too big to make decisions directly; they often create agencies designed to manage particular fields of human action. Specific agencies also exist for managing health care (e.g., national health services). Such agencies can manage health care directly or indirectly in a number of different ways. They can *pay*

for health services, partially or totally, directly or indirectly. They also can *provide* health services, partially or totally, directly or indirectly. They can force all citizens or some categories of citizens to prepare health insurance forms, or they can simply create incentives to subscribe to an insurance carrier. Hence a *national health service* (NHS) providing services or simply paying for them (e.g., à la Beveridge) or a *compulsory health insurance system* (à la Bismarck) may exist. Alternatively, an extremely complex system such as that in the United States can exist, where health insurance is voluntary but incentives exist to subscribe to an insurance carrier and where some citizens are covered by the federal government. In this sense, we can consider two great subjects: the *health care provider* and the *third party payer.* The study will then differ according to different perspectives and the "vocations" of different subjects. Private providers generally are willing to consider only their costs and benefits in order to maximize their profits; they will need information about how a treatment affects their workload, revenues, productivity, and availability of services, as well as logistic issues. The hospital budget and the opportunity costs of allocating resources to the therapy under examination are other important factors.

The *payer* naturally is concerned with budget constraints. Whether the payer is a health maintenance organization or a statutory or private health insurance organization, the costs of the services provided are carefully compared so as to select the most efficient treatment; this may not always be the most effective approach. This perspective of the payer is powerful in any health care provision scenario. The payer also can be a national health service, and it can acknowledge itself to be nothing more than an agency of society.

Increasingly, the *patient,* both as a decision-maker (i.e., as the payer of his/her own personal out-of-pocket expenses) and as a member of a pressure group, will desire insight into the consequences of his treatment. Factors to be considered are the nonreimbursable portion of treatment costs paid by the individual, quality of life, increased years of life, and independent functioning. Intangible costs, such as grief and discomfort, are difficult to measure but are obviously important to consider.

Once the audience and relevant issues have been defined, it is important to reach agreement as to the goals and objectives of the analysis. When defining the objective, bear in mind the potential uses of the economic evaluations for the audience. For example, a clear objective in assessing a growth factor indicated for neutropenia caused by chemotherapy would be to provide hospital pharmacists with the details of the impact of the drug on antibiotic consumption before assessing the drug's impact on reducing productivity losses. A study can be designed to assess alternative therapies when undertaking national price negotiations and to determine the reimbursement status or copayment level when deciding to include a product on local formularies or treatment guidelines or in improving prescribing decisions. For pharmaceutical companies, the advantages of one drug therapy over another will be of importance in convincing regulatory agencies of the value of the company's product, in allocating marketing budgets, in revamping a new product, and in determining the drug's price.

It also must be made clear why a study is needed, since this will determine the focus and limits of the study. This will then determine the type of study required. For instance, if an identical or nearly identical outcome is desired, the least expensive approach to this outcome can be reviewed through a cost-minimization study. Cost-benefit analyses measure absolute benefits of alternative programs such as medical complications or disability days avoided. Cost-effectiveness analyses relate to measuring resources used in achieving a single common effect, such as life-years gained. The value of a particular improvement in health status is quantified using cost-utility analyses. Even after considerable attention in the literature, and despite the availability of excellent texts outlining the differences between various pharmacoeconomic studies, the terms are frequently confused. In particular, the concepts of cost containment and efficiency (both technical and allocative), i.e., crudely, the rational use of scarce resources, are confused.

Once the audience perspective and the type of study have been decided on, any official requirements (e.g., formal guidelines) should be checked before designing the study. For instance, Germany's social security law states that all health services must be provided economically and that "the principle of economic efficiency should guide the behavior of providers and payers." If the group to whom the results will be presented has not drawn up formal requirements, the study can use other recognized guidelines as a model. Guidelines adopted by the U.S. Pharmaceutical Research and Manufacturers of America and/or the Food and Drug Administration have been discussed increasingly, with a wide base of approval.

THE MAJOR COMPONENTS OF A PHARMACOECONOMIC EVALUATION

All economic studies investigate the balance between inputs (e.g., the consumption of resources) and outcomes (e.g., improvements in the state of health of individuals and/or society).

INPUTS (COSTS)

Although the unit price of a drug is often a prime factor in decision-making, economic outcomes research provides a more comprehensive interpretation of cost. This is accomplished by determining the overall cost of a given diagnostic or therapeutic process from diagnosis until a final outcome is achieved. The various types of costs can be grouped under the following categories:

- direct medical costs,
- direct nonmedical costs, and
- indirect costs.

Direct medical costs

Interpretations of what belongs in each of these categories vary in the economic literature. *Direct medical costs* are defined as the resources used by a provider in the delivery of medical care. For example, direct medical costs for a hospital include (1) drugs, (2) laboratory tests, (3) medical supplies, (4) use of diagnostic equipment (e.g., magnetic resonance imaging, computed tomographic scans, and radiographs), (5) medical staff time for personnel such as physicians, nurses, pharmacists, physical therapists, and laboratory technicians, and (6) room and board – the cost of supplies, equipment, and personnel required for routine patient-related services such as food, laundry, and housekeeping.

These are examples of costs that can be related directly to patient care. Other costs of operating a hospital include plant maintenance and repairs, utilities, telephone service, accounting, legal fees, insurance, taxes, real estate costs, and interest expense. In general, most economic studies do not factor general operating costs into the dollar value assigned to the cost of resources expended for a given therapy.

Looking down the list of direct medical expenses, it is easy to see why length of stay is an important cost factor to hospitals, especially when payment is determined by diagnosis-related groups (DRGs). Costs such as room and board are directly tied to the length of stay, regardless of the reason. The cost of laboratory tests, supplies, and medical staff time vary with the medical condition being treated but are multiplied by the length of stay.

Since the introduction of DRGs, a common selling strategy has been to emphasize how a given technology such as a new antimicrobial drug can help shorten hospital stay. More recently, economic studies began to collect and analyze data linking specific therapeutic strategies to length of stay. Length of stay in hospital settings translates to the number of patient visits in a managed care settings. Although the specific items included under the category of direct medical costs will be slightly different in managed care organizations, the same principles of cost analysis apply. Drugs that achieve results quickly and predictably benefit not only the patient but also to the provider by reducing the number of patient visits. Every patient visit incurs provider resource costs that may not be reimbursed by a third-party payer. Drugs that minimize patient visits are clearly a cost savings for the health care organization.

Direct nonmedical costs

The economic literature generally defines *direct nonmedical costs* as out-of-pocket expenses paid by the patient for items outside the health care sector. This category includes such costs as (1) travel to and from the hospital, clinic, or doctor's office, (2) travel and lodging for family members who live elsewhere, (3) domestic help or home nursing services, (4) insurance copayments and premiums, and (5) treatment not covered by third-party payers.

Although these costs are generally classified as "nonmedical," to the patient they are real and often substantial costs of medical care. What makes them nonmedical is that they are not costs incurred by the health care provider and are somewhat difficult to measure. For example, a patient's inability to afford competent follow-up care at home may result in poor compliance with drug therapies and eventual treatment failure. This may lead to additional hospital stays or office visits, which affect the provider's bottom line. Moreover, a patient's inability to bear the unreimbursed cost of medications also may lead to poor compliance and costly complications. Finally, high transportation costs may lead to missed appointments for necessary follow-up visits, which can result in deterioration of a patient's medical condition and increased treatment costs for the provider.

Even though these costs may not be incurred directly by the provider, they can be used in selling situations by making the provider aware of their potential economic impact. It also may be possible to use these costs to encourage payers (e.g., employers, insurance companies) to discuss the use of a more cost-effective test with the health care provider.

Indirect costs

One definition of *indirect costs* is the overall economic impact of illness on a patient's life. These costs include (1) loss of earnings due to temporary, partial, or permanent disability, (2) unpaid assistance by family members in providing home health care, and (3) loss of income to family members who forfeit paid employment to remain at home and care for the patient.

Like direct nonmedical costs, indirect costs are real to the patient but abstract to the provider – but they may have an impact on the provider's direct medical costs. For example, patients who cannot earn income may not be able to pay their bills, including their medical bills. Economic hardship may result in poor compliance with drug therapies as patients reduce doses or fail to refill prescriptions to save money. The medical provider may have to bear the additional costs of managing complications. Economic hardship also may result in missed follow-up appointments, leading to the same types of problems for providers as described previously with direct nonmedical costs.

Note the overlap between quality of life and indirect costs. Both measures deal with the impact of disability. However, quality of life relates to the psychologic, physical, and/or social dimensions of disability, whereas indirect costs relate to its economic effects.

CONSEQUENCES AND OUTCOMES

Final states or outcomes can be *negative* (sometimes referred to as the "five D's"): death, disability (patient is permanently disabled and unable to return to work or school, perform household chores, etc.), discomfort (patient is in a constant state of moderate to high-level pain), dissatisfaction (patient is not satisfied with the course of treatment or services provided), and disease (patient's condition is not being controlled, resulting in frequent relapses, rehospitalizations, and expenditure of additional resources).

There are also *positive* outcomes; namely, the patient is cured; the patient is able to resume normal functions; the patient enjoys an improved or satisfactory quality of life; or the patient's medical condition is managed successfully or stabilized by continued drug therapy.

The use of outcomes research represents an important advance in medical economic analysis because of the relationship between the final state, or result, of diagnosis and therapy and overall cost-effectiveness. If one can demonstrate that a product achieves cost-effective positive outcomes, one increases the chances of selling that product.

AVERAGE, MARGINAL, AND JOINT COSTS

Most decisions in health care are not concerned with whether or not a service should be provided or whether or not a particular procedure should be undertaken; rather, such decisions center on how much of the service or procedure should be provided. That is, should existing levels of provision by expanded or contracted? For example, should the existing provision of day care for people with mental illness be expanded and, if so, by how much? What family planning services should be made available? How many patients presenting with head injuries should have computed tomograms? All these decisions require that attention be focused on marginal costs – that is, on the change in total costs resulting from a marginal change in activity.

In the short run there is often an important difference between the marginal costs of an activity and that activity's average cost, where the *average cost* is defined as the total costs divided by the total number of units of output

Table 90.2 Total, average, and marginal costs ($): an illustration

No. of patients treated	Total cost	Average cost	Marginal cost
10	4000	400	0
20	5000	250	100
30	6000	200	100
40	6800	170	80
50	7400	148	60

*In this example, each marginal cost is provided by the "rates": differences in total cost/differences in number of patients treated (e.g., 6800-6000/40-30=80)

(Tab. 90.2). An example is provided by a study of the cost-effectiveness of hypolipidemic treatment in the prevention of coronary heart disease. In this study, the marginal cost was calculated per life-year saved of continuing drug treatment for successive periods of 5 additional years for patients between 35 and 70 years of age. These calculations indicated large differences between average and marginal cost-effectiveness, since marginal costs increased quite steeply after 55 years of age.

Another context in which the distinction between average and marginal costs is important is in relation to duration of hospital stay of inpatients. Many new procedures have reduced the amount of time necessary for a patient to remain in hospital and thereby have yielded cost savings. When valuing these savings, however, it is important to keep in mind that using average costs per day generally will overstate the savings because the later days of a stay usually cost less than the earlier days. It is the marginal costs per day that is the relevant measure.

Another problem of cost measurement arises in connection with joint costs. Often a single production process can result in multiple outputs. For example, a single chemical analysis of a blood sample can diagnose the presence of many diseases. How should the cost be allocated to each diagnosis? Similarly, within a hospital setting, there are many common services (such as medical records, radiology, operating theaters, laundry, catering, and cleaning) that contribute to a number of specialties. Economic evaluation requires some method for allocating the joint costs of these services to individual programs or procedures. Several methods may be used to do this. Most of them use some physical unit of utilization, such as the number of laboratory tests, hours of operating theater use, or square feet of ward space, to apportion total laboratory, operating theater, and ward cleaning costs.

COSTS OF CAPITAL

Investments in buildings and equipment that yield a flow of services over a number of years give rise to capital costs. Generally, investment expenditure will be undertaken at the beginning of a project, but the use of items of capital equipment will generate annual capital costs over the lifetime of the asset. These costs have two components – namely, interest and depreciation. *Interest costs* should be included even if the asset was not acquired with borrowed money because tying up money in an item of capital equipment involves an opportunity cost, i.e., interest foregone. *Depreciation costs* arise because of the wear and tear that an asset receives through use and the consequent reduction in the length of its useful life.

Sometimes an item of capital expenditure is unique to a particular use and has little or no alternative use value (opportunity cost). In such cases, it is referred to as a *sunk cost*. A hospital building or an item of medical equipment, for example, may have considerable value in its existing use but little resale value. This can provide a powerful case for continuing to use existing assets instead of undertaking new investments because, in an economic evaluation, sunk costs should not be included among annual capital costs. In practice, this consideration is likely to be more important in the case of major capital developments than of individual procedures.

DISCOUNTING

The current (operating) costs associated with most projects can be expected to extend over a number of years into the future, but their time profiles may differ. In the case of many preventive procedures, such as treatment for hypertension, costs will be incurred regularly over a number of years. The alternative of no preventive treatment may well incur zero expenditure in the early years but incur the costs of surgery earlier than would otherwise have been the case. *Discounting* offers a means of standardizing different cost/time profiles so that total costs can be compared.

Discounting is based on the assumption that costs incurred in the immediate future are of greater importance than costs incurred in the distant future. This is so because earlier access to finance would permit investment at a positive rate of interest, thereby yielding a larger sum in the future (there is an opportunity cost) or because people and society attach more importance to current opportunities than to future ones (positive time preference). For these reasons, economic evaluation weights costs by a discount rate, according to the year in which they accrue, before adding them up and expressing total costs in present-value terms (values in the current year).

In essence, discounting is the reverse application of the more familiar compound interest formula. Instead of sums being calculated forward, they are discounted backward. Fortunately, the application of discounting does not require close familiarity with the formula because many finance and accounting textbooks include discount tables. These indicate the present values of the dollar at different discount rates.

Table 90.3 shows how present discounted values will vary for selected combinations of the discount rate and the years in which the costs accrue. Looking across the second row of the table, for example, shows that in the fifth year $ 1 will be worth 86 cents at a discount rate of

Table 90.3 Present value of $ 1

	Discount rate					
Year	3%	4%	5%	6%	7%	8%
1	0.9709	0.9615	0.9524	0.9434	0.9346	0.9259
5	0.8626	0.8219	0.7835	0.7473	0.7130	0.6806
10	0.7441	0.6756	0.6139	0.5584	0.5083	0.4632
15	0.6419	0.5553	0.4810	0.4173	0.3624	0.3152
20	0.5537	0.4564	0.3769	0.3118	0.2584	0.2145
25	0.4776	0.3751	0.2953	0.2330	0.1842	0.1460

3% but only 68 cents at a discount rate of 8%. The choice of the appropriate discount rate depends in part on the national recommendations. The U.K. Treasury's current recommended discount rate for public-sector projects in the United Kingdom is 6%. Given the sensitivity of the choice of discount rates, however, and the fact that the ranking of different projects with different time profiles could depend on the rate chosen, it is good practice to compute costs in terms of a range of discount rates.

Inflation

Most programs that extend over several years will be affected by inflation. It is important, however, to distinguish between changes in the general price level and changes in relative prices. In the case of general inflation, there will be no change in the relative cost of inputs (i.e., their opportunity costs remain constant). As such, all future inputs can be valued at current prices and discounted by a real (excluding inflationary effect) rate of interest. If, however, some input prices are expected to increase more than others, there will be relative changes in their opportunity costs, and these need to be taken into account. One way of doing this is to use the general rate of inflation as a benchmark and to adjust the future prices of individual inputs – upward or downward – by an amount that reflects the difference between their rate of inflation and the general rate. Thereafter, all costs once again should be discounted by the same real rate of interest.

MEASURING INDIRECT COSTS

The human capital approach

Early approaches to benefit valuation commonly were based on the concept of *human capital*. This concept is designed to convey the fact that human beings are similar to capital equipment (at least as far as their working lives are concerned) in the sense that they can be expected to yield a flow of productive activity in future years. If the value of this activity in any period of time is assumed to be equal to the individual person's rate of pay, then the benefits of health care can be measured in terms of the future flow of income that would otherwise have been forgone because of ill health. Because these calculations involve adding up a stream of income that accrues over a number of different years, the sum in each year must be time discounted to take into account the precise time profile of benefits.

The human capital approach has been applied in the valuation of health benefits in cases of both avoidable morbidity and mortality. However, there have been various criticisms. As one of the first attempts to place a monetary value on avoided mortality, it led to monetary values being placed on human life, and many people have strong ethical objections to such a valuation. In contrast, most economists think that implicit valuations are placed on human lives in a whole range of decisions about allocation of resources in the public sector and that the cost-benefit approach is simply being explicit about the process.

Other criticisms have centered on the use of rates of pay as a measure of value. Economic theory suggests that productivity is accurately measured only by rates of pay when certain conditions in the labor market are met. The widespread existence of restrictive practices and other forms of imperfections in the labor market means that these conditions often do not apply in practice. At the same time, valuing benefits in terms of rates of pay neglects the health benefits that accrue to people who are not employed, e.g., nonworking wives and retired people. It also ignores the nonfinancial costs of pain, suffering, and grief that are often associated with illness. However, from an economist's perspective, the main criticism of this approach is that it is not based on an individual person's valuations of benefits. Indeed, a third-party view is taken about people's "worth" to society in terms of their productive potential. This viewpoint is inconsistent with the prevailing view among economists that the individual person is the best judge of his own welfare.

Individuals' preferences and willingness to pay

The *observed preferences approach* involves observing individuals' behavior and using these observations as a basis for valuing benefits. One method of doing this is to observe the behavior of individuals toward risk and then to estimate the personal valuations implicit in this behavior. Some people accept "danger money" for undertaking work with an increased risk of injury or death, e.g., deep-sea divers. Others spend money on cars with enhanced safety features to reduce the risk of injury or death. Converting valuations associated with small changes in risk into full life valuation is not straightforward, but various techniques associated with "scaling risks" have been developed. On a practical level, however, one of the main disadvantages of this approach is the limited number of situations under which attitudes toward risk can be observed and measured. This has led to the development of other techniques, in which people are asked to state their preferences among specified choices in monetary terms. This is known as the *willingness-to-pay approach.*

In the context of health, the willingness-to-pay approach seeks to establish the value that people attach to health care outcomes by asking them how much they would be prepared to pay to obtain the benefits or to avoid the costs of illness. Because payment or compensation is not actually made, however, either interviews or postal questionnaires are normally used that are based on open-ended or discrete valuation questions. With open-ended questions, a form of bidding game resembling an auction is the most common approach. An opening bid is made that the respondent either accepts or rejects; thereafter, bids are either raised or lowered until the respondent's maximum willingness to pay is reached. With discrete questions, the respondent is presented with a series of prices and asked to offer a yes/no answer depending on his personal willingness to pay. This approach is less susceptible to starting point bias, which may cause the respondent's answers to be influenced by the starting bid, but there are a number of other forms of strategic and compliance bias that must be guarded against.

Applications of the willingness-to-pay approach to health care are still relatively rare, but some interesting studies have been undertaken. For example, in an early application of the approach, the investigators analyzed the willingness to pay for mobile coronary care units that would reduce the risk of death after a heart attack. Among other things, this study looked at a respondent's willingness to pay for a personal program, given various probabilities of heart attack and death, in comparison with their willingness to pay for a community program. Not surprisingly, perhaps, willingness to pay was greater for perceived personal benefits than it was for community benefits.

More recently, Thompson used willingness-to-pay methods to value the effect of a hypothetical cure on their state of health in 247 patients with rheumatoid arthritis enrolled in a randomized, controlled drug trial. During interviews, respondents were asked to think about the ways in which arthritis affected their lives and their families. They were then told to assume that there was a complete cure for their disease and asked how much they would be willing to pay for it. The precise question asked was, "What percentage of your family's (i.e., household's) total monthly income would you be willing to pay on a regular basis for a complete cure for arthritis?" Consistency of answers was checked by a follow-up question about how the family would manage to live on the remaining amount.

Using these methods, Thompson obtained a 96% response, and 84% of the responders gave answers that met predetermined criteria for plausibility. The results indicated that the average responder was willing to pay 22% of his household income to secure a cure for arthritis. This proportion did not vary with income.

In another study, Johannesson and colleagues examined willingness to pay for antihypertensive therapy. They achieved a response rate of 67% from an elderly population (mean age 64.4 years) comprising 481 patients at a primary health care center. A particular focus of this study was an investigation of the relative merits of an open-ended questionnaire compared with one using discrete yes/no questions. The authors concluded that open-ended questions do not work well in willingness-to-pay postal surveys. Discrete questions, on the other hand, led to a lower nonresponse rate and provided respondents with an easier valuation task. This approach indicated that people would be willing to pay between SKr 2500 and SKr 5000 per year (about £ 225-450) for antihypertensive therapy. The authors also concluded that although the results should be interpreted with caution, they indicated a large potential application for willingness-to-pay methods in the field of preventive health care.

Rushby investigated willingness to pay for improvements in the quality of life offered by heart pacemakers.

Respondents were asked to state their maximum willingness to pay to be free of specified symptoms associated with heart disease (e.g., shortness of breath, chest pain, dizziness, fainting, and palpitations). Groups of respondents included those with personal experience of the symptoms, those with experience of caring for patients, and those with no more experience of the symptoms than the general population. All groups, however, were asked to base their answers on hypothetical cases rather than on current experience. The answers indicated that the mean willingness to pay varied from £ 45.50 per month for heart palpitations to £ 70.67 per month for chest pain.

Donaldson applied willingness to pay in an attempt to value the benefits of continuing care accommodation for elderly people in the United Kingdom. The aim was to compare National Health Service (NHS) nursing homes with NHS hospital accommodations. A distinctive feature of the study was that relatives of respondents, not the residents themselves, were asked how much they thought the government should be willing to pay for the respective accommodations; 71% of respondents provided reliable valuations, and their answers indicated a clear preference for nursing home accommodation over hospital accommodation when the total willingness to pay of the two options was compared with their respective costs.

In a recent review of the application of willingness-to-pay studies, Morrison and Gyldmark argued that three criteria must be met if use of the approach is to be valid. First, given the uncertainty surrounding individual subjects' needs for health care, willingness-to-pay questions should ask how much a person is willing to pay as an insurance premium so that a given service would be available if needed. Second, expectations should be expressed in terms of probabilities; i.e., what is the probability of needing treatment and of its success? Third, representative samples of the population are necessary to establish the total willingness to pay of the relevant population. These authors concluded that few of the studies carried out to date meet these criteria and that there are other methodologic issues that require attention, among which is the link between willingness to pay and income.

FORMS OF PHARMACOECONOMIC EVALUATION

The most common methods employed by health economists are classic research designs such as cost-of-illness, cost-benefit, cost-effectiveness, cost-utility, cost-minimization, and quality-of-life analyses.

Cost-of-illness studies

In the economic literature one also will find references to cost of illness. Definitions vary, but generally, *cost of illness* refers to all the costs as they are borne by society. The cost of illness to society is reflected by such factors as loss of productivity in the work force and loss of income by the patient, which results in the loss of tax revenues and inability to purchase the goods and services that drive the economy. The important point is that everyone in society bears the cost of health care providers, patients, third-party payers, and business and industry.

Cost-of-illness studies typically are divided into two main categories: (1) core costs, i.e., those resulting directly from the illness, and (2) other related costs, including nonhealth costs of the illness. Within each category there are direct costs (for which payments are made) and indirect costs (for which resources are lost). Direct costs (e.g., expenditures for hospital and nursing home care, physician and other professional services, drugs, spectacles, and appliances) are generally estimated as the product of two components – number of services and unit prices or charges. For example, short-stay hospital days of care, by diagnosis, can be obtained in the United States from the National Hospital Discharge Survey conducted by the National Center for Health Statistics (NCHS), and expenses per patient day can be obtained from the Annual Survey of the American Hospital Association. Nursing home costs are estimated by multiplying the numbers of residents with the diagnosis by the annual charge for all residents as reported by the National Nursing Home Survey conducted periodically by NCHS. Costs of outpatient care by office-based physicians can be based on visit data from the National Ambulatory Care Survey, also conducted periodically by NCHS, and charge data for physicians can be obtained from the American Medical Association Annual Report on Physician Practice. Other direct medical and related costs are calculated similarly from other data sources. In other countries all these data sources have to be explored prior to undertaking a cost-of-illness analysis.

Indirect costs include morbidity and mortality costs. *Morbidity costs* are the value of reduced or lost productivity due to the disease in question and are estimated as the product of (1) mean earnings an individual would have accrued had he not been affected by the disease, disaggregated by age and gender, and (2) the number of days lost from work for the employed population or days lost in performing their main activity. If an individual had not died prematurely from the disease, he would have continued to be productive in future years. *Mortality costs* are the product of the number of deaths from the disease and the expected value of an individual's future earnings, with gender and age taken into account. This method of derivation considers life expectancy for different age and gender groups, the changing pattern of earnings at successive ages, the varying labor force participation rates, an imputed value for housekeeping services, and the appropriate discount rate to convert a stream of earnings into its present worth.

National surveys provide reasonably good information on the use of services for estimation of direct costs, but charge and cost data are less readily available and probably less reliable. Indirect costs depend on the discount rate used; the higher the discount rate, the lower are the final costs. If the results of different cost-of-illness studies are compared, special attention should be paid to the techniques used, the discount rate, the reference years, and the scope and recency of the data. Cost-of-illness studies are used by policymakers to justify budgets, to set priorities for funding in biomedical research, and to develop inter-

vention programs to ameliorate or prevent a disease. Researchers in this area have an obligation to present the methods in considerable detail so that users will be better able to assess their accuracy and to evaluate whether the results are fact or fiction.

Example of a cost-of-illness study: the case of ischemic heart disease in Switzerland

The objective of this study was (1) to assess the trend in the economic costs of the disease as a result of the more intensive utilization of health care services and more frequent use of new technologies and (2) to quantify the changes in economic costs to society resulting from the decreased mortality in the working population.

Methods A societal perspective was taken for a prevalence-based asssessment of the direct and indirect costs. Direct costs comprised of total resources consumed by outpatients and inpatients, whereas indirect costs included costs due to morbidity, premature death, and invalidity. The estimates of direct costs elements were derived from information on the average number of patients in outpatient care and the costs thereof. IMS data were used to estimate drug expenditures and the number of patients with ischemic heart disease in Switzerland. There were no existing statistics on the type and frequency of medical care in doctors' surgeries per visit. Thus, expert panels were established to estimate the average number of physician visits per year and the medical interventions per visit. The costs of the office visits, individual laboratory tests, chest radiographs, etc. were based on the official reimbursement tariffs in use throughout the country. The database of the Swiss National Hospital Association was used to identify hospitalized patients, their average length of stay, and the number of in-hospital deaths. The number of

Table 90.4 Costs of ischemic heart disease in Switzerland, 1993

Cost elements	$ Million per 10 000 population	Range ($ million per 10 000 population)	Percentage (%)
Outpatient care	4.1	4.1-4.4	41
Inpatient care	5.6	5.6-6.2	57
Rehabilitation	0.15	0.15-0.18	2
Total direct costs	9.9	9.9-10.8	100
Indirect costs, morbidity	3.4	3.1-3.4	30
Indirect costs, disability	2.7	2.7-3.1	24
Indirect costs, premature death	5.2	4.8-5.7	46
Total indirect costs	11.3	10.6-12.2	100
Total direct and indirect costs	21.2	20.5-23	

major interventions (e.g., balloon dilatations, coronary bypass operations) carried out was available from the Swiss Society of Cardiology, which regularly publishes the total number of procedures performed in the country. Information on individual cost elements was not generally available but could be obtained by extrapolating calculations from the Cantonal Hospital of St. Gallen. Cost data on rehabilitation were obtained directly from the administrators of the major rehabilitation centers in Switzerland.

The elements of indirect cost were evaluated using the human capital approach. Thus, productivity losses were calculated on the basis of the foregone incomes, assuming that loss of productivity is approximated by loss of wages. The current value of lifetime earnings foregone due to premature death was calculated using the generally accepted method of discounting (with a 4% discount rate). Absenteeism was derived from a representative database from the Swiss railroads. Information on partial and total disability was made available by the National Social Security office. In addition, the national statistics on income distributions and on labor force participation rates were included in the calculations. The algorithm used to obtain the value of foregone earnings lost due to premature death took into account that (1) the number of deaths due to ischemic heart disease depends on age, (2) incomes are a function of age, (3) today's value of possible future income is less than the nominal value, (4) patients dying of ischemic heart disease would not have necessarily lived for another 10, 20, or more years had they survived the disease, i.e., they may have died from other diseases, and (5) patients surviving the disease would not necessarily have returned to work.

Results The total cost of ischemic heart disease in Switzerland in 1993 amounted to 2.1 billion Swiss francs. This corresponded to US $ 1.42 billion (1993 dollars), taking into account the average exchange rate in 1993. The standardized costs were US $ 21 million per 10 000 population. The cost components are displayed in Table 90.4.

Example of a cost-of-illness study: the case of drug-related morbidity and mortality

Preventable drug-related morbidity and mortality represent a serious medical problem that urgently requires expert attention. The costs to society of the misuse of prescription medications, in terms of morbidity, mortality, and treatment, can be immense. To date, research has documented increased rates of hospitalization secondary to medication noncompliance and/or adverse drug effects. When medications are prescribed for patients for the treatment of disease, the full intent of all parties involved should be to achieve an optimal therapeutic outcome. *Optimal therapeutic outcome* has been defined as an absence of drug-related problems. A *drug-related problem* (DRP) is defined as an event or circumstance that involves a patient's drug treatment that actually or potentially interferes with the achievement of an optimal outcome.

Methods A conceptual model of drug-related morbidity and mortality was developed to estimate the associated costs in the ambulatory setting in the United States based primarily on the DRPs and negative therapeutic outcomes. Any one or a combination of these DRPs may occur in any given patient and may lead to treatment failures (TFs) and new medical problems (NMPs) as possible negative therapeutic outcomes. An absence of DRPs would represent the optimal therapeutic outcome. These potential negative outcomes were used as the basis for the conceptual model. However, because a TF and an NMP may occur in the same patient as a result of a number of DRPs, a third negative therapeutic outcome was included (i.e., a combination of a TF and an NMP) to make the possible therapeutic outcomes mutually exclusive. An example of a TF due to a DRP would be an unresolved infection following improper antibiotic selection; an NMP might be a rash that develops after starting antibiotic therapy. A combination of negative therapeutic outcomes might occur when an infection is treated with an improper antibiotic that causes a rash.

For patients experiencing a TF or an NMP due to DRPs, it was thought that one of eight subsequent events could occur as follows: (1) a revisit with a physician, (2) a further prescription medication, (3) an urgent care visit, (4) an emergency department visit, (5) a hospital admission, (6) a long-term care facility admission, (7) death, or (8) no further attention of a health care professional. These eight events were defined as the endpoints, or final resolutions, of negative therapeutic outcomes and, as such, are considered to be mutually exclusive (i.e., their respective probabilities would sum to 1.0).

To determine estimates of the probabilities of negative outcomes of drug therapy, a panel of pharmacists was surveyed. These individuals were selected based on their extensive clinical practice in an ambulatory care setting and recognition as leaders in pharmacy practice in the United States. The primary goals of each of their clinical practices were the identification, resolution, and prevention of DRPs. A standardized interview form was developed based on the cost-of-illness model described earlier.

Respondents were instructed to provide their estimate of the likelihood of the three negative therapeutic outcomes owing to drug therapy in patients in a typical general ambulatory health care setting in which they were not available to provide their current level of clinical practice. Respondents were then asked to estimate the percentage of patients who experienced each of the three negative therapeutic outcomes that would require further attention and use of additional health care resources.

The cost-generating components of therapeutic outcomes were identified, and these components were assigned a monetary value. Monetary values for relevant therapeutic outcomes were identified from previous published research reports and from available statistical reports. The perspective taken was that of a third-party payer, such as a managed care organization. Only those health care costs which were directly associated with the treatment of preventable drug-related morbidity and mortality were estimated.

Conditional probabilities for all therapeutic outcomes,

based on responses from the panel members, were inserted into the decision analysis model. The expected costs of drug therapy following a health care encounter under each scenario were calculated by "folding back" the decision tree. Folding back is the process of multiplying the cumulative conditional probabilities by the cost of the outcomes and then summing these values to determine the mean aggregate cost of the scenario. Expected cost is not a prediction of what will actually occur but is simply a weighted average of the possible outcomes.

Cost-of-illness analysis Health care utilization and associated costs owing to negative therapeutic outcomes in ambulatory populations were estimated. The number of revisits to physicians, additional prescriptions, emergency department visits, hospital admissions, long-term care admissions, and deaths resulting from negative therapeutic outcomes were calculated by multiplying the cumulative conditional probabilities for each outcome derived from the decision analysis model by the assumed number of physician visits. The direct cost of treating drug-related morbidity and mortality in the United States was then estimated by multiplying the number of health services used as a result of negative therapeutic outcomes by the estimated unit cost of each service. Calculations were made under the following assumptions: (1) an estimated 669 689 000 physician office visits annually, (2) 63.3% of office visits result in at least one medication ordered or supplied by the physician, and (3) 10% of initial prescriptions are never filled, leading to TFs or a combination of a TF and an NMP.

Results The *therapeutic outcomes* were as follows: According to the panel members, 23.4 ±13.2% (mean ± SD) of patients who receive drug therapy would experience a TF as a result of DRPs, 10.5 ± 5.4% would experience an NMP, and 6.5 ± 4.1% would experience a combination of a TF and an NMP. The panel members estimated that less than 60% of patients who were receiving medication would not have a DRP (i.e., would have an optimal outcome).

The *cost outcomes* were as follows: folding back the decision tree to merge the conditional probabilities and costs of all pathway outcomes produced the mean aggregate cost that was associated with health care encounters. The expected cost of a physician visit was $ 194 (95% confidence interval, $ 154-234). This cost figure has no intrinsic value but is simply the weighted mean cost of the entire pathway model (i.e., all possible outcomes).

When therapeutic outcomes resulting from drug therapy were modeled for the ambulatory population in the United States, the estimated cost that was associated with the management of drug-related morbidity and mortality was $ 76.6 billion annually. The largest component of the total cost comprised drug-related hospitalizations, i.e., an estimated 8.76 million admissions at a cost of $ 47.4 billion annually, or approximately 62% of the total cost. Based on 31.1 million hospital admissions in 1992, the model estimated that 28.2% of all hospital admissions were a result of drug-related morbidity and mortality.

Admissions to long-term care facilities represented the second largest component of the total cost of illness, with 3.15 million admissions at a cost of $ 14.4 billion. Visits to the physician resulting from DRPs exceeded 115 million, and these visits cost nearly $ 7.5 billion, whereas an additional 76.3 million prescriptions would be required to resolve TFs and NMPs, adding $ 1.93 billion to the total cost. This represents 17.3% of all physician office visits and 8.2% of all prescriptions that were estimated for 1992. The number of emergency department visits that resulted from drug-related morbidity represented 18.9% of an estimated 89.8 million emergency department visits in 1992.

Causes of preventable drug-related morbidity and mortality may be a result of inappropriate behavior, either noncompliance by patients or inappropriate prescribing and/or monitoring by health care professionals. As such, drug-related morbidity and mortality could be considered a "behavioral disease". Given this view, an estimate of the economic impact of the "disease" could be assessed by using cost-of-illness methods.

COST-MINIMIZATION ANALYSES

Cost-minimization analysis (CMA) is concerned with comparing the costs of different treatment modes that produce the same result. For example, this form of analysis could be used to compare the costs of two programs that involve minor surgery for adults. Both programs have the same outcome in terms of the surgical procedure, but the first might require the patient to stay overnight in the hospital, and the second might involve day surgery without necessitating overnight hospitalization. Given these two alternatives, the search would be for the least costly treatment. While we might be interested in the extent to which day surgery shifts cost from the institution to the patient, the main efficiency comparison would be on a cost per surgical procedure basis.

As far as pharmaceuticals are concerned, this type of study is used most frequently when a new drug is introduced into a therapeutic class that includes close competitors and no measurable therapeutic effect between them has been documented. When the cost of two interventions is being compared, cost-minimization analysis often assumes that the two interventions lead to the same health outcome. Studies of this nature should report evidence to support the contention that there are no differences in outcome or that any differences are trivial in nature. In most cases, however, the issue is more than simply that of cost alone. It is rare for two therapies that have the same indication to produce identical health outcomes in every respect.

Example of a cost-minimization analysis: the case of parenteral antibiotics

As an example of a well-conducted cost-minimization analysis, Foran and colleagues studied cost differences between antibiotic dosing frequencies. Results showed

Table 90.5 Evaluating the cost impact of iv antibiotic dosing frequencies

Pharmacy manufacturing process

Admixture labor

Admixture supplies
Labels
Container

Pharmacy complications
Admixture waste
Missing doses

Nursing administration

Administration labor

Administration supplies
Supply sets
NaCl 0.9%
Heparin flush
Alcohol wipes
Gloves

Administrative complications
Locate missing doses
Locate patient
Locate iv pump
Obtain additional supplies

that the average nonantibiotic cost associated with each administered dose was $ 3.35, based on labor and material costs associated with admixture and administration (Tab. 90.5, Fig. 90.2). An average of 4.6 minutes per dose saves nurses up to 23 minutes for each patient who receives an antibiotic administered once rather than six times daily over a 24-h period. The authors concluded that costs for admixture and administration should be considered in comparisons of combination therapy with monotherapy

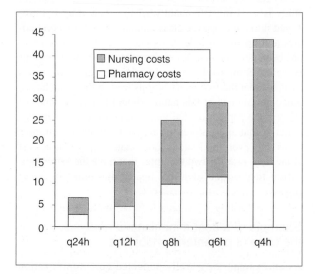

Figure 90.2 Rise in nursing and pharmacy cost when going from single (q24h) to multiple (6 per day, q6h) antibiotic doses.

when deciding between two therapeutically equivalent alternatives.

COST-BENEFIT ANALYSES

As applied to health care, cost-benefit analysis (CBA) measures all costs and benefits of competing therapies in terms of monetary units. Generally, a ratio of the discounted value of benefits to costs (the present value of both) is calculated for each competing therapy. The ratios for each of the competing therapies and for competing programs (e.g., intensive care unit versus new diagnostic equipment) can be readily compared. CBA has the shortcoming of requiring the assignment of a dollar value to life and to health improvements, including quality-of-life variables. This raises equal benefit issues as well as substantial measurement problems. CBA, for these reasons, has not been used widely in recent years for evaluating drug therapies.

Example of a cost-benefit analysis: the case of ceftriaxone in outpatients

Patients who participated in an outpatient iv therapy program designed to limit hospitalization for those who could be maintained on ceftriaxone at home were interviewed about costs and benefits. Of the 79 patients interviewed concerning 83 therapeutic episodes, 43.4% were able to perform their usual activities as soon as they began the program, 28.9% were restricted for part of the time, and 27.7% never resumed their usual activities. The 83 therapeutic episodes represent a total of 2409 outpatient days (mean 29.7, SD 17.7), 1406 of which represent unrestricted activities. Costs and benefits of the program were calculated separately for four employment groups: not employed, usually employed but not while on iv therapy, employed while on iv therapy with time off for follow-up visits, and employed while on iv therapy with no time off for follow-up required. The mean total benefit, weighted across all four groups, was $ 6588.14 (SD $ 3802.90) per patient. Mean weighted costs totaled $ 1768.02 (SD $ 1129.36). The overall weighted benefit-cost ratio was approximately 5:1. Although private insurers reimbursed 63% of the patients for all hospitalization costs, only 39% were fully covered for the follow-up physician visits required during outpatient therapy.

Income and monetary valuation of benefits

Valuing the benefits of health care interventions in terms of willingness to pay raises the problem that the amount people are willing to pay is often positively related to their level of income. The fact that a rich person is willing to pay £ 40 per week for a drug whereas a poor person is willing to pay only £ 10 per week is likely to reflect the value each of them attaches to money itself as well as the benefits of the drug to health.

This is a problem that bedevils all attempts to value benefits in monetary terms, both inside and outside the health sector, and it occurs when payment is actually made as well as when it is based on willingness-to-pay surveys. In some cases attempts have been made to overcome the problem by "weighting" benefits according to the income group of recipients, with lower income groups receiving larger weights, but this raises many practical problems in addition to the obvious one of calculating the appropriate scale of weights. Another approach is to take willingness-to-pay figures at their face value if the program under consideration requires only small expenditure in relation to a person's total income. If this is done, distortions that result from different valuations of money itself are likely to be minimized.

COST-EFFECTIVENESS ANALYSES

Cost-effectiveness analyses (CEAs) measure changes in the cost of all relevant treatment alternatives, namely, the differences in outcome in some natural unit such as actual lives saved, years of life saved, event prevented, or children immunized. CEAs also can be applied equally to cases where the outcome is in terms of quality of life. CEAs are useful in comparing alternative therapies that have the same outcome units (e.g., years of life expectancy or lives saved) but the treatments do not have the same effectiveness (i.e., one drug may lead to greater life expectancy). The measure compared is the cost of therapy divided by the units of effectiveness, and thus a lower number signifies a more cost-effective outcome.

This type of study has the advantage that it does not require the conversion of health outcomes to monetary units and thereby avoids equal benefit and other difficult issues involving the valuation of benefits. It has the disadvantage of not permitting comparisons across programs that have different endpoints. In other words, a drug whose function is aimed at reducing infant mortality cannot be compared with a drug designed to improve the functional status of senior citizens. Moreover, CEA cannot compare outcomes measured in clinical units with quality-of-life measures.

Example of a cost-effectiveness analysis: the case of quinolone treatment

This research project was completed under the auspices of the Drug Surveillance Network of the State University of New York at Buffalo. Pharmacists from over 50 institutions surveyed the use of ciprofloxacin as follow-up to parenteral therapy in 766 patients (see Chap. 38). All patients were hospitalized and were identified as possible candidates for early discontinuation of parenteral therapy in favor of switching to oral ciprofloxacin. The effects of ciprofloxacin on hospitalization and drug therapy were evaluated from prior experience with each clinical situation. Patients enrolled in the study had infections of the respiratory tract, skin or skin structure, bone and/or joint, or urinary tract. The median duration of antibiotic therapy prior to oral ciprofloxacin therapy ranged from 4 to 7.5 days. The median duration of ciprofloxacin therapy prior to discharge ranged from 2 to 4 days. The drug was well tolerated, and no drug-induced adverse events were noted. Only 7% of the patients had an unsatisfactory outcome on

oral ciprofloxacin and had to have parenteral therapy restarted.

However, since patients were only followed to discharge, it is possible that more patients could have failed as outpatients. It was estimated that more than 70% of patients would have continued to receive parenteral antibiotics and 10% would have been given an oral agent were ciprofloxacin not available. It was further estimated that nearly 17 000 parenteral doses were saved with a net reduction in expenditures of approximately US $ 187 000. Nearly 2270 hospital days were saved in 418 patients, yielding net savings of nearly US $ 800 000. The authors concluded that more aggressive intervention could yield additional savings.

COST-UTILITY ANALYSES

Cost-utility analysis (CUA) compares the added costs of therapy with the number of quality-adjusted life years gained. The quality adjustment weight is a utility value that can be measured as part of clinical trials or independently. The advantage of CUA is that therapies that produce different or multiple results can be compared.

Establishing utility values

As explained in the preceding section, the quality-adjusted life-year (QALY), which has been the standard measure of benefit thus far, is arrived at in each case by adjusting the length of time affected through the health outcome by the utility value (on a scale of 0 to 1) of the resulting health status. Many analysts are more comfortable with this measure of the consequence of medical care than with the use of money as the measure of benefits. CUA is an improvement over CEA because it can measure the effects of multiple outcomes (such as the impact of vaccines on both morbidity and mortality or the impact on both pain and physical functional status). Cost per QALY can be computed and compared across alternative treatment scenarios (Tab. 90.6).

Example of a cost-utiliy analysis: the case of intensive therapy in diabetes care

In 1983, the Diabetes Control and Complications Trial (DCCT), a multicenter, randomized controlled clinical trial, was initiated to compare the effects of intensive and conventional therapy in insulin-dependent diabetes mellitus (IDDM). The intensive therapy regimen was designed to achieve blood glucose levels as close to the nondiabetic range as possible with three or more daily insulin injections or treatment with an insulin pump, self-monitoring of blood glucose levels four times daily, and monthly outpatient visits with a multidisciplinary diabetes treatment team. Conventional therapy consisted of one or two insulin injections per day, daily self-monitoring, and quarterly visits with the diabetes treatment team. Intensive diabetes therapy delayed the onset and slowed the progression of the early complications of IDDM and reduced the occurrence of severe nonproliferative and proliferative retinopathy by 47%, microalbuminuria by 39%, clinical nephropathy by 54%, and clinical neuropathy by 60%. Compared with conventional therapy, DCCT intensive therapy consumed more resources and was substantially more expensive.

The purpose of this study was to answer two questions: if intensive therapy were implemented in all persons with IDDM in the United States who meet demographic and clinical eligibility criteria for enrollment in the DCCT, (1) what would the lifetime benefits and costs of intensive therapy be, and (2) would more costly intensive therapy be preferable to conventional therapy from the perspective of the health care system?

Method A Monte Carlo simulation model was developed to estimate the lifetime benefits and costs of conventional and intensive insulin therapy. Data were collected as part of the DCCT and supplemented with data from other clinical trials and epidemiologic studies. The model then was used to simulate the course of the patient's disease over his expected lifetime. The patient's course of retinopathy, nephropathy, and neuropathy was advanced in parallel and on an annual basis. At each point in time, an individual is in one of the five retinopathy health states, one of the four nephropathy health states, and one of the three neuropathy health states. The probability that a patient will advance to a more severe stage of disease in a given year depends on the patient's current state of health, treatment (i.e., conventional versus intensive therapy), and treatment duration.

Each year, after the patient's disease is advanced, the model determines whether the patient is alive or dead. If the patient is alive, the model cycles back to the step that advances the progression of disease. If the patient is dead, the next patient is selected from the hypothetical sample, age and disease characteristics are assigned, and the course of disease is simulated over the patient's expected lifetime. This process is repeated for each of the 10 000 individuals comprising the sample until all the patients have died. At the end of the simulation, the time spent in each of the treatments and health states and the time spent alive are calculated, costs are assigned, and means are calculated by treatment group.

Cost-of-illness analysis A health care system perspective for the CEA was adopted. This perspective considers all direct medical costs associated with disease, including those associated with inpatient care, outpatient care, medications, medical equipment, supplies, and laboratory tests. Direct nonmedical costs such as the costs of transportation, lodging, and family care arising from the disease were not included. Likewise, potential production losses arising from disease-related absence from work, long-term disability, and premature death were not included. The costs of conventional and intensive therapy were

Table 90.6 League table for various medical interventions[1]

Intervention	Cost per QALY
PKU screening	<0
Antepartum anti-D serum	1970
Continuous antidepressive pharmacotherapy	6600
Coronary bypass	6800
Treatment of severe hypertension	15 200
Treatment of mild hypertension	30 900
Coronary bypass for single-vessel disease in severe angina pectoris	58 700
Peritoneal dialysis	76 200
Dialysis in center	87 400

[1]Costs are expressed in US $. Values <0 indicated that the intervention is cost saving.

based on actual resources used in the DCCT, excluding research costs. Briefly, these costs include the cost of initiating intensive therapy on an inpatient basis and the annual costs associated with inpatient care, outpatient care, case-management services, self-care, and the adverse effects of therapy (i.e., hypoglycemia and weight gain). The cost of intensive therapy represents a weighted average of the costs of multiple daily injection (MDI) therapy and continuous sc insulin infusion (CSII) pump therapy and includes the cost of changing from one form of intensive therapy to the other. The resources used in the management of diabetic eye disease, kidney disease, and neuropathy were based on guidelines for care and consensus of the DCCT research group. The costs of blindness, [seve]re renal disease (ESRD), and amputation were [based on] Medicare reimbursement. All costs were reported in 199[?] US dollars. Both costs and effects were discounted at 3% per year.

Life-years gained were applied as the primary measure of effectiveness, and the following outcomes were tracked: sight years, ESRD-free years, amputation-free years, complication-free years, and quality-adjusted life-years (QALYs), which is a summary measure used to adjust length of life for quality of life. The value assigned to quality of life is defined as a health utility. To compute QALYs in the simulation, the following utilities were applied: 0.69 for blindness, 0.61 for ESRD, 0.80 for lower extremity amputation, 0.00 for death, and 1.00 for all other health states. Health utility values were assumed to be the same for comparable health states in both treatment groups. Patients with multiple complications were assigned the utility of the worst health state; e.g., a patient who was blind and had ESRD was assigned a health utility of 0.61.

Results Intensive therapy reduces the cumulative incidence of all the microvascular and neuropathic health states. For example, the simulation model predicts that 70% of conventional therapy patients and 30% of intensive therapy patients will develop proliferative retinopathy by age 70. The cumulative lifetime benefits of conventional and intensive therapy also can be described as the average number of years a patient will remain free from complications. For example, conventional therapy patients will experience an average of 49.1 years of sight, and intensive therapy patients will experience 56.8 years of sight. The difference in outcome between conventional and intensive therapies can be expressed as the average lifetime gain in disease-free years. On average, intensive therapy patients will experience 7.7 additional years of sight, 5.8 additional years free from ESRD, and 5.6 additional years free from lower extremity amputation compared with conventional therapy patients. If these gains in quality of life are extrapolated to the 120 000 persons with IDDM in the United States who meet DCCT eligibility criteria, then intensive therapy will result in approximately 920 000 years free from blindness, 691 000 years free from ESRD, and 678 000 years free from lower extremity amputation compared with conventional therapy. The complications include proliferative retinopathy, albuminuria, and neuropathy. Compared with conventional therapy patients, intensive therapy patients will, on average, gain 15.3 years of life free from any significant microvascular or neurologic complication.

Finally, the benefits of conventional and intensive therapy can be described in terms of survival. Conventional and intensive therapy patients live, on average, 56.5 and 61.6 years, respectively. Intensive therapy is thus associated with a 5.1-year increase in survival.

If this gain in length of life is extrapolated to the 120 000 persons with IDDM in the United States who meet DCCT eligibility criteria, intensive therapy will result in approximately 611 000 additional years of life.

The average lifetime costs associated with conventional and intensive therapy were calculated by accruing annual costs of therapy, adverse effects of therapy, and complications incurred by each patient over a lifetime in the simulation and by calculating the average for all the patients in each treatment group. The expected lifetime costs associated with intensive therapy were more than the expected lifetime costs associated with conventional therapy. Using a 3% discount rate, the expected lifetime cost per patient was $ 99 822 for intensive therapy and $ 66 076 for conventional therapy. This included the cost savings that accrue with intensive therapy from decreased long-term complications. On average, intensive therapy costs $ 33 746 more than conventional therapy per patient over a lifetime. If this additional cost per patient is extrapolated to the 120 000 persons with IDDM in the United States who meet DCCT eligibility criteria, intensive therapy will cost approximately $ 4.0 billion more than conventional therapy over the lifetime of this population.

If the additional benefits of intensive therapy, measured in terms of length of life, are compared with the incremental costs of intensive therapy and both benefits and costs are discounted at 3% per year, then intensive therapy costs $ 28 661 per year of life gained.

Implementing DCCT intensive therapy in the U.S. population with IDDM who meet DCCT eligibility criteria would improve both quality of life and length of life. Intensive therapy patients would have a better quality of life because they would experience fewer complications for a shorter time than conventional therapy patients. They would have a longer life because they would experience less renal disease than conventional therapy patients.

In addition, from a health care system perspective, intensive therapy represents a good monetary value for the investment. Intensive therapy costs $ 28 661 per year of life gained. When length of life is adjusted for quality of life, intensive therapy costs $ 19 987 per QALY gained. These ratios are in a range generally considered to be cost-effective and are similar to the cost-effectiveness ratios for other medical treatments that have been widely adopted in the United States.

THE QUALITY OF PHARMACOECONOMIC RESEARCH

In response to the exploding amount of pharmacoeconomic research, governments and other bodies have started to develop formal requirements and guidelines regarding pharmacoeconomic studies. Canada (the Province of Ontario) and Australia were in the forefront of health economic requirements. Guidelines also have been published recently by the Canadian Coordinating Office of Health Technology Assessment. Several European countries have begun formalizing their criteria for health economics studies. For instance, Germany's social security law states that all health services must be provided economically and that *the principle of economic efficiency should guide the behavior of providers and payers.* Portugal's laws state that patient copayment lists should be based on data from proven favorable cost-benefit ratios. Sweden's *Apoteksbolaget* welcomes the submission of economic evidence as one of the factors for determining fair prices for pharmaceuticals. The United Kingdom included a section on the role of cost-benefit and cost-effectiveness studies in the document addressing indicative prescribing schemes for general practitioners, and in June of 1994, the Department of Health and the Association of the British Pharmaceutical Industry (ABPI) published guidelines on good economic practice. In Finland, the Ministry of Social Affairs and the Social Insurance Institution will consider available economic evidence on reimbursement issues by the National Sickness Institute. In Switzerland, economic aspects of drug therapy regarding inclusions on the national positive list (*Spezialitätenliste*) are considered by the Federal Office of Social Insurance. In the United States recently, the DD MAC of the Food and Drug Administration has dealt with the problem of advertisement. Recently, consensus on the role and methods of cost-effectiveness analysis in health and medicine has been reached and published by a panel of experts convened by the US Public Health Service.

International medical journals are also producing guidelines or otherwise disclosing their policies regarding the submission of economic evaluations of medical technologies.

Since pharmaceutical manufacturers also have long been active in the field of pharmacoeconomics, they have been particularly concerned that the standards for

Table 90.7 Rank order of methodologies in terms of credibility, financial cost, and time to complete

Economic analysis integrated into a randomized, controlled clinical trial
Economic analysis integrated into case-control or cohort observational study
Model based on published RCT
Model based on published observational study
Model based on expert opinion
Model with unclear or incomplete source of data

their work are established so as to legitimize the results. Until recently, the industry has had to exercise great caution in using these studies, because the criteria were not clearly defined by the governmental bodies assessing them. It is vital for the industry that guidelines and protocols are adhered to in order to protect products and manufacturers from unsubstantiated claims against them. The Pharmaceutical Research and Manufacturers of America (PhRMA) has prepared a set of voluntary principles to guide its members in conducting and evaluating pharmacoeconomic research. Other working groups, including members of the industry, have been active in the field of producing voluntary guidelines or standards. Although this is not the complete list of all attempts to standardize methodologies and to offer common principles in the conduct of economic analyses, it does give an idea of the need for standardization in this rapidly growing field, i.e., pharmacoeconomics and health economics studies.

THE CHALLENGES FOR THE FUTURE

Further health economic studies will have to fulfill certain needs. These likely will be (1) establishment of a drug's effectiveness under real (everyday) conditions as opposed to clinical trial conditions, (2) determination of the real value of production losses and their proper measurement, (3) improved conditions for implementing vaccination programs, and (4) cost estimates for more ambitious programs. Furthermore, the adaptation of economic studies across countries will not be an easy task. Problem areas in this respect may be the choice of the perspective of the economic study, local practice patterns, and the customer structure for drug-purchasing decisions. In addition, patient preferences as well as the different sociodemographic structures, price levels, and vaccine effectiveness will have to be taken into consideration.

USING ECONOMIC ANALYSES IN DECISION MAKING

Just conducting pharmacoeconomic research is often not enough. What has to be done is to increase the impact of

such evaluations. A great deal of economic data already have been compiled but are not being used properly. Therefore, the challenge of the future lies also in using results and increasing the impact of these evaluations. One method, for example, is to involve decision makers in the planning of such studies. In the past, manufacturers have produced data and tried to convince decision makers to use their product, instead of working together with decision makers beforehand. It always should be noted that economic analysis and economic data are and will only represent one part of the information required for the decision process. The next step is to make decision makers aware of the usefulness of an economic evaluation. No matter who the decision maker is, the situation will not be improved if he or she is not confident that a better decision can be made based on the economic evidence. It is therefore extremely important to have the data available before a decision is made.

The next point is to make the community aware of the study by all means of publication and communication, preferably through channels that reach decision makers. This means that methodologies have to be reviewed in terms of their credibility, financial costs, and time to completion. Classifications such as those used, for example, in the Cochrane Collaboration also may be suitable for analyzing and rating the sources of economic evaluations. Table 90.7 lists a rank order of methodologies for assessing the credibility of economic evaluations. In those cases where economic studies cannot be combined with randomized, controlled studies, modeling techniques must be employed. However, good modeling practice must be used here. These criteria are also being used increasingly in the peer-review process by many biomedical journals.

INCREASING THE IMPACT OF PHARMACOECONOMIC STUDIES

The degree of impact of a study will be greater if the relevant decision makers are involved in the commissioning and/or conduct of the study. Thus, researchers must "sell" their research before it is started. Moreover, an economic study will only be one of various pieces of information available to decision makers, so researchers must aim to convince decision makers of the relevance of their work. In addition, the greater the number of relevant decision makers who are aware of the study, the greater is the possibility of impact. This will require that researchers disseminate their work appropriately, convincing decision makers of the need for making decisions based on efficiency. Preferably, the results of an economic study must be available prior to the health policy decision to be taken and must meet the criteria of high methodologic standards.

Despite certain methodologic challenges, pharmacoeconomic analyses will be critical to rational allocation of resources by manufacturers, providers, and payers. These analyses can help payers and providers make coverage and utilization decisions and help manufacturers document the value of their products. Rational use of new and established technologies is going to require increased technologic assessment, better assessment of patient preferences, and more rigorous economic evaluations. The benefits of such assessments, however, will be worth their cost.

THE LIMITATIONS OF PHARMACOECONOMICS

Pharmacoeconomics, however, will not solve all substantive issues. For instance, the results of a study may not be conclusive enough to improve the quality of decision making. Or the cost of gathering an extra piece of information may be far more than the extra benefit it gives the decision maker. In addition, it is vital to be aware that health care cannot be rationed using a simple economic calculation. There are always moral and ethical issues for society to take into consideration.

There is also a political danger associated with economic evaluations: They may become the "fourth hurdle" for registration of new products. Regulators not only may review data about a product's efficacy, safety, and quality but also may demand economic efficiency. This is already occurring in some countries.

There are, however, practical problems related to the introduction of a statutory requirement for economic appraisals. They may delay patient access to new technologies and reduce the returns to innovators. Because they are expensive and time-consuming, they could push up costs. Analysis of results may be challenged because there are no "gold standards" for conducting economic trials (see below) and many regulatory bodies do not (yet) have the expertise to properly review economic data. Nonetheless, many countries are moving toward statutory economic evaluations of new health care products.

COMMUNICATING THE RESULTS OF PHARMACOECONOMIC STUDIES

Greater awareness among the public of pharmacoeconomic issues, in particular about quality of life and indirect costs, can help to enlist support from patient organizations. This can be most successful when a patient organization is involved in the definition of a study's objective. With the increasing pressure for cost containment focusing on pharmaceutical expenditures as opposed to hospitalization and diagnostic costs, it is important for the pharmaceutical industry to provide evidence to both public authorities and insurance companies that somewhat higher drug costs can result in substantial overall savings. Careful assessment of the context in which a study operates dictates how that study will be designed and communicated and how persuasive the arguments will be found to be. A good example is Glaxo's sumatriptan study, in which economic justifications for the product's price included the indirect cost of migraine due to lost productivity. Because the relevance of that indirect cost – pro-

ductivity – was unresolved for European authorities, a strong thrust of the argument was rendered less effective.

Another important issue in communicating the results of an economic study is the choice of the correct communication channel, e.g., publication in newspapers, newsletters, scientific journals, mass media, or the lay press. Given the differing interests of the audience, only proper selection of a communication channel will determine whether the message reaches the people who ultimately make decisions and might appreciate the results of an economic evaluation. The importance of daily newspapers in acting as a mutiplier of scientific evidence even within the scientific community has been clearly demonstrated. However, although this channel seems attractive, this does not justify neglecting the publication of economic analyses in peer-reviewed scientific journals.

THE FUTURE RESEARCH AGENDA

The following economic evaluations are required for future policymaking in Europe:
1. *Comparative cost-of-illness studies.* The economic burden of diseases to society and third-party payers has to be demonstrated, preferably in comparison with other indications and/or medical conditions.
2. *Standard data set of economic variables.* Such a set of economic variables should be identified and defined in order to facilitate the conduct of socioeconomic evaluations across countries and among different research sites.
3. *Treatment algorithms.* Treatment algorithms must be identified and compiled.
4. *A core economic model.* The development of a core economic model for selected interventions that can be adapted easily to local/national settings would be a major step forward. This European economic model should be endorsed by local/national decision makers.
5. *A league table.* A league table specifically adapted for interventions across several countries must be elaborated. Such a league table should be based on pharmacoeconomic evaluations using a common methodology in order to make the results comparable and facilitate decision making.

In addition, a European database on drug reimbursement policies including economic assessments and epidemiologic data would be helpful for harmonizing and fostering future research and policy formulation. The database should be accessible to anyone who needs information.

The challenge for conducting more economic research in Europe not only is pressing but also is rewarding. It can be expected that this type of information will become an important cornerstone in health care policy formulation as a basis for better health care decision-making. This will be especially true for indications where an imminent public health impact can is expected.

Suggested readings

AMERICAN DIABETES ASSOCIATION. Standards of medical care for patients with diabetes mellitus. Diabetes Care 1994;17:616-23.

BARRIERE SL. Efficacy and cost effectiveness of oral ciprofloxacin. Pharmacoeconomics 1992;1:146-7.

CHALMERS I, HAYNES B. Reporting, updating, and correcting systematic reviews of the effects of health care. Br Med J 1994;309:862-5.

CLEMENS K, TOWNSEND, R, LUSCOMBE F, et al. Methodological and conduct principles for pharmacoeconomic research. Pharmacoeconomics 1995;8:169-74.

THE DIABETES CONTROL AND COMPLICATIONS TRIAL RESEARCH GROUP. Resource utilization and costs of care in the Diabetes Control and Complications Trial. Diabetes Care 1995;18:1468-78.

FORAN RM, BRETT J, WULF PH. Evaluating the cost impact of intravenous antibiotic dosing frequencies. DICP, Ann Pharmacother 1991;25:546-52.

JOHANNESSON et al. Cost-benefit analysis of nonpharmacological treatment of hypertension. J Intern Med 1991;230:307-12.

JOHNSON JA, BOOTMAN JL. Drug-related morbidity and mortality: a cost-of-illness model. Arch Intern Med 1995;155:1949-56.

MICHEL BC, AL MJ, REMME WJ, et al. Economic aspects of treatment with captopril for patients with asymptomatic left ventricular dysfunction in The Netherlands. Eur Heart J 1996;17:731-40.

OSTER G, EPSTEIN AM. Cost-effectiveness of antihyperlipemic therapy in the prevention of coronary heart disease. JAMA 1987;258:2381-7.

RUSSEL LB, GOLD MR, SIEGEL JE, et al. The role of cost-effectiveness analysis in health and medicine. JAMA 1996;276:1172-7.

SAGMEISTER M, GESSNER U, OGGIER W, et al. An economic analysis of ischaemic heart disease in Switzerland. Eur Heart J 1997;18:1102-9.

TASK FORCE ON PRINCIPLES FOR ECONOMIC ANALYSIS OF HEALTH CARE PRINCIPLES. Economic analysis of health care technology: a report on principles. Ann Intern Med 1995;123:61-70.

THOMPSON MS. Willingness to pay and accept risks to cure chronic disease. Am J Public Health 1986;76:392-6.

Outline of registration procedures in various nations, with an emphasis on Europe

Cristina Borghi, George Wade

In Europe, drug registration procedures[1] date back to Community Directives 65/65/EEC, 75/318/EEC, 75/319/EEC, and 87/22/EEC; in the United States, the procedures derive from the *Code of Federal Regulations* 39 FR 11680 29/3/74, revised in 1978, in 1979 with the new drug application (NDA) rewrite, in 1981 with reform of the new drug application process and a further new drug application rewrite in 1982, and finally, with the accelerated approval regulation in 1992.

Since then, the main objectives of regulators working in a global environment have been harmonization of the procedures to achieve a global dossier based on hard and reliable data on an optimal and justified patient population sample, and the implementation of additional rules and guidelines to make the process as transparent as possible.

From regulatory affairs to regulatory science

To reach such ambitious objectives, the regulatory affairs bodies have moved forward, slowly but efficiently, to regulatory science. Regulatory science aims at finding the most efficient and efficacious way to register a medicinal product usually containing a new active substance (NAS) approximately at the same time worldwide. Regulatory science also means building up a dossier based on clinically relevant information to be evaluated in full transparency and to be accepted worldwide. The harmonization process is helpful so as not to duplicate pharmacological and clinical studies–i.e., to avoid an unnecessary exposure of animals and patients to a new drug either if it does not work or if it has already demonstrated that it is efficacious in a patient population (comparable for demographic, clinical, and prognostic criteria) studied – in one or more countries.

To harmonize also means to reach an agreement on the entire drug development program and to use the same standardized procedures in conducting pharmaceutical, pharmacotoxicological, and clinical studies, applying globally shared guidelines on manufacturing, laboratory, and clinical practice, i.e., good manufacturing practice (GMP), good laboratory practice (GLP), and good clinical practice (GCP). These guidelines are aimed at producing homogeneous and complete documentation regarding the structure and format of every protocol to guarantee the transparency, reliability, and "real" existence of the data obtained in animals and patients. Additional guidelines in terms of diagnostic criteria, outcome measures, and key clinical issues to take into account during the clinical development of medicinal products in the different indications, aimed at producing sound scientific data accepted worldwide, are under development or have already been implemented.

The harmonization process: the international conference on harmonization

In parallel with implementation of the regulatory procedures, additional initiatives were rendered to facilitate the harmonization process through guidelines focused on the three major parts of the registration dossier: quality (chemistry and pharmacy), safety (preclinical models and studies), and efficacy (clinical studies, general rules, and specific guidelines for the most important indications).

Such an ambitious program has required a joint effort of all the parties involved in producing data for registration purposes (the pharmaceutical industry and related associations, hospital and university centers, and centers of excellence) and in evaluating those data (regulatory bodies).

In fact, since 1990, the International Conference on Harmonization of technical requirements for registration

---

[1] This chapter deals only with procedures for authorization of medicinal products for human use.

of pharmaceuticals for human use has been in operation, often called the ICH process or simply ICH. It is apparent that the context in which ICH works relates to "new" medicines arising from clinical research rather than established or generic medicines, although many of the quality guidelines are applicable in principle to generic products as well. ICH has the scope of producing harmonized guidelines recognized in the three main regions of the world where the pharmaceutical industry is well advanced and pharmaceutical medicines are used to treat large patient populations, i.e., Europe, the United States, and Japan, taking into account the existing guidelines already approved in these three areas.

ICH is a joint initiative involving both regulators and industry as equal partners in the scientific and technical discussion of the testing procedures required to ensure and assess the quality, safety, and efficacy of medicines.

There are six parties directly involved, as well as observers and the International Federation of Pharmaceutical Manufacturers Association (IFPMA), which represents the research-based pharmaceutical industry and other manufacturers of prescription medicines in 56 countries throughout the world.

The six parties involved include the following:

1. the European Commission - European Union (EU), based in Brussels, which represents the 15 members of the EU. The Commission is working to achieve a single market in pharmaceuticals that would allow free movement of products throughout the EU. The European Agency for the Evaluation of Medicinal Products (EMEA) has been established by the Commission in 1995 in London; it provides technical and scientific support for ICH activities through its Committee for Proprietary Medicinal Products (CPMP);
2. the European Federation of Pharmaceutical Industries' Associations (EFPIA), situated in Brussels, which has member associations in 16 countries in western Europe. Members are all from Europe's major research-based pharmaceutical companies;
3. the Ministry of Health and Welfare, Japan (MHW), which is responsible for the improvement and promotion of social welfare, social security, and public health. One of its nine bureaus is the Pharmaceutical Affairs Bureau with its Pharmaceutical and Cosmetic Division, responsible for the review and licensing of all medicinal products and cosmetics;
4. the Japan Pharmaceutical Manufacturers Association (JPMA), which has 90 member companies representing all the major research-based pharmaceutical manufacturers in Japan;
5. the U.S. Food and Drug Administration (FDA), which is the world's largest drug regulatory agency and is responsible for approval of all drug products used in the United States;
6. the Pharmaceutical Research and Manufacturers of America (PhRMA), which represents the research-based industry in the United States. This association

has 67 companies that are involved in the discovery, development, and manufacture of prescription medicines. There are also 24 research affiliates that conduct biological research related to the development of drugs and vaccines.

The ICH has its own Steering Committee, Expert Working Groups (EWGs), and a Secretariat, provided by IFPMA and situated in Geneva. The observers, associated with the process, act as a link with non-ICH countries and regions. The observers to ICH include:

1. the World Health Organization (WHO);
2. the European Free Trade Area (EFTA), represented at the ICH by Switzerland;
3. Canada, represented at the ICH by the Drug Directorate, Health Canada.

Each of the observer parties has a seat on the ICH Steering Committee.

In only few years we can easily say that most of the main guidelines on general topics (drug development, GMP, GLP, GCP, pharmacovigilance, pharmacotoxicology, etc.) and on specific medical indications have been implemented; therefore, a dossier can be filed easily in the European Union and in the United States at the same time with the same data, saving time and money and offering to physicians and patients medicinal products tested worldwide under a stringent and consolidated methodology that is agreed on globally.

EUROPEAN MEDICINAL PRODUCT APPROVAL AND POSTMARKETING ACTIVITIES: PROCEDURES

The main purpose of the rules governing medicinal products is to safeguard public health. These rules governing the authorization of medicinal products for human and veterinary use in the European Union currently comprise five volumes. Volume 2A, also called the *Notice to Applicants (NTA),* deals with procedures in general. It has no legal force, and therefore, in case of doubt, reference should be made to the appropriate community directives and regulations set out in Volume 1. The latest version of the *NTA* was published in 1998 and covers the operational procedures for applications of marketing authorization (MA) using community procedures, e.g., centralized, mutual recognition and referrals, as well as national procedures, according to the regulations in force.

PROCEDURES FOR MARKETING AUTHORIZATION

The NTA has been prepared in accordance with Article 6 of Regulation 2309/93/EEC and the Annex of Directive 75/318/EEC. This Notice represents the harmonized view of the members states and the EMEA on how the requirements of the directives and regulations may be met. A medicinal product may only be placed on the market in the European Union when a marketing authorization has been issued by the competent authority of a member state (MS) for its own territory (national authorization) or an authorization has been granted in accordance with Regulation 2309/93/EEC for the entire community (community authorization). For applications submitted after the January 1, 1995, the marketing authorization holder (MAH) must be established in the European Economic Area (EEA), which encompasses the European Union plus Norway, Iceland, and Liechtenstein. For medicinal products already on the market, this requirement to be established in the EEA will be applied at the time of 5-year renewal.

The rules foresee two types of authorizations: the *national authorization* and the *community authorization.* The national authorization has to be submitted to the competent authority of the member state where the product will be placed on the market. A marketing authorization is granted by that member state and is valid only for that member state. National authorizations may be granted for products containing "established" or new active substances (except biotechnology products; see below). The community authorization consists of an authorization that is valid within each of the 15 member states of the European Community. Two types of medicinal products can be authorized through this centralized procedure: medicinal products developed by means of one of the biotechnological processes referred to in Regulation 2309/93/EEC, Annex, Part A, for which this procedure has to be considered mandatory, and medicinal products listed in the Annex, Part B of the Regulation 2309/93 for which the marketing authorization holder can chose either this procedure or the mutual recognition one. It is apparent from this Annex that the whole context of community authorization currently relates to medicinal products that have some new or novel aspect, most probably arising from the research-based pharmaceutical industry. Established drugs in conventional dosage forms for established indications are currently not eligible. The application has to be submitted to the EMEA, and the marketing authorization is granted by the European Commission. The marketing authorization includes a single invented name for the medicinal product (brand name) and the international nonproprietary name (INN) of the active substance when available.

The rules foresee three types of community procedures:

1. the *community procedure* (or *centralized procedure*) for medicinal products that satisfy the criteria of the Annex to Regulation 2309/93/EEC. The application is submitted to the EMEA, which coordinates the scientific evaluation process. It receives an opinion from the main scientific committee of the EMEA, the Committee on Proprietary Medicinal Products (CPMP), consisting of delegates from each member state. This opinion is forwarded to the Commission, who prepares a decision on a community marketing authorization. This authorization is valid throughout the community and confers the same rights and obligations on each of the members states as a marketing authorization granted by that member state;

2. the *mutual recognition procedure* (or *decentralized*

procedure), which is a procedure introduced to coordinate the granting of marketing authorizations in more than one member state and which has been developed to facilitate access to the community market. The application has to be submitted to the reference member state (RMS), and the marketing authorization is granted by that member state and is mutually recognized by the concerned member states (CMSs) for which the marketing authorization has been requested. It is recommended that the same brand name be used in all member states; however, if a different brand name is to be used, the applicant has to give a justification to the competent authority. In cases where companies wish to market with a second brand name, then an application for a second authorization must be submitted;

3. the *community referrals,* which are procedures applied in cases of divergent decisions between member states or in cases of community interest. This is used during the mutual recognition procedure when a concerned member state considers that there may be a risk to public health. Then the matter is resolved by a binding community decision following a scientific evaluation of the issues involved within the EMEA and an opinion from the CPMP.

For reasons of completeness, it should be mentioned that there are two types of applications.

Stand-alone applications   There are two types of stand-alone applications: (1) *full applications,* which must be accompanied by the particulars and documents set out in the Article 4 of Directive 65/65/EEC, e.g., physicochemical, biological, or microbiological tests; pharmacological and toxicological studies; and clinical trials, and (2) *bibliographic applications,* where the constituent or constituents of the medicinal product have a well-established medicinal use, with recognized efficacy and an acceptable level of safety, documented by detailed references to published literature in accordance with Article 1 of Directive 75/318/EEC. The relevant application for marketing authorization may be submitted in accordance with Directives 65/65/EEC and 75/319/EEC as amended.

Abridged applications   Here, the results of pharmacological and toxicological tests or clinical trials are not required to be provided[2]. There are three types: (1) *informed consent* from a marketing authorization, where a holder refers to its dossier in case of an application for an essentially similar medicinal product (the application can only be submitted after the first MA has been granted); (2) the product is *essentially similar to a product authorized for 6 or 10 years* (generic) (evidence of the date of authorization for more than 6 to 10 years and confirmation that the medicinal product marketed in the

---

[2]The details and procedures to be followed are not described in this chapter; they can be found in the quoted directives and in the *Notice to Applicants.*

member states concerned should be provided in the applications); and (3) *new indication, different routes, or doses* (the results of appropriate pharmacological and toxicological tests and/or clinical trials must be provided).

In accordance with Directive 65/65/EEC, a marketing authorization for a medicinal product is granted for a period of 5 years, renewable on application at least 3 months before expiration.

Throughout the life of a medicinal product, the holder of the authorization is responsible for the product that circulates in the marketplace and is also required to take into account technical and scientific progress and to make the relative amendments, which must be approved by the competent authority prior to

their introduction. The marketing authorization holder may, in addition, wish to alter/improve the medicinal product or introduce an additional safeguard during the 5-year period. Such changes, or *variations,* should follow the procedures set out in the Commission Regulations No. 542/95 (community authorizations) or 541/95 (mutual recognition or ex-concertation or community referrals).

Mutual recognition

The *NTA* says at point 1 of Chapter 2, Vol. 2A (Mutual Recognition: Legal Basis and Purpose): "As of 1 January 1995, a pharmaceutical company wishing to market a medicinal product in more than one member state can use the mutual recognition procedure. This can be achieved

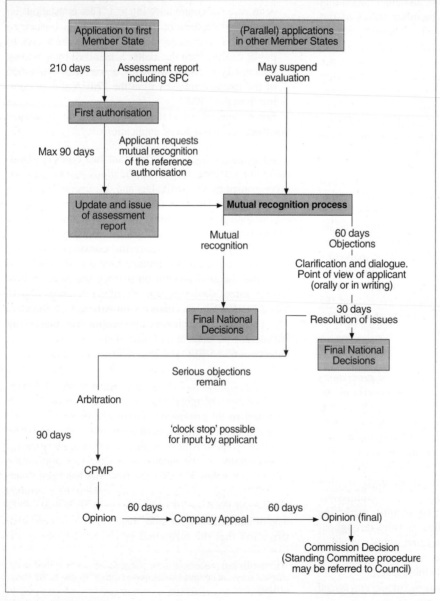

Figure A.1 Mutual recognition procedures(s).

by asking the second or subsequent member states to mutually recognize, within 90 days, the marketing authorization granted by the reference member state. Equally, member states may benefit from the assessment of another member state by mutual recognition even in cases where the company has not requested mutual recognition with its application. Again, a period of 90 days applies. Thus the rapid access to a single market, with the necessary safeguards for the protection of public health, can be obtained using the principle of mutual recognition, either at the request of the company or the member state."

The legal reference texts are in the Directives 65/65/EEC and 75/319/EEC as amended.

All medicinal products, with the exception of those which are subject to the centralized community authorization procedure (listed in Part A), can be authorized via this procedure. In general, if all goes well, it may be regarded as a speedy procedure.

There are two important new elements:

1. a member state can suspend the examination of an application that is currently under examination by another member state and recognize the decision of this latter member state;

2. in the event of disagreement between member state about one of the three main parts of the dossier, a scientific evaluation is undertaken by the CPMP, leading to a single decision binding on all member state—the arbitration procedure.

The procedure may be used for either stand-alone or abridged applications, provided the application is valid and meets the requirements of the legislation in force. Any subsequent variation must use the mutual recognition procedure. The same concept applies to medicinal products authorised by member states following an opinion of the CPMP given before January 1, 1995, i.e., the so-called "ex-concertation" products. The concertation procedure was the forerunner of today's centralised procedure. It was coordinated by the CPMP, there was a CPMP opinion, however the opinion was not binding and led to a series of national authorisation.

The procedure may be used more than once for subsequent applications to other member states for the same medicinal product. The dossier is the same, and the proposal for a summary of product characteristics (SPC) is identical to that authorized and updated for the approved variations. An arbitration that follows the usual procedure (see also Community Referrals) may be used in case of disagreement between member states.

The procedure leading to a mutual recognition is different in relation to which body initiates the mutual recognition: the member state or the marketing authorization holder (Fig. A.1). In the first case, when a member state is informed that an application for a medicinal product, submitted after January 1, 1995, is already under active examination in another member state (taken to be the reference member state), it may suspend the examination and wait for the assessment report prepared by the reference member state. In such cases, the concerned member state shall inform the reference member state, the CPMP, and the marketing authorization holder of its decision to suspend the application in question. The reference mem-

ber state, on the other hand, shall forward a copy of its assessment report to the concerned member state, which has 90 days to recognize (or refuse) the decision of the reference member state and the summary of product characteristics as approved by it. This kind of procedure allows for efficient use of resources and avoidance of duplication of effort. This possibility was not limited to the transitional period, from January 1, 1995 to January 1, 1998, but it also may be used today by member states for applications that are submitted in parallel to member states for medicinal products for which a marketing authorization has not yet been granted.

In the second case, the marketing authorization holder may request one or more member states to mutually recognize an authorization granted by a reference member state. An application is submitted to the competent authorities of the member state or states concerned, together with the information and the particulars referred to in Articles 4, 4a, and 4b of Directive 65/65/EEC as amended. The marketing authorization holder has to certify that all the dossiers filed as part of the procedure are identical.

Before submitting the application under the mutual recognition procedure, the marketing authorization holder must inform the reference member state that an application is going to be filed. A discussion with the reference member state is advised in order to gain agreement as to whether the dossier and the expert reports should be updated to be sure that all the relevant information is supplied according to current requirements and legislative and technical aspects. The reference member state should be reassured by the marketing authorization holder that the dossier submitted in other member states is identical to that on which it took its own decisions. When a national application is first submitted to eventually request a mutual recognition in other member state, it is advantageous to inform the reference member state in advance and to ask for advice and counsel. This also facilitates the availability of the assessment report in a short time frame. It is also advisable that the marketing authorization holder informs other member states regarding the application, particularly when the product is already authorized.

Since technology and science progress rather quickly, and consequently, new guidelines may have been issued, the marketing authorization holder is responsible for keeping the dossier and the expert report updated (see Presentation and Content of the Application Dossier), asking for the relative variations after a drug has been approved and on the market. The summary of product characteristics should be modified accordingly. When the dossier and the expert reports have been amended by the marketing authorization holder, the assessment report is either rewritten or updated to be consistent with the other documents produced by the company. The marketing authorization holder must ask the reference member state in writing to supply this newly written or updated assessment report (in accordance with Guidelines III/5447/94) no later than 90 days after receipt of the request. Arrangements for translations into a language understood in the CMS may be made by the reference member state, but the costs will be charged to the marketing authorization holder.

To summarize, the appropriate steps to be followed to get the marketing authorization through mutual recognition procedure consist of groups of several actions to be done: (1) before submitting the application; (2) when making the application; (3) after submission and before the marketing authorization; and (4) after the marketing authorization has been granted.

Before submitting the marketing authorization, the marketing authorization holder should ensure that: (1) the application is complete and updated appropriately (including the three expert reports); (2) the product will be regarded as a medicinal product in all concerned member states; (3) the medicinal product has been reviewed in accordance with the requirements of the directives; (4) adequate clinical data are available to support the claimed indications in the summary of product characteristics; (5) the requirements for "essential similarity" (product authorized in the European Union more than 6 or 10 years previously and marketed in the concerned member states) for the abridged applications have been met; (6) the dossiers in the reference and concerned member states are the same; (7) all the variations to the original authorization have been authorized by the reference member state in advance of the initiation of the procedure; and (8) the final texts of the approved summary of product characteristics and package leaflet are available in the national language of the reference member state and translated in those of all the concerned member states.

When making the application, the marketing authorization holder must submit an application to the competent authorities of each concerned member state and send a notification to the CPMP through the EMEA secretariat; it is required to give an assurance that the dossier is identical to that accepted by the reference member state or that any addition is identified and identical to that submitted in each concerned member state (including the summary of product characteristics); a European Union application format Part I should be included, and the national fees need to be paid; the application has to be sent to the officially designated address in each state; in addition, a copy of the application should be available to be sent to the reference member state on request and also, only in the event of arbitration, to the EMEA.

After submission and before marketing authorization, the application is checked for completeness of documentation, availability of translations, and fees paid by each concerned member state, according to an appropriate checklist published in the Notice to Applicants (Vol. 2A, Chap. 7). Any problem must be announced within 2 weeks to the reference member state and to the marketing authorization holder; the marketing authorization holder has 2 weeks as well to rectify the application; if there are different views among member states regarding the validity of the dossier, the matter can be discussed in the meeting of the mutual recognition facilitation group (MRFG). When all the concerned member states have confirmed receipt of the valid application, along with the assessment report written by the reference member state, the reference member state notifies all the concerned member states and the marketing authorization holder of the start of the 90-day evaluation period, starting from receipt of the confirmation from the last member state that the documentation has arrived. Normally, in accordance with Article 9.4 of Directive 75/319/EEC as amended, each member state should recognize the marketing authorization and the summary of product characteristics granted by the reference member state within 90 days; then it informs the other concerned member states, the CPMP, and the marketing authorization holder accordingly. In the event of a need for clarification of concerns and deficiencies regarding the quality of the data produced by the marketing authorization holder, or if a potential risk to public health has arisen in a member state, a dialogue starts between the reference member state and other concerned member states within the first 60 days of the evaluation period in order to allow time to resolve the issue. Divergent opinions are discussed first during the MRFG meetings and, eventually, during the CPMP meetings if an agreement cannot be reached (call for an arbitration).

After the marketing authorization has been granted, the benefit of mutual recognition of the marketing authorization carries through the life of the medicinal product. Thus the marketing authorization/dossier which has been harmonized continues to be consistent and identical in all the member states where the marketing authorization was granted. The dossier, consequently, has to be updated when necessary, taking into account the technical and scientific factors concerning quality, safety, and efficacy through the relative procedures of variations.

The marketing authorization is valid for 5 years. However, in order to synchronize the renewal dates in all the member states, the marketing authorization holder can apply for renewal before the scheduled date. Before filing for renewal, the holder is advised to liaise with the competent authority concerning the relevant documentation to be produced and the timetable. It must be stressed that to file for renewal at the same time in all the member states is a benefit that belongs to mutual recognition, and therefore, it is an optional procedure to be followed on a voluntary basis by the marketing authorization holder and the member states.

The documentation to be forwarded, 3 months before the marketing authorization expires, in order to secure the renewal consists of the updated Part I of the national renewal application form, a chronological list of variations approved, the periodic safety update report (PSUR), the agreed summary of product characteristics and the updated package leaflet and label texts (for national approval only), and the payment of the national fees, where relevant. The procedure for renewal also applies to products whose authorization was granted following a CPMP opinion before January 1, 1995 and it were converted to the mutual recognition procedure according to Directive 87/22/EEC i.e., the so-called ex-concertation products. In this latter case, the date of authorization by the first member state is used to calculate the starting date for the renewal.

The scope of this procedure is to provide a mechanism for the resolution of divergence of opinion between member states on serious grounds; e.g., the authorization of medicinal product may present a risk to public health. In this case, if serious doubts have been raised by a member state regarding the quality, safety, or efficacy of a product, a clarification has not been obtained during the mutual recognition procedure, and an agreement has not been reached during the MRFG meetings, a scientific evaluation of the matter would be undertaken by the CPMP in the EMEA, leading to an opinion from which the Commission would prepare a single decision on the area of disagreement that is binding on the member states. This decision would be adopted by a rapid procedure ensuring close cooperation between the Commission and member states. The instances where a disagreement could arise are set out in Directive 65/65/EEC as amended (suspension of examination, member state–initiated mutual recognition), Directive 75/319/EEC as amended (risk for public health, divergent decision, community interest, variation, protection of public health, previous concertation procedures, and pharmacovigilance), and Commission Regulation 541/95 on variations. The procedure to be followed is defined in Articles 13 and 14 of Directive 75/319/EEC as amended.

A standard operating procedure has been prepared by the EMEA to cover the mechanism of making referrals. Normally, the referral should be addressed to the CPMP, at the latest by day 90, by all the member states that wish to make it. These member states should notify the CPMP (secretariat of the EMEA) on which grounds they propose that the authorization of the medicinal product concerned may present a risk to public health. A copy has to be sent to the other member states and the marketing authorization holder, then the reference member state distributes a consolidated report of the issues for arbitration to be circulated, through the EMEA secretariat, to CPMP members to be discussed during their first scheduled meeting.

The content of the referral report consists of the product description (the latest agreed and available summary of product characteristics); a description of the scientific discussion undertaken during the mutual recognition procedure between the reference member state and the concerned member states, including a summary of other major issues already solved within the first 60 days of the procedure; a detailed description of discrepancies focused on the issues at arbitration and a proposal for question(s) to be addressed by the company; and the initial reference member state assessment report.

The committee considers the matter and issues an opinion within 90 days of the date of referral (Tab. A.1). This period may be extended or shortened in case of urgency. The procedure may be stopped only if the marketing authorization holder decides to withdraw the product from all European Union markets and if the CPMP agrees; otherwise, it continues to be discussed by the CPMP until the serious issue regarding public health has been resolved.

In case a positive opinion has been adopted by the CPMP (e.g., the committee states that the objections raised should not prevent the granting of marketing authorization), the final opinion with its annexes is then forwarded in the official European Union languages to the Commission, which issues a decision that is binding on all the member states. This decision must be implemented within 30 days of notification by the reference member state, the concerned member state, and all other member states where the product is on the market.

In case a negative opinion has been adopted by the CPMP, the EMEA secretariat informs the marketing

Table A.1 Timetable for the arbitration	
Day 1	• First meeting of the Committee following the referral to discuss the question(s) for arbitration and the appointment of the Rapporteur (Co-rapporteur?) • Questions to be addressed to the CPMP and the applicant:
clock stops	- For the Company to answer the list of questions raised by the CPMP
clock re-starts	- Submission of responses with translation of the RMS Assessment Report in English (where necessary) - Adoption at the CPMP of timetable for the rest of the procedure
Day 45	• Company submission of the translations in all official languages of the latest available SPC as achieved during mutual recognition • (Co-)Rapporteur(s) prepare a report on the written comments from the MAH together with the draft SPC to be annexed to the opinion
Day 60	• Comments from Committee members on the (Co-)Rapporteur(s)' assessment reports plus draft SPC as well as translation in all official languages • Need to have an oral explanation: (Co-)Rapporteur(s) and EMEA Secretariat to liaise • Discussion at the CPMP:
clock stops	- For the preparation of the oral explanation, if necessary
Day 90	• Oral explanation, if necessary • Adoption of the CPMP Opinion plus SPC

authorization holder about the terms of the opinion: i.e., the application does not satisfy the criteria for authorization; the proposed summary of product characteristics should be amended; the marketing authorization is subject to certain essential conditions; or the marketing authorization should be suspended, varied, or withdrawn. In the latter case, the company has 15 days to notify the EMEA of its intention to appeal and 60 days to indicate its grounds for appeal. Within 60 days of receipt of the grounds for appeal, the committee must reconsider its opinion and issue a statement on the subject. After completion of the appeal procedure, or if the applicant did not appeal, the opinion becomes final.

Centralized procedure

The scope of this procedure, set out in Council Regulation 2309/93/EEC, is to provide a mechanism for the authorization of medicinal products for which there is a single application, a single evaluation, and a single authorization allowing direct access to the single market of the European Community. To accomplish this community task, the regulation has established a European Agency for the Evaluation of Medicinal Products (EMEA), which is responsible for coordinating the resources at its disposal for the evaluation and supervision of medicinal products. The regulation, built up on the experience of the old concertation procedure (Council Directive 87/22/EEC), responds to the need to protect the public health within the European Community while also allowing rapid access to a single market for important new medicinal products.

The regulation relies on the fundamental requirement that the authorization of medicinal products should be based on objective scientific criteria of quality, safety, and efficacy of the concerned medicinal product. A marketing authorization granted under the centralized procedure is valid for the entire European Community market.

Two types of products fall within the scope of the regulation and are listed in the relative Annex: *Part A products,* i.e., medicinal products developed by means of biotechnological processes (e.g., recombinant DNA technology, genes coding for biologically active proteins, hybridoma, and monoclonal antibody techniques), for which the applicants are obliged to follow the centralized procedure and send their application to the EMEA, and *Part B products,* which are innovative medicinal products (e.g., new active substances or those presenting novel characteristics), for which the applicants may use either the centralized or the mutual recognition procedure.

Again, as mentioned earlier, it is apparent from Parts A and B of this Annex that the centralized procedure is currently only open to those medicinal products which have a new or novel feature and in general are classified as high-technology medicinal products.

The advantages of the centralized procedure may be summarized as follows: to get a marketing authorization equally valid in all 15 European Community member states, to undergo a transparent scientific evaluation procedure that involves all the member states who sit together in the CPMP meetings, to take advantage of good cooperation with the EMEA secretariat and the CPMP members involved during the whole evaluation process, and to take advantage of a consultation procedure to address the medicinal product development early in advance of presentation of the dossier, i.e., Scientific Advice. This latter point refers to Article 51j of the Regulation, which mentions that one of the tasks of the EMEA is "where necessary, [to advise] . . . companies on the conduct of the various tests and trials necessary to demonstrate the quality, safety, or efficacy of medicinal products." Normally, this advice is provided in the relative guidelines that the working parties write and discuss during their periodical meetings at the EMEA, adopted by the CPMP, and already published by the European Commission in the *Rules Governing Medicinal Products in the European Community,* Vol. 3. Scientific advice was originally given only for products eligible for the centralized procedure and in those circumstances where the pharmacopoeia monographs, CPMP guidelines, and previous guidelines do not already cover the points of concern or do not provide sufficient guidance. However, recent amendments to the procedure mean that such scientific advice is now available for all products. Since science develops quickly and the advice could have been given too early in the development of a product, an alternative approach to that advised may be appropriate. Therefore, in some cases, the company may choose not to fully comply with the advice, provided an explanation is given in the appropriate part of the dossier. For the same reasons mentioned earlier, any advice is not binding on the EMEA with regard to any future marketing application of the product concerned.

The procedure to be followed for the submission of a centralized application foresees subsequent steps according to the relevant standard operating procedures prepared by the EMEA secretariat and agreed on by the CPMP (1) before submitting the application, (2) when making the application, (3) after the submission, (4) before the Commission decision and marketing approval, and (5) after the marketing approval has been granted.

Before submitting the application, the applicants have the opportunity to meet with the EMEA secretariat and discuss procedural matters during the presubmission meetings. A notification of the intention to submit an application, along with a provisional date of filing, normally should be sent to the EMEA 6 months before submission. The notification should include a draft summary of product characteristics, a justification of the product's eligibility for the centralized procedure, a statement about whether the application is full or abridged, a statement on the appropriateness of granting a marketing authorization under exceptional circumstances, scientific advice received, a proposed classification for the supply of the medicinal product, the intention to present sensitive and confidential details relating to the manufacture of the active substance separately in a drug master file, any preference regarding the choice of Rapporteur and Co-Rapporteur, details of compliance with the requirements of Council Directive 90/220/EEC on the deliberate release into the environment of genetically modified organisms if relevant, the location(s) of manufacturer(s) of finished product and active substance, any request for fee waivers or reductions (i.e., in the case of so-called orphan medicinal products), and any difficulties or issues already identified that may require clarification or detailed consideration (e.g., multiple applications, trade name). The French words *Rapporteur* and *Co-Rapporteur* have been adopted in English to define the CPMP members who write the reports, or coordinate the evaluation, and report back to CPMP. When the notification is received, a member of the staff of the Human Medicines Evaluation Unit of the EMEA will be officially appointed as EMEA project manager, and the applicant will be notified of his or her identity. The project manager works in close cooperation with the Rapporteur and Co-Rapporteur, ensures that the applicant is kept fully informed of all the issues relating to the application, and acts as a liaison between the CPMP, EMEA, Rapporteur, Co-Rapporteur, and the applicant.

Approximately 3 months before the expected submission date, the CPMP appoints one of its member to act as a Rapporteur for coordination of the evaluation of the dossier, taking into account the preferences expressed by the applicant. A Co-Rapporteur may be appointed as well. The EMEA secretariat presents to the CPMP members the information they need to evaluate whether the product falls within the scope of either part A or part B of the Annex to the Regulation. At the time of the Co-Rapporteur's appointment, the EMEA checks, in liaison with competent national authorities, if the proposed trade name is acceptable or if it would raise any identifiable public health concern, for resolution 1 month thereafter. If the intended application is deemed to be admissible, the EMEA notifies the applicant of the names of the Rapporteur and Co-Rapporteur, the applicable fees, and the usual dossier requirements of the various CPMP members. The applicant is also invited to submit an electronic version of the draft summary of product characteristics, labeling, and package leaflet, which should have been standardized regarding headings, subheadings, and content according to the latest templates provided by the EMEA.

When making the application, the EMEA asks the applicant to provide by the agreed date of delivery of the application one full copy of the dossier, including the drug master file (if any), two copies of Part I (including one copy in each of the 11 official European Union languages of the draft summary of product characteristics, labeling, and package leaflet), along with a mock up or specimen of the sales presentation of the medicinal product. Further documentation is requested, according to Council Directive 90/220/EEC, if the product contains or consists of genetically modified organisms.

In addition, the applicant must provide evidence of establishment within the European Economic area, as well as documents showing its capacity to meet all the responsibilities required under community legislation, e.g., persons responsible for disseminating scientific information, pharmacovigilance, and batch recall in the event of a quality defect. In order to accelerate and facilitate the procedure, the applicant is invited to submit, in parallel with the EMEA, one full copy of the dossier to the Rapporteur and Co-Rapporteur.

The fees due should have been received by the EMEA before the evaluation procedure starts.

After submission, the EMEA project manager, within 10 working days following receipt of the dossier, validates the dossier regarding format and procedural aspects in cooperation, if needed, with the Rapporteur and Co-Rapporteur and any other person not directly related with evaluation of the dossier (e.g., GMP and GCP inspection, ad hoc expert group, Commission for legal aspects). In the case of a negative validation, the applicant is required to initiate another procedure, should a new complete dossier be submitted in the future.

In case of a positive outcome, the applicant is informed in writing and is invited to send a full or partial copy of the dossier to all other members of CPMP. The precise requirements of each CPMP member can be decided on an individual case-by-case basis and are not known until the next meeting of the CPMP, when members declare what they wish to see. A timetable for the start of the "clock" for the first evaluation phase is also decided at this meeting, and this timetable also enters into the EMEA's internal tracking system.

The scientific evaluation procedure starts as soon as the validation is over and the Rapporteur and Co-Rapporteur have confirmed that they have received the dossier and all the additional information that had been requested during the evaluation process. The EMEA shall ensure that the opinion of the CPMP is given within 210 days (Tab. A.2). Where it considers it necessary, the CPMP may ask for a preauthorization inspection of the manufacturing site(s), and this should be performed by a competent inspection team of the EMEA secretariat within the time frame of the scientific evaluation period.

During the evaluation period, the EMEA project manager works in strict cooperation with the Rapporteur and Co-Rapporteur, and he or she may liaise directly with the applicant for any additional information requested by the CPMP.

A preliminary assessment report is prepared by the Rapporteur and Co-Rapporteur within 70 days from the start of the procedure, and it is circulated to all the other CPMP members for comments, which should be received by day 100 by the Rapporteur, Co-Rapporteur, other CPMP members, and EMEA. The Rapporteur and Co-Rapporteur may consult, when needed, with additional experts in the specific medical field belonging to the list of national experts that each European Union country has put at disposal for this purpose in accordance with Article 53 of Council Regulation 2309/93/EEC. A summary of conclusions on the basis of the scientific data presented, including the comments of the other members, is prepared by the Rapporteur and Co-Rapporteur outlining the outstanding issues that the applicant has to address before receiving authorization. When the CPMP adopts this consolidated list of questions (day 120), the clock stops until the applicant sends his or her responses.

The applicant normally has to send the responses within 6 months. During this time frame, the applicant is advised to consult the Rapporteur and Co-Rapporteur and to liaise with the EMEA project manager to properly frame the answers. Should the 6-month time be too short to provide satisfactory answers, careful consideration should be given to withdrawing the application or formally requesting the CPMP to grant an extension to the time allowed for submitting a response. In addition to written responses, the applicant also may avail himself or herself of an oral explanation to the CPMP. The time limit set out in Article 6 of the regulation shall be suspended for the time allowed to the applicant to provide adequate additional information during the oral explanation.

Before day 210, the CPMP adopts its opinion in light of the final recommendation of the Rapporteur and Co-Rapporteur and further evidence presented at the oral explanation. The draft opinion is prepared by the EMEA secretariat (project manager) according to the latest information available, usually the day before the meeting. The final or "adopted" CPMP opinion, which may be favorable (positive) or unfavorable (negative), is, wherever possible, reached by scientific consensus or, when diver-

Table A.2 Timetable for the evaluation of a centralised application

Day	Action
1	Start of the procedure
70	Receipt of the Assessment Reports from (Co-)Rapporteur(s) by CPMP members of the EMEA. Rapporteurs also send assessment Reports to the applicant without confidential aspects (making it clear that id does not yet represent the position of the CPMP)
100	(Co-)Rapporteur(s), other CPMP members and EMEA receive comments from Members of the CPMP
115	Receipt of draft list of questions (including overall conclusions and overview of the scientific data) from (Co-)Rapporteurs by CPMP members and EMEA. (Co-)Rapporteurs transmit to CPMP members for internal use only the list of questions which have been left aside
120	CPMP validates the list of questions as well as the overall conclusions and review of the scientific data to be sent to the applicant by EMEA. (If needed updated position statement from (Co-)Rapporteurs on initial assessment). Clock stops
121	Submission of the response; restart of the clock (on 11 official dates per year). Submission of mock-ups in color for each presentation covering all Member States languages or language combinations
150	Common response Assessment Report from (Co-)Rapporteurs received by CPMP members and EMEA
170	Deadline for comments from CPMP Members back to (Co-)Rapporteurs
180	CPMP discussion and decision on the need for an oral explanation by the applicant. If oral explanation is needed, the clock is stopped to allow the applicant to prepare the oral explanation
181	Restart the clock and oral explanation
185	Final draft of English SPC, Leaflet and Labelling by applicant to the (Co-)Rapporteurs, EMEA and other CPMP Members
Before 210	CPMP opinion + CPMP draft Assessment Report
Day 5 at the latest after opinion	Applicant provides EMEA and CPMP members with all translations of SPC, labelling and package leaflets
Day 15 after opinion	Preparation by the applicant of final revised translations of SPC, labelling and package leaflets taking into account comments received by EMEA and CPMP
Day 20 at the latest cial after opinion	Applicant provides EMEA with final translations of SPC, labelling and package leaflets in all offi-languages of the EU. Final full color mock-ups covering all Member States should also be submitted
Before 240	Finalisation of CPMP Assessment Report to be transmitted to the applicant Transmission of opinion to the applicant, Commission and Member States in all languages
Before 300	Finalisation of EPAR in consultation with (Co-)Rapporteurs, CPMP and company (for confidentiality aspects)

gent positions have been expressed, by a majority. These divergent positions will be appended to the opinion.

In the event of a positive opinion, the following documents are annexed and/or appended to the opinion: (1) a summary of product characteristics (SPC), (2) manufacturing and/or importing conditions and conditions of the marketing authorization, (3) a package leaflet and text for the labels, (4) a classification for the supply of the medicinal product, (5) the CPMP assessment report, and (6) the divergent positions with their grounds, if any.

The opinion may be subject either to follow-up measures or adopted under exceptional circumstances. Should the CPMP want to record any follow-up measures, they will be included in the assessment report and referenced in a letter of undertaking signed by the applicant that will be annexed to it. Such follow-up measures usually relate to pharmaceutical quality aspects of the dossier (Part II). A timetable is also agreed on for the submission and evaluation of follow-up measures or specific obligations, and the relevant data are to be reviewed accordingly, including at least the annual reassessment of the risk-benefit profile of the product. In case of nonfulfillment of the follow-up measures or specific obligations, the CPMP will have to consider the possibility of taking appropriate action: variations or suspension or withdrawal of the marketing authorization.

In the event of a negative opinion, the EMEA informs the applicant, and the following documents are annexed and/or appended to the opinion: (1) the CPMP assessment report stating the reasons for its negative conclusions and (2) the divergent positions with their grounds, if any.

The applicant must notify of any intention to appeal within 15 days of receipt of the opinion. The grounds for appeal must be forwarded within 60 days to the EMEA, and the CPMP will reconsider within 60 days whether the opinion is to be revised.

Within 30 days after the positive opinion has been adopted by the CPMP, the translations of the opinion and its annexes or appendices in all 11 European Union languages must be finalized by the applicant. Throughout the evaluation procedure, and in particular, after validation, a regular check on the quality of translations (i.e., format and content, concerning mainly reliability, clarity, legibility, and patients' comprehension of the terms used in the package leaflet) will be carried out by the EMEA secretariat in cooperation with the member states. Then the opinion and the final translations will be sent to the European Commission for its legally binding decision. The Commission will prepare within 30 days a draft decision that is forwarded to the member states and the applicant, and each has 30 days to formulate its approval, rejection, or abstention. After this deadline, the whole documentation will be sent to the Standing Committee, and if the Standing Committee formulates a favorable opinion, in the following 30 days the Commission decision will be issued. The decision is effective from the moment it is signed and the member states and company concerned are notified.

If the Commission's draft decision does not meet with a favorable opinion (i.e., qualified majority), the matter is forwarded to the Council as a proposal for a Council deci-

sion. Within 3 months, either the proposal is adopted with a qualified majority or it is refused by simple majority; if the council does not make a decision, the commission adopts the proposed decision.

The most important outcome of the community authorization, which summarizes all the available updated information regarding the benefit-risk profile of the authorized medicinal product, is the product "literature," consisting of the summary of product characteristics, package leaflet, labeling, and presentation of the medicinal product. Therefore, the services of the Commission have prepared a guideline for information on medicinal products for human use authorized by the Community. This guideline applies to applications submitted to the EMEA after September 1, 1997. It has been prepared to describe how to comply with Directives 92/26/EEC and 92/27/EEC. The purpose of the guideline is to explain in detail and in a practical way why and how the literature should be standardized, coherent, and identical, apart from the language(s), in the different community states. It also provides rules for specimens or mock-ups of the outer packaging and of the immediate packaging of the medicinal product, together with the package leaflet. The only departure from the standardized and identical text that is allowed, according to national regulations, is in the so-called "blue box" (special area on one side of the package), where the price of the medicinal product, the reimbursement conditions, the legal status, and the identification and authenticity of the product may be indicated. Details of a local contact point for information may also be included here. Symbols and pictograms that are informative for the patient may be included in the labeling, provided that any element of a promotional nature is excluded.

After the marketing authorization has been granted, in accordance with Article 12 of Council Regulation and on request from any interested person, the EMEA shall make available the assessment report about the medicinal product by the Committee and the reasons for its opinion in favor of granting the marketing authorization, after deletion of any information of a commercially confidential nature. This document is called the *European Public Assessment Report* (EPAR).

The marketing authorization is valid for 5 years and is renewable for 5-year periods on application by the holder at least 3 months before expiration. The application should be accompanied by the fee to be paid (Council Regulation 297/95/EC) and by a dossier containing up-to-date information on pharmacovigilance in the form of completed periodic safety updates in accordance with Article 22 of Council Regulation 2309/93/EEC.

Variations

Throughout the life a medicinal product, the marketing authorization holder is responsible for the product that circulates in the marketplace and is also required to take into account technical and scientific progress and, eventually, to make the appropriate amendments to the product that have to be approved by the competent authorities. In addition, the holder may wish to alter/improve the medicinal product or to introduce a safeguard during one of the 5-year periods. Such changes or *variations* may involve administrative and/or more substantial changes, whose approval procedures have been in operation for some years in most member states. With the implementation of the new system for marketing authorization and in order to maintain the harmonization achieved and to guarantee that the changes do not give rise to public health concerns, two regulations have been introduced: 541/95/EEC and 542/95/EEC. The relative guidance and forms have been prepared for the operational aspects of the procedure to be followed for medicinal products approved by either mutual recognition or centralized procedure.

These variations to the marketing authorization have been categorized as follows:

- *type I variations:* these are listed in Annex 1 of the Regulation and concern an amendment to the contents of the documents as they existed at the moment the decision on the marketing authorization was signed. These variations, which often relate to pharmaceutical quality aspects, may be applied to "minor/administrative" rather than "substantial scientific" changes in the use of the product (e.g., content of the marketing authorization; name of the product or name/address of the holder; minor changes in the formulation, manufacturing, packaging, shelf-life extension, storage conditions, or test procedures; deletion of indication, route of administration, etc.);

- *type II variations:* these are listed in Annex 2 of the Regulation and concern any change to the documentation proposed by the marketing authorization holder that is not a type I variation and does not require a new application procedure. These variations may be applied to "major/scientific" changes of the relevant part of the dossier (Part I, administrative/summary of product characteristics; Part II, chemical/pharmaceutical/biological; Part III, pharmacotoxicological; Part IV, clinical). The type II procedure also applies to certain type I categories for the products covered by Directives 89/342/EEC (immunological), 89/381/EEC (blood products), 90/677/EEC (veterinary immunological), and 87/22/EEC (high-technology, list A) and by Council Regulation 2308/93 (Part A);

- *urgent safety restriction:* this is an interim or provisional change to product information by the marketing authorization holder restricting the indication(s), and/or dosage, and/or target species of the medicinal product or adding a contraindication and/or warning due to new information having a bearing on the safe use of the product. It requires implementation within 24 hours and must be followed by a type II variation.

Normally, a type I procedure is to be completed within 30 days. A type II procedure is to be completed within 90 days (which may be extended a further 60 days of clock off if supplementary information is required) for products authorized through the mutual recognition procedure and within 60 days (which may be extended a further 60 days or more) for products authorized through the centralized procedure.

The procedure for processing variations of products authorized through mutual recognition is slightly different from the one followed for products authorized through the centralized procedure. In the first case, the process is finalized with the joint cooperation between the reference member state, the concerned member states, and the applicant. For type I variations, the reference member state is required to fix the clock start date or stop date if supplementary information is required, to evaluate the grounds for refusal, and to refuse or approve the variation; the concerned member states may ask for amendments; and the applicant may request arbitration in case of divergent positions advising the reference member state, all concerned member states, and the EMEA of this within 10 days of receipt of the refusal. On the contrary, if the applicant has not received advice of grounds for non-acceptance of the variation from either from reference member state or any of the concerned member states 30 days after the clock starts, the variation may be implemented. For type II variations, the reference member state is required to fix the clock start dates, to request supplementary information (60 days clock off), to liaise with the applicant if a divergent position or refusal is likely so that the applicant has the opportunity to withdraw the variation application in all member states, to cooperate with the concerned member states, and in case of divergent positions, to participate in an arbitration procedure.

In the second case of the centralized procedure, the applicant liaises mainly with the EMEA (namely, for type I variations), which, through the CPMP, in certain cases for type I and for all type II variations nominates a Rapporteur and, if appropriate, a Co-Rapporteur. In principle, they would remain the same as for the evaluation of the application for marketing authorization. A project manager is appointed in all cases. The European Variation Application Form available from the EMEA has to be used. A separate application form has to be submitted for each variation, unless sequential variations are concerned. The applicant is advised to contact the EMEA secretariat at least 1 month before the intended date for submission, and he or she should consult with the EMEA to ascertain the best strategy when the applicant intends to submit more than one application. For type I variations, the application form should be accompanied by the data supporting the variation applied for; all the documents amended; if appropriate, amendments to be introduced in the Commission decision translated in the 11 European Union official languages; and the payment of the fee. In absence of any reaction from the EMEA within 30 days after the clock starts, the variation is deemed to have been accepted and can be implemented by the company. If the EMEA, in consultation with the CPMP, is of the opinion that the application cannot be accepted, it informs the company within 30 days, allowing the company a further 30 days to amend the application. Then the EMEA informs the commission of the variation to be made to the terms of marketing authorization.

For type II variations, the application form should be accompanied by the data supporting the variation applied for, all the documents amended, an addendum or an update assessment report, and the payment of the fee. After validation by the EMEA secretariat within 5 working days, the opinion is issued by the CPMP in the following 60 days, which may be extended by a further 60 days or more. In the case of a positive opinion, the EMEA informs the marketing authorization holder and the commission immediately and sends the commission the amendments to be made to the terms of marketing authorization accompanied by the relative documents. Where the CPMP delivers an unfavorable opinion, the appeal procedure can be activated within 15 days of receipt of the opinion by the applicant.

In the event of risk to public health (pharmacovigilance, preclinical safety, or quality signals), the holder of a marketing authorization may introduce provisional urgent safety restrictions that eventually may be introduced via a corresponding variation in the marketing authorization. The EMEA, Rapporteur, Co-Rapporteur, and member states must be informed immediately. If the EMEA has not raised any objections within 24 hours, the marketing authorization holder can implement the safety restrictions and submit an application for a type II variation without delay.

FORMAT FOR APPLICATIONS

Volume 2B of the *Notice to Applicants* provides guidance for compilation of the application dossier and is applicable for the centralized procedure and the national procedures, including mutual recognition. The requirements are set out in Directive 75/318/EEC as amended. The particulars and documents accompanying an application for marketing authorization pursuant to Article 4 of Council Directive 65/65/EEC shall be presented in four parts, in accordance with the requirements set out in the Annex.

All the data to be presented in the dossier may be shown as a pyramid, the apex being the summarized data and the lower layers the more detailed data, so that the very bottom consists of individual data for each different protocol and the paper trail documenting good clinical practice, testifying that data really exist, are reliable, and are available to all the parties involved (Fig. A.2).

Presentation and content of the application dossier

The community application dossier, which should be submitted in either a community or a national procedure, consists of administrative information and the necessary demonstration of quality, safety, and efficacy of the medicinal product.

This is presented in four parts:
• Part I: summary of the dossier;
• Part II: chemical/pharmaceutical/biological tests;
• Part III: toxicopharmacological tests;
• Part IV: clinical documentation.

Part I is further divided in three subsections. Part IA contains administrative data, packaging, samples, and manufacturing and marketing authorization applied for or obtained elsewhere. Part IB contains a summary of the product characteristics (SPC) and package leaflet. Part IC contains the expert reports and their annexes.

All these parts should be prepared according to a harmonized format, indicated in the relevant templates and guidelines. Part I is always required, even for abridged applications. Part IB must be in the language(s) of the member state concerned or in all community languages for centralized applications.

Part I is the most important part because it contains summaries of all the administrative and scientific data, and if it is well prepared, coherent, and clearly written according to the relative guidelines, it greatly facilitates the evaluation process. In particular, Directive 75/319/EEC as amended requires that the particulars and

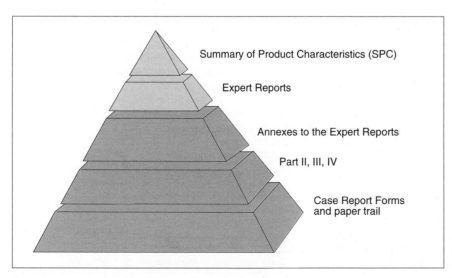

Figure A.2 Documentation necessary to obtain the marketing authorisation approval.

the documents submitted in the dossier are drawn up, signed, and dated by recognized experts. The place of issue should be mentioned, and attached to the expert report. There should be a brief (1-page) description of the expert(s): name(s), educational background, training, and occupation. The professional relationship of the expert to the applicant also should be declared.

There should be three expert reports, each related to the corresponding technical part of the dossier: chemical/pharmaceutical/biological, toxicopharmacological and clinical documentation. The scope of the expert reports is to provide a critical discussion of the properties of the product, covering quality, safety, and clinical aspects. The experts should be independent in their judgments, but they are expected to take and defend a clear position on the product in light of current scientific knowledge. Each report should contain the appropriate tabulations and a written summary, along with precise volume and page references to the specific studies or other relevant information contained in the study report tables and in the full dossier. Each report should be concise, clear, complete, and consistent with the updated scientific information and knowledge on the product, and each should take into consideration the different guidelines that already have been issued prior to commencement of the current tests, studies, and clinical trials. In particular, the experts should give valid justification of the statements in the proposed summary of product characteristics, taking into account the data submitted and the summary of product characteristics guideline.

The expert report summary should present only factual data. Repetition and duplication should be avoided either in the text or between the report and tabulations or written summary. Overview tables play a pivotal role, mainly for Parts III and IV. Therefore, applicants are strongly recommended to include them in the submission. A written summary for the relevant sections of Parts III and IV would facilitate and speed up either recognition by concerned member states in the mutual recognition procedure or evaluation by members of the Scientific Committee of the EMEA, the CPMP. The summary should be concise (e.g., the clinical summary should not be longer than 30 pages); in cases of complex dossiers, it could be necessary to present a larger summary (e.g., up to 100 pages).

In synthesis, the structure of each of the three expert reports should include (1) a critical assessment of the part concerned (II, III, or IV), which should be no longer than 10 pages for part II and 25 pages for Parts III and IV and which is obligatory, (2) the tabular formats, with the option to use alternative tabulations, which are obligatory, (3) a tabular overview, which is strongly recommended for parts III and IV, and (4) a written summary, which is recommended and which should be no longer than 30 pages for part II, 10 pages for part III, and 30 pages for part IV (up to 100 pages for a complex dossier).

Parts II, III, and IV are the technical sections of the entire documentation that applicants supply with the application form (part IA of the dossier). In Part IV, clin-

ical documentation, case report forms are always required, and applicants should be prepared to supply them normally within 48 hours but not later than 7 calendar days when the competent authority requests them.

The table of contents for an application for marketing authorization is presented in Table A.3. Part II is slightly different for radiopharmaceutical products, biological medicinal products, or products derived from biotechnology and herbal medicinal products.

The principles and detailed guidelines of good manufacturing practice (GMP), good laboratory practice (GLP), and good clinical practice (GCP) are applicable to all the processes, tests, and clinical trials used in performing the necessary studies to prepare the dossier for

Table A.3 Presentation of the application within the European Union: structure of the dossier*

Part I	**Summary of the dossier**
Part IA	Administrative data
Part IB	B1 Summary of product characteristics (SPC)
	B2 Proposal for packaging, labeling, and package leaflet
	B3 SPC already approved in the member States
Part IC	Expert reports
	C1 Chemical, pharmaceutical, and biological documentation
	C2 Toxicopharmacological (preclinical) documentation
	C3 Clinical documentation
Part II	**Concerning chemical, pharmaceutical, and biological documentation for chemical active substance(s)**
Part IIA	Composition
Part IIB	Method of preparation
Part IIC	Control of starting materials
Part IID	Control tests on intermediate products (if necessary)
Part IIE	Control tests on the finished product
Part IIF	Stability
Part IIH	Data related to the environmental risk assessment for products containing or consisting of genetically modified organisms (GMOs)
Part IIQ	Other information
Part III	**Toxicopharmacological documentation**
Part IIIA	Toxicity
Part IIIB	Reproductive function (fertility and general reproductive performance)
Part IIIC	Embryofetal and perinatal toxicity
Part IIID	Mutagenic potential
Part IIIE	Carcinogenic potential
Part IIIF	Pharmacodynamics
Part IIIG	Pharmacokinetics
Part IIIH	Local tolerance (where appropriate)
Part IIIQ	Other information
Part IIIR	Environmental risk assessment/ecotoxicity
Part IV	**Clinical documentation**
Part IVA	Clinical pharmacology
Part IVB	Clinical experience
Part IVQ	Other information

*Drawn from *Notice to Applicants*, Vol. 2B, 1988 edition.

registration purposes. The published directives, Council regulation, and harmonized guidelines must be followed. Any deficiency should be commented on and justified by the relevant expert.

Practicalities

The development of a medicinal product for registration purposes is a complex procedure, since protection of the public health is a major concern of the European Union. Therefore, the application for marketing authorization consists of a substantial body of documentation, often in excess of 100 volumes. Information technology can provide a fundamental contribution in the management of such a huge amount of data and information. However, a clear and direct strategy should be applied in medicinal product development right from the beginning in order not to be overcome by the information and the procedure itself. A high quality dossier increases the probability of authorisation, and saves time and money.

In order to succeed in preparing such a good-quality dossier the following simple suggestions are given to applicants:

1. start planning the development of a medicinal product from the summary of product characteristics you would like to see approved in the future;
2. secure the appropriate guidelines and follow them accurately;
3. ask for CPMP scientific advice, if needed, early during the development;
4. avoid duplication of studies and effort;
5. establish periodic checkpoints to review the data in the most objective fashion;
6. check to see if the aims of the development are feasible (as far as time and effort are concerned), according to the scientific findings obtained;
7. avoid premature applications, which eventually make the evaluation process longer and more difficult and result in a waste of time and money;
8. liaise properly and take advantage of the suggestions of the EMEA secretariat or national authorities as relevant;
9. make the right choice of experts;
10. take into account that the evaluation process in the hands of the assessors normally starts with the expert reports. If the reports are well structured, well written, simple, easy to read, reliable, and show hard data, the CPMP or national authorities will take less time to evaluate them;
11. consider that the CPMP assessment report for centralized applications is based on the Co-Rapporteur's reports, and the data in these reports often can be traced back to the company's original expert reports.
12. Remember that the EPAR for a centrally authorized product is derived from the CPMP assessment report. It follows that the information that will be available to the physician, the patient, and indeed the general public in the EPAR strongly depends on the quality of the data provided by the applicant in terms of content and presentation.

PROCEDURES FOR PHARMACOVIGILANCE

Pharmacovigilance is the scientific process by which companies and regulatory bodies identify and respond to safety issues after a marketing authorization has been granted. This involves the close monitoring of products on the market to ensure that the benefit-risk ratio established during the evaluation procedure is still favorable. If it is not, appropriate action must be taken to protect the public health.

In Europe, the parties involved in compliance with the obligations of law are the companies, the competent authorities of the member states, the European

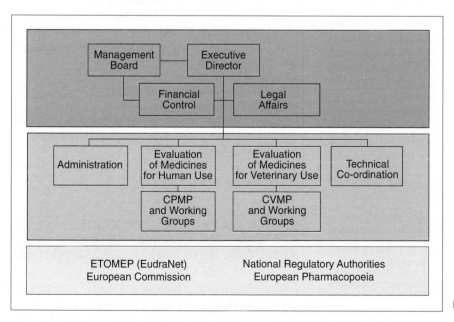

Figure A.3 Structure of the Agency.

Commission, and the EMEA, through the secretariat, the CPMP members, and the Pharmacovigilance Working Party (PhVWP) European physicians, working either at universities or in hospitals or their own practices (i.e., general practitioners) are the sources of the information.

The timing of reporting of adverse drug reaction[3] varies according to the type of report: *expedite reports* are aimed at serious reactions[4]; *nonexpedite reports* target nonserious reactions; and *signals* are aimed at potentially serious safety problems[5]. The pharmacovigilance community central system (EMEA and Commission) requires that all serious suspected reactions occurring within a member state and all serious unexpected reactions occurring in a third country, and noted by the national pharmacovigilance center, are reported directly to the EMEA and marketing authorization holder within 15 days of receipt. In case of centrally authorized medicinal products, it is the responsibility of the Agency to inform each member state of serious reports received from other member states.

For products that have national authorizations, the competent authority of the member state in which the authorization is held is responsible for pharmacovigilance and maintenance of that marketing authorization. At the European level the EMEA has a coordinating role promoting dialogue between member states through the CPMP and the PhVWP.

Under the terms of Article 12 of Directive 75/319/EEC as amended, a member state, the Commission, or a marketing authorization holder may refer a pharmacovigilance issue to the committees of the Agency whenever the interests of the Community are involved. Referrals result in consideration of the matter by the EMEA according to a specific procedure and time frame. The final CPMP opinion (withdrawal, suspension, variation, or no change) is translated and forwarded to the Commission, which prepares a decision that is binding on all concerned member states.

All other reports concerning nonserious reactions occurring within or outside the community should be summarized and commented on in the Periodic Safety Update Report (PSUR)[6], which must be sent to the EMEA (for products authorized by a centralized procedure) or to the competent authorities of the member states (for products authorized by a mutual recognition procedure) every 6 months during the first 2 years after approval and yearly thereafter.

The monitoring and control of signals by national pharmacovigilance centers are performed according to two methods of communication: rapid alert and nonurgent exchange of information. The purpose of the rapid alert

system is to alert with an appropriate degree of urgency the other member states and the Agency about pharmacovigilance data relating to medicinal products. The criteria for sending a rapid alert are the occurrence of serious drug hazard that could lead to the urgent suspension or withdrawal of the marketing authorization, the introduction of major contraindications, and restrictions in the indications or availability of a product. In case of urgency, the member state concerned may suspend the marketing of a medicinal product, provided the Agency and the other member states are informed, at the latest, on the following working day. Under normal circumstances, the concerned member state will transmit all relevant data about the alert to other member states and the Agency. The other member states will respond to the originating member state, the Agency, and the Commission within 7 days by providing the pertinent information and the responses to any specific questions. An assessment report will be prepared by the appointed Rapporteur and circulated to member states and the EMEA within 1 month of receipt of the information. This will be considered by the PhVWP and the CPMP, which will make a proposal for a common position and recommendation expressed in an opinion, to be forwarded to the Commission for a relative decision.

In the case of a nonurgent exchange of information, the system to be used will be infofax. A pharmacovigilance network called EudraWatch that links all the competent authorities of member states and the EMEA has been implemented by the EMEA. This computerized database greatly facilitates the exchange of data and the monitoring of suspected serious adverse drug reactions and safety data in general, resulting in a more efficient, less paper-dependent system for rapidly exchanging information that is the basis for making the appropriate reflections to take the right decisions.

The legal basis and procedures for conducting pharmacovigilance inside the European Union are set out in the following directives and regulations:
• Council Regulation 2309/93/EEC;
• Council Directive 75/319/EEC;
• Commission Regulation 540/95/EC (PSUR);
• Commission Regulation 542/95/EC (Variations; Urgent Safety Restrictions, USR).

In addition, the following guidelines have been implemented by the CPMP:
• *Notice to Applicants,* Vol. 9;
• CPMP/183/97 Conduct of Pharmacovigilance for Centrally Authorized Products;
• CPMP/PhVWP/175/95 Note for Guidance on Procedure for Competent Authorities on the Undertaking of Pharmacovigilance Activities;
• CPMP/SOP/PhVWP/005/96 Rapid Alert System (RAS) in Pharmacovigilance Conduction.

EUROPEAN MEDICINAL PRODUCT APPROVAL AND POSTMARKETING ACTIVITIES: ROLES AND RESPONSIBILITIES

Article 1 of Title 1 of Council Regulation 2309/93/EEC says: "The purpose of this regulation is to lay down

---

[3]Harmful and unintended reaction that occurs at doses normally used in man for prophylaxis, diagnosis, or treatment of disease or modification of a physiologic function.

[4]Death, life-threatening conditions, hospitalization or prolongation of existing hospitalization, persistent or significant disability/incapacity, congenital anomaly/birth defect.

[5]A series of unexpected or serious reactions or an increase in the reporting rate of a known adverse drug reaction report.

[6]PSUR is prepared by the applicant for all authorized medicinal products. It is intended to provide an updated summary of the worldwide safety experience of a medicinal product to competent authorities at defined times postauthorization.

Community procedures for the authorization and supervision of medicinal products for human and veterinary use and to establish a European Agency for the Evaluation of Medicinal Products." This regulation, however, has the scope to harmonize within the European Union the registration procedures without affecting the powers of member state authorities with regard to the price setting or their inclusion in the national formulary and modality for reimbursement by the National Health System.

The parties involved in the procedures for registration and postmarketing activities are the European Agency for Evaluation of Medicinal Products, which expresses its opinion through the CPMP; the European Commission, which actually formulates its decision which is binding on all member states; and the competent national authorities for products following the mutual recognition procedure. Other competent bodies or working groups belonging to the above-mentioned authorities support them in discussing and implementing additional notices or guidelines.

THE EUROPEAN AGENCY FOR THE EVALUATION OF MEDICINAL PRODUCTS (EMEA)

EMEA was established in 1993, and it has been seated in London since 1995. A global review has been scheduled for 2001.

Unlike the Food and Drug Administration in the United States, which has a permanent staff of thousands of persons dealing directly with evaluation and tracking of registration and postmarketing procedures and activities, the EMEA is a "virtual" Agency because it has a mainly coordinating role in facilitating scientific evaluations that are carried out by experts in member states. Thus the member states share the workload with the Agency secretariat, consisting of only about 160 temporary agents.

In fact, EMEA comprises:
- the CPMP, which is responsible for preparing a scientific opinion of the agency on any issue relating to the evaluation of medicinal products for human use;
- the CVMP (Committee for Proprietary Veterinary Products), which is responsible for preparing the opinion of the Agency on any question relating to the veterinary evaluation;
- a Secretariat, which provides technical and administrative support for the two committees and ensures appropriate coordination between them;
- an Executive Director, who is the legal representative of the Agency appointed by the Management Board and is responsible for the activities and all financial expenditures;
- a Management Board, which adopts the general report on the activities of the Agency for the previous year and its program for the coming year, as well as the budget.

The CPMP and CVMP may seek guidance on important questions of a general scientific or ethical nature.

According to the regulation, the tasks of the EMEA are:
- to advise companies on medicinal product development and research;
- to provide the member states and community institutions with the best possible scientific advice on quality, safety, and efficacy of medicinal products for human and veterinary use;
- to organize and provide a multinational scientific expertise using the existing national resources to achieve a single evaluation of medicinal products (via centralized or decentralized systems);
- to perform evaluations of centralized procedures through a speedy, transparent, and efficient process for the authorization, surveillance, and, where appropriate, withdrawal of products in the European Union;
- to provide arbitration for the decentralized procedure;
- to coordinate pharmacovigilance activities and member state inspections (GMP, GLP, and GCP);
- to create the necessary databases and telecommunication facilities to promote more rational drug use.

The critical success factors for EMEA since its establishment may be summarized as follows: the first success factor is the transparency and public access to EMEA documents, according to the rules set out during a workshop on this matter held in October 1997. These rules have been discussed and agreed on by a number of competent national authorities and representatives from a wide range of consumer, patient, pharmaceutical company, and media groups. Representatives of the European Ombudsman, European Parliament and U.S. Food and Drug Administration, together with the Nordic Council on Medicines, also participated in this workshop.

The second factor that signifies EMEA's success is its performance and quality-management activities, which consist of working groups inside the secretariat exploring new strategies and related activities to measure EMEA's performance, to improve the standard of its service, to evaluate the efficiency and costs of the system, and to enhance the quality of the system itself.

Another factor is EMEA's contacts with European institutions and interested parties and the participation in all meetings and working groups of the Commission's pharmaceutical committees for human and veterinary medicines, which are under the management of Directorate General Enterprise, formerly DG III. Contacts have been established with the new scientific committees of Directorate General XXIV to prevent possible overlap of activities with those of the EMEA scientific committees. Continuous contact with the European Parliament, in particular with the Committees on Environment, Consumer Protection, and Public Health, as well as the Committee on Budgets, is ongoing.

The EMEA also participated in the work of the European Pharmacopoeia as part of the European Union delegation. Interested parties, including representatives of consumer, patient, industry, and health care professional groups, are invited to the CPMP and CVPM quarterly meetings and to several EMEA meetings. A number of technical workshops on specific topics, e.g., scientific opinions, decision-making procedures, pharmacovigilance, and performance indicators, were organized with the interested parties in 1997, and these will continue.

International relations are increasing. In addition to the regular contacts and meetings with the ICH for the harmonization activities in the human and veterinary fields, EMEA started to establish strict cooperation contacts with Nordic Council of Medicine, the incoming members of the European Union (e.g., Iceland and Norway), national regulatory authorities of central and eastern European countries (CEECs), and national regulatory authorities of the new independent states of the former Soviet Union, under the auspices of the World Health Organization (WHO). In 1997, EMEA received a number of delegations from national authorities of other countries, including Australia, Canada, China, Hungary, Japan, Korea, New Zealand, and Ukraine. A meeting with Latin American national authorities also was hosted in 1997. More recently the EMEA has coordinated the Pan European Regulatory Forum in 1999 to assise Eastern European countries to align their regulatory practice with Europe.

Role and mission

EMEA plays an important role in guaranteeing good-quality logistical and administrative support to member states in tracking the important and vital activities of the evaluation procedures during the preapproval and maintenance phases of medicinal product authorizations and in the management of time frames. This has been performed since its establishment through an efficient organization and network of resources, such as CPMP members and national experts, and strict cooperation with the scientific and regulatory staffs belonging to national authorities.

The EMEA mission statement, contained in the Third General Report of 1997, is: "To contribute to protection and promotion of public and animal health by: mobilizing scientific resources from throughout the European Union to provide high-quality evaluation of medicinal products, to advise on research and development programs, and to provide useful and clear information to users and health professionals, developing efficient and transparent procedures to allow timely access by users to innovative medicines through a single European marketing authorization, controlling the safety of medicines for humans and animals, particularly through a pharmacovigilance network and the establishment of safe limits for residues in food-producing animals."

Structure

The EMEA is located at Canary Wharf between the City and the City Airport.

The structure (Fig. A.3) of EMEA includes:
• a Management Board, which consists of two representatives per member state, two representatives of the commission, and two representatives appointed by the European Parliament (present Chairman, Mr. Strachan Heppell);

• two Scientific Committees, responsible for formulating EMEA's opinion on any question relating to the evaluation of human (CPMP) or veterinary (CVMP) medicinal products. Each committee consists of two members appointed by each member state;
• a Secretariat.

The EMEA secretariat consists of:
• a Directorate (Executive Director, Mr. Fernand Sauer at the time of writing this article), who is responsible of all the activities and budget and sets objectives and priorities in cooperation with staff;
• an Administration Unit, which is responsible for personnel and support services (selection and recruitment, salary and benefits, training, facilities management, security, office equipment and supplies) and accounting (payment of expenditures, collection of fees, preparation of budget);
• the Unit for Evaluation of Medicines for Human Use, which is responsible for the management and follow-up of dossiers undergoing evaluation under the centralized procedure and arbitration under the decentralized procedure. It provides technical and administrative support for the CPMP. The unit is also directly involved in the ICH process, which brings together the regulatory authorities of Europe, the United States, and Japan in consultation with experts from the pharmaceutical industry of the three regions in order to eliminate redundant and duplicative technical requirements for registration, saving, eventually, effort, time, and money;
• the Unit for Evaluation of Medicines for Veterinary Use, which is responsible for activities related to the acceptance and processing of registration dossiers for veterinary medicines and advises on the maximum limits for residues in food-producing animals;
• the Technical Coordination Unit, which coordinates national inspections regarding GMP, GLP, and GCP. This unit is also responsible for document management (in the 11 European Union languages), publishing, archives, and mail services. The conference Service is responsible for the organization of meetings and travel arrangements for delegates. The information and technology sector is responsible for the installation of computers and local networks for national delegates via EUDRANET with the support of the Joint Research Center ETOMEP at Ispra (Italy).

PARTIES INVOLVED

A number of bodies take part in the process of safeguarding the public health. They are the European Commission and its staff, granting the final decisions binding on all member states and setting out the legislation proposals; the Committee for Proprietary Medicinal Products, which makes the evaluation of the scientific issues during the centralized procedure and maintenance period; the Mutual Recognition Facilitation Group, which helps the member states during the mutual recognition procedure; and the Working Parties on Quality, Safety, Efficacy, and Pharmacovigilance, which make proposals for the relative guidelines and offer their advice when needed. A number of *ad hoc* expert groups may also be convened to discuss specific issues. The EMEA supports and coordinates all the above activities in one form or another.

The European Commission and its Directorates General

The European Commission is the heart of the European Union's policymaking process. In fact, the other institutions derive from it much of their energy and purpose. It consists of 20 members (two from France, Germany, Italy, Spain, and the United Kingdom and one from each of the other member states) and 15000 staff who serve it. Its term of office is 5 years: from 1995 to 2000.

The Council and the European Parliament need a proposal from the Commission before they can pass legislation. European Union laws are mainly held up by Commission action, the integrity of a single market is preserved by the Commission, and development policies are sustained and managed by the Commission in cooperation with third countries.

The full Commission has to be approved by the European Parliament before its members can take office. Its members are obliged to be completely independent of their national governments and to act in the interest of the European Union, mediating conflicts of interests between member states when needed. With its staff of 15000, the Commission is the largest of the European Union's institutions. It is divided in 26 Directorates General (DGs) with an additional 15 or so specialized services.

The Commission's role identifies three distinct functions: (1) initiating proposals for legislation, (2) guarding the treaties, and (3) managing and executing European Union policies and international trade relationships. As far as medicinal product approval and maintenance are concerned, the Commission prepares decisions for approval, arbitration, or variations binding on all member states.

The Committee for Proprietary Medicinal Products

The CPMP is a scientific committee set up to facilitate the adoption of common decisions between member states on the authorization of medicinal products on the basis of scientific criteria of safety, quality, and efficacy. In addition, the members ensure an appropriate coordination between the tasks of EMEA and the work of competent national authorities.

The CPMP consists of 30 members and a chairman. Each member state nominates two members for a term of 3 years, which may be renewable. Appointees have to disclose their possible indirect interests in the pharmaceutical industry and state their scientific competence. During the meetings, they should act independently, using only their scientific skills. They may arrange to be accompanied by the experts, with established and proven experience in the assessment of medicinal products, belonging to the European list of about 2000 experts appointed by each member state.

The CPMP is responsible for formulating a scientifc opinion on any question concerning human medicinal products. It is assisted by working parties (see below) that provide advice on specific matters related to the quality, safety, and efficacy of medicinal products.

The CPMP is required to appoint one of its members to act as a Rapporteur for the coordination of the evaluation of each dossier, taking into account the applicant's preference; it also may appoint a second member as Co-Rapporteur. When preparing an opinion, each member of the CPMP uses his or her best efforts to reach a scientific consensus.

The CPMP meets every month (usually August excluded) to adopt opinions regarding either applications for centralized procedures or arbitration or any other scientific matter that is within its competence. Each meeting is expected to occupy one week per month. Meeting dates of the CPMP are published in advance to allow for planning for both the EMEA and to guide applicants for optimization of the time of submission of applications.

The provision of service by the Rapporteur or experts is governed by agreement between EMEA and the national competent authorities.

The Mutual Recognition Facilitation Group (MRFG)

This is an informal liaison group of member states that generally meets in London, at the same time that the CPMP meets, to discuss any important issue regarding mutual recognition procedures and the harmonization of any other regulatory procedures or questions with each of the national regulatory authorities.

Along with the MRFG meetings, break-out sessions are also organized under the responsibility of the reference member state to discuss applications and for resolving outstanding questions. During these meetings, a discussion and a sort of negotiation take place in an attempt to avoid, whenever possible, the arbitration procedure. The reference member state will inform the marketing authorization holder if representatives from the company should be available at the relevant meeting to aid in resolution of these issues.

During 1997, the MRFG created a validation report form, a response document form, and a procedure for handling postauthorization commitments. Introduction of the tracking system EudraTrack in October 1997 was a significant step forward because it allows more statistical information to be generated and made available monthly, improving the monitoring of procedures.

The working parties: quality, safety, efficacy, biotechnology, and pharmacovigilance

The Working Parties are groups of experts belonging either to the European expert list or to the national competent authorities, and they meet every month or every other month or on a different schedule in relation to the urgency of the support for which they are asked. They assist the CPMP, advising the committee on specific matters related to their competence and skills.

The joint CPMP/CVMP Quality Working Party (QWP) provides on request of the CPMP/CVMP a forum for dialogue and understanding between pharmaceutical experts to maintain a harmonized approach to quality issues and to eliminate national divergencies in assessing quality problems. Recently, representatives from the industry side have been asked to present an industry view on matters of interest. The Safety Working Party (SWP) provides a forum for dialogue and understanding on preclinical safety issues and methodological guidelines. The Efficacy Working Party (EWP) draws up and updates methodologic guidelines in established therapeutic areas and elaborates position papers on efficacy issues of developing clinical areas. The Biotechnology Working Party (BWP) advises the CPMP on any matter concerning biotech-derived products and biological products. It deals with centralized procedure applications and scientific questions of general interest. The Pharmacovigilance Working Party (PhVWP) provides a forum for dialogue and understanding between national authorities and EMEA on pharmacovigilance matters (i.e., harmonization of terminology, development of IT communication facilities, setting up of pharmacovigilance procedures in member states) and examines any questions related to drug hazards.

EUROPEAN MEDICINAL PRODUCT APPROVAL AND POST-MARKETING ACTIVITIES: *CORPUS LEGIS*

The fundamental legislation the applicants have to refer to is listed in Volume 1 of *The Rules Governing Medicinal Products in the European Union.* Any update or new legislation may be found in *The Official Journal of the European Communities.*

DIRECTIVES, REGULATIONS, AND QUALITY, SAFETY, AND EFFICACY GUIDELINES

Community law, adopted by the Council or by the Parliament and Council in the framework of a codecision procedure, may take the following forms:

- *regulations:* these are applied directly without the need for national measures to implement them.
- *directives:* these bind member states as to the objectives to be achieved while leaving the national authorities the power to choose the form and the means to be used.
- *decisions:* these are binding in all their aspects on those to whom they are addressed. A decision may be addressed to any or all member states, to undertakings, or to individuals.

- *recommendations and opinions:* these are not binding.

Community legislation, as well as the Council's common positions transmitted to the European Parliament, are published in *The Official Journal of the European Communities* in all the official languages. In addition to the law, there are nonbinding documents consisting of:

- a *Notice to Applicants* for marketing authorization describing the administrative procedures to be followed and the format for the application file (Vols. 2A and 2B of *The Rules Governing Medicinal Products in the European Union*);
- *guidelines on the Conduct of Quality, Safety, and Efficacy Studies* that must be carried out in support of an application for marketing authorization (Vol. 3 of *The Rules Governing Medicinal Products in the European Union*);
- a detailed *Guide to Good Manufacturing Practice* (Vol. 4 of *The Rules Governing Medicinal Products in the European Union*);
- a detailed *Guide to Drug Monitoring* (Vol. 9 of *The Rules Governing Medicinal Products in the European Union*).

BRIEF NOTES ON U.S. MEDICINAL PRODUCT APPROVAL AND POSTMARKETING ACTIVITIES: THE FOOD AND DRUG ADMINISTRATION (FDA) AND ITS PROCEDURES

In the United States, the regulations concerning medicinal product approval belong to the *Code of Federal Regulations* (CFR), which is a codification of the general and permanent rules published in the *Federal Register* by the executive departments and agencies of the federal government. The CFR is divided into 50 titles that represent broad areas subject to federal regulation. Each title is divided into chapters that usually bear the name of the issuing agency. Each chapter is further subdivided into parts covering specific regulatory areas, which, in turn, may be subdivided into subparts and sections. Each volume of the CFR is revised once each calendar year.

The title relative to the Food and Drug Administration is Title 21, and it is issued every year on April 1. The reference relative to new drug applications (NDA) for marketing authorization is Chapter I of Title 21, Part 314, "Applications for FDA Approval to Market a New Drug or an Antibiotic Drug" (50 FR 7493, Feb. 22, 1985, as amended at 57 FR 17981, Apr. 28, 1992).

The purpose of this part is to establish an efficient review process for the approval of drugs shown to be safe and effective and to establish an effective system for FDA surveillance of marketed drugs. The regulations apply to either applications or abbreviated applications. Three copies of the application are required: an archival copy, a review copy, and a field copy. The application is required to contain reports of all investigations of the drug product sponsored by the applicant and all other pertinent information. Guidelines on the format and content are available to assist applicants in their preparation. As far as the normal procedure to be followed is concerned, applicants are positively encouraged to meet with the FDA before submitting an application to discuss the presentation and the format of supporting information (pre-new drug application meeting). Once approval has been granted, the drug goes into the "Listed Drugs."

Relative to regulatory agencies in other Western countries, the FDA traditionally has been considered a conservative, risk-averse agency. Whereas European Union national authorities such as the United Kingdom's Medicine Control Agency and the EMEA itself rely on summary reports supplied by the applicant (expert reports), new drug review by the FDA typically involves careful scrutiny and reanalyses of "raw" company data. The table of contents of the application (see below), in fact, reflects this different attitude of the FDA as regards European regulatory bodies.

FULL APPLICATIONS[7]

The contents and format of the application are presented in Table A.4. The application form will contain the administrative data of the applicant and of the procedure (number if it is a resubmission, an amendment, or a supplement), the specifications of the drug and of the investigators, and the signatures. The index will contain the reference to volume and page number of each part of the dossier.

The summary will contain enough details (regarding chemistry, nonclinical pharmacology and toxicology, human pharmacokinetics, microbiology, and clinical data) that the reader may gain a good general understanding of the data and information contained in the application; tabular and graphic forms of the data are included. The summary may be used eventually by the FDA or the applicant to prepare the summary basis of approval document for public disclosure when the application is approved. The proposed text of the labeling, with the annotations to the information in the summary and technical sections that support the inclusion of each statement in the labeling, should be included. A brief description of the marketing history, mentioning the countries where the product already has been marketed or withdrawn for any reason related to safety or efficacy or the applications are pending, should be included. A concluding discussion underlying the risks and benefits and any proposed additional study or surveillance the applicant intends to conduct after approval will be present.

The technical sections are required to contain data and information in sufficient detail to permit the FDA to make a knowledgeable judgment. In the "Chemistry, Manufacturing, and Controls" section, the environmental impact will be discussed. The "Clinical" section will include all the available information from any source, foreign or domestic, including published and unpublished literature, even if relative to other indications. An integrated summary of the data demonstrating substantial evidence of effectiveness for the claimed indications, along with a

---

Table A.4 Presentation of the application for FDA approval to market a new drug or an antibiotic drug

1. Application Form

2. Index

3. Summary

4. Technical sections
   (a) Chemistry, manufacturing, and controls section
   (b) Nonclinical pharmacology and toxicology section
   (c) Human pharmacokinetics and bioavailability section
   (d) Microbiology section
   (e) Clinical data section
   (f) Statistical section

5. Samples and labeling

6. Case report forms and tabulations

7. Other

8. Patent information

9. Patent certification

10. Claiming exclusivity

11. Financial certification or disclosure statement

Table A.5 Presentation of an abbreviated application for FDA approval to market a new drug or an antibiotic drug

1. Application form

2. Table of contents

3. Basis for abbreviated new drug application submission

4. Conditions of use

5. Active ingredients

6. Route of administration, dosage form, and strength

7. Bioequivalence

8. Labeling

9. Case report forms and tabulations

10. Chemistry, manufacturing, and controls

11. Samples

12. Other

13. Patent certification

14. Financial certification or disclosure statement

---

[7]All the details are in Subpart B: Applications, Title 21, Part 314 (from 314.50, 314.54, 314.60, and 314.65).

summary and updates of safety information summarizing the risks and benefits, will be provided. The case report forms of each patient who died during the clinical trial or who did not complete the study because of an adverse event will be presented. The statistical section shall include the description and analysis of each controlled clinical trial and any other efficacy or safety data that have been presented with the application.

Samples shall be forwarded on FDA request and in sufficient quantity to perform all the necessary tests to the places indicated by the FDA. Copies of the label and all labeling, including the final printed ones, will be presented.

The case report form tabulations of the data of each patient from each adequate and well-controlled study, including the data from the earliest clinical pharmacology studies and tabulations of safety data from other clinical studies, have to be submitted.

The applicant may submit an amendment during the approval procedure, either according to his or her own wish or on FDA invitation. If it is a major amendment (e.g., significant new data or a reanalysis of previously presented data), the time frame for approval will be extended by the FDA accordingly, but for a period not longer than 180 days.

An applicant may at any time withdraw an application for a drug product that is not yet been approved by notifying in writing, without prejudice to refiling. A full application is required for a new indication or for other changes in a listed drug if investigations, other than bioavailability or bioequivalence studies, are essential to approval of the change.

ABBREVIATED APPLICATIONS[8]

Abbreviated applications may be submitted for drug products that are the same as a listed drug, that are duplicates, or which have been declared suitable for an abbreviated new application submission by the FDA through the petition procedures. Three copies of the application are required: an archival copy, a review copy, and a field copy. Guidelines on the format and content are available to assist applicants in their preparation.

The archival copy will include all the information listed in Table A.5. The application form and the table of contents will be roughly the same as for a full application. The basis for abbreviated application must refer to a listed drug that ordinarily would be the drug product selected as the reference standard for conducting bioequivalence testing. As far as points 4, 5, and 6 are concerned, a statement indicating that they will be the same as those already approved for the listed drug, along with the relative information, will be included. Sufficient information and data

will be presented to show that the drug product is bioequivalent to the reference listed drug.

ACCELERATED APPROVAL OF NEW DRUGS FOR SERIOUS OR LIFE-THREATENING ILLNESSES[9]

This procedure applies to certain new drug and antibiotic products that have been studied for their safety and effectiveness in treating serious or life-threatening illnesses and which provide meaningful therapeutic benefit to patients over existing treatments. The FDA may grant marketing approval on the basis of adequate well-controlled clinical trials proving an effect of the drug on a surrogate endpoint that is reasonably likely to predict clinical benefit or on a clinical endpoint other than survival or irreversible morbidity. The approval, in these circumstances, will be subject to the requirement that the applicant study the drug further to verify and describe on its clinical benefit where there is uncertainty as to the relation of the surrogate endpoint to clinical benefit or of the observed clinical benefit on ultimate outcome.

The FDA may conclude that the product reviewed according to this procedure can be used safely only if distribution or use is restricted. After completion of well-conducted postmarketing clinical trials, the FDA, on the basis of the data obtained, may determine that restriction is no longer necessary for the safe and effective use of a drug product. A notification is sent to the company, and then the drug product would be appropriate for approval under traditional procedures.

TIME FRAMES FOR REVIEWING FULL AND ABBREVIATED APPLICATIONS[10]

The reviewing process should not be longer than 180 days either for a full or an abbreviated application ("review clock"). During the review period, the applicant may withdraw an application or an abbreviated application and later resubmit it. The review clock may be extended by mutual agreement between the FDA and the applicant as a result of a major amendment.

In case of an application and an abbreviated antibiotic application, within 60 days after FDA receives the application, the agency will determine whether the application may be filed. Then the review process starts with the same time frames as for a new drug application or an abbreviated one.

During the course of reviewing, there is an efficient and documented communication (e.g., phone conversations, letters, or meetings) between the FDA and the applicant, according to the procedures described in a staff manual guide that is publicly available. In addition, during the evaluating period, a 90-day conference (approximately 90 days after the FDA receives the application) may constitute a good opportunity for the company to meet with FDA reviewing officials to discuss scientific and administrative issues. An end-of-review conference, at the conclusion of the FDA review, may

---

[8]All the details are in Subpart C: Abbreviated Applications, Title 21, Part 314 (from 314.92 to 314.94).
[9]All the details are in Subpart H: Accelerated Approval of New Drugs for Serious or Life-Threatening Illnesses, Title 21, Part 314.

---

[10]All the details are in Subpart D: FDA Action on Applications and Abbreviated Applications, Title 21, Part 314.

constitute another opportunity to meet with FDA officials. These conferences may constitute an appropriate forum to discuss and try to solve any possible dispute.

The FDA will review, according to the scheduled period, the application and send the applicant either an approval letter or an approvable letter or a letter of nonapproval. The approvable letter may serve, in most instances, as a mechanism for solving outstanding issues on drugs that are about to be approved and marketed. The approvable letter means a written communication from the FDA to the applicant approving an application, and the approval becomes effective on the date of issuance of this letter. The letter of nonapproval describes the deficiencies for which the agency believes the application may not be approved.

As far as the applications based solely on foreign data are concerned, they are valid if they meet the following US criteria for marketing approval: they are applicable to the US population and US medical practice; the studies have been conducted by clinical investigators with recognized competence; and the data meet the criteria of good clinical practice guidelines, which have been harmonized recently (CPMP/ICH/135/95). In this case in particular, applicants are encouraged to meet with agency officials in a presubmission meeting.

SUPPLEMENTS AND OTHER CHANGES TO AN APPROVED APPLICATION[11]

The applicant shall notify the FDA about each change in each condition established in an approved application beyond the variations already provided for in the application. The following circumstances are foreseen:
• supplements requiring FDA approval before the change is made;
• supplements for changes that may be made before FDA approval;
• changes described in the annual report (see the following paragraph).

POSTMARKETING SURVEILLANCE[12]

Applicants having an approved application are required to promptly review all adverse drug experience[13] information and data obtained or otherwise received from other sources, domestic or foreign, including those derived from commercial marketing experience, postmarketing clinical investigations, postmarketing epidemiologic/surveillance studies, reports in the scientific literature, and unpublished scientific papers. All serious unexpected adverse drug experiences

(alert reports and follow-ups of alert reports) occurring within the United States or abroad will be reported as soon as possible but in no case later than 15 calendar days after receipt of the information by the applicant.

A periodic adverse drug experience report, which includes any information not yet reported (alert reports and follow-ups), has to be submitted by the applicant at quarterly intervals for 3 years from the date of approval and then at annual intervals. Each report shall contain a narrative summary and analysis of the information in the report and an analysis of the 15-day alert reports, a FDA Form 3500A (adverse reaction report) for each adverse drug experience not yet reported, and a history of actions taken since the last report because of adverse drug experiences (e.g., labelling changes or studies initiated). The records of all adverse drug experiences known to the applicant shall be kept for 10 years.

The following other postmarketing reports have to be prepared by the applicant and sent to the FDA:
• *new drug application field alert report:* this consists of information concerning any incident that causes the drug product or its labelling to be mistaken for, or applied to, another article; any bacteriologic contamination; any change or deterioration in the distributed product; etc. The information must be provided by phone or other rapid communication;
• *annual report:* this consists of a summary of significant new information that might affect safety, effectiveness, or labelling of the drug product, along with the relative actions taken; the distribution data; the labelling; any chemistry, manufacturing, and control changes; nonclinical laboratory studies; clinical data (including all new published and unpublished information on every kind of pharmacoepidemiologic completed study or survey); and a status report (current status of any postmarketing studies performed by or on behalf of the applicant);
• *other reporting:* advertisements and promotional labelling, special reports, withdrawal of approved drug products from sale.

Just a short final comment on the most important differences in the philosophy and the evaluation strategy of the FDA in comparison with the EMEA. The FDA has a big staff, thousands of people employed, and they work in strict cooperation with the companies during the whole filing and reviewing period. The staff evaluates the dossier and, when necessary, makes a reanalysis of the data starting from the tabulations of each patient from each trial. This approach to evaluation has been described as working from a very basic level with raw data and moving up to reach an overview, i.e., a "bottom-up approach."

The EMEA has a small staff, less than 200 temporary agents, and its secretariat works in strict cooperation with CPMP members, who belong to the 15 member states. The CPMP relies on the (Co)-Rapporteur's reports, written by recognized scientists, and gives its opinion on the basis of these reports and on the dossier filed by the company, asking questions during the evaluation period in order to clarify the issues which it thinks need further details or expla-

---

[11]All the details are in Subpart B: Applications, Title 21, Part 314 (from 314.70 to 314.72).
[12]All the details are in Subpart B: Applications, Title 21, Part 314 (from 314.80 to 314.81).
[13]Any adverse event associated with the use of a drug in humans, whether or not considered drug related, including the following: an adverse event occurring in the course of the use of a drug product in professional practice, an adverse event occurring from drug overdose whether accidental or intentional, an adverse event occurring from drug abuse, an adverse event occurring from drug withdrawal, and any failure of expected pharmacologic action.

nation. This approach usually begins with a summary or general overview at a high level (i.e., the applicant's expert reports) and then moves down to see if the data support or contradict this view, i.e., a "top-down approach."

INTERNET ADDRESSES

- *http://www.cec.lu* (information regarding the European Commission).

- *http://www.eudra.org/emea.html.*
- *http://www2.eudra.org/; http://www4.eudra.org/* (information regarding EMEA and links related to EMEA: companies, authorities, other regulatory and scientific European and worldwide sites).
- *http://www.fda.org* (information regarding worldwide regulatory bodies).
- *http://rainfo.org* (information regarding worldwide regulatory bodies).
- *http://europa.eu.int/index.htm* (information regarding the European Union).
- *http://158.167.39.75/clxint/celex-en.html* (access to European Community legislation).

Abbreviations			
ATS =	Agency tracking system	IFPMA =	International Federation of Pharmaceutical Manufacturers Association
BWP =	Biotechnology Working Party		
CEECs =	Central and Eastern European Countries	INN =	International Non-Proprietary Name
CFR =	Code of Federal Regulations	JPMA =	Japan Pharmaceutical Manufacturers Association
CMS(s) =	Concerned Member States(s)		
CPMP =	Committee for Proprietary Medicinal Products	MA =	Marketing Authorisation
CVMP =	Committee for Proprietary Veterinary Products	MAH =	Marketing Authorisation Holder
DG(s) =	Directorate(s) General	MHW =	Ministry of Health and Welfare, Japan
EEA =	European Economic Area	MRFG =	Mutual Recognition Facilitation Group
EFPIA =	European Federation of Pharmaceutical Industries' Associations	MS(s) =	Member State(s)
		NAS =	New Active Substance
EFTA =	European Free Trade Area	NDA =	New Drug Application
EMEA =	European Agency for the Evaluation of Medicinal Products	NTA =	Notice to Applicants
		PhRMA =	Pharmaceutical Research and Manufacturers of America
EPAR =	European Public Assessment Report		
EU =	European Commission-European Union	PhVWP =	Pharmacovigilance Working Party
EWGs =	Expert Working Groups	PSUR =	Periodic Safety Update Report
EWP =	Efficacy Working Party	QWP =	Quality Working Party
FDA =	US Food and Drug Administration	RAS =	Rapid Alert system
GCP =	Good Clinical Practice	RMS =	Reference Member State
GLP =	Good Laboratory Practice	SPC =	Summary of Product Characteristics
GMP =	Good Manufacturing Practice	SWP =	Safety Working Party
ICH =	International Conference on Harmonisation of technical requirements for registration of pharmaceutical for human use	USA, US =	United States of America
		USR =	Urgent Safety Restrictions
		WHO =	World Health Organisation

COLOR ATLAS

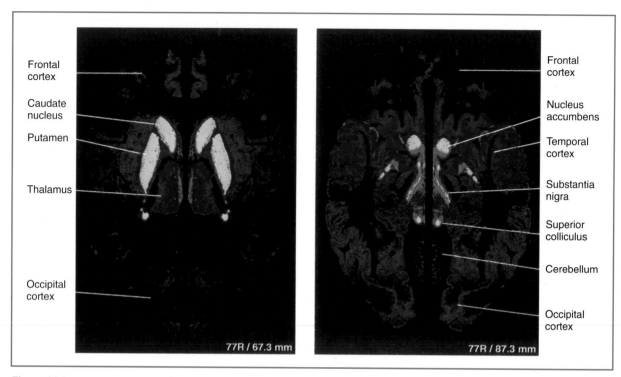

Figure 14.1 Distribution of D2-like dopamine receptors in the postmortem human brain. The illustrations demonstrate radioactivity accumulation in a section from a cryosectioned human brain hemisphere. The section was incubated with ^{125}I epidepride, a D2 dopamine receptor antagonist. (*Left*) D2 dopamine receptor densities in the basal ganglia, thalamus, and medial frontal cortex. (*Right*) D2 dopamine receptor densities in the nucleus accumbens, substantia nigra, superior colliculus, and tip of the temporal cortex (Used with permission from Hall H, Halldin C, Jerning E, et al. Autoradiographic comparison of [125I]epidepride and [125I]NCQ 298 binding to human brain extrastriated dopamine receptors. Nucl Med Biol 1997;24:389; and Sedvall G, Farde L. Chemical brain anatomy in schizophrenia. Lancet 1995;346:743.)

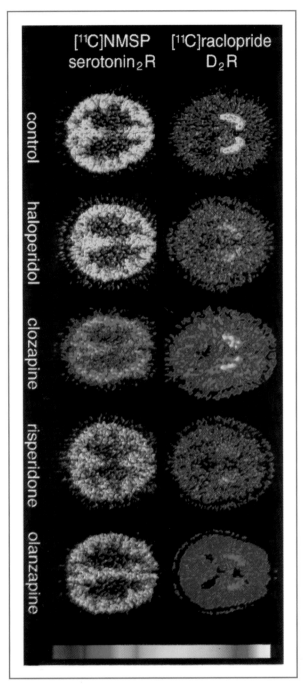

Figure 14.2 PET scan images demonstrating radioligand binding to dopamine D2 and serotonin 5-HT 2A receptors in the brain of an untreated schizophrenic patient and patients treated with chemically distinct types of antipsychotic drugs as indicated in the figure. Note the high D2 but not 5-HT 2A occupancy after haloperidol treatment but marked occupancy of both receptor subtypes by the atypical antipsychotic drugs.

INDEX